Spanish-English English-Spanish Pocket Medical Dictionary

Diccionario Médico de Bolsillo Español-Inglés Inglés-Español

First Edition

Onyria Herrera McElroy, Ph.D.
Lola L. Grabb, M.A.

Wolters Kluwer | Lippincott Williams & Wilkins
Health
Philadelphia · Baltimore · New York · London
Buenos Aires · Hong Kong · Sydney · Tokyo

Publisher: Julie K. Stegman
Senior Product Manager: Eric Branger
Managing Editor: Tiffany Piper
Graphic Artist: Susan Caldwell
Designer: Parkton Art Studio, Inc.
Compositor: Aptara, Inc.
Manufacturing Coordinator: Margie Orzech
Senior Marketing Manager: Zhan Caplan

DISCLAIMER

Care has been taken to confirm the accuracy of the information present and to describe generally accepted practices. However, the authors, editors, and publisher are not responsible for errors or omissions or for any consequences from application of the information in this book and make no warranty, expressed or implied, with respect to the currency, completeness, or accuracy of the contents of the publication. Application of this information in a particular situation remains the professional responsibility of the practitioner; the clinical treatments described and recommended may not be considered absolute and universal recommendations.

Printed in the United States of America.

Library of Congress Cataloging-in-Publication Data
McElroy, Onyria Herrera.

Spanish-English English-Spanish pocket medical dictionary = Diccionario médico de bolsillo español-inglés inglés-español / Onyria Herrera McElroy, Lola L. Grabb. – 1st ed.

p. ; cm.

Includes bibliographical references.

English and Spanish.

ISBN 978-0-7817-7951-7

1. Medicine–Dictionaries. 2. English language–Dictionaries–Spanish. 3. Medicine–Dictionaries–Spanish. 4. Spanish language–Dictionaries–English. I. Grabb, Lola L. II. Title.

[DNLM: 1. Medicine–Dictionary–English. 2. Medicine–Dictionary–Spanish. W 13 M478s 2008]

R121.M4882 2008

610.3—dc22   2008004324

CONTENTS / CONTENIDO

Contents / Contenido

PROLOGUE

More than a decade ago, our first medical-bilingual dictionary was addressed to English-speaking medical professionals to help them to establish better communication with their Spanish-speaking patients. Our effort has been received with enthusiasm by professionals who recognize that communication with patients in their language yields better results during physical examinations, in visits to a medical office, and during procedures.

Taking into consideration that patients are now participating more actively in their health care, our purpose in this new dictionary has been to design a concise bilingual dictionary, condensing the necessary information that will be most useful to health professionals who care for Spanish-speaking patients.

Spanish-English English-Spanish Pocket Medical Dictionary includes a medical glossary with medical phrases that are easy to understand by the general public, in which users can find: a Spanish-English, English-Spanish resource with notes on grammar and pronunciation; medical terms with clear definitions; signs and symptoms that patients can identify; dialogues between patient and their attending medical professional; descriptions of common sicknesses; emergency situations; information about nutrition and physical fitness; notes about the weather; and weights and measures. In this handy pocket dictionary the health care professionals will find the needed condensed information to establish communication with their Spanish-speaking patients.

Spanish-English English-Spanish Pocket Medical Dictionary also serves as a consulting work to readers that want to have a reference for a basic knowledge of English and Spanish grammar and pronunciation. Further, health care professionals from Latin America can use the dictionary as a tool to practice English, using the dictionary's specialized medical vocabulary and phrases.

O. H. M.
L. L. G.

PRÓLOGO

Hace más de una década, nuestro primer diccionario médico-bilingüe se dirigió a los profesionales de asistencia médica de habla inglesa para ayudarles a establecer comunicación con pacientes hispano parlantes. Nuestro esfuerzo ha sido recibido con entusiasmo por profesionales que reconocen la importancia de comunicarse con pacientes en su propia lengua. Les ha ayudado a obtener mejores resultados en reconocimientos físicos, en la aplicación de procedimientos y tratamientos en la asistencia diaria, y en la consulta médica.

Teniendo en cuenta que actualmente los pacientes demuestran una participación más activa en el estado de su salud, nuestro propósito ha sido diseñar un nuevo diccionario bilingüe de bolsillo, conciso, manuable, en el cual los usuarios puedan encontrar un recurso en el glosario español-inglés; inglés-español con notas de gramática y pronunciación, frases médicas; términos médicos con claras definiciones; signos y síntomas que los pacientes identifican; diálogos entre paciente y profesional médico; síntomas y descripciones de enfermedades comunes; situaciones de emergencia; información sobre la nutrición y acondicionamiento físico; notas sobre el tiempo, y pesos y medidas. En este manuable diccionario de bolsillo, los profesionales médicos encontrarán los recursos necesarios para comunicarse eficazmente con pacientes hispano-hablantes.

El nuevo *Diccionario Médico de Bolsillo, Español-Inglés, Inglés-Español* sirve de obra de consulta a lectores que deseen una información básica sobre la gramática y la pronunciación del inglés. Además, los profesionales de asistencia médica en países hispano-hablantes pueden usar el diccionario como instrumento de práctica del inglés haciendo uso del vocabulario médico especializado.

O. H. M.
L. L. G.

ACKNOWLEDGEMENTS

We wish to acknowledge and thank the following persons for their encouragement and helpful assistance during our work on this dictionary. To Albert Grabb, MD, Julius Pietrzak, MD, and Ana María López, MD, for their useful replies to our inquiries. To John H. McElroy, PhD, for copyediting advice. To Lauren McElroy, for valuable translations and proofreading. To Roseann D. Gonzalez, PhD, who has always been supportive of our work. And to Eric Branger, Tiffany Piper, and Julie Stegman at Lippincott Williams and Wilkins, who have worked so diligently in directing and producing the dictionary.

O. H. M.
L. L. G.

HOW TO USE THE DICTIONARY

MAIN ENTRIES

The main entries are printed in **boldface**, in slightly larger type than the rest of the text, set flush to the left hand margin. The main entry may consist of:

1. one word: **abdomen**
2. words joined by a hyphen: **cross-eyed**
3. descriptive phrases: **sympathetic nervous system**

The main entries are listed in alphabetical order according to the initial letter of the entry. Two kinds of entries appear: a) strictly medical words and b) common words related to general communication with patients.

When the main entry is a medical term, a simple definition is given. When the main entry has different meanings which are identified as the same part of speech, they are itemized numerically and labeled with an abbreviation if it is needed for clarification (1). If the main entry is a non-medical word or a common term, synonyms are used to define it. If a main entry has more than one meaning, a word or phrase between brackets is given, in italics, in the same language as the entry to clarify its meaning, or the entry is used in a phrase to clarify its use (2). We have listed new technical words designating programs, products, instruments, or treatments and defined them by following the general rules of language usage.

> (1) **absorption** *n.* absorción. 1. la acción de un organismo de absorber o pasar líquidos u otras sustancias; 2. ensimismación.

> (2) **fit** *n.* ataque, convulsión; *a.* [*suitable*] adecuado-a; *v.* [*to adjust to shape*] ajustar, encajar.

When there is a slight difference in the spelling of words with the same meaning, both spellings are entered together, and the most common one of the two is entered first (3).

> (3) **exophthalmia, exophthalmus** *n.* exoftalmia, exoftalmus, protrusión anormal del globo del ojo.

Only words that pertain to communication in a medical situation and to needs related to patients or medical personnel are included in the glossary.

SUBENTRIES

Subentries under main entries of medical words in the same language as the entry are printed in **boldface type** (4); subentries under main entries of common words and phrases and idiomatic expressions are printed in **boldface type** (5). A slash (/) separates the translation of the subentries from English to Spanish or Spanish to English, while a double space (__) stands for the main entry. Subentries generally are not defined. Their plural forms are indicated by adding **-s** or **-es** after the double space.

---

(4) **dislocation** *n.* luxación, desplazamiento de una articulación; **closed** ___ / ___ cerrada; **complicated** ___ / ___ complicada; **congenital** ___ / ___ congénita.

---

(5) **around** *prep.* cerca de; en; *adv.* alrededor de, cerca; a la vuelta; más o menos; ___ **here** / ___ aquí; *v.* **to look** ___ / buscar, **to turn** ___ / dar la vuelta; voltear; voltearse.

SYNONYMS

When an entry refers to a sickness which is known by more than one name, only one definition is given. The abbreviation *V.* (See) will guide the reader to the term defined (6).

---

(6) **chickenpox** *n.* varicela. *V.* **varicella.**

PARTS OF SPEECH

All main entries, simple or combined, are identified as to part of speech. When the main entry has more than one word, the combined phrase is also identified (7).

---

(7) **robust** *a.*
role model *n.*
radioactive iodine excretion test *n.*

The meanings of a word used as more than one part of speech are indicated in the following order of forms: **noun** *n.*; **adjective** *a.*; **verb** *v.*; **irregular verb** *vi.*; **reflexive verb** *vr.*; **adverb** *adv.* (2).

In the English section of the dictionary, the glossary includes nouns, adjectives, infinitives of verbs, the past participle (classified as an adjective), comparatives and superlatives, prepositions, and adverbs. Idiomatic expressions involving the main entry are included following the definitions. Other parts of speech such as pronouns and verb forms can be found in the grammar section of the dictionary.

In the Spanish section, nouns and adjectives are identified by their gender *(m., f.)*. In the English section, the translations into Spanish of nouns and adjectives indicate their gender (masculine or feminine) by adding the feminine ending **-a**, accordingly, to nouns and adjectives ending in **-o** that are inflected. In example (8) **rápido-a** means that the masculine is **rápido**, and the feminine is **rápida.** When the adverb is indicated by the ending **-mente,** it means that this ending has to be added to the feminine ending of the adjective, or when the adjective ends in a consonant.

---

(8) **fast** *n. ayuno; a. (speedy)* rápido-a; ligero-a; **color** ___ / resistente a un colorante; *v. (not to eat anything)* ayunar; **to break one's** ___ / dejar de ayunar; *adv.* aprisa; rápidamente; **to walk** ___ / andar ___ ; ___**asleep** / profundamente dormido-a.

HOMOGRAPHS AND EPONYMS

When entries are spelled alike but have a different classification (homographs), the part of speech is indicated by its corresponding abbreviation. Definitions follow separated by semicolons without using numerals, as is the case when the entry has the same classification regarding part of speech (9).

(9) **mucoid** *n.* mucoide, glucoproteína similar a la mucina; *a.* de consistencia mucosa.

Eponyms are entered alphabetically according to last names (10).

(10) **Babinski's reflex** *n.* reflejo de Babinski, dorsiflexión del dedo gordo al estimularse la planta del pie.

PLURALS

Irregular plurals in English, and the plurals of Latin and Greek nouns used in medical terminology, are indicated in parentheses after the entry (11) and (12).

(11) **woman** *n.* (*pl.* **women**) mujer.

(12) **septum** *L.* (*pl.* **septa**) septum, tabique o membrana que divide dos cavidades o espacios.

Consult the grammar section of the dictionary to find the rules that apply to the formation of plurals in each language.

CAPITALIZATION

Most entries in English begin with a lowercase. Capitalization is used in eponyms and trade names of medications; names of plants and animals are capitalized, printed in italics, and given in the singular if referring to the genus, and in the plural if referring to the class, order, family, or phylum (13).

(13) *Salmonella n. Salmonela,* género de bacterias de la familia *Enterobacteriaceae* que causan fiebres entéricas, otras infecciones gastrointestinales y septicemia.

COMMUNICATION WITH PATIENTS

This section is provided to facilitate easy interchange between the patient and the health care personnel assisting them. The health care professional has the advantage to select the areas that correspond to their field of expertise before interviewing patients.

APPENDICES

The appendices offer in their clear information a comprehensive resource to health care professionals and patients. The appendices contain dialogues based on systems and specialties, signs and symptoms, diagnosis, major diseases, medical phrases, and practical expressions used in daily-life communication related to health care issues.

ILLUSTRATIONS

The reader will find the small illustrations throughout the vocabulary sections useful and informative on organs and parts of the human body. The charts and the illustrations serve as a visual resource for vocabulary practice of new medical terms in the two languages, English and Spanish.

USO DEL DICCIONARIO

ENTRADAS PRINCIPALES

Las entradas principales aparecen impresas en letra **negrita** formando el margen izquierdo. La entrada principal puede consistir en:

1. una sola palabra: **abdomen**
2. una palabra compuesta: **intra-abdominal**
3. una frase descriptiva: **cuello uterino**

Las entradas principales siguen un orden alfabético de acuerdo con la primera letra de la palabra. Hay dos tipos de entradas: (a) palabras estrictamente médicas, (b) palabras del lenguaje común necesarias para la comunicación con los pacientes.

Cuando la entrada principal es un vocablo médico, a éste le sigue una definición simple que señala los aspectos más importantes del mismo. Si el vocablo tiene más de una acepción para una misma parte de la oración (sustantivo, adjetivo, etc.), a cada acepción se le atribuye un número y una abreviatura adicional para mayor claridad (1). Cuando la entrada principal es un vocablo común, no médico, se hace uso de sinónimos para traducirla. Si tiene más de un significado, se hace uso de alguna palabra o frase entre corchetes ([]), en bastardilla y en el mismo idioma de la entrada, para aclarar su significado, o se emplea la misma entrada en una frase para aclarar su uso. (2). En algunos casos incluimos nuevas palabras técnicas que designan programas, productos, instrumentos y tratamientos; estas palabras están definidas de acuerdo con las reglas generales del uso del idioma.

> (1) **absorción** *f.* absorption, uptake. 1. taking up of fluids and other substances by an organism; 2. self-centeredness.

> (2) **apagar** *v.* [*luces*] to turn off; [*fuego*] to put out.

En algunos casos, cuando hay una pequeña diferencia en la forma escrita de dos palabras con el mismo significado, ambas palabras se presentan en la misma entrada, y se registra primero la palabra de uso más común (3).

> (3) **fibrocístico-a, fibroquístico-a** *a.* fibrocystic, cystic and fibrous in nature; **enfermedad __ de la mama** / __ disease of the breast.

En el glosario de este diccionario se han incluido solamente términos relacionados con una situación médica, ya sea para la comunicación con los pacientes o para la atención a sus necesidades.

ENTRADAS SUBALTERNAS

Las entradas subalternas que aparecen bajo la entrada principal están impresas en letra **negrita** si están en el mismo idioma que ésta; asimismo, ya refiriéndose a la terminología no médica o a expresiones idiomáticas en el mismo. Una línea inclinada (/) separa la traducción del español al inglés y del inglés al español en las entradas subalternas, y un doble guión (__) sustituye la entrada principal; el plural se indica con una **-s** o con **-es** después del doble guión. Las entradas subalternas generalmente no se definen (4).

(4) **cuidado** *m.* care, attention; ___ **intensivo** / intensive___ ; ___ **postnatal** / postnatal ___; **estar al ___de** / to be under the ___ of; **tratar con,** ___ / to handle with ___.
febril *a.* febrile, having a body temperature above normal, convulsiones ___ -es / convulsions.

SINÓNIMOS

Cuando un término médico tiene más de un nombre, solamente se define uno de los términos; la abreviatura *V.* (Véase) en la entrada del otro término, guia al lector a la entrada que aparece definida (5).

(5) **glucopenia** *f. V.* **hipoglicemia.**

PARTES DE LA ORACIÓN

Después de cada entrada, consistente ésta de una o de más palabras, se indica la parte correspondiente de la oración (6).

(6) **emulsión** *f.*
enajenamiento mental *m.*
brazalete de identificación *m.*

Cuando una misma entrada tiene más de una clasificación como parte de la oración, se sigue el siguiente orden: **nombre** *m., f.*; **adjetivo** *a.*; **verbo** *v.*; **verbo irregular** *vi.*; **verbo reflexivo** *vr.*; **adverbio** *adv.* Las terminaciones **-a** y **-mente** indican la terminación que se añade a la entrada para formar el adjetivo y el adverbio respectivamente (7).

(7) **elástico** *m.* elastic; **-a** *a.* elastic, that can be returned to its original shape after being extended or distorted. **natural** *a.* natural; **-mente** *adv.* naturally.

En la sección del diccionario en español, el glosario incluye sustantivos, adjetivos, infinitivos de verbos, el participio pasado (clasificado como adjetivo), preposiciones y adverbios. Las expressiones idiomáticas aparecen como entradas subalternas a continuación de las definiciones. Otras partes de la oración, pronombres y distintas formas de los verbos aparecen en la sección de gramática del diccionario.

En la sección del diccionario en español, los sustantivos y adjetivos se identifican por su género (*m.,f.*). En la sección en inglés, la traducción de sustantivos y adjetivos al español indica el género de los mismos (masculino o femenino) mediante el uso de la terminación **-a** añadida a los sustantivos y adjetivos terminados en **o** (8).

(8) **métrico-a** *a.* metric, rel. to meter or the metric system.

HOMÓGRAFOS Y EPÓNIMOS

Cuando a una misma entrada se le atribuye más de una clasificación (términos homógrafos) cada parte de la oración se indica con su correspondiente abreviatura, y las definiciones siguen a cada clasificación, separadas por un punto y coma pero sin asignarles números como se hace en los casos en que un mismo término tiene más de una acepción pero mantiene la misma clasificación (véanse ejemplos 1 y 7). Los epónimos están registrados alfabéticamente por apellido (9).

> (9) **Babinski, reflejo de** *m.* Babinski's reflex, dorsiflexion of the big toe on stimulation of the sole of the foot.

PLURALES

Los plurales de vocablos incorporados del latín y del griego, así como los plurales irregulares, se indican entre paréntesis a continuación de la entrada (10).

> (10) **septum** *L.* (pl. **septa**) septum, partition between two cavities.

En la sección de gramática del diccionario se encuentran las reglas que gobiernan la formación de los plurales en cada idioma.

LETRAS MAYÚSCULAS

La mayoría de las entradas en inglés y en español aparecen en letra minúscula. Las letras mayúsculas se usan en los epónimos y en nombres comerciales de medicinas. Los nombres de plantas y animales se presentan con letra mayúscula, en bastardilla, en singular si se refieren al género y en plural si se refieren a la clase, orden, familia o filo (11).

> (11) ***Salmonela*** *f. Salmonella,* a gram-negative bacteria of the *Enterobacteriaceae* that causes enteric fever, gastrointestinal infection and septicemia.

COMUNICACIÓN CON LOS PACIENTES

El propósito de esta sección es de facilitar la comunicación oral entre los pacientes y el personal de salud que le asiste. Los profesionales de salud tienen la ventaja de seleccionar en los diálogos, frases médicas y vocabulario general el área correspondiente a su campo de especialización y aplicar sus conocimientos al caso que estudien o a las necesidades de cada paciente.

APÉNDICES

Los apéndices ofrecen al profesional de salud y a sus pacientes una información clara y fácil de comprender que incluye diálogos elaborados de acuerdo con sistemas y especialidades, síntomas, diagnósticos, fases médicas, nociones de enfermedades prominentes y expresiones usadas en la vida diaria que corresponden a problemas de salud.

ILUSTRACIONES

Los usuarios del diccionario encontrarán que las ilustraciones y cuadros que aparecen a través del vocabulario les servirán de instrumentos útiles para el aprendizaje del vocabulario de los órganos y partes del cuerpo humano. Además, estos objetos visuales serán un medio para el reconocimiento de términos médicos en los dos idiomas, inglés y español.

ABBREVIATIONS / ABREVIATURAS

ENGLISH		SPANISH	
a.	adjective	*a.*	adjetivo
abbr.	abbreviation	*abr.*	abreviatura
adv.	adverb	*adv.*	adverbio
approx.	approximate	*aprox.*	aproximadamente
art.	article	*art.*	artículo
aux	auxiliary	*aux.*	auxiliar
Cast.	Castilian	*Cast.*	castellano
comp.	comparative	*comp.*	comparativo
cond.	conditional	*cond.*	condicional
conj.	conjunction	*conj.*	conjunción
cu.	cubic	*cu.*	cúbico
dem.	demonstrative	*dem.*	demostrativo
esp.	especially	*esp.*	especialmente
f	feminine	*f.*	femenino
		fam.	familiar
Fr.	French	*Fr.*	francés
form.	formal pronoun		
gen.	generally	*gen.*	generalmente
Gr.	Greek	*Gr.*	griego
gr.	grammar	*gr.*	gramática
H.A.	Hispanic America	*H.A.*	Hispanoamérica
imp.	imperative	*imp.*	imperativo
impf.	imperfect	*impf.*	imperfecto
ind.	indicative	*ind.*	indicativo
indef.	indefinite	*indef.*	indefinido
inf.	infinitive	*inf.*	infinitivo
infl.	inflammation	*infl.*	inflamación
int.	interjection	*int.*	interjección
interr.	interrogative	*interr.*	interrogativo
L.	Latin	*L.*	latín
m.	masculine	*m.*	masculino
Mex.	Mexico	*Mex.*	México
Mex.A.	Mexican- American	*Mex.A.*	Mexicano-americano
n.	noun	*n.*	nombre
neut.	neuter	*neut.*	neutro
obj.	object	*obj.*	objeto
pop.	popular	*pop.*	popular
pp.	past participle	*pp.*	participio de pasado
p.p.	present participle	*p.p.*	participio de presente
pref.	prefix	*pref.*	prefijo
prep.	preposition	*prep.*	preposición
pres.	present	*pres.*	presente
pret.	preterite	*pret.*	pretérito
pron.	pronoun	*pron.*	pronombre
psych.	psychology	*psic.*	psicología
ref.	reflexive	*ref.*	reflexivo
rel.	relative	*rel.*	relativo

ENGLISH		SPANISH	
subj.	subjunctive	*subj.*	subjuntivo
sup.	superlative	*sup.*	superlativo
surg.	surgery	*cirg.*	cirugía
U.S.A.	United States of America	*E.U.A.*	Estados Unidos de América
usu.	usually	*usu.*	usualmente
V.	see	*V.*	véase
v.	verb	*v.*	verbo
vi.	irregular verb	*vi.*	verbo irregular
vr.	reflexive verb	*vr.*	verbo reflexivo

SPANISH SOUNDS / SONIDOS DEL ESPAÑOL

The Spanish alphabet has four more characters than the English alphabet: **ch, ll, ñ, rr.** When alphabetizing Spanish words those words beginning with **ch, ll,** and **ñ,** follow words that begin in **c, l,** and **ñ.** The letter **rr** never begins a word.

Learning to Pronounce Spanish

English equivalents given for Spanish sounds are only approximate.

1. Spanish Vowel Sounds / Sonidos vocálicos en español

a, e, i, o, u and sometimes **y** are single sounds pronounced always clearly whether they are a stressed vowel or not. A tendency by English speakers to slur over the unstressed vowels is a habit that should not be done when Spanish vowels are pronounced. Spanish vowel sounds are short. There are only five vowel sounds in Spanish.

VOWEL / VOCAL	SOUND / SONIDO	EXAMPLE / EJEMPLO	MEANING / SIGNIFICADO
a	ah as in *father*	*a*meba* (ah-meh-bah)	ameba
e	eh as in *let*	acn*é* (ahk-neh)	acne
i	ee as in *see*	anem*i*a (ah-neh-mee-ah)	anemia
o	oh as in *spoke*	call*o* (kah-yoh)	callus
u	oo as in *cool*	ac*ú*stica (ah-coos-tee-kah)	acoustics

The stressed syllable is indicated in bold. Example of vowels are indicated in italics.
*Although these two words are written alike, in the English word the **e** is pronounced like the Spanish **i**.

Note / Nota: The **y** is pronounced like the vowel **i** when it is by itself or at the end of a word: **y** / and; **I** am / Yo soy (pronounced as in boy).

Mute Vowel u and Consonant h / La vocal muda u y la consonante h.

The **u** is only mute when placed after **g** or **q** preceding **e** or **i** in the syllables **gue, gui.** If **u** has a dieresis (two dots over the **ü**) it is sounded. Examples: silent **u: guitarra** (ghee-tah-rrah); sounded **u: ungüento (oon-goo-ehn-toh).**

The consonant **h** is never pronounced in Spanish. The vowel **u** sounds when indicated by a diéresis.

Diphthongs / Diptongos

A diphthong is a combination of two vowels in a syllable. A dipthong is made by two vowels, one of the vowels can be a strong vowel (**a, e, o**) and the other a weak vowel (**i, [y],** or **u**), or two weak vowels. Two strong vowels together do not form a diphthong. When the combination is that of a strong vowel and a weak vowel, the strong vowel is stressed; if the diphthong is formed by two weak vowels, the second vowel is stressed.

STRONG AND WEAK VOWELS FORMING A DIPHTHONG:

ai	au	ia	ua
ai-re air	**au**-sente absent	**via**-ble viable	**cua**-dro picture
ei	eu	ie	ue
rei-no kingdom	**eu**-fórico euphoric	**rie**sgo risk	**bue**-no good
oi	oy	ey	uo
oi-go I hear	voy	**rey**	**cuo**-ta

2. CONSONANT SOUNDS THAT DIFFER MOST FROM ENGLISH.

Sonidos de las consonantes que más difieren de los sonidos en inglés.

The consonant example is given in bold. / La consonante usada como ejemplo aparece en letra negrita.

LETTER / LETRA	APPROX. ENGLISH SOUND / SONIDO APROX. EN INGLÉS	WORD, PRONUNCIATION AND MEANING / PALABRA, PRONUNCIATION Y SIGNIFICADO
c before e, i (Cast.)	**th** as in *think* (Castillian Spanish)	**cír**culo (**theer**-koo-loh) / circle
c before e, i (H.A.)	**s** as in *sick*	**c**entro (**sehn**-troh) / center
c before a, o, u	**k** as in *cancer*	**cán**cer (**kahn**-sehr) / cancer
ch	**ch** as in *check*	le**che** (leh-**cheh**) / milk
d between vowels	like **th** in *weather*	me**d**io (meh-**dee**-oh) / half
d after n or l	like **d** in *dart*	don**d**e (dohn-**deh**) / where
g before e, i	harsher than **h** in *hemoglobin*	**g**ermen (**her**-men) / germ
gue, gui	hard **g** as in *guest*	**gui**sado[a] (**ghee**-sah-doh) / stew
güe, güi	**gwe** as in *Gwen*	un**güe**nto[b] (oon-**goo-en**-toh) / **ointment**
h[c]	always silent as in *hour*	**h**ora (oh-rah) / hour
j	more forcefully than in *ham*	**j**amón (**hah**-mohn) / ham
ll (Cast.)	**lli** as in *million*	mi**lló**n (mee-**llohn**) / million

Spanish Sounds / Sonidos del español

LETTER / LETRA	APPROX. ENGLISH SOUND / SONIDO APROX. EN INGLÉS	WORD, PRONUNCIATION AND MEANING / PALABRA, PRONUNCIATION Y SIGNIFICADO
ll (H.A.)	same as **y** in *yes*	**ll**ón (mee-yohn)
ñ	**ny** as in *canyon*	mu**ñ**eca (moo-nyeh-kah) / wrist
p	not aspirated, less explosive than in *patient*	**p**aciente (pah-see-enh-teh) / patient
q	always pronounced as **k**	**qu**eso[d] (keh-soh) / cheese
r	1 . initial: multiple thrill, roll **r** more than in *diarrhea*	**r**euma (reh-oo-mah) / rheum
r	2. not initial, sound produced by tip of the tongue against the alveolar ridge	ci**r**ugía / surgery
rr	same as initial **r**	dia**rr**ea (deeah-reh-ah) / diarrhea
v as in b labial	as in *bowl*	**v**acuna (bah-koo-nah) (bacuna) / vaccine
x	**ks, gs** as in *oxygen*	o**x**ígeno /oxygen / e**x**celente (egseh-**lehn**-teh) / excellent
y	same as **y** in *yes* / like **j** in *injection*	**y**eso (yeh-soh) / plaster / in**y**ección (een-yek-seeohn) / injection
y	by itself or at the end of a word, like **e** in *me*	so**y** (soh-eeh) / **I am**
z (Cast.)	like **th** in *thumb*	**z**umo (thoo-moh) /juice
z (H.A.)	as **s** in *soft*	**z**umbido (soom-bee-doh) / buzz

[a] Silent u. la u muda
[c] sounded in English. la u pronunciada.
[c] the letter h is never pronounced in Spanish. La letra h no se pronuncia nunca en el español.
[d] Silent u.

Note/Nota: The pronunciation of the words in parentheses is the pronunciation of the word in Latin America. The descriptions of sounds in this chart are approximations and do not indicate exact equivalence between English and Spanish sounds.

Letter B: **b** and **v** have the same sound in Spanish. Try to pronounce the **b** in *bacteria*. Imitate this same sound of the **b** or **v** in other Spanish words. After **m** or **n** the sound of the **b** is more like the English **b** as in *imbecil*, or in *invasive*, words that are very similar in Spanish: *imbécil* (eem-**beh**-seehl) stressed in the syllable **be**, and *invasivo* (een-bah-**seeh**-boh) stressed in the syllable **si.**

Letter C: **c** sounds like **k** or "hard" **c**, as in *cat*, when preceding **a, o, u,** as in *cancer*. This "hard" sound of **c** is not aspirated. Pronounce *cavidad* (kah-bee-**dahd**) as in *cavity; costo* (**kohs**-toh) cost; *cuatro* (**kooah**-troh) four. **c** has a different pronunciation when placed before **e** or **i** as in *centro* (**sehn**-troh) center, as pronounced in Latin America; *círculo,* with a **th** sound as in *think* (**theer**-coo-loh) as pronounced in Castillian.

Letter CH: Pronounce **ch** as in *child, leche* (**leh**-sheh).

Note. The Royal Academy of the Spanish Language has ruled since 1994 that **ch** and **ll** are considered combinations of letters of the alphabet (called *dígrafas);* for alphabetization purposes only.

Letter G: g placed before **a, o, u** has a gutural sound as in *gasp, gota* (**goh**-tah) drop, **g** has a different pronunciation when placed before **e** or **i**, in that case it sounds like a harsher **h**, as in *hemoglobin, género* (**heh**-neh-roh) gender.

Letter J: j is pronounced more forcefully than in *ham* as in *jarabe* (jah-**rah**-beh) syrup.

Letter Q: q is always pronounced as **k**, or **c** as in *cut, queso* (**keh**-soh) cheese; or *quiste* (**kees**-teh) cyst, **q** is always followed by a silent **u.**

Letter R: r inicial and **rr** in the middle of a word has a multiple thrill as in *hemorrhage / hemorragia* (eh-moh-**rrah**-heeah). Remember that the **h** is always silent. **r** in the middle, or at the end of a word is pronounced as in *heart, mirar* (meeh-**rahr**) to look.

Letter Ñ: ñ (n with a tilde), pronounce this letter as ny in *canyon, niño* (**neeh**-nyoh) child.

Letter LL: ll is pronounced approximately like in *million,* as in *millón* (meeh-**llóhn**) in Castillian, and like *yes* in Latin America (meeh-**yóhn**).

Letter X: x its approximate sounds are **ks, gs**, as in *oxygen, oxígeno* (ohg-**see**-heh-noh) placed between vowels. It is pronounced like **s** before consonants, as in *see, extraño,* (ehs-**trah**-gnoh) strange.

Letter Y: y with the same sound as **y** in *yes, yeso* (**yeh**-soh) chalk, and like the vowel **i** by itself as the conjunction **y** (meaning and).

Letter Z: z same sound as **th** in *thumb* in Castillian, *zumo* (**thooh**-moh) juice, or like *see* in Latin America, (**sooh**-moh).

3. Rules of Syllabication in Spanish / División de palabras en sílabas.

A Spanish word has as many syllables as it has vowels or diphthongs.

1. The consonants **b, c, f, g, p, t**, combine with **l** or **r** to form a syllable with the following vowel. The letter **d** also combines with **r** but it does not with the letter **l**.

b	c	f
blan-co (**blahn**-coh) white	**cla**-se (**clah**-seh) class	**fla**-co (**flah**-coh) thin, lanky

g	p	
glu-**co**-sa (glooh-**coh**-sah) glucose	**pla**-ca (**plah**-cah), plate, plaque	

c	b	d
cre-ma (**creh**-mah) cream	**bra**-vo (**brah**-voh) brave	**dra**-ma (**drah**-mah) drama

f	g	p
frá-gil (**frah**-geel) fragile	**gran**-de (**grahn**-deh) big	**pre**-cio (**preh**-seeoh) price

t
trau-ma (**trahooh**-mah) trauma

2. Any consonant following another (except the combinations described above) mark a division between syllables.
   parte: par-**te** (**pahr**-teh), part
   bronquitis: bron-**qui**-tis (brohn-**keeh**-teehs), bronchitis
   pulso: **pul**-so (**pool**-soh), pulse
3. The vowels that make up a dipthong are never separated:
   malaria: ma-**la**-ria (mah-**lah**-reeah), malaria
   tifoidea: ti-**foi**-dea (tee-pho-heeh-deh-hah) typhoid
   serie: **se**-rie (**seh**-reeeh) series
4. An accent over a weak vowel (**i** or **u**) dissolves the dipthong and forms a separated syllable:
   anatomía: a-na-to-**mí**-a (ah-nah-toh-**mee**-ah) anatomy
   oído: o-**í**-do (oh-**eeh**-doh) ear
5. Consecutive strong vowels are separated, forming different syllables:
   monitoreo: mo-ni-to-re-**o** (moh-nee-toh-**reh**-oh), monitoring
6. A vowel followed by a consonant at the beginning of a word can make a syllable by itself if the consonant forms a syllable with a following vowel, or if it is part of a combination described in (1).
   inexperiencia: **i**-nex-pe-rien-cia (e-negs-peh-**reehn**-see-ah) inexperience
   aplicación: **a**-pli-ca-ción (ah-pleeh-cah-**seeohn**) application

Rules of Accentuation / Reglas de acentuación

STRESS / ACENTO TÓNICO O FUERZA DE VOZ.

Stress is the emphasis given to a certain syllable in a word. The stress establishes a change between different words. (The stress is on the syllable in bold.)

IN-GRE-SAR
This word has three syllables; in-gre-**sar** is a verb infinitive. All infinitives in Spanish have the stress on the last syllable.
ingre**sa**do in-gre-**sa**-do The stress falls on the syllable **-sa.**
The patient is admitted. / El paciente es in-gre-**sa**-do.
ingresar and *ingresado* follow the rules of accentuation:

ENDING / TERMINACIÓN	STRESS / ACENTO	EXAMPLE /EJEMPLO
vowel: **a e i o u**	next-to-the-last syllable	ingres**a**do (in-gre-**sa**-do)
consonant: **n** or **s**	next-to-the-last syllable	in**gre**san (in-**gre**-san)
consonant other than **n** or **s**	on the last syllable	ingre**sar** (in-gre-**sar**)

WHERE SHOULD A WRITTEN ACCENT MARK BE PLACED?

Any words that do not comply wth the above rules require a written **accent mark / acento escrito** over the vowel as in: café, atención, **rí**gido.

A written accent mark is also used to distinguish two words of different meaning that are written alike, such as demonstrative adjectives, demonstrative pronouns, interrogatives, and relative pronouns.

adjective	**pronoun**
this patient / este paciente	this one / **éste**

Adjective: This patient is admitted today / este paciente es ingresado hoy
Pronoun: This one will be admitted tomorrow / **éste** (this one) será admitido mañana

interrogative what? / ¿qué?	**relative pronoun** that / que
What patient? / ¿**Qué paciente?**	The patient that will be admitted
	El paciente **que** (that) será admitido

Other words that require an accent to differentiate them are:

> yes / **sí** to make a difference from if / **si**;
> **dé** / give, a command, and the preposition **de** / of;
> he / **él** and the / **el** the definitive article;
> the subject pronoun you (familiar) **tú** /, and your / **tu** possessive adjective.

Punctuation / Punctuación

(.) puntos	(ü) diérisis
(;) punto y coma	(*) asterisco
(:) dos puntos	(-) guión
(¿) interrogación abierta	(_) raya
(?) interrogación cerrada	() paréntesis
(i) admiración abierta	(" ") comillas
(!) admiración cerrada	(. . .) puntos suspensivos

ENGLISH SOUNDS/ SONIDOS DEL INGLÉS

A difernica del español, en el que cada letra tiene un sonido más o menos definido, en inglés una misma letra puede tener más de una pronunciación y es esa la mayor dificultad que la persona hispanoparlante confronta al tratar de aprender la pronunciación de la lengua inglesa. La mayoría de los textos lingüísticos recurren al uso de algún alfabeto fonético que sirve de clave para la pronunciación. Para los efectos de este diccionario nos hemos limitado a dar una sencilla orientación que ayude al lector a pronunciar aquellas letras y sonidos que más diferen de la pronunciación en español y que, por lo tanto, presentan mayor dificultad al hispanoparlante. Debemos señalar que esta presentación simplificada de las letras en inglés no abarca todas las posibilidades; las excepciones a las reglas generales son muy numerosas.

El alfabeto inglés tiene veintiséis letras: cinco vocales y veintiuna consonantes. La letra **y**, como en español, puede ser vocal (se pronuncia como la **i** en español) **remedy** / remedio, o puede ser una consonante (se pronuncia como la **y** en *ya*) como en **yes** / sí.

Vocales / Vowels

Las vocales en inglés tienen generalmente dos sonidos, uno breve o corto y otro largo. La e puede además ser muda al final de la palabra.

[*Sonido breve o corto*: Ocurre generalmente cuando la vocal es seguida por una consonante en la misma sílaba.]

LETRA	PALABRA EN INGLÉS	SONIDO APROXIMADO EN ESPAÑOL
a	**nap** / siesta	sonido intermedio entre la a de mano y la e de pesa.
	call / llamada	**bo**ca (gen. en palabras que terminan en **ll**).
e	**bed** / cama	frente.
	late / tarde	muda (gen. ocurre al final de la palabra).
i	**chill** / enfriamiento	sonido intermedio entre la **i** y la **e** en español.
o	**compare** / comparar	comparar
	hot / caliente	sonido intermedio entre la **a** y la **o** en español.
	move / mover	cura
u	**drug** / droga	sonido intermedio entre la **o** y la **u** en español.
	full / lleno	tú

[*Sonido largo*: Ocurre generalmente cuando la vocal es la vocal final de una sílaba o cuando va seguida de una e muda o de una e muda y una consonante. Es un sonido vocálico demorado en el cual algunas veces una vocal sencilla tiene un sonido diptongado.]

a	**basic** / básico	**ley**
e	**he** /él	**sí**
i	**bite** / picadura	hay
o	**dose** / dosis	sonido equivalente al sonido del diptongo **ou** en español.
oo	**blood** / sangre	poro
	book / libro	cura
u	**putrid** / pútrido	ciudad, combinación equivalente al sonido de **iu** en español

Diptongos / Diphthongs

ew: Sonido en inglés corresponde al sonido **iu**:

few / varios	ci**u**dad

ou: Sonido semejante al diptongo **au** en español o sonido breve semejante **a** la **o** en español:

mouth / boca	ca**u**sa
bought / compró	d**o**sis

Consonantes / Consonants

El alfabeto inglés tiene dos consonantes que casi no se usan en español, la **k** y la **w**; la **ñ**, en cambio, no existe en el alfabeto inglés **y** las letras **ch**, **ll**, y **rr** no se consideran caracteres propios, sino combinación de dos letras (letra *dígrafa*). En general, la pronunciación de la mayoría de las consonantes es semejante en ambos idiomas, aunque en inglés la pronunciación de las mismas es más explosiva.

Consonantes y letras dígrafas que más difieren de la pronunciación española

CONSONANTES	PALABRA EN INGLÉS	SONIDO APROXIMADO EN ESPAÑOL
b	Sonido semejante a la **b** initial en español; es muda en algunas palabras cuando precede a la letra **t**. *Sonido aproximado en español*	
	bacillus / bacilo	**b**acilo
	doubt / duda	(muda)
ch	Presenta varios sonidos según su posición en la palabra.	
	child / niño	**ch**ico
	cholera / cólera	**c**ólera
	machine / máquina	**sh**shsh! (*semejante al sonido que se emplea para indicar silencio*)

English Sounds/ Sonidos del inglés

CONSONANTES	PALABRA EN INGLÉS	SONIDO APROXIMADO EN ESPAÑOL
g	Cuando le sigue una **e** o una **i** tiene un sonido semejante a la **y** en español (*sonido suave*). Esta regla tiene por excepción las palabras monosílabas.	
	general / general	**y**eso (*sonido africado*)
	giant / gigante	**y**eso (*sonido africado*)
	girl / muchacha	**g**ota
	En casi todas las otras situaciones, tiene el mismo sonido que la **g** fuerte en español.	
	gastric / gástrico	**g**ástrico
	gram / gramo	**g**ramo
	guide / guía	**g**uía
gh	En medio de la palabra, esta combinación de letras es generalmente muda.	
	daughter / hija	
h	Sonido aproximado al de la **j** en español, pero algo más suave.	
	hemorrhage / hemorragia	**j**arabe
j	Sonido semejante a la **y** en español.	
	jejunum / yeyuno	**y**ey**u**no (*con africación*)
ll	Sonido igual al de la **l** sencilla.	
	generally / generalmente	genera**l**mente
kn	La **k** es muda.	
	knee / rodilla	**n**uez
mm	Sonido igual a la **m** simple.	
	immunology / inmunología	a**m**eba
ph	Sonido de **f**.	
	pharmacy / farmacia	**f**armacia
r	Sonido articulado en inglés sin trino y con la lengua situada más hacia atrás de la boca y la parte anterior curvada hacia el paladar sin tocarlo.	
	surgery / cirugía	ci**r**ugía
rr	Sonido igual al del la **r** sencilla.	
	hemorrhage / hemorragia	ci**r**ugía
s	Sonido semejante a la **s** sorda en español en la mayoría de los vocablos.	
	consult / consultar	con**s**ulta
	sperm / esperma	e**s**perma
	Sonido semejante a la **s** sonora de mismo o desde cuando está entre vocales o antes de la consonante **m**.	
	disease / enfermedad	mi**s**mo
	metabolism / metabolismo	de**s**de
	Al final de la palabra, puede tener sonido de **s** o de **z** en inglés.	
	yes / sí	**s**í
	is / es	(*sonido de z en inglés*)

English Sounds/ Sonidos del inglés

CONSONANTES	PALABRA EN INGLÉS	SONIDO APROXIMADO EN ESPAÑOL
s	Cuando está seguida del diptongo **io**, tiene sonido semejante al de la **y** (*sonido de consonante*), muy exagerado, o al de la **j** en francés como en **J**ean. **lesion** / lesión	leyó
	Cuando está seguida de la vocal **u**, tiene un sonido semejante a la **sh** en inglés. **sure** / seguro	**sh**shsh (*como cuando se está silenciando a alguien*)
ss	Sonido igual al de la **s** en español. **class** / clase	clase
th	Tiene dos sonidos: (1) parecido a la **d**; (2) parecido a la **z** castellana. **this** / este **therapy** / terapia	de**d**o **z**apato (*con ceceo castellano*)
w	Sonido semejante al de la **u** en español como en la palabra h**u**eso. **weight** / peso	h**u**eso
z	Sonido semejante al que se hace para imitar el zumbido de una abeja. **zero** / cero	**zz**zz. . .

Acentuación de las palabras en inglés

El acento gráfico no existe en inglés. Las reglas a seguir son pocas, pero tienen muchas excepciones.

1. Las palabras de dos sílabas se acentúan generalmente en la penúltima sílaba:
   swollen / hinchado
   abscess / abceso
2. Palabras a las que se le hayan anadido sufijos o prefijos retienen el acento en la misma sílaba acentuada de la raíz o palabra básica:
   normal: abnormal / anormal
   coloration: discoloration / descoloración
3. Palabras de tres o más sílabas generalmente tienen una sílaba que se acentúa más enfáticamente y otra sílaba que lleva un acento menos pronunciado:
   rapidly / **rá**pidamente

Punctuation / Puntuación

(.) period	(-) the dash
(,) comma	() parentheses
(;) semicolon	(" ") quotation marks
(:) colon	([ ]) brackets
(?) the question mark*	(') apostrophe
(!) the exclamation point*	(*) asterisk

*En inglés los signos de interrogación y admiración se usan solamente al final de la oración.

ORTHOGRAPHIC CHANGES AND COGNATES / CAMBIOS ORTOGRÁFICOS Y COGNADOS

Orthographic Changes / Cambios ortográficos

English / Inglés	Spanish / Español	English / Inglés	Spanish / Español
cc	c	accommodate	acomodar
cc[1]	cc before e and i	accessory	accesorio
		accident	accidente
ch	c	character	carácter
ch before e and i	qui	chemistry	química
		chiropractor	quiropráctico
comm-	com-	commissure	comisura
im-	in-	immersion	inmersión
qu	cu	quart	cuarto
r[2]	l	paper	papel
es[3]	special	especial	
		gastrospasm	gastroespasmo
ph	f	phlebitis	flebitis
pn[4]	pn or n	pneumonia	pneumonía, neumonía
ps	ps or s	psychology	psicología, sicología
rh	r	rheumatic	reumático
th	t	therapy	terapia
y[5]	i	typhoid	tifoidea

[1] In Spanish words only two double consonants are used; **cc** and **nn.** The **ll** and **rr** are considered to be single characters in the Spanish alphabet.
En español sólo hay dos consonantes dobles: **cc** y **nn.** La **ll** y la **rr** se consideran letras en el alfabeto español.

[2] May change to **l** at the end of a word.
Puede cambiar a **l** al final de palabra.

[3] Only before consonants **p** and **t**, including compound words.
Sólo delante de las consonantes **p** y **t** incluso en palabras compuestas.

[4] **pn** and **ps** may drop the initial **p** in Spanish.
En español se puede omitir la **p** inicial en las palabras que comienzan en **pn** o **ps.**

[5] When **y** is not at the end of the word.
Cuando la **y** no es final.

Orthographic Changes and Cognates / Cambios ortográficos y cognadas

	EXAMPLES	EJEMPLOS
1. There are only two double consonants in Spanish words: **cc** and **nn**		acción accidente innovación
2. Change **mm** to **m** except when preceded by **i**	communicate communication	comunicar comunicación
3. **ch** changes to **c**, except when it is before **e** or **i**, then it changes to **qu**	mechanic choleric chimera chemotherapy	mecánico colérico quimera quimioterapia
4. Drop the **h-** inside words except in **alcohol**[a]	therapy authorization hemorrhage	terapia autorización hemorragia
5. **ph** becomes **f** The **ph** at the beginning or in the middle of a word corresponds to **f** in Spanish.	pharmacy phase diphtheria	farmacia fase difteria
6. Drop one **-s**. There are no words with double **ss** in Spanish.	necessity dissect fissura	necesidad disecar fisura
7. English words that begin in **s** + **consonant** have corresponding Spanish words beginning in **es-**.	special scene scan	especial escena escán
8. The **y** in the middle of a word may change to **-í**.	crystal syphilis trypsin	cristal sífilis tripsina
9. **Add -a** to words ending in **-gram**: gram + **-a** = **grama.**	diagram	diagrama
10. The suffix **-um** drops and is substituted by **-o** in Spanish.	stadium pendulum rostrum	estadio péndulo rostro
11. The suffix **-osis** referring[b] to condition or disease, remains the same in Spanish.	dermatosis lymphocytosis anisocytosis	dermatosis linfocitosis anisocitosis

[a] and other words of Arabic origin.
[b] Spanish nouns ending in -osis are feminine.

	EXAMPLES	EJEMPLOS
12. **-ty** becomes **-dad**	fideli**ty**	fideli**dad**
Many words in English ending in **-ty** have a corresponding Spanish word ending in **-dad**.	communi**ty**	comuni**dad**
	reali**ty**	reali**dad**
13. **-ous** becomes **-oso** or **-osa**	vigor**ous**	vigor**oso**
For many words ending in **-ous** in English, the corresponding word in Spanish ends in **-oso** or **osa**	numer**ous**	numer**oso**
	por**ous**	por**oso**
14. **-tion** becomes **-ción** in Spanish	educa**tion**	educa**ción**
	communica**tion**	comunica**ción**
	administra**tion**	administra**ción**

15. **Exact cognates.**
Words in Spanish and English that are spelled exactly the same way, have the same root, and mean the same are called exact cognates: **control, factor, local.**
However, there are other cognates that have similar or the same spelling and are misleading, because the meaning could be different: **real** can be translated **real** or **royal; actual** can mean **current; asistir** can be translated as **to attend** or **to help;** while **atender** in Spanish means to **pay attention** or **to take care of.**

Cognates / Cognados

Cognates are words related in origin, that is, words that have the same origin as other words in another language. The spelling of a word (noun, adjective, or verb) may be identical or almost the same as the other language's word. Cognates follow spelling rules, and may have equivalent endings in both languages. The terminology made up of the "new" terms found, are words made by combining prefixes, roots (stems) and suffixes of Greek and Latin origin. Spelling changes took place in the stem of the word, new word endings were added to the Latin or Greek words, which were substituted by derivatives proper to the many languages of the users.

You will find in the following pages some of the variations that have occurred to scientific terms and in common English and Spanish words. These two languages, English and Spanish, have as many as seventy-five percent of scientific words that are common to each other, called **cognates / cognados.** By using the examples of cognates given in the following list and the rules employed in the English words for transformation into Spanish, you will learn to build your own additional vocabulary.

Equivalences in Endings, English / Spanish

ENGLISH	SPANISH	ENGLISH	SPANISH
-ent	-ente	accident	accidente
-ine	-ina	morphine	morfina
-ment	-mento	instrument	instrumento
-ide	-uro	chloride	cloruro

Adjective Endings

ENGLISH	SPANISH	ENGLISH	SPANISH
-ive	-ivo, -iva	active	activo (*m.*), activa (*f.*)
-nal	-no, -na	internal	interno (*m.*), interna (*f.*)
-id	-ido	liquid	líquido (*m.*), líquida (*f.*)
-ct	-cto, -cta	perfect	perfecto (*m.*), perfecta (*f.*)

Verb Endings

ENGLISH	SPANISH	ENGLISH	SPANISH
-ce	-zar	commence	comenzar
-iate	-iar	affiliate	afiliar
-ish	-ecer	establish	establecer
-ize	-izar	cauterize	cauterizar

Orthographic Changes and Cognates / Cambios ortográficos y cognados

List of Cognates and Their Pronunciations in Spanish—Words
That Have the Same or Similar Spelling[a]

COGNATES	SPANISH PRONUNCIATION
anasarca *f.* anasarca	ah-nah-**sahr'**-kah
abdominal *a.* abdominal	ahb-doh-mee-**náhl'**
abulia *n.* abulia	ah-**boo'**-leeah
acarina *f.* acarina	ah-kah-**ree'**-nah
accidente *m.* accident	ahk-see-**dehn'**-te
acidosis *f.* acidosis	ah-see-**doh'**-sees
bismuto *m.* bismuth	bees-**moo**-toh
benzocaína *f.* benzocaine	behn-zoh-kah-**ee'**-nah
bradicardia *f.* bradycardia	brah-dee-**cahr'**-deeah
cervix[b] *m.* cervix	**sehr'**-beegs
cisterna *f.* cistern	sees-**tehr'**-nah
clavícula *f.* clavicle	klah-**beeh'**-cooh-lah
colon *m.* colon	**koh'**-lohn
color *m.* color	koh-**lohr'**
coma *m.* coma	**koh'**-mah
comensal *m.* commensal	koh-mehn-**sahl**
compacta *a.* compact	kohm-**pahk**-tah
control *m.* control	kohn-**trohl**
gama *f.* gamma	**gah**-mah
gástrico *a.* gastric	**gáhs**-tree-coh
glándula *f.* gland	**gláhn**-doo-lah

[a] The stressed syllable in the Spanish words is indicated by **bold** and the symbol (').
[b] **Cervix**, a Latin word used in anatomy in both English and Spanish, is pronounced very similarly in both languages. Do not confuse this word, translated as **cuello uterino** (part of the uterus), with the term **cerviz**, nape of the neck.

COGNATES	SPANISH PRONUNCIATION
glaucoma *m.* glaucoma	glahoo-**koh**-mah
gluten *m.* gluten	**gloo**-tehn
hepatitis *f.* hepatitis	eh-pah-**tee**-tees
hospital *m.* hospital	ohs-pee-**tahl'**
hematoma *m.* hematoma	eh-mah-**toh'**-mah
infantil *a.* infantile	eehn-fahn-**teel'**
infección *f.* infection	een-fehk-**seeohn'**
influenza *f.* influenza	een-flooh**ehn'**-zah
lámina *f.* lamina	**lah'**-mee-nah
lanugo *a.* lanugo	lah-**noo'**-goh
medicamento *m.* medicament	meh-dee-kah-**mehn'** -toh
nasal *a.* nasal	nah-**sahl'**
neonatal *a.* neonatal	neh-oh-**nah'**-tahl
neoplasia *f.* neoplasia	neh-oh-**plah'**-seeah
normal *a.* normal	nor-**mahl'**
nuclear *a.* nuclear	noo-kleh-**ahr'**
osmosis *f.* osmosis	ohs-**moh'**-sees
orolingual *a.* orolingual	oh-roh-leen-**gooahl'**
pectoral *a.* pectoral	pehk-toh-**rahl'**
persona *f.* persona	pehr-**soh'**-nah
placenta *f.* placenta	plah-**sehn'**-tah
pneumonia[c] *f.* pneumonia	nehoo-moh-**neeah'**
podagra *f.* podagra	poh-**dah'**-grah
región *f.* region	reh-hee-**ohn'**
renal *a.* renal	reh-**nahl'**
repulsión *f.* repulsion	reh-pool-**seeohn'**

Orthographic Changes and Cognates / Cambios ortográficos y cognados

COGNATES	SPANISH PRONUNCIATION
saliva *f.* saliva	sah-**lee'**-bah
semicircular *a.* semicircular	seh-mee-seer-coo-**lahr'**
senil *a.* senile	seh-**neel'**
sensorial *a.* sensoreal	sehn-soh-**reeahl'**
serositis *f.* serositis	she-roh-**see'**-tees
sexual *a.* sexual	sehg-**sooahl'**
simple *a.* simple	**seem'**-pleh
soda *a.* soda	**soh'**-dah
superior *a.* superior	soo-peh-**reeohr'**
temporal *a.* temporal	tehm-poh-**rahl'**
tenia *f.* tenia	**teh'**-neeah
tensión *f.* tension	tehn-see**óhn'**
trauma *m.* trauma	**trahw'**-mah

Brief Notes on Spanish Grammar

Notas breves de gramática española

THE SPANISH ARTICLE: DEFINITE AND INDEFINITE / EL ARTÍCULO ESPAÑOL: DEFINIDO E INDEFINIDO

Articles (definite or indefinite) precede the noun. Spanish articles agree with the noun in gender and number. Forms of the definite article in the masculine and feminine: singular and plural. The Spanish article, like the English article, precedes the noun.

THE DEFINITE ARTICLE (THE) / EL ARTÍCULO DEFINIDO

	MASCULINE	*FEMININE*
singular	el	la
plural	los	las

Placing the definite article with feminine nouns:

the American doctor / **la** doctora americana
the artery / **la** arteria
the arteries / **las** arterias

With masculine nouns:

the sick boy / **el** niño enfermo
the sick boys / **los** niños enfermos

Singular feminine nouns which begin with stressed **a-** or **ha-** are preceded by the masculine form **el**.

the water / **el** agua
the speech / **el** habla.

The contraction **al** and **del** takes place when **a** / to, precedes **el**; and **de** / of, precedes **el**.

to the boy / **al** niño
of the boy / **del** niño
whose? / ¿de quién?
the medicine **of** the boy / la medicina **del** niño

THE INDEFINITE ARTICLE / EL ARTÍCULO INDEFINIDO

	FEMININE	*MASCULINE*
singular	a / **una**	a / **uno**
plural	some / **unas**	some / **unos**

With a feminine noun:

a tablet / **una tableta**
some tablets / **unas tabletas**

3

With a masculine noun:

> a small thermometer / **un termómetro pequeño**
> some small thermometers / **unos termómetros pequeños**

In the first two examples the nouns tablet / **tableta**, a feminine noun, and thermometer / **termómetro**, a masculine noun, determine the gender and number of the article that precedes them. Descriptive adjectives that follow the nouns, show their agreement in gender and number with the noun. The same agreement on article and noun is shown in the examples using the indefinite article.

GENDER / GÉNERO

NOUN GENDER / GÉNERO DEL NOMBRE

Spanish nouns are masculine or feminine, there are no neuter nouns. Nouns referring to female beings are classified as feminine. Objects are also given a gender. Most of the feminine nouns end in –**a**, but there are other endings that characterize feminine nouns. The exception to the rule is the noun **día** which, although it ends in –**a**, is a masculine noun. Nouns ending in –**ma -pa -ta** of Greek origin are also masculine with the exception of **flema** (phlem), which is a feminine noun. Those nouns are preceded by masculine articles. Examples: el mapa, el poeta, el planeta; un mapa, un poeta, un planeta.

Endings of Feminine Nouns / Terminaciones de nombres femeninos

ENDING / TERMINACIÓN	EXAMPLE / EJEMPLO	EXCEPTION / EXCEPCIÓN
-ad	truth **verdad**	–
-ión	education **educación**	airplane **avión**
-is	colitis **colitis**	–
-ud	health **salud**	–
-umbre	habit **costumbre**	–

Nouns referring to masculine beings, days of the week, and names of languages, and others are usually classified as masculine with the ending –**o**. The exception to the rule is **mano** which is a feminine noun.

Endings of Masculine Nouns / Terminaciones de nombres masculinos

ENDING	EXAMPLE	EXCEPTION
-ma	symptom **síntoma**	phlegm (**la**) **flema**
-pa	map **mapa**	
-ta	planet **planeta**	
-or	doctor **doctor**	–

ADJECTIVES GENDER / GÉNERO DE LOS ADJETIVOS

Adjectives are used in both the masculine and feminine genders. Change the ending **-o** of a masculine adjective to **-a** to form the feminine.

> the good boy / **el niño bueno**
> the good girl / **la niña buena**

Add **-a** to an adjective of nationality ending in consonant to form the feminine. Drop the accent of the last syllable before adding the feminine ending. However, the stress remains on the vowel.

> Englishman / **inglés**
> English woman / **inglesa**

Adjectives that end in **-e** or in a consonant remain with the same form for both the masculine and feminine forms.

> an urgent call / **una llamada urgente**
> an urgent case / **un caso urgente**
> an easy test / **una prueba fácil**
> an easy work / **un trabajo fácil**

Adjectives ending in **-án, -ón, -or** (except comparatives), add **-a** to form the feminine. The accent drops when the feminine ending is added.

> lazy / **haragán, haragana**

The adjective may follow or precede the noun, however, nouns and adjectives are inflected alike.

PLURAL OF NOUNS AND ADJECTIVES / EL PLURAL DE NOMBRES Y ADJETIVOS

add	- *s*	if the word ending is an unaccented vowel or dipthong, or stressed *é*:
		system / **sistema** systems / **sistemas**
		coffee / **café** coffees / **cafés**
add	**-es**	if the adjective ends in a consonant:
		special / **especial** specials / **especiales**
add	**-es**	if it ends in **z**, change **z** to **c** before addding **-es**:
		light / **luz** lights / **luces**

The plural is indicated in nouns ending in **–s** by the preceding article. The singular form does not change. The days of the week (except Saturday / el sábado and Sunday / el domingo) are examples.

> Monday / **el lunes**   Mondays / **los lunes**
> Thursday / **el jueves**   Thursdays / **los jueves**

5

ADJECTIVES PRECEDING THE NOUN / ADJETIVOS QUE PRECEDEN AL NOMBRE

POSSESSIVE ADJECTIVES / ADJETIVOS POSESIVOS

Possessive adjectives precede the noun, and show agreement in gender and number with the thing possessed (a noun they modify). The following forms precede the noun.

ENGLISH / INGLÉS	*SPANISH / ESPAÑOL*	
SINGULAR	*SINGULAR*	*PLURAL*
my	**mi**	**mis**
your (fam.)	**tu**	**tus**
your, his, her, its;	**su**	**sus**
our	**nuestro-a**	**nuestros,-as**
your (fam. Cast.)	**vuestro-a**	**vuestros,-as**
your, their	**su**	**sus**

our test / **nuestra prueba**	our diet / **nuestra dieta**
your cases / **tus casos**	our hospital / **nuestro hospital**

To clarify **su** (which can refer to more than one possessor), substitute **su** by using the preposition **de** + the subject pronoun. "Su conteo sanguíneo es normal" (his blood count is normal) can also be said "el conteo sanguíneo **de él** es normal."

Her test was easy.   **Su prueba fue fácil.   La prueba de ella fue fácil.**

DEMONSTRATIVE ADJECTIVES / ADJETIVOS DEMOSTRATIVOS

Demonstratives can be adjectives or pronouns. Demonstrative adjectives precede the noun. Demonstrative pronouns always have a written accent, demonstrative adjectives do not.

Masculine	**Feminine**
SINGULAR this / **este**	SINGULAR this / **esta**
this sick man **este hombre enfermo**	this medication **esta medicina**
PLURAL these / **estos**	PLURAL these / **estas**
these sick men **estos hombres enfermos**	these medications **estas medicinas**
SINGULAR that / **ese**	SINGULAR that / **esa**
that sick man **ese hombre enfermo**	that medication **esa medicina**
PLURAL those / **esos**	PLURAL those / **esas**
those sick men **esos hombres enfermos**	those medications **esas medicinas**
SINGULAR that / **aquel**	SINGULAR that / **aquella**
that case (farther, in distance or time) **aquel caso**	that medication (farther in distance or time) **aquella medicina**
PLURAL those / **aquellos**	PLURAL those / **aquellas**
those cases **aquellos casos**	those medications **aquellas medicinas**

SUPERLATIVES / SUPERLATIVOS

ADJECTIVES / ADJETIVOS	SUPERLATIVE (FOR COMPARISONS) / SUPERLATIVOS EN COMPARACIONES
low / **bajo**	(the) lowest / **(el) (la) inferior**
good / **bueno**	(the) better, best / **(el) (la) mejor**
bad / **malo**	(the) worst / **(el) (la) peor**
large / **grande**	(the) greater, greatest / **(el) (la)mayor**
mayor / **oldest**	(the) oldest, older / **(el) (la) mayor**
small / **pequeño**	(the) smaller, smallest, younger /**(el) (la) menor**
youngest / **menor**	(the) youngest, younger / **(el) (la) menor**

The **absolute superlative** refers only to a quality possesed by a person or object in a high degree, without comparison to others. The ending *-ísimo-a,* is added to the radical of the adjective to form the absolute superlative.

ADVERBS / ADVERBIOS

An adverb modifies an adjective or a verb, not a noun.

> The hospital is much closer. / El hospital está **más cerca**.
> How do you feel today, better? / ¿Cómo se siente hoy, **mejor**?
> Better than yesterday. / **Mejor** que ayer.

ADVERBS		SUPERLATIVES	
well / **bien**	best, better / **mejor**	is well / **está bien**	is better / **está mejor**
bad, badly / **mal**	worse, worst / **peor**	is well / **está bien**	is worse / **está peor**
much / **mucho**	more, most / **más**	knows too much / **sabe mucho**	
little / **poco**	less, least / **menos**	a little / **un poco**	a little less / **un poco menos**

LIST OF ADVERBS / LISTA DE ADVERBIOS

abajo below, down	**se encuentra abajo**	it is below
adelante forward, ahead	**siga adelante**	go ahead
afuera outside	**se queda afuera**	remains outside
ahora, ahorita now, shortly	**ahora vengo**	I am coming immediately
algo something, somewhat	**es algo parecido**	it is somewhat alike
a la moda in fashion, new	**está siempre a la moda**	he, she is always in style

apenas hardly, scarcely	**apenas lo reconoció**	hardly recognized him
arriba up, higher	**arriba del estómago**	higher than the stomach
atrás behind	**atrás del corazón**	behind the heart
a tiempo in, on time	**llega a tiempo**	arrives on time
bastante enough	**bastante grande**	big enough

PRONOUNS / PRONOMBRES

A pronoun is a word that takes the place or is used instead of a noun.

DEMONSTRATIVE PRONOUNS / PRONOMBRES DEMOSTRATIVOS

Demonstrative pronouns are used when referring to a noun which is unexpressed. Demonstrative pronouns always have a written accent.

	SINGULAR	*PLURAL*
Masculine	**éste, ése, aquél**	**éstos, ésos, aquéllos**
Feminine	**ésta, ésa, aquélla**	**éstas, ésas, aquéllas**

SUBJECT PRONOUNS / PRONOMBRES PERSONALES

Subject pronouns tell who is performing the action of the verb. Subject pronouns are used in Spanish for clarification and emphasis. They are not used as commonly as in English since the verb in Spanish indicates person and number. The familiar pronoun of the second person singular **tú** is used when speaking to a friend, relative or a child. The plural form **vosotros, -as** is rarely used in Hispanic América, where **ustedes** is used for the plural of **tú**. There is no translation in Spanish for the English subject pronoun **it**. **It** as a subject of a verb is not translated either.

> It is imposible. / No es posible.
> It is I. / Soy yo.

DIRECT OBJECT PRONOUNS / PRONOMBRES DE OBJETO DIRECTO

A direct object pronoun is used instead of a noun object of the verb.

> Do you see the letter? Yes, I see **it**. / ¿Ve **la** letra ? Sí, **la** veo.

INDIRECT OBJECT PRONOUNS / PRONOMBRES DE OBJETO INDIRECTO

An indirect object pronoun is used instead of a noun indirect object of the verb. Placement of object pronouns before a conjugated verb: ind.o.p. + d.o.p. + verb. (indirect object pronoun + direct object pronoun + verb)

> Do you give the medication to her? ¿**Le** da la medicina a ella?
> Yes, I gave it to her. Sí, **se la** di.(if **le** precedes **la** or **lo** it changes to **se**).

In the example, ¿Le da la medicina a ella? la **medicina** is the direct object of the verb, and corresponds to the pronoun **la**, answering the question, What did you give her? Her corresponds to **le**, indirect object pronoun. Sí, se la dí. / Yes, I gave it to her.

OBJECT PRONOUNS ATTACHED TO AN INFINITIVE / PRONOMBRES DE OBJETO AÑADIDOS A UN INFINITIVO

When a personal pronoun is the object of the verb infinitive as in:

> You want to buy it (the medication) for me. Quiere comprármela.
> You want to buy the medication for me. Quiere comprar la medicina para mí.

> "Me" (same word in Spanish, pronounced meh) is the indirect object pronoun. (ind.o.p.)
> Quiere **comprarme** la medicina. Quiere **comprármela.**
> A direct object pronoun substitutes the noun **la medicina**. *la* (d.o.p).

Order to follow: Attach to the infinitive the indirect object pronoun preceding the direct object pronoun. The same rules are observed with affirmative (usted) commands: ¡cómpresela! (buy it! for her); or with only a direct object: Example: the house, buy it! ¡cómprela! With both direct and indirect object pronouns: Tell it to him! ¡dígaselo! (*se* substituted *le*, referring to *to him*)

In the affirmative commands above, a stress falls in the third syllable from the end so a written accent mark is needed.

REFLEXIVE PRONOUNS / PRONOMBRES REFLEXIVOS

A reflexive pronoun is used when the subject acts upon itself. The forms **me, te, nos, os,** are also used in the reflexive, meaning myself, yourself, ourselves, yourselves. For the other persons **se** is used, meaning yourself (for **usted**), herself, and himself for the singular forms; yourselves (for **ustedes**), and themselves for the plural form. In Spanish the possessive is not used when referring to parts of the body. The reflexive indicates that it is referring to the subject's own body.

> She washes her hands / Ella **se** lava las manos
> The patient washed his hands. /El paciente **se** lavó las manos.

Reflexive Pronouns and the Reflexive Verb Levantarse / Pronombres reflexivos y el verbo reflexivo levantarse

PERSONAL PRONOUN	REFLEXIVE PRONOUN	INDICATIVE, PRESENT TENSE
I / **yo**	myself / **me**	I get up / **me levanto**
you / **tú** (familiar)	yourself / **te**	you get up / **te levantas**
you / **usted** (formal)	yourself / **se**	you get up / **usted se levanta**
he / **él**	himself / **se**	he gets up / **él se levanta**
she / **ella**	herself / **se**	she gets up / **ella se levanta**
we / **nosotros**	ourselves / **nos**	we get up / **nos levantamos**
we / **nosotras**	ourselves / **nos**	we get up / **nosotras nos levantamos**
you / **vosotros** (familiar)	yourselves / **os**	you get up / **vosotros os levantáis**
you / **vosotras** (familiar)	yourselves / **os**	you get up / **vosotras os levantáis**
you / **ustedes** (formal)	yourselves / **se**	you get up / **ustedes se levantan**
they / **ellos**	themselves / **se**	they get up / **ellos, se levantan**
they / **ellas**	themselves / **se**	they get up / **ellas se levantan**

RELATIVE PRONOUNS / PRONOMBRES RELATIVOS

Relative pronouns (that, which, whom, whose / **que, cual, quien, cuyo**) introduce an adjective clause that can be used as a direct object, the object of a preposition, and clarifying an antecedent.

> The medicine **(that)** you took. / La medicina **que** usted tomó.
> The patient, **of whom** I spoke today. / El paciente de **quien** hablé hoy

PERSONAL PRONOUNS, SINGULAR / PRONOMBRES PERSONALES, DE OBJETO DIRECTO E INDIRECTO, SINGULAR

SUBJECT PRONOUN	DIRECT OBJECT PRONOUN	INDIRECT OBJECT PRONOUN
I / **yo**	me / **me**	to me, for me / **me**
You / **tú**	you / **te**	to you, for you / **te (se)**
You / **usted**	you / **lo, la**	to you, for you / **le**
He / **él**	him / **lo**	to him, for him / **le (se)**
She / **ella**	her / **la**	to her, for her / **le (se)**

Note: **me, te, nos** and **os,** can be used as direct or indirect object pronouns and reflexive pronouns.

PERSONAL PRONOUNS, PLURAL / PRONOMBRES PERSONALES, DE OBJETO DIRECTO E INDIRECTO, PLURAL

SUBJECT PRONOUN	DIRECT OBJECT PRONOUN	INDIRECT OBJECT PRONOUN
we / **nosotros**	us / **nos**	to us / **nos**
you / **ustedes**	you / **los, las**	to you, for you / **les**
they / **ellos**	them / **los**	to them, for them / **les**
they / **ellas**	them / **las**	to them, for them / **les**

Mismo, used as an adjective, means –self, same.

> the same patient / el **mismo** paciente
> the same nurse / la **misma** enfermera

Mismo, used as a pronoun, has an emphatic tone.

> Ella **misma** da la medicina al paciente. / She herself gives the medication to the patient.
> Él **mismo** estaba por la noche aquí. / He himself was here during the night.

VERBS / VERBOS

In Spanish the action expressed by a verb refers either to **a fact** or to a condition in the mind of the speaker involving some **doubt, wish, hope** or **possibility**. A verb may also express a **command** or **request for action**. The indicative mood indicates facts, while the subjunctive mood (gen. in the dependent clause) indicates something that is **uncertain, doubtful, wishful** or **hopeful**, stated or implied in the main clause. The subjunctive is more frequently used in Spanish than it is in English. It is seldom used in the main clause, except to take the place of a command.

Indicative: Expressing reality, knowledge, and belief.

> **I speak** to the doctor. / **Hablo** con el medico.
> Yes, **I know** where the hospital is. / Sí, **yo sé** donde está el hospital

Subjunctive: Expressing in a dependent clause, a wish or desire, possibility, doubt, or something which is not a fact,

> **I hope** that **you feel better.** / **Espero** que usted **se sienta** mejor.

Imperative: Giving a command or making a request

> **Take** the medication in the morning. / **Tome** la medicina por la mañana.

Subjunctive: uncertainty

> **I doubt** that she is feeling better. / **Dudo** que ella se sienta major.

The affirmative command of the familiar **tú** is the same form of the third person singular of the present. **¡Habla!** Pedro; **¡Escuchame!** (Listen to me). Verbs with irregular forms: Venir **(ven),** salir **(sal),** tener **(ten). ¡Ven** aquí! (Come here) **¡Ten** cuidado! (Be careful!); **¡Sal** de ahí! (Get out!).

TWO SPANISH VERBS MEANING TO BE / DOS VERBOS CON EL MISMO SIGNIFICADO, EN INGLÉS

SER

Indicative (present tense)

soy, eres, es
somos, sois, son

SER expresses the permanent or inherent

Profession: José es medico.
Religion: José es católico.
Telling time: José, ¿Qué hora es? Son las ocho de la mañana.
Origin: José es de California.
Identity: ¿Quién es su padre?
Quality by nature: José y yo somos optimistas.
Ownership: ¿De quién es el libro? Es de Juan. (Whose book? Is John's.)
What things are made of: La casa es de madera.
Location of an event: El concierto es en el auditorio
A chronic condition: Carlos es asmático.

ESTAR

Indicativo (tiempo presente)

estoy, estás, está
estás, estamos, están

ESTAR expresses temporary or occasional

Temporary condition: El niño está enfermo.
Location: Carmen está en el hospital con su niño.
Casual expression: ¿Cómo está? Está mejor.
Change in weather: Está lloviendo. (It is raining.)
Emotional state: Estoy triste. (I am sad.)
Asking for the date: ¿A cómo estamos?
Answering: Estamos a diez de febrero.
An action in progress: ¿Qué estás haciendo? Estoy escribiendo. (What are you doing? I am writing.)
Any location except for events: Estoy en el hospital.
Giving directions: ¿Dónde está el hospital? Está cerca, a dos cuadras. (Where is the hospital? It is close, two blocks away.)

REGULAR VERBS FORMATION / FORMACIÓN DE LOS TIEMPOS DE VERBOS REGULARES

The infinitive form of Spanish verbs end in -ar (to cure / curar), -er (to eat / comer), or -ir (to admit / admitir). Most Spanish verbs ends in -ar, and the majority of infinitives ending in -ar are regular verbs. The letters preceding the infinitive ending are the root or stem of the verb. Root of curar> cur-; comer> com-; admitir> admit-. The tenses of regular verbs, except the future and the conditional (when the whole infinitive is used), are formed by adding endings to the root.

Present Indicative: Endings of Regular Verbs / Presente de Indicativo: Terminaciones de verbos regulares

Infinitive Ending –ar

SINGULAR	HABLAR (HABL+)	PLURAL	HABLAR (HABL+)
Yo -o	Yo hablo	Nosotros -amos	Nosotros hablamos
Tú -as	Tú hablas	Vosotros -áis	Vosotros habláis
Usted, él, ella -a	Usted, él, ella habla	Ustedes, ellos, ellas -an	Ustedes, ellos, ellas hablan

Infinitive Ending -er

SINGULAR	COMER (COM+)	PLURAL	COMER (COM+)
Yo -o	Yo como	Nosotros -emos	Nosotros comemos
Tú -es	Tú comes	Vosotros -éis	Vosotros coméis
Usted, él, ella -e	Usted, él, ella come	Ustedes, ellos, ellas -en	Ustedes, ellos ellas comen

Note: Verbs with infinitive ending **–ir** take the same endings as those ending in **–er**, except for the first person plural that ends in **–imos**, as in vivir / **vivimos**; and the second person (vosotros) **–ís** as in **vivís**. (This form is hardly used in Latin America.). The endings of the present, imperfect and the preterit are added to the root to form those tenses. The endings of the conditional and future are added to the complete infinitive.

Imperfect Indicative: Endings of Regular Verbs / Indicativo Tiempo Imperfecto: Terminaciones de verbos regulares

Infinitive Ending –ar

SINGULAR	HABLAR (HABL+)	PLURAL	HABLAR (HABL+)
Yo -aba	Yo hablaba	Nosotros -ábamos	Nosotros hablábamos
Tú -abas	Tú hablabas	Vosotros -abais	Vosotros hablabais
Usted, él, ella -aba	Usted, él, ella hablaba	Ustedes, ellos, ellas -aban	Ustedes, ellos, ellas hablaban

Note: First and third person singular have the same verb form.

13

Infinitive Ending -er

SINGULAR	COMER (COM+)	PLURAL	COMER (COM+)
Yo -ía	Yo comía	Nosotros -íamos	Nosotros comíamos
Tú -ías	Tú comías	Vosotros -íais	Vosotros comíais
Usted, él, ella -ía	Usted, él, ella comía	Ustedes, ellos, ías -fan	Ustedes, ellos, ellas comían

Note: First and third person singular have the same endings in both the present and the imperfect.

Preterit Indicative: Endings of Regular Verbs / Pretérito de Indicativo: Terminaciones de verbos regulares

Infinitive Ending –ar

SINGULAR	HABLAR (HABL+)	PLURAL	HABLAR (HABL+)
Yo -é	Yo hablé	Nosotros -amos	Nosotros hablamos
Tú -aste	Tú hablaste	Vosotros -ásteis	Vosotros hablásteis
Usted, él, ella -ó	Usted, él, ella habló	Ustedes, ellos, ellas -aron	Ustedes, ellos, ellas hablaron

Infinitive Ending -er

SINGULAR	COMER (COM+)	PLURAL	COMER (COM+)
Yo -í	Yo comí	Nosotros -imos	Nosotros comimos
Tú -iste	Tú comiste	Vosotros -isteis	Vosotros comísteis
Usted, él, ella -ió	Usted, él, ella comió	Ustedes, ellos, ellas -ieron	Ustedes, ellos, ellas comieron

Infinitive Ending -ir

SINGULAR	VIVIR (VIV+)	PLURAL	VIVIR (VIV+)
Yo -í	Yo viví	Nosotros -imos	Nosotros comimos
Tú -iste	Tú viviste	Vosotros -isteis	Vosotros vivísteis
Usted, él, ella -ió	Usted, él, ella vivió	Ustedes, ellos, ellas -ieron	Ustedes, ellos, ellas vivieron

Future Indicative: Endings of Regular Verbs / Futuro de Indicativo: Terminaciones de verbos regulares

Infinitive Ending –ar

SINGULAR	HABLAR (HABL+)	PLURAL	HABLAR (HABL+)
Yo -é	Yo hablaré	Nosotros -emos	Nosotros hablaremos
Tú -as	Tú hablarás	Vosotros -éis	Vosotros hablareis
Usted, él, ella -á	Usted, él, ella hablará	Ustedes, ellos, ellas -aron	Ustedes, ellos, ellas hablarán

Note: Verb infinitives ending in -er and -ir add the same endings as -ar verbs to their forms in the singular and plural.

Conditional (Simple Tense): Endings of Regular Verbs / Condicional simple: Terminaciones de verbos regulares

Infinitive Ending –ar

SINGULAR	HABLAR (HABL+)	PLURAL	HABLAR (HABL+)
Yo -ía	Yo hablaría	Nosotros -íamos	Nosotros hablaríamos
Tú -ías	Tú hablarías	Vosotros -íaia	Vosotros hablaríais
Usted, él, ella -ía	Usted, él, ella hablaría	Ustedes, ellos, ellas -ían	Ustedes, ellos, ellas hablarían

Note: Verb infinitives ending in -er and -ir add the same endings as -ar verbs to their forms in the singular and plural.

Present Subjunctive: Endings of Regular Verbs / Presente de Subjuntivo: Terminaciones de verbos regulares

Infinitive Ending –ar

SINGULAR	HABLAR (HABL+)	PLURAL	HABLAR (HABL+)
Yo -e	Yo hable	Nosotros -emos	Nosotros hablemos
Tú -es	Tú hables	Vosotros -éis	Vosotros habléis
Usted, él, ella -e	Usted, él, ella hable	Ustedes, ellos,ellas -en	Ustedes, ellos, ellas hablen

15

Note: The vowel *e* is predominant in the conjugated forms.

Infinitive Ending -er

SINGULAR	COMER (COM+)	PLURAL	COMER (COM+)
Yo -a	Yo coma	Nosotros -amos	Nosotros comamos
Tú -as	Tú comas	Vosotros -áis	Vosotros comáis
Usted, él, ella -a	Usted, él, ella coma	Ustedes, ellos, ellas -an	Ustedes, ellos, ellas coman

Note: The vowel *a* is predominant in the conjugated forms.

Verbs with infinitive ending -ir take the same endings as those ending in -er (vivir: viva, vas, viva; vivamos, viváis, vivan).

PRESENT PARTICIPLE / PARTICIPIO DE PRESENTE

Formation of the Present Participle / Formación del participio de presente

The present participle is also known as a gerund. The gerund has the ending **–ing** in English. To form the present participle in Spanish do as follows:

drop the **–ar** ending of the infinitive and add **–ando**
    e.g. **curar** cur + **-ando** > **curando**

drop the **–er** ending of the infinitive and add **–iendo**;
    e.g. **comer** com +**-iendo** > **comiendo**

drop the **–ir** ending of the infinitive and add **–iendo**
    e.g. **admitir** admit+ **-iendo** >**admitiendo**

The most common irregular present participles (p.p.) (gerund)

ENDING IN -IENDO		ENDING IN -YENDO	
to sleep **dormir**	durmiendo	to fall **caer**	cayendo
to die **morir**	muriendo	to believe **creer**	creyendo
to ask for **pedir**	pidiendo	to destroy **destruir**	destruyendo
to be able **poder**	pudiendo	to read **leer**	leyendo
to come **venir**	viniendo	to listen **oír**	oyendo
to tell **decir**	diciendo	to bring **traer**	trayendo

Uses of the Present Participle / Usos del participio de presente

When the verb estar is used with the present participle in the progressive form, it refers to an action that continues happening, in the present, past or in the future.

> *Present:* The surgeon is operating on the patient. / El cirujano **está operando** al paciente.
>
> *Past:* The surgeon was operating on the patient. / El cirujano **estaba operando** al paciente.
>
> *Future:* The surgeon will be operating on the patient on Monday. / El cirujano **estará operando** al paciente el lunes.

With verbs of motion, (to go / **ir**; to run / **correr**; to walk / **andar**; to come / **venir**; to return / **volver**; to follow, to continue / **seguir**) to qualify an action in progress.

> The nurse continued working. / La enfermera seguía **trabajando**.

With the verb **ir** + a present participle to express the equivalent of "to go on" in English, or to do something gradually.

> The patient will continue to improve (gradually) little by little. / El paciente **irá mejorando** poco a poco. (future of ir + p.p. of mejorar / to improve)

Acting as an adverb.

> He was a long time improving / Pasó mucho tiempo **mejorando.**

PAST PARTICIPLE / PARTICIPIO DE PASADO

Formation of the Past Participle / Formación del participio de pasado

Drop the **–ar** ending and add **–ado** to the root. **operar** to operate	**operar** oper + -ado>operado
Drop the **–er** ending of the infinitive and add –ido to the root. **beber** to drink	**beber** beb + -ido > bebido
Drop the –ir ending of the infinitive and add **–ido** **subir** to climb, to go up	**subir** sub+ -ido >subido

Uses of the Past Participle / Usos del participio de pasado

The past participle acts like an adjective. The past participle is used with **ser** to express the passive voice. It can end in **–o** or **–a**, since it agrees with the subject in gender and number.

> The patient is operated on by the surgeon. / El paciente es **operado** por el cirujano. The patient was examined by her doctor. / La paciente era **examinada** por su médico.

The past participle is used more frequently with the auxiliary verb **haber** to form the perfect tenses. As a part of a verb form, it always ends in **–o**.

> We have examined the patient./ **Hemos examinado** a la paciente.

Note: See Appendix C for the conjugation of perfect tenses and a selection of irregular verbs.

Notas breves de gramática inglesa

Brief Notes on English Grammar

EL NOMBRE O SUSTANTIVO / THE NOUN

GÉNERO / GENDER

Los nombres o sustantivos en inglés se clasifican en masculinos, femeninos y neutros. El género de cosas inanimadas es generalmente neutro.

Femenino	nombre de mujer o animal hembra
	la mujer / **the woman**
Masculino	nombre de hombre o animal varón
	el hombre / **the man**
Neutro	nombres de cosas, concretas o abstractas
	la inyección / **the shot;** el dolor / **the pain**

En ciertos nombres se distingue el género por medio de las palabras; hembra / **female,** varón / **male,** o por niño / **boy** y niña / **girl.**

enfermera / **female nurse**   enfermero / **male nurse**
bebita / **baby girl**   bebito / **baby boy**

Note: En este diccionario se ha incorporado la palabra **person** / persona a palabras como **chairman,** cambiada a **chairperson,** para evitar el uso exclusivo del masculino en nombres que pueden referirse al sexo masculino o femenino.

NÚMERO / NUMBER

El plural de los nombres

Añada **-s** para formar el plural de la mayor parte de los nombres.

síntoma / **symptom**   síntomas / **symptoms**

Añada **-es** si la palabra termina en **ch, h, sh, ss, x, u o.**

punto quirúrgico / **stitch**   puntos quirúrgicos / **stitches**
fogaje / **hot flash**   fogajes / **hot flashes**
absceso / **abscess**   abscesos / **abscesses**
reflejo / **reflex**   reflejos / **reflexes**
mosquito / **mosquito**   mosquitos / **mosquitoes**

Añada **-es** si la palabra termina en **y;** cambie la **y** por **i.**

deformidad / **deformity**   deformidades / **deformities**

Añada **-es** si la palabra termina en **f** o **fe;** cambie la **f** por **v.**

vida / **life**   vidas / **lives**
hoja / **leaf**   hojas / **leaves**

PLURALES IRREGULARES MÁS COMUNES EN INGLÉS / MOST COMMON IRREGULAR PLURALS IN ENGLISH

SINGULAR	PLURAL	SINGULAR	PLURAL
diente / **tooth**	dientes / **teeth**	hombre / **man**	hombres / **men**
mujer / **woman**	mujeres / **women**	niño / **child**	niños / **children**
pie / **foot**	pies / **feet**	piojo / **louse**	piojos / **lice**
ratón / **mouse**	ratones / **mice**		

EL CASO POSESIVO DE LOS NOMBRES / THE POSSESSIVE OF NOUNS

El caso posesivo de los nombres en inglés se forma invirtiendo el orden del caso posesivo en español.

> Poseedor + ' (apóstrofe) + **s** + nombre de lo que posee

> la enfermedad de la mujer / **the woman's illness**

Los nombres que terminan en **-s** y los nombres plurales añaden solamente un apóstrofe al final de la palabra.

> Poseedor + ' (apóstrofe) + nombre de lo que posee

> la opinión de los doctores / **the doctors' opinion**

Comparativo de igualdad de los nombres

> Singular: **as much** + nombre + **as**

> Ella tiene tanta fiebre hoy como ayer. / She has **as much** fever today **as** yesterday.

> Plural: **as many** + nombre + **as**

> Ella tiene tantos síntomas hoy como ayer. / She has **as many** symptoms today **as** yesterday.

EL ARTÍCULO / THE ARTICLE

Los artículos en inglés son invariables en género y número.

EL ARTÍCULO DEFINIDO / THE DEFINITE ARTICLE

el, la, los, las / **the**	el hospital / **the hospital**
	la medicina / **the medicine**
	los riñones / **the kidneys**
	las recetas / **the prescriptions**

El artículo definido se omite en inglés cuando:

1. el sustantivo es un nombre común que expresa una idea general.
   Las medicinas ayudan / medicines are helpful
2. precede a los títulos de Sr., Sra. y Srta., o a cargos dignatarios o profesionales.
   El Sr. Jones / **Mr. Jones;** el Dr. Jones / **Dr. Jones**

EL ARTÍCULO INDEFINIDO / THE INDEFINITE ARTICLE

un, una / **a**	una píldora / **a pill**
	un laboratorio / **a laboratory**
	una unión / **a union**
	un eufemismo / **a euphemism**
	una hora / **an hour**
un, una / **an**	un accidente / **an accident**

1. **a:** Se emplea delante de las palabras que empiezan con consonante o con la vocal **u**, o el diptongo **eu** cuando éste se pronuncia como la letra **y**.
2. **an:** Se emplea delante de palabras que empiezan con una vocal o una **h** muda.

USOS DEL ARTÍCULO INDEFINIDO / USES OF THE INDEFINITE ARTICLE

1. Con nombres que designan el empleo o la profesión después del verbo **to be.**

   Ella es enfermera. / **She is a nurse.**

2. En generalizaciones sobre especies o clases precediendo a un nombre en singular; si el nombre está en plural el artículo se omite.

   El mosquito puede transmitir enfermedades. / **A mosquito can transmit disease.**
   Los antibióticos son indispensables. / **Antibiotics are indispensable.**

Nota: El plural del artículo indefinido **unos, unas,** se traduce al inglés como **some:**

   unas indicaciones preventivas / **some preventive indications**
   unos procedimientos quirúrgicos / **some surgical procedures**

EL ADJETIVO Y EL ADVERBIO / THE ADJECTIVE AND THE ADVERB

Los adjetivos en inglés generalmente preceden al nombre y son invariables en género y número. Los adjetivos demostrativos son una excepción a esta regla, ya que cambian del singular al plural de acuerdo con el nombre que modifican.

FORMACIÓN DEL ADVERBIO / HOW ADVERBS ARE FORMED

1. Los adverbios de modo que en español terminan generalmente en **-mente,** se forman en inglés añadiendo la terminación **-ly** al adjetivo.

> frecuente / **frequent**   frecuentemente / **frequently**

2. Si el adjetivo en inglés termina en **-ble**, la **e** se convierte en **y**.

> posible / **possible**   posiblemente / **possibly**

3. Si el adjetivo en inglés termina en **-ic**, el adverbio se forma añadiendo la terminación **-ally.**

> crónico / **chronic**   crónicamente / **chronically**

COMPARACIÓN DE LOS ADJETIVOS Y ADVERBIOS / COMPARATIVE FORMS OF ADJECTIVES AND ADVERBS

Tanto los adjetivos como los adverbios admiten grados de comparación.

1. Los monosílabos y algunos bisílabos cortos añaden la terminación -er y -est a la forma positiva:

a.	frío / **cold**	más frío / **colder**	(el)(la) más frío-a / **the coldest**
adv.	despacio / **slow**	más despacio / **slower**	(el)(la) más despacio / **the slowest**

2. Palabras que terminan en **-y** cambian la **-y** en **i** y añaden **-er** y **-est** para formar el comparativo y el superlativo, respectivamente:

a.	contento-a / **happy**	más contento-a / **happier**	(el)(la) más contento-a / **the happiest**
adv.	temprano / **early**	más temprano / **earlier**	(el)(la) más temprano-a / **the earliest**

3. El resto de los adjetivos y adverbios forman el comparativo de superioridad y el superlativo anteponiendo las palabras **more** y **most.**

a.	doloroso-a / **painful**	más doloroso-a / **more painful**	(el)(la) más doloroso-a / **the most painful**
adv.	frecuentemente / **frequently**	más frecuentemente / **more frequently**	(el)(la) más frecuentemente / **the most frequently**

4. El comparative y el superlativo de inferioridad se forma anteponiendo las palabras **less** y **least.**

a.	contagioso-a / **contagious**	menos contagioso-a / **less contagious**	(el)(la) menos contagioso-a / **the least contagious**
adv.	frecuentemente / **frequently**	menos frecuentemente / **less frequently**	(el)(la) menos frecuentemente / **the least frequently**

5. El comparativo de igualdad se forma usando la palabra **as** antes y después del adjetivo y del adverbio.

as+adjetivo+**as**	tan infeccioso como / **as infectious as**
as+adverbio+**as**	tan temprano como / **as early as**

Adjetivos comunes con comparativos y superlativos irregulares / Adjectives with Irregular Comparatives and Superlatives

malo / **bad**	peor / **worse**	(el)(la) peor / **the worst**
bueno / **good**	mejor / **better**	(el)(la) mejor / **the best**
poco / **little**	menos / **less**	(el)(la) menos / **the least**
mucho / **much, many**	más / **more**	(el)(la) más / **the most**

Adverbios comunes con comparativos y superlativos irregulares

lejos / **far**	más lejos / **farther**	(el)(la) más lejos / **the farthest**
poco / **little**	menos / **less**	menor / **the least**
much / **mucho**	más / **more**	mayor / **the most**
bien / **well**	mejor / **better**	(el)(la) mejor / **the best**

PRONOMBRES Y ADJETIVOS / PRONOUNS AND ADJECTIVES

PRONOMBRES PERSONALES / SUBJECT PRONOUNS

1. Los pronombres personales nominativos, es decir, los que sirven de sujeto, nunca se omiten en inglés:

> (Yo) Tengo dolor / **I have a pain; I am in pain.**

El pronombre **I** (yo) siempre se escribe con mayúscula en inglés.

Pronombres personales / Subject Pronouns

PERSONAL	SINGULAR	PLURAL
1a.	I	we
2a.	you	you
3a. (*m.*)	he	they
3a. (*f.*)	she	they
3a. (*neut.*)	it	they

2. El pronombre (objeto directo) siempre precede al pronombre (objeto indirecto). El pronombre que actúa de objeto indirecto va precedido por un preposición (**to, from, for, of**).

> Me las dio. / She gave **them to me**.

Cuando el objeto directo es un nombre y el objeto indirecto es un pronombre, el pronombre precede al objeto directo.

> La enfermera me dio las instrucciones / **The nurse gave me the instructions.**

Pronombres como complemento / Pronouns as a Complement

PERSONA	SINGULAR	PLURAL
1a.	me	us
2a.	you	you
3a. (*m.*)	him	them
3a. (*f.*)	her	them
3a. (*neut.*)	it	them

3. Además de actuar como sujeto o complemento, el pronombre personal en inglés puede también ser reflexivo cuando el complemento es la misma persona que el sujeto:

Él **se** curó a **sí** mismo. / He cured **himself.**

Pronombres reflexives / Reflexive Pronouns

PERSONA	SINGULAR	PLURAL
1a.	myself	ourselves
2a.	yourself	yourselves
3a. (*m.*)	himself	themselves
3a. (*f.*)	herself	themselves
3a. (*neut.*)	itself	themselves

PRONOMBRES Y ADJETIVOS DEMOSTRATIVOS / DEMONSTRATIVE PRONOUNS AND ADJECTIVES

Los demostrativos son los únicos adjetivos que cambian del singular al plural de acuerdo con el número del nombre que modifican.

ADJETIVOS DEMOSTRATIVOS / DEMONSTRATIVE ADJECTIVES

este	esta	**this**
estos	estas	**these**
ese	esa	**that**
aquel	aquella	**that**
esos	esas	**those**
aquellos	aquellas	**those**

esta enfermedad / **this disease**
estas enfermedades / **these diseases**
esa pastilla / **that pill**

PRONOMBRES DEMOSTRATIVOS / DEMONSTRATIVE PRONOUNS

éste, ésta, esto	**this one, this**
éstos, éstas	**these**
ése, ésa, eso	**that one, that**
aquél, aquélla, aquello	**that one, that**
ésos, ésas	**those**
aquéllos, aquéllas	**those**

Tome ésta. / **Take this one.**
Tome éstas. / **Take these.**

Ése es mejor. / **That one is better.**
Es aquélla. / **It is that one.**

PRONOMBRES Y ADJETIVOS POSESIVOS / POSSESSIVE ADJECTIVES AND PRONOUNS

PERSONA	ADJETIVO	PRONOMBRE
Sing. 1a.	my	mine
2a.	your	yours
3a. (*m.*)	his	his
3a. (*f.*)	her	hers
3a. (*neut.*)	its	its
Plur. 1a.	our	ours
2a.	your	yours
3a.	their	theirs

mi paciente / **my patient**
sus síntomas / **her symptoms**
La medicina es mía. / **The medicine is mine.**
El problema es nuestro. / **The problem is ours.**

Nota: En inglés el adjetivo posesivo se emplea con las partes del cuerpo: Me lastimé el brazo. / **I hurt my arm.**

PRONOMBRES Y ADJETIVOS INTERROGATIVOS / INTERROGATIVE ADJECTIVES AND PRONOUNS

INTERROGATIVOS / INTERROGATIVES

¿quién?, ¿quiénes?	who?
¿de quién?, ¿de quiénes?	whose?
¿a quién?, ¿a quiénes?	whom?
¿qué?, ¿cuál?, ¿cuáles?	what, which?

¿Quién está enfermo? / **Who is ill?**
¿De quién es la receta? / **Whose prescription is it?**
¿A quién vio ella? / **Whom did she see?**
¿Qué medicina prefiere? / **Which medicine do you prefer?**
¿Qué recomendó el doctor? / **What did the doctor recommend?**
¿Cuál recomendó el doctor? / **Which one did the doctor recommend?**
De esos antibióticos, ¿cuáles prefiere? / **Of those antibiotics, which do you prefer?**

PRONOMBRES RELATIVOS / RELATIVE PRONOUNS

que, el cual, la cual, el que, la que, lo que, los que, las que	**that**
que, quien, el cual, la cual, el que, etc.	**which**
quien, que, el cual, la cual, etc.	**who**
que, quien, el cual, la cual, etc.	**whom**
de quien, cuyo, del cual, de la cual, etc.	**whose**

el jarabe que (ella) tomó / **the cough syrup that she took**
la medicina que se recetó / **the medicine which was prescribed**
el paciente que está esperando / **the patient who is waiting**
el paciente que (a quién) la enfermera atiende / **the patient whom the nurse is helping**
el paciente cuya radiografía necesita el doctor / **the patient whose x-rays the doctor needs**

Nota: Las terminaciones **-ever** y **-soever** se añaden a **who, which,** y **what** para formar los pronombres relativos compuestos **whoever** / quienquiera, **whichever** / cualquiera y **whatever** / quienquiera o cualquiera.

PRONOMBRES Y ADJETIVOS INDEFINIDOS MÁS COMUNES / MOST COMMON INDEFINITE ADJECTIVES AND PRONOUNS

all	todo	**many**	muchos
another	otro	**nobody**	nadie
any	cualquiera	**none**	ninguno, ninguna
anybody	cualquiera	**no one**	nadie
anyone	cualquiera	**nothing**	nada
anything	cualquier cosa, algo	**one**	uno-a
both	ambos, ambas	**other**	otro-a
each (one)	cada (uno), cada cual	**some**	algunos, algunas
everybody	todos	**somebody**	alguien
everyone	todos	**someone**	alguien
everything	todo	**something**	algo
few	pocos		
a few	unos pocos		

EL VERBO / THE VERB

FORMAS DEL VERBO / FORMS OF THE VERB

INFINITIVO	*PASADO*	*PARTICIPIO*	*GERUNDIO*
curar / to heal	healed	healed	healing
comer / to eat	ate	ate	eating
Infinitivo / Infinitive		El verbo precedido de la preposición to: examina / **to examine**	
Presente / Present		La misma forma verbal del infinitivo sin la preposición **to** precedida del pronombre correspondiente: yo examino / **I examine** nosotros examinamos / **we examine**	
Pasado / Past		El infinitivo + la terminación **-d** o **-ed** yo examiné / **I examined** nosotros examinamos / **we examined**	
Participio pasado / Past Participle		La misma forma verbal que el pasado: examinado / **examined**	
Participio de presente / Present Participle		El infinitivo + **-ing**: examinando / **examining**	

Nota: Para formar el pasado o el participio de verbos regulares se añade la terminación **-ed** al infinitivo. Las variaciones a esta regla son las siguientes.

a. Si el infinitivo termina en **e**, se añade **-d** (die, di**ed**).
b. Si el infinitivo termina en la letra **y** precedida de una consonante, se cambia la **y** por **i** antes de añadir **-ed** (try, tr**ied**).
c. Si el infinitivo termina en consonante precedida de una vocal y la sílaba final lleva el énfasis, se dobla la consonante antes de añadir **-ed** (permit, permit**ted**).

Nota: Para formar el gerundio se añade la terminación **-ing** al infinitivo; **to drink** / beber; **drinking** / bebiendo. Las variaciones a esta regla son las siguientes:

a. Si el infinitivo termina en **-e** precedida de una consonante, la **e** se pierde antes de añadir la terminación **-ing** (arise, arising).
b. Si el infinitivo termina en **ie**, la **ie** se sustituye por la letra **y** antes de añadir **-ing** (l**ie**, l**y**ing).
c. En algunos verbos se dobla la consonante antes de añadir **-ing** si la sílaba final del infinitivo lleva el énfasis (spit, spit**ting**), excepto en verbos terminados en **h, w, e** y **y**, los cuales no doblan la consonante al formar el gerundio **to chew** / masticar; **chewing** / masticando.

TIEMPOS DEL VERBO / TENSES OF THE VERB
TIEMPOS SIMPLES / SIMPLE TENSES

to cough / toser

Presente / Present	yo toso / **I cough**
Pasado (pretérite e imperfecto) / Past	yo tosí, tosía / **I coughed**
Futuro / Future	yo toseré / **I will, shall cough**

El imperfecto se traduce al inglés con las formas **used to** o **would** para indicar una acción repetida indefinida-mente o habitualmente en el pasado.

Yo tomaba la medicina todos los días. / **I used to take the medicine every day.**

El futuro de todas las personas se forma con el verbo auxiliar **will** o **shall,** que precede a la forma del verbo en todos los tiempos.

Tomaré la medicina. / **I will take the medicine.**

TIEMPOS COMPUESTOS / COMPOUND TENSES

Los tiempos compuestos se forman con el verbo auxiliar haber / **to have.** (Véase la conjugación del verbo **to have** al final de la explicación del verbo.)

Perfecto / Present perfect	yo he tosido / **I have coughed**
Pluscuamperfecto / Past perfect	yo había, hube tosido / **I had coughed**
Futuro anterior / Future perfect	yo habré tosido / **I will, I shall have coughed**

Nota: Además de los seis tiempos indicados, todos los verbos tienen una forma progresiva que indica una acción continuada dentro de la configuración del tiempo a que se refieren. Se forma con el verbo auxiliar estar / **to be,** seguido del participio presente (gerundio). (Véase la conjugación del verbo **to be** al final de la explicación del verbo.)

Presente	yo estoy tosiendo / **I am coughing**
Pasado	yo estaba, estuve tosiendo / **I was coughing**
Futuro	yo estaré tosiendo / **I will, shall be coughing**
Perfecto	yo he estado tosiendo / **I have been coughing**
Pluscuamperfecto	yo había, hube estado tosiendo / **I had been coughing**
Futuro anterior	yo habré estado tosiendo / **I will, shall have been coughing**

MODOS DEL VERBO / MOODS OF THE VERB
INDICATIVO / INDICATIVE

Yo toso / **I cough.**

La oración interrogativa, negativa y enfática se forma con el verbo auxiliar **to do.** (Véase la conjugación del verbo al final de la explicación del verbo.)

Interrogación	¿Tose usted por las mañanas? / **Do you cough in the morning?**
Negación	No toso durante el día. / **I do not cough during the day.**
Énfasis	Toso mucho por las noches. / **I do cough a lot at night.**

Nota: El verbo **to do** también se emplea para dar énfasis a la respuesta de sí o no a una pregunta:

¿Tose mucho? / **Do you cough much?**   Sí toso. / **Yes, I do.**
                                          No toso. / **No, I do not.**

IMPERATIVO / IMPERATIVE

Tosa, por favor. / **Cough please.**

CONJUGACIÓN DE UN VERBO REGULAR / CONJUGATION OF A REGULAR VERB

preparar / to prepare

INFINITIVO	PARTICIPIO	GERUNDIO
preparar / **to prepare**	preparado / **prepared**	preparando / **preparing**

Indicativo / Indicative

PRESENTE / PRESENT

yo preparo / **I prepare**	nosotros preparamos / **we prepare**
Ud. prepara, tú preparas / **you prepare**	vosotros preparáis, ustedes preparan / **you prepare**
él, ella prepara / **he, she, it prepares**	ellos, ellas preparan / **they prepare**

PRETÉRITO / IMPERFECTO / PAST

preparé, preparaba / **I prepared**	preparamos, preparábamos / **we prepared**
preparó, preparaba, preparaste, preparabas / **you prepared**	prepararon, preparaban, preparasteis, preparabais / **you prepared**
preparó, preparaba / **he, she, it, prepared**	prepararon, preparaban / **they prepared**

FUTURO / FUTURE

prepararé / **I will, shall prepare**	prepararemos / **we will, shall prepare**
preparará, prepararás / **you will prepare**	prepararéis, prepararán / **you will prepare**
preparará / **he, she, it will prepare**	prepararán / **they will prepare**

PERFECTO / PERFECT

he preparado / **I have prepared**	hemos preparado / **we have prepared**
ha preparado, has preparado / **you have prepared**	habéis, han preparado / **you have prepared**
ha preparado / **he, she, it has prepared**	han preparado / **they have prepared**

PLUSCUAMPERFECTO / PAST PERFECT

había preparado / **I had prepared**	habíamos preparado / **we had prepared**
había, habías preparado / **you had prepared**	habíais, habían preparado / **you had prepared**
había preparado / **he, she, it had prepared**	habían preparado / **they had prepared**

FUTURO ANTERIOR / FUTURE PERFECT

habré preparado / **I will, shall have prepared**	habremos preparado / **we will, shall have prepared**
habrá, habrás preparado / **you will have prepared**	habréis, habrán preparado / **you will have prepared**
habrá preparado / **he, she, it will have prepared**	habrán preparado / **they will have prepared**

Imperativo / Imperative

prepara (tú), prepare (usted), preparad (vosotros), preparen (ustedes, ellos)	**prepare**
preparemos (nosotros)	**let's prepare**

En inglés no existe la distinción entre el **tú** familiar y el **usted** formal. La segunda persona del singular es siempre **you**. La segunda persona del plural (**vosotros** y **ustedes**) tiene igualmente una sola forma, que se traduce también como **you**. La tercera persona singular del presente es la única forma verbal que difiere de las demás al tomar la terminación **-s.**

Excepciones del inglés:
a. Si el verbo en el infinitivo termina en **-s, -x, -z, -ch,** o **-sh**, se añade **-es**; alcanzar / **to reach;** he, she, it **reaches.**
b. Si el verbo termina en **-z**, precedida por una sola vocal, la **z** se dobla y se añade **-es**; preguntar / **to quiz;** he, she, it **quizzes.**
c. Si el verbo termina en **y**, precedida de consonante, la **y** cambia a **i** y se añade **-es**; llevar / **to carry;** he, she, it **carries.**

CONJUGACIÓN DE LOS VERBOS AUXILIARES / CONJUGATION OF AUXILIARY VERBS

haber / to have

INFINITIVO	PARTICIPIO	GERUNDIO
haber / **to have**	habido / **had**	habiendo / **having**

Indicativo / Indicative

PRESENTE / PRESENT

yo he / **I have**	nosotros hemos / **we have**
Ud. ha, tú has / **you have**	vosotros habéis, ustedes han / **you have**
él, ella ha / **he, she, it has**	ellos han / **they have**

PRETÉRITO / IMPERFECTO / PAST

hube, había / **I had**	hubimos, habíamos / **we had**
hubo, había, hubiste, habías/ **you had**	hubisteis, habíais, hubieron, habían / **you had**
hubo, había / **he, she, it had**	hubieron, habían / **they had**

FUTURO / FUTURE

habré / **I will, shall have**	habremos / **we will, shall have**
habrá, habrás / **you will have**	habréis, habrán / **you will have**
habrá / **he, she, it will have**	habrán / **they will have**

Nota: Para formar los tiempos compuestos se añade el participio de pasado **had** a las formas simples: **I have had, I had had, I will, shall have had.**

ser, estar / to be

INFINITIVO	PARTICIPIO	GERUNDIO
ser / **to be**	sido / **been**	siendo / **being**

PRESENTE / PRESENT

yo soy / **I am**	nosotros somos / **we are**
Ud. es, tú eres / **you are**	vosotros sois, ustedes son / **you are**
él, ella es / **he, she, it is**	ellos, ellas son / **they are**

PRETÉRITO / IMPERFECTO / PAST

fui, era / **I was**	fuimos, éramos / **we were**
fue, era, fuiste, eras / **you were**	fuisteis, erais, fueron, eran / **you were**
fue, era / **he, she, it was**	fueron, eran / **they were**

FUTURO / FUTURE

seré / **I will, shall be**	seremos / **we will, shall be**
será, serás / **you will be**	seréis, serán / **you will be**
será / **he, she, it will be**	serán / **they will be**

Nota: Para formar los tiempos compuestos se usan las formas simples del verbo auxiliar **to have** y el participio de **to be: been. I have been; I had been; I will, shall have been.**

hacer / to do

El verbo **to do** no existe como verbo auxiliar en español; por lo tanto, las formas **do, does** y **did** en oraciones interrogativas, negativas y enfáticas no tienen traducción al español.

INFINITIVO	PARTICIPIO	GERUNDIO
hacer / **to do**	hecho / **done**	haciendo / **doing**

PRESENTS / PRESENT

yo hago / **I do**	nosotros hacemos / **we do**
Ud. hace, tú haces / **you do**	vosotros hacéis, ustedes hacen / **you do**
él, ella hace / **he, she, it does**	ellos, ellas hacen / **they do**

PRETÉRITO / IMPERFECTO / PAST

hice, hacía / **I did**	hicimos, hacíamos / **we did**
hiciste, hacías / **you did**	hicisteis, hacíais, hicieron, hacían / **you did**
hizo, hacía / **he, she, it did**	hicieron, hacían / **they did**

FUTURO / FUTURE

haré / **I will, shall do**	haremos / **we will, shall do**
hará, harás / **you will do**	haréis, harán / **you will do**
hará / **he, she, it will do**	harán / **they will do**

Nota: Para formar los tiempos compuestos se usan las formas simples del verbo auxiliar **to have** y el participio de **to do, done: I have done, I had done, I will, shall have done.**

Imperativo / Imperative

haz (tú), haga (usted), haced (vosotros), hagan (ustedes, ellos)	**do**
hagamos (nosotros)	**let us do**

Subjuntivo / Subjunctive

El modo subjuntivo se emplea en inglés con mucha menos frecuencia que en español, y para los efectos de este diccionario, no lo hemos incluido.

Spanish-English
Glossary

Glosario español-inglés

a

a *abr.* **absoluto** / absolute; **acidez** / acidity; **acomodación** / accommodation; **alergia** / allergy; **anterior** / anterior; **aqua** / aqua; **arteria** / artery.

a *prep.* [*hacia*] to, **voy __ la farmacia** / I am going to the drugstore; [*dirección*] to, __ **la derecha** / to the right; __ **la izquierda** / to the left; [*hora*] at, **voy__ las tres** / I'm going at three o'clock; [*frecuencia*] a, per, **tres veces al día** / three times a day.

abajo *adv.* below, down.

abandonar *vt.* to abandon, to neglect.

abarcar *vt.* to contain, to include; __ **mucho** / to cover a lot of ground.

abasia *f.* abasia, uncertainty of movement.

abastecer *vt.* to supply.

abastecimiento *m.* supply; **artículos para __** / supplies.

abatido-a *a.* depressed, dejected.

abdomen *m.* abdomen; *pop.* belly; __ **de péndulo** / pendulous __; __ **escafoideo** / scaphoid __ See illustration on page 40.

abdominal *a.* abdominal, rel. to the abdomen; **cirugía __** / __ surgery; **cavidad __** / __ cavity; **disnea __** / __ dysnea; **distensión __** / __ distention; **fístula __** / __ fistula; **punción __** / __ puncture; **respiración __** / __ breathing; **retortijón, torsón __** / __ cramp; **rigidez __** / __ rigidity; **traumatismos __ -es** / __ injuries; **vendaje __** / __ bandage.

abdominocentesis *f.* abdominocentesis, abdominal puncture.

abdominoplastia *f.* abdominoplasty, plastic surgical repair of the abdominal wall.

abducción *f.* abduction; separation.

abducente *f.* abducent, that separates; **músculo __** / __ muscle.

abeja *f.* bee.

aberración *f.* aberration. 1. deviation from the norm; __ **cromática** / chromatic __; 2. mental disorder; __ **mental** / mental __ .

aberrante *a.* aberrant, departing from the usual course; wandering.

abertura *f.* opening.

abetalipoproteinemia *f.* abetalipoproteinemia, rare inherited condition characterized by the absence or deficiency of betalipoproteins in fat metabolism.

abierto-a *a. pp.* of **abrir,** open.

abiotrofia *f.* abiotrophy, premature loss of vitality.

ablación *f.* ablatio, ablation, detachment, removal; __ **de la placenta** / __ placentae; __ **de la retina** / __ retinae.

ablandar *vt.* to soften.

abofetear *vt.* to slap.

abortivo *m.* abortifacient, stimulant to induce abortion.

aborto *m.* abortion, miscarriage. See table on page 258.

abotonar *vt.* to button up.

abrasión *f.* abrasion, damage to or wearing away of a surface by injury or friction; **círculo de __** / __ collar, circular trace left on the skin by gunpowder.

abrasivo-a *a.* abrasive, rel. to or that causes abrasion.

abrazadera *f.* brace.

abrazo *m.* hug, embrace.

abreviatura *f.* abbreviation.

abrigarse *vr., vi.* to put on warm clothing; to keep warm.

abrigo *m.* overcoat; cover; **buscar __** / to look for shelter.

abrir *vt.* to open; __ **de nuevo** / to reopen.

abrochar *vt.* to fasten.

abrumar *vt.* to overwhelm; to tax.

abrupción de la placenta *f.* abruptio placentae, premature detachment of the placenta.

abrupto-a *a.* abrupt, brusque.

absceso *m.* abscess, accumulation of pus gen. due to a breakdown of tissue. See table on page 40.

absoluto-a *a.* absolute, unconditional.

absorbente *a.* absorbent.

absorber *vt.* to absorb, to take in.

absorción *f.* absorption, uptake. 1. taking up of fluids and other substances by an organism; __ **bucal** / mouth __; __ **cutánea** / cutaneous __; __ **entérica** / intestinal __; __ **estomacal** / stomach __; __ **externa** / external __; __ **parenteral** / parenteral __; __ **percutánea** / percutaneous __; 2. self-centeredness.

abstenerse

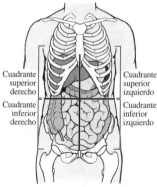

Cuadrantes abdominales:
mostrando los órganos dentro de cada cuadrante

Absceso	Abscess
agudo	acute
alveolar	alveolar
crónico	chronic
cutáneo	cutaneous
de drenaje	drainage
de la raíz	radicular
de la uña	paronychial
de las amígdalas	peritonsilar
de las encías	gingival
de sutura	suture
dental	dental
enquistado	encysted
facial	facial
fecal	fecal
folicular	follicular
hepático	hepatic
mamario	mammary
mastoideo	mastoid
óseo	osseous
pancreático	pancreatic
pélvico	pelvic
pulmonar	pulmonary
tubárico	tubo-ovarian

abstenerse *vr., vi.* to abstain, to refrain; ___ de relaciones sexuales / ___ from sexual intercourse.

abstinencia *f.* abstinence, voluntary restraint.
abuelo-a *m., f.* grandfather; grandmother.
abulia *f.* abulia, loss of will power; ___ cíclica / cyclic ___ .
abultado-a *a.* bulky, massive; swollen.
abundancia *f.* abundance.
aburrido-a *a.* bored.
aburrirse *vr.* to become bored.
abusado-a *a.* abused; beyond the limits.
abusar *vt.* to abuse, to mistreat.
abuso *m.* abuse, overuse; ___ de medicamento / overuse of medication; ___ emocional / emotional ___; ___ físico / physical ___; ___ verbal / verbal ___ .
acalasia *f.* achalasia, inability to relax, esp. in reference to the sphincter muscles.
acantoma *m.* acanthoma, benign tumor of the skin.
acantosis *f.* acanthosis, skin condition manifested by thick and warty growth.
acapnia *f.* acapnia, state produced by a decrease of carbon dioxide in the blood.
acariasis *f.* acariasis, skin disease caused by acarids.
ácaro *m.* acarid, parasite, mite.
acatalepsia *f.* acatalepsy, deterioration of mental abilities.
acatarrarse *vr.* to catch a cold.
acceso *m.* 1. access, attack, seizure; ___ de asma / an asthma attack; 2. entrance.
accesorio *m.* accessory; nervio ___ / ___ nerve.
accidentado-a *m., f.* an injured person.
accidental *a.* accidental, unexpected.
accidente *m.* accident; ___ automovilístico / car ___; ___ de trabajo / work-related ___; ___ de tráfico / traffic ___; propenso as ___ / prone; víctima de un ___ / casualty.
acción *f.* action.
aceite *m.* oil; ___ de hígado de bacalao / cod liver ___; ___ de jojoba / jojoba ___; ___ de oliva / olive ___; ___ de palmito / palm ___; ___ de ricino / castor ___; ___ de soya / soy ___; ___ graso / fatty ___ .
acento *m.* accent.
acentuar *vt.* to accentuate, to emphasize.
aceptable *a.* acceptable; consumo diario ___ / ___ daily intake.
aceptación *f.* acceptance.
acera *f.* sidewalk.

acerca (de) *adv.* about, concerning; ___ **de eso** / about that.

acercar *vt.* to bring closer; **acercarse vr.** to approach, to get close.

acertado-a *a.* right; **un diagnóstico** ___ / a correct diagnosis.

acetábulo *m.* acetabulum, hip socket.

acético-a *a.* acetic, sour, rel. to vinegar or its acid.

acetilcolinesterasa *m.* acetycholinisterasa, enzyme present in several tissues such as in blood cells, nerve cells, and muscles.

acetona *f.* acetone, fragrant substance used as a solvent and found in excessive amount in diabetic urine.

acetonemia *f.* acetonemia, excess acetone in the blood.

acetonuria *f.* acetonuria, excess acetone in the urine.

achaque *m.* ailment, infirmity.

achicar *vt.* to reduce.

acidemia *f.* acidemia, excess acid in the blood.

acidez *f.* acidity, sourness.

ácido *m.* acid; ___ **acético** / acetic ___; ___ **ascórbico** / ascorbic ___; ___ **bórico** / boric ___; ___ **butírico** / butyric ___; ___ **clorogénico** / chlorogenic ___; ___ **cólico** / cholic ___; ___ **desoxirribonucleico** / deoxyribonucleic ___; ___ **fólico** / folic ___; ___ **gástrico** / gastric ___; ___ **láctico** / lactic ___; ___ **nicotínico** / nicotinic ___; ___ **nucleico** / nucleic ___; ___ **para-amino benzoico** / para-amino benzoic ___; ___ **resistente** / ___ fast; ___ **ribonucleico** / ribonucleic ___; ___ **salicílico** / salicylic ___; ___**-s grasos** / fatty ___ -s; ___ **sulfónico** / sulfonic ___; ___ **sulfúrico** / sulfuric ___; **a prueba de** ___ / ___ proof; -*a a.* bitter.

ácido clorhídrico, hidroclórico *m.* hydrochloric acid, a constituent of gastric juice.

ácido glicocólico *m.* glycocholic acid, a compound of glycine and cholic acid.

ácido glucurónico *m.* glucuronic, glycuronic acid, acid that acts as a disinfectant in human metabolism.

ácido hialurónico *m.* hyaluronic acid, acid present in the substance of the connective tissue that acts as a lubricant and connecting agent.

acidos grasos omega *m., pl.* omega fatty acids.

acidosis *f.* acidosis, excessive acidity in the blood and tissues of the body; ___ **diabética** / diabetic ___; ___ **metabólica** / metabolic ___ .

acidosis respiratoria *f.* respiratory acidosis, affliction caused by retention of carbon dioxide due to hypoventilation.

ácido úrico *m.* uric acid, a product of protein breakdown present in the blood and excreted in the urine.

acinesia *f.* akinesia, acinesia, partial or total loss of movement.

aclaramiento *m.* clearance, elimination of a given substance from the blood plasma of the kidneys.

aclimatarse *vr.* to acclimate; to get used to a condition or custom; to adjust.

acloropsia *f.* achlropsia, inability to distinguish the color green.

acné *f.* acne, inflammatory skin condition; ___ **rosácea** / ___ rosacea; ___ **vulgar o común** / ___ vulgaris, common acne.

acolia *f.* acholia, absence of bile.

acomodación *f.* accomodation, adaptation; the state of adapting to something; ___ **de un nervio** / nerve ___; ___ **histológica** / histologic ___; ___ **negativa** / negative ___; ___ **positiva** / positive ___; **amplitud de** ___ / amplitude of ___; **jerarquía de** ___ / range of ___ .

acomodación del ojo *f.* eye accommodation, coordination process of the eye muscles and the lens to enable the eye to focus in near objects.

acompañante *m., f.* companion.

acompañar *vt.* to accompany.

acondicionamiento *m.* conditioning; ___ **físico** / physical fitness.

acondroplasia *f.* achondroplasia, dwarfism, congenital osseous deformity.

aconsejar *vt.* to advise, to recommend; ___ **mal** / to misguide.

acontecer *v.* to transpire, to occur.

acordar *vi.* to agree; **acordarse** / *vr.* to remember, to recall.

acortar *vt.* to shorten.

acosamiento *m.* harassment.

acosar *vt.* to harass.

acostado-a *a.* reclining; lying down.

acostar *vt.* to lay down, to put to bed; **acostarse** / *vr.* to go to bed, to lie down; **hora de** ___ / bedtime.

acostumbrarse *vr.* to get used to.

acre *a.* acrid, sour.

acreción *f.* accretion, growth; accumulation.

acreditado-a *a.* accredited, certified.

acreditar *vt.* to credit, to accredit, to certify.

acrocianosis *f.* acrocyanosis, Raynaud's disease, bluish discoloration and coldness of the extremities due to a circulatory disorder gen. brought about by exposure to cold or by emotional stress.

acrodermatitis *f.* acrodermatitis, infl. of the skin of hands and feet; ___ **crónica atrófica** / ___ chronica atrophicans.

acrofobia *f.* acrophobia, excessive fear of heights.

acromasia *f.* achromasia, lack or loss of pigmentation in the skin, characteristic of albinos.

acromático-a *a.* achromatic, lacking in color.

acromatopsia *f.* achromatopsia, color blindness.

acromegalia *f.* acromegaly, chronic disease common in middle age, manifested by progressive enlargement of the bones of the extremities and of certain head bones, gen. caused by a malfunction of the pituitary gland.

acromion *m.* acromion, part of the scapular bone of the shoulder.

acropustulosis *f.* acropustulosis, pustular eruptions of the hands and feet, often a form of psoriasis.

acrotismo *m.* acrotism, absence or imperceptibility of the pulse.

actina *f.* actin, protein in muscle tissue that together with myosin makes possible muscle contraction.

activar *vt.* to activate.

actividad *f.* activity; ___ **mental** / mental ___.

actividades de resistencia *f.* endurance activities.

actividades de la vida diaria *f.* activities of daily living.

activo-a *a.* active.

actual *a.* actual, present, true, real; **-mente** *adv.* currently.

actuar *v.* to act.

acuclillarse *vr.* to squat.

acumulación *f.* accumulation; pile, heap.

acuoso-a *a.* aqueous; **humor** ___ / ___ humor; **intoxicación** ___ / water intoxication, condition caused by excessive retention of water in the body.

acupuntura *f.* acupuncture, method of inserting needles into specific points of the body as a means of relieving pain.

acústico-a *a.* acoustic, rel. to sound or hearing.

Adán, nuez de *f.* Adam's apple.

adaptabilidad *f.* adaptability; compliance. 1. the ease with which a substance or structure can change its shape, such as the ability of an organ to distend; 2. the degree to which a patient follows a prescribed regimen.

adaptación *f.* adaptation, adjustment.

adaptar *v.* to adapt, to fit, to accommodate; **adaptarse** *vr.* to adapt oneself.

Addison, enfermedad de *f.* Addison's disease, insufficiency or nonfunction of the adrenal glands.

adecuado-a *a.* adequate, suitable.

adelantado-a *a.* advanced, ahead; **por** ___ / in advance.

adelantar *vt.* to advance, to move ahead; ___ **la fecha** / to move up the date.

adelante *adv.* forward, ahead; **más** ___ / later on; **de hoy en** ___ / from now on.

adelanto *m.* improvement, progress.

adelgazar *vi.* to lose weight, to get thin.

además *adv.* besides, in addition.

adenectomía *f.* adenectomy, removal of a gland.

adenitis *f.* adenitis, infl. of a gland.

adenoacantoma *m.* adenoacanthoma, slow-growing cancer of the uterus.

adenocarcinoma *m.* adenocarcinoma, malignant tumor arising from a gland and organ.

adenocistoma *m.* adenocystoma, benign gland tumor formed by cysts.

adenofibroma *m.* adenofibroma, benign fibrous glandular tumor seen in the breast and uterus.

adenoide *m.* adenoid, glandlike; accumulation of lymphatic tissue located in the throat behind the nose.

adenoidectomía *f.* adenoidectomy, excision of the adenoid.

adenoiditis *f.* adenoiditis, infl. of the adenoid.

adenoma *m.* adenoma, glandlike tumor; ___ **acidófilo** / acidophil ___; ___ **adrenocortical** / adrenocortical ___; ___ **basófilo** / basophil ___; ___ **bronquial** /

bronchial __; __ **de la mama** / __ of the breast; __ **embrional** / embryonal __; __ **folicular** / follicular __; __ **hepático** / hepatic __; __ **renal cortical** / renal cortical __; __ **sebáceo** / sebaceous __; __ **tóxico** / toxic __ .

adenomatosis *f.* adenomatosis, condition by which there are large glandlike growths.

adenomioma *m.* adenomyoma, benign tumor usu. seen in the uterus.

adenopatía *f.* adenopathy, a lymph gland disease.

adenosarcoma *m.* adenosarcoma, malignant tumor.

adenosis *f.* adenosis, enlargement of a gland.

adenovirus *m.* adenovirus, a group of viruses that can cause respiratory tract infections, such as the common cold.

adentro (de) *adv.* inside; inside of.

adherencia *f.* adhesion, attachment.

adherir *vt.* to adhere, to attach.

adhesivo-a *a.* adhesive.

adicción *f.* addiction, dependency, propensity; **dejar la** __ / *pop.* [*droga*] to kick the habit.

adictivo *m.* addictive, rel. to or causing addiction.

adicto-a *a.* addicted, physically or psychologically dependent on a substance such as alcohol or a narcotic.

adiós *int.* goodbye.

adiposito *m.* adipocyte, adipose cell.

adiposo-a *a.* adipose, fatty; **cirrosis** __ / __ cirrhosis; **corazón** __ / __ heart; **hernia** __ / __ hernia; **riñón** __ / __ kidney; **tejido** __ / __ tissue.

adjetivo *m.* adjective.

adjuntar *vt.* to enclose; to include.

adjutor *m.* adjuvant, helper; substance added to a medication to heighten its action.

administración *f.* administration, management.

administrador-a *m., f.* administrator, manager.

admisión *f.* admission.

admitir *v.* to admit.

ADN recombinante *n.* recombinant DNA, alteration of the DNA in the laboratory by which the genes from one organism are transplanted or spliced to another organism.

adolescencia *f.* adolescence, puberty.

adolescente *m., f.* adolescent.

adolorido-a *a.* sore.

adopción *f.* adoption.

adoptar *v.* to adopt.

adormecer *vi.* to put to sleep, [*un nervio*] to deaden; **adormecerse** *vr.* to drowse.

adrenal *a.* adrenal, suprarenal.

adrenalectomía *f.* adrenalectomy, removal of the adrenal gland.

adrenalina *f.* adrenaline, epinephrine, hormone secreted by the adrenal medulla, commonly used as a cardiac stimulant.

adrenérgicos *m., pl.* adrenergic, blocking agents, rel. to drugs that mimic the actions of the sympathetic nervous system.

adrenocorticotropina *f.* adrenocorticotropin, hormone secreted by the pituitary gland that has a stimulating effect on the adrenal cortex.

aducción *f.* adduction. 1. movement toward the midline of the body or toward a limb or part; 2. movement toward a common center.

aductor-a *a.* adductor, a muscle that draws a part towards the median line.

adueñarse *vr.* to take possession.

adulteración *f.* adulteration, changing from the original.

adulterado-a *a.* adulterated, changed from the original; **no** __ / unadulterated.

adulterar *vt.* to adulterate, to change the original.

adulto-a *a.* adult.

adverbio *m. gr.* adverb.

adverso-a *a.* adverse, unfavorable.

adyacente *a.* adjacent, next to.

aeróbic *f.* aerobics, a system of physical fitness combining calisthenics and a dance routine intended to promote cardiovascular endurance.

aeróbico-a *a.* aerobic, 1. rel. to an aerobe; 2. rel. to an exercise coordinated as a physical activity; **baile** __ / __ dance; **ejercicio** __ / __ exercise; 3. that lives or occurs in the presence of oxygen.

aerobio *m.* aerobe, organism that requires oxygen to live.

aeroembolismo *m.* aeroembolism, condition caused by a release of bubbles of nitrogen into the blood gen. due to a sudden change in atmospheric pressure; *pop.* the bends.

aeroenfisema *m.* aeroemphysema, condition caused by a sudden ascent in space without adequate decompression; *pop.* the chokes.

aerofagia *f.* aerophagia, excessive swallowing of air.

aerogénico-a *a.* aerogenic, gas-producing.

afán *m.* eagerness, desire.

afasia *f.* aphasia, inability to coordinate word and thought in speaking. ___ **atáxica** / ataxic ___; ___ **amnésica** / amnesic ___ .

afebril *a.* afebrile, without fever.

afección *f.* affection, fondness; condition, sickness.

afectar *v.* to affect; to cause change.

afeitar *vt.* to shave; **afeitarse** *vr.* to shave oneself.

afeminado *a.* effeminate.

aferente *a.* afferent, that moves in a direction toward a center, as in certain arteries, veins, vessels, and nerves.

afinidad *f.* affinity; similarity.

afligido-a *a.* afflicted, distressed, sorrowful, grief-stricken, troubled.

aflojar *vt.* to loosen, to slacken; **aflojarse** *vr.* to become weak; to lose courage.

afonía *f.* aphonia, loss of voice due to an affliction of the larynx.

afónico-a *a.* aphonic, without voice or sound.

afrodisíaco *m.* aphrodisiac, any agent that arouses sexual desire.

afrontar *vt.* to confront.

afta *f.* aphtha, a small ulcer, sign of fungal infection of the oral mucosa.

afuera *adv.* outside.

agacharse *vr.* to bend; to stoop, to squat.

agallas *f. pl.* tonsils; *pop.* **tener** ___ / to have guts, to be bold.

agalorrea *f.* agalorrhea, cessation or lack of milk in the breasts.

agammaglobulinemia *f.* agammaglobulinemia, deficiency of gamma globulin in the blood.

agenesia, agenesis *f.* agenesia, agenesis. 1. congenital failure of an organ to grow or develop; 2. sterility or impotence.

agente *m.* agent, factor.

agentes citotóxicos *m., pl.* cytotoxic agents, chemical compounds used in chemotherapy to destroy cancerous cells.

ágil *a.* agile, nimble; mentally sharp.

agilidad *f.* agility; ___ **mental** / mental ___ .

agitado-a *a.* agitated, restless.

agitar *vt.* to stir up, to shake; ___ **la botella** / to shake the bottle **agitarse** *vr.* to become agitated or excited.

aglomeración *f.* agglomeration.

aglutinación *f.* agglutination, the act of binding together.

aglutinante *m.* agglutinant, agent or factor that holds parts together during the healing process.

agnosia *f.* agnosia, disorder or incapacity due to a cerebral lesion by which the person suffers a total or partial loss of the senses and does not recognize familiar persons or objects; ___ **visual** / visual ___ .

agobiar *v.* to weigh down; to burden.

agorafobia *f.* agoraphobia, fear of being alone in a wide open space.

agotado-a *a.* exhausted, tired.

agotador-a *a.* exhausting, tiring.

agotamiento *m.* exhaustion, extreme fatigue; wasting.

agotar *vt.* to exhaust; ___ **todos los recursos** / to ___ all means.

agradecer *vt.* to be grateful, to be thankful.

agrafia *f.* agraphia, loss of ability to write due to a brain disorder.

agrandamiento *m.* enlargement.

agrandar *v.* to enlarge.

agranulocitosis *f.* agranulocytosis, acute condition caused by the absence of leukocytes in the blood.

agregar *vt.* to add.

agresivo-a *a.* aggressive, hostile.

agriarse *vr.* to turn sour.

agrietado-a *a.* chapped; **labios** ___-s / ___ lips; **manos** ___-as / ___ hands.

agua *f.* water; **abastecimiento de** ___ / ___ supply; ___ **alcanforizada** / camphor julep; ___ **corriente o de pila** / tap ___; ___ **de rosa** / rose ___; ___ **helada** / ice ___; ___ **oxigenada** / hydrogen peroxide; **bolsa de** ___ **caliente** / hot ___ bottle; **cama de, colchón de** ___ / ___ bed; **contaminación del** ___ / ___ pollution; **ingestión o toma de** ___ / ___ intake; **purificación del** ___ / ___ purification; **soluble en** ___ / ___ soluble.

aguado-a *a.* watered down.

aguantar *vt.* to hold; to endure.

agudo-a *a.* acute, piercing, sharp.

aguja *f.* needle; ___ **hipodérmica** / hypodermic ___ .

agujero *m.* hole.

ahí *adv.* there.

ahijado-a *m., f.* godchild.

ahogamiento *m.* drowning.

ahogar *vi.* to drown; to smother, to extinguish; **ahogarse** *vr.* to drown oneself; to choke.

ahora *adv.* now, presently.

ahorcarse *vr.* to hang oneself.

ahorita *adv.* right away.

ahorrar *vt.* to save; to spare; ___ **tiempo** / ___ time.

aire *m.* air, wind; breath; ___ **acondicionado** / ___ conditioned; ___ **contaminado, viciado** / ___ pollution; ___ **de ventilación** / ventilated ___; ___ **respiratorio** / tidal ___ ; **bolsa de** ___ / ___ pocket; **burbujas de** ___ / ___ bubbles; **cámara de** ___ / ___ chamber; **conducto de** ___ / airway, air passage; **enfriado por** ___ / ___ -cooled; **falta de** ___ / ___ hunger; **falto de** ___ / shortness of breath.

airear *v.* to aerate, to ventilate. 1. to saturate a liquid with air; 2. to change the venous blood into arterial blood in the lungs; 3. to circulate fresh air.

aislamiento *m.* isolation, of a patient or patients to avoid contagion. ___ **conductual** / behavioral ___; ___ **infeccioso** / infectious ___; ___ **por exclusión** / exclusion ___; ___ **protector** / protective ___; **sala de** ___ / ___ ward.

aislar *vt.* to isolate.

ajustado-a *a.* tight-fitting; adjusted.

ajuste *m.* adjustment, fit; ___ **oclusivo** / oclussive ___.

alar *a.* rel. or similar to a wing.

alargado-a *a.* elongated, as the digestive tract.

alarma *f.* alarm; danger signal; ___ **de fuego** / fire ___ .

alarmante *a.* alarming.

alberca *f.* swimming pool; pond; tank.

albinismo *m.* albinism, lack of pigment in the skin and hair.

albino-a *m., f.* albino, person afflicted with albinism.

albúmina *f.* albumin, protein component.

albuminuria *f.* albuminuria, presence of albumin or globulin in the urine.

alcalemia *f.* alkalemia, excess of alkalinity in the blood.

alcaloide *m.* alkaloid, one of a group of organic, basic substances found in plants.

alcalosis *f.* alkalosis, physiological disorder in the normal acid-base balance of the body.

alcance *m.* reach; span; **al** ___ **de** / within ___; ___ **de movimiento** / range of motion.

alcanfor *m.* camphor, camphor julep.

alcohol *m.* alcohol; ___ **etílico** / ethyl ___ .

alcohólico-a *m., f.* an alcoholic; **abstinencia** ___ / ___ withdrawal; **detoxificación** ___ / ___ detoxification; **privación** ___ / ___ withdrawal

alcoholismo *m.* alcoholism, excess intake of alcohol.

aldosterona *f.* aldosterone, hormone produced by the adrenal gland.

aldosteronismo *m.* aldosteronism, anomaly caused by excessive secretion of aldosterone.

alelo, alelomorfo *m.* allele, any one of a series of two or more genes situated at the same place in homologous chromosomes that determine alternative characteristics in inheritance.

alentar *vt.* to encourage, to reassure.

alérgenos *m., pl.* allergens, term for any antigen that induces an allergic or hypersensitive response. See table on page 264.

alergia *f.* allergy.

alérgico-a *a.* allergic; **reacción** ___ / ___ reaction; **rinitis** ___ / ___ rhinitis.

alergista *m., f.* allergist.

alerta *a.* alert, vigilant, being alert.

aleteo *m.* flutter, cardiac arrhythmia characterized by fast auricular contractions that simulate the flutter of the wings of birds; ___ **auricular** / atrial, auricular ___; ___ **ventricular** / ventricular ___; ___ **y fibrilación** / ___ and fibrillation.

alexia *f.* alexia, inability to understand the written word.

alfiler *m.* pin.

alfombra *f.* rug.

algodón *m.* cotton.

algoritmo *m.* algorithm, arithmetical and algebraic method used in the diagnosis and treatment of a disease.

aliento *m.* 1. breath; **mal** ___ / bad ___; **sin** ___ / out of breath 2. encouragement.

aligeramiento *m.* lightening, descent of the uterus into the pelvic cavity in the final stage of pregnancy.

aligerar *vt.* to lighten, to ease.

alimentación *f.* feeding, alimentation, nourishment; ___ **enteral** / enteral ___; ___ **forzada** / forced ___; ___

intravenosa / intravenous ___; ___ **por
sonda** / tube ___; ___ **rectal** / rectal ___;
horario de ___ / feeding schedule;
requisitos de la ___ / food
requirements.
alimentar *vt.* to nourish, to feed.
alimenticio-a *a.* alimentary,
nourishing; **aditivos** ___**-s** / food
additives; **intoxicación** ___ / food
poisoning; **tracto** ___ / ___ tract.
alimento *m.* food, nourishment,
nutrient; ___ **dietético** / dietetic ___; ___
orgánico / organic ___; ___ **sano** /
health ___; ___**-s enriquecidos** /
supplements; **manipulación de** ___**-s** /
___ handling.
alinfocitosis *f.* alymphocytosis,
abnormal decrease of lymphocytes.
aliviado-a *a.* relieved, alleviated.
aliviar *vt.* to relieve, to alleviate; [*un
dolor*] to lessen.
alivio *m.* relief; ¡qué ___ ! / what a
relief!
allí *adv.* there.
almacenamiento *m.* storage; [toma]
captura y ___ / uptake
and ___ .
almidón *m.* starch, main form of storage
of carbohydrates.
almohada *f.* pillow.
almohadilla *f.* pad.
almorzar *vi.* to have lunch.
almuerzo *m.* lunch.
alógeno-a *a.* allogenic, having a
different genetic constitution from
others belonging to the same species;
células ___ **-as** / ___ cells; **sistema** ___ /
___ system.
aloinjerto *m.* allograft,
homoinjection.
alojamiento *m.* lodging.
alojar *v.* to lodge; to accommodate.
alopecia *f.* alopecia, loss of hair.
alquilar *v.* to rent.
alrededor *adv.* around, about.
alteración *f.* alteration. 1. a change;
2. changing; making different;
cualitativa / qualitative ___; ___
cuantitativa / quantitative ___ .
alterar *v.* to alter, to change.
alternar *v.* to alternate.
alternativa *f.* alternative, option.
alto riesgo *m.* high risk; ___ **de
contaminación** / ___ of contamination;
___ **de infección** / ___ of infection;
___ **de lesión** / ___ of injury; ___ **de
violencia** / ___ of violence.
altura *f.* height.

alucinación, alucinamiento *f., m.*
hallucination, subjective perception not
related to a real stimulus; ___ **auditiva**
/ auditory ___ , imaginary perception of
sound; ___ **gustativa** / gustatory ___ ,
imaginary perception of taste; ___
motora / motor ___ , imaginary
perception of body movements; ___
olfativa / olfactory ___ , imaginary
perception of odors; ___ **táctil** / haptic
___ , imaginary perception of pain,
temperature or other skin sensation.
alucinar *v.* to hallucinate.
alucinógeno *m.* hallucinogen, drug
that produces hallucinations, such as
LSD, peyote, or mescaline.
alucinosis *f.* hallucinosis, state of
persistent hallucinations; ___
alcohólica / alcoholic ___ , extreme fear
accompanied by auditory
hallucinations.
alumbramiento *m.* parturition, the act
of giving birth.
alveolar *a.* alveolar, rel. to an alveolus.
alveolitis *f.* alveolitis. 1. infl. of lung's
alveoli; 2. infl. of a tooth socket. ___
alérgica extrínseca / extrinsic allergic
___; ___ **fibrosa crónica** / chronic
fibrosing ___; ___ **fibrosa criptogénica** /
cryptogenic fibrosing ___; ___
pulmonar aguda / acute pulmonary
___ .
alvéolo *m.* alveolus, cavity; ___
pulmonar / air sac.
alzar *vi.* to raise, to lift; **alzarse /** *vr.* to
raise oneself, to get up.
Alzheimer, enfermedad de *f.*
Alzheimer's disease, presenile
dementia.
amable *a.* kind, nice.
amamantar *v.* to nurse, to suckle, to
breast-feed.
amar *v.* to love.
amargado-a *m., f.* a bitter person; *a.*
[*persona*] bitter.
amargar *vi.* to make bitter; **amargarse**
vr., vi. to become bitter.
amargo-a *a.* bitter.
amarillento-a *a.* yellowish.
amarillo-a *a.* yellow. **atrofia** ___ **del
hígado** / ___ atrophy of the liver; **fibras**
___ / ___ fibers; **fiebre** ___ / ___ fever.
amarrar *v.* to tie, to fasten, to bind.
amarre *m.* fastening, binding; ___ **de las
trompas** / tubal ligation.
amasadura, amasamiento *f. v.,
m.* kneading, methodical rubbing and
pressing of muscles.

amastia *f.* amastia, absence of breasts.

amaurosis *f.* amaurosis, blindness without apparent change in the eye, attributed to an injury in the brain.

amaurótico-a *a.* amaurotic, rel. to amaurosis.

ambarino-a *a.* amber-colored.

ambidextro *a.* ambidextrous.

ambiente *m.* environment, ambiance, setting.

ambivalencia *f.* ambivalence.

ambliopía *f.* amblyopia, diminished vision.

ambos-as *a.* both.

ambulación temprana *f.* early ambulation.

ambulancia *f.* ambulance.

ambulante, ambulatorio-a *a.* ambulant, ambulatory.

ameba *m.* amoeba, ameba, one-celled organism.

amebiano-a *a.* amebic, rel. to amebae.

amebiasis *f.* amebiasis, infection by amebae.

amenaza *f.* threat; menace.

amenorrea *f.* amenorrhoea, absence of menstrual period.

americano-a *a.* American.

ametropía *f.* ametropia, poor vision due to an anomaly or disturbance in the refractive powers of the eye.

amígdalas *f. pl.* amygdalae, tonsils.

amigdalitis *f.* tonsillitis, infl. of the tonsils.

amigdalotomía *f.* tonsillectomy, removal of the tonsils.

amigo-a *m., f.* friend.

amiloide *a.* amyloid, starch-like protein. **degeneración** ___ / ___ degeneration; **enfermedad** ___ / ___ sickness; **nefrosis** ___ / ___ nephrosis; **riñón** ___ / ___ kidney.

amiloidosis *m.* amyloidosis, accumulation of amyloid in different tissues of the body.

amina *f.* amine, one of the basic compounds derived from ammonia.

aminoácido *m.* amino acid, an organic metabolic compound that is the end product of protein and necessary for the growth and development of the human body.

amistad *f.* friendship.

amitosis *f.* amitosis, direct division of the nucleus and cell, without the changes in the nucleus that occur in the ordinary process of cell reproduction.

amnesia *f.* amnesia, loss of memory.

amniocentesis *m.* amniocentesis, puncture of the uterus to obtain amniotic fluid.

amnios *m.* amnion, membranous sac surrounding the embryo in the womb.

amnioscopía *f.* amnioscopy, use of the amnioscope to visualize the fetus through the amniotic fluid.

amnioscopio *m.* amnioscope, endoscope used in the study of the amniotic fluid.

amniótico-a *a.* amniotic, rel. to the amnion; **fluido** ___ / ___ fluid; **saco** ___ / ___ sac.

amoldamiento *m.* molding, adjustment of the head of the fetus to the shape and size of the birth canal.

amoníaco *m.* ammonia.

amoniuria *f.* ammoniuria, excretion of urine containing ammonia.

amor *m.* love.

amor propio *m.* self-esteem.

amoratado-a *a.* black and blue, bruised.

amorfo-a *a.* amorphous, without shape.

amparar *vt.* to protect; to shelter.

ampicilina *f.* ampicillin, semisynthetic penicillin.

ampolla *f.* blister, bulla.

ámpula *f.* ampule, vial, small glass container.

amputación *f.* amputation.

amputar *vt.* to amputate.

Amsler, gráfico de *m.* Amsler graphic, chart useful in revealing signs of macular degeneration.

anabólico-a *a.* anabolic, rel. to anabolism; **esteroides** ___-s / ___ steroids.

anabolismo *m.* anabolism, cellular process by which simple substances are converted into complex compounds; constructive metabolism.

anaerobio *m.* anaerobe, germ that multiplies in the absence of air or oxygen.

anafase *f.* anaphase, a stage in cell division.

anafiláctico-a *a.* anaphylactic, rel. to anaphylaxis.

anafilaxis *f.* anaphylaxis, extreme allergic reaction; hypersensitivity.

anal *a.* anal; **fístula** ___ / ___ fistula.

analgésico *m.* analgesic, pain reliever.

análisis *m.* analysis, test, assay; ___ **de acumulación** / accumulation ___; ___

de aminoácido / amino acid ___; **___ de huevos y parásitos en las heces fecales** / ___ of eggs and parasites in the stools; **de la mordida** / bite ___; **___ del aliento** / breath ___; **cefalométrico** / cephalometric ___; **del character** / character ___; **___ cualitativo** / qualitative ___; **cuantitativo** / quantitative ___; **___ de costos** / cost ___; **___ de datos** / data ___; **___ de orina** / urinalysis; **___ del pelo** / hair ___; **___ gástrico** / gastric ___; **___ de los sueños** / dream ___ .

analizar vt. to analyze, to examine.

anaplasia f. anaplasia, lack or loss of differentiation of cells.

anaquel m. shelf; shelf-like structure.

anaranjado-a a. orange.

anasarca f. anasarca, generalized infiltration of edema fluid in subcutaneous connective tissue.

anastomosis f. anastomosis, creation of a passage or communication between two or more organs; inosculating.

anastomosis ileoanal f. ileoanal anastomosis, removal of the colon and the inner lining of the rectum.

anatomía f. anatomy, science that studies the structure of the human body and its organs; **___ macroscópica** / gross ___ , rel. to structures that can be seen with the naked eye; **___ topográfica** / topographic ___ , rel. to a specific area of the body.

anatómico-a a. anatomic, anatomical, rel. to anatomy.

ancianidad f. old age.

anciano-a m., f. old man, old woman.

andador m. walker, device used to help a person walk.

andar vi. to walk; to go; **___ con cuidado** / to be careful.

andrógeno m. androgen, masculine hormone; a. androgenic, rel. to the male sexual characteristics.

androginoide a. androgynous, having both male and female characteristics.

anejos, anexos m. pl. adnexa, appendages, such as the uterine tubes.

anemia f. anemia, insufficiency of blood cells either in quality, quantity or in hemoglobin content; **___ aplástica** / aplastic ___ , highly deficient production of blood cells; **___ de glóbulos falciformes** / sickle cell ___; **___ hemorrágica o hemolítica** / hemorrhagic, hemolytic ___ ,

progressive destruction of red blood cells; **___ hipercrómica** / hyperchromic ___ , abnormal increase in the hemoglobin content; **___ hipocrómica y microcítica** / hypochromic and microcytic ___ , small-sized blood cells and insufficient amount of hemoglobin; **___ macrocítica** / macrocytic ___ , large-sized blood cells, pernicious anemia; **___ por deficiencia de hierro** / iron deficiency ___ .

anemia macrocítica n. macrocytic anemia, type of anemia presenting a large number of macrocytes.

anergia f. anergy. 1. asthenia, lack of energy; 2. reduction or lack of response to a specific antigen.

anestesia f. anesthesia; **___ con hipotension controlada** / hypotensive ___; **___ en silla de montar** / saddle block ___; **___ endotraqueal** / endotracheal ___; **___ epidural** / epidural ___; **___ general intravenosa** / general intravenous ___; **___ general por inhalación** / general ___ by inhalation; **___ general por intubación** / general ___ by intubation; **___ intercostal** / intercostal ___; **___ local** / local ___; **___ por hipnosis** / hypnosis ___; **___ tópica** / topical ___; **___ témica** / thermic ___; **___ raquídea** / spinal ___; **___ regional** / regional ___.

anestesiar v. to anesthetize.

anestésico m. anesthetic.

anestesiólogo-a m., f. anesthesiologist.

aneurisma m. aneurysm, dilation of a portion of the wall of the artery; **___ aórtico** / aortic ___; **___ cerebral** / cerebral ___; **___ desecante** / dissecting ___; **___ falso** / false ___; **___ fusiforme** / fusiform ___; **___ saculado** / berry ___; **___ verdadero** / true ___ .

aneurisma de la arteria coronaria m. coronary artery aneurysm, gen. caused by atherosclerosis, inflammatory processes, or a coronary fistula.

aneurismal a. aneurysmal, rel. to an aneurysm.

aneurismectomía f. aneurysmectomy, excision of an aneurysm.

anfetamina f. amphetamine, type of drug used as a stimulant of the nervous system.

angiitis f. angiitis, infl. of blood or lymph vessel.

ansiedad

angina *f.* angina, painful constrictive sensation; **___ inestable** / unstable **___**; **___ intestinal** / intestinal **___** , acute abdominal pain caused by insufficient blood supply to the intestines; **laríngea** / laryngeal **___** , infl. of the throat; **___ pectoris** / **___** pectoris, chest pain caused by insufficient blood supply to the heart muscle.

angiocardiografía *f.* angiocardiography, x-ray of the heart chambers.

angioespasmo *m.* angiospasm, prolonged contraction of a blood vessel.

angiogénesis *f.* angiogenesis, the development of the vascular system.

angiografía *f.* angiography, x-ray of the blood vessels after injection of a substance to show their outline; **___ de resonancia magnética** / magnetic resonance **___**.

angiografía coronaria *f.* coronary angiography, images of the circulation of the myocardium taken with a contrast medium, and gen. done through catheterization of each of the coronary arteries.

angiograma *m.* angiogram; visualization of a blood vessel obtained after injecting a radiopaque substance.

angioma *m.* angioma, benign vascular tumor.

angioneurótico *m.* angioneurotic, rel. to angioneurosis.

angioplastia *f.* angioplasty, plastic surgery of the blood vessels; **___ coronaria percutánea** / percutaneous coronary **___**; **___ periférica percutánea** / percutaneous peripheral **___**.

angioplastia transluminal percutánea *f.* percutaneous transluminal angioplasty, process of dilating an artery or vessel by using a balloon that is inflated by pressure.

angiosarcoma *m.* angiosarcoma, a rare malignant neoplasm most often found in soft tissues.

angiotensina *f.* angiotensin, a family of peptides of known and similar sequence, produced by enzymatic action of renin.

angiotensinógeno *m.* angiotensinogen, a protein that when activated by the enzyme renin causes

the blood vessels to constrict and raises the blood pressure.

angloparlante *m., f.* English speaker.

ángulo *m.* angle.

angustia *f.* anguish, distress.

angustiado-a *a.* distraught, distressed.

angustiarse *vr.* to be distressed, to feel anguish.

anhidrasa *f.* anhydrase, enzyme that catalyzes the removal of water from a compound; **inhibidores de ___ carbónica** / carbonic **___** inhibitors.

anhidrosis *f.* anhidrosis, diminished secretion of sweat.

anillo *m.* ring, margin, verge; **___ anal** / anal verge.

animar *v.* to animate, to cheer up; **animarse** *vr.* to become more lively.

ánimo *m.* spirit; **estado de ___** / mood; **no tener ___** / to be without motivation.

animosidad *f.* animosity, rancor.

anisocitosis *f.* anisocytosis, unequal size of red blood cells.

anisocoria *f.* anisocoria, a condition in which the two pupils are not of equal size. **___ central-simple** / simple-central **___**; **___ esencial** / essential **___**; **___ fisiológica** / physiologic **___**; **___ simple** /simple **___** .

ano *m.* anus.

anoche *adv.* last night.

anodino *m.* anodyne, pain reliever; **-a** / *a.* insipid.

anomalía, anormalidad *f.* anomaly, abnormality, irregularity.

anorexia *f.* anorexia, disorder characterized by total lack of appetite.

anoréxico-a *a.* 1. lacking appetite. *n.* 2. person affected with anorexia nervosa.

anormal *a.* abnormal, irregular.

anosmia *f.* anosmia, lack of the sense of smell.

anovulación *f.* anovulation, cessation of ovulation.

anoxemia *f.* anoxemia, insufficient oxygen in the blood.

anoxia *f.* anoxia, lack of oxygen in body tissues. **___ anémica** / anemic **___**; **___ de altitud** / altitude **___**; **___ de estancamiento** / stagnant **___**; **___ del neonato** / **___** neonatorum.

anquilosis *f.* ankylosis, immobility of an articulation.

ansiedad *f.* anxiety, anguish, state of apprehension or excessive worry;

ansioso-a

estados de ___ / ___ disorders; **neurosis de** ___ / ___ neurosis.

ansioso-a *a.* anxious, apprehensive.

anteayer *adv.* the day before yesterday.

antebrazo *f.* forearm.

antecubital *a.* antecubital, preceding the elbow.

anteflexión *f.* anteflexion, bending forward.

antemano *adv.* beforehand.

antemortem *adv.* antemortem, before death.

antenatal *a.* antenatal, that occurs or is formed before birth.

anteojos *m. pl.* eyeglasses; binoculars.

antepasados *m. pl.* ancestors.

antepié *m.* ball of the foot.

anterior *a.* preceding, previous; [*tiempo*] before, pre-existing; [*posición*] ___ **ventral** / ventral ___ .

anteroposterior *a.* anteroposterior, from front to back.

antes *adv.* before, sooner; ___ **de** / before, prior to; ___ **de las comidas** / ___ meals; **lo** ___ **posible** / as soon as possible.

anteversión *f.* anteversion, turned toward the front.

antiácido *m.* antacid, acidity neutralizer.

antiadrenérgico *m.* antiadrenergic, adrenergic blocking agents, antagonistic to the action of sympathetic or other adrenergic nerve fibers.

antialérgico *m.* antiallergic, drug used to treat allergies.

antiarrítmico-a *a.* antiarrhythmic, that can prevent or be effective in the treatment of arrhythmia; **agentes** ___**-s** / cardiac depressants.

antiartrítico-a *a.* antiarthritic, rel. to medication used in the treatment of arthritis.

antibiótico *m.* antibiotic, antibacterial drug; ___ **antineoplásico** / antineoplastic ___; ___ **bactericida** / bactericidal ___; ___ **de amplio espectro** / broad spectrum ___ .

anticarcinógeno *m.* anticarcinogen, drug used in the treatment of cancer.

anticoagulante *m.* anticoagulant, substance used in the prevention of blood clotting.

anticolinérgico-a *a.* anticholinergic, that rel. to the blockage of the impulses of the parasympathetic nerves.

anticonceptivo *m.* contraceptive; **-a** / *a.* that acts as a contraceptive; ___ **oral** / oral ___; **drogas** ___**-s** / anovulatory drugs; **injerto** ___ / ___ implant.

anticonvulsante, anticonvulsivo *m.* anticonvulsant, medication used to prevent fits or convulsions.

anticuerpo *m.* antibody, protein substance produced by lymph tissue in response to the presence of an antigen; ___ **monoclónico** / monoclonal ___ , derived from hybridoma cells; ___**-s de reacción cruzada** / cross reacting ___ -s.

antidepresivo *m.* antidepressant, medication or process used in the treatment of depression.

antidiarreico *m.* antidiarrheal.

antidiurético *m.* antidiuretic, drug that decreases urine secretion; **hormona** ___ / ___ hormone.

antídoto *m.* antidote, substance used to neutralize a poison; ___ **universal** / universal ___ .

antiemético *m.* antiemetic, medication used to treat nausea.

antiespasmódico *m.* antispasmodic, drug used in the treatment of spasms.

antígeno *m.* antigen, toxic substance which stimulates formation of antibodies; ___ **carcinoembriogénico** / carcinoembryogenic ___ .

antígeno B *m.* B antigen, protein present in the erythrocytes' membranes that could cause a serious reaction in a transfusion.

antihipertensivo *m.* antihypertensive, medication to lower elevated blood pressure.

antihistamínico *m.* antihistamine, medication used in the treatment of some allergies.

antiinflamatorio *m.* anti-inflammatory, agent used to treat inflammations.

antineoplástico *m.* antineoplastic, drug that controls or destroys cancer cells.

antipirético *m.* antipyretic, agent that reduces fever.

antiprurítico *m.* antipruritic, medication used to reduce itching.

antiséptico *m.* antiseptic, agent that destroys bacteria.

antisuero anafiláctico *m.* anaphylactic antiserum.

antitóxico *m.* antitoxin, neutralizer of the effects of toxins.

antitoxina *f.* antitoxin, antibody that has a neutralizing effect on a given poison introduced in the body by a microorganism; ___ **diftérica** / diphtheria ___; ___ **tetánica** / tetanus ___ .

antivirósico *m.* antiviral, agent that stops the action of a virus.

antracosis *f.* anthracosis, lung condition due to prolonged inhalation of coal dust.

ántrax *m.* anthrax, virus caused by the agent *cutaneous anthrax*. The *Bacillus anthracis* develops in infected animals through the skin. Humans suffering from anthrax experience symptoms of hemorrhage and serous effusions in several organ cavities and lethargy; it is not transmissible by contact, but if transmitted by air can cause fatal pneumonia. **cerebral** / cerebral ___; ___ **cutáneo** / cutaneous ___ .

antro *m.* antrum, any cavity semi-closed, particulary one with bony walls; ___ **auris** / ___ auris; ___ **cardíaco** / ___ cardiacum; ___ **folicular** / follicular ___; ___ **mastoideo** / ___ mastoideum; ___ **maxilar** / maxillary ___; ___ **pilórico** / ___ pyloricum; ___ **timpánico** / tympanic ___ .

antropoide *a.* anthropoid, of human resemblance.

anuria *f.* anuria, lack of urine production due to kidney malfunction.

año *m.* year; ___**s perdidos de vida potencial** / ___s of potential life lost.

aorta *f.* aorta, major artery originating from the left ventricle; ___ **ascendente** / ascending ___; **cayado de la** ___ / aortic arch; **coartación o compresión de la** ___ / coarctation of the ___; **descendente** / descending ___ .

aórtico-a *a.* aortic, rel. to the aorta; **válvula semilunar** ___ / ___ semilunar valve.

aortocoronaria *a.* aortocoronary, rel. to the aorta and coronary arteries.

aortografía *f.* aortography, outline of the aorta on an x-ray.

aparato digestivo *m.* digestive system.

aparato eléctrico *m.* electrical appliance.

aparente *a.* apparent, manifest, patent, visible.

apatía *f.* apathy, lack of interest.

apellido *m.* surname, family name.

apenado-a *a.* grieved.

apenas *adv.* barely; no sooner than; as soon as.

apendectomía *f.* appendectomy, removal of the appendix.

apéndice *m.* appendix.

apendicitis *f.* appendicitis, infl. of the appendix.

apendicular *a.* appendicular, rel. to the appendix.

apesadumbrado-a *a.* mournful, grieved.

apetito *m.* appetite.

ápice *m.* apex, the upper or base point of an organ.

apio *m.* celery.

aplanar *vt.* to flatten.

aplasia *f.* aplasia, failure of organ development.

aplastamiento *m.* squashing, crushing.

aplastar *v.* to crush, to squash.

aplazar *vi.* to postpone, to put off.

aplicador *m.* applicator; ___ **de algodón** / cotton ___ .

aplicar *vt.* to apply.

apnea *f.* apnea, temporary arrest of breathing; ___ **del sueño** / sleep ___ , intermittent apnea that occurs during sleep.

aponeurosis *f.* aponeurosis, connective tissue that attaches the muscles to the bones and to other tissue.

apoplejía *f.* apoplexy, stroke, cerebrovascular accident.

apósito *m.* dressing. 1. clean or sterile application of material, to a wound for protection, absorbency, drainage, etc. 2. adhesive absorbent dressing. ___ **amarrado** / tie-over ___; ___ **antiséptico** / antiseptic ___; ___ **apretado** / pressure ___; ___ **cambiado** / removable ___; ___ **desechable** / removable ___; ___ **fijo** / fixed ___; ___ **humedecido** / wet ___; ___ **oclusivo** / occlusive ___; ___ **seco** / dry ___ .

apoyar *vt.* to back, to support; **apoyarse** *vr.* to lean on.

apoyo *m.* backing, support.

apraxia *f.* apraxia, lack of muscular coordination and movement.

aprendizaje *m.* learning. 1. generic term for the relatively permanent change in behavior that occurs as a result of practice or experience; 2. act of acquisition of knowledge; ___ **cognitivo** / cognitive ___; ___ **dependiente de estado** / state-dependent ___; ___ **incidental** /

incidental __; **latente** / latent __;
__ **pasivo** / passive __ .

apretado-a *a.* tight.

apretar *vt.* to tighten, to squeeze, to
press down.

aprisa *adv.* fast.

aprobar *vt.* to approve; to accept.

apropiado-a *a.* appropriate, adequate.

aprovechar *v.* to make use of; to take
advantage of.

aproximado-a *a.* approximate; **-mente**
adv. approximately.

aptitud *f.* aptitude, capacity, ability;
prueba de __ / __ test.

apto-a *a.* competent, apt.

apurado-a *a.* in a hurry; in difficulty.

apurarse *vr.* to hurry.

apuro *m.* need; hurry; **estar en un __** /
to be in trouble.

aquí *adv.* here; **por __** / this way.

aquietar *v.* to calm down.

Aquiles, tendón de *m.* Achilles
tendon, the tendon that originates in the
muscles of the calf and attaches to the
heel.

aracnoide *m.* arachnoid, weblike
membrane that covers the brain and
spinal cord.

araña *f.* spider; __ **viuda negra** / black
widow __ .

arañar *v.* to scratch.

arañazo *m.* scratch.

árbol *m.* 1. anatomical structure
resembling a tree; 2. tree; __
bronquial / bronchial __; __
genealógico / genealogical __ .

arcadas *f., pl.* retching, spasmodic
abdominal contractions that precede
vomiting.

arco *m.* arch. __ **carotídeo** / carotid __;
__ **del paladar** / palate __; __ **plantar**
/ plantar __ .

arder *vt.* to have a burning feeling; to
burn.

ardor *m.* ardor, burning feeling; __ **en el
estómago** / heartburn.

arenilla *f.* minute, sandlike particles.

arenoso-a *a.* sandy.

aréola *f.* areola, circular area of a
different color around a central point.

Argyll Robertson, pupila de *f.*
Argyll Robertson's pupil, a pupil of the
eye that accommodates to distance but
does not react to the refraction of
light.

arma química *f.* chemical weapon,
chemical substances that can be
delivered by warfare to cause death or
severe harm to humans, animals, and
plants.

armazón *f.* frame, supportive structure.
__ **de tracción en garra** / claw type
traction __ .

aroma *m.* aroma, pleasant smell.

aromático-a *a.* aromatic, rel. to an
aroma.

arquetipo *m.* archetype, original type
from which modified versions evolve.

arraigado-a *a.* deep-rooted.

arrancar *vt.* to tear off; to pull out.

arrebato *m.* fit; temporary insanity.

arreflexia *f.* areflexia, absence of
reflexes.

arreglado-a *a.* in order; neat; fixed.

arreglo *m.* settlement, agreement.

arrenoblastoma *m.* arrhenoblastoma.

arrepentido-a *a.* repentant, regretful.

arrepentirse *vr. vi.* to regret; to
repent.

arriba *adv.* above, upstairs; **de __ a
abajo** / from top to bottom.

arriesgado-a *a.* risky.

arriesgar *vt.* to risk, to imperil;
arriesgarse *vr.* to take a risk.

arritmia *f.* arrhythmia, irregular
heartbeats.

arrodillarse *vr.* to kneel.

arrojar *vt.* to throw up, to vomit.

arroz *m.* rice.

arruga *f.* wrinkle.

arrugado-a *a.* wrinkled.

arsénico *m.* arsenic; **envenenamiento
por __** / __ poisoning.

arteria *f.* artery; vessel carrying blood
from the heart to tissues throughout the
body; __ **innominada** / innominate
__ .

arterial *a.* arterial, rel. to the arteries;
enfermedades __ -es oclusivas / __
occlusive diseases; **sistema __** / __
system.

arterioesclerosis *f.* arteriosclerosis,
hardening of the walls of the arteries.

arteriografía *f.* arteriography, x-ray of
the arteries.

arteriograma *m.* arteriogram,
angiogram of the arteries; __ **cerebral
o carótico** / cerebral or carotid __; __
mesentérico / mesenteric __; __
periférico / peripheral __; __ **renal** /
renal __ .

arteriola *f.* arteriole, minute artery
ending in a capillary.

arterioplastia *f.* arterioplasty, surgical
procedure to repair or reconstruct an
artery.

arteriotomía f. arteriotomy, opening of an artery.

arteriovenoso-a a. arteriovenous; rel. to an artery and a vein; **anastomosis** ___ **quirúrgica** / ___ shunt, surgical; **fístula** ___ / ___ fistula; **malformaciones** ___ -as / ___ malformations.

arteritis f. arteritis, infl. of an artery.

articulación f. joint, articulation. 1. joint between two or more bones; ___ **cartilaginosa** / cartilagenous ___; ___ **chasqueante** / snapping ___; ___ **condiloidea** / condyloid ___; ___ **de la cabeza de la cadera** / ___ of head of hip; ___ **de la cadera** / hip ___; ___ **de la falange** / phalangeal ___; ___ **de la mandíbula** / mandibullar ___; ___ **de la mano** / ___ of hand; ___ **de la pelvis** / pelvic ___; ___ **de la rodilla** / knee ___; ___ **del carpo**/carpal ___; ___ **del codo** / elbow ___; ___ **del hombro** / shoulder ___; ___ **del oído** / of ear bones; ___ **del pie** / foot ___; ___ **del tobillo** / ankle ___; ___ **femuropatelar** / femuropatellar ___; ___ **fibrosa** / fibrous ___; ___ **inestable** / flail ___; ___ **inmóvil** / immovable ___; ___ **interarticular** / interarticular ___; ___ **intercarpales** / intercarpal ___; ___ **interfalange** / interphalangeal ___; ___ **neurocentral** / neurocentral ___; ___ **petrooccipital** / petrooccipital; ___ **radioulnar** / radioulnar ___; ___ **rotatoria**/pivot ___; ___ **seudoartrosis**/ false ___; ___ **sinovial** / synovial ___; ___ **tibiofibular** / tibiofibular ___; 2. articulation, distinctive and clear pronunciation of words in speech.

articulaciones del metatarso falangial f., pl. joints of the phalangeal metatarsus, rel. to the metatarsus and the toes.

artículo m. article.

artificial a. artificial, substituting that which is natural; **fecundación** ___ / ___ impregnation, fecundation; **respiración** ___ / ___ respiration.

artrítico-a a. arthritic, rel. to or suffering from arthritis.

artritis f. arthritis, infl. of an articulation or joint; ___ **aguda** / acute ___; ___ **coronaria reumatoide** / rheumatoid coronary ___; ___ **crónica** / chronic ___; ___ **degenerativa** / degenerative ___; ___ **hemofílica** / hemophilic ___; ___ **reumatoidea** / rheumatoid ___; ___ **traumática** / traumatic ___ .

artrodesis f. arthrodesis. 1. fusion of the bones of a joint; 2. artificial ankylosis.

artograífa f. arthography, X-ray of a joint.

artroplastia f. arthroplasty, reparation of a joint or building of an artificial one.

asbesto m. asbestos.

asbestosis f. asbestosis, chronic infection of the lungs caused by asbestos.

ascariasis f. ascariasis, intestinal infection caused by a worm of the genus *Ascaris*.

ascárido m. ascaris, type of worm commonly found in the intestinal tract.

ascendiente m. ascendent, ancestor.

ascitis f. ascites, accumulation of fluid in the peritoneal cavity.

asco m. nausea; disgust, loathing; **dar** ___ / to produce nausea.

aseado-a a. clean, tidy.

asear vt. to clean; **asearse** vr. to clean oneself.

asegurar vt. to assure; **asegurarse** vr. to make sure.

asentaderas f. pl. buttocks.

asepsia f. asepsia, total absence of germs.

aséptico-a a. aseptic, sterile.

asexual a. asexual, having no gender; **reproducción** ___ / ___ reproduction.

asfixia f. asphyxia, suffocation; ___ **fetal** / ___ fetalis.

asfixiarse vr. to asphyxiate, to suffocate.

así adv. like this; ___ **que** / therefore.

asiento m. seat, space upon which a structure rests.

asilo m. nursing home, shelter; ___ **para ancianos** / ___ for the aged.

asimilación f. assimilation. 1. integration of digested materials from food into the tissues; 2. restructuring and modification of received information and experiences into a cognitive structure.

asinergia f. asynergia, lack of coordination among normally harmonious organs.

asintomático-a a. asymptomatic, without symptoms.

asistencia f. 1. assistance, care, help; ___ **medico-sanitaria** / health and medical ___; ___ **social** / welfare; ___ **social a la infancia** / child welfare; **recibir** ___ / to be on relief; 2. attendance.

asistente

asistente *m., f.* attendant, assistant.
asistir *vt.* to attend; to help.
asistolia *f.* asystole, asystolia, absence of heart contractions.
asma *m.* asthma, allergic condition that causes bouts of short breath, wheezing, and edema of the mucosa; ___ **cardíaca** / cardiac ___ .
asmático-a *a.* asthmatic, rel. to or suffering from asthma.
asociado-a *m., f.* associate.
aspartamo *m.* aspartame, low calorie sweetener.
aspartato *m.* aspartate, a salt or ester of aspartic acid.
aspartato amino transferasa *m.* aspartate amino transferase, diagnostic aid in viral hepatitis and in myocardial infarction.
aspecto *m.* appearance, aspect.
aspereza *f.* roughness, harshness.
Asperger, syndrome de *m.* Asperger's disorder, characterized by impairment in social skills, pedantic speech, superficial interests, however having a normal IQ.
aspergilosis *f.* aspergillosis, infection caused by the fungi *Aspergillus hyphae* that gen. affects the sense of hearing.
áspero-a *a.* rough, harsh; **piel** ___ / ___ skin.
aspersión nasal *f.* the act of using nasal spray.
aspiración *f.* aspiration, inhalation.
aspirar *vt.* to breathe in, to inhale; ___ **por la mucosa nasal** / to snort.
aspirina *f.* aspirin, a derivative of salicylic acid.
astigmatismo *m.* astigmatism, defective curvature of the refractive surfaces of the eye.
astilla *f.* splinter.
astrágalo *m.* astragalus, ankle bone.
astringente *m.* astringent, agent that has the power to constrict tissues and mucous membranes.
astrocitoma *f.* astrocytoma, brain tumor.
asustado-a *a.* frightened, startled.
asustar *vt.* to frighten, to scare; **asustarse** *vr.* to become frightened.
ataque *m.* attack, fit, stroke, bout, seizure; ___ **cardíaco** / heart ___ .
ataraxia *f.* ataraxia, impassiveness.
atareado-a *a.* busy.
ataúd *m.* coffin, casket.

atavismo *m.* atavism, inherited trait from remote ancestors.
ataxia *f.* ataxia, deficiency in muscular coordination; ___ **sifilítica** / tabes dorsal.
atelectasia *f.* atelectasis, partial or total collapse of a lung.
atención *f.* attention; care; courtesy; ___ **a largo plazo** / long term ___; ___ **de especialidad** / specialty ___; ___ **del neonato** / newborn ___; ___ **dirigida** / managed ___; ___ **domiciliaria** / home ___; **falta de** ___ / lack of ___; ___ **holística** / holistic ___; ___ **intraparto** / intrapartum ___; ___ **médica** / medical care; ___ **médica laboral** / occupational ___; **prestar** ___ / to pay ___; ___ **temporal** / respite ___; ___ **sanitaria preventiva** / preventive health ___ .
atender *v.* to attend, to look after; to pay attention.
atenuación *f.* attenuation, rendering less virulent.
aterectomía coronaria *f.* coronary atherectomy, removal of obstructions from the coronary artery by use of a cardiac catheter.
ateroma *f.* atheroma, fatty deposits in the intima of an artery.
atetosis *f.* athetosis, infantile spasmodic paraplegia.
atleta *m.* athlete.
atlético-a *a.* athletic.
atmósfera *f.* atmosphere.
atmósferico-a *a.* atmospheric.
atolondrado-a *a.* confused, bewildered.
atolondramiento *m.* confusion, bewilderment.
atomizador *m.* atomizer.
átomo *m.* atom.
atonía *f.* atony, lack of normal tone, esp. in the muscles.
atontado-a *a.* stunned, stupefied.
atopía *f.* atopy, type of allergy considered as having a hereditary tendency.
atorarse *vr.* to gag, to choke.
atormentar *vt.* to torment.
atrás *adv.* behind; **ir hacia** ___ / to go backwards.
atrasado-a *a.* backward, late, behind; ___ **mental** / mentally retarded.
atravesar *vt.* to cross; to go through; ___ **la calle** / ___ the street.
atresia *f.* atresia, congenital absence or closure of a body passage.
atreverse *vr.* to dare, to take a chance.

54

atrevido-a *a.* daring; insolent.

atrial *a.* atrial, rel. to an atrium; **defecto septal** __ / __ septal defect.

atribuir *vt.* to attribute; to confer.

atrio *m.* atrium. 1. cavity that is connected to another structure; 2. upper chamber of the heart that receives the blood from the veins.

atrioventricular, auriculoventricular *a.* atrioventricular, auriculoventricular, rel. to an atrium and a ventricle of the heart; **nudo** __ / __ node; **orificio** __ / __ orifice.

atrofia *f.* atrophy, deterioration of cells, tissue, and organs of the body; __ **artrítica** / arthritic __; __ **alveolar** / alveolar __; __ **amarilla aguda hepática** / acute yellow __ of the liver; __ **cerebelosa** / cerebellar __; __ **cerebelar de tipo nutricional** / nutritional type cerebellar __; __ **cerebral progresiva** / progressive cerebral __; __ **de sistema múltiple** / multiple system __; __ **epiléptica** / epileptic __; __ **infantil músculo-espinal progresiva** / infantile progressive spinal-muscular __; __ **macular primaria de la piel** / primary macular __ of skin; __ **muscular espinal juvenil** / juvenile spinal muscular __; __ **muscular isquémica** / ischemic muscular __; __ **macular** / macular __; __ **neurogénica** / neurogenic __; __ **periodontal** / periodontal __; __ **postmenopáusica** / postmenopausal __; __ **senil** / senil __.

atropina *f.* atropine sulphate, agent used as a muscle relaxer, esp. applied to the eyes to dilate the pupil and paralyze the ciliary muscle during eye examination.

atún *m.* tuna fish.

aturdido-a *a.* confused, stunned.

aturdimiento *m.* confusion, bewilderment.

audición *f.* audition, sense of hearing; **pérdida de la** __ / hearing loss.

audífono *m.* hearing aid.

audiograma *m.* audiogram, instrument that records the degree of hearing.

auditivo-a, auditorio-a *a.* auditory, rel. to hearing; **conducto** __ / __ canal; **nervio** __ / __ nerve; **tapón** __ / ear plug.

aumentar *v.* to increase, to augment, to magnify; __ **de peso** / to gain weight.

aumento *m.* increase.

aún *adv.* still, yet; __ **cuando** / even though.

aunque *conj.* although.

aura *f.* aura, sensation preceding an epileptic attack.

aurícula *f.* auricle. 1. the outer visible part of the ear; 2. either of the two upper chambers of the heart.

auricular *m.* earphone; *a.* 1. rel. to the sense of hearing; 2. rel. to an auricle of the heart.

auscultación *f.* auscultation, the act of listening to sounds arising from organs such as the lungs and the heart for diagnostic purposes.

auscultar *v.* to auscultate, to examine by auscultation.

ausencia *f.* absence.

autismo *m.* autism, behavioral disorder manifested by extreme self-centeredness; __ **infantil** / infantile __.

autístico-a *a.* autistic, suffering from or rel. to autism.

autoclave *f.* autoclave, an instrument for sterilizing by steam pressure.

autóctono-a *a.* native, autochthonous, indigenous.

autodigestión *f.* autodigestion, digestion of tissues by their own enzymes and juices.

autógeno-a *a.* autogenous, produced within the individual.

autoinfección *f.* autoinfection, infection by an agent from the same body.

autoinjerto *m.* autograft, autogenous implant taken from another part of the patient's body.

autoinmunización *f.* autoimmunization, immunity resulting from a substance developed within the affected person's own body.

autoinoculable *a.* autoinoculable, susceptible to a germ from within.

autólogo-a *a.* autologous, derived from the same individual.

automatismo *m.* automatism, behavior not under voluntary control.

automedicación *f.* self-medication.

autónomo-a *a.* autonomic, autonomous, that functions independently; **sistema nervioso** __ / __ nervous system.

autoplastia *f.* autoplasty, implantation of an autograft.

autopsia *f.* autopsy, postmortem examination of the body.

autorización *f.* authorization.

autorizar *vi.* to authorize.

autosugestión *f.* autosuggestion, self-suggested thought.

autotrasfusión *f.* autotransfusion, transfusion of an individual's own blood.

autotrasplante *m.* autotransplant, autologous graft.

auxilio *m.* aid, help; **primeros ___-s /** first ___ .

avena *f.* oats; **harina de ___ /** oatmeal.

aventado-a *a.* bloated.

aventarse *vr.* to become bloated.

aversión *f.* aversion, dislike.

aviso *m.* notice; **dar ___ /** to notify.

avispa *f.* wasp; **picadura de ___ /** sting.

avispón *m.* hornet.

avitaminosis *f.* avitaminosis, disorder caused by a lack of vitamins.

avivar *v.* to liven up; to strengthen.

avulsión *f.* avulsion, removal or extraction of part of a structure.

axial *a.* axial, rel. to the axis.

axila *f.* axilla, armpit.

axilar *a.* axillary, rel. to the axilla.

axis *m.* axis, imaginary central line passing through the body or through an organ.

ayer *adv.* yesterday.

Ayerza, síndrome de *m.* Ayerza's syndrome, syndrome manifested by multiple symptoms, esp. dyspnea and cyanosis, gen. as a result of pulmonary deficiency.

ayuda *f.* help; **sin ___ /** unassisted.

ayudante *m., f.* helper.

ayudar *v.* to help, to assist.

ayunar *v.* to fast.

ayuno *m.* fast.

azoospermia *f.* azoospermia, lack of spermatozoa in the semen.

azotemia *f.* azotemia, excess urea in the blood.

azúcar *m.* sugar, carbohydrate consisting essentially of sucrose; ___ **de la uva /** grape ___ , dextrose.

azufre *m.* sulfur.

azul *a.* blue; **mal ___ / ___** baby.

azul de metileno *m.* methylene blue, crystalline powder of a greenish blue color that is used as an antidote for cyanide and carbon monoxide poisoning.

b

---

b *abr.* bacilo / bacillus; **bucal** / buccal.

babear *v.* to slobber.

Babinski reflejo de *m.* Babinski's reflex, dorsiflexion of the big toe when the sole of the foot is stimulated.

bacilar *a.* bacillary, rel. to bacillus.

bacilemia *f.* bacillemia, presence of bacilli in the blood.

bacilo *m. bacilli* bacillus rod-shaped bacteria; **___ de Calmette-Guérin /** Calmette-Guérin bacillus, bacile bilié; **___ de Koch** / Koch's **___ ,** *Mycobacterium tuberculosis;* **___ de la fiebre tifoidea** / typhoid **___ ,** Salmonella typhi; **portador de ___ -s /** bacilli carrier.

baciluria *f.* bacilluria, presence of bacilli in the urine.

bacín *m.* basin, large bowl; bedpan.

bacitracina *f.* bacitracin, antibiotic effective against some staphylococci.

bacteremia *f.* bacteremia, presence of bacteria in the blood.

bacteria *f.* bacterium; germ.

bacteriano-a *a.* bacterial; **infecciones ___ -s /** **___** infections; **endocarditis ___ / ___** endocarditis; **pruebas de sensibilidad ___ / ___** sensitivity tests.

bactericida *m.* bactericide, agent that kills bacteria.

bacteriógeno *a.* bacteriogenic. 1. of bacterial origin; 2. that produces bacteria.

bacteriolisina *f.* bacteriolysin, antibody that destroys bacterial cells.

bacteriólisis *f.* bacteriolysis, the destruction of bacteria.

bacteriología *f.* bacteriology, the study of bacteria.

bacteriológico-a *a.* bacteriologic, bacteriological, rel. to bacteria.

bacteriólogo-a *m., f.* bacteriologist, specialist in bacteriology.

bacteriostasis *f.* bacteriostasis, condition by which growth and multiplication of bacteria is inhibited.

bacteriuria *f.* bacteriuria, presence of bacteria in the urine.

baipás *m.* bypass; surgically created alternate channel or route; derivación. **___ aortoilíaco** / aortoiliac **___ ; ___**

aortorrenal / aortorenal **___ ; ___ cardiopulmonar** / cardiopulmonary **___ ; ___ coronario** / coronary **___ ; ___ extracraneal-intracraneal /** extracranial-intracranial **___ ; ___ o derivación aortocoronaria** / aortocoronary **___ ; ___ jejonoileal /** jejunoileal **___ ;** *v.* to move new flow of fluids from one body part to another through a diversionary channel.

bajar *vt.* [*escaleras*] to go down; [*movimiento*] to lower; **___ de peso** / to lose weight; **___ el brazo** / to lower the arm.

bajo-a *a.* low, short; **presión ___ / ___** blood pressure; **bajo** *prep.* under; **___ observación / ___** observation; **___ tratamiento / ___** treatment.

bala *f.* bullet; **herida de ___ / ___** wound.

balance *m.* balance, equilibrium, quantities and concentrations of parts and fluids that normally constitute the human body; **___ acidobásico /** acid-base **___ ; ___ hídrico** / fluid **___ .**

balance de agua *m.* water balance, the equilibrium between intake and excretion of liquids.

balanceado-a *a.* balanced; in a state of equilibrium.

balanitis *f.* balanitis, an infl. of the glans penis, gen. accompanied by infl. of the prepuce.

balanopostitis *f.* balanoposthitis, infl. of the glans penis and prepuce.

balanza *f.* balance, scale, device to measure weights.

baldado-a *a.* maimed, crippled.

balón *m.* balloon; **___ insuflable / ___** tamponade.

banco *m.* bank; bench.

bañar *vt.* to bathe. **bañarse** *vr.* to take a bath.

baño *m.* bath, bathroom; **___ aceitado /** oil **___ ; ___ antipirético** / antipyretic **___ ,** to reduce fever; **___ aromático /** aromatic **___ ; ___ cinetoterapéutico /** kinetotherapeutic **___ ; ___ completo /** full **___ ; ___ con esponja** / sponge **___ ; ___ con inmersión** / immersion **___ ; ___ de agua caliente** / hot **___ ; ___ de agua fría** / cold **___ ; ___ de agua tibia** / warm **___ ; ___ de asiento caliente** / Sitz **___ ,** from the waist down; **___ de remolino /** whirlpool **___ ; cuarto de ___ /** bathroom; **papel de ___** / toilet tissue.

barba *f.* beard.

barbilla *f.* chin, the tip of the chin.

barbituratos

barbituratos *m.* barbiturates, derivatives of barbituric acid.
barbitúrico *m.* barbiturate, hypnotic and sedative agent.
bario *m.* barium, ingested suspension of barium sulfate to be used as a contrast medium in a radiography of the hypopharynx and the esophagus.
barorreceptor *m.* baroreceptor, a sensory nerve ending that reacts to changes in pressure.
barrera *f.* barrier, obstacle.
barriga *f.* belly; **dolor de __** / __ ache.
barrigón-a *a. pop.* pot-bellied.
barro *m.* blackhead, pimple; mud.
bartolinitis *f.* bartholinitis, infl. of Bartholin's vulvovaginal gland.
Bartolino, glándula de *f.* Bartholin's vulvovaginal gland.
basal *a.* basal, pertaining or close to a base; **enfermedad de los ganglios __ -es** / __ ganglia disease; **metabolismo __** / __ metabolic rate.
base *f.* base, foundation.
basial, basilar *a.* basal, basilar, rel. to a base.
básico-a *a.* basic.
bastante *a.* sufficient, enough.
bastardo-a *m., f.* bastard; *a.* bastard, illegitimate.
bastón *m.* cane.
bastoncillo *m.* rod; __ **-s y conos** / __ -s and cones, sensitive receptors of the retina.
batalla *f.* battle, struggle.
batallar *vt.* to struggle.
bazo *m.* spleen, vascular lymphatic organ situated in the abdominal cavity; __ **accesorio** / accessory __ .
bebé *m.* baby, infant.
beber *vt., vi.* to drink.
bebida *f.* beverage; **dado a la __** / heavy drinker.
beligerante *a.* belligerent.
Bell, parálisis de *f.* Bell's palsy, paralysis of one side of the face caused by an affliction of the facial nerve.
belladona *f.* belladonna, medicinal herb whose leaves and roots contain atropine and related alkaloids.
bello-a *a.* beautiful.
Benedict, prueba de *f.* Benedict's test, chemical analysis to determine the presence of sugar in the urine.
beneficiado-a *a.* beneficiary.
beneficio *m.* benefit; **asignación de __** / allocation of __; __ **-s de asistencia social** / welfare __ -s.

benigno-a *a.* benign.
béquico *m.* cough medicine.
beriberi *m.* beriberi, endemic neuritis caused by a deficiency of thiamine in the diet.
besar *vt.* to kiss.
beso *m.* kiss.
bestialidad *f.* bestiality, sexual relations with an animal.
bezoar *m.* bezoar, concretion found in the stomach or the intestines constituted by elements such as hair or vegetable fibers.
biberón *m.* baby bottle; **suplemento con __** / bottle propping.
bicarbonato *m.* bicarbonate, a salt of carbonic acid.
bicarbonato de sodio *m.* baking soda.
bíceps *m.* biceps muscle.
bicicleta *f.* bicycle; __ **estacionaria** / stationary __ .
bicipital *a.* bicipital. 1. rel. to the biceps muscle; 2. having two heads.
bien *adv.* well; **todo va o está __** / all is well; **me siento __** / I feel fine.
bienestar *m.* well-being, welfare, solace.
bienvenida *f.* welcome.
bifocal *a.* bifocal, having two foci.
bifurcación *f.* bifurcation, division into two branches or parts.
bigeminal *a.* bigeminal, occurring in pairs.
bigote *m.* moustache.
bilabial *a.* bilabial, having two lips.
bilateral *a.* bilateral, having or rel. to two sides.
bilharziasis *f.* bilharziasis, schistosomiasis.
biliar *a.* biliary, rel. to the bile, to the bile ducts, or to the gallbladder; **ácidos y sales __ -es** / __ acids and salts; **conductos __ -es** / bile ducts; **cálculo __** / gallstone; **enfermedades de los conductos __ -es** / __ tract diseases; **obstrucción del conducto __** / __ duct obstruction; **pigmentos __ -es** / __ pigments.
bilingüe *a.* bilingual.
biliosidad *f.* biliousness, disorder manifested by constipation, headache, and indigestion due to excess secretion of bile.
bilioso-a *a.* bilious, excess bile.
bilirrubina *f.* bilirubin, a red pigment of the bile.

bilirrubinemia *f.* bilirubinemia, presence of bilirubin in the blood.

bilirrubinuria *f.* bilirubinuria, presence of bilirubin in the urine.

bilis *f.* bile, gall, bitter secretion stored in the gallbladder.

binario-a *a.* binary, consisting of two of the same.

bioensayo *m.* bioassay, sampling the effect of a drug on an animal to determine its potency.

biología *f.* biology, the study of live organisms; __ **celular** / cellular __; __ **molecular** / molecular __ .

biológico-a *a.* biologic, biological, rel. to biology; **análisis** __ / __ assay; **control** __ / __ control; **evolución** __ / __ evolution; **guerra** __ / __ warfare; **indicador** __ / __ indicator; **inmunoterapia** __ / __ immunotherapy; **semivida** __ / __ half-life; **siquiatría** __ / __ psychiatry.

biólogo-a *m., f.* biologist.

biopsia *f.* biopsy, procedure to remove sample tissue for diagnostic examination; __ **abierta por excisión** / open __ by excision; __ **con cepillo** / brush __; __ **de aguja fina** / fine needle __; __ **de espécimen cuneiforme** / specimen wedge __; __ **de la arteria temporal** / temporal artery __; __ **de la mama** / __ of the breast; __ **de la médula ósea** / bone marrow __; __ **del cuello uterino** / __ of the cervix; __ **del ganglio vigilante** / sentinel node __; __ **del nódulo linfático** / __ of lymph nodes; __ **endoscópica** / endoscopic __; __ **muscular** / muscle __; __ **por ablación** / __ by ablation; __ **por aspiración** / aspiration __ ; needle __; __ **por excisión** / excision __; __ **por incisión** / incision __ .

bioquímica *f.* biochemistry, the chemistry of living organisms.

biosíntesis *f.* biosynthesis, formation of chemical substances in the physiological processes of living organisms.

bípedo *m.* biped, two-legged animal.

bisabuelo-a *m., f.* great-grandfather; great-grandmother.

bisexual *a.* bisexual. 1. having gonads of both sexes, (**intersexual**) hermaphrodite; 2. having sexual relations with both sexes.

bisinosis *f.* bissinosis, obstructive airway disease suffered by workers of unprocessed cotton, flax, or hemp, caused by reaction to the dust that may include endotoxin from bacterial contamination. Known as "Monday morning asthma" or "cotton-dust asthma."

bisturí *m.* scalpel, surgical knife.

Bitot, manchas de *f., pl.* Bitot spots, small triangular gray spots that appear in the conjunctiva and are associated with a deficiency of vitamin B.

bizco-a *a.* cross-eyed.

biznieto-a *m., f.* great-grandson; great-grand daughter.

bizquera *f.* squint, the condition of being cross-eyed, strabismus.

Blalock-Tausig, operación de *f.* Blalock-Tausig operation, surgery to repair a congenital malformation of the heart.

blanco *m.* target. 1. an object or area at which something is directed; 2. a cell or organ that is affected by a particular agent such as a drug or a hormone; 3. the color white. *-a / a.* white.

blancuzco-a *a.* whitish.

blando-a *a.* soft, bland.

blastomicosis *f.* blastomycosis, infectious fungal disease.

blefaritis *f.* blepharitis, infl. of the eyelid.

blefarocalasis *f.* blepharochalasis, relaxation of the skin of the upper eyelid due to loss of interstitial elasticity.

blefaroplastia *f.* blepharoplasty, plastic surgery of the eyelids.

blefaroplejía *f.* blepharoplegia, paralysis of the eyelid.

blenorragia *f.* blennorrhagia. 1. discharge of mucus; 2. gonorrhea.

bloqueado-a *a.* blocked, obstructed.

bloqueador *m.* blocker, __ **de canal cálcico, antagonista cálcico** / calcium channel __ .

bloqueo *m.* block, stoppage, obstruction; __ **atrioventricular** / heart __ , atrioventricular, interruption in the A-V node; __ **de rama** / heart __ , bundle-branch; __ **ganglionar** / ganglionic __; __ **interventricular** / heart, __ interventricular; __ **senoatrial** / heart __ , sinoatrial.

bobo-a *m., f.* fool, simpleton; *a.* silly, foolish.

boca *f.* mouth; __ **abajo** / face-down; __ **arriba** / face-up; **por la** __ / by mouth, orally.

boca de trinchera *f.* trench mouth, infection with ulceration of the mucous membranes of the mouth and the pharynx.

bocado *m.* mouthful, bite.

bochorno *m.* embarrassment.

bocio *m.* goiter, enlargement of the thyroid gland; __ **coloide endémico** / endemic, colloid __; __ **congénito** / congenital __; __ **exoftálmico** / exophthalmic __; __ **móvil** / wandering __; __ **tóxico** / toxic __ .

bofetada *f.* slap.

bola *f.* ball; __ **adiposa** / fat pad; __ **de pelo** / hair __ , a type of bezoar.

bolo *m.* bolus. 1. a specific amount of a given substance administered intravenously; 2. dose in a rounded mass given to obtain an immediate response; 3. mass of soft consistency ready to be ingested; __ **alimenticio** / alimentary __; **infusión en __** / __ infusion.

bolsa *f.* sac; bag; handbag, pouch, pocket; __ **amniótica** (*de aguas*) / amniotic __; __ **de agua caliente** / hot water bottle; __ **de hielo** / icepack; __ **eléctrica** / heating pad.

bomba *f.* pump; __ **de angioplastia** / angioplasty __; __ **desmontable** / detachable __; __ **gástrica** / stomach __; __ **intravenosa** / intravenous __; __ **oxigenadora** / oxygenator __ .

bomba-balón *f.* balloon-pump. 1. an expandable device used to support several body structures; 2. an inflatable device used for widening or stretching a blood vessel.

bombear *v.* to pump; __ **hacia afuera** / to __ out.

bombeo *m.* pumping; __ **del corazón** / heart __; __ **estomacal** / stomach __ .

bombilla *f.* light bulb.

bondadoso-a *a.* kind.

bonito-a *a.* pretty.

boquiabierto-a *a.* open-mouthed.

borato de sodio *m.* borax.

borde *m.* border, rim, edge; __ **bermellón** / vermillion __; the exposed pink margin of a lip.

bordeando *a.* bordering.

borracho-a *a.* drunk.

borradura, borramiento *f. m.* effacement, obliteration of an organ, such as the cervix during labor.

borrar *v.* to erase, scrape; wipe out.

bostezar *vi.* to yawn.

bostezo *m.* yawn; yawning.

botella *f.* bottle.

boticario-a *m., f.* druggist, pharmacist.

botiquín *m.* medicine cabinet; __ **de primeros auxilios** / first aid kit.

botón *m.* button; __ **para llamar** / call __ .

botulismo *m.* botulism, food poisoning caused by a toxin that grows in improperly canned or preserved foods.

BRCA 1 y BRCA 2 acronym of the gene of the mammary cancer and ovarian cancer, specific inherited genes that when having mutations can become a high cancerous risk. It is advisable to women with family history of mammary or ovarian cancer to undergo the BRCA analysis tests to detect the mutations that can cause mammary cancer before fifty years of age and later with higher risk at age seventy. The alterations or mutations also present a high risk in developing ovarian cancer in women before the age of seventy.

bracero *m.* farmhand; laborer.

bradicardia *f.* bradycardia, abnormally slow heart beat.

bradipnea *f.* bradypnea, abnormally slow respiration.

braguero *m.* truss, binding device used to keep a reduced hernia in place; brace; __ **de cuello** / neck __ .

Braille, sistema de lectura *m.* Braille reading system, a method of writing and printing of raised dots that distinguishes letters, numbers, and punctuation and enables the blind to read by touching.

braquial *a.* brachial, rel. to the arm; **músculo __** / __ muscle.

braquiocefálico-a *a.* brachiocephalic, rel. to the arm and the head.

brazalete de identificación *m.* identification bracelet.

brazo *m.* arm.

bregma *m.* bregma, the point in the skull at the junction of the sagittal and coronal sutures.

breve *a.* brief; short; **en __** / in short, briefly.

Bright, enfermedad de *f.* Bright's disease. glomerulonephritis.

brillante *a.* bright.

bromidrosis *f.* bromhidrosis, fetid perspiration.

bromo, bromuro *m.* bromide, nonmetallic element, member of the halogen group, very irritating to mucous membranes. It is used as an oxidant and antiseptic.

broncoalveolar *a.* bronchoalveolar, *Syn.* **bronchovesicular**.

broncoconstricción *f.* bronchoconstriction, diminution in the caliber of a bronchus.

broncodilatación *f.* bronchodilation, dilation of a bronchus.

broncodilatador *m.* bronchodilator, agent that dilates the caliber of a bronchus; **-a;** *a.* **agentes** ___ **-es /** ___ agents.

broncoesofagoscopía *f.* bronchoesophagoscopy, examination of the bronchi and esophagus with an instrument.

broncoespasmo *m.* bronchospasm, spasmodic contraction of the bronchi and bronchioles.

broncoespirometría *f.* bronchospirometry, process of measuring the ventilatory function of each lung by using a bronchospirometer.

broncofibroscopía *f.* bronchofibroscopy, test done with a flexible fiberoptic bronchoscope for diagnostic purposes, or to remove foreign bodies from the bronchi.

broncógeno-a *a.* bronchogenic, rel. to or originating in the bronchus. **carcinoma** ___ **/** ___ carcinoma; **quiste** ___ **/** ___ cyst.

broncografía *f.* bronchography, x-ray of the tracheobronchial tree using an opaque medium in the bronchi.

broncolito *m.* broncholith, a bronchial calculus.

bronconeumonía *f.* bronchopneumonia, acute infl. of the bronchi and the alveoli of the lungs.

broncopulmonar *a.* bronchopulmonary, rel. to the bronchi and the lungs; **ganglios linfáticos** ___ **-es /** ___ lymph nodes; **lavado** ___ **/** ___ lavage.

broncoscopía *f.* bronchoscopy, inspection of the bronchi with a bronchoscope.

broncoscopío *m.* bronchoscope, instrument to examine the interior of the bronchi; ___ **de fibra óptica /** fiberoptic ___; ___ **con láser /** laser ___ .

broncostomía *f.* bronchostomy, surgical formation of a new opening into a bronchus.

broncotomograma *m.* bronchotomogram, image taken using computerized tomography of the upper respiratory track from the trachea to the lower inferior bronchi.

broncovesicular *a.* bronchovesicular, rel. to the bronchi and alveoli, esp. in regard to the sounds heard in auscultation. *Syn:* **bronchoalveolar**.

bronquial *a.* bronchial, rel. to the bronchi; **adenoma** ___ **/** ___ adenoma; **árbol** ___ **/** ___ tree; **arco** ___ **/** ___ arch; **asma** ___ **/** ___ asthma; **bloqueo** ___ **/** ___ blockage; **espasmo** ___ **/** ___ spasm; **estenosis** ___ **/** ___ stenosis; **fisura** ___ **/** ___ cleft; **glándulas bronquiales /** ___ glands; **lavado** ___ **/** ___ lavage; **lesion del plexo** ___ **/** ___ plexus injury; **venas bronquiales /** ___ veins.

bronquiectasia *f.* bronchiectasis, chronic dilation of the bronchi due to an inflammatory disease or obstruction.

bronquio *m. bronqus* bronchus, part of the trachea, passageway of the respiratory tract. Both of the bronchi (right and left) resemble the branches of a tree as they subdivide in smaller passageways and are called bronchioli or conducting tubes. ___ **intermedio /** intermediate ___; ___ **lobar /** lobar ___; ___ **lobar izquierdo /** left lobar ___; ___ **principal /** main ___; ___ **principal derecho /** right main ___; ___ **principal izquierdo /** left main ___; ___ **superior a una arteria /** eparterial ___; **impacto mucoso** ___ **/** mucoid impaction of the ___ .

bronquiocele *m.* bronchiocele, a localized dilation of a bronchus.

bronquiolitis *f.* bronchiolitis, infl. of the bronchioles.

bronquiolo *m.* bronchiole, one of the small branches of the bronquial tree.

bronquitis *f.* bronchitis, infl. of the bronchial tubes.

brotar *v.* to flare up.

brote *m.* flare-up, outburst, outbreak, reddening of the skin due to a lesion, infection, or allergic reaction.

brucelosis *f.* brucellosis, Mediterranean fever, undulant fever, disease caused by bacteria obtained through contact with infected animals or their by-products.

Bruck, enfermedad de *f.* Bruck disease, sickness manifested in imperfect osteogenesis, joint ankylosis, and muscular atrophy.

brusco-a *a.* abrupt, rude.

bruto-a *a.* stupid; rough.

bucal *a.* buccal, rel. to the mouth; **antiséptico __** / mouthwash; **higiene __** / oral hygiene; **por vía __** / by mouth.

buche *m.* mouthful; **un __ de agua** / a __ of water.

bucolabial *a.* buccolabial, rel. to the lips and the cheeks.

bueno-a *a.* good, kind; **buenas noches** / [*saludo*] good evening, [*despedida*] good night; **buenas tardes** / good afternoon; **buenos días** / good morning; **de buena fé** / in good faith.

bulbo *m.* bulb, circular or oval expansion of a tube or cylinder; **__ piloso** / hair __ .

bulbo raquídeo *m.* medulla oblongata, the most vital part of the brain, the lower portion of the brain stem.

bulbouretral *a.* bulbourethral, rel. to the bulb of the urethra and the penis.

bulimia *f.* bulimia, hyperorexia, exaggerated appetite.

bulto *m.* lump; swelling; bundle, package.

bunio *m.* bunion, swelling of the bursa on the first joint of the big toe.

burbuja *f.* bubble.

burdo-a *a.* coarse; rough.

buril *m.* burr, type of drill used to make openings in bones or teeth.

bursa *f.*, *L.* bursa, saclike cavity containing synovial fluid, situated in tissue areas where friction would otherwise occur; **__ del tendón calcáneo** / Achille's __; **__ poplitea** / popliteal __ .

bursitis *f.* bursitis, infl. of a bursa.

buscar *vi.* to look for, to search.

búsqueda *f.* search; pursuit.

búster *m.* booster shot, reactivation of an original immunizing agent.

busto *m.* bust.

buzo *m.* diver.

buzón *m.* mailbox.

C

C *abr.* **caloría** / calorie; **centígrado** / centigrade; **carbono** / carbon; **Celsius** / Celsius.

c cobalt / cobalto; **cocaína** / cocaine; **contracción** / contraction.

cabalgamiento *m.* [*fracturas*] overriding, the slipping of one part of the bone over the other.

caballero *m.* gentleman.

caballo *m.* horse.

caballo de fuerza *m.* horsepower, a unit of power.

cabecear *vt., vi.* to nod; to drop one's head as when snoozing; *pop.* to nod off.

cabecera *f.* head of a bed or table.

cabellera *f.* head of hair.

cabello *m.* hair.

caber *vi.* to fit into something; to have enough room.

cabestrillo *m.* sling, bandage-like support. ___ **de restricción** / restraining ___; ___ **de rodilla** / knee ___; ___ **de suspensión** / suspension ___ .

cabeza *f.* head; **caída de la** ___ / ___ drop; **traumatismo del cráneo, golpe en la** ___ / ___ injury; **apoyo de** ___ / ___ rest; **asentir con la** ___ / to nod one's head.

cabezón-a *a.* big-headed; stubborn.

caca *f.* excrement; childish term for excrement.

cachete *m.* cheek.

cadáver *m.* cadaver, corpse.

cadena *f.* chain; **reacción en** ___ / ___ reaction; **sutura en** ___ / ___ suture.

cadera *f.* hip; **articulación de la** ___ / ___ joint; ___ **de resorte** / snapping; **dislocación congenita de la** ___ / congenital ___ dislocation; **restitución total de la** ___ / total ___ replacement.

cadmio *m.* cadmium, a bivalent metal similar to tin.

caducidad *f.* 1. expiration date; 2. old age.

caer *vi.* to fall; *caerse vr.* to fall down; ___ **muerto** / to drop dead.

café *m.* coffee.

cafeína *f.* caffeine, alkaloid present chiefly in coffee and tea used as a stimulant and diuretic.

cafetería *f.* cafeteria.

caída *f.* fall.

caído-a *a., pp.* of caer, fallen.

caja torácica *f.* thoracic cage.

cajero-a *m., f.* cashier.

calambre *m.* cramp, painful contraction of a muscle; ___ **muscular localizado** / Charley horse.

calamina *f.* calamine, astringent and antiseptic used for skin disorders.

calavera *f.* skull.

calcáneo *m.* calcaneus, heel bone.

calcáreo-a *a.* calcareous, rel. to lime or calcium.

calcemia *f.* calcemia, presence of calcium in the blood.

calcetines *m.* socks.

calciferol *m.* calciferol, derivative of ergosterol, vitamin D_2.

calcificación *f.* calcification, hardening of organic tissue by deposits of calcium salts.

calcificado-a *a.* calcified.

calcinosis *f.* calcinosis, presence of calcium salts in the skin, subcutaneous tissues, or other organs.

calcio *m.* calcium; **antagonista del** ___ / ___ antagonist.

calcitonina *f.* calcitonin, a hormone secreted by the thyroid gland.

calciuria *f.* calciuria, presence of calcium in the urine.

cálculo *m.* calculus, [*pl.* calculi], stone; ___ **biliar** / biliary ___ , gallstone; ___ **de cistina** / cystine ___; ___ **de fibrina** / fibrin ___; ___ **de oxalato de calcio** / calcium oxalate ___; ___ **urinario** / urinary ___ .

calefacción *f.* heating system; heat.

calendario *m.* calendar.

calentamiento *m.* [*acondicionamiento físico*] warm-up.

calentar *vt.* to heat; **calentarse** / *vr.* to warm oneself up.

calentura *f.* fever, temperature.

calenturiento-a *a.* feverish.

calibre *m.* caliber, the diameter of a tube or canal.

caliceal *a.* caliceal, rel. to the calix.

calicreína *f.* kallicrein, an inactive enzyme present in blood, plasma, and urine, that when activated acts as a powerful vasodilator.

calidad *f.* quality, property.

caliente *a.* hot, warm.

caliuresis *f.* kaliuresis, kaluresis, increased urinary excretion of potassium.

callo *m.* callus, composite mass of tissue.

calma

calma *f.* calm; calmness; **tener ___** / to be calm.

calmado-a *a.* calm, serene, tranquil, peaceful.

calmante *m.* sedative, tranquilizer; *a.* soothing, mitigating.

calmar *v.* to calm down, to soothe; **calmarse** *vr.* to become calm.

calmodulina *f.* calmodulin, calcium-binding protein that intervenes in cellular processes.

calor *m.* heat; warmth; **___ de conducción** / conductive ___; **___ de convección** / convective ___; **___ seco** / dry ___; **hace ___** / it is hot; **pérdida de ___** / ___ loss; **tener ___** / to be hot.

caloría *f.* calorie, a heat unit, commonly referred to as the energy value of a particular food.

calórico-a *a.* caloric, rel. to the energy value of food; **ingestión ___** / ___ intake.

calostro *m.* colostrum, fluid secreted by the mammary glands before the secretion of milk.

calva *f.* bald crown of the head.

calvaria *f.* calvaria, superior portion of the cranium.

calvicie *f.* calvities, baldness.

calvo-a *a.* bald, without hair.

callado-a *a.* quiet, low-key.

callar *v.* to hush, to silence; **callarse** *vr.* to become quiet.

calle *f.* street.

callo, callosidad *m., f.* callus, corn.

calloso-a *a.* callous, rel. to a callus.

calzoncillos *m., pl.* men's underpants; shorts.

cama *f.* bed; **al lado de la ___** / at bedside; **estar en ___** / to be bedridden; **guardar ___** / to stay in bed, bedrest; **ocupación de ___-s** / ___ occupancy; **orinarse en la ___** / bedwetting; **recluido en ___** / bed-confined; **ropa de ___** / bedclothes.

cámara *f.* 1. chamber, cavity; **___ acuosa** / aqueous ___; **___ anterior** / anterior ___; **___ hiperbárica** / hyperbaric ___; **___ -s oculares** / ___ -s of the eye; 2. photographic camera.

cambiar *vt.* to change; **cambiarse** *vr.* to change clothes.

cambio *m.* change; [*posición*] shift.

camilla *f.* stretcher.

caminar *v.* to walk; to hike.

caminata *f.* a walk; a hike.

camisa *f.* shirt; **___ de fuerza** / straightjacket.

camiseta *f.* men's undershirt; T-shirt.

camisón *m.* nightgown.

campanilla *f.* úvula, epiglottis.

campo *m.* field. 1. area or open space; 2. specialization; **___ de bajo aumento** / low-power ___; **___ marginal** / fringe ___; **___ neuromagnético** / neuromagnetic ___; **___ visual** / visual ___ .

cana *f.* gray hair.

canal *m.* canal, channel, trough, groove, tubular structure; **___ del parto** / birth ___; **___ femoral** / femoral ___; **___ inguinal** / inguinal ___; **___ radicular** / root ___ .

canalículo *m.* canaliculus, small channel; **___ biliar** / biliary ___, between liver cells; **___ lacrimal, lagrimal** / lacrimal ___ .

cancelar *vt.* to cancel, to annul.

canceloso-a *a.* cancellous, spongy, resembling a lattice.

cáncer *m.* cancer, tumor; **___ colorectal** / colorectal ___; **___ incipiente** / early ___; **fases o etapas en relación a la extensión del ___** / ___ staging; **grado de malignidad del ___** / ___ grading; **supervivientes de ___** / ___ survivors.

cáncer embrional *m.* embryonal carcinoma, malignant tumor of the testis.

cancerofobia *f.* cancerophobia, morbid fear of cancer.

canceroso-a *a.* cancerous, rel. to or afflicted by cancer.

candidiasis *f.* candidiasis, skin infection caused by a yeastlike fungus.

canilla *f.* shinbone; tibia.

cannabis *L.* cannabis, marijuana, plant whose leaves have a narcotic or hallucinatory effect when smoked.

canoso-a *a.* gray-haired.

cansado-a *a.* tired, weary.

cansancio *m.* tiredness, fatigue.

cansar *vt.* to tire; **cansarse** *vr.* to get tired.

cantidad *f.* quantity.

canto *m.* canthus. 1. angles at the corner of the eyes formed by the joining of the external and internal eyelids on both sides of the eye; 2. edge, rim.

cánula *f.* cannula, tube through which fluid and gas are put into the body.

canulación *f.* cannulation, the act of introducing a cannula through a vessel or duct; **___ aórtica** / aortic ___ .

capa *f.* layer; **___ del cuello uterino** / cervical layer.

capacidad f. capacity. 1. ability to contain; ___ **de difusión de los pulmones** / diffusion ___ of the lungs; ___ **de memoria** / memory storage ___; ___ **de reserva** / reserve ___; ___ **de sustención** / carrying ___; ___ **inspiratoria** / inspiratory ___; ___ **oxigenadora de la sangre** / oxygen ___ of blood; ___ **vital** / vital ___; 2. qualification, competence.

capaz a. able, capable.

capilar m. capillary, small blood vessel; ___ **arterial** / arterial ___, tiny channels carrying arterial blood; ___ **linfático** / lymph ___, minute vessels of the lymphatic system; ___ **venoso** / venous ___, small channels carrying venous blood; a. resembling hair.

capitelum L. capitellum. 1. hair bulb; 2. part of the humerus.

capítulo m. chapter.

caprichoso-a a. capricious; stubborn.

cápsula f. capsule, membranous enclosure.

cápsula articular n. capsular ligament, fibrous structure lined with synovial membrane surrounding the articulations.

caquexia f. cachexia, a grave condition showing great loss of weight and general weakness.

cara f. face; ___ **de luna** / moon ___, round, puffy face usu. characteristic of an individual who has been under steroid treatment for a long period of time; **peladura de** ___ / ___ peeling; coloq. **estiramiento de** ___ / facelift.

carácter m. 1. character; 2. quality, nature; 3. actor, actress. **tener buen** ___ / to be good-natured; **tener mal** ___ / to be ill-tempered.

característico-a a. characteristic.

carbohidrato m. carbohydrate, organic substance composed of carbon, hydrogen, and oxygen such as starch, sugar, and cellulose.

carbón m. coal.

carbonatado-a a. carbonated.

carbono m. carbon; ___ **radioactivo** / ___ radioactive ___; **dióxido de** ___ / ___ dioxide; **monóxido de** ___ / ___ monoxide

carboxihemoglobina f. carboxyhemoglobin, a combination of carbon monoxide and hemoglobin that impairs the transportation of oxygen in the blood.

carbunco m. carbuncle, large boil of the skin that discharges pus.

carcinogénesis f. carcinogenesis, production of cancer.

carcinógeno m. carcinogen, cancer producing substance; a. **carcinógeno-a** carcinogenic.

carcinoma m. carcinoma, cancer derived from living cells of organs. See table on page 287.

carcinoma anaplástico maligno m. anaplastic undifferentiated carcinoma, carcinoma manifested mainly in the lung.

carcinoma in situ m. carcinoma in situ, localized tumor cells that have not invaded adjacent structures.

carcinoma microcelular no diferenciado m. oat cell carcinoma, fast growing malignant tumor formed by small epithelial cells clustered very close together.

carcinoma maligno de transición m. transitional cell carcinoma, gen found in the bladder, ureter, or renal pelvis.

carcinomatosis f. carcinomatosis, cancer that has spread throughout the body.

carcinosarcoma m. carcinosarcoma, malignant neoplasm with mixed characteristics of carcinoma and sarcoma.

cardíaco-a a. cardiac, rel. to the heart; **ápex** ___ / ___ apex; **arritmia** ___ / ___ arrhythmia; **asma** ___ / ___ asthma; **ataque** ___ / heart attack; **aurícula** ___ / heart atrium; **auscultación** ___ / ___ examination; **cateterización** ___ / ___ catheterization; **edema** ___ / ___ edema; **esfínter** ___ / ___ sphincter; **estimulación** ___ **artificial** / ___ pacing, artificial; **frecuencia** ___ / heart rate; **gasto o rendimiento** ___ / heart output; **generador del impulso** ___ / ___ impulse generator; **insuficiencia** ___, **ventricular derecha** / heart failure, right-sided; **insuficiencia** ___, **ventricular izquierda** / heart failure, left-sided; **insuficiencia o fallo** ___ **congestivo** / heart failure, congestive; **masaje** ___ / ___ massage; **paro** ___ / heart arrest, standstill; **reanimación** ___ / ___ resuscitation; **reflejo** ___ / heart reflex; **ruptura** ___ / ___ rupture; **taponamiento** ___ / ___ tamponade; **tonos o ruidos** ___ / ___ sounds.

cardioangiograma *m.* cardioangiogram, image by x-rays of the blood vessels and the chambers of the heart taken after injecting a dye.

cardiectomía *f.* cardiectomy; 1. removal of the heart; 2. removal of the upper part of the stomach.

cardioespasmo *m.* cardiospasm, contraction or spasm of the cardia.

cardiogénico *a.* cardiogenic, of cardiac origin; **choque __ / __** shock.

cardiografía *f.* cardiography, recording of the movements of the heart by a cardiograph.

cardiograma *m.* cardiogram, electrical tracing of the impulses of the heart.

cardiología *f.* cardiology, the study of the heart.

cardiólogo-a *m., f.* cardiologist, specialist in cardiology.

cardiomegalia *f.* cardiomegaly, enlarged heart.

cardiomiopatía *f.* cardiomyopathy, a disorder of the heart muscle; __ **alcohólica** / alcoholic __; __ **congestiva** / congestive __; __ **dilatada** / dilated __; __ **hipertrófica** / hypertrophic __; __ **hipertrófica familiar** / familial hypertrophic __; __ **idiopática** / idiopathic __; __ **postpartum** / postpartum __; __ **primaria** / primary __; __ **restrictiva** / restrictive __; __ **secundaria** / secondary __ .

cardiopatía *f.* cardiopathy, heart disease; __ **por hipertensión** / hypertensive __ .

cardiopulmonar *a.* cardiopulmonary, rel. to the heart and the lungs; **máquina __** / heart-lung machine; **puente __** / __ bypass; **resucitación, reanimación __** / __ resuscitation.

cardiovascular *a.* cardiovascular, rel. to the heart and blood vessels; **insuficiencia __** / __ insufficiency.

cardioversión *f.* cardioversion, the act of restoring the heart to a normal sinus rhythm by electrical countershock.

carditis *f.* carditis, infl. of the heart.

carecer *vi.* to lack.

caries *f.* caries. 1. progressive destruction of bone tissue; __ **distal** / distal __; __ **de fissura** / fissure __; 2. dental cavity.

cariñoso-a *a.* affectionate.

cariólisis *f.* karyolysis, breakdown of the nucleus of a cell.

caritativo-a *a.* charitable.

carmesí, carmín *m.* carmine.

carne *f.* 1. meat; __ **asada** / roast beef; __ **de carnero** / lamb; __ **de puerco** / pork; __ **de ternera** / veal; 2. flesh, muscular tissue of the body.

carnívoro-a *a.* carnivorous, that eats meat.

carnosidad *f.* carnosity, fleshy excrescence.

caro-a *a.* expensive, costly.

carótida *f.* carotid, main artery of the neck; **arterias __ -s** / __ arteries; **seno de la __** / __ sinus; **síncope del seno de la __** / __ sinus syncope.

carotina *f.* carotene, yellow-red pigment found in some vegetables that converts into vitamin A.

carpo *m.* carpus, portion of the upper extremity between the hand and the forearm.

cartílago *m.* cartilage, elastic, semihard tissue that covers the bones.

carúncula *f.* caruncle, small, irritated piece of flesh; __ **uretral** / urethral __.

casa *f.* house, home; __ **de socorro** / first aid station.

casado-a *a.* married.

cáscara *f.* peel, shell.

cáscara sagrada *f.* cascara sagrada, the bark of Rhamus purshiana shrub, commonly used to treat chronic constipation.

caseína *f.* casein, the main protein found in milk.

casi *adv.* almost.

caso *m.* case, a specific instance of disease; __ **ambulatorio** / ambulatory __; **presentación de un __** / __ reporting; **en __ de** / in __ of; **hacer __** / to pay attention; **no viene al __** / it is irrelevant.

caspa *f.* dandruff; dander.

castigar *vt.* to punish.

casual *a.* casual, accidental.

casualidad *f.* chance; **de __** / by __; **por __** / by __.

catabolismo *m.* catabolism, cellular process by which complex substances are converted into simpler compounds; destructive metabolism.

catalepsia *f.* catalepsy, a condition characterized by loss of voluntary muscular movement and irresponsiveness to any outside stimuli, gen. associated with psychological disorders.

catalítico-a *a.* catalytic.

célula T8 supresora

catalizador *m.* catalyst, an agent that stimulates a chemical reaction.

cataplexia *f.* cataplexy, sudden loss of muscular tone caused by an exaggerated emotional state.

catarata *f.* cataract, opacity of the lens of the eye; ___ **anular** / annular ___; ___ **blanda** / soft ___; ___ **cerúlea** / blue ___; ___ **completa** / complete ___; ___ **congénita** / congenital ___; ___ **congénita diabética** / congenital diabetic ___; ___ **eléctrica** / electric ___, caused by high power electric current; ___ **madura** / mature ___; ___ **negra** / black ___; ___ **senil** / senile ___; ___ **verde** / green ___.

catarral *a.* rel. to catarrh.

catarro *m.* catarrh, cold, sniffle; ___ **de pecho, bronquial** / chest cold.

catarsis *f.* catharsis, purification. 1. purging the body of chemical or other material; 2. therapeutic liberation of anxiety and tension.

catártico *m.* cathartic, laxative; **-a** / *a.* cathartic, rel. to catharsis.

catatonía *f.* catatony, a phase of extreme negativism in schizophrenia in which the patient does not speak, remains in a fixed position, and resists any attempts to activate his or her movement or speech. The same symptoms are present in other mental conditions.

catecolaminas *f., pl.* catecholamines, amines such as norepinephrine, epinephrine, and dopamine that are produced in the adrenal glands and have a sympathomimetic action.

categoría *f.* category; quality.

catéter *m.* catheter, a rubber or plastic tube used to drain fluid from a body cavity such as urine from the bladder, or to inject fluid, as in cardiac catheterization.

catéter permanente *m.* in-dwelling catheter.

cateterización *f.* catheterization, insertion of a catheter.

cateterizar *vi.* to catheterize, to insert a catheter.

catgut *f.* catgut, type of surgical suture made from the gut of some animals.

causa *f.* cause, reason; ___ **actual** / existing ___; ___ **constitucional** / constitutional ___; ___ **de factor predisponente** / predisposing ___; ___ **específica** / specific ___; ___ **inmediata** / proximate ___; ___ **necesaria** / necessary ___; **sin** ___ / unreasonable.

causalgia *f.* causalgia, burning pain in the skin.

causar *vt.* to cause.

cáustico *m.* caustic, substance used to destroy tissue.

cauterización *f.* cauterization, burning by application of a caustic, heat, or electric current.

cauterizar *vt.* to cauterize, to burn by application of heat or electric current.

cava *f.* cava, hollow organ, cavity. vena cava.

caverna *f.* cavern, cave, pathological cavity or depression.

cavernoso-a *a.* cavernous, having hollow spaces.

cavidad *f.* cavity, hole; ___ **abdominal** / abdominal ___; ___ **-es cardíacas: auricular y ventricular** / heart chambers; ___ **-es craneales** / cranial cavities; ___ **pelviana** / pelvic ___; ___ **torácica** / thoracic ___.

cecostomía *f.* cecostomy, surgical opening into the cecum.

cefalea, cefalalgia *f.* cephalea, cephalalgia, headache.

cefálico-a *a.* cephalic, rel. to the head.

cefalorraquídeo-a *a.* cerebrospinal.

cefalosporina *f.* cephalosporin, wide spectrum antibiotic.

ceguera, cequedad *f.* blindness; ___ **al color** / color ___; ___ **nocturna** / night ___; ___ **verde** / green ___; ___ **roja** / red ___.

ceja *f.* eyebrow.

celíaco-a *a.* celiac, rel. to the abdomen.

celiotomía *f.* celiotomy, laparotomy.

célula *f.* cell, structural unit of all living organisms. See illustration on page 68. See table on page 290.

célula de microglia *f.* microglia cell, small intestinal migrating cell of the nervous system.

célula T4 cooperadora *f.* T cell also called CD4.

célula T8 citotóxica *f.* cytotoxic T-cell, also called CD8, carries out functions by destroying antigens, and attacks and eliminates cells infected by viruses, parasites and fungi.

célula T reguladora *f.* T Cell regulator directing other cells of the immune system to do special functions having an effect of controlling aberrant immune responses.

célula T8 supresora *n.* T8 Cell suppressor, a group of cells with a

celular

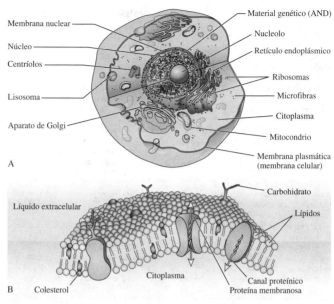

La célula: (A) La célula y los organillos; (B) Célula típica de un animal y membrana plasmática

function to inhibit the immune response.

celular *a.* cellular, rel. to the cell; **agua** __ / __ water; **compartimentos** __-es / __ compartments; **crecimiento** __ / __ growth; **tejido** __ / __ tissue.

celulitis *f.* cellulitis, infl. of connective tissue.

celulosa *a.* cellulose.

central, céntrico-a *a.* central; **sistema nervioso** __ / __ nervous system.

centrífugo-a *a.* centrifugal, going from the center outward.

centrípeto-a *a.* centripetal, going from the outside towards the center.

centro *m.* 1. center; 2. middle, core.

Centro de control de enfermedades *m.* Center for Disease Control.

ceño *m.* brow; **fruncir el** __ / to frown.

cepa *f.* strain, group of microorganisms within a species or variety characterized by some particular quality.

cepillo *m.* brush; __ **de dientes** / toothbrush.

cera *f.* wax. 1. beeswax; 2. waxy secretion of the body; __ **depilatoria** / depilatory __ .

cerca *f., adv.* near; **de aquí** / close by.

cercanía *f.* vicinity.

cercano-a *a.* close; neighboring, proximate.

cerebelo *m.* cerebellum, posterior brain mass; **enfermedades del** __ / cerebellar diseases.

cerebeloso-a *a.* cerebellous, rel. to the cerebrum.

cerebral *a.* cerebral, rel. to the brain; **apoplejía** __ / cerebrovascular accident; **concusión o conmoción** __ / __ concussion; **corteza** __ / __ cortex; **edema** __ / __ edema; **embolismo y trombosis** __ / __ embolism and thrombosis; **hemorragia o infarto** __ / __ hemorrhage or infarct; **muerte** __ / brain death; **trauma** __ / brain injury; **tronco** __ / brain stem; **tumor** __ / brain tumor.

cerebro *m.* brain, cerebrum, portion of the central nervous system contained within the cranium that is the chief

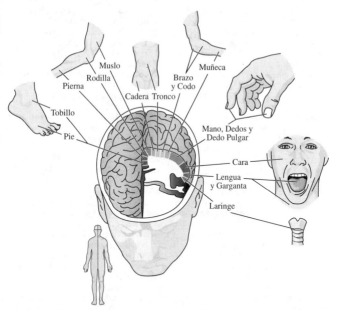

Labels on illustration: Muslo, Rodilla, Pierna, Muñeca, Brazo y Codo, Cadera, Tronco, Tobillo, Pie, Mano, Dedos y Dedo Pulgar, Cara, Lengua y Garganta, Laringe

Partes del cerebro: lóbulo frontal

regulator of body functions; __ **medio** / midbrain; **escán del __ (gammagrama)** / __ scan. See illustration on this page.

cerebroespinal, cefalorraquídeo-a *a.* cerebrospinal, rel. to the brain and the spinal cord; **eje** __ / __ axis; **líquido** __ / __ fluid; **meningitis** __ / __ meningitis; **presión** __ / __ pressure.

cerebrovascular *a.* cerebrovascular, rel. to the blood vessels of the brain.

cero *m.* zero.

ceroso-a *a.* waxy.

cerrado-a *a.* closed.

cerrar *vi.* to close; __ **con llave** / to lock.

certero-a *a.* accurate.

certeza *f.* certainty; accuracy.

certificado *m.* certificate; __ **de defunción** / death __ .

cerumen *m.* cerumen, wax that builds up in the ear; __ **impactado** / impacted __ .

cerveza *f.* beer.

cervical *a.* cervical. 1. rel. to the cervix; **dilatador** __ / __ dilator; 2. rel. to the area of the neck; **displasia** __ / __ dysplasia; **erosión** __ / __ erosion; **pólipo** __ / __ polyp.

cerviz *f.* nape of the neck.

cesar *v.* to cease, to stop.

cesárea *f.* cesarean section.

cese *m.* stoppage.

cesio *m.* cesium, metallic element belonging to the group of alkaline metals.

cetoacidosis *f.* ketoacidosis, acidosis caused by an increase in ketone bodies in the blood.

cetoaciduria *f.* ketoaciduria, acidosis caused by an increase in ketone bodies in the blood.

cetogénesis *f.* ketogenesis, production of acetone.

cetonemia *f.* ketonemia, concentration of ketone bodies in the plasma.

cetosa *f.* ketose.

cetosis *f.* ketosis, excessive production of acetone as a result of incomplete metabolism of fatty acids; acidosis.

ch *f.* fourth letter of the Spanish alphabet.

chalación *f.* chalazion, meibomian cyst, a cyst of the eyelid.

chancro *m.* chancre, the primary lesion of syphilis.

chancroide *m.* chancroid, a nonsyphilitic venereal ulcer.

chaparro-a *a. Mex.* short person.

chaqueta *f.* jacket.

charla *f.* chat.

charlatán-a *m., f.* charlatan, a quack, someone claiming knowledge and skills he or she does not have.

chasquido *m.* snap, sharp brief sound related to the abrupt opening of the cardiac valve, gen. the mitral valve; __ de apertura / opening __ .

chata *f.* bedpan.

cheque *m.* check.

chequear *vt.* to check, to verify.

chequeo *m.* checkup, complete medical examination.

Cheyne-Stokes, respiración de *f.* Cheyne-Stokes respiration, respiration manifested by alternating periods of apnea of increased frequency and depth, gen. associated with disorders of the neurologic respiration center.

chicano-a *a. pop.* (U.S.) Mexican-American.

chícharo *m.* green pea.

chichón *m.* bump on the head.

chico-a *m., f.* young boy; young girl; *a.* small.

chiflado-a *a. pop.* crazy, nuts.

chile *m.* hot pepper.

chinche *f.* bedbug.

chiquito-a *a.* small.

chochera *f.* senility.

chocho-a *a.* senile.

chocolate *m.* chocolate.

choque *m.* 1. shock; an abnormal state, gen. following trauma, in which insufficient flow of blood through the body can cause reduced cardiac output, subnormal temperature, descending blood pressure and rapid pulse; __ alérgico / allergic __; __ anafiláctico / anaphylactic __; __ eléctrico / electric __; __ séptico / septic __; 2. collision.

chorizo *m.* sausage.

chorrear *vt.* to drip; to spout.

chorro *n.* jet, spurt; stream.

chueco-a *a.* crooked, bent.

chupar *v.* to suck; to absorb; **chuparse el dedo** / thumb sucking.

churre *m.* dirt, grime.

cianocobalamina *f.* cyanocobalamin, vitamin B_{12}, complex of cyanide and cobalamin used in the treatment of pernicious anemia.

cianosis *f.* cyanosis, purplish blue discoloration of the skin, often as a result of cardiac, anatomic or functional abnormalities.

cianótico-a *a.* cyanotic, rel. to or afflicted by cyanosis.

cianuro *m.* cyanide; **envenenamiento por __ / __** poisoning.

ciática *f.* sciatica, neuralgia along the course of the sciatic nerve.

cibernética *f.* cybernetics, the study of biological systems such as the brain and the nervous system by electronic means.

cicatriz *f.* scar.

cicatrización *f.* cicatrization, scarring.

cicatrizante *m.* cicatrizant, agent that aids the healing process of a wound.

cicatrizar *vt.* to scar, the healing process of a wound.

ciclamato *m.* cyclamate, artificial sweetening agent.

ciclitis *f.* cyclitis, infl. of the ciliary body.

ciclo *m.* cycle, recurring period of time; __ **gravídico** / pregnancy __ .

ciclofosfamida *f.* cyclophosphamide, antineoplastic drug also used as an immunosuppressive agent in organ transplants.

ciclofotocoagulación *f.* cyclophotocoagulation, photocoagulation through the pupil with a laser, gen. used in glaucoma.

ciclosporina *f.* cyclosporine, immunosuppressive agent used in organ transplant.

ciclotomía *f.* cyclotomy, incision through the ciliary body of the eye.

ciego-a *m., f.* blind person; *a.* blind.

ciego *m.* cecum. 1. cul-de-sac lying below the terminal ileum forming the first part of the large intestine; 2. any cul-de-sac structure.

cielo *m.* sky.

cien, ciento *a., m.* a hundred.

ciencia *f.* science; __ **médica** / medical __; **a __ cierta** / for sure.

científico-a *m., f.* scientist; *a.* scientific.

cierto-a *a.* certain, true; **por __** / as a matter of fact.

cifosis *f.* kyphosis, exaggerated posterior curvature of the thoracic spine.

cifótico-a *a.* kyphotic, suffering from or rel. to kyphosis.

cigarrillo, cigarro *m.* cigarette, cigar.

cigoma, zigoma m. zygoma, osseous prominence at the point where the temporal and malar bones join.

cigomático-a a. zygomatic, rel. to the zygoma; **arco __ / __ arch; hueso __ / __ bone.**

cigoto m. zygote, the fertilized ovum, cell resulting from the union of two gametes.

ciliar a. ciliary, rel. to or resembling the eyelash or eyelid.

cilíndrico-a a. cylindrical.

cilindro m. cylinder. 1. geometrical form resembling a column; 2. cylindrical lens; 3. cylindrical renal cast; __ **epithelial** / epithelial __; __ **hemático** / blood cast __.

cilindro granuloso m. [renal] granular cast, urinary cylinder seen in degenerative or inflammatory nephropathies.

cilio m. cilium, eyelid.

cima f. summit, top.

cimetidina f. cimetidine, antacid used in the treatment of gastric and duodenal ulcers.

cimiento m. foundation, base.

cinc m. zinc.

cinconismo m. cinchonism. quininism.

cineangiografía f. cineangogiography, moving pictures of a radiopaque substance as it goes through the blood vessels.

cinerradiografía f. cineradiography, x-ray of an area in motion.

cinesioterapia f. kinesiotherapy, treatment involving physical exercises or specific movements.

cinesis f. kinesis, term used to designate physical movements in general, including those that result as a response to a stimulus such as light.

cinestesia f. kinesthesia, sensorial experience, sense and perception of a movement.

cinética f. kinesics, the study of the body and its static and dynamic positions as a means of communication.

cinético-a a. kinetic, rel. to movement or what causes it.

cinta magnética f. audiotape.

cinto m. belt; waistband.

cintura f. waist; waistline.

cinturón m. girdle; wide belt; __ **escapular o torácico** / thoracic __ .

circuito m. circuit.

circulación f. circulation; **mala __ / poor __; __ periférica** / peripheral __ .

círculo m. circle, a round figure or structure.

circuncidar v. to circumcise.

circuncisión f. circumcision, removing part or all of the prepuce.

circundar v. to encircle, to surround.

circunferencia f. circumference.

circunstancia f. circumstance; __ -s **atenuantes** / mitigating __ -s.

circunvolución f. gyrus, elevated portion of the cerebral cortex; __ -es **de Broca** / __ , Broca's, third, frontal or inferior; __ **frontal, superior** / __ , frontal, superior; __ -es **occipitales** / __ , occipital first, superior.

cirrosis f. cirrhosis, progressive disease of the liver characterized by interstitial infl. and associated with failure in the function of hepatocytes and resistance to the flow of blood through the liver; __ **alcohólica** / alcoholic __; __ **biliar** / biliary __.

cirugía f. surgery; the branch of medicine that treats diseases, malformations, and injuries and restores or reconstructs body structures through operative procedures. See table on page 470.

cirugía citoreductiva f. cytoreductive surgery, surgery that reduces a tumor that cannot be removed completely.

cirugía laparoscópica f. laparoscopic surgery, surgery through a laparoscope.

cirugía torácica asistida por video f. video-assisted thoracic surgery, thoracic surgery performed using endoscopic cameras, optical systems, and display screens.

cirujano-a m., f. surgeon, specialist in surgery.

cistadenocarcinoma m. cystadenocarcinoma, carcinoma and cystadenoma.

cistadenoma m. cystadenoma, adenoma that has one or more cysts.

cistectomía f. cystectomy, total or partial resection of the urinary bladder.

cisterna f. cistern, a closed space that serves as a reservoir or receptacle.

cístico-a a. cystic, rel. to the gallbladder or the bladder.

cistinuria f. cystinuria, excessive cystine in the urine.

cistitis f. cystitis, infl. of the urinary bladder characterized by frequent urination accompanied by pain and burning.

cistocele *m.* cystocele, hernia of the bladder.

cistofibroma *f.* cystofibroma, fibroma in which cysts or cyst-like formations have developed.

cistograma *m.* cystogram, x-ray of the bladder using air or a contrasting medium.

cistolitotomía *f.* cystolithotomy, removal of a stone by cutting into the bladder.

cistoscopía *f.* cystoscopy, inspection of the bladder through a cystoscope.

cistoscopio *m.* cystoscope, tube-shaped instrument used to examine the bladder and the urethra.

cistostomía *f.* cystostomy, creation of an opening into the bladder for drainage.

cisura *f.* cleft, elongated opening; fissure.

cita *f.* appointment; **hacer una __** / to make an __; **tener una __** / to have an __.

citolisis *f.* cytolysis, destruction of living cells.

citolítico-a *a.* cytolytic, having the power to dissolve or destroy a cell.

citología *f.* cytology, the science that deals with the nature of cells.

citomegálico-a *a.* cytomegalic, characterized by abnormally enlarged cells.

citomegalovirus *m.* cytomegalovirus, any of a group of herpes viruses that causes cellular enlargement and is the causative agent of cytomegalic inclusion disease.

citómetro *m.* cytometer, a device used for counting and measuring blood cells.

citopenia *f.* cytopenia, deficiency of cellular elements in the blood.

citoplasma *m.* cytoplasm, protoplasm of a cell with the exception of the nucleus.

citotoxicidad *f.* cytotoxicity, the capacity of an agent to destroy certain cells.

citotoxina *f.* cytotoxin, toxic agent that damages or destroys cells.

citrato *m.* citrate, salt of citric acid.

cítrico-a *a.* citric, citrous.

cítula *f.* cytula, term used to define the ovum or small impregnated cell.

ciudadanía *f.* citizenship.

ciudadano-a *m., f.* citizen.

clara *f.* the white of the egg.

claridad *f.* clarity, brightness.

clarificación *f.* clarification.

clarificar *vt.* to clarify.

claro-a *a.* clear.

clase *f.* class, sort, kind.

clasificación *f.* classification.

clasificar *vt.* to classify, to sort out.

claudicación *f.* claudication, limping; **__ intermitente** / intermittent __ .

clavícula *f.* clavicle, collarbone.

clavo *m.* nail, slender rod of metal or bone used to fasten together parts of a broken bone; **__ ortopédico** / orthopedic pin.

cleptomanía *f.* kleptomania, morbid compulsion to steal.

clima *m.* climate.

climatérico-a *a.* climacteric, rel. to menopause in women and to a period of sexual decline in men.

clímax *m.* climax. 1. crisis in an illness; 2. sexual orgasm.

clínica *f.* clinic, a health-care facility; **__ de consulta externa** / outpatient __ .

clínico-a *a.* clinical. 1. rel. to a clinic; 2. rel. to direct observation of patients; **cuadro __** / __ picture; **curso __** / __ progress; **ensayos __ -s** / __ trials; **historia __**, **expediente médico** / __ history; **procedimiento __** / __ procedure.

clisis *f.* clysis, the act of supplying fluid to the body by other means than orally.

clitoridectomía *f.* clitoridectomy, excision of the clitoris.

clítoris *m.* clitoris, small protruding body situated in the most anterior part of the vulva.

cloaca *f.* cloaca. 1. common opening for the intestinal and urinary tracts in the early development of the embryo; 2. sewer.

cloasma *f.* chloasma, skin discoloration seen during pregnancy.

clono *m.* 1. clonus, a series of rapid and rhythmic contractions of a muscle; 2. clone, an individual derived from a single organism through asexual reproduction.

clorambucil *m.* chlorambucil, a form of nitrogen mustard used to combat some forms of cancer.

cloranfenicol m. chloramphenicol, chloromycetin, antibiotic esp. effective in the treatment of typhoid fever.

clorhidria f. chlorhydria, excess acidity in the stomach.

cloro m. chlorine, gaseous element used as a disinfectant and bleaching agent.

clorofila f. chlorophyll, green pigment in plants by which photosynthesis takes place.

cloroquina f. chloroquine, a compound used in the treatment of malaria.

clorosis f. chlorosis, type of anemia usu. seen in women and gen. associated with iron deficiency.

clorpromacina f. chlorpromazine, tranquilizing and antiemetic agent.

cloruro m. chloride, a compound of chlorine.

coaglutinación f. coagglutination, group agglutination.

coaglutinina f. coagglutinin, agglutinate that affects two or more organisms.

coagulación f. coagulation, clot; ___ **diseminada intravascular** / disseminated intravascular ___; **propiedad de** ___ / blood clotting ability; **tiempo de** ___ / blood ___ time.

coagulante m. coagulant, that which causes or precipitates coagulation.

coagular v. to coagulate, to clot.

coágulo m. coagulation, clot.

coagulopatía f. coagulopathy, a disease or condition that affects the coagulation mechanism of the blood.

coartación f. coarctation, stricture; compression.

cobarde a. coward.

cobija f. cover, blanket.

cobrar vt. to charge; to collect.

cobre m. copper.

coca f. coca, plant from which cocaine is extracted.

cocaína f. cocaine, addictive narcotic alkaloid derived from coca leaves.

coccidioidomicosis f. coccidioidomycosis, valley fever, endemic respiratory infection in the southwestern United States, Mexico, and parts of South America.

coccigodinia f. coccygodynia, pain in the region of the coccyx.

cóccix m. coccyx, last bone at the bottom of the vertebral column.

cocer vi. to cook; to stew; ___ **a fuego lento** / to simmer.

cociente m. quotient; ___ **de inteligencia** / intelligence ___ .

cocimiento m. concoction made of medicinal herbs.

cocinado-a a. cooked; **bien** ___ / well-done.

cóclea f. cochlea, spiral tube that forms part of the inner ear.

coco m. 1. coccus, bacteria; 2. coconut; **agua de** ___ / ___ milk.

cocoa f. cocoa.

coche m. automobile.

cochinada f. filthy act; dirty trick; filth.

cochino-a m., f. pig; a. filthy.

codeína f. codeine, narcotic analgesic.

codo m. elbow; ___ **de tenista** / tennis ___; **coyuntura del** ___ / ___ joint.

coenzima f. coenzyme, a substance that enhances the action of an enzyme.

coerción f. duress, coercion; **bajo** ___ / under ___ .

coger vt. to take, to grasp; to get; ___ **un resfriado** / to catch a cold.

cognado m. cognate. 1. that which is of the same nature; 2. word that derives from the same root.

cognición f. knowledge, the act of knowing.

cognitivo-a a. cognitive, rel. to knowledge.

cogote m. nape, back of neck.

cohabitar v. to live together.

coherente a. coherent.

cohesión f. cohesion, the force that holds molecules together.

cohibido a. inhibited; uneasy.

coincidencia f. coincidence.

coito m. coitus, sexual intercourse.

cojear v. to limp.

cojera f. lameness.

cojinete m. cushion.

cojo-a a. lame, crippled.

cola f. 1. glue; **inhalar** ___ / to sniff ___; 2. tail.

colaborar v. to collaborate.

colágeno m. collagen, the main supportive protein of skin, bone, tendon, and cartilage.

colangiografía f. cholangiography, x-ray of the biliary ducts.

colangitis f. cholangitis, infl. of the biliary ducts.

colapso m. collapse, failure; ___ **cardiovascular** / cardiovascular failure; ___ **circulatorio** / circulatory failure; ___ **nervioso** / nervous breakdown; ___ **parcial del pulmón** / partial lung ___ .

colar vt. to strain; to sift.
colateral a. collateral. 1. indirect, subsidiary, or accessory to the principal; 2. rel. to a side branch of a nerve axon or blood vessel.
colaterización coronaria f. coronary collaterization, expontaneous growth of new blood vessels around cardiac regions with restricted blood flow.
colcha f. cover, coverlet.
colecistectomía f. cholecystectomy, removal of the gallbladder.
colecistitis f. cholecystitis, infl. of the gallbladder.
colecistoduodenostomía f. cholecistoduodenostomy, anastomosis of the gallbladder and the duodenum.
colecistogastrostomía f. cholecystogastrostomy, anastomosis of the gallbladder and the stomach.
colecistografía f. cholecystography, x-ray of the gallbladder by administration of a dye, orally or by injection.
colectar, coleccionar vt. to collect.
colectomía f. colectomy, excision of part or all of the colon.
colédoco m. choledochus, common bile duct, formed by the union of the hepatic and cystic ducts.
coledocoduodenostomía f. choledochoduodenostomy, anastomosis of the choledochus and the duodenum.
coledocoyeyunostomía f. choledochojejunostomy, anastomosis of the common bile duct and the jejunum.
colegio m. school.
colelitiasis f. cholelithiasis, presence of stones in the gallbladder or in the common bile duct.
colemia f. cholemia, presence of bile in the blood.
cólera f. cholera. 1. acute infectious disease characterized by severe diarrhea and vomiting; 2. anger, rage.
colestasis f. cholestasis, biliary stasis.
colesteatoma m. cholesteatoma, a tumor containing cholesterol, found most commonly in the middle ear.
colesterol m. cholesterol, component of animal oils, fats, and nerve tissue, a precursor of sex hormones and adrenal corticoids; __ **alto** / high __; **reductor de** __ / __ reducer.

colgajo m. flap, detached tissue.
cólico m. colic, acute spasmodic abdominal pain.
colirio m. colyrium, liquid medicinal preparation for the eye.
colitis f. colitis, infl. of the colon; __ **crónica**/chronic __; **espasmódica** / spasmodic __; __ **mucomembranosa** / pseudomembranous __; __ **mucosa** / mucous __; __ **ulcerativa** / ulcerative __ .
colmena f. beehive.
colocar vt. to place, to set; **colocarse** vr. to position oneself.
colodión m. collodion, liquid substance used to cover or protect skin cuts.
coloide m. colloid, gelatin-like substance produced by some forms of tissue decay.
colon m. colon, the portion of the intestine extending from the cecum to the rectum; __ **ascendente** / ascending __; __ **descendente** / descending __; **neoplasma del** __ / colonic neoplasm.
colonia f. colony, a group of bacteria in a culture, all derived from the same organism.
colónico-a a. colonic, rel. to the colon.
colonoscopía f. colonoscopy, examination of the inner surface of the colon through a colonoscope.
colonoscopio m. colonoscope, instrument used to examine the colon.
color m. color. __ **-es complementarios** / complementary __ s; __ **estructural** / structural __; __ **-es extrínsecos** / extrinsic __; __ **-es intrínsecos** / intrinsic __; __ **primario** / primary __; __ **puro** / pure __; __ **reflejado** / reflected __; __ **saturado** / saturated __; __ **simple** / simple __; **confusión de** __ / __ confusion; **percepción del** __ / __ perception; **tono de** __ / __ tone. See table on page 75.
colorado-a a. red; **ponerse** __ / to blush.
colorante m. dye, stain.
colorimétrico-a a. rel. to color; **guía** __ / color index.
colorrectal a. colorectal, rel. to the colon and rectum, or to the entire large bowel.
colostomía f. colostomy, creation of an artificial anus; **bolsa de** __ / __ bag.
colpitis f. colpitis, infl. of the vaginal membrane.

Colores	Colors
amarillo	yellow
ámbar	amber
anaranjado	orange
azul	blue
blanco	white
carmelita	brown
cenizo	ashen
cetrino	greenish yellow
gris	gray
morado, púrpura	purple, black and blue
pardo	brown
negro	black
rojizo	reddish
rojo	red
rosáceo	pinkish
verde	green

colporrafía f. colporrhaphy, suture of the vagina.

colposcopía f. colposcopy, examination of the vagina and the cervix through a colposcope.

columna, espina vertebral f. spinal column, osseous structure formed by thirty-three vertebrae that surround and contain the spinal cord.

coluria f. choluria, presence of bile in the urine.

coma m. coma, state of unconsciousness.

comadrona f. woman who specializes in the health of women during pregnancy, delivery, and postpartum, midwife.

comatoso-a a. comatose, rel. to or in a state of coma; **estado** __ / __ state.

combatir v. to combat, to fight.

combinación f. combination.

combinar v. to combine.

comedón m. blackhead, comedo.

comedor m. dining room.

comensal m. commensal, host, organism that benefits from living within or on another living organism without either benefiting or harming it.

comenzar vi. to commence, to begin.

comer v. to eat; **dar de** __ / to feed.

comestible m. food; a. edible.

cometer v. to commit.

comezón f. itch.

comida f. food; meal; **hora de** __ / meal time.

comienzo m. beginning; start.

comilón-a a. big eater.

comisura f. commissure, coming together of two parts, such as the labial angles.

comisurotomía f. commissurotomy, incision of the fibrous bands of a commissure, such as the labial angles or the commissure of a cardiac valve.

como adv. how, as; __ **quiera** / as you wish; conj. like, as; __ **no** / of course; prep. about; **está** __ **a (una milla)** / it is about (a mile) away; __ **a (las ocho)** / about (eight o'clock).

cómodo-a a. comfortable.

compacto-a a. compact.

compadecer v. to pity; **compadecerse** vr. to feel sorry for; __ **a sí mismo** / self-pity.

compadre m. godfather; close friend.

compañero m. companion, mate.

comparación f. comparison.

comparar v. to compare.

compartir v. to share.

compatible a. compatible.

compensación f. compensation. 1. that which makes up for a defect or counterbalances some deficiency; 2. defense mechanism; 3. remuneration.

competente a. competent, qualified, able to perform well.

complejo m. complex, a series of related mental processes that affect behavior and personality; __ **de castración** / castration __; __ **de culpa** / guilt __; __ **de Edipo** / Oedipus __ , morbid love of a son for the mother; __ **de Electra** / Electra __ , morbid love of a daughter for the father; __ **de inferioridad** / inferiority __; **-a** a. complicated; intricate.

complementar v. to supplement.

complemento m. complement, a serum protein substance that destroys bacteria and other cells with which it comes into contact.

complexión f. complexion, appearance of the facial skin.

complicación f. complication.

complicar vt. to complicate; **complicarse** vr., to become difficult; to become involved, to get entangled.

componente m. component.

componer vt. [una fractura] to set; to put together; to heal, to restore.

composición f. composition.

comprar v. to buy, to purchase.

comprender v. to understand.

compresa f. compress, pack; ___ fría / cold ___ .

compresión f. compression, exertion of pressure on a point of the body.

comprimidos m., pl. pills.

comprobar vt. to prove, to verify.

comprometer v. to compromise; **comprometerse** vr. to commit oneself; to compromise, to become involved.

compromiso m. commitment, obligation.

compuesto m. compound.

compulsivo-a a. compulsive.

computadora f. computer.

común a. common; **nombre** ___ / ___ name; **no** ___ / uncommon; **por lo** ___ / gen; **sentido** ___ / ___ sense.

comunicación f. communication.

comunicación privilegiada f. privileged communication, such as that between a doctor or psychotherapist and a patient; it is the patient's privilege to keep this information confidential.

comunicar vt. to communicate, to inform; **comunicarse** vr. to communicate with.

comunidad f. community.

con prep. with, by; ___ **frecuencia** / frequently; ___ **mucho gusto** / gladly; ___ **permiso** / excuse me; ___ **regularidad** / regularly.

cóncavo-a a. concave, hollowed.

concebir vi. to conceive.

concentración f. concentration. 1. increased strength of a fluid by evaporation; 2. the act of concentrating.

concentrado-a a. concentrated; ___ **en sí mismo-a** / self-conscious.

concentrar vt. to concentrate; **concentrarse** vr. to concentrate oneself.

concepción f. conception.

concepto m. concept, idea.

concha f. shell; that which resembles a shell.

conciencia f. consciousness; conscience, state of awareness.

conciso-a a. concise.

concluir vi. to conclude; to infer.

conclusión f. conclusion.

concreción f. concretion, hardening, solidification.

concretio cordis L. concretio cordis, partial or complete obliteration of the pericardial cavity due to chronic constrictive pericarditis.

concreto-a a. concrete.

concusión f. concussion, trauma gen. caused by a head injury and manifested at times by dizziness and nausea; ___ **cerebral** / cerebral ___; ___ **de la médula espinal** / spinal ___ .

condensar vt. to condense, to make something more dense.

condición f. condition, quality; ___ **anterior** / preexisting ___; ___ **sin diagnosticar** / undiagnosed ___ .

condicionar vt. to condition, to train.

cóndilo m. condyle, rounded portion of the bone usu. present at the joint.

condiloma f. condyloma, warty growth usu. found around the genitalia and the perineum.

condimentado-a a. spicy.

condón m. condom, contraceptive device.

condral a. chondral, of a cartilaginous nature.

condritis f. chondritis, infl. of a cartilage.

condromalacia f. chondromalacia, abnormal softening of cartilage.

condrosarcoma m. chondrosarcoma, malignant tumor formed by cartilage cells.

conducir vt. to conduct; to drive.

conducta f. conduct, behavior.

conducto m. duct, conduit; ___ **eyaculatorio** / ejaculatory ___; ___ **lacrimal** / lacrimal ___ . See Table on this page.

conducto lacrimal n. tear duct.

conectar vt. to connect; to switch on.

conejillo de Indias m. guinea pig.

Conducto	Duct
biliar	biliary
cístico	cystic
colédoco	common bile
de Müeller	mullerian
de Wolff	wolffian
deferente	deferent
excretorio	excretory
eyaculatorio	ejaculatory
hepático	hepatic
lacrimal, lagrimal	lacrimal
linfático	lymphatic
nasolagrimal	nasolacrimal
seminal	seminal
seminífero	seminiferous tubule

conexión *f.* connection.
conexión con el expediente médico *f.* medical record linkage. 1. any information that connects the patient with his or her medical history; 2. collection of data from the medical history of a patient provided by different sources; 3. any data of a participating patient in a clinical study that can reveal his or her identity as a participating subject.
conferencia *f.* conference, lecture, meeting.
confiar *v.* to entrust, to trust.
confidencial *a.* confidential; **comunicación o información** __ / privileged communication or information.
confidencialidad *f.* confidentiality.
confinado-a, *a.* confined.
confirmación *f.* confirmation.
confirmar *v.* to confirm.
conflicto *m.* conflict.
confluencia *f.* confluence, meeting point of several channels.
conformar *v.* to conform, to adapt; **conformarse** *vr.* to resign oneself.
confortar *v.* to comfort.
confundido-a, confuso-a *a.* confused, at a loss; **estar** __ / to be at a loss.
confundir *v.* to confuse, to mix up; **confundirse** *vr.* to be or to become confused.
confusión *f.* confusion.
congelación *m.* freezing; **corte por** __ / frozen cut; **punto de** __ / __ point; **secar por** __ / freeze-dry; **sección por** __ / frozen section, thin specimen of tissue that is frozen quickly and aids in diagnosing malignancies.
congelado-a *a.* frozen; __ **al instante** / quick-frozen.
congelar *v.* to freeze; **congelarse** *vr.* to become frozen.
congénito-a *a.* congenital, existing since birth; ingrown.
congestión *f.* congestion, excessive accumulation of blood in a given body part or organ. __ **activa** / active __; __ **funcional** / functional __; __ **pasiva** / passive __; __ **venosa** / venous __.
congestionado-a *a.* congested.
conización *f.* conization, removal of a cone shaped tissue such as the mucosa of the cervix.

conjugar *vi.* to conjugate.
conjuntiva *f.* conjunctiva, delicate mucous membrane covering the eyelids and the anterior surface of the eyeball; __ **bulbar** / bulbar __; __ **palpebral** / palpebral __ .
conjuntivitis *f.* conjunctivitis, infl. of the conjunctiva; __ **aguda contagiosa** / acute contagious __; __ **alérgica** / allergic __; __ **catarral** / catarrhal __; __ **crónica** / chronic __; __ **epidémica** / epidemic __; __ **folicular** / follicular __; __ **hemorrágica** / hemorrhagic __; __ **infantil purulenta** / infantile purulent __; __ **vernal** / vernal __; __ **viral** / viral __ .
conjuntivitis vernal o primaveral *f.* vernal or primaveral conjunctivitis, bilateral conjunctivitis accompanied by itching, most likely caused by allergy.
conjunto *m.* whole, sum of parts; a set; **en** __ / as a whole.
conminuto-a *a.* comminuted, broken in many small fragments as in a fracture.
cono *m.* cone, cells that together with the rods are the visual cells of the retina.
conocer *vi.* to know; to know about; **conocerse** *vr.* to know each other; to know oneself.
conocimiento *m.* 1. consciousness; **perder el** __ / to lose __; 2. knowledge; **no tener** __ **de** / to be unaware of.
conque *conj.* so, so then.
consanguíneos *m.* blood relatives.
consciencia, conciencia *f.* conscience.
consciente *a.* conscious, aware.
consecuencia *f.* consequence; aftermath; **a** __ **de** / as a result of.
conseguir *vi.* to obtain, to get.
consejero-a *m., f.* counselor.
consejo *m.* counsel, advice.
consenso *m.* consensus.
consentimiento *m.* consent, permission; __ **informado** / informed consent, voluntary permission given by the patient or guardian to perform a medical procedure or study after understanding all the different aspects involved in the procedure.
consentir *vi.* to consent, to permit; to pamper.
conservación *f.* conservation, preservation.

consideración f. consideration; regard.

considerado-a a. considerate.

consistencia f. consistency.

consistente a. consistent, stable.

consolar v. to console, to comfort.

constante a. constant, invariable.

constitución f. constitution, physical makeup.

constituir vi. to constitute.

consulta f. consultation; consulting room; __ **particular** / private practice; **horas de** __ / office hours.

consultar vt. to consult, to confer.

consultor-a m., f. consultant, person who acts in an advisory capacity.

consultorio m. doctor's office; consulting room.

consumir vt. to consume; **consumirse** vr. to waste away.

consunción f. consumption, wasting, general emaciation of the body, as seen in patients with tuberculosis.

contacto m. contact; __ **inicial** / initial __; **lentes de** __ / __ lenses.

contado-a a. numbered; scarce; **al** __ / cash.

contagiar vt. to transmit, to pass on, to infect.

contagio m. contagion, communication of disease.

contagioso-a a. contagious, communicable.

contaminación f. contamination.

contaminar v. to contaminate.

contar vt. to count; to tell; __ **con** / to rely on.

contener vt. to contain; **contenerse** vr. to restrain oneself, to hold back.

contenido m. content.

contento-a a. happy, content, pleased.

conteo m. count; __ **globular o de células sanguíneas** / blood cell __ .

contestar v. to answer.

continencia f. continence, abstinence, or moderation.

continuación f. continuation.

continuar vt. to continue.

continuidad f. continuity.

contra prep. against.

contracción f. contraction, temporary shortening, as of a muscle fiber; __ **de fondo** / deep __; __ **de hambre** / hunger __; __ **espasmódica** / twitching; __ **ulterior** / after- __ .

contracepción f. contraception, birth control.

contraceptivo m. contraceptive; **métodos** __ **-s** / methods of contraception.

contráctil a. contractile, having the capacity to contract.

contractura f. contracture, prolonged or permanent involuntary contraction.

contraer vt. to contract, [una enfermedad] to catch a sickness; **contraerse** vr. to be reduced in size, to shrink up, to crumple up.

contragolpe m. countercoup, lesion that occurs as a result of a blow to the opposite point.

contraindicación f. contraindication.

contraindicado-a a. contraindicated.

contrariado-a a. upset.

contrariar vt. to disappoint, to upset.

contrario-a a. contrary; **al** __ / on the __; **de lo** __ / otherwise.

contrarrestar v. to counter, to oppose.

contrastar v. to contrast.

contraste m. contrast; **medio de** __ / __ medium.

contraveneno m. counterpoison, antidote.

contribución f. contribution.

control m. control.

controlar vt. to control, to regulate; **controlarse** vr. to control oneself.

contusión f. contusion, bruise.

convalecencia f. convalescence, period of time between an illness and the return to health.

convaleciente a. convalescent.

conveniente a. convenient, handy.

conversación f. conversation.

conversión f. conversion, 1. change, transformation; 2. transformation of an emotion into a physical manifestation.

convertir vi. to convert; **convertirse** vr. to become.

convexo-a a. convex.

convulsión f. convulsion, violent involuntary muscular contraction; __ **febril** / febrile __; __ **jacksoniana** / Jacksonian __; __ **tónico-clónica** / tonic-clonic __ .

convulsivo-a a. convulsive, rel. to convulsions; **actividad** __ / seizure activity.

cooperación f. cooperation.

cooperar vi. to cooperate.

cooperativo-a a. cooperative.

coordinación f. coordination; **falta de** __ / lack of __ .

coordinar v. to coordinate.

copa f. cup.
copia f. copy, imitation.
copiar v. to copy; to imitate.
copioso-a a. copious, abundant.
coproemoliente m. stool softener.
coprofagia f. coprophagy, disorder that drives a person to eat feces.
cópula f. copulation, sexual intercourse.
coqueluche m. whooping cough.
cor L. cor, heart; ___ **errante** / ___ mobile; ___ **juvenil** / ___ juvenum; ___ **pulmonar** / ___ pulmonale.
coraje m. courage; anger.
corazón m. heart; hollow, muscular organ situated in the thorax that maintains the circulation of blood; **anormalidades congénitas del** ___ / congenital ___ diseases; **bloqueo del** ___ / ___ block; **bulbo del** ___ / bulbus cordis; **hipertrofia del** ___ / ___ hypertrophy; **latido del** ___ / heartbeat; **operación a** ___ **abierto** / open ___ surgery; **ruido del** ___ / ___ sound; **trasplante del** ___ / ___ transplant; **válvula del** ___ / ___ valve.
corazón artificial m. artificial heart, instrument or device that pumps blood with the same capacity as a normal heart.
cordal a. **muela** ___ / wisdom tooth.
cordectomía f. cordectomy, excision of a vocal cord.
cordón m. cord, any elongated, rounded structure; ___ **espermático** / spermatic ___.
cordón umbilical m. umbilical cord, structure that connects the fetus with the placenta during the gestation period.
cordotomía f. cordotomy, an operation to cut certain sensory fibers in the spinal cord.
cordura f. sanity.
corea f. chorea, Huntington's disease, St. Vitus' dance, nervous disorder manifested by involuntary, rapid, and jerky, but well-coordinated movements of the limbs or facial muscles.
coriocarcinoma m. choriocarcinoma, malignant tumor found primarily in the testicle and the uterus.
corion m. 1. chorion, one of the two membranes that surround the fetus; 2. corium, dermis or true skin.
coriza f. coryza, acute or chronic rhinitis; runny nose.
córnea f. cornea, transparent membrane on the anterior surface of the eyeball. **injerto de la** ___ / corneal grafting.

córneo-a a. corneous, callous.
cornete nasal m. nasal concha.
cornezuelo de centeno m. ergot, fungus used in dry form or as an extract to induce uterine contractions or stop hemorrhaging after delivery.
coroides f. choroid membrane, membrane that supplies blood to the eye.
coroiditis f. choroiditis, infl. of the choroid.
coronamiento m. crowning. 1. the stage of childbirth when the head of the fetus has entered completely the vulvar ring; 2. recovering of the prepared natural tooth with a chosen dental material as a veneer.
coronario-a a. coronary, encircling in the manner of a crown; **aneurisma de la arteria** ___ / ___ artery bypass; **arteria** ___ / ___ artery; **desviación** ___ / ___ bypass; **trombosis** ___ / ___ thrombosis; **unidad de atención** ___ / ___ care unit; **vasoespasmo** ___ / ___ vasospasm.
corpulento-a a. corpulent, stout, robust.
corpus m. corpus, the human body.
corpus callosum L. corpus callosum, the great commissure of the brain.
corpúsculo m. corpuscle, bud, small mass.
corpus luteum L. corpus luteum, yellow body, yellow glandular mass in the ovary that is formed by a ruptured follicle and produces progesterone.
correa f. strap, belt.
correctivo-a m., f. corrective; antidote.
correcto-a a. correct; accurate.
corregir vi. to correct, to rectify.
correo m. mail.
correr v. to run, to jog.
corriente f. current, stream, flow of fluid, air, or electricity along a conductor; **al** ___ / current, up-to-date; a. current.
corromperse vr. to be affected with putrefaction, to be tainted.
corrosivo m. corrosive, agent that causes destruction of living cells.
cortado-a a. cut, incised.
cortadura f. cut, slit.
cortar v. to cut, to incise; **cortarse** vr. to cut one-self.
corte m. cut, slit; ___ **transversal** / transection.
corteza f. cortex, the outer layer of an organ; ___ **suprarrenal** / adrenal ___; ___ **cerebral** / cerebral ___.

Corti, órgano de *m.* Corti's organ, the organ of hearing by which sound is perceived.

cortical *a.* cortical, rel. to the cortex.

corticoide, corticosteroide *m.* corticoid, corticosteroid, a steroid produced by the adrenal cortex.

corticotropina *f.* corticotropin, hormonal substance of adrenocorticotropic activity.

cortisol *m.* cortisol, hormone secreted by the adrenal cortex.

cortisona *f.* cortisone, glycogenic steroid derived from cortisol or produced synthetically.

corto-a *a.* short; ___ **de vista** / nearsighted.

cosmético *m.* cosmetic.

cosquillas *f., pl.* tickle, tickling; **hacer** ___ / to tickle; **tener** ___ / to be ticklish.

cosquilleo *m.* tingling or prickling sensation, tickling.

costado *m.* side, flank; **al** ___ / to the ___ .

costal *a.* costal, rel. to the ribs.

costalgia *f.* costalgia, neuralgia, pain in the ribs.

costar *vi.* to cost; ___ **trabajo** / to be difficult.

costilla *f.* rib. 1. one of the bones of twelve pairs that form the thoracic cage; 2. chop, a cut of meat.

costo *m.* cost; ___ **de vida** / ___ of living.

costoclavicular *a.* costoclavicular, rel. to the ribs and the clavicle.

costocondritis *f.* costochondritis, infl. of one or more costal cartilages.

costoso-a *a.* costly, expensive.

costovertebral *a.* costovertebral, rel. to the angle of the ribs and the thoracic vertebrae.

costra *f.* crust, scab; ___ **láctea** / cradle cap.

costumbre *f.* custom, habit; **tener la** ___ / to be in the habit of.

cotidiano-a *a.* quotidian, that occurs every day; **malaria** ___ / ___ malaria.

cowperitis *f.* cowperitis, infl. of Cowper's gland.

coxa *f.* coxa, hip.

coxa magna *f.* coxa magna, abnormal widening of the head of the femur.

coxa valga *f.* coxa valga, hip deformity resulting in abnormal angulation of the femoral shaft away from the midline of the body.

coxa vara *f.* coxa vara, hip deformity resulting in abnormal angulation of the femoral shaft toward the midline of the body.

coxalgia *f.* coxalgia, pain in the hip.

coyuntura *f.* joint; articulation.

craneal *a.* cranial, rel. to the cranium; **fractura** ___ / skull fracture.

craneales, nervios *m., pl.* cranial nerves, each of the twelve pairs of nerves connected to the brain; **I. olfatorio** / olfactory; **II. óptico** / optic; **III. motor ocular común** / oculomotor; **IV. troclear** / trochlear; **V. trigémino** / trigeminal; **VI. motor ocular externo, abducente** / abducent; **VII. facial** / facial; **VIII. auditivo** / auditory; **IX. glosofaríngeo** / glossopharyngeal; **X. neumogástrico, vago** / vagus; **XI. espinal** / accessory; **XII. hipogloso** / hypoglossal.

cráneo *m.* cranium, skull, braincase, the bony structure of the head that covers the brain; **base del** ___ / cranial base.

craneofaringioma *m.* craniopharingioma, malignant brain tumor seen esp. in children.

craneotomía *f.* craniotomy, trepanation of the cranium.

craurosis *f.* kraurosis, atrophy and dryness of the mucous membranes of the vulva.

creación *f.* creation.

crear *vt.* to create.

creatina *f.* creatine, component of muscular tissue important in the anaerobic phase of muscular contraction.

creatinina *f.* creatinine, end product of the metabolism of creatine present in urine; **depuración de la** ___ / ___ clearance, volume of plasma that is clear of creatinine.

crecer *vi.* to grow; ___ **hacia adentro** / to grow inward.

crecido-a *a.* grown; large.

crecimiento *m.* growth.

crecimiento cero de población *m.* zero population growth, a demographic condition during a certain period of time, in which a population is stable, neither increasing nor diminishing.

crédito *m.* credit.

creer *vi.* to believe; to think.

crema *f.* cream, ointment.

cremastérico *a.* cremasteric, rel. to the cremaster muscle of the scrotal wall.

creosota *f.* creosote, antiseptic, oily liquid used as an expectorant.
crepitación *f.* crepitation, crackling; __ **pleural** / pleural __ .
cresta *f.* crest. 1. a bony ridge; 2. the peak of a graph.
cretinismo *m.* cretinism, congenital hypothyroidism due to severe deficiency of the thyroid hormone.
cretino-a *m., f.* cretin, person afflicted with cretinism.
crianestesia *f.* cryanesthesia. 1. anesthesia applied by means of localized refrigeration; 2. loss of ability to perceive cold.
crimen *m.* crime.
criminal *m.* criminal; felon.
criocirugía *f.* cryosurgery, destruction of tissue through the application of intense cold.
criógeno *a.* cryogenic, that which produces low temperatures.
crioglobulina *f.* cryoglobulin, a serum globulin that crystallizes spontaneously at low temperatures.
crioscopía *f.* cryoscopy, testing and determining the freezing point of a fluid, gen. blood or urine as a sample, and comparing it with that of distilled water.
crioterapia *f.* cryotherapy, therapeutic treatment using a cold medium.
cripta *f.* crypt, small tubular recess.
criptococosis *f.* cryptococcosis, a systemic fungal infection that may affect different organs of the body, esp. the brain.
criptorquidia, criptorquismo *f., m.* cryptorchism, failure of a testis to descend into the scrotum.
crisis *f.* crisis, turning point in a disease; __ **de identidad** / identity __; __ **nerviosa** / nervous breakdown.
crisoterapia *f.* chrysotherapy, treatment with gold salts.
cristalino *m.* crystalline lens, lens of the eye behind the pupil; **-a** *a.* crystalline, transparent.
cristaloideo-a *a.* crystalloid, resembling crystal.
cromático-a *a.* chromatic, rel. to colors.
cromatina *f.* chromatin, portion of the cell nucleus that stains more readily.
cromocito *m.* chromocyte, a colored or pigmented cell.

cromógeno *m.* chromogen, a substance that produces color.
cromosoma *m.* chromosome, part of the nucleus of the cell that contains the genes.
cromosoma x *m.* X-chromosome, differential chromosome that determines the female sex characteristics.
cromosoma y *m.* Y-chromosome, differential chromosome that determines the male sex characteristics.
cromosómico-a *a.* chromosomic, rel. to the chromosome; **aberraciones** __ **-s** / chromosome aberrations.
crónico-a *a.* chronic, of long duration, prolonged effect.
cronológico-a *a.* chronological, rel. to the sequence of time.
cruel *a.* cruel.
cruento-a *a.* bloody.
crup *m.* croup, infl. of the larynx in children, usu. accompanied by hoarse coughing, fever, and difficulty in breathing; **espasmódico** / spasmodic __ .
crus *L.* crus, leg or a structure resembling one; __ **del cerebro** / cerebral __ .
Cruz Roja Internacional *f.* International Red Cross, international organization for medical assistance.
cruzar *vi.* to cross.
cuadrante *m.* quadrant, 90°, one-fourth of a circle.
cuadrar *vt.* to square; to fit.
cuadriceps *m.* quadriceps, four-headed muscle, extensor of the leg.
cuadriplegia *f.* quadriplegia, paralysis of the four extremities.
cuajado-a *a.* curdled; **leche** __ / __ milk.
cuajar *vt.* to curdle; **cuajarse** *vr.* to congeal, to thicken.
cuajo *m.* curd.
cualidad *f.* quality.
cualitativo-a *a.* qualitative, rel. to quality; **prueba** __ / __ test.
cualquier-a *a.* any.
cuantitativo-a *a.* quantitative, rel. to amount.
cuanto, cúanto-a *a., adv.* how much, how many; ¿ __ **tiempo?** / how long?; __ **antes** / as soon as possible; **en** __ / as soon as; **en** __ **a** / in regard to; **unos** __ **-s** / a few.
cuarentena *f.* quarantine, period during which a restraint is put on the

cubeta

movement of persons or animals to prevent the spread of a disease.

cubeta *f.* basin.

cubierta *f.* covering, sheath, shield; ___ **entérica** / enteric coated.

cubierto-a *a., pp.* of **cubrir,** covered.

cúbito *m.* cubitus, ulna, the inner, long bone of the forearm.

cubreboca *m.* surgical mask.

cubrir *v.* to cover, to drape as with a sterilized cloth.

cucaracha *f.* cockroach.

cuclillas (en) *adv.* in a squatting position.

cucharita *f.* teaspoon; ___ **de cafe** / cochleare parvum, a tea spoonful.

cuello *m.* neck; collar. 1. part that joins the head and the trunk of the body; 2. area between the crown and the root of a tooth.

cuello uterino *m.* cervix, uterine neck; cervix uteri; **dilatación del** ___ / dilation of the cervix; **incompetencia del** ___ / cervical incompetence.

cuentacélulas *m.* cell counting device.

cuerdas vocales *f., pl.* vocal chords, main organ of the voice; ___ **superiores o falsas** / false ___; ___ **inferiores o verdaderas** / true ___ .

cuerdo-a *a.* sane; wise.

cuerno *m.* horn.

cuerpo *m.* body; ___ **-s extraños** / foreign bodies. See illustration on this page.

cuerpo amarillo *m.* yellow body; corpus luteum.

cuerpos cetónicos, acetónicos *m., pl.* ketone bodies, known as acetones.

cuestión *f.* question; issue, matter.

cuestionario *m.* questionnaire.

cuidado *m.* care, attention; ___ **bajo custodia** / custodial care; ___ **intensivo** / intensive ___; ___ **postnatal** / postnatal ___; ___ **prenatal** / prenatal ___; ___ **primario** / primary ___; **estar al** ___ **de** / to be under the ___ of; **negación de** ___ / refusal of ___; **nivel de** ___ **satisfactorio** / reasonable ___; **tratar con** ___ / to handle with care.

cuidadoso-a *a.* careful, mindful.

cuidar *v.* to take care, to look after.

cul-de-sac *Fr.* cul-de-sac. 1. blind pouch, cavity closed on one end; 2. rectouterine pouch.

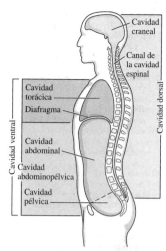

Cavidades del cuerpo: vista lateral

culdoscopía *f.* culdoscopy, viewing of the pelvic and abdominal cavity with a culdoscope.

culebra *f.* snake.

culebrilla *f.* the shingles, herpes zoster, herpes-like cutaneous disease.

culero *m.* diaper.

culpa *f.* guilt; fault, blame; **tener la** ___ / to be at fault.

culpar *v.* to blame.

cultivo *m.* culture, artificial growth of microorganisms or living tissue cells in the laboratory; ___ **de orina** / urine ___; ___ **de sangre** / blood ___; ___ **de tejido** / tissue ___; **medio de** ___ / ___ medium.

cuna *f.* crib, cradle, bassinet.

cunilinguo-a *a.* cunnilingus, rel. to the practice of oral stimulation or manipulation of the clitoris.

cuña *f.* wedge; bedpan.

cuñado-a *m., f.* brother-in-law; sister-in-law.

cúpula *f.* dome.

cura *f.* 1. cure; *m.* 2. priest.

curable *a.* curable, healable.

curación *f.* cure; healing process.

curanderismo *m.* faith healing.

curandero *m.* faith healer, medicine man, shaman.

curar *v.* to cure, to heal.

curare *m.* curare, venom extracted from various plants used to provide muscle relaxation during anesthesia.

curativo-a *a.* curative, having healing properties.

cureta *f.* curette, scoop-like instrument with sharp edges used for curettage.

curetaje *m.* curettage, scraping of a surface or cavity with a sharp-edged instrument; __ **uterino** / D&C, dilation and curettage of the uterine cavity.

curita *f.* bandaid.

curso *m.* course; direction.

curva *f.* curve, bend.

curvatura *f.* curvature, deviation from a straight line.

Cushing, síndrome de *m.* Cushing's syndrome, adrenogenital syndrome manifested by obesity and muscular weakness gen. associated with an excessive production of cortisol.

custodia *f.* custody; **bajo __ del estado** / ward of the state.

cutáneo-a *a.* cutaneous, rel. to the skin; **absorción __** / __ absorption; **glándulas __-s o sebáceas** / __ glands; **manifestaciones __ -s** / skin manifestations; **pruebas __ -s** / skin tests; **úlcera __** / skin ulcer.

cutícula *f.* cuticle, outer layer of the skin.

cutis *m.* cutis, complexion, skin.

cutis colgante *m.* sagging facial skin.

d

d *abr.* densidad / density; **difunto** / deceased; **dosis** / dose.

dacriadenitis *f.* dacryadenitis, infl. of the lacrimal gland.

dacrioadenectomía *f.* dacryoadenectomy, removal of a lacrimal gland.

dacriocistectomía *f.* dacryocystectomy, surgical removal of the lacrimal sac.

dacriocistitis *f.* dacryocystitis, infl. of the lacrimal sac.

dacriocisto *m.* dacryocyst, internal lacrimal sac.

dacrioestenosis *f.* dacriostenosis, stricture of the lacrimal sac.

dacriorrea *f.* dacryorrhea, excessive flow of tears.

dactilitis *f.* dactylitis, infl. of a finger or toe.

dáctilo *m.* dactyl, finger or toe.

dactilogía *f.* dactylology, sign language.

dactilografía *f.* dactylography, study of fingerprints.

dactiloscopia *f.* dactyloscopy, study of fingerprints for the purpose of identification.

dado-a *a. pp.* de **dar**, given; ___ **a** / ___ to; ___ **que** / ___ that.

daltonismo *m.* daltonism, defective perception of the colors red and green.

danazol *m.* danazol, Deprancol, Danocrine, synthetic hormone that suppresses the action of the anterior pituitary.

dañado-a *a.* hurt; [*comida*] spoiled; tainted.

dañar *vt.* to harm; to hurt; to injure.

dañino-a *a.* harmful; noxious.

daño *m.* harm, [*to an object*] damage, hurt; *v.* **hacer** ___ / to harm, to hurt; **no hace** ___ / it doesn't hurt.

daños y perjuicios *m., pl.* damages.

dar *vi.* to give; to minister; ___ **a luz** / to give birth; ___ **de alta** / discharge from the hospital; ___ **de comer** / to feed; ___ **el pecho** / to breast-feed; ___ **lugar a** / to cause; **darse** / *vr.* to give oneself; ___ **por vencido** / to give up; ___ **prisa** / to hurry.

dartos *m.* dartos, a layer of smooth muscle fibers found beneath the skin of the scrotum.

Darvon *m.* Darvon, trade name for dextro propoxyphene hydrochloride, an oral analgesic.

Darwin, teoría de *f.* Darwinism, theory of the origin and perpetuation of species through the action of natural selection on variations that occur by chance.

dátil *m.* date.

dato *m.* fact, piece of information.

de *prep.* of, from; [*posesión*], **los rayos-x ___ la paciente** / the patient's x-rays; [*contenido*] **bicarbonato ___ sodio** / sodium bicarbonate; [*procedencia*] **vengo ___ la consulta /** I am coming from the doctor's office.

debajo *adv.* underneath; ___ **de** / under; **por ___** / beneath.

débil *a.* debilitated, weak, feeble.

debilitante *a.* debilitating, rel. to a sickness that causes weakness.

debilitar *v.* to weaken; **debilitar(se)** *vr.* to feel weaker.

decaer *vi.* to weaken; [*en ánimo*] to decline.

decaído-a *a.* dispirited, dejected.

decaimiento *m.* dejection.

decalcificación *f.* decalcification, loss or reduction of lime salts from bones or teeth.

decapsulación *f.* decapsulation, incision and extirpation of a capsule.

deceleración *f.* deceleration; diminished velocity, such as of heart frequency.

decepción *f.* deceit; layer of uterine endometrium that is shed during menstruation.

decidido-a *a.* decided; determined.

decidir *vi.* to decide; **decidirse** *vr.* to make up one's mind.

decidua *f.* decidua, mucous membrane of the uterus that develops during pregnancy and is discharged after delivery.

deciduo-a *a.* deciduous, of a temporal nature.

decir *vt.* to say; to tell; **querer ___** / to mean.

decisión *f.* decision, resolution.

decorticación *f.* decortication, removal of part of the cortical surface of an organ such as the brain.

decrépito-a *a.* decrepit, worn with age.

decúbito *m.* decubitus, lying down position; ___ **dorsal** / dorsal ___, on the back; ___ **lateral** / lateral ___, on the side ; ___ **prono** / ventral ___; ___ **supino** / dorsal ___; ___ **ventral** / ventral ___, on the stomach; **radiografía en** ___ **lateral** / lateral ___ x-ray film.

dedalera *f.* foxglove, common name for Digitalis purpurea.

dedo *m.* finger; toe; **caída de los** ___ **-s del pie** / toe drop; ___ **del pie** / toe; ___ **en garra, en martillo** / hammer, mallet finger or toe; ___ **en palillo de tambor** / clubbing; ___ **gordo** / hallux; ___ **índice** / index ___, forefinger; ___ **meñique** / little ___; ___ **pulgar** / thumb; **desviación de un** ___ / valgus; **separación de un** ___ / varus.

deducción *f.* deduction, to reason from the general to the particular.

deducir *vi.* to deduce, to infer.

defecación *f.* defecation, bowel movement.

defecar *vt.* to defecate.

defectivo-a *a.* defective.

defecto *m.* defect; blemish; ___ **congénito** / congenital ___ .

defectuoso-a *a.* defective, faulty.

defensa *f.* defense, resistance to a disease; ___ **propia** / self-___; **mecanismo de** ___ / ___ mechanism.

deferente *a.* deferent, conveying away from.

defibrilación *f.* defibrillation, the act of changing an irregular heart beat to a normal rhythm.

deficiencia *f.* deficiency; ___ **de lactasa** / lactase ___; ___ **de galactocinasa** / galactokinasa ___; **enfermedad por** ___ / ___ disease; ___ **mental** / mental ___; ___ **mineral** / mineral ___ .

deficiente *a.* deficient, wanting.

definición *f.* definition.

definitivo-a *a.* definitive, final; **diagnosis** ___ / ___ diagnosis; **-mente** *adv.* definitely.

deflexión *f.* deflection, diversion; unconscious diversion of ideas.

deforme *a.* deformed.

deformidad *f.* deformity, irregularity, a congenital or acquired malformation.

defunción *f.* demise, death.

degeneración *f.* degeneration, deterioration.

degeneración macular *f.* macular degeneration, eye disease in which the macula is pregressively destroyed, impairing central vision.

deglución *f.* deglutition, the act of swallowing.

degradación *f.* degradation, reducing a chemical compound to a simpler one.

dehidroandrosterona *f.* dehydroandrosterone, previously known as dehydroepiandrosterone, androgenic steroid found in the urine.

dehidrocolesterol *m.* dehydrocholesterol, skin substance that becomes vitamin B complex by the action of the sun's rays.

dehidrocorticosterona *f.* dehydrocorticosterone, steroid found in the adrenal cortex.

dehiscencia *f.* dehiscence, splitting open of a wound.

déjá vu *Fr.* déjá vu, an illusory impression of having seen or experienced a new situation before.

dejadez *f.* lassitude, neglect, carelessness.

dejar *v.* to leave; to let, to allow; ___ **dicho** / ___ word; ___ **órdenes** / ___ orders; ___ **de** / to stop from, to quit.

del contraction of the *prep.* **de** and the *art.* **el.**

delante *adv.* in front; before.

delgado-a *a.* thin, slender, slim.

delgaducho-a *a.* thin; delicate.

delicado-a *a.* delicate, tender.

delicioso-a *a.* delicious.

delicuescencia *f.* deliquescence, condition of a substance when it becomes liquified by absorption of water from the air.

deligación *f.* deligation, art of applying ligatures or binders.

delimitación *f.* delimitation, process of marking the limits or circumscribing.

delincuencia *f.* delinquency; ___ **juvenil** / juvenile ___ .

delincuente *a.* delinquent.

delirante *a.* delirious, raving.

delirar *vi.* to be delirious, to rave.

delirio *m.* delirium, temporary mental disturbance marked by hallucinations and distorted perceptions; ___ **agudo** / acute ___; ___ **crónico** / chronic ___; ___ **de control** / ___ of control; ___ **de grandeza** / ___ of grandeur; ___ **de negación** / ___ of negation; ___ **de persecución** / persecution complex; ___ **tremens** / ___ tremens, a form of alcoholic psychosis.

deltoideo-a

deltoideo-a *a.* deltoid. 1. rel. to the deltoid muscle that covers the shoulder; 2. shaped like a triangle.

delusión *f.* delusion, false beliefs.

demacrado-a *a.* gaunt, wasted.

demanda *f.* demand; **alimentación por __ / __** feeding.

demás *adv.* besides; that which is beyond a certain measure; **lo __ /** the rest.

demasiado-a *a.* excessive; *adv.* too much.

demencia *f.* dementia, dementia praecox, insanity; esquizofrenia; **__ alcohólica /** alcoholic __; **__ orgánica /** organic __; **__ senil /** senile __ .

demente *a.* demented, one suffering from dementia.

Demerol *m.* Demerol, meperidine hydrochloride, trade name for an analgesic drug with properties similar to morphine.

demora *f.* delay.

demorar *v.* to delay; **demorarse** *vr.* to be delayed, to take too long.

demostración *f.* demonstration.

demostrar *vt.* to demonstrate; to prove.

demulcente *m.* demulcent, agent that soothes and softens the skin or mucosa.

dendrita *f.* dendrite, protoplasmic prolongation of the nerve cell that receives the nervous impulses.

dengue *m.* dengue fever, acute febrile and infectious disease caused by a virus and transmitted by the *Aedes* mosquito.

denominación *f.* denomination, name.

densidad *f.* density; **__ del vapor /** vapor __; **__ óptica /** optic __; **__ ósea /** bone __; **__ urinaria /** urinary __ .

denso-a *a.* dense; thick.

dentado-a *a.* dentiform, toothed; 1. having projections like teeth on the edge; 2. shaped like a tooth.

dentadura *f.* teeth; **__ postiza /** denture.

dental, dentario-a *a.* dental, rel. to the teeth; **absceso __ / __** abscess; **anquilosis __ / __** ankylosis; **arco __ / __** arch; **bulbo __ / __** bulb; **cavidad __ / __** cavity; **cirujano __ / __** surgeon; **cuidado __ / __** care; **esmalte __ / __** enamel; **folículo __ / __** follicle; **hilo __ / __** floss; **implante __ / __** implant; **inclusión __ / __** inclusion; **impacción __ / __** impaction; **impresión __ / __** impression; **placa dentaria / __**

plaque; **salud pública __ / __** public health; **sarro __ / __** tartar; **servicios de salud __ / __** health services; **técnico __ / __** technician; **técnico en profiláctica __ / __** hygienist; **uso de hilo __ /** flossing.

dentición *f.* dentition, time when children's teeth are cut; **__ primaria /** primary __, first teeth; **__ secundaria o dientes permanentes /** secondary __, permanent teeth.

dentilabial *a.* dentilabial, rel. to the teeth and the lips.

dentina *f.* dentin, calcified tissue that constitutes the larger portion of the tooth.

dentinogénesis *f.* dentinogenesis, formation of dentin.

dentista *m., f.* dentist; **__ de niños /** pedodontist.

dentoide *a.* dentoid, tooth-shaped.

dentro *adv.* within; **por __ /** inside.

denudación *f.* denudation, deprival of a protecting surface by surgery, trauma, or pathologic change.

deoxihemoglobina *f.* deoxyhemoglobin, reduced form of hemoglobin that occurs when the oxihemoglobin looses oxygen.

dependencia *f.* dependence, subordination.

depender *vi.* to depend; to rely.

dependiente *m., f.* dependent; **drenaje __ / __** drainage; **edema __ / __** edema; **personalidad __ / __** personality.

despersonalización *f.* depersonalization, a state of mind in which the subject loses the feeling of his/her own identity in relation to members of groups that he/she is associated with.

depigmentación *f.* depigmentation, partial or complete loss of pigment.

depilación *f.* depilation, removal of hair by the roots.

depleción *f.* depletion; 1. the act of draining; 2. the removal of accumulated liquids or solids to an excess; **__ de fluido /** fluid __; **__ de líquidos del cuerpo, deshidratación / __** of body liquids, dehydration; **__ de potasio, hipopotasemia /** potassium __, hypopotassemia; **__ salina /** saline __ .

deporte *m.* sports; athletics.

deposición *f.* bowel movement; **__ -es blandas o acuosas /** loose bowels.

depositar *vt.* to deposit.

depósito *m.* deposit; precipitate.

depravación *f.* depravation, perversion.

depravado-a *a.* depraved, corrupt; perverted.

depresión *f.* depression. 1. state of sadness and melancholia accompanied by apathy; 2. cavity.

depresor *m.* depressor. 1. agent used to lower an established level of function or activity of the organism; __ **de lengua** / tongue __; 2. tranquilizer; -a *a.* producing or rel. to depression.

deprimente *n.* depressing.

deprimido-a *a.* depressed, downcast.

depuración *f.* depuration, purification.

depurar *vt.* to depurate, to purify.

derecha *f.* right hand side; **a la __** / to the right

derecho-a *a.* straight, erect; *adv.* straight, straight ahead.

derecho *m.* right; the study of law; **los __-s del paciente** / the patient's __-s; **tener __** / to have the __ .

derecho a rehusar tratamiento *m.* the right to refuse treatment.

derecho a tratamiento *m.* right to treatment, the patient's right to receive adequate treatment by a medical facility that has assumed responsibility for the patient's care.

derivación *f.* derivation, bypass; 1. shunt, alternate or lateral course that occurs through anastomosis or through a natural anatomical characteristic; __ **aortocoronaria** / aortocoronary bypass; __ **aortoilíaca** / aortoiliac bypass; __ **portacava** / portacaval shunt; 2. origin or source of a substance.

derivación de flujo lento *f.* low-flow shunt.

dermabrasión *f.* dermabrasion, procedure to remove acne scars, nevi or fine wrinkles of the skin.

dermalgia, dermatalgia *f.* dermalgia, dermatalgia, pain in the skin.

dermático-a *a.* dermal, dermatic, rel. to the skin.

dermatitis *f.* dermatitis, infl. of the skin; __ **actínica** / actinic __, produced by sunlight or ultraviolet light; __ **alérgica** / allergic __; __ **atópica** / atopic __; __ **eritematosa** / erythematous __; __ **gangrenosa** / gangrenous __; __ **medicamentosa** / medicinal __; __ **ocupacional,**

industrial / __ occupational; __ **papillaris capilliti** / papillaris capilliti __; __ **por contacto** / contact __; __ **seborréica** / seborrheic __ .

dermatofitosis *f.* dermatophytosis, athlete's foot, fungal infection of the skin caused by a dermatophyte.

dermatolisis *f.* dermatolysis, loss or atrophy of skin due to sickness.

dermatología *f.* dermatology, the study of skin diseases.

dermatólogo *m.* dermatologist, specialist in dermatology.

dermatomicosis *f.* dermatomycosis, infl. of the skin by fungi.

dermatomiositis *f.* dermatomyositis, disease of the connective tissue manifested by edema, dermatitis, and infl. of the muscles.

dermatoneurosis *f.* dermatoneurosis, any cutaneous eruption or rash due to emotional stimuli.

dermatoplastia *f.* dermatoplasty, surgery of the skin.

dermatosífilis *f.* dermatosyphilis, skin manifestation of syphilis.

dérmico-a *a.* dermic, rel. to the skin.

dermis *f.* dermis, skin.

dermitis *f.* dermitis, infl. of the skin.

dermoflebitis *f.* dermophlebitis, infl. of superficial veins.

dermoideo-a *a.* dermoid, resembling skin; **quiste __** / __ cyst, congenital, usu. benign.

desabrido-a *a.* tasteless; insipid.

desabrigado-a *a.* underclothed; too exposed to the elements.

desacostumbrado-a *a.* unaccustomed.

desacuerdo *m.* disagreement.

desadvertidamente *adv.* inadvertently; unintentionally.

desafortunado-a *a.* unfortunate, unlucky.

desagradable *a.* disagreeable, unpleasant.

desagradecido-a *a.* ungrateful.

desahogarse *vr., vi.* to release one's grief; *pop.* to let out steam.

desalentar *v., vi.* to discourage; **desalentarse** *vr.* to become discouraged.

desangramiento *m.* excessive bleeding.

desangrarse *vr.* to bleed excessively.

desanimado-a *a.* downhearted, discouraged.

desaprobar *vi.* to disapprove; to refute.

desarrollado-a *a.* developed.

desarrollar *v.* [*síntomas*] to develop; to grow.

desarrollo *m.* development; growth; ___ **infantil** / child ___; ___ **físico** / physical ___; ___ **psicomotor y físico** / psychomotor and physical ___ .

desarrollo motor *n.* motor development.

desarticulación *f.* disarticulation, separation or amputation of two or more bones from one joint.

desarticulado-a *a.* disarticulated, rel. to a bone that has been separated from its joint.

desaseo *m.* uncleanliness.

desasosiego *m.* uneasiness, unrest.

desastre *m.* disaster.

desatendido-a *a.* unattended.

desatinado-a *a.* lacking good judgment, wild.

desayunar *v.* to have breakfast.

desayuno *m.* breakfast.

desbridamiento *m.* debridement, removal of foreign bodies or dead or damaged tissue, esp. from a wound.

descafeinado-a *a.* decaffeinated.

descalcificación *f.* decalcification. 1. loss of calcium salts from a bone; 2. removal of calcareous matter.

descalzo-a *a.* barefooted.

descamación *f.* desquamation, the act of shedding scales from the epidermis.

descansado-a *a.* rested, refreshed.

descanso *m.* rest, tranquility.

descarado-a *a.* impudent, shameless.

descarga *f.* discharge, excretion.

descendente *a.* descending.

descendiente *a.* descendant, offspring.

descentrado-a *a.* decentered, not centered.

descoloramiento *m.* discoloration.

descolorido-a *a.* discolored, washed out.

descompensación *f.* decompensation, inability of the heart to maintain adequate circulation.

descomponerse *vr.*, *vi.* to decompose.

descompresión *f.* decompression, lack of air or gas pressure as in deep-sea diving; **cámara de** ___ / ___ chamber; ___ **quirúrgica** / surgical ___; **enfermedad por** ___ / ___ sickness *pop.* the bends.

desconcierto *m.* uncertainty, confusion.

desconectar *v.* to disconnect; to switch off.

descongelación *f.* thawing.

descongelar *v.* to defrost; to thaw.

descongestionante *m.* decongestant.

descongestionar *v.* to decongest.

descontaminación *f.* decontamination, the process of freeing the environment, objects, or persons from contaminated or harmful agents such as radioactive substances.

descontinuado-a *a.* discontinued, suspended.

descontinuar *vt.* to discontinue.

describir *vt.* to describe.

descripción *f.* description.

descrito-a *a. pp.* de **describir**, described.

descubierto-a *a. pp.* de **descubrir**, uncovered.

descubrir *vi.* to discover; to uncover.

desde *prep.* since, from; ___ **ahora en adelante** / from now on; ___ **hace (una semana, un mes)** / it has been (a week, a month) since; ___ **luego** / of course.

desear *vt.* to wish, to desire.

desecación *f.* desiccation, drying, draining.

desecado-a *a.* desiccated, dried up.

desecante *m.* desiccant, substance that causes dryness.

desechable *a.* disposable.

desechar *vt.* to discard, to cast aside.

desecho *m.* waste; ___ **de efectos medicos** / medical ___ .

desencadenamiento *m.* trigger, impulse that initiates other events; **puntos de** ___ / ___ points.

desencadenar *vt.* to trigger, to initiate a succession of events.

desencajado-a *a.* disengaged; disjointed; gaunt.

desenlace *m.* outcome, conclusion.

desensibilizar *v.* to desensitize, to diminish or annul sensibility.

deseoso-a *a.* desirous, eager.

desequilibrado-a *a.* imbalanced; ___ **mental** / mentally ___ .

desequilibrio *m.* imbalance; ___ **degenerativo** / degenerative ___; ___ **hidroelectrolítico** / hydroelectrolytic ___; ___ **hormonal** / hormonal ___ .

desesperado-a *a.* desperate, despairing, despondent.

desfallecer *vi.* to faint; to become weak.

desfervescencia f. defervescence, period of fever decline.

desfibrilación f. defibrillation, action of returning an irregular heartbeat to its normal rhythm.

desfibrilador m. defibrillator, electrical device used to restore the heart to a normal rhythm.

desfiguración, desfiguramiento m., f. defacement; disfigurement.

desgarradura, desgarro m., f. tear, laceration.

desgaste m. wearing down.

desgrasar vt. to degrease, to remove the fat.

deshidratado-a a. dehydrated, free of water.

deshidratar vt. to dehydrate, eliminate water from a substance.

deshidratarse vr. to dehydrate, to lose liquid from the body or tissues.

deshumectante m. dehumidifier, device to diminish humidity.

desigual a. uneven; unlike, unequal.

desinfección f. disinfection.
1. process of extensive cleansing and elimination of pathogens; 2. cleaning for the purpose of daily control of disposal of contaminated organisms, and elimination of microorganisms as done in hospitals.

desinfestación f. desinfestation, thorough cleaning and elimination of parasites, rodents, and pests that could bring infestation.

desinfectante m. disinfectant, agent that kills bacteria.

desinfectar vt. to disinfect.

desinflamar v. to reduce or remove an inflammation.

desintegración f. disintegration; decomposition.

deslizamiento m. slipping; sliding.

deslumbramiento m. glare.
1. blurring of the vision with possible permanent damage to the retina; 2. intense light.

desmayarse vr. to faint, to pass out; to swoon.

desmayo m. fainting.

desmembración, desmembradura f. dismemberment.

desmielinación, desmielinización f. demyelination, demyelinization, loss or destruction of the myelin layer of the nerve.

desmineralización f. demineralization, loss of minerals from the body, esp. the bones.

desmoma f. desmoma, tumor of the connective tissue.

desmosis f. desmosis, disease of the connective tissue.

desnaturalización f. denaturation, change of the usual nature of a substance as by adding methanol or acetone to alcohol.

desnervado-a a. denervated, deprived of nerve supply.

desnivel m. unevenness.

desnudarse vr. to undress.

desnudo-a a. naked, bare.

desnutrido-a a. undernourished, malnourished, underfed.

desodorante m. deodorant.

desodorizar vi. to deodorize, to remove fetid or unpleasant odors.

desorden m. disorder, abnormal condition of the body or mind.

desordenado-a a. disorderly, unorganized.

desorganización f. disorganization.

desorganizado-a a. disorganized, unstructured.

desorientado-a a. disoriented, confused.

desosificación f. deossification, loss or removal of minerals from the bones.

desoxicorticosterona f. deoxycorticosterone, steroid hormone produced in the cortex of the adrenal glands that has a marked effect on the metabolism of water and electrolytes.

desoxigenación f. deoxygenation, process of removing oxygen.

desoxigenado-a a. deoxygenated, lacking oxygen.

despacio adv. slow, slowly.

despejado-a a. clear, cloudless; [persona] smart, vivacious.

despellejarse vr. to peel; to shed skin.

desperdiciar vt. to waste, to squander.

desperdicio m. waste.

despersonalización f. depersonalization, loss of identity.

despierto-a a., pp. de **despertar,** awake; diligent.

despigmentación f. depigmentation, abnormal change in the color of skin and hair.

despiojamiento m. delousing, freeing the body from lice.

desplazamiento

desplazamiento *m.* 1. displacement;
___ **del cristalino** / dislocation of the
lens; 2. transfer of emotion from the
original idea or situation to a different
one.

desplazar *vi.* to displace.

despliegue *m.* display, exhibition.

desprender *vt.* to loosen, to unfasten;
desprenderse *vr.* to become loose.

desprendimiento *m.* detachment,
separation.

desproporción *f.* disproportion.

desproporcionado-a *a.*
disproportionate.

después *adv.* after, afterward.

despuntado-a *a.* [*instrumento*]
blunt.

destapar *v.* to uncover.

destemplanza *f.* distemper,
indisposition, any disorder with a
general feeling of discomfort.

desteñir *vi.* to fade; **desteñirse** *vr.* to
become faded.

destetado-a *f.* weanling.

destetar *v.* to wean, to adjust an infant
to a form of nourishment other than
breast or bottle feeding.

destete *m.* delactation, discontinued
breastfeeding; weaning.

destilado-a *a.* distilled; **agua** ___ / ___
water.

destorsión *f.* detorsion, detortion.
1. surgical correction of a testicular or
intestinal torsion; 2. correction of the
curvature or malformation of a
structure.

destoxicación, destoxificación
f. detoxification, reduction of the toxic
quality.

destreza *f.* skill.

destruido-a *a.* destroyed; exhausted,
physically or emotionally.

desunión *f.* disengagement.
1. emergence of the fetal head from
the vulva; 2. separation.

desvalido-a *a.* destitute, helpless,
handicapped.

desvanecerse *vr. vi.* to black out; to
swoon.

desvelado-a *a.* unable to sleep,
wakeful.

desvelarse *vr.* to stay awake at night.

desvelo *m.* insomnia.

desventaja *f.* disadvantage; diminished
capacity.

desvestir *vi.* to strip; **desvestirse** *vr.* to
undress.

desviación, desvío *f., m.* deviation,
shunt. 1. departure from the established
path; 2. mental
aberration.

desviar *v.* to shunt, to change course;
desviarse *vr.* to deviate.

detalle *m.* detail.

detección *f.* detection; ___ **temprana** /
early detection.

detener *vi.* to detain, to stop.

deterioración, deterioro *f., m.*
deterioration, wear, decay.

deteriorarse *vr.* to deteriorate.

determinación *f.* determination;
decision; resolution; ___ **propia** /
self- ___ .

determinado-a *a.* determined,
strong-minded; [*una prueba*] proven.

determinante *m.* determinant,
prevailing element; *a.* rel. to a
prevailing element or cause.

determinar *vt.* to determine.

detestar *v.* to hate, to abhor.

detrás (de) *adv.* behind, in back of.

detrito *m.* debris, detritus, residue of
disintegrating matter.

detrusor *m.* detrusor, muscle that expels
or projects outward.

deuteranopía *f.* deuteranopia,
blindness to the color green.

devitalizar *vt.* to devitalize, to
debilitate; to deprive from vital force.

devolución *f.* devolution. catabolismo.

devolver *vt.* to return, to give back.

Dexedrina *f.* Dexedrine, amphetamine
type drug that stimulates the nervous
system.

dextrocardia *f.* dextrocardia,
dislocation of the heart to the right.

dextrómano-a *m.* dextromanual,
person who gives preference to the use
of the right hand.

dextrosa *f.* dextrose, form of glucose
in the blood popularly called grape
sugar.

dextroversión *f.* dextroversion, turn to
the right.

día *m.* day; **de** ___ / daytime, daylight;
(dos, tres) veces al ___ / (two, three)
times a ___ ; **todo el** ___ / all ___ .

diabetes *f.* diabetes, a disease
manifested by excessive urination. This
term is often used in reference to
diabetes mellitus.

diabetes insípida *f.* diabetes
insipidus, type of diabetes caused by a
deficiency in antidiuretic hormone.

dicigótico-a

diabetes mellitus *f.* diabetes mellitus, diabetes caused by insufficient production or use of insulin and resulting in hyperglycemia and glycosuria; __ **con dependencia de insulina** / insulin-dependent __; __ **sin dependencia de insulina** / noninsulin-dependent __ .

diabético-a *a.* diabetic, rel. to or suffering from diabetes; **angiopatías** __ **-s** / __ angiopathies; **choque** __ / __ **shock**; **coma** __ / __ **coma**; **inestable** / brittle __; **dieta** __ / __ diet; **neuropatía** __ / __ neuropathy; **retinopatía** __ / __ retinopathy.

diabetógrafo *m.* diabetograph, instrument used to determine the proportion of glucose in the urine.

diacetemia *f.* diacetemia, presence of diacetic acid in the blood.

diacetilmorfina *f.* diacetylmorphine, heroin.

diáfisis *f.* diaphysis, shaft or middle part of a long, cylindrical bone such as the humerus.

diaforesis *f.* diaphoresis, excessive perspiration caused by a high body temperature due to strenuous physical exercise or to high heat.

diafragma *m.* diaphragm. 1. muscle that separates the thorax and the abdomen; 2. contraceptive device.

diagnosticar *vt.* to diagnose.

diagnóstico, diagnosis *m. f.* diagnosis, determination of the patient's ailment; __ **computado** / computer __; __ **de imágenes por medios radioactivos** / __ imaging; __ **diferencial** / differential __; **equivocado o erróneo** / misdiagnosis; __ **físico** / physical __; __ **propio** / autodiagnosis; **errores de** __ / diagnostic errors.

diagonal *a.* diagonal.

diálisis *f.* dialysis, procedure used to filter and eliminate waste products from the blood of patients with renal insufficiency; **aparato de** __ [**riñón artificial**] / __ machine; __ **peritoneal** / peritoneal __ .

dializado *m.* dialysate, the part of the liquid that goes through the dializing membrane in dialysis; **-a** *a.* dialyzed, having been separated by dialysis.

dializador *m.* dialyzer, device used in dialysis.

dializar *vt.* to dialyze.

diámetro *m.* diameter.

Diana, complejo de *m.* Diana's complex, adoption by a woman of masculine characteristics and conduct.

diapasón *m.* diapason, U-shaped metal device used to determine the degree of deafness.

diapédesis *f.* diapedesis, passage of blood cells, esp. leukocytes, through the intact walls of a capillary vessel.

diapositiva *f.* slide.

diario-a *a.* daily; **-mente** *adv.* daily.

diarrea *f.* diarrhea; __ **del viajero** / traveler's __; __ **disentérica** / dysenteric __; __ **emocional** / emotional __; __ **estival** / summer __; __ **infantil** / infantile __; __ **licentírica** / lienteric __; __ **mucosa** / mucous __; __ **nerviosa** / nervous __; __ **pancreática** / pancreatic __; __ **purulenta** / purulent __ .

diastasa *f.* diastase, enzyme that acts in the digestion of starches and sugars.

diastasis *f.* diastasis. 1. separation of normally attached bones; 2. the rest period of the cardiac cycle, just before systole.

diástole *f.* diastole, dilation period of the heart during which the cardiac chambers are filled with blood.

diastólico-a *a.* diastolic, rel. to the diastole; **presión** __ / __ pressure, the lowest pressure point in the cardiovascular system.

diatermia *f.* diathermy, application of heat to body tissues through an electric current.

diatesis *f.* diathesis, organic disposition to contract certain diseases; __ **hemorrágica** / hemorrhagic __; __ **reumática** / rheumatic __ .

diatrizoato de meglumina *m.* diatrizoate meglumine, radiopaque substance used to visualize arteries and veins of the heart and the brain as well as the gallbladder, kidneys, and urinary bladder.

diazepam *m.* diazepam, Valium, drug used as a tranquilizer and muscle relaxer.

diccionario *m.* dictionary.

dicigótico-a *a.* dizygotic, rel. to twins derived from two separate fertilized ova.

dicloxacilina

dicloxacilina *f.* dicloxacillim sodium, semi-synthetic penicillin used against gram-positive organisms.

dicotomía *f.* dichotomy, dichotomization, process of dividing into two parts.

dicromatismo *m.* dichromatism, the property of presenting two different colors.

dicrómico-a *a.* dichromic, rel. to two colors.

dicroto-a *a.* dicrotic, having two pulse beats for each heartbeat.

didelfo-a *a.* didelphic, rel. to a double uterus.

didimitis *f.* orquiditis, orquitis.

diembrionismo *m.* diembryony, production of two embryos from a single egg.

diencéfalo *m.* diencephalon, part of the brain.

dienestrol *m.* dienestrol, synthetic nonsteroid estrogen.

diente *m.* tooth (*pl.* teeth); ___ **desviado** / wandering ___; ___ **impactado** / impacted ___; ___ **incisivo** / incisor; ___ **molar** / wall ___; ___ **no erupcionado** / unerupted ___; ___ **-s deciduos, de leche** / deciduous teeth, baby teeth; ___ **-s permanentes** / permanent teeth; ___ **-s postizos** / denture; ___ **-s secundarios** / second teeth.

diestro-a *a.* dexter, rel. to the right side; righthanded.

dieta *f.* diet; ___ **alta en fibra** / high fiber ___; ___ **alta en residuos (fibras celulosas)** / high-residue ___; ___ **baja en grasa** / low in fat ___; ___ **balanceada** / balanced ___; ___ **blanda** / bland ___; ___ **diabética** / diabetic ___; ___ **hospitalaria** / ward ___; ___ **libre de gluten** / gluten-free ___; ___ **líquida** / liquid ___; ___ **macrocítica** / macrocytic ___; ___ **para bajar de peso** / weight reduction ___; ___ **rica en calorías** / high-calorie ___; ___ **sin sal** / salt-free

dieta de eliminación *f.* elimination diet, diet that results from eliminating those nutrients that can produce an allergic reaction on the patient.

dietética *f.* dietetics, the science of regulating diets to preserve or recuperate health.

dietético-a *a.* dietetic, rel. to diets.

dietilamida de ácido lisérgico *f.* lysergic acid diethylamide, LSD.

dietilestilbestrol *m.* diethylstilbestrol, synthetic estrogen compound.

dietista *m., f.* dietitian, nutrition specialist.

diezma *f.* decimation, high mortality rate.

difalo *a.* diphallus, partial or complete duplication of the penis.

difásico-a *a.* diphasic, that occurs in two different stages.

difenhidramina *f.* diphenhydramine, Benadryl, antihistamine.

diferencia *f.* difference.

diferenciación *f.* differentiation, distinction of one substance, disease, or entity from another.

diferencial *a.* differential, rel. to differentiation.

diferente *a.* different.

diferir *vi.* to disagree.

difícil *a.* difficult.

dificultad *f.* difficulty.

difonía *f.* diphonia, double voice.

difracción *f.* diffraction, the breaking up of a ray of light into its component parts when it passes through a glass or a prism; **patrón de** ___ / ___ pattern.

difteria *f.* diphtheria, acute infectious and contagious disease caused by the bacillus *Corynebacterium diphtheriae* (Klebs-Loffler bacillus) characterized by the formation of false membranes esp. in the throat; **antitoxina contra la** ___ / ___ antitoxin.

difterotoxina *f.* diphtherotoxin, toxin derived from cultures of diphtheria bacillus.

difunto-a *a.* deceased.

difusión *f.* diffusion. 1. the process of becoming widely spread; 2. dialysis through a membrane.

difuso-a *a.* diffused; extended; **absceso** ___ / ___ abscess; **lesión extensa** ___ / ___ injury; **mastocitosis cutánea** ___ / ___ cutaneous mastocytosis.

digerible, digestible *a.* digestible.

digerido-a *a.* digested; **no** ___ / undigested.

digerir *vt.* to digest.

digestión *f.* digestion, transformation of liquids and solids into simpler substances that can be absorbed easily by the body; ___ **gástrica** / gastric ___; ___ **intestinal** / intestinal ___; ___ **pancreática** / pancreatic ___ .

digestivo *m.* digestant, digestive, an agent that assists in the digestive process.

digitalis *f.* digitalis, cardiotonic agent obtained from the dried leaves of Digitalis purpurea; **intoxicación por** __ / __ toxicity, poisoning

digitalización *f.* digitalization, therapeutic use of digitalis.

digitiforme *a.* finger-shaped.

dígito *m.* digit, digitus, finger or toe.

digitoxina *f.* digitoxin, cardiotonic glycoside obtained from *Digitalis purpurea* used in the treatment of congestive heart failure.

digoxina *f.* digoxin, cardiotonic glycoside obtained from *Digitalis purpurea* used in the treatment of cardiac arrhythmia.

dihidroestreptomicina *f.* dihydrostreptomycin, antibiotic derived from and used more commonly than streptomycin as it causes less neurotoxicity.

dilatación *f.* dilation, stretching; normal or abnormal enlargement of an organ or orifice; __ **de la pupila** / __ of the pupil.

dilatador *m.* dilator, stretcher. 1. muscle that on contraction dilates an organ; 2. device used to enlarge cavities or an opening; __ **de Hegar** / Hegar's __, used to enlarge the cervical canal.

dilatar *vt.* to dilate, to expand.

dilaudid *m.* dilaudid, opium-derived drug that can produce dependence.

diluente *m.* diluent, agent that has the property of diluting.

diluir *vt.* to dilute; __ **con agua** / to water down; **sin** __ / undiluted.

dimetilsulfóxido *m.* dimethyl sulfoxide, analgesic and anti-inflammatory agent.

dimetría *f.* dimetria, double uterus.

diminuir, disminuir *vt.* to diminish.

diminuto-a *a.* minute, very small.

dimorfismo *m.* dimorphism, occurring in two different forms; __ **sexual, hermafroditismo** / sexual __, hermaphrodism.

dina *f.* dyne, unit of force needed to accelerate one gram of mass one centimeter per second.

dinámica *f.* dynamics, the study of organs or parts of the body in movement.

dinámico-a *a.* dynamic.

dinamómetro *m.* dynamometer. 1. instrument used to measure muscular strength; 2. device that determines the magnifying power of a lens.

dinero *m.* money.

dioptómetro *m.* dioptometer, instrument used to measure ocular refraction.

dióptrica *f.* dioptrics, the science that studies the refraction of light.

dióptrico-a *a.* dioptric, rel. to the refraction of light.

Dios *m.* God.

dióxido de carbono *m.* carbon dioxide.

diplacusia *f.* diplacusis, hearing disorder characterized by the perception of two tones for every sound produced.

diplejía *f.* diplegia, bilateral paralysis; __ **espástica** / spastic __; __ **facial** / facial __ .

diplocoria *f.* diplocoria, double pupil.

diploe *m.* diploe, spongy layer that lies between the two flat compact plates of the cranial bones.

diploide *a.* diploid, having two sets of chromosomes.

diplópagos *m.* diplopagus, conjoined twins, each with fairly complete bodies but sharing some organs.

diplopía *f.* diplopia, double vision.

dipsógeno *m.* dipsogen, thirst-causing agent.

dipsomanía *f.* dipsomania, recurring, uncontrollable urge to drink alcohol.

dirección *f.* direction; address.

directo-a *a.* direct, in a straight line; uninterrupted; **-mente** *adv.* directly.

directrices *f.* guidelines.

dirigir *vt.* to direct; to guide.

disacusia, disacusis *f.* dysacusia, dysacousis, difficulty in hearing.

disafea *f.* dysaphia, impaired sense of touch.

disartria *f.* dysarthria, unclear speech due to impairment of the tongue or any other muscle related to speech.

disasimilación *f.* disassimilation, destructive metabolism.

disautonomía *f.* dysautonomy, hereditary disorder of the autonomic nervous system.

disbarismo *m.* dysbarism, condition caused by decompression.

disbasia *f.* dysbasia, difficulty in walking gen. caused by nervous lesions.

disbulia *f.* dysbulia, inability to concentrate.

discefalia *f.* dyscephalia, malformation of the head and the facial bones.

discinesia *f.* dyskinesia, inability to perform voluntary movements.

disciplina *f.* discipline, strict behavior.

disco *m.* disk; __ **desplazado** / slipped __; __ **óptico** / optic __; **ruptura de** __ / __ rupture.

discógeno-a *a.* discogenic, rel. to an intervertebral disk.

discografía *f.* x-ray of a vertebral disk following injection of a radiopaque substance.

discoide *a.* discoid, shaped like a disk.

discordancia *f.* discordance, the absence of a genetic trait in one of a pair of twins.

discoria *f.* dyscoria, abnormal shape of the pupil.

discrasia *f.* dyscrasia, synonym of disease.

discrepancia *f.* discrepancy.

discriminación *f.* discrimination, differentiation of race or quality.

discriminar *vt.* to discriminate.

discusión *f.* discussion, argument, debate.

diseminación *f.* dissemination, spreading.

diseminado-a *a.* disseminated, spread out over a large area.

disentería *f.* dysentery, painful infl. of the intestines, esp. of the colon, gen. caused by bacteria or parasites and accompanied by diarrhea; __ **amebiana** / amebic __; __ **bacilar** / bacillary __ .

disentir *vi.* to disagree, to have an opposite view.

diseño *m.* design; **drogas de** __ / __ drugs; **estrógeno por** __ / __ estrogen.

disestesia *f.* dysesthesia, impaired sense of touch.

disfagia *f.* dysphagia, difficulty in swallowing; __ **esofágica** / esophageal __; __ **orofaríngea** / oropharyngeal __ .

disfasia *f.* dysphasia, speech impairment caused by a brain lesion.

disfonía *f.* dysphonia, hoarseness.

disforia *f.* dysphoria, severe depression.

disfrutar *vt.* to enjoy.

disfuncional *a.* dysfunctional.

disgenesia *f.* dysgenesis, malformation.

disgerminoma *m.* dysgerminoma, malignant tumor in the ovary.

dishidrosis *f.* dyshidrosis, anomaly of the sweating function.

dislalia *f.* dyslalia, speech impairment due to functional anomalies of the speech organ.

dislexia *f.* dyslexia, reading disorder, sometimes hereditary or caused by a brain lesion.

dislocación, dislocadura *f.* dislocation, displacement; __ **cerrada** / closed __, simple; __ **complicada** / complicated __; __ **congénita** / congenital __ .

dislocado-a *a.* dislocated

dismenorrea, dismenia *f.* dysmenorrhea, painful and difficult menstruation.

dismetría *f.* dysmetria, impaired ability to control range of movement in a coordinated fashion.

disminución *f.* diminution, reducing process; __ **de lágrimas** / __ of tears; __ **del rendimiento urinario** / urine output __; __ **de saliva** / saliva __ .

disminuir *vi.* to diminish, to reduce, to lessen. __ **la dosis** / to reduce the dosage.

dismiotonía *f.* dysmyotonia, abnormal muscular tonicity.

dismnesia *f.* dysmnesia, impaired memory.

dismorfismo *m.* dysmorphism, capacity of a parasite or agent to change its shape.

disnea, dispnea *f.* dispnoea, dyspnea, shortness of breath; __ **paroxística nocturna** / paroxysmal nocturnal dyspnea; __ **por esfuerzo** / exertional __ .

disneico-a *a.* dyspneic, rel. to or suffering from dyspnea.

disociación *f.* dissociation, split. 1. the action and effect of separating; 2. decomposition of a molecular aggregate in a simpler one; 3. unconscious split of personality, a characteristic of schizophrenia; __ **atrial** / __ atrial; __ **atrioventricular** / __ atrioventricular; __ **de la personalidad** / split personality; __ **del sueño** / sleep __; __ **pupilar** / pupillar __; __ **visual quinética** / visual-kinetic __ .

disoluble *a.* dissoluble.

disolución *f.* dissolution, decomposition; death.

disolvente *m.* dissolvent; *a.* capable of being dissolved.

disolver *vi.* to dissolve, to liquify.

disonancia *f.* dissonance, combination of tones that produces an unpleasant sound.

disosmia *f.* dysosmia, impaired smell.

disostosis *f.* dysostosis, abnormal bone growth.

dispareunia *f.* dispareunia, painful coitus.

disparidad *f.* disparity, inequality.

dispensar *vt.* to dispense, to distribute.

dispensario *m.* dispensary, a place that provides medical assistance and dispenses medicines and drugs.

dispepsia *f.* dyspepsia, indigestion characterized by irregularities in the digestive process such as eructation, nausea, acidity, flatulence, and loss of appetite.

dispermia *f.* dyspermia, pain on ejaculation.

dispigmentación *f.* dyspigmentation, abnormal change in the color of the skin and hair.

displasia *f.* dysplasia, abnormal development of the tissues; __ cervical / cervical __ .

displásico-a *a.* rel. to dysplasia.

disponer *vt.* to arrange, to prepare.

disponibilidad *f.* availability.

disponible *a.* available.

disposición *f.* disposition, tendency to acquire certain disease.

dispositivo *m.* device, mechanism; __ intrauterino / intrauterine __ .

dispraxia *f.* dyspraxia, pain or difficulty in performing coordinated movements.

disrreflexia *f.* dysreflexia, disruption of the autonomic nervous system causing reactions and stimuli to be inappropriate and out of order.

disrritmia *f.* dysrhythmia, any alteration of a rhythm.

distal *a.* distal, farthermost away from the beginning or center of a structure.

distancia *f.* distance.

distasia *f.* dystasia, difficulty in maintaining a standing position.

distensibilidad *f.* distensibility, capacity of a structure to be extended, dilated, or enlarged in size.

distensión *f.* distension, distention, dilation; __ gaseosa / gas __ , resulting from accumulation of gas in the abdominal cavity.

distinguido-a *a.* [*persona o característica*] distinguished.

distinguir *vi.* to distinguish, to differentiate.

distinto-a *a.* different.

distobucal *a.* distobuccal, rel. to the distal and buccal surfaces of a tooth.

distocia *f.* dystocia, difficult labor.

distoclusión *f.* distoclusion, defective closure, irregular bite.

distonía *f.* dystonia, defective tonicity, esp. muscular.

distorsión *f.* distorsion, bending or twisting out of shape.

distracción *f.* distraction. 1. separation of the surfaces of a joint without dislocation; 2. inability to concentrate or fix the mind on a given experience.

distribución *f.* breakdown, distribution; __ detallada / detailed __.

distribuir *vt.* to distribute.

distrofia *f.* dystrophy, degenerative disorder caused by defective nutrition or metabolism.

distrofia muscular *f.* muscular dystrophy, slow, progressive muscular degeneration.

disuelto-a *a. pp.* de **disolver,** dissolved.

disulfiram *m.* disulfiram, Antabuse, drug used in the treatment of alcoholism.

disuria *f.* dysuria, difficult urination.

diuresis *f.* diuresis, increased excretion of urine.

diurético *m.* diuretic, agent that causes increased urination; *pop.* water pill.

divergencia *f.* divergence, spreading apart, separation from a common center.

divergente *a.* divergent, moving in different directions.

diverticulectomía *f.* diverticulectomy, removal of a diverticulum.

diverticulitis *f.* diverticulitis, infl. of a diverticulum.

divertículo *m.* diverticulum, pouch or sac that originates from a hollow organ or structure.

diverticulosis *f.* diverticulosis, presence of diverticula in the colon; __ vesical / vesical __ .

divertirse *vr.*, *vi.* to have fun.

dividido-a *a.* divided.

dividir *vt.* to divide, to disunite; to split.

divorciado-a *a.* divorced.

doblarse vr. to bend; __ hacia adelante / __ forward; __ hacia atrás / __ backward.

doble m. double; a. double; __ útero / __ uterus.

docena f. dozen.

doctor-a m., f. doctor.

documentación f. documentation.

doler vi. to be in pain; to ache.

dolicocefálico-a a. dolichocephalic, having a narrow, long head.

dolor m. pain; __ agudo / acute __; __ cólico / colicky __; __ constante / constant __; __ de oído / earache __; __ fuerte / strong __; __ leve / mild __; __ localizado / localized __; __ opresivo / oppressive __; __ oprimente / pressing __; __ penetrante / penetrating __; __ profundo / deep __; __ quemante / burning __; __ referido / __ referred; __ sordo / dull __; __ sujetivo / subjective __.

doloroso-a a. painful.

doméstico-a a. domestic.

dominante a. dominant, predominant; características __ -s / __ characteristics.

donación f. donation.

donante m. donor; tarjeta de __ / __'s card.

donante universal m. universal donor, individual belonging to blood group O or whose blood can be given to persons belonging to any other of the AB blood groups with minimal risk of complication.

donde adv. where.

dondequiera adv. anywhere; everywhere.

Donovanía granulomatosis f. Donovania granulomatosis, Donovan's body, bacterial infection that affects the skin and the mucous membranes of the genitalia and the anal area.

dopado pp. of **dopar**, doping, to estimate the potency of a drug dose.

dopamina f. dopamine, substance synthesized by the adrenal glands that increases blood pressure and is gen. used in shock treatment.

Doppler, técnica de f. Doppler's technique, based in the fact that the frequency of the ultrasonic waves changes when these are reflected in a moving surface.

dormido-a a. asleep; profundamente __ / sound __ .

dormir vi. to sleep; **dormirse** vr. to fall asleep.

dorsal a. dorsal, rel. to the back; fisura o corte __ / __ slit.

dorsalgia f. dorsalgia, backache.

dorsiflexión f. dorsiflexion, bending backward.

dorso m. dorsum, posterior part, such as the back of the hand or the body.

dorsocefálico-a a. dorsocephalic, rel. to the back of the head.

dorsodinia f. dorsodynia, pain in the muscles of the upper part of the back.

dorsoespinal a. dorsospinal, rel. to the back and the spine.

dorsolateral a. dorsolateral, rel. to the back and the side.

dorsolumbar a. dorsolumbar, rel. to the lower thoracic and upper lumbar vertebrae area of the back.

dosis, dosificación f. dose. 1. the giving of medication or other therapeutic agents in prescribed amounts; 2. in nuclear medicine, quantity of radiopharmaco given; __ acumulada / cumulative __; __ curativa / curative __; __ de absorción / absortion __; __ de bolo, intravenosa / bolus __, intravenous; __ de exposición / exposure __; __ de la médula ósea / bone marrow __; __ de reducción / reduction __; __ de refuerzo / booster __; __ dermal / skin __; __ diaria / daily __; __ dividida / divided __; __ efectiva / effective __; __ equivalente / equivalent __; __ individual / unit __; __ inicial / initial __; __ integral / integral __; __ máxima / maximal __; __ mínima letal / minimal lethal __; __ mínima reactiva / minimal reacting __; __ óptima / optimum __; __ preventiva / preventive __; __ subletal / sublethal __, of insufficient amount to cause death; __ terapéutica / therapeutic __; __ tolerada / tolerance __; __ umbral / threshold __, minimal dose needed to produce an effect; máxima __ permitida / maximal permissible __; máxima __ tolerable / maximum tolerated __ .

Douglas, placa (saco) de m. Douglas cul-de-sac, peritoneal pouch between the uterus and the rectum.

Down, síndrome de m. Down syndrome, chromosomal abnormality that causes physical deformity and moderate to severe mental retardation.

dramamina *f.* dramamine, antihistamine used in the prevention and treatment of motion sickness.

dramatismo *m.* dramatism, pompous behavior and language, gen. seen in mental disorders.

drapetomanía, dromomanía *f.* drapetomania, dromomania, abnormal impulse to wander.

drástico *m.* drastic, strong cathartic; **-a** *a.* extreme, very strong.

drenaje *m.* drainage, outlet; __ **abierto** / open __; __ **postural** / postural __, that allows drainage by gravity; **tubo de** __ / __ tube.

drenar *v.* to drain, to draw off fluid or pus from a cavity or an infected wound.

droga *f.* drug; medication; **abuso de la** __ / __ abuse; **anomalías causadas por la** __ / __ anomalies; __ **adictiva** / dependence producing __; __ **de acción prolongada** / long-acting __; __ **neuroléptica** / neuroleptic __, causing symptoms similar to those manifested by nervous diseases; **entregarse a la** __ / to become __ addicted; **resistencia microbiana a la** __ / __ resistance, microbial.

drogadicción *f.* drug addiction.

drogadicto-a *m., f.* drug addict.

dromotrópico-a *a.* dromotropic, that affects the conductibility of muscular and nervous fibers.

dúctulo *m.* ductule, a very small conduit; *a.* ductile, allowing deformation without breaking.

ductus *m.* ductus, duct.

ducha *f.* douche, jet of water applied to the body for medicinal or cleansing effects; shower; *vr.* **darse una** __, **ducharse** / to shower.

duda *f.* doubt.

dudar *v.* to doubt, to question.

dudoso-a *a.* doubtful.

duela *f.* fluke, parasitic worm of the *Trematoda* family; __ **hepática** / liver __; __ **intestinal** / intestinal __; __ **pulmonar** / lung __; __ **sanguínea** / blood __ .

dulce *a.* sweet.

dulces *m. pl.* [*golosinas*] sweets.

dulcificante *m.* sweetener.

duodenal *a.* duodenal, rel. to the duodenum.

duodenectomía *f.* duodenectomy, partial or total excision of the duodenum.

duodenitis *f.* duodenitis, infl. of the duodenum.

duodeno *m.* duodenum, essential part of the alimentary tract situated between the pylorus and the jejunum.

duodenoenterostomía *f.* duodenoenterostomy, anastomosis between the duodenum and the small intestine.

duodenoscopía *f.* duodenoscopy, endoscopic examination of the duodenum.

duodenostomía *f.* duodenostomy, opening into the duodenum through the abdominal wall to alleviate stenosis of the pylorus.

duodenotomía *f.* duodenotomy, incision of the duodenum.

duodenoyeyunostomía *f.* duodenojejunostomy, creation of a communication between the duodenum and the jejunum.

durabilidad *f.* durability; duration.

durable *a.* durable, lasting.

duración *f.* duration; continuation.

duramadre, duramáter *f.* dura mater, the outer membrane that covers the encephalum and the spinal cord.

durante *prep.* during; lasting; __ **los días de invierno** / __ winter days.

durar *v.* to last; to endure.

dureza *f.* hardness.

duro-a *a.* hard, firm.

E *abr.* **emetropía** / emmetropia; **enema** / enema; **enzima** / enzyme.

e *conj.* and.

ebrio-a *a.* drunk.

ebullición *f.* ebullition, boiling; **punto de __** / boiling point.

echar *vt.* to throw; **__ una carta** / to mail a letter; **__ una mirada** / to give a look; **echarse** *vr.* [food] **echarse a perder** / to go bad.

Echinococcus *L.* Echinococcus. equinococo.

Echo, virus *m.* echovirus, any of a group of viruses found in the gastrointestinal tract, associated with meningitis and enteritis.

eclampsia *f.* eclampsia, toxic, convulsive disorder that usu. occurs near the end of pregnancy or right after delivery.

eco *m.* echo, repercussion of sound.

ecocardiografía *f.* echocardiography, diagnostic procedure that uses sound waves (ultrasound) to visualize the internal structures of the heart; **__ transesofágica** / transesophageal __ .

ecocardiograma *m.* echocardiogram, ultrasonic record obtained by an echocardiography.

ecoencefalografía *f.* echoencephalography, diagnostic procedure that sends sound waves (ultrasound) to the brain structure and records the returning echoes.

ecografía *f.* echography, ultrasonografía.

ecograma *m.* echogram, graphic representation of an echography.

ecolalia *f.* echolalia, disorder manifested by involuntary repetition of words spoken by another person.

ecología *f.* ecology, the study of plants and animals and their relationship to the environment.

ecológico-a *a.* ecological; **sistema __** / __ system.

económico-a *a.* economical, economic.

ecosistema *f.* ecosystem, ecologic microcosm.

ectasia *f.* ectasia, ectasis, expansion of a part of an organ.

ectópico-a *a.* ectopic, rel. to ectopia.

ectoplasma *m.* ectoplasm, external membrane surrounding the cell cytoplasm.

ectropión *m.* ectropion, eversion of the margin of a body part, such as the eyelid.

ecuador *m.* equator, imaginary line that divides a body in two equal parts.

eczema, eccema *m.* eczema, inflammatory, noncontagious skin disease.

edad *f.* age; **__ cronológica** / chronological __; **de __ avanzada** / elderly; **mayor de__** / __ of consent; **menor de __** / under __, a minor.

edad gestacional *f.* gestational age, estimated age of a fetus counted by weeks of gestation.

edema *m.* edema, abnormal amount of fluid in the intercellular tissue; **__ angioneurótico** / angioneurotic __; **__ cardíaco** / cardiac __; **__ cerebral** / cerebral __; **__ de fóvea** / pitting __; **__ dependiente** / dependent __; **__ pulmonar** / pulmonary __ .

educación *f.* education.

educar *vt.* to educate.

efectividad *f.* effectiveness.

efectivo-a *a.* effective; **en __** / cash; **-mente** *adv.* in effect, actually.

efecto *m.* effect, impression; result; **__ secundario** / side __ .

efector *m.* effector, nerve ending that produces an efferent action on muscles and glands.

efedrina *f.* ephedrine, adrenalinelike drug used chiefly as a bronchodilator.

eferente *a.* efferent, centrifugal, that pulls away from the center.

efervescente *a.* effervescent, that produces gas bubbles.

efluente *a.* effluent, flowing out.

efusión *f.* effusion, escape of fluid into a cavity or tissue; **__ pericardial** / pericardial __; **pleural** / pleural __ .

ego *m.* ego, the self, human consciousness.

egocéntrico-a *a.* egocentric, self-centered.

egoísmo *m.* selfishness, self-centeredness.

egoísta *m., f.* selfish person; *a.* selfish.

egomanía *f.* egomania, excessive self-esteem.

egreso *m.* output; [*dar de alta*] discharge; **sumario de __** / discharge summary.

eje *m.* axis.

ejemplo *m.* example.

ejercer *vi.* [*una profesión*] to practice; [*autoridad*] to exercise.

ejercicio *m.* exercise; **__ activo** / active **__**; **__ aeróbico** / aerobic **__**; **__ correctivo** / corrective **__**; **__ de respiración profunda** / deep-breathing **__**; **__ físico** / physical **__**; **__ isométrico** / isometric **__**; **__ isotónico** / isotonic **__**; **__ para adelgazar** / reducing **__**; **__ pasivo** / passive **__** .

elástico *m.* elastic; **-a** *a.* elastic, that can be returned to its original shape after being extended or distorted; **tejido __** / **__ tissue**.

electivo-a *a.* elective, optional; **terapia __** / **__ therapy**; **cirugía __** / **__ surgery**

electricidad *f.* electricity.

eléctrico-a *a.* electric, electrical; **corriente __** / **__ current**.

electrocardiograma *m.* electrocardiogram, graphic record of the changes in the electric currents produced by the contractions of the heart muscle; **__ de esfuerzo** / exercise **__** .

electrocauterización *m.* electrocauterization, destruction of tissues by an electric current.

electrocirugía *f.* electrosurgery, use of electric current in surgical procedures.

electrochoque *m.* electroshock, electroconvulsive therapy, treatment of some mental disorders by applying an electric current to the brain.

electrodiagnosis *f.* electrodiagnosis, the use of electronic devices to use for diagnostic purposes.

electrodo *m.* electrode, a medium between the electric current and the object to which the current is applied.

electroencefalografía *f.* electroencephalography, registering of the electrical currents produced in the brain.

electrofisiología *f.* electrophysiology, the study of the relationship between physiological processes and electrical phenomena.

electroforesis *f.* electrophoresis, movement of coloidal particles suspended in a medium charged with an electric current that separates them, such as occurs in the separation of proteins in plasma.

electrólisis *f.* electrolysis, destruction or disintegration by means of an electric current.

electrólito *m.* electrolyte, ion that carries an electrical charge.

electromagnético-a *a.* electromagnetic.

electromiografía *f.* electromyography. 1. recording of muscular activity for diagnostic use; 2. any type of study done in a recording studio including studies on neurologic conduction.

electromiograma *m.* electromyogram, graphic report obtained by electromyography.

electrónico-a *a.* electronic; **monitoreo fetal __** / **__ fetal monitoring**.

electroretinograma *n.* electroretinogram, graphic recording of the electric activity of the retina.

electroversión *f.* cardioversion, termination of a cardiac dysrhythmia by electric means.

elefantiasis *f.* elephantiasis, chronic disease produced by obstruction of the lymphatic vessels, hypertrophy of the skin and subcutaneous cellular tissue, affecting most frequently the legs and scrotum.

elegible *a.* eligible, qualified for selection.

elegir *vt.* to elect, to choose.

elemental *a.* elemental; rudimentary.

elemento *m.* element.

elemento radiactivo *m.* radioactive element.

elevación *f.* elevation.

elevado-a *a.* elevated, raised.

elevador *m.* elevator. 1. surgical device used for lifting a sunken part or for elevating tissues; 2. elevator.

eliminar *vt.* to eliminate; to discard waste from the body.

elixir *m.* elixir, aromatic, sweet liquor containing an active medicinal ingredient.

emaciado-a *a.* excessively thin.

embalsamamiento *m.* embalming, treatment of a dead body to retard its decay.

embarazada *a.* pregnant.

embarazo *m.* pregnancy; ___ **de probeta** / test-tube ___; ___ **ectópico** / ectopic ___, extrauterine; ___ **falso** / false ___, enlargement of the abdomen simulating pregnancy; ___ **intersticial** / interstitial ___, located in the part of the uterine tube within the wall of the uterus; ___ **múltiple** / multiple ___, more than one fetus in the uterus at the same time; ___ **prolongado** / prolonged ___, beyond full term; ___ **subrogado** / surrogate ___; ___ **tubárico** / tubal ___, when the egg develops in the Fallopian tube; ___ **tuboabdominal** / tuboabdominal ___; **prueba del ___** / ___ test.

embarazo ampular *m.* ampular pregnancy. *Syn.* **embarazo tubular**.

embarazo tubárico *n.* tubal pregnancy, fallopian pregnancy, situated near the mid portion of the oviduct.

embolia, embolismo *f., m.* embolism, sudden obstruction of a cerebral artery by a loose piece of clot, plaque, fat, or air bubble; ___ **cerebral** / cerebral ___, stroke; ___ **gaseosa** / air ___; **embolismo pulmonar** / pulmonary ___ .

embolia amniótica *f.* amniotic fluid embolism usually occurring during labor, complication of the gestational cycle that can cause death.

émbolo *m.* embolus, clot of blood or other material that when traveling through the blood-stream becomes lodged in a vessel of lesser diameter.

embriología *f.* embryology, study of the embryo and its development up to the moment of birth.

embrión *m.* embryo, primitive phase of an organism from the moment of fertilization to about the second month.

embudo *m.* funnel.

emergencia *f.* emergency, urgency *Syn.* **urgencia**; ___ **de nacimiento repentino** / sudden childbirth ___; ___ **de un caso extremo** / ___ of an urgent case; ___ **de intervención quirúrgica** / surgical ___; ___ **de una traqueotomía** / ___ of a tracheotomy; **línea telefónica de ___** / ___ / hotline; **servicios de ___** / ___ medicine.

emético *m.* emetic, agent that stimulates vomiting.

emigración, migración *f.* emigration, escape, such as of leukocytes, through the walls of capillaries and small veins.

eminencia *f.* eminence, prominence or elevation such as on the surface of a bone.

emisión *f.* emission, discharge; ___ **seminal nocturna** / wet dream, involuntary emission of semen during sleep.

emitir *vt.* to emit, to expel; to issue.

emoción *f.* emotion, intense feeling.

emocional, emocionante *a.* emotional, rel. to emotion.

emoliente *a.* emollient, soothing to the skin or mucous membrane.

empachado-a *a.* suffering from indigestion.

empacho *m.* indigestion.

emparejar *vt.* to match, to pair off.

empaste *m.* [*dientes*] filling.

empatía *f.* empathy, understanding and appreciation of the feelings of another person.

empeine *m.* instep, arched medial portion of the foot.

empeorar *v.* to worsen; **empeorarse** *vr.* to get worse.

empezar *vt.* to begin, to start.

empiema *f.* empyema, presence of pus in a cavity, esp. the pleural cavity.

empírico-a *a.* empiric, empirical, based on practical observations.

empleado-a *m., f.* employee.

empleo *m.* employment, job.

emprender *vt.* to undertake.

empujar *vt.* to push, to press forward.

empujón *m.* push, shove.

emulsión *f.* emulsion, distribution of a liquid in small globules throughout another liquid.

en *prep.* in, on, at; ___ **el hospital** / in the hospital; ___ **la mesa** / on the table; ___ **casa** / at home.

enajenación mental *m.* derangement, mental disorder.

enajenamiento *m.* conversion disorder, the process by which repressed emotions are translated into physical manifestations.

enamorarse *vr.* to fall in love; ___ **de** / ___with.

enanismo *m.* dwarfism, impaired growth of the body caused by hereditary or physical deficiencies.

enano-a *m., f.* dwarf, individual who is undersized in relation to the group to which he or she belongs; ___ **acondroplástico-a** / achondroplastic ___; ___ **asexual** / asexual ___; ___

infantil / infantile ___; ___
micromélico-a / micromelic ___ .
encadenamiento *m.* linkage.
encadenar *vt.* to link; to chain.
encajamiento *m.* engagement.
encantis *n.* encanthis, small growth at the inner angle of the eyelid.
encapsulado-a *a.* enclosed in a capsule; walled-off.
encefalalgia *f.* encephalalgia, intense headache.
encefálico-a *a.* encephalic, rel. to the encephalon.
encefalinas *f.* enkephalins, chemical substances produced in the brain.
encefalitis *f.* encephalitis, infl. of the brain; ___ **alérgica experimental** / experimental allergic ___; ___ **bacteriana** / bacterial ___; ___ **del recién nacido** / neonatorum ___; ___ **epidémica** / epidemic___; ___ **equina del este** / eastern equine ___; ___ **equina del oeste** / western equine ___; ___ **herpética** / herpes ___; ___ **infantil** / infantile ___; ___ **letárgica** / lethargic ___; ___ **piogénica** / pyogenica; ___ **purulenta** / purulent ___; ___ **severa hemorrágica** / acute hemorrhagic ___; ___ **severa, necronizante** / acute necrotizing ___; ___ **supurativa** / suppurative ___ .
encéfalo *m.* encephalon, portion of the nervous system contained in the cranium.
encefalocele *m.* encephalocele, protrusion of brain matter through a congenital or traumatic defect in the skull.
encefalograma *m.* encephalogram, X-ray examination of the brain.
encefaloma *m.* encephaloma, brain tumor.
encefalomalacia *f.* encephalomalacia, softening of the brain.
encefalomielitis *f.* encephalomyelitis, infl. of the brain and the spinal cord.
encefalopatía *f.* encephalopathy, any disease or malfunction of the brain.
encender *vi.* [*una bombilla*] to switch on; [*un fuego*] to kindle.
encerar *v.* to wax, to treat or rub the skin with wax.
encerrar *vt.* to enclose; **encerrarse** *vr.* to lock oneself up.
encía *f.* gum.

encigótico-a, enzigótico-a *a.* enzygotic, rel. to twins developed from the same fertilized ovum.
encima *adv.* on, upon, on top of.
encinta *a.* pregnant.
enclenque *a.* emaciated; feeble.
encogerse *vr.* to shrink.
enconarse *vr.* to fester, to become ulcerated.
encondroma *f.* enchondroma, tumor that develops within a bone.
encontrar *vt.* to encounter, to find; **encontrarse** *vr.* to meet with someone; to find.
encopresis *f.* encopresis, incontinence of feces.
encuesta *f.* inquest, official investigation, survey.
endarteritis *f.* endarteritis, infl. of the lining of an artery.
endémico-a *a.* endemic, endemical, rel. to a disease that remains for an indefinite length of time in a given community or region; **área** ___ / ___ area; **enfermedad** ___ / ___ sickness.
endentado-a *a.* serrated, teethlike projection.
enderezar *vt.* to straighten out.
endocardio *m.* endocardium, the serous inner lining membrane of the heart.
endocarditis *f.* infl. of the endocardium; ___ **bacteriana** / bacterial ___; ___ **constrictiva** / constrictive ___; ___ **infecciosa** / infectious ___; ___ **maligna** / malignant ___; ___ **mucomenbranosa** / mucomembranous ___; ___ **reumática** / rheumatic ___; ___ **tuberculosa** / tuberculous ___ .
endocardio *m.* endocardium, serose interior membrane of the heart.
endocervicitis *f.* endocervicitis, infl. of the glands and the epithelium of the cervix and the uterus.
endocervix *m.* endocervix, mucous membrane of the cervix.
endocrino-a *a.* endocrine, rel. to internal secretions and the glands that secrete them; **glándulas** ___ -s / endocrine glands, glands that secrete hormones directly into the bloodstream.
endocrinología *f.* endocrinology, the study of the endocrine glands and the hormones secreted by them.
endocrinólogo *m.* endocrinologist.
endodermo *m.* endoderm, the innermost of the three layers of the embryo.

endofítico *a.* endophytic, rel. to an invasive tumor growing internally.

endoflebitis *f.* endophlebitis, infl. of the intima of a vein.

endoftalmitis *f.* endophthalmitis, infl. of the interior tissues of the eyeball, which can be caused by an allergic reaction, a reaction to a drug, or a bacteriologic infection; serious redness of the eye, a probable infection, that in some cases has pus. Other symptoms are vomiting, fever and headache; __ facoanafiláctica / __ phacoanaphylactic; __ **granulomatosa** / granulomatous __; __ **nodosa** / __ nodosa.

endógeno-a *a.* endogenous; **infección** __ / __ infection.

endometrial *a.* endometrial, rel. to the endometrium; **biopsia** __ / __ biopsy; **quiste** __ / __ cyst.

endometrio *m.* endometrium, inner mucous membrane of the uterus.

endometriosis *f.* endometriosis, disorder by which endometrial-like tissue is found in areas outside the uterus.

endometritis *f.* endometritis, infl. of the mucous membrane.

endomiocarditis *f.* endomyocarditis, infl. of the internal layers of the heart, the endocardium, and the myocardium.

endomorfo *m.* endomorph, person whose body is more heavily developed in the torso than in the limbs.

endoprótesis *f.* stent, device used for supporting tubular structures that are being joined.

endorfinas *f.* endorphins, chemical substances produced in the brain that have the property of easing pain.

endoscopía *f.* endoscopy, examination of a cavity or conduit using an endoscope.

endoscopio *m.* endoscope, instrument used to examine a hollow organ or cavity.

endosteo *m.* endosteum, cells located in the central medullar cavity of the bones.

endostio *m.* endosteum, tissue that covers the medullar cavity of the bone.

endotelio *m.* endothelium, thin layer of cells that form the inner lining of the blood vessels, the lymph channels, the heart, and other cavities.

endotoxemia *f.* endotoxemia, presence of endotoxins in the blood.

endotoxina *f.* endotoxin, venous toxin-free after the organism dies; with less potency than the exotoxin; the infected person may have symptoms of fever, chills, and shock.

endotraqueal *a.* endotracheal, within or through the trachea; **tubo __ con manguito** / __ tube, cuffed.

endulzar *vt.* to sweeten.

endurecer *vt.* to harden; **endurecerse** *vr.* to become hardened.

endurecimiento *m.* hardening.

enema *f.* enema; __ **de bario** / barium __; __ **de contraste doble** / double-contrast __ .

energía *f.* energy, the capacity to work, to move, and to exercise with vigor; __ **cinética** / kinetic __; __ **de activación** / __ of activation; __ **de fusión** / fusion __; __ **interna** / internal __; __ **latente** / latent __; __ **nuclear** / nuclear __; __ **nutritiva** / nutritional __; __ **potencial** / potential __; __ **química** / chemical __; __ **síquica** / psychic __; __ **solar** / solar __; __ **total** / total __ .

enérgico-a *a.* energetic, vigorous.

enfadar *vt.* to make angry, to upset; **enfadarse** *vr.* to become angry.

enfermar *v.* to cause disease; **enfermarse** *vr.* to become ill, to get sick.

enfermedad *f.* sickness, illness, disease, infirmity; **control de __ -es contagiosas** / communicable control; __ **africana aguda del sueño** / acute African sleeping __; __ **ambulante** / walking __; __ **biliar** / gall __; __ **cardíaca** / cardiac disease; __ **concomitante** / companion __; __ **de la altura** / high altitude sickness, caused by diminished oxygen; __ **de los buzos** / decompression __; __ **de la membrano hialina** / hyaline membrane disease, respiratory disease of the newborn; __ **de los mineros** / coal miner's __; __ **de red o cadena** / heavy chain __; __ **de viajeros** / motion __; __ **funcional** / functional __, of unknown origin; __ **ósea** / bone __; __ **por radiación** / radiation __; __ **pulmonar crónica obstructiva** / chronic obstructive pulmonary disease; __ **renal** / renal __; __ **respiratoria crónica** / chronic respiratory __; __ **sanguínea** / blood __; __ **venérea** / venereal __; **licencia por __** / sick leave.

enfermería *f.* infirmary, a place used for treatment of the sick.

enfermero-a *m., f.* nurse; **asistente de __ /** orderly; **__ anestesista /** __ anesthetist; **__ de cirugía /** scrub __, surgical __; **__ de salud pública /** community or public health __; **__ graduado-a /** trained __; **__ práctico-a /** practical __; **__ privado-a /** private duty __; **__ registrado-a /** registered __; **jefe-a de __ -s /** chief or head __ .

enfermizo-a *a.* sickly; predisposed to become ill.

enfermo-a *m., f.* sick person; **cuidado de __ -s /** nursing.

enfisema *m.* emphysema, chronic lung condition that causes distension of the small air sacs (alveoli) in the lungs and atrophy of the tissue between them, impairing the respiratory process.

enfocar *vi.* to focus.

enfrente *adv.* across from; in front of.

enfriar *vt.* to cool down.

engordar *vi.* to gain weight; to get fat.

engorroso-a *a.* cumbersome, troublesome.

engrama *f.* engram. 1. permanent mark or trace left in the protoplasm by a passing stimulus; 2. a latent permanent picture produced by a sensorial experience.

engurgitado-a *a.* engorged, distended by excess of liquid.

enjabonar *vt.* to soap; **enjabonarse** *vr.* to soap oneself.

enjambrazón *f.* swarming, the act of multiplying or spreading, such as bacteria over a culture.

enjuagar *vt.* to rinse; **enjuagarse** *vr.* to rinse oneself out.

enjuague *m.* rinse, mouthwash.

enoftalmia *f.* enophthalmos, receded eyeball.

enojado-a *a.* angry, fretful.

enojar *vt.* to anger; **enojarse** *vr.* to get angry.

enorme *a.* enormous, huge.

enquistado-a *a.* encysted, enclosed in a sac or cyst.

enriquecido-a *a.* enriched; of increased value.

ensangrentado-a *a.* bloody, stained with blood.

ensayo *m.* assay.

enseñar *v.* to teach; to show; to instruct.

ensimismado-a *a.* absorbed in thought, pensive.

ensuciar *v.* to dirty; to defecate.

entablillar *v.* to splint.

entamebiasis *f.* entamebiasis, infestation by an ameba.

ente *m.* entity, being.

entender *vt.* to understand, to comprehend.

enteralgia *f.* enteralgia, neuralgia of the intestine.

entérico-a, enteral *a.* enteral, rel. to the intestine; **alimentación __ /** nutrition; **cubierta __ /** __ coated.

enteritis *f.* enteritis, infl. of the intestine, esp. the small intestine.

entero-a *a.* whole; undiminished; **__ mente /** *adv.* totally.

enterocele *n.* enterocele, a hernial protrusion through a defect in the rectovaginal or vesicovaginal pouch.

enteroclisis *f.* enteroclysis, irrigation of the colon.

enterococo *m.* enterococcus, a streptococcus that inhabits the intestinal tract.

enterocolitis *f.* enterocolitis, infl. of both the large and small intestine.

enteropatía *f.* enteropathy, any anomaly or disease of the intestines.

enterostomía *f.* enterostomy, opening or communication between the intestine and the abdominal wall skin; **revisión de una __ /** __ revision.

enterotoxina *f.* enterotoxin, a toxin produced by or originating in the intestines.

enterovirus *m.* enterovirus, a group of viruses that infect the human gastrointestinal tract, and can cause respiratory diseases and neurological anomalies.

enterrar *vt.* to bury.

entibiar *vt.* to make lukewarm.

entierro *m.* burial.

entonces *adv.* then, at that time.

entorno *m.* environment, setting, ambiance.

entrar *vi.* to go in; to come in.

entre *prep.* between.

entrenamiento *m.* training.

entropía *f.* entropy, in thermodynamics, diminished capacity to convert internal energy into work.

entropión *m.* entropion, inversion or turning inward such as that of the eyelid.

entuerto *m.* afterbirth pains.

entumecido-a *a.* numb.

entumecimiento *m.* numbness; torpor.

enucleación *f.* enucleation, removal of a tumor or a structure.

enuresis, enuresia *f.* enuresis, incontinence; bed-wetting; ___ **nocturna** / nocturnal ___ .

envejecer *vi.* to grow old.

envejecido-a *a.* grown old, looking old.

envenenado-a *a.* poisoned.

envenenamiento *m.* poisoning.

envenomación *m.* envenomation, the act of injecting by stinging, biting, or any other designed apparatus or form, a poisonous material or venom to a victim.

enviudar *vi.* to become a widow or a widower.

envoltura *f.* pack, cold or hot wrapping.

enyesar *vt.* to make a cast using plaster of Paris; to plaster.

enzima *f.* enzyme, protein that acts as a catalyst in vital chemical reactions; ___ **mucomembranosa** / mucomembranous ___ ; ___ **tuberculosa** / ___ tuberculous; **grupos de ___ -s** / enzyme groups.

eosina *f.* eosin, insoluble substance used as a red dye for coloring tissue in microscopic studies.

eosinofilia *f.* eosinophilia, presence of a large number of eosinophilic leukocytes in the blood.

eosinófilo-a *a.* eosinophilic, that stains readily with eosin.

epéndimo *m.* ependyma, membrane that lines the ventricles of the brain and the central canal of the spinal cord.

ependimoma *f.* ependymoma, a tumor of the central nervous system that contains fetal ependymal cells.

epicardio *m.* epicardium, visceral surface of the pericardium.

epicondilitis humeral lateral *f.* lateral humeral epycondilitis, *pop.* tennis elbow.

epicóndilo *m.* epicondyle, a projection or eminence above the condyle of a bone.

epidemia *f.* epidemic, disease that affects a large number of people in a region or community at the same time.

epidémico-a *a.* epidemic; **brote ___ /** ___ outbreak.

epidemiología *f.* epidemiology, the study of epidemic diseases.

epidérmico-a *a.* epidermal, epidermic, rel. to the epidermis.

epidermis *f.* epidermis, external epithelial covering of the skin.

epidermoide *m.* epidermoid, tumor that contains epidermal cells; *a.* 1. resembling the dermis; 2. rel. to a tumor that has epidermal cells.

epidermólisis *f.* epidermolysis, loosening of the epidermis.

epididimitis *f.* epididymitis, infection and infl. of the epididymis.

epidídimo *m.* epididymis, a duct along the back side of the testes that collects the sperm from the testicle to be transported by the vas deferens to the seminal vesicle.

epidural *a.* epidural, situated above or outside of the dura mater.

epífisis *f.* epiphysis, the end of a long bone, usu. wider than the diaphysis.

epifisitis *f.* epiphysitis, infl. of an epiphysis.

epífora *f.* epiphora, watering of the eye.

epigástrico-a *a.* epigastric, rel. to the epigastrium; **reflejo ___ /** ___ reflex.

epigastrio *m.* epigastrium, upper back portion of the abdomen.

epiglotis *f.* epiglottis, cartilage that covers the entrance to the larynx and prevents food or liquid from entering during swallowing.

epiglotitis *f.* epiglottitis, infl. of the epiglottis and adjacent tissues.

epilación *f.* epilation, removal of hair by electrolysis.

epilepsia *f.* epilepsy, grand mal, neurological disorder, gen. chronic and in some cases hereditary, manifested by periodic convulsions and sometimes by loss of consciousness.

epilepsia jacksoniana *f.* Jacksonian epilepsy, partial epilepsy with loss of consciousness.

epiléptico-a *m., f.* person affected with epilepsy; *a.* epileptic, rel. to or suffering from epilepsy; **ataque o crisis ___ /** ___ seizure; **ausencia ___ /** absentia epileptica, momentary loss of consciousness during an epileptic seizure; **demencia ___ /** ___ dementia; **espasmo ___ /** ___ spasm.

epinefrina *f.* epinephrine. *See* **adrenalina**

epiploico-a *a.* epiploic, rel. to the epiploon; **foramen ___ /** ___ foramen, opening that connects the greater and the lesser peritoneal cavities.

epiplón *m.* epiploon, [omentum] a fold of peritoneum passing from the stomach and covering the intestines.

episiotomía f. episiotomy, incision of the perineum to avoid tearing during parturition.

episodio m. episode, non-regulated event as part of a physical or mental condition, or both, and that manifests itself in some illnesses such as epilepsy.

epispadias m. epispadias, abnormal congenital opening of the male urethra on the upper surface of the penis.

epistaxis f. epistaxis, nosebleed.

epitelial a. epithelial, rel. to the epithelium.

epitelio m. epithelium, the outer layer of mucous membranes; __ ciliado / ciliated __; __ columnar / columnar __; __ cuboidal / cuboidal __; __ de transición / transitional __; __ escamoso / squamous __; __ estratificado / stratified __ .

epitelioma f. epithelioma, carcinoma consisting mainly of epithelial cells.

epitelización f. epithelization, growth of epithelium over an exposed surface, such as a wound.

Epsom, sales de f. Epsom salts, magnesium sulfate, used as laxative.

Epstein-Barr, virus de m. Epstein-Barr virus, virus thought to be the causative agent of infectious mononucleosis.

epúlide gravida f. epulis gravidarum, pyogenic granuloma of the gums that can result during pregnancy.

equilibrado-a a. balanced.

equilibrio m. equilibrium. 1. the condition of being evenly balanced between opposite forces or effects. An object is in state of equilibrium if forces acting upon it are in equilibrium; 2. a state of apparent repose sometimes indicated by two opposing arrows that refer to two balanced chemical reactions in opposite directions at the same speed; 3. balancing, a method to produce a balance in the body aligning energy by manipulating certain parts of the body.

equimosis f. ecchymosis, bruise, gradual blue-black discoloration of the skin due to blood filtering into the cellular subcutaneous tissue.

equinasia f. echinacea, herb used to reduce inflammation.

equinococo m. echinococcus, a genus of tapeworm.

equinococosis f. echinococcosis, infestation by echinococcus; __ hepática / hepatic __; __ pulmonar / pulmonary __ .

equinovaro m. equinovarus, congenital deformity of the foot.

equipo m. equipment, provision, accessories.

equivalencia f. equivalence.

equivalente a. equivalent.

equivocación f. mistake, error.

equivocado-a a. mistaken, in error.

equivocarse vr.; vi. to make a mistake; to be in error; to miscalculate.

erección f. erection, state of rigidity or hardening of erectile tissue when it is filled with blood, such as the penis.

eréctil a. erectile, capable of erection or dilation.

ergonomía f. ergonomics, branch of ecology that studies design and operations of machines and the physical environment as related to humans.

ergotamina f. ergotamine, alkaloid used chiefly in the treatment of migraine headaches.

ergotismo m. ergotism, chronic poisoning due to excessive intake of ergot.

erisipela f. erysipelas, cutaneous infection of cellulites by the streptococcus B-hemolytic characterized by a reddish or brown eruption, defined in size; __ ambulante / ambulant __; __ interna / internum __; __ migrante / migrant __; __ pustulosa / __ pustulosum; __ quirúrgica / surgical __ .

eritema f. erythema, redness of the skin due to congestion of the capillaries; __ de los pañales / diaper rash; __ solar / sunburn.

eritematoso-a a. erythematic, erythematous, rel. to erythema.

eritremia f. erythremia, increase of red blood cells due to an excessive production of erythroblasts by the bone marrow.

eritroblasto m. erythroblast, primitive red blood cell.

eritroblastosis f. erythroblastosis, excessive number of erythroblasts in the blood.

eritrocito m. erythrocyte, red blood cell made in the bone marrow that serves to transport oxygen to tissues; **índice de sedimentación de** __-s / __ sedimentation rate.

eritrocitopenia *f.* erythrocytopenia, deficiency in the number of erythrocytes present in the blood.

eritrocitosis *f.* erythrocytosis, increase in the number of erythrocytes in the blood.

eritroide *a.* erythroid, reddish.

eritroleucemia *f.* erythroleukemia, malignant blood disease caused by abnormal growth of both red and white blood cells.

eritromelia *f.* erythromelia, cutaneous disorder of the lower extremities with erythema of unknown origin and atrophy of the skin.

eritromelalgia *f.* erythromelalgia, disorder involving the extremities, characterized by paroxysmal attacks of severe burning pains, reddening, sweating, most common in middle age.

eritromicina *f.* erythromycin, antibiotic used chiefly in infections caused by gram-positive bacteria.

eritrón *m.* erythron, system formed by erythrocytes circulating in the blood and the organ from which they arise.

eritropoyesis *f.* erythropoiesis, red blood cell production.

eritropoyetina *f.* erythropoietin, a non-dialyzable protein that stimulates red blood cell production.

erógeno-a *a.* erogenous, that which produces erotic sensations; **zona __ / __ zone.**

erosión *f.* erosion, the act of wearing out or away.

erosivo-a *a.* erosive, that causes erosion.

erótico-a *a.* erotic, rel. to eroticism or having the power to arouse sexual impulses.

erotismo *m.* eroticism, erotism, lustful sexual impulses.

erradicar *vt.* to eradicate, to remove, to extirpate.

errante, errático-a *a.* wandering, deviating from the normal course; **exantema __ / __ rash; neumonía __ / __ pneumonia.**

error *m.* error, mistake.

error innato en el metabolismo *m.* innate error in metabolism, an anomaly in the metabolism that results from an inherited defect, such as it occurs in galactosemia and in Tay-Sachs disease, among others.

eructación *f.* eructation, belching.

eructar, erutar *v.* to eructate, to belch.

eructo, eruto *m.* eructation, belch.

erupción *f.* eruption, rash, skin outbreak; **escamosa** / squamous **__; __ maculopapular** / maculopapular __ .

escafoide *a.* scaphoid, shaped like a boat, esp. in reference to the bone of the carpus or the tarsus.

escala *f.* scale; **__ de diferenciación** / range.

escaldadura *f.* scald, skin burn caused by boiling liquid or vapor.

escalera *f.* staircase; ladder; **__ de escape** / fire escape.

escalofrío *m.* chill, a cold, shivering sensation.

escalpelo, escarpelo *m.* scalpel, surgical blade, dissecting knife.

escán *m.* scan, the process of producing an image of a specific organ or tissue by means of a radioactive substance that is injected as a contrasting element; **__ cardíaco** / heart __; **__ de la tiroides** / thyroid __; **__ de los huesos** / bone __; **__ del cerebro** / brain __; **__ pulmonar** / lung __ .

escáner *m.* scanner, exploratory device.

escán radioisótopo *m.* radioisotope scanning, scan that makes use of radioisotopes for theurapeutic of diagnostic purposes.

escápula *f.* scapula, shoulder blade.

escara *f.* eschar, dark-colored scab or crust that forms in the skin after a burn.

escarificación *f.* scarification, the act of producing a number of small superficial scratches or punctures on the skin.

escarlatina *f.* scarlatina, scarlet fever, an acute contagious disease characterized by fever and a bright red rash on the skin and tongue.

escatología *f.* scatology. 1. the study of feces; 2. a morbid preoccupation with feces and filth.

escintigrafía *f.* scintigraphy, diagnostic test that uses radioisotopes to obtain a bidimensional image of the distribution of a radiopharmaceutical in a designed area of the body.

escintilación *f.* scintillation, a visual sensation of seeing flashes of light.

escintilador *m.* scintillator.

escirro *m.* scirrhus, hard cancerous tumor.

escirroso-a *a.* scirrhous, hard, rel. to a scirrhus.

escleritis f. scleritis, infl. of the sclera.

esclerodermia m. scleroderma, a chronic illness that can cause atrophy of the skin, more common in middle aged women than in men.

escleroma m. scleroma, a hardened, circumscribed area of granulation tissue in the skin or in the mucous membrane.

esclerosis f. sclerosis, progressive hardening of organs or tissues; ___ **arterial** / arterial ___; ___ **de Alzheimer** / Alzheimer's ___; ___ **lateral amiotrófica** / amyotrophic lateral ___ .

esclerosis múltiple f. multiple sclerosis, slow, progressive disease of the central nervous system caused by a loss of the protective myelin covering the nerve fibers of the brain and spinal cord.

esclerosis tuberosa f. tuberous sclerosis, familial disease manifested by convulsive seizures, progressive mental deficiency, and multiple tumor formations in the skin and the brain.

escleroterapia f. sclerotherapy, the process of injecting chemical solutions to treat varices in order to produce sclerosis.

esclerótica f. sclera, sclerotica, the hard, white exterior part of the eye made of fibrous tissue.

esclerótico-a a. sclerotic, rel. to or afflicted by sclerosis.

escoliosis f. scoliosis, pronounced lateral curvature of the spine.

escorbuto m. scurvy, disease caused by lack of vitamin C and manifested by anemia, bleeding gums, and a general state of inanition.

escotoma m. scotoma, area of lost or diminished vision within the visual field.

escotopía f. scotopia, adjustment to nocturnal vision.

escotópico-a a. scotopic, rel. to scotopia; **visión** ___ / ___ vision.

escrito-a a. pp. of **escribir**, written.

escrófula f. scrofula, tuberculosis of the lymphatic glands.

escrofuloderma m. scrofuloderma, a type of scrofula with skin lesions.

escrotal a. scrotal, rel. to the scrotum.

escroto m. scrotum, the sac surrounding and enclosing the testes.

escrutinio m. scrutiny; screening.

escudo m. shield, a protective covering.

escupir v. to spit.

esencia f. essence; indispensable quality.

esencial a. essential, indispensable.

esfenoidal a. sphenoidal, rel. to the sphenoid bone.

esfenoides m. sphenoid bone, large bone at the base of the skull.

esfera f. sphere. 1. a structure shaped like a globe or ball; 2. sociological environment.

esferocito m. spherocyte, sphere-shaped erythrocyte.

esferocitosis f. spherocytosis, presence of spherocytes in the blood.

esférula f. spherule, minute sphere.

esfigmomanómetro m. sphygmomanometer, instrument for determining blood pressure.

esfínter m. sphincter, circular muscle that opens and closes an orifice.

esfinteroplastia f. sphincteroplasty, plastic surgery of a sphincter muscle.

esfinterotomía f. sphincterotomy, cutting of a sphincter muscle.

esfuerzo m. effort; ___ **coordinado** / teamwork; ___ **excesivo** / overexertion, strain; **prueba de** ___ / stress test.

esguince m. sprain. See **torcedura**.

eslabón m. link.

esmalte m. enamel, hard substance that covers and protects the dentin of a tooth.

esmegma m. smegma, thick cheesy substance secreted by sebaceous glands, esp. seen in the external genitalia.

esofagectomía f. esophagectomy, excision of a portion of the esophagus.

esofágico-a a. esophageal, rel. to the esophagus; **cintigrafía** ___ / ___ scintigraphy; **dilatación** ___ / ___ dilatation; **disfagia** ___ / ___ dysphagia; **espasmo** ___ / ___ spasm; **obstrucción** ___ / ___ obstruction.

esofagitis f. esophagitis, infl. of the esophagus.

esófago m. esophagus, portion of the alimentary tract between the pharynx and the stomach.

esofagodinia f. esophagodynia, pain in the esophagus.

esofagogastritis f. esophagogastritis, infl. of the stomach and the esophagus.

esofagogastroduodenoscopía f. esophagogastroduodenoscopy, examination of the esophagus, the stomach, and the duodenum by means of an endoscope.

esofagogastroscopía *f.*
esophagogastroscopy, endoscopic
examination of the esophagus and the
stomach.

esofagoscopía *f.* esophagoscopy,
interior inspection of the esophagus by
using an endoscope.

esoforia *f.* esophoria, crossed
eyes, inward deviation of the
eyes.

esotropía *f.* esotropia.

espacio *m.* space, area.

espalda *f.* back; **dolor de __ /**
backache.

español *m.* [*idioma*] Spanish; [*nativo-a*]
Spanish; **-a** *a.* Spanish.

esparadrapo *m.* adhesive tape.

esparcido-a *a.* spread out; scattered.

espárrago *m.* asparagus.

espasmo *m.* spasm, twitch, involuntary
muscular contraction.

espasmódico-a *a.* spasmodic, rel. to
spasms; **crup __ / __** croup.

espasticidad *f.* spasticity, increase in
the normal tension of a muscle
resulting in stiffness and difficult
movement.

espástico-a *a.* spastic. 1. resembling,
or of the nature of spasms; 2. afflicted
with spasms.

especia *f.* spice.

especial *a.* special, especial, unique;
-mente *adv.* specially.

especialidad *f.* specialty. See table on
this page.

especialista *m., f.* specialist.

especialización *f.* specialization.

específico-a *a.* specific; determined;
precise; **no __ /** nonspecific.

espécimen *m.* specimen, sample.

espectro *m.* spectrum. 1. range of
activity of an antibiotic against a
variety of microorganisms; 2. series of
images resulting from the refraction of
electromagnetic radiation; 3. series of
colors of refracted sunlight that can be
seen with the naked eye or with the
help of a sensitive instrument.

espectro electromagnético *m.*
electromagnetic spectrum.

espéculo *m.* speculum, instrument used
for dilating a conduit or cavity; __
rectal / proctoscope.

espejo *m.* mirror.

espejuelos *m. pl.* eyeglasses,
spectacles; __ **bifocales /** bifocal __;
__ **para leer /** reading __; __
trifocales / trifocal __ .

Especialidades	Specialties
anestesiología	anesthesiology
cirugía cardiotorácica	cardiothoracic surgery
cirugía general	general surgery
cirugía plástica	plastic surgery
dermatología	dermatology
gastroenterología	gastroenterology
medicina de emergencia o de urgencia	emergency medicine
medicina general	family practice
medicina interna	internal medicine
medicina nuclear	nuclear medicine
nefrología	nephrology
neurología	neurology
neurocirugía	neurosurgery
obstetricia y ginecología	obstetrics and gynecology
oftalmología	ophthalmology
oncología	oncology
ortopedia	orthopedics
otolaringología	otolaryngology
patología	pathology
pediatría	pediatrics
perinatología	perinatology
psiquiatría	psychiatry
radiología	radiology
urología	urology

espera *f.* wait; **salón de __ /** waiting
room.

esperma *f.* sperm, semen; **conteo
disminuído de __ /** reduced __ count;
donante de __ / __ donor.

esperma de ballena *m.* whale
sperm, called in Spanish spermaceti, a
lipid substance extracted from the head
of a whale.

espermaticida, espermicida *m.*
spermatocide, spermicidal, agent that
destroys spermatozoa; *a.*
spermatocidal, that kills spermatozoa.

espermático-a *a.* spermatic; rel. to
sperm or semen.

espermatocele *m.* spermatocele, a
cystic tumor of the epididymis
containing spermatozoa.

espermatogénesis *f.*
spermatogenesis, the process of
formation and development of
spermatozoa.

espermatozoide *m.* sperm cell; the male sperm that fertilizes the female egg.

espermaturia *f.* spermaturia, semen discharged into the urine.

espermiograma *m.* spermiogram, evaluation of spermatozoa as an aid to determine sterility.

espesar *vt.* to thicken; to condense; **espesarse** *vr.* to become thicker; to become condensed.

espeso-a *a.* thick, condensed.

espesor *m.* thickness, consistency.

espica *f.* spica, a type of bandage.

espícula *f.* spicule, a body shaped like a small needle.

espicular *a.* spicular, needle-shaped.

espiga *f.* spike, sharp rise in a curve, such as in the tracing of brain waves.

espín *m.* spin, auricular rotation; *v.* to gyrate, to extend, to prolong.

espina *f.* spina; thorn; fishbone.

espina bífida *f.* spina bifida, congenital anomaly of the spine with a gap; __ oculta / __ occulta, without protrusion, gen. at the lumbar level.

espina dorsal *f.* columna. columna vertebral.

espinal *a.* spinal, rel. to the spine or the spinal cord; **atrofia muscular** __ / __ muscular atrophy; **canal** __ / __ canal; **choque** __ / __ shock; **fusión** __ / __ fusion; **médula** __ / __ cord; **nervio accesorio** __ / __ accessory nerve; **nervios** __-es / __ nerves; **punción** __ / __ puncture.

espinazo *m.* spine, *pop.* backbone.

espinilla *f.* 1. blackhead; 2. shinbone, anterior edge of the tibia.

espirar *v.* to exhale.

espíritu *m.* spirit. 1. alcoholic solution of a volatile substance; 2. soul; **tranquilidad de** __ / peace of mind.

espiritual *a.* spiritual, rel. to the soul; **cura** __ / __ healing.

espirometría *f.* spirometry, the act of measuring the breathing capacity through the use of a spirometer.

espirómetro *m.* spirometer, device used to measure the amount of inhaled and exhaled air.

espiroqueta *f.* spirochete, spinal microorganism that belongs to the order *Spirochaetales* that includes the syphilis causing agent.

espiroquetósico-a *a.* spirochetal, rel. to spirochetes.

esplácnico-a *a.* splanchnic, rel. to or that reaches the viscera; **nervios** __ -s / __ nerves.

esplenectomía *f.* splenectomy, excision of the spleen.

esplénico-a *a.* splenic, rel. to the spleen; **infarto** __ / __ infarction.

esplenitis *f.* splenitis, infl. of the speen.

esplenoportografía *f.* splenoportography, x-ray of the splenic and portal veins following injection of a radiopaque dye into the spleen.

esplenorrenal *a.* splenorenal, rel. to the spleen and the kidneys; **derivación** __ / __ shunt, anastomosis of the splenic veins or artery to the renal vein, esp. used in the treatment of portal hypertension.

espolón *m.* spur, pointed projection, as of a bone; __ **calcáneo** / calcaneal __ .

espondilitis *f.* spondylitis, infl. of one or more vertebrae.

espondilitis anquilosa *f.* ankylosing spondylitis, arthritis of the spine, resembling rheumatoid arthritis.

espondilólisis *f.* spondylolysis, dissolution or destruction of a vertebra.

espondilolistesis *f.* spondylolisthesis, forward displacement of one vertebra over another, usu. the fourth lumber over the fifth or the fifth over the sacrum.

espondilopatía *f.* spondylopathy, any disease or disorder of a vertebra.

espondilosis *f.* spondylosis. 1. vertebral ankylosis; 2. any degenerative condition affecting the vertebrae.

esponja *f.* sponge.

esponjar *v.* to sponge, to soak with a sponge.

espontáneo-a *a.* spontaneous.

espora *f.* spore, unicellular reproductive cell.

esporádico-a *a.* sporadic, occurring irregularly.

esporicida *m.* sporicide, agent that destroys spores.

esposo-a *m., f.* husband; wife.

esprue *m.* sprue, chronic disease that affects the ability to absorb dietary gluten.

espulgar *vt.* to cleanse of lice or fleas.

esputo *m.* sputum, spittle; __ **sanguinolento** / bloody __ .

esqueleto *m.* skeleton, the bony structure of the body.

esquina *f.* corner.

esquirla *f.* bone splinter.

esquistosoma m. Schistosoma, blood fluke, a trematode larva that enters the blood through the digestive tract or through the skin by contact with contaminated water.

esquistosomiasis f. schistosomiasis, infestation with blood flukes.

esquizofrenia f. schizophrenia, a breaking down of the mental functions with different psychotic manifestations such as delusion, withdrawal, and distorted perception of reality.

esquizofrénico-a a. schizophrenic, rel. to or suffering from schizophrenia.

esquizoide a. schizoid, resembling schizophrenia.

estabilidad f. stability, permanence.

estabilizar vt. to stabilize, to eliminate fluctuations.

estable a. stable, nonfluctuating.

establecer vt. to establish.

estación f. station. 1. status of condition; 2. stopping place such as a nurse's station; 3. season of the year.

estacionario-a a. stationary, in a fixed position.

estadificación f. staging, classification in the process of the degree of an illness. ___ **clínica** / clinical ___ .

estadío m. stage or transition period during the evolution of an illness.

estado m. state, condition; ___ **asmaticus** / status asthmaticus; ___ **crepuscular** / twilight ___; ___ **de gestación** / pregnancy; ___ **nutricional** / nutritional ___ .

estado epiléctico m. status epilepticus, repeated epileptic episodes without regaining consciousness between attacks.

estafilococemia f. staphylococcemia, presence of staphylococci in the blood.

estafilocócico-a a. staphylococcal, staphylococcic, rel. to or caused by staphylococci; **infecciones** ___ / ___ infections.

estafilococo m. staphylococcus, any pathological micrococci; **intoxicación alimentaria por** ___ **-s** / staphylococcal food poisoning.

estafilotoxina f. staphylotoxin, toxin produced by staphylococci.

estancación, estancamiento m., f. stagnation, lack of movement or circulation in fluids.

estancia f. stay; ___ **breve en el hospital** / short ___ in the hospital.

estándar a. standard, normal established way; **atención o cuidado** ___ / ___ of care; **desviación** ___ / ___ deviation; **error** ___ / ___ error; **procedimiento** ___ / ___ procedure.

estandarización f. standardization, uniformity; normalcy.

estapedectomía f. stapedectomy, excision of the stapes of the ear to improve hearing.

estar vi. to be; ___ **de guardia** / to be on call.

estasis f. stasis, stagnation of a body fluid such as blood or urine.

estático-a a. static, without movement.

estatura f. stature, height.

estatutorio n. statutory.

este m. [punto cardinal] east; **al** ___ **de** / to the ___ of; **esta** a. this; **estos-as** pl. / these; **éste-a** dem. pron. / this, this one; **éstos-as** pl. / these; **esto** neut. / this, this one.

esteatorrea f. steatorrhea, excess fat in the stool.

estenosado-a a. stenosed, rel. to stenosis.

estenosis f. stenosis, constriction or abnormal narrowing of a passageway; ___ **aórtica** / aortic ___; ___ **espinal** / spinal ___; ___ **pilórica** / pyloric ___; ___ **traqueal** / tracheal ___ .

estepaje m. steppage, alteration in the gait as a result of the pendular fall of the foot forcing the lifting of the knee and flexing the muscle over the pelvis.

éster m. ester, compound formed by the combination of an organic acid and alcohol.

estereotaxia f. stereotaxis, technique used in neurological procedures to locate with precision an area in the brain.

estereotipia f. stereotype, a type that represents a whole group.

estereotípico-a a. stereotypic, rel. to a stereotype.

esterificación f. esterification, transformation of an acid into ester.

estéril a. sterile. 1. aseptic, free of germs; 2. incapable of producing offspring.

esterilidad f. sterility. 1. the condition of being sterile; 2. inability to reproduce.

esterilización f. sterilization. 1. procedure to prevent reproduction; 2. total destruction of microorganisms; ___ **por calor** / thermosterilization; ___

por gas / gas ___; ___ **por vapor** / steam ___.
esterilizador m. sterilizer.
esterilizar vt. to sterilize.
esternal a. sternal, rel. to the sternum; **punción** ___ / ___ puncture.
esternalgia f. sternalgia, pain in the sternum.
esternón m. sternum, breastbone, the frontal bone in the middle of the thorax.
esternotomía f. sternotomy, cutting through the sternum.
esteroide a. steroid, rel. to steroids.
esteroides m. steroids, complex organic compounds that resemble cholesterol and of which many hormones such as estrogen, testosterone, and cortisone are made.
estertor m. rale, stertor, an abnormal rattle-like sound heard on auscultation; ___ **agónico** / death rattle; ___ **áspero** / coarse; ___; ___ **crepitante** / crepitant ___; ___ **crujiente** / crackling ___; ___ **húmedo** / moist ___; ___ **roncus** / rhonchus ___, rattling in the throat; ___ **seco** / dry ___ .
estetoscopio m. stethoscope, instrument used for auscultation.
estigma m. stigma. 1. a specific sign of a disease; 2. a mark or sign on the body.
estilete m. style, stylet, stylus; [cirugía] flexible probe.
estimado m. estimate, evaluation.
estimulación f. stimulation; motivation.
estimulador cardíaco m. pacemaker.
estimulante m. stimulant, agent that incites a reaction; pop. upper.
estimular vt. to stimulate; to motivate, to animate to action, to boost, to prompt.
estímulo m. stimulus, agent or factor that produces a reaction; ___ **condicionado** / conditioned ___; ___ **subliminal** / subliminal ___ .
estíptico m. styptic, agent with astringent power.
estirado-a a. extended, elongated.
estirar vt. to stretch, to extend.
estirón m. stretch, forceful pull.
estoma m. stoma, artificial permanent opening, esp. in the abdominal wall.
estómago m. stomach, sac-like organ of the alimentary canal; ___ **en cascada** / cascade ___; ___ **en bota de vino** / leather bottle ___; **lavado de** ___ / ___ pumping.

estomatitis f. stomatitis, infl. of the mucosa of the mouth; ___ **aftosa** / aphthous ___ .
estornudar vi. to sneeze.
estornudo m. sneeze.
estrabismo m. strabismus, squint, abnormal alignment of the eyes due to muscular deficiency.
estradiol m. estradiol, steroid produced by the ovaries.
estrangulación f. strangulation. 1. asphyxia or suffocation gen. caused by obstruction of the air passages; 2. constriction of an organ or structure due to compression.
estrangulado-a a. strangulated; constricted.
estratificación f. stratification; arrangement in layers.
estratificado-a a. stratified, arranged in layers; **epitelio** ___ / ___ epithelium.
estrato m. stratum, layer.
estrechamiento m. narrowing; tightness.
estrechar vt. to make narrower.
estrechez, estrechura f. stricture, narrowness, closeness.
estrecho-a a. narrow.
estreñido-a a. constipated; hard bound.
estreñimiento m. constipation; infrequent or incomplete bowel movements.
estreptococcemia f. streptococcemia, blood infection caused by the presence of streptococci.
estreptocócico-a a. streptococcal, rel. to or caused by streptococci; **infecciones** ___ **-s** / ___ infections.
estreptococo m. streptococcus, organism of the genus Streptococcus.
estreptomicina f. streptomycin, antibiotic drug used against bacterial infections.
estrés m. stress.
estría f. stria, streak.
estriado-a a. striated, striate, marked by streaks; **músculo** ___ / ___ muscle.
estribo m. stapes, the innermost of the auditory ossicles shaped like a stirrup.
estricnina f. strychnine, highly poisonous alkaloid.
estricturotomía f. stricturotomy, the cutting of strictures.
estridor m. stridor, whoop, harsh sound during respiration such as following an attack of whooping cough.

estrinización *m.* estrinization, epithelial changes of the vagina due to stimulation by estrogen.

estrógeno *m.* estrogen, female sex hormone produced by the ovaries; __ **por diseño** / __ by design; **receptor de** __ / __ receptor.

estroma *m.* stroma, the supporting tissue of an organ.

estrona *f.* estrone, oestrone, estrogenic hormone.

estropear *v.* to spoil; to damage; to cripple.

estructura *f.* structure; order.

estudiante *m., f.* student.

estudiar *v.* to study.

estudio *m.* study.

estudios cruzados *m., pl.* cross studies.

estupefaciente *m.* stupefacient. 1. agent causing stupor; 2. narcotic analgesic that alters the physiological conditions and produces euphoria.

estupidez *f.* stupidity, foolishness.

estúpido-a *a.* stupid, foolish.

estupor *m.* stupor, daze, state of lethargy.

etapa *n.* stage; __ -s de la enfermedad / __ of the illness.

etapas del parto *f., pl.* stages of labor. First, stage uterine contractions; second, stage dilation of the cervix; third, stage expulsion of the infant, expulsion of the placenta and membranes.

éter *m.* ether, chemical liquid used as a general anesthetic through inhalation of its vapor.

eternal, eterno-a *a.* eternal.

ética *f.* ethics, norms and principles that rule professional conduct.

etileno *m.* ethylene, anesthetic.

etiología *f.* etiology, branch of medicine that studies the cause of diseases.

etiológico-a *a.* etiologic, rel. to etiology.

etmoidectomía *f.* ethmoidectomy, removal of ethmoid cells or part of the ethmoid bone.

etmoideo-a *a.* ethmoid, sievelike; **seno** __ / __ sinus, air cavity within the ethmoid bone.

etmoides *m.* ethmoid bone, spongy bone located at the base of the cranium.

eubolismo *m.* eubolism, normal metabolism.

eucalipto *m.* eucalyptus tree.

euforia *f.* euphoria, an abnormal or exaggerated state of well-being.

eugenesia *f.* eugenics, the science that deals with improving and controling procreation to achieve more desirable hereditary characteristics.

eunuco *m.* eunuch, castrated male.

euploidia *f.* euploidy, complete set of chromosomes.

Eustaquio, trompa de *m.* Eustachian tube, part of the auditory conduit.

eutanasia *f.* euthanasia, mercy killing.

eutiroideo-a *a.* euthyroid, rel. to the normal function of the thyroid gland.

evacuación *f.* evacuation. 1. act of emptying or evacuating esp. the bowels; 2. the act of making a vacuum.

evacuante *m.* evacuant, an agent that stimulates bowel movement.

evacuar *vt.* to evacuate, to empty; to void.

evaginación *f.* evagination, protrusion of some part or organ from its normal position.

evaluación *f.* evaluation, assessment, rating, score; weighing the physical and mental state and capabilities of an individual; __ **clínica** / clinical assessment; __ **del estado de salud** / health assessment; __ **del proceso evolutivo** / follow-up assessment.

evaluar *vt.* to evaluate.

evanescente *a.* evanescent, of brief duration.

evaporación *f.* evaporation, conversion of a liquid or a solid into vapor.

eventración *f.* eventration, partial protrusion of the intestine through an opening in the abdominal wall.

eversión *f.* eversion, outward turning, esp. of the mucosa surrounding a natural orifice.

evidencia *f.* evidence, manifestation; [*legal*] evidence; testimony.

evisceración *f.* evisceration, removal of the viscera or contents of a cavity; disembowelment.

evitar *vt.* to avoid.

evolución *f.* evolution, gradual change.

evulsión *f.* evulsion, tearing away, pulling out.

exacerbación *f.* exacerbation, increase in the severity of a symptom or disease.

exacto-a *a.* exact; **-mente** *adv.* exactly.

exageración *f.* exaggeration.

exaltación *f.* exaltation, state of jubilation.

examen *m.* exam, examination; evaluation; investigation; __ **físico completo** / complete physical checkup.

examinar *vt.* to examine, to view and study the human body to determine a person's state of health; to look into, to investigate.

exantema *f.* exanthema. 1. cutaneous rash, sign of an acute viral or coccal disease as in scarlet fever or measles; 2. cutaneous eruption; __ **epidémico** / epidemic __; __ **keratoideo** / keratoid __; __ **súbito** / __ subitum.

exasperado-a *a.* exasperated.

exceder *vt.* to exceed; to outweigh; to surpass; **excederse** *vr.* to go too far, *pop.* to go overboard.

excéntrico-a *a.* eccentric, odd, different from the norm.

excepción *f.* exception, outside of the rule; **a __ de** / with the __ of.

excepto *prep.* except.

excesivo-a *a.* excessive, too much.

exceso *m.* excess; **en __** / excessively.

excisión *f.* excision, removal, ablation.

excitación *f.* excitation, reaction to a stimulus.

excitado-a *a.* excited, worked up.

excitante *m.* stimulant, *pop.* upper; *a.* stimulating, exciting.

excitar *vt.* to stimulate; to provoke.

excoriación *f.* excoriation, abrasion of the skin.

excrecencia *f.* excrescence, tumor protruding from the surface of a part or organ.

excreción *f.* excretion, elimination of waste matter.

excremento *m.* excrement, feces.

excreta *f.* excreta, all waste matter of the body.

excretar *vt.* to excrete, to eliminate waste from the body.

excusa *f.* excuse.

excusado *m.* outside toilet; privy.

exfoliación *f.* exfoliation, shedding or peeling of tissue.

exhalación *f.* exhalation, the act of breathing out.

exhalar *vt.* to exhale.

exhausto-a *a.* exhausted, fatigued.

exhibición *f.* exhibition.

exhibicionismo *m.* exhibitionism, obsessive drive to expose one's body, esp. the genitals.

exhibicionista *m., f.* exhibitionist, one who practices exhibitionism.

exhumación *f.* exhumation, disinterment.

exigir *vi.* to demand; to require.

existente *a.* existent, on hand.

existir *vi.* to exist, to be.

éxito *m.* success; good result.

exocrino-a *a.* exocrine, rel. to the external secretion of a gland.

exoftalmia *f.* exophthalmia, exophthalmos, exophthalmus, abnormal protrusion of the eyeball.

exoftálmico-a *a.* exophthalmic, rel. to or suffering from exophthalmia.

exógeno-a *a.* exogenous, originating outside the organism.

exostosis *f.* exostosis, cartilaginous osseus hypertrophy that projects outward from a bone, or the root of a tooth.

exotoxina *f.* exotoxin, toxic substance secreted by bacteria.

exotropía *f.* exotropia, a type of strabismus, outward turning of the eyes due to muscular imbalance.

expandir *vt.* to expand, to dilate; **expandirse** *vr.* to become expanded.

expansión *f.* expansion, extension.

expectoración *f.* expectoration, the expulsion of mucus or phlegm from the lungs, trachea or bronchi.

expectorante *m.* expectorant, an agent that stimulates expectoration.

expediente *m.* medical record; file; **sumario del __** / summary of hospital records.

experiencia *f.* experience, knowledge gained by practice.

experimental *a.* experimental, rel. to or known by experiment.

experimentar *v.* to experiment.

experimento *m.* experiment.

experto-a *m., f.* expert.

expiración *f.* expiration, termination; death.

expirar *vt.* 1. to expel breathing air; 2. to expire, to die.

explicación *f.* explanation; interpretation.

explicativo-a *a.* explanatory.

exploración *f.* exploration, search, investigation, scanning.

exploratorio-a *a.* exploratory, rel. to exploration.

expresión *f.* expression, facial appearance.

expresividad *f.* expressivity, degree of manifestation of a given hereditary trait in the individual that carries the conditioning gene.

exprimir *vt.* to squeeze; to extrude.

expuesto-a *a. pp.* of **exponer,** exposed.

expulsión *f.* expulsion; __ de la placenta / __ of the placenta; __ del recién nacido / __ of the infant.

exsanguinación *f.* exsanguination, severe blood loss.

exsanguinotransfusión *f.* exsanguino-transfusion, exchange transfusion, gradual and simultaneous withdrawal of a recipient's blood with transfusion of a donor's blood.

éxtasis *m.* ecstasy, trance accompanied by a pleasurable feeling.

extendedor *m.* stretcher.

extender *vt.* to extend, to stretch out; **extenderse** *vr.* to spread out.

extendido-a *a.* extended; widespread.

extensión *f.* extension, prolongation, straightening of a contracted finger or limb or aligning a dislocated or fractured bone.

extensor-a *a.* extensor, having the property of extending.

extenuado-a *a.* extenuated, exhausted.

exterior *a.* exterior.

exteriorizar *v.* to exteriorize, to temporarily expose a part or organ.

externo-a *a.* external, outer.

extinción *f.* extinction, cessation.

extinguir *vt.* to extinguish, to put out.

extirpación *f.* extirpation, removal of a part or organ.

extirpar *vt.* to eradicate, to remove, to excise, to enervate.

extra *a.* extra, extraordinary, additional.

extracción *f.* extraction, the process of removing, pulling, or drawing out.

extracelular *a.* extracellular, occurring outside a cell.

extracorporal *a.* extracorporeal, occurring outside the body.

extracto *m.* extract, a concentrated product; __ **alcohólico** / alcoholic __; __ **alérgico** / allergic __; __ **de**

belladona / belladonna __; __ **equivalente** / equivalent __; __ **líquido** / fluid __; __ **hidroalcohólico** / hydroalcoholic __ .

extradural *a.* extradural. *See* **epidural**.

extraer *vt.* to extract, to remove.

extrañarse *vr.* to wonder, to question.

extraño-a *a.* extraneous. 1. unrelated to or outside an organism; 2. strange, rare; 3. foreign.

extraocular *a.* extraocular, outside the eye.

extrapancreático *a.* extrapancreatic, not connected with the pancreas.

extrasístole *f.* extrasystole, arrhythmic beat of the heart; *pop.* skipped beat.

extrauterino *a.* extrauterine, that occurs or is found outside the uterus.

extravasado-a *a.* extravasated, rel. to the escape of fluid from a vessel or organ into the surrounding tissue.

extravascular *a.* extravascular, outside a vessel.

extremidad *f.* extremity. 1. the end portion; 2. a limb of the body; **amputación de una** __ / limb amputation; **rigidez de una** __ / limb rigidity.

extremo-a *a.* extreme, excessive.

extrínseco-a *a.* extrinsic, that comes from without; **músculo** __ / __ muscle.

extrovertido-a *a.* extroverted, excessive manifestation and attention outside the self.

extrusion *f.* extrusion, expulsion.

extubación *f.* extubation, removal of a tube, as the laryngeal tube.

exuberante *a.* exuberant, excessive proliferation; overabundant.

exudación *f.* exudation. *See* **exudado**.

exudado *m.* exudate, inflammatory fluid such as pus or serum.

eyaculación *f.* ejaculation, sudden and rapid expulsion, such as the emission of semen.

eyacular *v.* to ejaculate, to expel fluid secretions such as semen.

eyección *f.* ejection, throwing out with force.

f

F *abr.* Fahrenheit / Fahrenheit.
f *abr.* fallo / failure; **femenino** / feminine; **fórmula** / formula; **función** / function.
faceta *f.* facet, facette *Fr.* small, smooth area on the surface of a hard structure such as a bone.
facial *a.* facial, rel. to the face; **arteria** __ / __ artery; **axis** __ / __ axis; **canal** __ / __ canal; **espasmo** __ / __ spasm; **hemiplejía** __ / __ hemiplegia; **huesos** __ -es / __ bones; **nervios** __ -es / __ nerves; **parálisis** __ / __ paralysis; **reflejo** __ / __ reflex; **tic** __ / __ tic; **vena** __ / __ vein.
facies *f. facies* expression or appearance of the face; __ **inexpresiva** / masklike __; __ **leontina** / __ leontina.
fácil *a.* easy; **-mente** / *adv.* easily.
facilitar *vt.* to facilitate, to make easier.
facioplastia *f.* facioplasty, plastic surgery of the face.
facioplejía *f.* facioplegia, facial paralysis.
factor *m.* factor, element that contributes to produce an action; __ **angiogenético tumoral** / tumor angiogenetic __; __ **antihemofílico** / antihemophilic __; __ **de coagulación de la sangre** / clotting __; __ **de crecimiento epidérmico** / epidermic growth __; __ **de crecimiento fibroblástico** / fibroblast growth__; __ **dominante** / dominant __; __ **liberador** / releasing __; __ **Rh** [ehrreh-ahcheh] / Rh __; __ **reumatoide** / rheumatoid __ .
facultad *f.* faculty. 1. capability to perform a normal function; 2. professional staff.
facultativo-a *a.* facultative. 1. not obligatory, voluntary; 2. of a professional nature; **asistencia** __ **médica** / professional medical help; **cuidado** __ / professional care.
Faget, signo de *m.* Faget, sign of, low point in relation to the present high temperature.
fagocito *m.* phagocyte, cell that ingests and destroys microorganisms or other cells and foreign particles.

fagocitosis *f.* phagocytosis, the process of ingestion and digestion by phagocytes.
Fahrenheit, escala de *f.* Fahrenheit scale, a temperature scale with a freezing point of water at 32° and a normal boiling point at 212°.
faja *f.* girdle; band.
falange *f.* phalanx, any of the long bones of the fingers or toes.
fálico-a *a.* phallic, rel. to or resembling the penis.
fallecer *vi.* to die, to pass away.
fallecimiento *m.* death.
fallo *m.* failure; insufficiency; __ **cardíaco** / heart __; __ **renal** / renal __; __ **respiratorio** / respiratory __ .
Fallot, tetralogía de *f.* tetralogy of Fallot, congenital deformity of the heart involving defects in the great blood vessels and the walls of the heart chambers.
falo *m.* phallus, the penis.
Falopio, trompas de *f.* Fallopian tubes, tubes leading from the uterus to the ovaries.
falso-a *a.* false, untrue; **anemia** __ / __ anemia; **aneurisma** __ / __ aneurysm; **anquilosis** __ / __ ankylosis; **articulación** __ / __ joint; **blefaroptosis** __ / __ blepharoptosis; **costillas falsas** __ / ribs; **cuerdas vocales** __ / __ vocal chords; **divertículo** __ / __ diverticulum; **embarazo** __ / __ pregnancy; __ **negativo** / __ negative; __ **positivo** / __ positive; **hematuria** __ / __ hematuria; **hermafroditismo** __ / __ hermaphroditism; **imagen** __ / __ image; **lumen** __ / __ lumen; **membrana** __ / __ membrane; **neuroma** __ / __ neuroma; **poliposis adenomatosa** __ / __ adenomatous polyposis; **sutura** __ / __ suture; **síndrome** __ **de la memoria** / __ memory syndrome.
falta *f.* lack, fault, error; __ **de alimentos** / __ of food; __ **de orientación** / __ of orientation; **sin** __ / without fail; for sure.
faltar *vt.* to be lacking or wanting; to be absent.
famélico-a *a.* famished.
familia *f.* family; **práctica de** __ / __ practice; **terapia de** __ / __ therapy.

familiar *m.* family member; *a.* familiar, familial; **bocio** __ / __ goiter; **degeneración macular pseudoinflamatoria** __ / __ pseudoinflammatory macular degeneration; **descendencia** __ / kinship; **disautonomía** __ / __ dysautonomy; **escrutinio** __ / __ screening; **hipercolesteremia** __ / __ hypercholesteremia; **ictericia** __ / __ jaundice; **neuropatía amiloide** __ / __ amyloid neuropathy; **parálisis periódica** __ / __ periodic paralysis; **poliposis adenomatosa** __ / __ adenomatous polyposis; **tendencia** __ / __ tendency.

Fanconi, síndrome de *m.* Fanconi's syndrome, congenital hypoplastic anemia.

fantasía *f.* fantasy, the use of the imagination to transform an unpleasant reality into an imaginary, satisfying experience.

fantoma *m.* phantom. 1. mental image; 2. a transparent model of the human body or any of its parts.

faringe *f.* pharynx, part of the alimentary canal extending from the base of the skull to the esophagus.

faríngeo-a *a.* pharyngeal, rel. to the pharynx.

faringitis *f.* pharyngitis, infl. of the pharynx.

farmacéutico-a *m., f.* pharmacist, specialist in pharmacy.

farmacia *f.* pharmacy, drugstore.

farmacocinética *f.* pharmacokinetics, the study *in vivo* of the metabolism and action of drugs.

farmacodependencia *f.* drug dependence.

farmacodinamia *f.* pharmacodynamics, the study of the effects of medication.

farmacología *f.* pharmacology, the study of drugs and their effect on living organisms.

farmacólogo-a *m., f.* pharmacologist, pharmacist, specialist in pharmacology.

farmacopea *f.* pharmacopeia, a publication containing a listing of drugs and formulas as well as information providing standards for their preparation and dispensation.

fascia *L.* fascia, fibrous connective tissue that envelops the body beneath the skin and encloses muscles, nerves, and blood vessels; __ **aponeurótica** / aponeurotic __, provides muscle protection; __ **de Buck** / Buck's __, covers the penis; __ **de Colles** / Colle's __, inner layer of the perineal fascia; __ **lata** / lata __, protects the muscles of the thigh; __ **transversalis** / transversalis __, between the transversalis muscle of the abdomen and the peritoneum; **injerto de una** __ / __ graft.

fascial *a.* fascial, rel. to a fascia.

fasciectomía *f.* fasciectomy, partial or total removal of a fascia.

fasciodesis *f.* fasciodesis, procedure to adhere a tendon to a fascia.

fascioplastia *f.* fascioplasty, plastic surgery of a fascia.

fasciotomía *f.* fasciotomy, incision or partition of a fascia.

fascitis *f.* fascitis, infl. of a fascia.

fase *f.* phase, stage; __ **terminal** / terminal __ .

fásico-a *a.* phasic, rel. to a phase.

fastidioso-a *a.* fastidious, in bacteriology, rel. to complex nutritional demands.

fatal *a.* fatal, deadly, mortal.

fatalidad *f.* fatality.

fatiga *f.* fatigue, extreme tiredness.

fatigarse *vr., vi.* to become fatigued, to get tired.

favor *m.* favor, good deed.

faz *f.* face.

febril *a.* febrile, having a body temperature above normal; **convulsiones** __ -es / __ convulsions.

fecal *a.* fecal, containing or rel. to feces; **absceso** __ / __ abscess; **examen** __ / __ examination; **fístula** __ / __ fistula.

fecalito *m.* fecalith, intestinal concretion of fecal material.

fecaloma *m.* fecaloma, tumor-like accumulation of feces in the colon or rectum.

fecaluria *f.* fecaluria, presence of fecal material in the urine.

fecha *f.* [*día, mes o año*] date; __ **de defunción** / __ of death; __ **del espécimen** / specimen __ or sample __; __ **de nacimiento** / birth __; __ **de vigencia** / effective __ .

fécula *f.* starch.

fecundación *f.* fecundation, the act of fertilizing.

fecundidad *f.* fecundity, fertility.

felino-a *a.* feline, rel. to or resembling a cat.

feliz *a.* happy; felicitous.

femenino-a *a.* feminine.

feminidad *f.* femininity; **complejo de ___ / ___** complex.

feminismo *m.* feminism.

feminización *f.* feminization, development of feminine characteristics.

femoral *a.* femoral, rel. to the femur; **arco ___ profundo / deep ___** arch; **arteria ___ / ___** artery; **arteria nutricional ___ / ___** nutrient artery; **canal ___ / ___** canal; **capa ___ / ___** sheath; **hernia ___ / ___** hernia; **nervio ___ / ___** nerve; **triángulo ___ / ___** triangle; **vena ___ / ___** vein.

femorotibial *a.* femorotibial, rel. to the femur and the tibia; **capilar___ / ___** capillary; **membrana ___ / ___** membrane.

fémur *m.* femur, the thighbone.

fenestración *f.* fenestration. 1. creation of an opening in the inner ear to restore lost hearing; 2. the act of perforating.

fénico, fenol *a.* phenic, carbolic.

fenobarbital *m.* phenobarbital, barbiturate used as a hypnotic or sedative.

fenómeno *m.* phenomenon. 1. objective symptom of a disease; 2. event or manifestation); 3. *pop.* freak.

fenotipo *m.* phenotype, characteristics of a species produced by the environment and heredity.

fermentación *f.* fermentation, splitting a complex compound into simpler ones by the action of enzymes or ferments.

fermento *m.* ferment, the product of fermentation.

ferroproteína *f.* ferroprotein, protein combined with a radical containing iron.

ferruginoso-a, ferrugíneo-a *a.* ferruginous. 1. that contains iron; 2. that has the color of oxidated iron.

fértil *a.* fertile, fruitful.

fertilidad *f.* fertility, fruitfulness.

férula *f.* splint, device made of any material such as wood, metal, or plaster, used to immobilize or support a fractured bone or a joint.

fetal *a.* fetal, rel. to the fetus; **circulación ___ / ___** circulation; **desperdicio / ___** wastage; **distocia ___**
/ ___ dystocia; **hidropesía ___ / ___** hydrops; **latido del corazón ___ / ___** heart tone; **medicina ___ / ___** medicine; **membrana ___ / ___** membrane; **muerte ___ / ___** death; **monitorización ___ / ___** monitoring; **placenta ___ / ___** placenta; **retardo del crecimiento ___ / ___** growth retardation; **síndrome de aspiración ___ / ___** aspiration syndrome; **viabilidad ___ / ___** viability.

fetidez, fetor *f., m.* stench, offensive odor.

fétido-a *a.* fetid, having a very bad odor.

feto *m.* fetus, phase of gestation between three months and the moment of birth; **presentación frontal del ___ / brow** presentation of ___ .

fetometría *f.* fetometry, estimate of the size of the fetus before birth, esp. of the head.

fetoscopía *f.* fetoscopy, antenatal inspection of the fetus by introducing a fetoscope transabdominaly in the mother's womb with the purpose of diagnosis.

fetoscopio *m.* fetoscope, instrument used to visualize the fetus *in utero* to facilitate prenatal diagnosis.

fibra *f.* fiber, filament; **___ -s amarillas / yellow ___ -s; ___ -s ópticas / fiberoptics.

fibrilación *f.* fibrillation. 1. involuntary or abnormal muscular contraction; **___ auricular / atrial, auricular ___,** irregular movement of the atria; **___ ventricular / ___** ventricular; 2. formation of fibrils.

fibrilación-aleteo *f.* flutter-fibrillation, auricular activity that shows signs of flutter and fibrillation.

fibrilar *a.* fibrillar, fibrillary, rel. to a fibril; **astrocito ___ / ___** astrocyte; **contracciones ___ -es / ___** contractions.

fibrilla *f.* fibril, a very small fiber.

fibrina *f.* fibrin, insoluble protein that is essential to the coagulation of blood.

fibrinogenemia *f.* fibrinogenemia, presence of fibrinogen in the blood.

fibrinogénico-a *a.* fibrinogenic, fibrinogenous, that produces fibrin.

fibrinógeno *m.* fibrinogen, protein present in blood plasma that converts into fibrin during blood clotting.

fibrinólisis *f.* fibrinolysis, the dissolution of fibrinogen by the action of enzymes.

fibrinoso-a

fibrinoso-a *a.* fibrous, fibrinous, of the nature of fibers; **bronquitis** __ / __ bronchitis; **inflamación** __ / __ inflammation; **pericarditis** __ / __ pericarditis; **pleuresía** __ / __ pleurisy; **pólipo** __ / __ polyp.

fibrinuria *f.* fibrinuria, presence of fibrin in the urine.

fibroadenoma *f.* fibroadenoma, a benign tumor composed of fibrous and glandular tissue.

fibroblasto *m.* fibroblast, a cell from which connective tissue develops.

fibrocartílago *m.* fibrocartilage, a type of cartilage in which the matrix contains a large amount of fibrous tissue.

fibrocístico-a, fibroquístico-a *a.* fibrocystic, cystic and fibrous in nature; **enfermedad __ de la mama** / __ disease of the breast.

fibrocondroma *m.* fibrochondroma, benign tumor made of fibrous and cartilaginous connective tissue.

fibroide *a.* fibroid, rel. to or of a fibrinous nature; **adenoma** __ / __ adenoma; **catarata** __ / __ cataract.

fibrolipoma *m.* fibrolipoma, tumor that contains fibrous and adipose tissue.

fibroma *m.* fibroma, a benign tumor composed of fibrous tissue.

fibromatosis *f.* fibromatosis, production of multiple fibromas on the skin or the uterus.

fibromialgia *f.* fibromyalgia, generalized chronic condition which results in pain and rigidity in the muscles and in the soft tissues.

fibromioma *m.* fibromyoma, tumor that contains muscular and fibrous tissue.

fibromuscular *a.* fibromuscular, of a fibrous and muscular nature; **displasia** __ / __ dysplasia.

fibroneuroma *m.* fibroneuroma, tumor of the conjunctive tissue of the nerves.

fibroplasia *f.* fibroplasia, formation of fibrous tissue as seen in the healing of a wound; **__ retrolental** / retrolental __.

fibrosarcoma *m.* fibrosarcoma, malignant tumor of fusiform cells, collagen, and reticulin fibers. Syn. **neurofibroma.**

fibrosis *f.* fibrosis, abnormal formation of fibrous tissue; **__ cística** / cystic __; **__ intersticial del pulmón** / diffuse interstitial pulmonary __; **__ proliferativa** / proliferative __; **__ pulmonar** / pulmonary __; **__ retroperitoneal** / retroperitoneal __ .

fibroso-a, fibrinoso-a *a.* fibrous, fibrinous. 1. rel. to or of the nature of fibrin; **anquilosis** __ / __ ankylosis; **articulación** __ / __ joint; **bocio** __ / __ goiter; **defecto cortical** __ / __ cortical defect; **degeneración** __ / __ degeneration; **tejido** __ / __ tissue; **tubérculo** __ / __ tubercle; 2. threadlike.

fibular *a.* fibular, rel. to the fibula; **arteria** __ / __ artery; **vena** __ / __ vein.

ficticio *a.* fictitious, false.

fidelidad *f.* fidelity; loyalty.

fiebre *f.* fever; **ampollas de __** / blisters; **__ de conejo** / rabbit __, tularemia; **__ de origen desconocido** / __ of unknown origin; **__ del heno** / hay __; **__ de trinchera** / trench __; **__ entérica** / enteric __, intestinal; **__ familiar del Mediterráneo** / familiar Mediterranean __; **__ intermitente** / intermittent __; **__ ondulante** / undulant __, brucellosis; **__ recurrente** / relapsing __; **__ remitente** / remittent __; **__ reumatoidea** / rheumatoid __; **__ tifoidea** / typhoid __; **tener __** / to run a temperature.

fiebre aftosa *f.* aphthous fever, foot and mouth disease, illness caused by a virus found in ruminants and pigs that can be transmitted to humans, and is characterized by an eruption of small vesicles in the tongue and fingers.

fiebre amarilla *f.* yellow fever, endemic disease of tropical areas, transmitted by the bite of a female mosquito, *Aedes aegypti*, and manifested by fever, jaundice, and albuminuria.

fiebre del valle *f.* valley fever, coccidiomicosis.

fiebre manchada de las Montañas Rocosas *f.* Rocky Mountain spotted fever, acute febrile disease caused by a germ transmitted by infected ticks.

fiebre Q *f.* Q fever, acute illness contracted from infected animals by *Coxiella burnetti*.

fiebre reumática *f.* rheumatic fever, a fever that gen. follows a streptococcal infection manifested by acute generalized pain of the joints, often with cardiac arrythmia and renal disorders as residual effects.

figura *f.* form, shape; figure.

fijación *f.* fixation. 1. immobilization; 2. the act of focusing the eyes directly upon an object; 3. the act of being strongly attached to a particular person or object; 4. interruption of the development of the personality before reaching maturity.

fijar *v.* to fix, to affix, [*una fractura*] to set.

film *m.* film; thin layer.

filtrar *v.* to strain; **filtrarse** *vr.* to filter through, to filtrate.

filtro *m.* filter, any device used to strain liquids.

fimbria *f.* fimbria. 1. fingerlike structure; 2. appendage of certain bacteria; ___ **ovárica** / ovarian ___; ___ **de la trompa de Falopio** / ___ of the uterine tube; ___ **del hipocampo** / hippocampal ___ .

fimosis *f.* phimosis, narrowness of the orifice of the prepuce that prevents its being drawn back over the glans penis.

fin *m.* end, conclusion; **¿con qué ___?** / for what purpose?; **a ___ de** / in order to.

final *m.* end; **al ___** / at the end; *a.* final, conclusive.

fingir *vi.* to fake, to malinger.

Finney, operación de *f.* Finney operation, gastroduodenostomy that creates a large opening to ensure that the stomach empties fully.

fino-a *a.* fine, as opposed to thick or coarse.

firma *f.* signature.

firmar *v.* to sign, to subscribe.

física *f.* physics, the study of matter and its changes.

físicamente *adv.* physically, referring to the body as opposed to the mind.

físico *m.* 1. physique, appearance, figure; **-a** *m.,* 2. physicist, specialist in physics; *a.* fisico-a, physical, rel. to the body and its condition; **examen ___** / ___ examination; **terapia ___** / ___ therapy.

fisiología *f.* physiology, the study of the physical and chemical processes affecting organisms.

fisión *f.* fission, a breaking up into parts; ___ **nuclear** / nuclear ___ .

fisioterapia *f.* physiotherapy, treatment by means of physical manipulation and agents such as heat, light, and water.

fisonomía *f.* physiognomy, facial features.

fístula *f.* fistula, abnormal passage from a hollow organ to the skin or from one organ to another; ___ **arteriovenosa** / arteriovenous ___; ___ **biliar** / biliary ___; ___ **del ano** / anal ___ .

fistulectomia *f.* fistulectomy, surgical removal of a fistula.

fistulización *f.* fistulization, pathological or surgical formation of a fistula.

fisura *f.* fissure, cleft, a longitudinal opening.

fitobezoar *m.* phytobezoar, a concretion of undigested vegetable fiber that forms in the stomach or intestine.

flácido-a *a.* flaccid, limber, lax.

flaco-a *a.* very thin, lanky.

flagelado-a *a.* flagellated, provided with flagella.

flageliforme *a.* flagelliform, shaped like a whip.

flagelo *m.* flagellum, prolongation or tail in the cells of some protozoa or bacteria.

flanco *m.* flank, loin, part of the body situated between the ribs and the upper border of the ilium.

flato *m.* flatus, gas or air in the stomach or intestines.

flatulencia *f.* flatulence, condition marked by distention and abdominal discomfort due to excessive gas in the gastrointestinal tract.

flebitis *f.* phlebitis, infl. of a vein.

flebolito *m.* phlebolith, phlebolite, a calcareous deposit in a vein.

flebotomía *f.* phlebotomy, venotomy, incision into a vein for the purpose of drawing blood.

flegmasia *f.* phlegmasia, inflammation.

flegmasia cerúlea dolorosa *f.* milk leg, phlegmasia cerulea dolens, thrombosis of one of the veins of the leg, gen. the femoral vein, that is manifested by acute pain, infl., cyanosis and edema, and that can cause a severe circulatory problem.

flema *f.* phlegm. 1. thick mucus; 2. one of the four humors of the body.

flemático-a *a.* phlegmatic. 1. that produces phlegm; 2. apathetic.

flemón *m.* phlegmon, an infl. of the cellular tissue.

flexibilidad *f.* flexibility, pliability, the capability to flex.

flexión *f.* flexion, flexure, the act of bending.

flexionar *vt.* to flex, to bend.

flexor *m.* flexor, a muscle that can flex a joint.

flexura *f.* flexure, fold, curvature, bend; __ esplénica / splenic __, left curvature of the colon; __ hepática / hepatic __, right curvature of the colon; __ sigmoidea / sigmoid __, curved part of the colon that precedes the rectum.

flogosis *f.* phlogosis.flegmasia.

flojera *f.* weakness.

flojo-a *a.* weak, flaccid; sluggish.

flora *f.* flora, group of bacteria within a given organ; __ intestinal / intestinal __ .

flotadores *m.* floaters, visual spots.

flotante *a.* floating, free, not adhered.

fluctuación *f.* fluctuation, wavering, wavelike movements produced by vibrations of body fluids on palpation.

fluído *m.* fluid, liquid; __ amniótico / amniotic __; __ cefalorraquídeo / cerebrospinal; __ extracelular / extracellular __; __ extravascular / extravascular __; __ intersticial / interstitial __; __ intracelular / intracellular __; __ seminal / seminal __; __ seroso / serous __; __ sinovial / synovial __ .

fluir *vi.* to flow.

flujo *m.* flow, flux. 1. large amount of fluid discharge from a cavity or surface of the body; __ laminar / laminar __; __ turbulento / turbulent __; medidor de __ / flowmeter; 2. the rush of blood or liquid; 3. menstruation.

flúor *m.* fluorine, gaseous chemical element.

fluorescente *a.* fluorescent, rel. to fluorescence; anticuerpo __ / __ antibody; técnica del anticuerpo __ / __ treponemal antibody absorption test.

fluoridación *f.* fluoridation, fluoridization, addition of fluorides to water.

fluoroscopía *f.* fluoroscopy, examination of tissues and structures of the body using the fluoroscope.

fluoroscopio *m.* fluoroscope, instrument that makes x-rays visible on a fluorescent screen.

fluorosis *f.* fluorosis, excess fluoride content.

fluoruro *m.* fluoride, combination of fluorine with a metal or a metalloid.

fobia *f.* phobia, abnormal irrational fear.

focal *a.* focal, rel. to focus.

foco *m.* focus, the main point or principal spot.

fofo-a *a.* flabby, soft.

fogaje *m.* hot flash.

folicular *a.* follicular, rel. to a follicle; fase __ / __ phase.

foliculitis *f.* folliculitis, infl. of a follicle, usu. in reference to a hair follicle.

folículo *m.* follicle, sac or pouchlike secretory depression or cavity; __ atrésico / atretic __; __ de Graaf, ovárico / Graafian, ovaric __; __ gástrico / gastric __; __ piloso / hair __; __ tiroideo / thyroid __ .

folleto *m.* pamphlet, brochure.

fomento *m.* hot compress.

fomes *L. fomites* fomes, an element that can absorb and transmit infectious agents.

fondillo *m.* buttocks.

fondo *m.* bottom; __ del ojo / eyeground.

fonética *f.* phonetics, the study of speech and prounciation.

fonético-a *a.* phonetic, rel. to the voice and articulated sounds.

foniatra *m., f.* phoniatrist, specialist in voice treatment.

fonograma *m.* phonogram, a graphic that indicates the intensity of a sound.

fonoscopio *m.* phonoscope, a device that registers heart sounds.

fontanela *f.* fontanel, fontanelle, soft spot in the skull of a newborn that closes as the cranial bones develop; caída de la __ / fallen __.

foramen *m.* foramen, orifice, passage, opening; __ intervertebral / intervertebral __; __ óptico / optic __; __ oval / oval __ ; __ sacrociático mayor / sciatic, greater __ ; __ yugular / jugular __ .

fórceps *m.* forceps, a surgical, tonglike instrument used to grasp, pull, or manipulate tissues or body parts.

forense *a.* forensic, rel. to the courts; laboratorio __ / __ laboratory; médico __ / __ physician.

forma *f.* form, shape; established manner of doing something; __ frustrada / forme fruste; *Fr.,* an aborted or atypical form of a disease.

formación *f.* formation, the manner in which something is arranged.

formaldehído *m.* formaldehyde, antiseptic.

Frohlich, síndrome de

formar *v.* to form, to shape.
formicación *f.* formication, skin sensation comparable to one produced by crawling insects.
fórmula *f.* formula, a prescribed way or model.
formulario *m.* 1. form, [*planilla*] blank; 2. formulary, prescription tablet, a book of formulas.
fórnix *m.* fornix, vaultlike structure such as the vagina.
fortalecer *vt.* to fortify, to strengthen.
fortificar *vt.* to fortify.
forúnculo *m.* boil.
fosa *f.* fossa, cavity, depression, hole; __ **etmoidal** / ethmoid __; __ **glenoidea** / glenoid __; __ **interpenduncular** / interpenduncular __; __ **mandibular** / mandibular __; __ **nasal** / nasal __; __ **navicular** / navicular __; __ **supraclavicular** / supraclavicular __; __ **yugular** / jugular __ .
fósforo *m.* phosphorus.
fotocoagulación *f.* photocoagulation, localized tissue coagulation by an intense controlled ray of light or laser beam, esp. used in surgery of the eye.
fotodermatitis *m.* photodermatitis, abnormal reaction of the skin to ultraviolet rays or to the sun.
fotoquimpoterapia *m.* photoquimotherapy, drug treatment that reacts to ultraviolet rays or to the sun.
fototerapia *f.* phototherapy, light therapy, exposure to sun rays or to an artificial light for therapeutic purposes.
fóvea *f.* fovea, small depression, esp. used in reference to the central fossa of the retina.
fracaso *m.* failure; **neurosis del __** / __ neurosis.
fracción *f.* fraction, separable part of a unit.
fractura *f.* fracture, breaking or separation of a bone; __ **abierta** / open __; __ **cerrada** / closed __; __ **conminuta** / comminuted __; __ **completa** / complete __; __ **con luxación** / dislocation __; __ **con hundimiento** / depressed __; __ **de línea fina** / hairline __; __ **en caña o tallo verde** / greenstick __; __ **en cuña** / wedge __; __ **en mariposa** / butterfly __; __ **en martillo** / mallet __; __ **en T** / T __; __ **espiral** / spiral __; __ **impactada** / impacted __; __ **incompleta** / incomplete __; __

patológica / pathologic __; __
perforante / perforating __; __ **por avulsión** / avulsion __; __ **por compresión** / compression __; __ **por estallamiento** / blow-out __; __ **por herida de bala** / gunshot __; __ **por sobrecarga** / stress __ . See table on page 343.
fracturar *v.* to fracture, to break a bone.
frágil *a.* fragile, brittle; breakable.
fragilidad *f.* fragility, disposition to tear or break easily.
frazada *f.* blanket.
frecuencia *f.* frequency; rate; **con __** / frequently; __ **cardíaca fetal** / baseline fetal heart __; __ **de filtración** / filtration __; __ **de goteo** / drip __; __ **del pulso** / pulse __; __ **glomerular** / glomerular __; __ **intrínseca** / intrinsic __; __ **respiratoria** / breathing __ .
frecuente *a.* frequent; **-mente** *adv.* frequently.
frémito *m.* fremitus, a vibration that can be detected during auscultation or on palpation, such as the chest vibrations during coughing.
frenectomía *f.* frenectomy, removal of the frenum.
frenillo *m.* frenum of the tongue; **con __** / tongue-tied.
frente *f.* forehead, brow; *prep.* in front; **en __ de** / in __ of; __ **a __** / face to face; __ **a** / across from.
frenulum *f.* frenulum, frenum, small membranous fold that limits the movement of an organ or part.
fresa *f.* bur, burr. 1. [*dental*] dental drill; __ **de fisura** / fissure __; 2. strawberry; **marca en __** / __ mark.
fresco *m.* refreshing air; **hace __** / it is cool.
freudiano-a *a.* Freudian, rel. to the doctrines of Sigmund Freud, Viennese neurologist, father of psychoanalysis, (1856–1939).
fricción *f.* friction, rub; __ **de alcohol** / alcohol rub; **roce de __** / __ rub.
frigidez *f.* frigidity, coldness, inability to respond to sexual arousement.
frigoterapia *f.* frigotherapy, therapy by using cold.
frijol *m.* bean.
frío-a *a.* cold; [*persona*] without warmth or affection; **hace __** / it is cold.
friolento-a *a.* chilly; too sensitive to cold.
Frohlich, síndrome de *m.* Frohlich's syndrome, adiposogenital

121

dystrophy, manifested by obesity and sexual infantilism.

frontal *a.* frontal, rel. to the forehead; **hueso** __ / __ bone; **músculo** __ / __ muscle; **senos** __ -es / __ sinuses.

frotar *v.* to rub; __ **suavemente** / to stroke.

frote *m.* rub. 1. friction; massage; 2. sound heard on ausculation, produced by two dry surfaces rubbing against each other.

frotis *m.* smear, sample of blood or a secretion for the purpose of microscopic study.

fructosa *f.* fructose, sugar of fruits; levulose; **intolerancia a la** __ / __ intolerance.

fructosuria *f.* fructosuria, presence of fructose in the urine.

frustrado-a *a.* frustrated.

fuente *f.* 1. source, origin; 2. fountain.

fuera *adv.* out, outside; **estar** __ / to be __ or away; __ **de sí** / beside oneself; **hacia** __ / outward.

fuerte *a.* strong, vigorous; hard.

fuerza *f.* force, strength; power; __ **catabólica** / catabolic __; __ **de gravedad** / __ of gravity; **no tengo** __ / I feel weak.

fulguración *f.* fulguration, use of electric current to destroy or coagulate tissue.

fulminante *a.* fulminant, appearing suddenly and with great intensity, esp. in reference to a disease or pain.

fumador-a *m., f.* person who smokes heavily.

fumador-a pasivo-a *m., f.* passive smoker, person who does not smoke but is exposed to other people smoking, thus inhaling the emanating smoke.

fumante *a.* fuming, that gives forth a visible vapor.

fumar *v.* to smoke.

fumigación *f.* fumigation, extermination, or disinfection through the use of vapors.

fumigante *m.* fumigant, agent used in fumigation.

función *f.* function.

funcional *a.* functional, having practical use or value.

funcionar *v.* to function, to work.

funda *f.* pillowcase; covering.

fungemia *f.* fungemia, presence of fungi in the blood.

fungicida *m.* fungicide, agent that destroys fungi.

fungistasis *f.* fungistasis, the action of thwarting the growth of fungi.

fungitóxico-a *a.* fungitoxic, that causes a toxicity in fungi.

fungoso-a *a.* fungous, fungal, rel. to fungi.

funicular *a.* funicular, rel. to the umbilical or spermatic chord.

funiculitis *f.* funiculitis, infl. of the spermatic chord.

furioso-a *a.* furious, frantic.

furosemida *f.* furosemide, diuretic agent.

furunculosis *f.* furunculosis, condition resulting from the presence of boils.

fusión *f.* fusion, the act of melting; __ **nuclear** / nuclear __ .

futuro *m.* future; *a.* **futuro-a** future.

ganglios basales

g

g *abr.* **género** / gender; **glucosa** / glucose; **gramo** / gram; **grano** / grain.
gabinete *m.* cabinet.
Gaenslen, examen de *m.* Gaenslen sign, test, procedure used to determine sacroiliac dysfunction.
gafas *f.* spectacles, eyeglasses.
gago-a *m., f.* stutterer.
gaguear *vi.* to stutter.
galactagogo, galactógeno *m.* galactagogue, agent that stimulates the flow of milk.
galactasa *f.* galactase, enzyme present in milk.
galactocele *m.* galactocele, breast cyst containing milk.
galactoforitis *f.* galactophoritis, infl. of the lacteal ducts.
galactografía *f.* galactography, x-ray of the mammary ducts.
galactopoyesis *f.* galactopoyesis, production of milk.
galáctoro-a *a.* galactophorous, that conducts or carries milk.
galactorrea *f.* galactorrhea. 1. milk secretion or discharge resembling milk; 2. continuation of milk secretion at intervals after the period of lactation has ended.
galactosa *f.* galactose, monosaccharide derived from lactose by the action of an enzyme or mineral acid; **catarata __** / __ cataract.
galactosemia *f.* galactosemia, congenital absence of the enzyme necessary to convert galactose to glucose and its derivatives.
galactosuria *f.* galactosuria, milk-like urine due to the presence of galactose.
galactoterapia *f.* galactotherapy. 1. the treatment of breast-fed infants by the administration of medication to the nursing mother; 2. therapeutic use of milk in the diet.
galacturia *f.* galacturia, milk-like urine.
galope *m.* gallop, cardiac rhythm resembling the gallop of a horse that indicates heart failure; **ritmo de __** / __ rhythm.
galvánico-a *a.* galvanic, rel. to galvanism; **batería __** / __ battery;

célula __ / __ cell; **corriente __** / __ current.
gama *f.* range; **__ de colores** / color __.
gameto *m.* gamete, 1. any sperm cell, sexual cell, masculine or feminine; 2. ovum or sperm.
gametocito *m.* gametocyte, a cell that divides to produce gametes.
gamma globulina *f.* gamma globulin, a class of antibodies produced in the lymph tissue or synthetically.
gammagrama *m.* scintiscan, a two-dimensional image representation of the interior distribution of a radiopharmaceutical in a previously selected area for diagnostic purposes.
gamofobia *n.* gamophobia, fear of marriage.
gamopatía *f.* gammopathy, disorder manifested by an excessive amount of immunoglobulins due to an abnormal proliferation of lymphoid cells.
gana *f.* desire, inclination; **de buena __** / willingly; **de mala __** / unwillingly; **tener __ -s de** / to desire, to want to.
gancho *m.* hook; clasp; **-s** [*dental*] braces.
gangliectomía, ganglionectomía *f.* gangliectomy, ganglionectomy, excision of a ganglion.
ganglio *m.* ganglion, collection of nerve cells resembling a knot; **__ basal** / basal __; **__ carotídeo** / carotid __; **__ celíaco** / celiac __ .
ganglioctomía *f.* ganglioctomy, excision of a ganglion.
ganglioglioma *m.* ganglioglioma, tumor with a large number of ganglionic cells.
ganglioma *m.* ganglioma, tumor of a ganglion, esp. a lymphatic ganglion.
ganglión *m.* ganglion, a cystic tumor that develops in a tendon or an aponeurosis, often seen in the wrist, the heel or the knee.
ganglionar *a.* ganglionic, rel. to a ganglion; **bloqueo __** / __ blockade.
ganglioneuroma *m.* ganglioneuroma, benign tumor composed by ganglionic neurons.
ganglionitis *f.* gangionitis, infl. of a ganglium.
ganglios basales *m. pl.* basal ganglia, gray matter localized in the

gangrena

low portion of the brain stem that takes part in muscular coordination.

gangrena *f.* gangrene, local death, destruction and putrefaction of body tissue due to interrupted blood supply.

gangrenoso-a *a.* gangrenous, rel. to gangrene.

Gardner, síndrome de *m.* Gardner's syndrome. 1. multiple polyps of the colon associated with risk of colon carcinoma; 2. soft-tissue tumors of the skin.

garganta *f.* throat, the area of the larynx and the pharynx; anterior part of the neck; **dolor de __ / sore __ .**

gárgara, gargarismo *f., m.* gargarism, gargle, gargling, rinsing of the throat and the mouth; **hacer __ -s /** to gargle.

gargolismo *m.* gargoylism, hereditary condition characterized by skeletal abnormalities and sometimes mental retardation.

garra *f.* claw; **mano en __ / __ hand; pie en __ / __ foot.**

garrapata *f.* tick, bloodsucking acarid that transmits specific diseases; **picadura de __ / __ bite.**

garrotillo *m.* croup.

gas *m.* gas; **__ -es arteriales /** arterial blood **__ -es; __ -es en la sangre /** blood **__-es; __ lacrimógeno /** tear **__; __ mostaza /** mustard **__; __ neurotóxico /** nerve **__ .**

gasa *f.* gauze; **compresa de __ / __** compress; **__ antiséptica /** antiseptic **__ .**

gaseoso-a *a.* gaseous, of the nature of gas.

gasto *m.* [*cardíaco*] output; costs, expense(s); expenditure; waste; **__ cubiertos /** covered **__ .**

gastralgia *f.* gastralgia, stomach ache.

gastrectomía *f.* gastrectomy, removal of part or all of the stomach.

gástrico-a *a.* gastric, rel. to the stomach; **alimentación __ / __** feeding; **arteria __ -s / __** arteries; **derivación __ / __** by-pass; **digestión __ / __** digestion; **fístula __ / __** fistula; **glándulas __ / __** glands; **jugo __ / __** juice; **lavado __ / __** lavage; **vaciamiento __ / __** emptying; **vértigo __ / __** vertigo.

gastritis *f.* gastritis, infl. of the stomach; **__ aguda /** acute **__; __ crónica /** chronic **__ .**

gastroanálisis *m.* gastric analysis, analysis of the stomach contents.

gastrocele *m.* gastrocele, stomach hernia.

gastrocnemio *m.* gastrocnemius, large calf muscle.

gastrocolitis *f.* gastrocolitis, infl. of the stomach and the colon.

gastrocolostomía *f.* gastrocolostomy, anastomosis of the stomach and the colon.

gastroduodenal *a.* gastroduodenal, rel. to the stomach and the duodenum.

gastroduodenitis *f.* gastroduodenitis, infl. of the stomach and the duodenum.

gastroduodenoscopía *f.* gastroduodenoscopy, visual examination of the stomach and the duodenum with an endoscope.

gastroectasia *f.* gastroectasis, gastroectasia, dilation of the stomach.

gastroenteritis *f.* gastroenteritis, infl. of the stomach and the intestine.

gastroenterocolitis *f.* gastroenterocolitis, infl. of the stomach and the small intestine.

gastroenterología *f.* gastroenterology, the study of the gastrointestinal tract.

gastroenterostomía *f.* gastroenterostomy, anastomosis of the stomach and the small bowel.

gastroesofágico-a *a.* gastroesophageal, rel. to the stomach and the esophagus; **enfermedad de reflujo __ / __** reflux disease; **hernia __ / __** hernia.

gastroespasmo *m.* gastrospasm, spasmodic contractions of the stomach walls.

gastrogavage *m.* gastrogavage, artificial feeding into the stomach through a tube.

gastrohepatitis *f.* gastrohepatitis, infl. of the stomach and the liver.

gastroileostomía *f.* gastroileostomy, anastomosis of the stomach and the ileum.

gastrointestinal *a.* gastrointestinal, rel. to the stomach and the intestine; **decompresión __ / __** decompression; **examen __ superior /** upper **__ examination; sangramiento __ / __** bleeding; **tracto __ / __** tract.

gastrolitiasis *f.* gastrolithiasis, calculi in the stomach.

gastrolito *m.* gastrolith, stomach concretion.

gastromegalia *f.* gastromegaly, enlargement of the stomach.

gastroplicación *f.* gastroplication, suture of a stomach wall to reduce its size. **Sin.** gastrorrafia.

gastrorrafía *f.* gastrorrhaphy, suture or perforation of the stomach.

gastrorragia *f.* gastrorrhagia, hemorrhaging from the stomach.

gastroscopía *f.* gastroscopy, examination of the stomach and the abdominal cavity with a gastroscope.

gastroscopio *m.* gastroscope, endoscope for visualizing the inside of the stomach.

gastrosquisis *f.* gastroschisis, congenital fissure in the abdominal wall due to a rupture of the amniotic membrane.

gastroyeyunostomía *f.* gastrojejunostomy, anastomosis of the stomach and the jejunum.

gatear *vi.* to crawl on all fours, such as babies.

Gauss, signo de *m.* Gauss sign, marked mobility in the uterus in early pregnancy.

gemelo-a *m., f.* twin, either of two offspring born of the same pregnancy; __ **dicigótico-a** / dizygotic __; __ **encigótico-a** / enzygotic __; __ **fraternal** / fraternal __; __ **idéntico-a** / identical __; __ **monocigótico-a** / monozygotic __; __ **siamés, siamesa** / Siamese __; __ **verdadero-a** / true __.

gemido *m.* groan, moan.

gemir *vi.* to groan, to moan.

gen, gene *m.* gene, basic unit of hereditary traits; __ **dominante** / dominant __; __ **letal** / lethal __; __ **ligado al sexo** / sex-linked __; __ **recesivo** / recessive __ .

generación *f.* generation, procreation. 1. the act of creating a new organism; 2. the whole body of individuals born within a time span of approximately thirty years.

general *a.* general; **estado** __ / __ condition; **tratamiento** __ / __ treatment; *adv.* **-mente** generally.

generalización *f.* generalization.

genérico-a *a.* generic, rel. to the gender; **nombre** __ / __ name, not protected by a trademark.

género *m.* 1. gender, sex of an individual; **identidad de** __ / __ identity; **papel de** __ / __ role; 2. genus, a category of biological classification.

génesis *f.* genesis, origin, beginning; reproduction.

genética *f.* genetics, branch of biology that studies heredity and the laws that govern it; __ **médica** / medical __ .

genético-a *a.* genetic, rel. to heredity or genetics; **acondicionamiento** __ / __ fitness; **amplificación** __ / __ amplification; **asesoramiento** __ / __ counseling; **asociación** __ / __ association; **carga** __ / __ load; **cartografía** __ / __ mapping; **determinante** __ / __ determinant; **división** __ / __ splicing; **droga** __ / __ drug; **epidemiología** __ / __ epidemiology; **ingeniería o construcción** __ / __ engineering; **marcador** __ / __ marker; **patrón** __ / __ code; **sustrato** __ / __ substratum.

geniculado-a *a.* geniculate. 1. bent as the knee; 2. rel. to the ganglion of the facial nerve.

genicular *a.* genicular, rel. to the knee.

genital *a.* genital, rel. to the genitals; **ambigüedad** __ / __ ambiguity; **cordón** __ / __ cord; **corpúsculos** __ / __ corpuscles; **fase** __ / __ phase; **herpes** __ / __ herpes; **surco** __ / __ furrow; **tracto** __ / __ tract; **verruga** __ / __ wart.

genitales *m. pl.* genitals, genitalia, reproductive organs; *pop.* privates; __ **externos** / __ externalia.

genitourinario-a *a.* genitourinary, rel. to the reproductive and urinary organs.

genocidio *m.* genocide, systematic extermination of an ethnic or social group of people.

genodermatosis *f.* genodermatosis, genetic condition of the skin.

genoma *m.* genome, the complete basic haploid set of chromosomes of an organism.

genómico-a *a.* genomic, rel. to a genome; **clon** __ / __ clone.

genotipo *m.* genotype, the basic genetic constitution of an individual.

gente *f.* people, persons in general.

genuflexión *f.* genuflexion, bending of the knee.

genu valgum *L.* genu valgum, abnormal inward curvature of the knees that begins at infancy as a result of osseus deficiency, *pop.* knock-knee.

genu varum *L.* genu varum, abnormal outward curvature of the knees, *pop.* bowleg.

geofagia, geofagismo *f., m.* geophagia, geophagism, geophagy, propensity to eat soil or similar substances.

geográfico-a *a.* geographic; showing natural, physical or superficial signs; **atrofia retinal** ___ / ___ retinal atrophy; **queratitis** ___ / ___ keratitis.

geriatra *m., f.* geriatrician, specialist in geriatrics.

geriatría *f.* geriatrics, a branch of medicine that deals with the problems of aging and the treatment of diseases and ills of old age.

germen *m.* germ. 1. microorganism or bacteria, esp. one that causes disease; 2. a substance that can develop and form an organism.

germicida *m.* germicide, germicidal, agent that destroys germs.

germinal *a.* germinal, rel. to or of the nature of germs; **célula** ___ / ___ cell; **disco** ___ / ___ disk; **epitelio** ___ / ___ epithelium; **localización** ___ / ___ localization.

germinoma *m.* germinoma, neoplasm of germinal cells in the testis or ovaries.

gerundio *m., gr.* gerund, the present participle of the verb.

gestación *f.* gestation, childbearing, pregnancy; ___ **abdominal** / abdominal ___; ___ **abdominal secundaria** / abdominal secundary ___; ___ **ectópica** / ectopic ___; ___ **intersticial** / interstitial ___; ___ **multiple** / multiple ___; ___ **prolongada** / prolonged ___; ___ **secundaria** / secondary ___; ___ **tubárica** / tubal ___; ___ **tubo-ovárica** / tubo-ovarian ___; ___ **uterotubárica** / uterotubaric ___ .

gestacional *a.* rel. to gestation; **edad** ___ / fetal estimated age.

Gestalt *m.* Gestalt, a configuration, model or experience consisting of elements unified as a whole with properties not derivable by summation of its parts.

gesticular *v.* to gesticulate, to communicate or express by means of gestures or signs.

Ghon, foco, lesión, tubérculo de *m.* Ghon's primary lesion, tubercule, first tubercular lesion in children.

giardiasis *f.* giardiasis, common intestinal infection with *Giardia lamblia* that spreads by contaminated food or water or through direct contact.

gibosidad *f.* gibbosity, the condition of having a hump.

giboso-a *a.* gibbous, humpbacked.

gigante *m.* giant; *a.* giant, unnaturally large; **célula** ___ / ___ cell; **tumor de células** ___ -s / ___ cell tumor.

gigantismo *m.* gigantism, excessive development of the body or some of its parts; ___ **acromegálico** / acromegalic ___; ___ **eunocoide** / eunochoid ___; ___ **normal** / normal ___ .

Gilles de la Tourette, síndrome de *m.* Tourette syndrome, a childhood disease affecting boys more frequently than girls, thought to be of a neurological nature and manifested by muscular anomalies; sometimes accompanied at puberty by involuntary uttering of obscenities and swearing.

gimnasia, gimnástica *f.* gymnastics.

ginandroide *a.* gynandroid, having enough hermaphroditic characteristics to give the appearance of the opposite sex.

ginecología *f.* gynecology, the study of the female reproductive organs.

ginecológico-a *a.* gynecologic, gynecological, rel. to gynecology.

ginecólogo-a *m., f.* gynecologist, specialist in gynecology.

ginecomastia *f.* gynecomastia, excessive development of the mammary glands in the male.

gingiva *L.* gingiva, gum, tissue around the neck of the teeth.

gingival *a.* rel. to the gums.

gingivectomía *f.* gingivectomy, resection of the gingiva.

gingivitis *f.* gingivitis, infl. of the gums.

girar *vt.* to rotate, to revolve.

glande *m.* glans, gland-like mass located at the distal end of the penis (glans penis), or clitoris (glans clitoridis).

glándula *f.* gland, an organ that secretes or excretes substances that have specific functions or that eliminate products from the organism; ___ **inflamada** / swollen ___; ___ **pituitaria** / pituitary ___; ___ **-s salivales** / salivary ___ -s.

glándulas endocrinas *f., pl.* endocrine glands, glands that secrete hormones directly absorbed into the blood or lymph such as the gonads, the pituitary and adrenal glands.

glándulas exocrinas *f., pl.* exocrine glands, glands that discharge their secretion through a duct, such as the mammary and sweat glands.

Glanzmann, trombastenia de *f.* Glanzmann's thrombasthenia, rare congenital disease caused by platelet abnormality.

Glasgow, escala de *f.* Glasgow's scale, instrument used to evaluate the degree of coma.

glaucoma *m.* glaucoma, eye disease caused by intraocular hypertension that results in hardening of the eye, atrophia of the retina, and sometimes blindness; __ **absoluto** / absolutum __ , final stage of acute glaucoma; __ **infantil** / infantile __ , between birth and three years of age; __ **juvenil** / juvenile __ , in older children and young adults without enlargement of the eyeball.

glenohumeral *a.* glenohumeral, rel. to the humerus and the glenoid cavity; **articulación** __ / __ joint; **ligamentos** __ **-es** / __ ligaments.

glenoideo-a *a.* glenoid, socket-like cavity; **cavidad** __ / __ cavity; **fosa** __ / __ fossa.

glicemia, glucemia *f.* glycemia, concentration of glucose in the blood.

glicerina, glicerol *f.* glycerine, glycerol, an alcohol found in fats.

glicina *f.* glycine, a nonessential amino acid.

glicógeno, glucógeno *m.* glycogen, polysaccharide usu. stored in the liver that converts into glucose as needed.

glicogenólisis, glucogenólisis *f.* glycogenolysis, the breakdown of glycogen into glucose.

glicólisis *f.* glycolysis, breakdown of sugar into simpler compounds.

glicosuria *f.* glycosuria. glucosuria.

glioblastoma *f.* glioblastoma, a type of brain tumor.

gliocistoma *m.* gliocystoma, type of cerebral tumor.

glioma *m.* glioma, malignant brain tumor composed of neuroglia cells.

glioneuroma *f.* glioneuroma, a glioma combined with a neuroma.

gliosarcoma *m.* gliosarcoma, glioma abundant in fusiform cells of sarcoma.

globular *a.* globular, spherical.

globulina *f.* globulin, one of a class of simple proteins that is insoluble in water but soluble in moderately concentrated salt solutions; **gamma** __ / gamma __ , a family of proteins capable of carrying antibodies; __ **antilinfocítica** / antilymphocyte __ , immunosuppressant.

globulina de enlace esteroide córtico suprarrenal *f.* corticosteroid-binding globulin.

globulinuria *f.* globulinuria, presence of globulin in the urine.

globus *L.* globus, spheric body; __ **histérico** / __ hystericus, sensation of having a lump in the throat.

glomerular *a.* glomerular, rel. or resembling a glomerulus; cluster-like; **índice de filtración** __ / __ filtration rate; **nefritis** __ / __ nephritis; **quiste** __ / __ cyst.

glomérulo *m.* glomerulus, collection of capillaries in the shape of a tiny ball, present in the kidney.

glomeruloesclerosis *f.* glomerulosclerosis, degenerative process within the renal glomeruli that occurs in renal arteriosclerosis and diabetes.

glomerulonefritis *f.* glomerulonephritis, Bright's disease, infl. of the kidney glomeruli.

glomo *m.* glomus, small mass of arterioles rich in nerve supply and connected directly to veins.

glosa *f.* glossa, tongue.

glosalgia *f.* glossalgia, pain in the tongue.

glosectomía *f.* glossectomy, partial or total excision of the tongue.

glositis *f.* glossitis, infl. of the tongue; __ **aguda** / acute __ , associated with stomatitis.

glosodinia *f.* glossodynia. glosalgia.

glosofaringeo *a.* glossopharyngeal, relative to the pharynx and the tongue.

glotis *f.* glottis, opening in the upper part of the larynx between the vocal cords; vocal apparatus of the larynx.

glucagón *m.* glucagon, one of the two hormones produced by the islets of Langerhans that increase the concentration of glucose in the blood having an anti-inflammatory effect.

glucagonoma *a.* glucagonoma, malignant tumor secreting glucagon.

glucocorticoide

glucocorticoide *a.* glucocorticoid, adrenal cortical hormones active in protecting against stress and affecting carbohydrate and protein metabolism.

glucofilia *f.* glycophilia, the propensity to develop hyperglycemia when even a small amount of glucose is ingested.

glucofosfato deshidrogenasa *m.* glucose-6-phosphate dehydrogenase, enzyme found in the liver and kidney, important in the conversion of glyceryl to glucose.

glucogénesis *f.* glucogenesis, formation of glucose from glycogen.

glucolítico-a *a.* glycolytic, that disintegrates or digests sugars.

glucoproteína *f.* glycoprotein, a protein belonging to a compound made of linked carbohydrates of which mucins, amyloid and mucoid are the most important.

glucorraquia *f.* glycorrhachia, presence of glucose in the cerebrospinal fluid.

glucosa *f.* glucose, dextrose, the main source of energy for living organisms; **nivel de ___ en la sangre** / blood level of ___; **prueba de tolerancia a la ___** / ___ tolerance test.

glucósido *m.* glucoside, glycoside, natural or synthetic compound that liberates sugar upon hydrolysis.

glucosuria *f.* glucosuria, glycosuria, abnormal amount of sugar in the urine; **___ diabética** / diabetic ___; **___ pituitaria** / pituitary ___; **___ renal** / renal ___.

gluten *m.* gluten, albuminoid vegetable matter.

glúteo-a *a.* gluteal, rel. to the buttocks; **pliegue ___** / ___ fold; **reflejo ___** / ___ reflex.

gnatoplastia *f.* gnathoplasty, plastic surgery of the jaw.

gnosia *f.* gnosia, ability to perceive and recognize people and things.

golpe *m.* blow; bruise; bang; **___ en la cabeza** / ___ to the head.

golpear *vt.* to beat, to hit.

goma *f.* 1. gumma, syphilitic tumor; 2. gum rubber; [*de borrar*] eraser; glue.

gónada *f.* gonad, a gland that produces sex cells (gametes). In males the gonads are the testes, in females, the ovaries.

gonadal *a.* gonadal, rel. to a gonad gland; **disgenesia ___** / ___ dysgenesis, malformation.

gonadectomía *f.* gonadectomy, excision of a sexual gland.

gonadotropina *f.* gonadotropin, gonad stimulating hormone; **___ coriónica** / chorionic ___, present in the blood and the urine of the female during pregnancy and used in the pregnancy test; **hormona que estimula la secreción de ___** / ___ releasing hormone.

gonalgia *f.* gonalgia, pain in the knee.

gonartritis *f.* gonarthritis, infl. of the knee joint.

goniopuntura *f.* goniopuncture, puncture of the anterior chamber of the eye as a means to treat glaucoma.

goniotomía *f.* goniotomy, procedure to relieve congenital glaucoma.

gonococcemia *f.* gonococcemia, presence of gonococci in the blood.

gonocócico-a *a.* gonococcal, rel. to gonococci; **artritis ___** / ___ arthritis; **conjuntivitis ___** / ___ conjunctivitis.

gonococo *m.* gonococcus, microorganism of the species *Neisseria gonorrhoeae* that causes gonorrhea.

gonorrea *f.* gonorrhea, highly contagious catarrhal bacterial infection of the genital mucosa, sexually transmitted.

gonorreico-a *a.* gonorrheal, rel. to gonorrhea; **artritis ___** / ___ arthritis; **oftalmia ___** / ___ ophthalmia.

gota *f.* gout. 1. a hereditary disease caused by a defect in uric acid metabolism; 2. drop, a very small portion of a liquid.

goteo *m.* drip, dripping; **___ postnasal** / postnasal ___.

gotero *m.* dropper; **___ para los ojos** / eye ___.

gotica *f.* droplet.

gracias *f. pl.* thanks; **muchas ___** / thank you very much.

grado *m.* [*temperatura*] degree; [*evaluación*] grade. 1. measurement or standard evaluation; 2. in cancer pathology, indication of the stage of the disease.

Graefe, operación de *f.* Graefe operation. 1. cataract operation by incision of the sclera, separation of the capsula and iridectomy; 2. iridectomy for glaucoma.

Graefe, signo de *m.* Graefe sign, failure of the upper eyelid to follow the downward movement of the eyeball.

guardian

gráfica, gráfico *f., m.* graph, chart, diagram.

grafología *f.* graphology, the study of handwriting as an indication of an individual's character, also used as an aid in diagnosis.

Gram, método de *m.* Gram's method, a system of coloring bacteria for the purpose of identifying them on analysis.

gramicidina *f.* gramicidin, antibacterial substance produced by *Bacillis brevis*, active locally against gram-positive bacteria.

gramnegativo *m.* gram-negative, bacteria or tissue that loses coloration when subjected to Gram's method.

grampositivo *m.* gram-positive, bacteria or tissue that retains coloration when subjected to Gram's method.

granulación *f.* granulation, round, small, fleshy masses that form in a wound.

granular, granuloso-a *a.* granular, made up or marked by grains; **cilindro** ___ / ___ cast, urinary cast seen in degenerative and inflammatory nephropathy; **conjunctivitis** ___ / ___ conjunctivitis; **córtex** ___ / ___ cortex; **distrofia** ___ **de la córnea** / ___ corneal dystrophy; **leucocito** ___ / ___ leukocyte; **oftalmia** ___ / ___ ophthalmia; **retículo endoplásmico** ___ / ___ endoplasmic reticulum; **tumor celular** ___ / ___ cell tumor.

gránulo *m.* granule, small grain or particle; ___ **acidófilo** / acidophil ___ , a stain with acid dyes; ___ **basófilo** / basophil ___ , a stain with basic dyes.

granulocito *m.* granulocyte, leukocyte containing granules.

granulocitopenia *f.* granulocytopenia, deficiency in the number of granulocytes in the blood.

granulocitosis *f.* granulocytosis, excessive increase of granulocytes in the blood.

granuloma *m.* granuloma, tumor or neoplasm of granular tissue; ___ **de cuerpo extraño** / foreign body ___; ___ **infeccioso** / infectious ___; ___ **inguinal** / inguinal ___; ___ **ulcerativo de los genitales** / venereum ___ .

granulomatoso-a *a.* granulomatous, with the characteristics of a granuloma; **colitis** ___ / ___ colitis; **encefalomielitis** ___ / ___ encephalomyelitis; **enteritis**

___ / ___ enteritis; **inflamación** ___ / ___ inflammation.

granulosa *f.* granulosa, ovarian membrane of epithelial cells; **tumor de células de la** ___ / ___ cell tumor; **tumor de la** ___ **teca** / ___ teca cell tumor.

grapar *vt.* to staple; surgical procedure.

grasa *f.* fat, adipose tissue; ___ **saturada** / saturated ___ .

grasiento-a, grasoso-a *a.* fatty, greasy; **degeneración** ___ / ___ degeneration.

gratificación *f.* gratification, reward.

gratificar *vi.* to gratify, to reward.

gratis *adv.* gratis, free.

grave *a.* critically ill; of a serious nature.

Grave, enfermedad de *f.* Grave's disease, exophthalmic goiter.

gravedad *f.* gravity. 1. seriousness; **estado de** ___ / critical condition; ___ **específica** ___ gravity; 2. force of gravity.

grávida *f.* gravida, pregnant woman.

grieta *f.* crevice, cleft, fissure; ___ **-s en las manos** / chapped hands.

gripe *f.* grippe, flu; ___ **asiatica** / Asiatic flu.

gris *a.* gray; **catarata** ___ / ___ cataract; **columnas** ___ **-es** / ___ columns; **degeneración** ___ / ___ degeneration; **fibras** ___ **-es** / ___ fibers; **hepatización** ___ / ___ hepatización; **induración** ___ / ___ induration; **sustancia** ___ / ___ matter.

gris, materia o sustancia *f.* gray matter, highly vascularized gray tissue of the central nervous system made up primarily of nerve cells and unmyelinated nerve fibers.

gritar *v.* to scream, to cry out.

grosero-a *a.* gross, coarse.

grosor *m.* thickness; density.

grueso-a *a.* heavy; thick.

grupo *m.* group, cluster; team, an associated group; ___ **de soporte, de apoyo** / support ___ .

grupo sanguíneo *m.* blood group, the different types of human erythrocytes, genetically determined and differentiated immunologically; ___ **RH** / Rh ___ .

guanetidina *f.* guanethidine, agent used in the treatment of hypertension.

guardar *v.* to put away; to keep.

guardería infantil *f.* nursery; children's day care center.

guardián *m.* guardian; custodian.

guayaco *m.* guaiac, substance used in tests as a reagent to detect the presence of blood.

guayacol *m.* guaiacol, antiseptic; expectorant.

guiar *v.* to guide, to direct.

Guillain-Barre, síndrome de *m.* Guillain-Barre syndrome, rare neurological disease evidenced by ascending paralysis that starts in the extremities and can rapidly include the respiratory muscles causing respiratory failure.

gusano *m.* earthworm, maggot, caterpillar; __ **nematodo que infecta los pulmones** / lungworm; __ **plano** / flatworm, intestinal worm.

gustación *f.* gustation, the sense of taste.

gustar *v.* to like, to enjoy; to taste.

gustativo-a *a.* gustatory, rel. to taste; **agnosia** __ / __ agnosia; **aura** __ / __ aura; **hiperhidrosis** __ / __ hyperhidrosis; **rinorrea** __ / __ rhinorrhoea.

gusto *m.* the sense of taste; taste; **buen** __ / good taste; **mal** __ / bad taste.

gutapercha *f.* gutta-percha, dried and purified latex of some trees that is used in medical and dental treatments.

gutural *a.* guttural, pronounced in the throat.

h

H *abr.* **heroína** / heroin; **hidrógeno** / hydrogen; **hipermetropía** / hypermetropia; **hipodérmico-a** / hypodermic.

h *abr.* **hora** / hour; **horizontal** / horizontal.

hábil, habilidoso-a *a.* able, skillful.

habilidad *f.* ability, aptitude.

habitación *f.* room.

hábito *m.* habit. ___ -s sanitarios / health ___ .

habla *m.* [*locución*] speech; **defecto del** ___ / ___ defect; **patología del** ___ / ___ pathology; **trastorno del** ___ / ___ disorder.

hablar *v.* to speak.

hacer *vt.* to do, to make; ___ **caso** / to mind, to pay attention; ___ **daño** / to harm or hurt; ___ **hincapié** / to emphasize; ___ **lo mejor posible** / to do one's best.

hacia *prep.* towards; ___ **acá** / this way; ___ **allá** / that way; ___ **adelante** / forward; ___ **atrás** / backwards.

hachís *m.* hashish, euphoria producing narcotic extracted from marijuana.

halar *v.* to pull.

halitosis *f.* halitosis, bad breath.

hallazgos *m., pl.* findings, results of an investigation or inquiry.

hallux valgus *L.* hallux valgus, inward turning of the big toe.

hallux varus *L.* hallux varus, separation of the big toe from the others.

hamartoma *m.* hamartoma, nodule simulating a tumor, usu. benign.

hambre *m.* hunger; **tener** ___ / to be hungry.

hambriento-a *a.* hungry, starved, famished.

Hanot, enfermedad de *f.* Hanot's disease, hypertrophic cirrhosis of the liver accompanied by jaundice; biliary cirrhosis.

Hansen, enfermedad de *f.* Hansen's disease. *See* **leprosy**.

haploide *a.* haploid, a sex cell that has half the number of chromosomes characteristic of the species.

hartarse *vt.* to do, to overeat, to stuff oneself.

hasta *prep.* until; up to; as far as; ___ **ahora** / heretofore, so far; ___ **aquí** / up to this point; ___ **luego** / goodbye, see you later.

haustrum *L.* haustrum, cavity or pouch, esp. in the colon.

hay *v.* there is, there are; ___ **que** / it is necessary; **no** ___ **remedio** / it can't be helped.

haz *m.* bundle; ___ **ascendente** / ascending tract.

heces *f., pl.* feces.

Heimlich, maniobra de *f.* Heimlich maneuver, technique applied to force the expulsion of a foreign body that is blocking the passage of air from the trachea or pharynx.

helado *m.* ice cream; *a.* **heladosa** frozen.

helio *m.* helium, gaseous inert chemical element mixed with air or oxygen to be used in the treatment of some respiratory disorders.

helioterapia *f.* heliotherapy, sunbathing as therapy.

helmintiasis *f.* helminthiasis, intestinal infection with worms.

helminticida *m.* helminthicide, agent that kills parasites; vermicide.

helminto *m.* helminth, worm found in the human intestines.

hemaglutinación, hemoaglutinación *f.* hemagglutination, agglutination of red cells.

hemaglutinina, hemoaglutinina *f.* hemaglutinin, antibody that causes agglutination of red cells.

hemangioma *m.* hemangioma, benign tumor formed by clustered blood vessels that produce a reddish birth mark.

hemangiosarcoma *m.* hemangiosarcoma, malignant tumor of the vascular tissue.

hemartrosis *f.* hemarthrosis, extravasation into a joint cavity.

hematemesis *f.* hematemesis, vomiting of blood.

hematerapia, hemoterapia *f.* hematherapy, hemotherapy, therapeutic use of blood.

hemático *m.* drug used in the treatment of anemia; *a.* **hemático-a** rel. to blood; **biometría** ___ / complete blood count (CBC).

hematocolpos *m.* hematocolpos, retention of menstrual blood in the vagina due to an imperforated hymen.

hematócrito *m.* hematocrit.
1. centrifuge that is used for separating cells and particles in the blood from the plasma; 2. the volume percentage of erythrocytes in the blood.

hematología *f.* hematology, the study of the blood and the organs that intervene in its formation.

hematológico-a *a.* hematologic, hematological, rel. to blood; **estudios __ -s /** __ studies.

hematológicos, valores **hemoglobina** / hemoglobin; **promedio de eritrocitos** / hematocrit; **pH de la sangre arterial** / arterial blood pH; **sedimentación de eritrocitos** / erythrocyte sedimentation; **tiempo de coagulación** / coagulation time; **tiempo parcial de tromboplastin** / partial thromboplastin time; **tiempo de protrombina** / prothrombin time; **tiempo de sangramiento** / bleeding time.

hematólogo-a *m., f.* 1. hematologist, specialist in hematology; 2. a specialist in diagnostic blood tests and treating blood diseases.

hematoma *m.* hematoma, localized collection of blood that has escaped from a blood vessel into an organ, space, or tissue; **__ pélvico** / pelvic __; __ **subdural** / subdural __, under the dura mater.

hematopoyesis, hemopoyesis *f.* hematopoiesis, hemopoiesis, formation of blood.

hematoquiste *m.* hematocyst; 1. bloody cyst; 2. hemorrhage within a cyst.

hembra *f.* the female of a species.

hemianopia, hemanopsia *f.* hemianopia, hemanopsia, loss of vision in one half of the visual field of the left or right eye, or of both.

hemicolectomía *f.* hemicolectomy, removal of one half of the colon.

hemihipertrofia *f.* hemihypertrophy, hypertrophy of one half of the body.

hemilaminectomía *f.* hemilaminectomy, removal of the vertebral lamina on one side.

hemiparálisis *f.* hemiparalysis, paralysis of one side of the body.

hemiparesia, hemiparesis *f.* hemiparesia, hemiparesis, paralysis affecting one side of the body.

hemiplejía *f.* hemiplegia, paralysis of the side of the body opposite to the affected cerebral hemisphere. __ **alternante** / alternating __; __ **cerebral** / cerebral __; __ **cruzada** / crossed __; __ **doble** / double __; __ **espástica** / spastic __; __ **facial** / facial __ .

hemipléjico-a *a.* hemiplegic, affected or rel. to hemiplegia.

hemisferio *m.* hemisphere, half of a spherical structure or organ.

hemitiroidectomía *f.* hemithyroidectomy, surgical removal of one lobe of the thyroid gland.

hemobilia *f.* hemobilia, bleeding in the bile ducts.

hemoclasis, hemoclasia *f.* hemoclasis, hemoclasia, rupture, [*hemolysis*] dissolution or other type of destruction of red blood cells.

hemoconcentración *f.* hemoconcentration, concentration of red blood cells due to a decrease of liquid elements in the blood.

hemocromatosis *f.* hemochromatosis, iron storage disease, bronze diabetes, disorder of iron metabolism due to excess deposition of iron in the tissues accompanied by anomalies such as bronze skin pigmentation, cirrhosis of the liver, diabetes mellitus, and malfunction of the pancreas.

hemocultivo *m.* blood culture.

hemodiálisis *f.* hemodialysis, dialysis process used to eliminate toxic substances from the blood in cases of acute renal disorders.

hemodializador *m.* hemodializer, artificial kidney machine used in the dialysis process.

hemodilución *f.* hemodilution, increase in the proportion of plasma to red cells in the blood.

hemodinamia *f.* hemodynamics, the study of the dynamics of blood circulation.

hemofilia *f.* hemophilia, inherited disease characterized by abnormal clotting of the blood and propensity to bleed.

hemofílico-a *m., f.* hemophiliac, person who suffers from hemophilia; *a.* hemophiliac, rel. to or suffering from hemophilia.

hemofobia *f.* hemophobia, pathologic fear of blood.

hemoglobina *f.* hemoglobin, important protein element of the blood that gives its red color and participates in the transportation of oxygen; **índice corpuscular de** ___ / mean corpuscular ___ .

hemoglobinemia *f.* hemoglobinemia, presence of freed hemoglobin in the plasma.

hemoglobinuria *f.* hemoglobinuria, presence of hemoglobin in the urine. ___ **de la postparturienta** / postparturient ___; ___ **en malaria** / malarial ___; ___ **epidémica** / epidemic ___; ___ **intermitente** / intermittent ___; ___ **paroxística fría** / paroxysmal cold ___; ___ **paroxística nocturna** / paroxysmal nocturnal ___ .

hemograma *m.* hemogram, graphic representation of the differential blood count.

hemólisis *f.* hemolysis, rupture of erythrocytes with release of hemoglobin into the plasma; ___ **del recién nacido** / hemolytic disease of the newborn, gen. caused by incompatibility of the Rh factor; ___ **inmune** / immune ___; ___ **venenosa** / venomous ___ .

hemolítico-a *a.* hemolytic, rel. to or that causes hemolysis; **anemia** ___ / ___ anemia, red cells that rupture easily due to a congenital condition caused by toxic agents; **trastorno** ___ / ___ disorder.

hemolito *m.* hemolith, concretion in a blood vessel.

hemopneumotórax *m.* hemopneumothorax, accumulation of blood and air in the pleural cavity.

hemoptisis *f.* hemoptysis, bloody expectoration.

hemorragia *f.* hemorrhage, profuse bleeding; ___ **cerebral** / cerebrovascular accident; ___ **intracraneana** / intracranial ___; ___ **intraventricular** / intraventicular ___; ___ **nasal** / nasal ___; ___ **oculta** / concealed ___; ___ **petequial** / petechial ___; ___ **puerperal** / postpartum ___ .

hemorrágico-a *a.* hemorrhagic, rel. to hemorrhage.

hemorroide(s) *f.* hemorrhoid, pile, a mass of dilated veins in the inferior anal or rectal wall; ___ **de prolapso** / prolapsed ___, that protrudes outside the anus; ___ **externa** / external ___, outside the anal sphincter; ___ **interna** / internal ___, hidden, proximal to the anorectal line.

hemorroidectomía *f.* hemorrhoidectomy, removal of hemorrhoids.

hemosálpinx *m.* hemosalpinx, accumulation of blood in the fallopian tubes.

hemosiderina *f.* hemosiderin, insoluble iron compound stored in the body for use in the formation of hemoglobin as needed.

hemosiderosis *f.* hemosiderosis, hemosiderin deposit in the liver and the spleen.

hemostasia, hemostasis *f.* hemostasis, cessation of bleeding, natural or otherwise.

hemóstato *m.* hemostat, a surgical clamp or a medication used to suppress bleeding.

hemotórax *m.* hemothorax, blood in the pleural cavity.

heparina *f.* heparin, anticoagulant.

heparinizar *vi.* heparinize, to avoid coagulation by the use of heparin.

hepatectomía *f.* hepatectomy, removal of a part or all of the liver.

hepático-a *a.* hepatic, rel. to the liver; **circulación** ___ / liver circulation; **cirrosis** ___ / liver cirrhosis; **coma** ___ / ___ coma; **conducto** ___ / ___ duct; **fallo** ___ / liver failure; **lesión** ___ / liver damage; **lóbulos o subdivisiones** ___ -s / ___ lobes; **manchas** ___ -s / liver spots; **pruebas funcionales** ___ -s / liver function tests; **venas** ___ -s / ___ veins.

hepatitis *f.* hepatitis, infl. of the liver; ___ **amébica** / amebic ___; ___ **colestásica** / cholestatic ___; ___ **crónica activa** / chronic active ___; ___ **crónica persistente** / chronic persistent ___; ___ **epidémica** / epidemic ___; ___ **inducida por droga** / drug-induced ___; ___ **infecciosa** / infectious ___; ___ **no A-no B** / non A-non B ___, linked to blood transfusion; ___ **sérica** / serum ___; ___ **tipo A, viral** ___ / type A, viral ___; ___ **tipo B, viral** / type B, viral ___ .

hepatoentérico-a *a.* hepatoenteric, rel. to the liver and the intestines.

hepatoesplenomegalia *f.* hepatosplenomegaly, enlargement of the liver and the spleen.

hepatolenticular *a.* hepatolenticular, rel. to the lenticular nucleus of the eye and the liver; **degeneración** ___ / ___ degeneration.

hepatologia *f.* hepatology, the study of the liver.

hepatólogo-a *m., f.* hepatologist, specialist in liver diseases.

hepatomegalia *f.* hepatomegaly, enlargement of the liver.

hepatorrenal *a.* hepatorenal, rel. to the liver and the kidneys; **síndrome __ /__** syndrome.

hepatotoxicidad *f.* hepatotoxicity, the propensity of a medication or toxic product to harm the liver.

hepatotoxina *f.* hepatotoxin, toxin that destroys liver cells.

heredado-a *a.* inherited.

hereditario-a *a.* hereditary, inherited.

herencia *f.* heredity, inheritance, transmission of genetic traits from parents to children; __ **familiar** / heredofamilial, rel. to a disease or condition that is inherited.

herida *f.* wound, injury; __ **contusa** / contused __ , subcutaneous lesion; __ **de perforación** / puncture __; __ **de bala** / gunshot __; __ **penetrante** / penetrating __ .

herido-a *a.* wounded; hurt.

hermafrodita *f.* hermaphrodite, an individual that has both ovaric and testicular tissue combined in the same organ or separately.

hermano-a *m., f.* brother; sister, sibling.

hermético-a *a.* hermetic, airtight.

hernia *f.* hernia, abnormal protrusion of an organ or viscera through the cavity wall that encloses it; __ **escrotal** / scrotal __ , that descends into the scrotum; __ **estrangulada** / strangulated __ , obstructing the intestines; __ **femoral** / femoral __ , protruding into the femoral canal; __ **hiatal** / hiatus __ , protruding through the esophagic hiatus of the diaphragm; __ **incarcerada** / incarcerated __ , frequently caused by adherences; __ **inguinal** / inguinal __ , protruding from the viscera into the inguinal canal; __ **lumbar** / lumbar __ , in the loin; __ **por deslizamiento** / sliding __ , of the colon; __ **reducible** / reducible __ , that can be treated by manipulation; __ **umbilical** / umbilical __ , occuring at the navel; __ **ventral** / ventral __ , protrusion through the abdominal wall; **saco de la __** / hernial sac, peritoneal sac into which the hernia descends.

herniación *f.* herniation, development of a hernia.

herniado-a *a.* herniated, hernial, rel. to or having a hernia; **bolsa __ / __** sac; **disco __ / __** disk.

herniografía *f.* herniography, x-ray of a hernia with the use of a contrasting medium.

hernioplastia *f.* hernioplasty, surgical reparation of a hernia.

herniorrafía *f.* herniorrhaphy, reparation or reconstruction of a hernia.

heroína *f.* heroin, diacetylmorphine, addictive narcotic derived from morphine; **adicto-a a la __** , **heroinómano-a** / __ addict.

herpangina *f.* herpangina, infectious disease (epidemic in the summer) that affects the mucous membranes of the throat.

herpes *m.* herpes, inflammatory, painful viral disease of the skin manifested by the formation of small, clustered, blisterlike eruptions; __ **genital** / genitalis; __ **ocular** / ocular __; __ **simple** / __ simplex, simple vesicles that keep recurring in the same area of the skin; __ **zóster [culebrilla]** / __ zoster; *pop.* shingles, painful eruption along the course of a nerve.

herpético-a *a.* herpetic, rel. to herpes or similar in nature.

heterogéneo-a *a.* heterogeneous, dissimilar, not alike.

heteroinjerto *m.* heterograft, graft that comes from a donor of a different species or type than that of the recipient.

heterólogo-a *a.* heterologous.
   1. formed by foreign cell tissue;
   2. derived or obtained from a different species.

heteroplasia *f.* heteroplasia, presence of tissue in areas foreign to its normal location.

heteroplastia *f.* heteroplasty, transplant of tissue from an individual of a different species.

heteroplástico-a *a.* heteroplastic, rel. to heteroplasia.

heterosexual *a.* heterosexual, attracted to the opposite sex.

heterosexualidad *f.* heterosexuality.

heterotopia *f.* heterotopia, displacement or deviation of an organ or part of the body from its normal position.

hético-a *a.* hectic, febrile.

hialinización *f.* hyalinization, degenerative process by which functioning tissue is replaced by a firm, glasslike material.

hialino-a *a.* hyaline, glasslike, or almost transparent; **cilindro** ___ / ___ cast, found in the urine.

hiatus *m.* hiatus, opening, orifice, fissure.

hibernoma *m.* hibernoma, benign tumor localized in the hip or the back.

híbrido-a *a.* hybrid, resulting from the crossing of different species of animals or plants.

hibridoma *m.* hybridoma, hybrid cell capable of producing a continuous supply of antibodies.

hidátide *m.* hydatid, cyst found in tissues, esp. in the liver.

hidatídico-a *a.* hydatid, rel. to a hydatid; **enfermedad** ___ / ___ disease, echinococcosis; **quiste** ___ / ___ mole, uterine cyst that produces hemorrhaging.

hidradenitis *f.* hidradenitis, infl. of the sweat glands.

hidramnios *m.* hydramnion, excess of amniotic fluid.

hidrartosis *f.* hydrarthrosis, effusion of a serous fluid into a cavity.

hidratado-a *a.* hydrated, that is moist or contains water.

hidratar *v.* to hydrate, to combine a body with water.

hídrico-a *a.* hydric, rel. to water.

hidrocefalia *f.* hydrocephaly, hydrocephalus, abnormal accumulation of cerebrospinal fluid within the ventricles of the brain.

hidrocele *m.* hydrocele, an accumulation of serous fluid esp. in the vaginal tunic of the testes.

hidrocelectomía *f.* hydrocelectomy, removal of a hydrocele.

hidrocortisona *f.* hydrocortisone, corticosteroid hormone produced by the adrenal cortex.

hidrofobia *f.* hydrophobia. 1. fear of water; 2. rabies, nervous disorder transmitted by an infected animal.

hidrógeno *m.* hydrogen; **concentración de** ___ / ___ concentration.

hidrólisis *f.* hydrolysis, dissolution of a compound by the action of water.

hidromielia *f.* hydromyelia, increase of fluid in the central canal of the spinal cord.

hidronefrosis *f.* hydronephrosis, distension of the renal pelvis and calices due to obstruction.

hidropesía, hidropsia *f.* hydropsy, dropsy, accumulation of serous fluid in a cavity or cellular tissue.

hidrópico-a *a.* hydropic, rel. to hydropsy.

hidrosálpinx *m.* hydrosalpinx, accumulation of watery fluid in the fallopian tubes.

hidrosis *f.* hidrosis, hydrosis, abnormal sweating.

hidroterapia *f.* hydrotherapy, therapeutic use of applied external water in the treatment of diseases.

hidrotórax *m.* hydrothorax, collection of fluid in the pleural cavity without inflammation.

hidrouréter *m.* hydroureter, abnormal distension of the ureter due to obstruction.

hiel *f.* bile; gall.

hierro *m.* iron.

hifema *f.* hyphema, bleeding in the anterior chamber of the eye.

hígado *m.* liver, largest gland of the body, located in the upper right part of the abdominal cavity. It secretes bile, stabilizes and produces sugar, enzymes, and cholesterol, and eliminates toxins from the body.

higiene *f.* hygiene, the study and practice of health standards; ___ **dental** / dental ___; ___ **mental** / mental ___; ___ **oral** / oral ___; ___ **pública** / public ___ .

higiénico-a *a.* hygienic, sanitary; rel. to hygiene; **absorbente** ___ / sanitary napkin.

higienista *m., f.* hygienist, specialist in hygiene; ___ **dental** / dental ___ , technician in dental profilaxis.

higroma *m.* hygroma, liquid containing sac.

hijastro-a *m., f.* stepson; stepdaughter.

hijo-a *m., f.* son; daughter.

hilio *m.* hilum, hilus, depression or opening in an organ from which blood vessels and nerves enter or leave.

himen *m.* hymen, membranous fold that partially covers the entrance of the vagina.

himenectomía *f.* hymenectomy, excision of the hymen.

himenotomía *f.* hymenotomy, incision in the hymen.

hinchado-a *a.* swollen, bloated.

hinchazón *f.* swelling.

hioides *m.* hyoid bone, horseshoe-shaped bone situated at the base of the tongue.

hipalgesia, hipalgia *f.* hypalgia, diminished sensitivity to pain.

hiperacidez *f.* hyperacidity, excessive acidity.

hiperactividad *f.* hyperactivity, excessive activity; *psych.,* excessive activity manifested in children and adolescents, usu. accompanied by irritability and inability to concentrate for any length of time.

hiperalbuminosis *f.* hyperalbuminosis, excess albumin in the blood.

hiperalimentación *f.* hyperalimentation, supplemental intravenous feeding; ___ **intravenosa / parenteral** ___ .

hiperbilirrubinemia *f.* hyperbilirubinemia, excessive bilirubin in the blood.

hipercalcemia *f.* hypercalcemia, excessive amount of calcium in the blood.

hipercalemia, hiperpotasemia *f.* hyperkalemia, hyperpotasemia, abnormal elevation of potassium in the blood.

hipercapnia *f.* hypercapnia, excessive amount of carbon dioxide in the blood.

hipercinesia *f.* hyperkinesia, abnormal increase of muscular activity.

hipercloremia *f.* hyperchloremia, excess of chlorides in the blood.

hipercloridia *f.* hyperchlorhydria, excessive secretion of chloric acid in the stomach.

hipercoagulabilidad *f.* hypercoagulability, abnormal increase in the coagulability of the blood.

hipercromático-a *a.* hyperchromatic, having excessive pigmentation.

hiperemesis *f.* hyperemesis, excessive vomiting.

hiperemia *f.* hyperemia, excessive blood in an organ or part.

hiperesplenismo *m.* hypersplenism, exacerbation of spleen function.

hiperestesia *f.* hyperesthesia, abnormal increased sensitivity to sensorial stimuli.

hiperglucemia *f.* hyperglycemia, excessive amount of sugar in the blood, such as in diabetes.

hiperglucosuria *f.* hyperglycosuria, excessive amount of sugar in the urine.

hiperhidratación *f.* hyperhydration, abnormal increase of water content in the body.

hiperhidrosis *f.* hyperhidrosis, excessive perspiration.

hiperinsulinismo *m.* hyperinsulinism, excessive secretion of insulin in the blood resulting in hypoglycemia.

hiperlipemia *f.* hyperlipemia, excessive amount of fat in the blood.

hiperlipidemia *f.* hyperlipidemia, excess of lipids in the blood.

hipermenorrea *f.* hypermenorrhea, heavy period, excessive and long menstruation.

hipermetropía *f.* hypermetropia, farsightedness, visual defect in which the rays of light come to focus behind the retina making distant objects better seen than closer ones.

hipermovilidad *f.* hypermobility, excessive mobility.

hipernatremia *f.* hypernatremia, excessive amount of sodium in the blood.

hipernefroma *m.* hypernephroma, Grawitz tumor, neoplasm of the renal parenchyma.

hiperopía *f.* hyperopia. hypermetropia.

hiperópico-a *a.* farsighted.

hiperorexia *f.* hyperorexia, excessive appetite.

hiperosmia *f.* hyperosmia, increased sensitivity of smell.

hiperostosis *f.* hyperostosis, excessive growth of a bony tissue.

hiperpirexia *f.* hyperpyrexia, abnormally high body temperature.

hiperpituitarismo *m.* hyperpituitarism, excessive activity of the pituitary gland.

hiperplasia *f.* hyperplasia, excessive proliferation of normal cells of tissues.

hiperpnea *f.* hyperpnea, increase in the depth and rapidity of breathing.

hiperreflexia *f.* hyperreflexia, exaggerated reflexes.

hipersalivación *f.* hypersalivation, excessive secretion of saliva.

hipersecreción *f.* hypersecretion, excessive secretion.

hipersensibilidad *f.* hypersensibility, excessive sensitivity to the effect of a stimulus or antigen.

hipertensión *f.* hypertension, high blood pressure; ___ **benigna** / benign ___; ___ **esencial** / essential ___; ___

maligna / malignant ___; ___ **portal** / portal ___; ___ **renal** / renal ___ .

hipertenso-a *a.* hypertensive, rel. to or suffering from hypertension.

hipertermia maligna *f.* malignant hyperthermia, onset of high fever that can reach 106°F or 41°C. *Sin.* **hiperpirexia fulminante**.

hipertiroidismo *m.* hyperthyroidism, excessive activity of the thyroid gland.

hipertónico-a *a.* hypertonic, rel. to increased tonicity or tension.

hipertrofia *f.* hypertrophy, abnormal growth or development of an organ or structure; ___ **cardíaca** / cardiac ___ , enlarged heart; ___ **compensadora** / compensatory ___ , resulting from a physical defect.

hipertropía *f.* hypertropia, a form of strabismus.

hiperuricemia *f.* hyperuricemia, excessive amount of uric acid in the blood.

hiperventilación *f.* hyperventilation, extremely rapid and deep inspiration and expiration of air.

hiperviscosidad *f.* hyperviscosity, excessive viscosity.

hipervolimia *f.* hypervolimia, abnormal increase in the volume of circulating blood.

hipnosis *f.* hypnosis, an artificially induced passive state during which the subject is responsive to suggestion.

hipnoterapia *f.* hypnotherapy, therapeutic treatment through hypnosis.

hipnotizar *vi.* to hypnotize, to put a subject under hypnosis.

hipo *m.* hiccups, involuntary contraction of the diaphragm and the glottis.

hipoadrenalismo *m.* hypoadrenalism, condition caused by diminished activity of the adrenal gland.

hipoalbuminemia *f.* hypoalbuminemia, low level of albumin in the blood.

hipocalcemia *f.* hypocalcemia, low amount of calcium in the blood.

hipocalemia, hipopotasemia *f.* hypokalemia, hypopotassemia, deficiency of potassium in the blood.

hipocampo *m.* hippocampus, curved elevation localized in the inferior horn of the lateral ventricle of the brain.

hipocapnia *f.* hypocapnia, deficiency of carbon dioxide in the blood.

hipociclosis *f.* hypocyclosis, deficiency in eye accommodation; ___

ciliar / ciliary ___ , weakness of the ciliary muscle; ___ **lenticular** / lenticular ___ , rigidity of the crystalline lens.

hipocinesia *f.* hypokinesia, diminished motor movement.

hipoclorhidria *f.* hypochlorhydria, deficiency of hydrochloric acid in the stomach, which can be a manifestation of cancer or anemia.

hipocolesteremia *f.* hypocholesteremia, diminished presence of cholesterol in the blood.

hipocondríaco-a *a.* hypochondriac, rel. to or suffering from hypochondria.

hipocondrio *m.* hypochondrium, upper abdominal region on either side of the thorax.

hipocromía *f.* hypochromia, abnormally pale erythrocytes.

hipodérmico-a *a.* hypodermic, beneath the skin.

hipofaringe *f.* hypopharynx, portion of the pharynx situated under the upper edge of the epiglottis.

hipofibrinogenemia *f.* hypofibrinogenemia, low content of fibrinogen in the blood.

hipofisectomía *f.* hypophysectomy, removal of the pituitary gland.

hipófisis *f.* hypophysis, pituitary gland, epithelial body situated at the base of the sella turcica.

hipofunción *f.* hypofunction, deficiency in the function of an organ.

hipogammaglobulinemia *f.* hypogammaglobulinemia, low level of gamma globulin in the blood; ___ **adquirida** / acquired ___ , manifested after infancy.

hipogastrio *m.* hypogastrium, anterior, middle and inferior portion of the abdomen.

hipoglicemia, hipoglucemia *f.* hypoglycemia, abnormally low level of glucose in the blood.

hipoglicémico-a, hipoglucémico-a *a.* hypoglycemic, rel. to or that produces hypoglycemia.

hipoglosal *a.* hypoglossal, rel. to the hyoid bone and the tongue.

hipogloso *m.* hypoglossus, muscle of the tongue that has retractive and lateral action; hypoglossal nerve; **-a** *a.* hypoglossal, beneath the tongue.

hipoinsulinismo *m.* hypoinsulinism, deficient insulin secretion in the blood. *See* **diabetes mellitus**.

hipolipoproteinemia *f.* hypolipoproteinemia, increase in the lipoprotein of the blood.

hiponatremia *f.* hyponatremia, sodium deficiency in the blood.

hipopituitarismo *m.* hypopituitarism, pathological condition due to diminished secretion of the pituitary gland.

hipoplasia *f.* hypoplasia, defective, or incomplete development of an organ or tissue.

hipoplástico-a *a.* hypoplastic, rel. to or suffering from hypoplasia.

hiporreflexia *f.* hyporeflexia, weak reflexes.

hipospadias *m., f.* hypospadias, congenital anomaly by which the wall of the urethra remains open in different degrees in the undersurface of the penis. In the female the urethra opens into the vagina.

hipotálamo *m.* hypothalamus, portion of the diencephalon situated beneath the thalamus at the base of the cerebrum.

hipotensión *f.* hypotension, low blood pressure.

hipotermia *f.* hypothermia, low body temperature.

hipótesis *f.* hypothesis, a proposition to be proven by experimentation; ___ **nula** / null ___ .

hipotiroideo-a *a.* hypothyroid, rel. to or suffering from hypothyroidism.

hipotiroidismo *m.* hypothyroidism, condition due to a deficiency in the production of thyroxin.

hipotónico-a *a.* hypotonic. 1. rel. to a deficiency in muscular tonicity; 2. having a lower osmotic pressure as compared to another element.

hipotrombinemia *f.* hypothrombinemia, deficiency of thrombin in the blood, which can cause a propensity to bleed.

hipoventilación *f.* hypoventilation, reduction of air entering the alveoli.

hipovolemia *f.* hypovolemia, decreased volume of blood in the body.

hipoxemia, hipoxia *f.* hypoxemia, hypoxia, diminished availability of oxygen to the blood.

hirsutismo *m.* hirsutism, excessive growth of hair in areas where there is usually no growth, esp. in women.

hirviente *a.* boiling; **agua** ___ / ___ water.

histamina *f.* histamine, substance that acts as a dilator of blood vessels and stimulates gastric secretion.

histerectomía *f.* hysterectomy, partial or total removal of the uterus; **abdominal** / abdominal ___ , through the abdomen; ___ **total** / total ___ , removal of the uterus and the cervix; ___ **vaginal** / vaginal ___ , through the vagina.

histerectomía abdominal completa *f.* total abdominal hysterectomy.

histeria *f.* hysteria, extreme neurosis.

histérico-a *a.* hysteric, hysterical, rel. to or suffering from hysteria.

histerosalpingografía *f.* hysterosalpingography, x-ray of the uterus and fallopian tubes after injecting a radiopaque substance.

histerosalpingooforectomía *f.* hysterosalpingoophorectomy, excision of the uterus, ovaries, and oviducts.

histeroscopía *f.* hysteroscopy, endoscopic examination of the uterine cavity.

histerotomía *f.* hysterotomy, incision of the uterus.

histidina *f.* histidine, amino acid essential in the growth and restoration of tissue.

histiocito *m.* histiocyte, large interstitial phagocytic cell of the reticuloendothelial system.

histocompatibilidad *f.* histocompatibility, state in which the tissues of a donor are accepted by the receiver; **complejo de** ___ **mayor** / major ___ complex.

histoplasmina *f.* histoplasmin, substance used in the cutaneous test for histoplasmosis.

histoplasmosis *f.* histoplasmosis, respiratory disease caused by the fungus *Histoplasma capsulatum*.

Hodgkin, enfermedad de *f.* Hodgkin's disease, malignant tumors in the lymph nodes and the spleen.

hoja *f.* leaf; [*de papel o metal*] sheet; ___ **clínica** / medical chart.

hola *int.* hi, hello.

holístico-a *a.* holistic, rel. to a whole or unit.

holocrino-a *a.* holocrine, rel. to the sweat glands.

holodiastólico-a *a.* holodiastolic, rel. to a complete diastole.

holografía *f.* holography, tridimensional representation of a figure by means of a photographic image.

hombre *m.* man, male.

hombro *m.* shoulder, the union of the clavicle, the scapula, and the humerus; __ **rigido** / frozen __.

homeopatía *f.* homeopathy, cure by means of administering medication diluted in minute doses that are capable of producing symptoms of the disease being treated.

homocigótico-a *a.* homozygotic, homozygous, rel. to twins that develop from gametes with similar alleles in regard to one or all characters.

homofobia *f.* homophobia, fear of or revulsion regarding homosexuals.

homofóbico-a *a.* fearful of or having an aversion to homosexuals.

homogéneo-a *a.* homogeneous, similar in nature.

homoinjerto *m.* homograft, transplant from a subject of the same species or type.

homólogo-a *a.* homologous, similar in structure and origin but not in function.

homosexual *a.* homosexual, sexually attracted to persons of the same sex.

homúnculo-a *m., f.* homunculus, dwarf with no deformities and with proportionate parts of the body.

hondo-a *a.* deep.

hongo *m.* fungus; mushroom; __ **venenoso** / toadstool.

honorario *m.* fee, charges; __ -s **razonables** / reasonable charges.

hora *f.* hour, time; **a cada** __ / hourly; __ **de acostarse** / bedtime; **¿qué** __ **es?** / what time is it?; **a qué** __ / at what time?

horario *m.* schedule; timetable.

hormigueo *m.* tingling sensation.

hormona *f.* hormone, natural chemical substance in the body that produces or stimulates the activity of an organ; __ **del crecimiento** / growth __; __ **estimulante** / stimulating __; __ **antidiurética** / antidiuretic __; __ **liberadora de gonadotropina** / gonadropin-releasing __.

hormona eritropoyética *f.* erythropoietic hormone, any protein

hormone that participates in the formation of erythrocytes.

hormona luteinizante *f.* luteinizing hormone produced by the anterior pituitary gland. It stimulates the secretion of sex hormones by the testis (testosterone) and the ovaries (progesterone) and also acts in the formation of sperm and ova.

hormona paratiroidea *f.* parathormone, parathyroid hormone, a hormone that regulates calcium in the body.

hormonal *a.* hormonal, rel. to or acting like a hormone; **receptor** __ / hormone __; **terapia** __ / hormone therapy.

Horner, sindrome de *m.* Horner's syndrome, sinking of the eyeball with accompanying eye and facial disorders due to paralysis of the cervical sympathetic nerve.

horquilla *f.* fourchette, posterior junction of the vulva.

hospedar *v.* to host; to lodge.

hospicio *m.* hospice, nursing facility.

hospital *m.* hospital.

hospitalizacion *f.* hospitalization.

hospitalizar *vi.* to hospitalize.

hoy *adv.* today; **de** __ **en adelante** / from now on; __ **en dia** / nowadays.

hoyo *m.* pit, hole.

hoyuelo *m.* dimple, dimple sign; small hole.

huérfano-a *m., f.* orphan.

huesecillo *m.* bonelet.

hueso *m.* bone; __ **compacto** / hard __; __ **esponjoso** / spongy __; __ **quebrado** / fractured __ .

huésped *m.* [*parasito*] host; **defensas del** __ / __ defenses; __ **definitivo** / definitive __; guest.

huesudo-a *a.* bony.

huevo *m.* egg, ovum, female sexual cell; **cáscara de** __ / eggshell; **clara de** __ / __ white; __ **duro** / hard-boiled ; __ **frito** / fried __; __ **pasado por agua** / soft-boiled __; **yema de** __ / __ yolk.

humano-a *a.* human; humane; rel. to humanity.

humectante *m.* humidifier, device that controls and maintains humidity in the air within a given area.

humedad *f.* humidity.

humedecer *v.* to moisten, to dampen.

húmero *m.* humerus, long bone of the upper arm.

humo *m.* smoke.

humor *m.* humor. 1. any liquid form in the body; ___ **acuoso** / aqueous ___ , clear fluid in the eye chambers; ___ **cristalino** / crystalline ___ , substance that constitutes the lens of the eye; ___ **vítreo** / vitreous ___ , clear, semifluid substance between the lens and the retina; 2. secretion; 3. disposition, mood; **buen** ___ / good ___; **estar de** **buen** ___ / to be in a good ___; **estar de mal** ___ / to be in a bad mood; **mal** ___ / bad ___ .

Huntington, corea de *f.* Huntington's chorea. corea, neurodegenerative disorder characterized by spasmodic movements of the limbs and dementia.

huy! *int.* ouch!

i

I *abr.* **iodo, yodo** / iodine.

iátrico-a *a.* iatric, rel. to medicine, the medical profession, or physicians.

iatrogénico-a, iatrógeno-a *a.* iatrogenic. yatrogénico, yatrógeno; **pneumotórax** __ / __ pneumothorax; **transmisión** __ / __ transmission.

ibuprofen *m.* ibuprofen, anti-inflammatory, antipyretic, and analgesic agent used in the treatment of rheumatoid arthritis.

ictericia *f.* jaundice, disorder caused by excessive bilirubin in the blood and manifested by a yellow-orange coloring of the skin and other tissues and fluids of the body; __ **del neonato** / icterus gravis neonatorum; __ **hemolítica** / hemolytic __; __ **hepatocvelular** / hepatocellular __; __ **retentive** / retentive __ .

ictérico-a *a.* icteric, jaundiced, or rel. to jaundice.

icterohepatitis *f.* icterohepatitis, hepatitis associated with jaundice.

icterus *L.* icterus. *See* **ictericia.**

icterus gravis *L.* icterus gravis, acute, yellow atrophy of the liver.

icterus neonatorum *L.* icterus neonatorum, jaundice of the newborn.

ictiosis *f.* ichthyosis, dry and scaly skin.

ictus *L.* ictus, sudden attack.

id *m.* id. 1. name given by Freud to the real unconscious where tendencies of autopreservation and instincts reside; 2. in psychiatry, one of the three divisions of the psyche; 3. -id, suffix denoting secondary eruptions of the skin that appear in areas away from the primary infection.

idea *f.* idea, concept, thought; __ **fija** / fixed __, idée fixe.

ideación *f.* ideation, process by which ideas are formed; __ **paranoide** / paranoid __ .

idéntico-a *a.* 1. identical, same; 2. rel. to twins that result from the fertilization of only one ovum.

identidad *f.* identity, self-recognition.

identificación *f.* identification, unconscious process of identifying oneself with another person or group and assuming its characteristics.

identificar *vi.* to identify.

idioma *m.* language.

idiopatía *f.* idiopathy, disease or morbid state of unknown origin.

idiopático-a *a.* 1. rel. to idiopathy; 2. of a spontaneous nature. **aldosteronismo** __ / __ aldosteronism; **fibrosis pulmonar** __ / __ pulmonary fibrosis; **estenosis subglótica** __ / __ subglottic stenosis; **hipercalcemia** __ **de los niños** / __ hypercalcemia of children; **neuralgia** __ / __ neuralgia.

idiosincracia *f.* idiosyncrasy. 1. set of individual characteristics; 2. an individual's own reaction to a given action, idea, medication, treatment or food.

idiota *m., f.* idiot, fool; __ **"savant"** / idiot savant.

idiotez *f.* idiocy, mental deficiency.

ignorante *a.* ignorant.

ignorar *v.* to ignore.

igual *a.* equal, even, same; **-mente** *adv.* equally.

igualar *v.* to equate.

ileal *a.* ileal, rel. to the ileum; **arterias** __ **-es** / __ arteries; **orificio** __ / __ orifice; **prueba** __ / __ patch; **uréter** __ / __ ureter; **venas** __ **-es** / __ veins.

ileectomía *f.* ileectomy, total or partial surgical removal of the ileum.

ileítis *f.* ileitis, infl. of the ileum; __ **regional** / regional __ .

ileocecal *a.* ileocecal, rel. to the ileum and the cecum; **válvula** __ / __ valve.

ileocecostomía *f.* ileocecostomy, surgical anastomosis of the ileum to the cecum.

ileocolitis *f.* ileocolitis, infl. of the mucous membrane of the ileum and the colon.

ileocolostomía *f.* ileocolostomy, surgical anastomosis from the ileum to the colon.

íleon *m.* ileum, distal portion of the small intestine extending from the jejunum to the cecum; **desviación quirúrgica del** __ / ileal bypass.

ileoproctostomía *f.* ileoproctostomy, anastomosis of the ileum and the rectum.

ileosigmoidostomía *f.* ileosigmoidostomy, anastomosis of the ileum and the sigmoid colon.

ileostomía *f.* ileostomy, anastomosis of the ileum and the anterior abdominal wall.

ileotransversostomía f.
ileotransversostomy, anastomosis of
the ileum and the transverse colon.

ilíaco-a a. iliac, rel. to the ilium; **colon**
___ / ___ colon; **cresta** ___ /
hueso ___ / ___ bone; **músculo** ___ / ___
muscle.

ilimitado-a a. unlimited, boundless.

iliolumbar a. iliolumbar, rel. to the iliac
and lumbar regions; **arteria** ___ / ___
artery; **vena** ___ / ___ vein.

ilion m. ilium, hip bone.

ilusión f. illusion, false interpretation of
sensory impressions.

iluso-a a. deluded.

imagen f. image; ___ **de espejo** / mirror
___; ___ **del cuerpo** / body ___; ___
directa / direct ___; ___ **doble** / double
___; ___ **eléctrica** / electric ___; ___
invertida / inverted ___; ___ **latente** /
latent ___; ___ **óptica** / optic ___; ___
radiográfica / radiographic ___; ___
real / real ___; ___ **virtual** / virtual ___ .

imagen virtual f. virtual image.

**imágenes por resonancia
magnética** f., pl. magnetic
resonance imaging, procedure based in
the quantitative analysis of the chemical
and biological structure of a tissue.

imágenes por ultrasonido f. pl.
ultrasound imaging, creation of images
of organs or tissues through the use of
reflex techniques (echogram).

imaginar vt. to imagine.

imán m. magnet, a body that has the
property of attracting iron.

imbécil m., f. imbecile. a. imbecilic,
stupid.

imbricado-a a. imbricate, imbricated,
in layers.

imitación f. imitation.

impacción f. impaction. 1. the
condition of being lodged or wedged
within a given space; 2. impediment of
an organ or part.

impacientarse vr. to become
impatient.

impaciente a. impatient.

impactado-a a. impacted; **diente** ___ /
___ tooth.

impalpable a. impalpable, incorporeal,
intangible.

impedido-a a. impeded, handicapped.

imperdible m. safety pin.

imperfección f. imperfection; defect.

imperforado-a a. imperforate,
abnormally closed; **himen** ___ / ___
hymen.

impermeable a. impermeable, not
allowing passage, such as fluids;
waterproof.

impétigo m. impetigo, bacterial skin
infection marked by vesicles that
become pustular and form a yellow
crust on rupturing; ___ **contagioso** /
___ contagious; ___ **del nenonato** / ___
neonatorum; ___ **vulgar** / ___ vulgaris.

implantar vt. to implant; to insert.

implante m. implant, any material
inserted or grafted into the body.

implosión f. implosion. 1. violent
collapse inward as it occurs in the
evacuation of a vessel; 2. method to
treat a fear caused by a phobia.

importante a. important.

imposible a. impossible.

impotencia f. impotence, inability to
have or maintain an erection.

impotente a. impotent, rel. to or
suffering from impotence.

impráctico-a a. impractical.

impregnar vt. to impregnate; to
saturate.

imprescindible a. indispensable.

imprevisto-a a. unexpected,
unforeseen.

impúbero-a a. below the age of
puberty.

impulso m. drive, thrust; sudden
pushing force; ___ **cardíaco** / cardiac
___; ___ **excitante** / excitatory ___; ___
inhibitorio / inhibitory ___; ___
nervioso / nervous ___; ___ **vital** / élan
vital.

inaccesible a. inaccessible.

inaceptable a. unacceptable.

inactividad f. inactivity; ___ **física** /
physical ___ .

inadaptado-a a. maladjusted, unable
to adjust to the environment or to
endure stress.

inadecuado-a a. inadequate.

inanición f. inanition, starvation,
hunger.

inanimado-a a. inanimate, without
animation, lacking life.

inarticulado-a a. inarticulate.
1. unable to articulate words or
syllables; 2. disjointed.

incansable a. tireless, untiring.

incapacitado-a a. disabled; unable.

incapaz a. incapable, unable.

incentivo m. incentive.

incertidumbre f. uncertainty.

incesto m. incest.

incidencia f. incidence.

incipiente *a.* incipient, just coming into existence.

incisión *f.* incision; surgical cut.

incisura *f.* slit; notch.

inclinación *f.* slant, slope, tilt; inclination, predisposition.

inclusión *f.* inclusion, the act of enclosing one thing in another; **cuerpos de __** / **__ bodies**, present in the cytoplasm of some cells in cases of infection

incoherente *a.* incoherent.

incoloro-a *a.* colorless; achromatic.

incómodo-a *a.* uncomfortable; annoyed.

incompatible *a.* incompatible.

incompleto-a *a.* incomplete, unfinished.

inconsciencia *f.* unconsciousness, impaired consciousness or the loss of it; unawareness.

inconsciente *a.* unconscious. 1. that has lost consciousness; 2. that does not respond to sensorial stimuli.

incontinencia *f.* incontinence, inability to control the emission or expulsion of urine or feces; **__ fecal** / fecal __; **__ intestinal** / bowel __; **__ por rebozamiento** / __ overflow; **__ por reflejo** / reflex __; **__ urinaria** / urinary __; **__ urinaria de esfuerzo** / __ urinary stress.

incontinente *a.* incontinent, rel. to incontinence.

incorporar *vt.* to incorporate, to include.

incrustación *f.* 1. incrustation, formation of a crust or scab; 2. inlay.

incubación *f.* incubation. 1. latent period of a disease before its manifestation; **período de __** / __ period; 2. care of a premature infant in an incubator.

incubadora *f.* incubator, device used to keep optimal conditions of temperature and humidity, esp. in the care of premature infants.

incudectomía *f.* incudectomy, excision of the incus.

incurable *a.* incurable, not subject to healing.

incus *L.* incus, small bone of the middle ear.

indeseable *a.* undesirable.

indicado-a *a.* indicated; appropriate.

indicador *m.* marker, indicator.

índice *m.* rate, index; mean; **__ de aborto** / abortion __; **__ de edad específica** / age specific __; **__ de letalidad de casos** / case fatality __; **__ de mortalidad, de mortandad** / death __; **__ de mortinatalidad** / birth-death rate; **__ de natalidad** / birth __; **__ de natalidad cero** / zero population growth; **__ de reproducción** / gross reproduction __; **__ medio (de)** / average flow __ .

indifferención *f.* undifferentiation.

indígena *m., f.* native, aboriginal; *a.* indigenous.

indigestarse *vr.* to suffer from indigestion.

indigestión *f.* indigestion, maldigestion.

indirecto-a *a.* indirect; **bilirubina reactiva __** / __ reacting bilirubin; **division nuclear __** / __ nuclear division; **fractura __** / __ fracture; **inmunofluorescencia __** / __ immunofluorescence; **laringoscopía __** / __ laryngoscopy; **prueba de hemaglutinación __** / __ hemagglutination test; **transfusión __** / __ transfusion; **visión __** / __ vision.

indispensable *a.* indispensable, necessary.

indispuesto-a *a.* indisposed, ill; upset.

individual *a.* individual.

individuo *m.* individual, person; fellow.

inducción *f.* induction, action or effect of inducing.

inducido-a *a.* induced.

inducir *vt.* to induce; to force; to provoke.

induración *f.* induration, the process of hardening such as it happens to soft tissues as with the mucous membranes.

inercia *f.* inertia, stillness; lack of activity.

inervación *f.* innervation, distribution of nerves or nervous energy in an organ or area.

inestabilidad *f.* instability.

inestable *a.* unstable, fluctuating; **angina __** / __ angina; **vejiga __** / __ bladder.

infancia *f.* infancy, period of time from birth to one or two years of age; early age.

infantil *a.* 1. rel. to infancy; 2. childish; **acropustulosis __** / __ acropustulosis; **atrofia muscular espinal __** / __ spinal muscular atrophy; **autismo __** / __ autism; **conjuntivitis purulenta __** / __ purulent conjunctivitis; **eczema __** / __ eczema; **escorbuto __** / __

infantilismo

scurvy; **hipotiroidismo** __ / __ hypothyroidism; **osteomalacia** __ / __ osteomalacia.

infantilismo *m.* infantilism, infantile characteristics carried into adult life.

infarto *m.* infarct, infarction, necrosis of a tissue area due to a lack of blood supply; __ **blando** / bland __; __ **cardíaco** / myocardial __; __ **cerebral** / cerebral __; __ **hemorrágico** / hemorrhagic __; __ **pulmonar** / pulmonary __.

infección *f.* infection, invasion of the body by pathogenic microorganisms and the reaction of tissue to their presence and effect; __ **inicial o primaria** / initial or primary __; __ **intrahospitalaria** / hospital acquired __; __ **aerógena** / airborne __; __ **aguda** / acute __; __ **contagiosa** / contagious __; __ **crónica** / chronic __; __ **de hongos** / fungus __; __ **hídrica** __ waterborne __; __ **inicial o primaria** / __ initial or primary; __ **masiva** / massive __; __ **piógena** / pyogenic __; __ **secundaria** / secondary __; __ **sistémica** / systemic __; __ **subclínica** / subclinical __.

infección oportunista *f.* opportunistic infection, caused by an organism, gen. harmless, that can become pathogenic when resistance to disease is impaired, such as occurs in AIDS.

infeccioso-a *a.* infectious, rel. to an infection; **agente** __ / __ agent; **enfermedad** __ / __ disease.

infectado-a *a.* infected.

infectar *vt.* to infect; **infectarse** *vr.* to become infected.

infectivo-a *a.* infectious.

infecundo-a *a.* sterile; barren.

inferior *a.* inferior, lower; **esfínter esofágico** __ / lower esophageal sphincter; **extremidad** __ / lower extremity.

inferir *vt.* to infer, to surmise.

infertilidad *f.* infertility, inability to conceive or procreate.

infestación *f.* infestation, invasion of the body by parasites.

infibulación *f.* infibulation, female circumcision.

infiltración *f.* infiltration, the accumulation of foreign substances in a tissue, organ, or cell.

inflación *f.* inflation, distension.

inflamación *f.* inflammation, reaction of a tissue to injury.

inflamatorio-a *a.* inflammatory, rel. to inflammation; **enfermedad** __ **de los intestinos** / __ bowel disease.

inflexión *f.* inflection, inflexion, the act of bending inward.

influenza *f.* influenza, acute contagious viral infection of the respiratory tract.

información *f.* information.

informar *vt.* to inform; **informarse** *vr.* to become informed.

informe *m.* report; account.

informe de consentimiento *m.* informed consent.

infraclavicular *a.* infraclavicular, under the clavicle.

infracostal *a.* infracostal, area below the rib.

infrarrojo-a *a.* infrared; **rayos** __ **-s** / __ rays.

infundíbulo *m.* infundibulum, funnel-like structure. 1. structure shaped like a funnel; 2. any one of the divisions of the renal pelvis; 3. short extension of the right ventricle from which the pulmonary artery begins.

infusión *f.* infusion. 1. slow gravitational introduction of fluid into a vein; 2. the steeping of an element in water to obtain its soluble active principles; __ **salina** / saline __.

ingerir *vi.* to ingest, to take in.

ingestión *f.* ingestion, the amount of liquids and substances taken into the body by mouth or parenterally; __ **calórica** / caloric __.

ingle *f.* groin.

ingresar *vi.* [*en un hospital*] to be admitted.

inguinal *a.* inguinal, rel. to the groin; **anillo** __ / __ ring; **canal** __ / __ canal; **hernia** __ / __ hernia; **ligamento** __ / __ ligament.

ingurgitado-a *a.* engorged, distended by excess fluid.

inhabilidad *f.* inability, incapacity.

inhabilidad de desarrollo *f.* developmental disability, loss or impairment of an acquired function due to pre- or postnatal events, such as the acquisition of language, a social or motor skill.

inhalación *f.* inhalation, aspiration; the act of drawing air or other vapor into the lungs; __ **de humo** / smoke __.

inhalación pasiva de humo *f.* passive smoking, the act of inhaling

inmunosupresión

smoke that comes from a person smoking nearby.

inhalante *m.* inhalant, medication administered by inhalation.

inhalar *vt.* to inhale, to draw in air or vapor.

inherente *a.* inherent, innate, natural to an individual or thing.

inhibición *f.* inhibition, interruption or restriction of a process.

inhibidor *m.* inhibitor, agent that causes inhibition; **___ de fusión /** fusion **___** .

inicial *a.* initial.

iniciar *v.* to initiate, to start.

injertar *vt.* to graft, to implant.

injerto *m.* graft, implant, inlay, any tissue or organ used for transplanation or implantation.

inmaduro-a *a.* immature.

inmediato-a *a.* immediate, close; *adv.* **-mente;** immediately.

inmersión *f.* immersion, submersion of a body in a liquid.

inminente *a.* imminent, about to happen.

inmóvil *a.* immobile, motionless.

inmovilizar *vt.* to immobilize.

inmune *a.* immune, resistant to contracting a specific disease; **adherencia ___ / ___** adherence; **adsorción ___ / ___** adsorption; **complejo ___ / ___** complex; **parálisis ___ / ___** parálisis; **respuesta ___ / ___** response.

inmunidad *f.* immunity. 1. condition of the organism to resist a particular antigen by activating specific antibodies; 2. resistance to contracting a specific disease; **___ activa /** active **___; ___ adoptiva /** adoptive **___; ___ adquirida /** acquired **___; ___ antivírica /** antiviral **___; ___ antiviral /** antiviral **___; ___ artificial /** artificial **___; ___ bacteriófaga /** bacteriophage **___; ___ concomitante /** concomitant **___; ___ de grupo /** group **___; ___ general /** general **___; ___ innata /** innate **___; ___ maternal /** maternal **___; ___ nata /** inborn **___; ___ natural /** natural **___; ___ pasiva /** passive **___** .

inmunización *f.* immunization, making the organism immune to a given disease. See table on page 369.

inmunizar *vt.* to immunize.

inmunoanálisis *m.* immunoassay, the process of identifying a substance by its capacity to act as an antigen and antibody in a tissue; **___ enzimático /** enzyme **___** .

inmunocompetencia *f.* immunocompetency, the process of becoming immune following exposure to an antigen.

inmunocomprometido-a *a.* immunocompromised, rel. to a person with a deficient immunologic system.

inmunodeficiencia *f.* immunodeficiency, inadequate cellular immunity reaction that diminishes the ability to respond to antigenic stimuli; **enfermedad grave de ___ combinada /** severe combined **___** disease.

inmunoestimulante *m.* immunostimulant, agent that can stimulate an immune response.

inmunógeno *m.* immunogen, stimulator that produces an antibody; *a.* immunogenic; that produces immunity; **___ específico /** targeted **___** .

inmunoglobulina *f.* immunoglobulin. 1. one of a group of proteins of animal origin that participates in the immune reaction; 2. one of the five types of gamma globulin capable of acting as an antibody.

inmunología *f.* immunology, the study of the body's response to bacteria, virus, or any other foreign invasion, such as transplanted tissue or organ.

inmunológico-a *a.* immunologic, rel. to immunology; **competencia ___ / ___** competence; **deficiencia ___ / ___** deficiency; **mecanismo ___ / ___** mechanism; **parálisis ___ / ___** paralysis; **prueba ___ del embarazo / ___** pregnancy test; **realce ___ / ___** enhancement; **respuesta o reacción ___ / ___** immune response; **tolerancia ___ / ___** tolerance.

inmunólogo-a *m., f.* immunologist, specialist in immunology.

inmunoproteína *f.* immunoprotein, protein that acts as an antibody.

inmunoquimioterapia *f.* immunochemotherapy, combined process of immunotherapy and chemotherapy used in the treatment of some malignant tumors.

inmunoreacción *f.* immunoreaction, immune reaction between antigens and antibodies.

inmunosupresión *f.* immunosuppression, diminishing or

inmunoterapia

preventing the body's normal immune response to foreign matter.

inmunoterapia *f.* immunotherapy, prevention or treatment of a disease using passive immunization of agents such as serum or gamma globulin.

inmunotrasfusión *f.* immunotransfusion, transfusion of blood from a donor that has been afflicted by the same specific infection as the recipient.

innato-a *a.* inborn; congenital; ingrown.

innecesario-a *a.* unnecessary.

inoculable *a.* inoculable, that can be transmitted by inoculation.

inoculación *f.* inoculation, immunization, administration of a serum, vaccine, or some other substance to increase immunization to a given disease.

inocular *vt.* to inoculate, to administer an inoculation.

inóculo *m.* inoculum, substance that is inoculated.

inocuo-a *a.* innocuous, that does no harm.

inodoro *m.* toilet, commode; **-a** / *a.* odorless.

inofensivo-a *a.* harmless.

inoperable *a.* inoperable, lacking potential for surgical treatment.

inoportuno-a *a.* untimely, inopportune.

inorgánico-a *a.* inorganic, independent of living organisms.

inotrópico-a *a.* inotropic, affecting the intensity or energy of muscular contractions.

inquieto-a *a.* uneasy, restless, jumpy.

inquietud *f.* unrest, restlessness.

inscribirse *v.* to register.

insecticida *m.* insecticide.

insecto *m.* insect.

inseguridad *f.* insecurity.

inseminación *f.* insemination, fertilization of an ovum.

insensible *a.* insensible, without sensibility.

inserción *f.* insertion. 1. the act of inserting; 2. the place where a muscle attaches to the bone.

insertar *v.* to insert.

inservible *a.* useless, unserviceable.

insidioso-a *a.* insidious, rel. to a disease that develops gradually and subtly without warning or early symptoms.

in situ *L.* in situ. 1. in its normal place; 2. that does not extend beyond the place of origin.

insoluble *a.* insoluble, that does not dissolve.

insomne *a.* insomnia, insomnious, rel. to or suffering from insomnia.

insomnio *m.* insomnia, inability to sleep.

insoportable *a.* unbearable.

inspección *f.* inspection.

inspiratorio-a *a.* inspiratory, rel. to inspiration; **capacidad __ / __** capacity; **estridor __ / __** stridor; **reserva de volumen __ / __** reserve volume.

instilación *f.* instillation, dripping of a liquid into a cavity or onto a surface.

instintivo-a *a.* instinctive.

instinto *m.* instinct.

institución *f.* institution, establishment; **__ benéficial** / charity **__** .

insuficiencia *f.* insufficiency, lacking; **__ cardíaca** / heart failure; **__ coronaria** / coronary **__**; **__ hepática** / hepatic **__**; **__ mitral** / mitral **__**; **pulmonar-valvular** / pulmonary valvular **__**; **__ renal** / renal **__**; **respiratoria** / respiratory **__**; **suprarrenal** / adrenal **__**; **__ valvular** / valvular **__**; **__ venosa** / venous **__** .

insuficiencia coronaria *f.* coronary insufficiency, deficiency in coronary circulation with risk of suffering pain caused by angina, thrombosis, or atheroma that can result in a myocardial infarct.

insuficiente *a.* insufficient.

insuflar *vt.* to insufflate, to blow air, powder, gas, or vapor into a tube, cavity, or organ of the body.

insufrible *a.* insufferable, unbearable.

ínsula *f.* insula, central lobe of the cerebral hemisphere.

insulina *f.* insulin, hormone secreted by the pancreas; **pompa de __ / __** pump; **resistente a la __ / __** resistant.

insulinemia *f.* insulinemia, excess amount of insulin in the blood.

insulinochoque *m.* insuline shock, severe hypoglycemia that is manifested by sweating, shaking, anxiety, vertigo, diplopia, and can be followed by delirium, convulsions, and collapse.

insulinodependiente *a.* insulin-dependent.

insulinogénesis *f.* insulinogenesis, production of insulin.

integración *f.* integration. 1. anabolic activity; 2. the process of combining into a being or total entity.

inteligencia *f.* intelligence.

intensidad *f.* intensity.

intensificar *vt.* to intensify.

intensivo-a *a.* intensive.

intenso-a *a.* intense.

interacción *f.* interaction; ___ **de medicamentos** / drug ___ .

intercalado-a *a.* intercalated, situated or placed between two parts or elements.

intercostal *a.* intercostal, between two ribs; **espacio** ___ / ___ space; **membranas** ___ **-es** / ___ membranes; **nervios** ___ / ___ nerves.

intercurrente *a.* intercurrent, that appears during the course of another disease modifying it in some way.

interdigitación *f.* interdigitation, interlocking of parts like the fingers of folded hands.

interferona *f.* interferon, a natural protein released by cells exposed to viruses that can be used in the treatment of infections and neoplasms.

interfibrilar *a.* interfibrillar, between fibrils.

interlobitis *f.* interlobitis, infl. of the pleura that separates two pulmonary lobules.

interlobular *a.* interlobular, occurring between lobules of an organ.

intermitente *a.* intermittent, not continuous; **pulso** ___ / ___ pulse; **ventilación** ___ **bajo presión positiva** / ___ positive-pressure ventilation.

internacional *a.* international; **unidad** ___ / ___ unit, accepted measured amount of a substance as defined by the International Conference of Unification of Formulae.

internado *m.* internship.

internalización *f.* internalization, unconscious process by which an individual adopts the beliefs, values, and attitudes of another person or of the society in which she or he lives.

internista *m., f.* physician specializing in internal medicine.

interno-a *m., f.* intern; *a.* internal, inside the body; **hemorragia** ___ / ___ bleeding.

interrogatorio *m.* questioning.

intersticial *a.* interstitial, rel. to spaces within an organ, cell, or tissue; **cistitis**

___ / ___ cystitis; **crecimiento** ___ / ___ growth; **embarazo** ___ / ___ pregnancy; **enfermedad** ___ / ___ disease; **enfisema** ___ / ___ emphysema; **fluido** ___ / ___ fluid; **gastritis** ___ / ___ gastritis; **hernia** ___ / ___ hernia; **nefritis** ___ / ___ nephritis; **hormona** ___ **estimulante de células** / ___ cell stimulating hormone.

intersticios *m., pl.* interstices, intervals or small spaces.

intértrigo *m.* intertrigo, irritating dermatitis that occurs between or under the folds of the skin.

intervalo *m.* interval, period of time.

intervención *f.* intervention, any action taken to improve the health or change the course of a disease.

interventricular *a.* interventricular, between the ventricles; **defecto del tabique** ___ / ___ septal defect; **tabique** ___ **del corazón** / ___ septum.

intervertebral *a.* intervertebral, between the vertebrae; **disco** ___ / ___ disk.

intestinal *a.* intestinal, rel. to the intestines; **desviación quirúrgica** ___ / ___ bypass surgery; **flora** ___ / ___ flora; **jugo** ___ / ___ juice; **obstrucción** ___ / ___ obstruction; **perforación** ___ / ___ perforation.

intestino *m.* intestine, the alimentary canal extending from the pylorus to the anus; ___ **delgado** / small ___; ___ **grueso** / large ___; ___ **medio del embrión** / midgut.

íntima *f.* intima. 1. the innermost of the three layers of a blood vessel; 2. the innermost layer of several organs or parts.

intolerancia *f.* intolerance, inability to withstand pain or the effects of drugs.

intorsión *f.* intorsion, rotation of the eye inwards.

intoxicación *f.* intoxication; poisoning, food poisoning, toxic state produced by the intake of a drug or toxic substance; ___ **de pescado** / fish poisoning. See table on page 375.

intra-abdominal *a.* intra-abdominal, within the abdominal cavity.

intra-aórtico-a *a.* intra-aortic, within the aorta.

intra-arterial *a.* intra-arterial, within an artery.

intra-articular *a.* intra-articular, within an articulation or joint.

intracapsular *a.* intracapsular, within a capsule.

intracelular *a.* intracellular, within a cell.

intracraneal *a.* intracranial, within the cranium.

intracutáneo-a *a.* intracutaneous, within the dermis.

intrahepático-a *a.* intrahepatic, within the liver; **colestasis __ del embarazo** / __ cholestasis of pregnancy.

intralobular *a.* intralobular, within a lobule.

intraluminal *a.* intraluminal, within the lumen of a tube.

intramuscular *a.* intramuscular, within a muscle.

intranquilidad *f.* restlessness, uneasiness.

intranquilo-a *a.* restless, uneasy.

intraocular *a.* intraocular, within the eye; **implante __ / __** implant; **presión __ / __** pressure.

intraoperatorio-a *a.* intraoperative, within the time frame of a surgical procedure.

intraóseo-a *a.* intraosseous, within the bone substance.

intrarrenal *a.* intrarenal, within the kidney; **fallo __ / __** failure.

intrauterino-a *a.* intrauterine, within the uterus; **dispositivo __ / __** device, coil.

intravenoso-a *a.* intravenous, within a vein; **alimentación __ / __** feeding; **infusión __ / __** infusion; **inyección __ / __** injection.

intraventricular *a.* intraventricular, within a ventricle.

intrínseco-a *a.* intrinsic, inherent; **factor __ / __** factor, protein normally present in the gastric juice of humans.

introducir *vt.* to introduce.

introductor, intubador *m.* introducer, intubator, device used to intubate.

introitus *L.* introitus, an entrance or opening to a canal or cavity.

introspección *f.* introspection, self-analysis.

introversión *f.* introversion, the act of turning one's interests inward with diminished interest in the outside world.

introvertido-a *m., f.* introvert; *a.* rel. to introversion.

intubación *f.* intubation, insertion of a tube into a conduit or cavity of the body.

intuición *f.* intuition.

intumescencia *f.* intumescence, thickening.

intususcepción *f.* intussusception, invagination of one part of the intestine into the lumen of the adjoining part causing obstruction.

in utero *L.* in utero, within the uterus.

invaginación *f.* invagination, process of inclusion of one part into another.

invaginar *v.* invaginate, to introduce one part of a structure into another part of the same structure.

invalido-a *m., f.* invalid; *a.* crippled; void.

invasión *f.* invasion, the act of invading.

invasivo-a, invasor-a *a.* invasive, rel. to a germ or substance that invades adjacent tissues; **procedimiento no __** / non __ procedure.

inversión *f.* inversion, process of turning around; **__ de cromosomas /** __ of chromosomes; **__ del utero /** __ of the uterus; **__ paracéntrica /** paracentric __; **__ pericéntrica /** pericentric __; **__ visceral /** visceral __ .

inverso-a, invertido-a *a.* inverse, inverted.

investigación *f.* research; **__ clínica /** clinical __; **__ de laboratorio /** laboratory __ .

invisible *a.* invisible, that cannot be seen with the naked eye.

in vitro *L.* in vitro, rel. to laboratory tests or biological experimentation occurring outside the living body esp. in a test-tube; **fertilización __ / __** fertilization.

in vivo *L.* in vivo, within the body of living organisms.

involución *f.* involution, a retrogressive change.

involucrado-a *a.* involved; **estar __ /** to be __ ; to become __ .

involuntario-a *a.* involuntary.

inyección *f.* injection, shot; **__ de depósito /** deposit __; **__ de refuerzo /** booster shot; **__ de insulina /** insulin __; **__ de prueba /** test __; **__ de sensibilización /** sensitizing __; **__ hipodérmica subcutánea /** hypodermic __; **__ intraarticular /** intraarticular __; **__ intradérmica /** intradermic __; **__ intrafecal /**

intrafecal ___; ___ **intravenosa /** intravenous ___; ___ **selectiva /** selective ___ .

inyectar v. to inject, to introduce fluid in a tissue, cavity, or blood vessel with an injector.

inyector m. injector, device used to inject; syringe.

iodo, yodo m. iodine, nonmetallic element used as a germicide and as an aid in the development and function of the thyroid gland.

ión m. ion, an atom or group of atoms carrying a charge of electricity.

ionización f. ionization, dissociation of compounds into their constituent ions; **radiación por** ___ / ionizing radiation.

ipeca, jarabe de, m. syrup of ipecac, an emetic and expectorant agent.

ipsolateral a. ipsolateral, on the same side.

ir vi. to go; **irse** vr. to go away, to leave.

iridectomía f. iridectomy, removal of a part of the iris.

iridencleisis f. iridencleisis, surgical intervention to reduce intraocular pressure.

iridología f. iridology, study of the changes suffered by the iris during the course of an illness.

iris m. iris, contractile membrane situated between the lens and the cornea in the aqueous humour of the eye which regulates the entrance of light.

iritis f. iritis, infl. of the iris.

irracional a. irrational.

irradiación f. irradiation, therapeutic use of radiation.

irreducible a. irreducible, that cannot be reduced.

irregular a. irregular.

irrigar vt. to irrigate, to wash out.

irritable a. irritable, that reacts to a stimulus.

irritante m. irritant, an irritation-causing agent.

iscuria f. ischuria, retention or suspension of urine.

isla f. island, isolated piece of tissue or group of cells.

islote m. islet, group of isolated cells of a different structure from the one of surrounding cells.

isométrico-a a. isometric, of equal dimensions; **ejercicio** ___ / ___ exercise.

isometropía f. isometropia, same refraction on both eyes.

isoniacida f. isoniazid, antibacterial medication used in the treatment of tuberculosis.

isostenuria f. isosthenuria, renal insufficiency.

isotónico-a a. isotonic, having equal tension.

isótopo m. isotope, one of a group of chemical elements that present almost identical qualities but differ in atomic weight.

isquemia f. ischemia, lack of blood supply to a given part of the body; ___ **silenciosa /** silent ___ .

isquemia miocárdica f. myocardial ischemia, deficiency of blood supply to the heart due to obstruction of the coronary arteries.

isquemico-a a. ischemic, rel. to or suffering from ischemia; **ataque** ___ **transitorio /** transient ___ attack, temporary stoppage of blood supply to the brain.

isquion m. ischium, posterior part of the pelvis.

istmectomia f. isthmectomy, excision of the middle part of the thyroid.

istmo m. isthmus. 1. narrow conduit that connects two cavities or two larger parts; 2. constriction between two parts of an organ or structure; ___ **del encéfalo /** ___ of the encephalon; ___ **del tubo auditivo /** ___ of auditory tube; ___ **del útero /** ___ of the uterus; ___ **de la aorta /** aortic ___; ___ **de la faringe /** pharyngeal ___; ___ **de la trompa de Eustaquio /** ___ of the Eustachian tube; ___ **de la trompa de Falopio /** ___ of the Falopian tube; ___ **de las fauces /** ___ of the fauces

ixodes L. genus that includes ticks and other acarids.

ixodiasis f. ixodiasis, cutaneous lesions due to the bite of a certain type of tick.

izquierda f. left; left hand; **a la** ___ / to the ___ .

izquierdo-a a. left.

jabón *m.* soap.
Jackson, epilepsia de *f.* Jackson's epilepsy, partial epilepsy without loss of consciousness.
jadeo *m.* panting, gasping, shortness of breath; wheeze.
Jaeger, examen de *m.* Jaeger test, chart of lines with different types and sizes of letters used to determine visual acuity.
jalea *f.* jelly; ___ **anticonceptiva** / contraceptive ___; ___ **vaginal** / vaginal ___ .
jamais vu *Fr. jamais vu*, the perception of familiar surroundings as a new experience.
jamás *adv.* never, ever.
jaqueca *f.* severe headache.
jarabe *m.* syrup; ___ **de ipecacuana** / ipecac syrup; ___ **para la tos** / cough.
jeringa, jeringuilla *f.* syringe; ___ **de aguja hueca** / hollow needle ___; ___ **con tubo de cristal** / glass cylinder ___; ___ **desechable** / disposable ___; ___ **hipodérmica** / hypodermic ___ .
jimaguas *m., pl. Cuba* twins.
joroba *f.* hump.
jorobado-a *m., f.* hunchback; crooked. *a.* hunchbacked; crooked.

joven *m., f.* (**el joven, la joven**) young person; *a.* young.
jovencito-a *a.* youngster.
juanete *m.* bunion, hallux valgus.
juego *m.* play, activity organized or spontaneous for the purpose of entertainment.
jubilado-a *m., f.* retiree; *a.* retired.
jugo *m.* juice; ___ **gástrico** / gastric ___; ___ **intestinal** / intestinal ___; ___ **pancreático** / pancreatic ___; ___ **de ciruela** / prune ___; ___ **de manzana** / apple ___; ___ **de naranja** / orange ___; ___ **de piña** / pineapple ___; ___ **de tomate** / tomato ___; ___ **de toronja** / grapefruit ___; ___ **de uva** / grape ___; ___ **de zanahoria** / carrot ___ .
juntar *v.* to join, to gather together.
juntura *f.* joint, juncture.
juramento *m.* oath; ___ **hipocrático** / Hippocratic ___ , medical oath.
jurisprudencia médica *f.* medical jurisprudence, the law as applied to the practice of medicine.
Jurkat, células de *f., pl.* Jurkat cells, line of T cells that is used in immunology investigations.
juvenil *a.* juvenile; **artritis** ___ / ___ arthritis; **catarata** ___ / ___ cataract; **delincuencia** ___ / ___ delinquency; **dermatitis plantar** ___ / ___ plantar dermatitis; **epilepsia mioclónica** ___ / ___ myoclonic epilepsy; **principio de diabetes** ___ / ___ on-set diabetes; **periodontitis** ___ / ___ periodontitis.
juventud *f.* youth.

k

K *abr.* **potasio** / kalium, potassium.

k *abr.* **kilogramo** / kilogram.

kala-azar *m.* kala-azar, *Hindi* black fever, visceral infestation by a protozoa.

Kanner, síndrome de *m.* Kanner syndrome, child autism.

Kaposi, enfermedad de *f.* Kaposi's disease, malignant neoplasm found on the skin of the lower extremities of adult males, very prevalent among individuals suffering from AIDS.

Karvonen, método de *m.* Karvonen method, a sequence to calculate the widest spectrum of cardiac rate during physical tolerance tests.

Katz, fórmula de *f.* Katz formula, formula to obtain the medium velocity of the sedimentation of erythrocytes.

Kawasaki, enfermedad de *f.* Kawasaki disease, acute febrile child disease, characterized by symptoms of conjunctivitis, lesions of the mouth, redness, infl. and peeling of the skin in hands and feet. These symptoms distinguish this disease from others such as scarlet fever and toxic shock syndrome.

Kegel, ejercicios de *m., pl.* Kegel exercises, activity that consists in alternating contractions and relaxation of the perineal muscles for better control of incontinence.

Kelly, operación de *f.* Kelly operation. 1. subtotal abdominal hysterectomy; 2. surgical procedure to correct urinary incontinence placing sutures in the vagina under the bladder neck.

kernicterus *m.* kernicterus, type of jaundice found in the newborn.

kerosen, kerosene *m., f.* kerosene.

Klebsiella *m.* Klebsiella, gram-negative bacilli associated with respiratory and urinary tract infections.

Klebs-Löffler, bacilo de *m.* Klebs-Löffler bacillus, the diphtheria bacillus.

Koch, bacilo de *m.* Koch's bacillus, *Mycobacterium tuberculosis* the cause of tuberculosis in mammals.

Koplic, manchas de *f.* Koplic spots, small whitish spots surrounded by a red ring that appear in the inner cheek during the early stage of the measles.

Krukenberg, tumor de *m.* Krukenberg's tumor, malignant tumor of the ovary, gen. bilateral and frequently secondary to malignancy in the gastrointestinal tract.

Kussmaul, respiracion de *f.* Kussmaul's breathing, deep and gasping respiration seen in cases of diabetic acidosis.

kwashiorkor *m.* kwashiorkor, severe protein deficiency seen in infants after weaning, esp. in tropical and subtropical areas.

l *abr.* **letal** / lethal; **ligero** / light.

L *abr.* **litro** / liter.

laberintectomía *f.* labyrinthectomy, excision of a labyrinth.

laberíntico-a *a.* labyrinthine, rel. to a labyrinth; **arteria** ___ / ___ artery; **fístula** ___ / ___ fistula; **nistagmo** ___ / ___ nystagmus; **punto** ___ / ___ punctum; **vena** ___ / ___ vein; **vértigo** ___ / ___ vertigo.

laberintitis *f.* labyrinthitis. 1. acute or chronic infl. of the labyrinth; 2. internal otitis.

laberinto *m.* labyrinth, maze. 1. communicating channels of the internal ear that function in relation to hearing and to body balance; 2. channels and cavities that communicate forming a system.

labial *a.* labial, rel. to the lips; **férula** ___ / ___ splint; **glándulas** ___ -es / ___ glands, situated between the labial mucosa and the orbicular muscle of the mouth; **hernia** ___ / ___ hernia; **oclusión** ___ / ___ occlusion; **ramas del nervio mentoniano** ___ / branches of the ___ mental nerve; **venas** ___ -es / ___ veins.

labihendido-a *a.* harelipped.

lábil *a.* labile, unstable, fragile, changeable or easily altered.

labio *m.* labios lip. 1. fleshy border; 2. lip-like structure; ___ **s mayores y menores de la vagina** / *sing.* labia majora and labia minora of the vagina.

labiocorea *f.* labichorea, chronic spasm of the lips that cause language disorders.

labio leporino *m.* harelip, cleft lip, congenital anomaly at the level of the upper lip, caused by faulty fusion of the upper jaw and the nasal processes; **cirugía del** ___ / ___ suture.

laboratorio *m.* laboratory; ___ **de trabajo** / workshop.

laboratorista *m., f.* medical laboratory technician.

laborioso-a *a.* labored, laborious; difficult.

laceración *f.* laceration; tear.

lacrimal, lagrimal *a.* lacrimal, lachrymal, rel. to tears or to tear ducts; **conducto** ___ / ___ duct; **hueso** ___ / ___ bone; **saco** ___ / ___ sac.

lacrimógeno-a *a.* lachrymogenous, that produces tears.

lactancia, lactación *f.* lactation, secretion of milk; ___ **materna** / breast-feeding.

lactante *m., f.* infant, approx. from birth to 12 months.

lactar *v.* to nurse; to suckle.

lactasa *f.* lactase, intestinal enzyme that hydrolizes lactose producing dextrose and galactose.

lácteo-a *a.* lacteal, rel. to milk; **productos** ___ -s / dairy products.

lactífero-a *a.* lactiferous, that secretes and conducts milk; **conductos** ___ / ___ ducts.

lactógeno *m.* lactogen, agent that stimulates the production or secretion of milk.

lacto-ovovegetariano-a *m., f.* lacto-ovovegetarian, person whose diet consists of vegetables, eggs, and dairy products.

lactosuria *f.* lactosuria, presence of lactose in the urine.

lacto-vegetariano-a *a.* lacto-vegetarian, that follows a diet of vegetables and dairy products.

lactosa, lactina *f.* lactose, lactin, milk sugar; **intolerancia a la** ___ / ___ intolerance, characterized by gastrointestinal disorders.

lado *m.* side; **al** ___ / alongside; **al** ___ **de** / next to; **de** ___ / sideways.

lágrima *f.* tear.

lagrimal *a.* lacrimal, lachrymal, rel. to tears or to the lacrimal apparatus; **aparato** ___ / ___ apparatus; **arteria** ___ / ___ artery; **canículo** ___ / ___ caniculus; **fosa** ___ / ___ fosa; **glándula** ___ / ___ gland; **nervio** ___ / ___ nerve; **papila** ___ / ___ papilla; **punto** ___ / ___ punctum; **vena** ___ / ___ vein.

lagrimoso-a *a.* tearful.

laguna *f.* lacuna, small cavity or depression such as those found in the brain.

Lamaze, método de *m.* Lamaze technique or method, method of natural childbirth by which the mother is trained in techniques of breathing and relaxation that facilitate the process of delivery.

lamentar *vt.* to regret; **lamentarse** *vr.* to lament, to complain; **lamento mucho** / I am very sorry.

lámina *f.* lamina, thin sheath or layer; __ **anterior clásica de la córnea** / __ limitans anterior cornea; __ **basal de la coroide** / __ basalis choroidae; __ **del arco vertebral** / __ arcus vertebrae; __ **elástica posterior de la córnea** / __ limitans posterior corneae; __ **multiforme del cortex del cerebro** / __ cerebral cortex multiformis.

laminectomía *f.* laminectomy, removal of one or more vertebral laminae.

laminilla *f.* lamella. 1. thin layer; 2. disk that is inserted in the eye to apply a medication.

lámpara *f.* lamp; __ **de hendidura** / slit __; __ **infrarroja** / infrared __; **luz de una** __ / lamplight.

lanceta *f.* lancet, lance, surgical instrument.

lancinante *a.* lancinating, rel. to an acute, piercing pain.

Landsteiner, clasificación de *f.* Landsteiner's classification, differentiation of blood types: O-A-B-AB.

lanolina *f.* lanolin, purified substance obtained from lamb's wool and used in ointments.

lanugo *m.* lanugo, soft fine hair that covers the body of the human fetus.

laparocele *m.* laparocele, abdominal hernia.

laparoscopía *f.* laparoscopy, examination of the peritoneal cavity with a laparoscope.

laparoscopio *m.* laparoscope, instrument used to visualize the peritoneal cavity.

laparotomía *f.* laparotomy, incision and opening of the abdomen.

lápiz *m.* pencil.

laringe *f.* larynx. 1. part of the respiratory tract situated in the upper part of the trachea; 2. voice organ.

laringectomía *f.* laryngectomy, removal of the larynx.

laríngeo-a *a.* laryngeal, rel. to the larynx; **estenosis** __ / __ stenosis; **papilomatosis** __ / __ papillomatosis; **prominencia** __ / __ prominence; **red** __ / __ web; **reflejo** __ / __ reflex, cough produced by irritation of the larynx; **síncope** __ / __ syncope; **ventrículo** __ / __ ventricle.

laringitis *f.* laryngitis, infl. of the larynx.

laringoespasmo *m.* laryngospasm, spasm of the laryngeal muscles.

laringofaringe *f.* laryngopharynx, inferior portion of the larynx.

laringofaringitis *f.* infl. of the larynx and the pharynx.

laringoplastia *f.* laryngoplasty, plastic reconstruction of the larynx.

laringoscopia *f.* laryngoscopy, examination of the larynx; __ **directa** / direct __, by means of a laryngoscope; __ **indirecta** / indirect __, by means of a mirror.

laringoscopio *m.* laryngoscope, instrument used to examine the larynx.

larva *f.* larva, maggot, early stage of some organisms such as insects.

larvicida *m.* larvicide, agent that exterminates larvae.

láser *m.* laser. 1. acronym for Light Amplification by Stimulated Emission of Radiation; 2. micro-surgical scalpel used in the cauterization of tumors; **canonización por** __ / __ canonization; **coagulación por** __ / __ coagulation.

laser, rayos de *m., pl.* laser beams, radiation rays applied for the purpose of destroying tissue or separating parts.

LASIK *abbr.* LASIK, laser assisted in-situ keratomileusis.

lasitud *f.* lassitude, languor.

lastimado-a *a.* injured, hurt.

lastimadura *f.* injury, hurt.

latencia *f.* latency, the condition of being latent; **período de** __ / __ period.

latente *a.* latent, present but not active; with no apparent symptoms or manifestations.

lateral *a.* lateral, rel. to a side.

lateroflexión *f.* lateroflexion, lateral flexion.

látex *m.* latex, substance derived from a seed plant that contains an element of natural rubber; in many cases it can be an allergen.

latido *m.* beat; throb; __ **del corazón** / heart __; __ **ectópico** / ectopic __ .

lavabo *m.* washstand, basin.

lavado *m.* lavage, enema, irrigation of a cavity; __ **broncopulmonar** / bronchopulmonary __ ; __ **bronquial** / bronchial washing.

lavamanos *m.* washstand, washbowl.

lavaojos *m.* eyecup.

lavar *vt.* to wash; **lavarse** *vr.* to wash oneself.

lavativa *f.* enema.

laxante *m.* laxative, mild physic.

Leber, enfermedad de *f.* Leber disease, hereditary type of atrophy that causes degeneration of the optic nerve and that affects males.

leche *f.* milk; __ **condensada** / condensed __; __ **cuajada** / curd milk; __ **de magnesia** / milk of magnesia; __ **descremada** / skim __; __ **en polvo** / dry milk; __ **evaporada** / evaporated __; __ **hervida** / boiled __; __ **materna** / mother's __; __ **pasteurizada** / pasteurized __ .

lecitina *f.* lecithin, essential substance in the metabolism of fats found in animal tissue, esp. in the nervous tissue.

legal *a.* legal, legitimate, according to the law; **ceguera** __ / __ **blindness**; **medicina** __ / __ medicine; **pleito** __ / lawsuit.

Legionarios, enfermedad de los *f.* Legionnaires disease, serious infectious disease that could be lethal and is characterized by pneumonia, a dry cough, muscular ache, and sometimes gastrointestinal symptoms.

leiomioma *m.* leiomyoma, benign tumor of essentially smooth muscular tissue.

leiomiosarcoma *f.* leiomyosarcoma, combined tumor of leiomyoma and sarcoma.

lejía *f.* lye, bleach; **envenenamiento por** __ / __ poisoning.

lejos *adv.* far, afar; **de** __ / __ away; **desde** __ / from afar.

Lenegre, síndrome de *f.* Lenegre syndrome, fibrosis of the intracardiac conductive system that is gen. characterized as idiopathic fibrosis of the atrioventricular nodule.

lengua *f.* 1. tongue, lingua; **depresor de** __ / __ depressor; 2. language; __ **materna** / native __ .

lengua geográfica *f.* geographic tongue, tongue characterized by bare patches surrounded by thick epithelium, resembling a geographic map.

lenguaje *m.* language; __ **hablado** / spoken __ .

lente *m.* lens; __ **acromático** / achromatic __; __ **bicóncavo** / biconcave __; __ **cilíndrico** / cylindrical __; __ **de aumento** /

magnifying glass; __ **-s bifocales** / bifocal __; __ **-s de contacto** / contact lens; __ **-s intraoculares** / __ implantation, intraocular; __ **-s trifocales** / trifocal __ .

lentes correctores *m., pl.* corrective lenses.

lentiginosis *f.* lentiginosis, presence of a large number of lentigos.

léntigo *m.* lentigo, skin macule; __ **maligno** / malignant __; __ **múltiple** / multiple __; __ **senil** / senile __ .

lento-a *a.* slow; sluggish, inactive; **-mente** *adv.* slowly.

lepra *f.* leprosy, Hansen's disease, infectious disease caused by the *Mycobacterium leprae* and characterized by more or less severe skin lesions.

leprecaunismo *m.* leprechaunism, hereditary condition with characteristics of dwarfism accompanied by mental and physical retardation, endocrine disorders, and susceptibility to infections.

leproso-a *m., f.* leper, person suffering from leprosy.

leptomeninges *f.* leptomeninges, the thinnest of the cerebral membranes: the pia madre and the arachnoid.

leptomeningitis *f.* leptomeningitis, infl. of the leptomeninges.

lesbiana *f.* lesbian, homosexual female.

lesión *f.* injury, lesion, contusion, wound; __ **de latigazo** / whiplash; __ **degenerative** / degenerative __; __ **depresiva** / depressive __; __ **difusa** / diffuse __; __ **funcional** / functional __; __ **periférica** / peripheral __; __ **precancerosa** / precancerous __; __ **sistémica** / systemic __; __ **traumática** / traumatic __; __ **vascular** / vascular __ .

letal *a.* lethal, mortal, that causes death; **dosis** __ / __ dose; **factor** __ / __ factor; **gene** __ / __ gene; **mutación** __ / __ mutation.

letargo *m.* lethargy, torpor.

leucaferesis *f.* leukapheresis, separation of leukocytes from a patient's blood and transfusion of the treated blood back into the patient.

leucemia *f.* leukemia, blood cancer; __ **aleucémica** / aleukemic __; __ **crónica** / chronic __; __ **eosinofílica** / eosinophilic __; __ **granulocítica crónica** / chronic granulocytic __; __ **linfocítica** / lymphocytic __; __

ligamento

mieloide crónica / chronic myeloid
___; ___ **monocítica** / monocytic ___ .
leucemoide *a.* leukemoid, with
leukemia-like signs and symptoms.
leucina *f.* leucine, amino acid that is
essential to the growth and metabolism
of humans.
leucinuria *f.* leucinuria, presence of
leucine in the urine.
leucoblasto *m.* leukoblast, immature
leukocyte.
leucocis *f.* leucosis, abnormal
formation of leukocytes.
leucocito *m.* leukocyte, white blood
cell, element of the blood important in
the defensive and reparative functions
of the body; ___ **acidófilo** / acidophil
___ , that changes color with acid dye;
___ **basófilo** / basophil ___ , that changes
color with basic dye; ___ **eosinofílico** /
eosinophilic ___ , that stains readily
with eosin; ___ **linfoide** / nongranular
lymphoid ___; ___ **neutrófilo** /
neutrophil ___ , that has an affinity for
neutral stains; ___ **polimorfonucleado** /
polymorphonuclear ___ , having
multilobed nuclei.
leucocitosis *f.* leukocytosis, an
abnormally increase of leukocytes in the
blood, gen. occurring during severe
infections; ___ **absoluta** / absolute ___;
___ **mononuclear** / mononuclear ___;
___ **polinuclear** / polynuclear ___; ___
relativa / relative ___ .
leucocoria *f.* leukokoria, leucocoria,
white appearance of the pupil due to a
cataract.
leucoencefalopatía *f.*
leucoencephalopathy, white matter
changes first discovered in children
suffering from leukemia, associated
with radiation and chemotherapy
lesions.
leucopatía *f.* leukopathia, albinism,
lack of pigmentation.
leucopenia *f.* leukopenia, below
normal number of leukocytes in the
blood.
leucorrea *f.* leukorrhea, whitish vaginal
discharge.
leucotriquia *f.* leukotrichia, white hair.
levadura *f.* yeast, leaven. 1. minute
fungi capable of producing fermentation;
2. a source of protein and vitamin.
levantamiento *m.* lift, the act of
lifting.
levantar *v.* to raise, to lift, to pull up;
levantarse *vr.* to get up.

levodopa *f.* levodopa, L. dopa, chemical
substance used in the treatment of
Parkinson's disease.
ley *f.* law; ___ **del buen Samaritano** /
good Samaritan ___ , legal protection to
a professional who gives aid in an
emergency.
liberación *f.* liberation.
líbido *m.* libido. 1. sexual impulse,
conscious or unconscious; 2. in
pychoanalysis, the force or energy that
determines human behavior.
libidinoso-a *a.* libidinous, rel. to the
libido.
Libman-Sacks, enfermedad de
f. Libman-Sacks endocarditis,
Libman-Sacks syndrome, non-bacterial
verrucose endocarditis that is
associated with disseminated
erythematous lupus.
libre *a.* free; **asociación** ___ / ___
association.
librería *f.* bookstore.
libreta *f.* notebook.
libro *m.* book.
licopenemia *f.* lycopenemia, increase
of lycopene in the blood that results in
a yellow-orange color of the skin.
licopina *f.* lycopene, vegetable pigment
abundant in tomatoes and carrots.
licor *m.* liquor; 1. watery solution that
contains a medicinal substance; 2.
general term used for some body fluids.
lidocaína *f.* lidocaine, anesthetic.
lientería *f.* lientery, diarrhea which
shows particles of non-digested food.
Liga de la Leche, La *f.* La Leche
League, an organization that promotes
breast-feeding.
ligadura *f.* ligature, tie, affixture;
linkage.
ligamento *m.* ligament. 1. bands of
connective tissue fibers that protect the
joints; ___ **acromioclavicular** /
acromioclavicular ___ , extending from
the clavicle to the acromion; ___
alveolodentario / alveolo-dental ___;
___ **ancho uterino** / broad uterine ___ ,
peritoneal fold that extends laterally
from the uterus to the pelvic wall; ___
anococcígeo / anococcygeal ___; ___
braquicubital / brachiocubital ___;
capsular / capsular ___; **desgarre del**
___ / ___ tear; ___ **esternoclavicular** /
sternoclavicular ___; ___ **gastrocólico** /
gastrocholic ___; ___ **glosoepiglótico** /
glossoepiglotic ___; ___
hepatoduodenal / hepatoduodenal ___;

ligar

___ **iliofemoral** / iliofemoral ___; ___
largo del plantar / long plantar ___; ___
palmar / palmar ___; ___ **radiocubital** /
radiocubital ___; ___ **trapezoide** /
trapezoid ___; ___ **Y,** ___ iliofemoral /
Y ligament, iliofemoral ___; 2.
protective band of fascia and muscles
that connect or support viscerae.

ligar *vi.* to tie, to apply a ligature; to
attach; ___ **las trompas** / ___ the
tubes.

ligazón *f.* binding, bandage.

ligero-a *a.* light, slight; *adv.* **-mente**
lightly, slightly.

limar *v.* to file; to smooth.

límbico-a *a.* limbic, marginal; **sistema**
___ / ___ system, group of cerebral
structures.

limbo *m.* limbus, the edge or border of a
part; ___ **de la córnea** / ___ cornea.

liminal *a.* liminal, almost imperceptible.

limitación *f.* limitation; restriction.

limitado-a *a.* limited, restricted;
movimiento ___ / restricted motion.

limitar *v.* to limit, to restrict.

límite *m.* limit; ___ **de asimilación** /
assimilation ___; ___ **de percepción** /
___ of perception; ___ **de saturación** /
saturation ___ .

limpiar *vt.* to clean; to wipe; *vr.*
limpiarse, to clean oneself.

limpieza *f.* cleaning; cleanliness.

limpio-a *a.* clean.

linaje *m.* pedigree, ancestral line of
descent.

lindo-a *a.* pretty.

línea *f.* line; wrinkle; guide.

linfa *f.* lymph, clear fluid found in
lymphatic vessels.

linfadenectomía *f.*
lymphadenectomy, removal of
lymphatic channels and nodes.

linfadenitis *f.* lymphadenitis, infl. of
the lymphatic ganglia.

linfadenopatía *f.* lymphadenopathy,
any disease affecting the lymph nodes;
___ **axilar** / axillary ___; ___ **biliar** /
portal ___; ___ **cervical** / cervical ___;
___ **generalizada** / generalized ___; ___
mediastínica / mediastinal ___; ___
supraclavicular / supraclavicular ___ .

linfangiectasis *f.* lymphangiectasis,
dilation of the lymphatic vessels.

linfangioma *m.* linfangioma, simple
tumor composed of lymphatic vessels;
___ **cavernoso** / cavernous ___ .

linfangitis *f.* lymphangitis, infl. of the
lymphatic vessels.

linfático-a *a.* lymphatic, rel. to lymph;
ganglios ___ **-s** / lymph nodes; **sistema**
___ / ___ system.

linfedema *m.* lymphedema, edema
caused by blockage of the lymph
vessels.

linfemia *f.* lymphemia, high number of
lymphocytes or its precursors or both in
the circulating blood.

linfoblasto *m.* lymphoblast, early stage
of a lymphocyte.

linfoblastoma *m.* lymphoblastoma,
malignant lymphoma formed by
lymphoblasts.

linfocito *m.* lymphocyte, lymphatic cell;
___ **B** / B cell, important in the
production of antibodies

linfocitopenia, linfopenia *f.*
lymphocytopenia, lymphopenia,
diminished number of lymphocytes in
the blood.

linfocitos T *m., pl.* T cells,
lymphocytes differentiated in the
thymus that direct the immunological
response and alert the B cells to
respond to antigens; ___ **inductores,
(ayudantes)** / helper ___ , enhance
production of antibody forming cells
from B cells; ___ **citotóxicos** / cytotoxic
___ , kill foreign cells (as in rejection of
transplanted organs); ___ **supresores** /
suppressor ___ , suppress production of
antibody forming cells from B cells.

linfocitosis *f.* lymphocytosis, excessive
number of lymphocytes in the blood.

linfogranuloma venéreo *f.*
lymphogranuloma venereum, viral
disorder that may lead to elephantiasis
of the genitalia and rectal stricture.

linfogranulomatosis *f.*
lymphogranulomatosis. *See* **Hodgkin,
enfermedad de.**

linfoma *m.* lymphoma, any neoplasm of
the lymphatic tissue.

linfopenia, linfocitopenia *f.*
lymphopenia, lymphocytopenia,
diminished number of lymphocytes in
the blood.

linforreticular *a.* lymphoreticular, rel.
to reticuloendothelial cells of the
lymph nodes.

linfosarcoma *m.* lymphosarcoma,
malignant neoplasm of the lymphoid
tissue.

lingual *a.* lingual, rel. to the tongue.

linimento *m.* liniment, liquid substance
for external use.

lino *m.* linen.

lío *m.* mess, confusion.

liofilización *f.* freeze-drying.

lipectomía *f.* lipectomy, removal of fat tissue; __ **submental** / submental __ , under the chin.

lipemia *f.* lipemia, abnormal presence of fat in the blood.

lipidemia *f.* lipidemia, excess lipids in the blood.

lípido *m.* lipid, lipide, organic substance that does not dissolve in water but is soluble in alcohol, ether, or chloroform.

lipoartritis *f.* lipoarthritis, infl. of fatty tissues in the knee.

lipodistrofia *f.* lipodystrophy, metabolic disorder of fats; __ **cefalotorácica** / cephalothoracic __; __ **insulínica** / insulin __; __ **intestinal** / intestinal __ .

lipofuscinosis *f.* lipofuscinosis, abnormal storage of any of a group of adipose pigments.

lipólisis *f.* lipolysis, decomposition of fat.

lipoma *m.* lipoma, adipose tissue tumor.

lipomatosis *f.* lipomatosis. 1. condition caused by excessive accumulation of fat in a given area; 2. multiple lipomas.

lipoproteínas *f., pl.* lipoproteins, proteins combined with lipid compounds that contain a high concentration of cholesterol; __ **de alta densidad** / high-density __; __ **de densidad baja** / low-density __ .

liposarcoma *m.* liposarcoma, malignant tumor containing fatty elements.

liposis *f.* liposis, obesity, excessive accumulation of fat in the body.

liposoluble *a.* liposoluble, that dissolves in fatty substances.

liposucción *f.* liposuction, process of extracting fat by high vacuum pressure.

lipuria *f.* lipuria, presence of lipids in the urine.

liquen *m.* lichen, noncontagious papular skin lesion; __ **de urticaria** / __ urticatus; __ **escleroso atrófico** / __ sclerosus and atrophicus; __ **escrofularia** / __ scrofulosorum; __ **plano** / __ planus; __ **ulcerativo** / __ erosive.

líquido *m.* fluid, liquid; __ **amniótico** __ / amniotic __; __ **articular** / joint __; __ **cefalorraquídeo** / cerebrospinal __; __ **corporal** / body __; __ **espeso** / heavy liquid; __ **extracelular** / extracellular liquid; __ **intersticial** / interstitial __; __

intracelular / intracellular __; __ **peritoneal** / peritoneal __; __ **seminal** / seminal liquid; __ **sérico** / serous __; __ **sinovial** / synovial __ .

lisiado-a *a.* crippled.

lisina *f.* lysin, antibody that dissolves or destroys cells or bacteria.

lisinógeno *m.* lysinogen, agent with the property of producing lysine.

lisis *f.* lysis. 1. destruction or dissolution of red cells, bacteria, or any antigen by lysin; 2. gradual cessation of the symptoms of a disease.

lista *f.* list; __ **de accidentados** / casualty __ .

litiasis *f.* lithiasis, formation of calculi, esp. in the biliary and urinary tracts.

litio *m.* lithium, metallic element used as a tranquilizer in severe cases of psychosis.

litotomía *f.* lithotomy, incision in an organ or conduit to remove stones.

litotripsia *f.* lithotripsy, crushing of calculi present in the kidney, ureter, bladder, or gallbladder.

litotriturador *m.* lithotriptor, machine or device used to crush calculi; __ **extracorporal con ondas de choque** / extracorporeal shock wave __ .

lituresis *f.* lithuresis, sandy urine.

livedo *m.* livedo, a stain in the skin, often blue or purple like in a bruise.

lividez *f.* lividity, discoloration resulting from the gravitation of blood; __ **cadavérica** / postmortem lividity.

llaga *f.* sore, ulcer, blain.

llegada *f.* arrival; coming.

llenar *v.* to fill; to complete.

lleno-a *a.* full, complete.

llevar *v.* to carry; to take; to transport; __ **puesto** / to be wearing; __ **a cabo** / to carry out; **llevarse** / *vr.* to take away; __ **a cabo** / to take place; __ **bien** / to get along well; __ **mal** / not to get along.

llorar *v.* to cry.

lobar *a.* lobar, rel. to a lobe; **pulmonía** __ / __ pneumonia.

lobectomía *f.* lobectomy, excision of a lobe.

lobotomía *f.* lobotomy, incision of a cerebral lobe to correct certain mental disorders; __ **completa** / complete __; __ **izquierda anterior** / left lower __; __ **parcial** / partial __ .

lobular *a.* lobular, rel. to a lobule; **neoplasia** __ / __ neoplasia.

lobulillo

lobulillo *m.* lobule, small lobe.
lóbulo *m.* lobe, rounded, well-defined portion of an organ.
local *a.* local, rel. to an isolated area, such as local anesthesia; **aplicación** ___ / ___ application; **reaparición** ___ / ___ recurrence.
localización *f.* localization, location. 1. reference to the point of origin of a sensation; 2. determination of the origin of an infection or lesion.
loción *f.* lotion.
loco-a *m., f.* insane person; *a.* mad, insane.
locomoción *f.* locomotion.
locular *a.* locular, loculated, rel. to loculus.
lóculo *m.* loculus, small cavity.
locura *f.* madness, insanity, lunacy.
locus *L.* locus, localization of a gene in a chromosome.
logamnesia *f.* logamnesia, sensorial aphasia, inability to recognize written or spoken words.
lógico-a *a.* logic, logical; reasonable.
logopeda *m., f.* speech-language pathologist.
logopedia *f.* speech pathology.
logoplejía *f.* logoplegia, paralysis of the organs of speech.
lombriz *f.* earthworm; ___ **intestinal** / pinworm, belly worm; ___ **solitaria** / tapeworm.
lonche *m., H.A.* lunch, midday meal.
longevidad *f.* longevity. 1. long duration of life; 2. life span.
longitud *f.* length.
loquios *m.* lochia, bloody, serosanguineous discharge from the uterus and the vagina during the first few weeks after delivery.
lordosis *f.* lordosis, abnormally increased curvature of the lumbar spine; saddle back.
Lou Gehrig, enfermedad de *f.* Lou Gehrig disease, amyotrophic lateral sclerosis; progressive muscular atrophy.
lubricante *m.* lubricant, oily agent that when applied diminishes friction between two surfaces; ___ **oleaginoso** / oil-based ___ .
luchar *v.* to struggle; to fight.
lucidez *f.* lucidity, mental clarity.
lugar *m.* place, space; **en ___ de** / in ___ of; **fuera de ___** / out of ___; **tener ___** / to take ___ .
lumbago *m.* lumbago, pain in the lower portion of the back.

lumbar *a.* lumbar, rel. to the part of the back between the thorax and the pelvis; back; **nervio ___** / ___ nerve; **plexus ___** / ___ plexus; **punción ___** / ___ puncture, spinal tap; **vértebras ___ -es** / ___ vertebrae.
lumen *m.* lumen. 1. space in a cavity, conduit, or organ; 2. unit of light.
luminal *a.* luminal, rel. to light in a conduit or canal.
luminiscencia, luminosidad *f.* luminescence, luminosity, emission of light without production of heat.
luna *f.* moon.
lunar *m.* mole; blemish; *a.* rel. to the moon.
lunático-a *m., f.* lunatic, crazy person.
lupus *L.* lupus, chronic skin disease of unknown origin that causes degenerative local lesions; ___ **anticoagulante** / anticoagulant ___; ___ **eritematoso discoide** / ___ erythematous, discoid, disease that causes irritation of the skin and is characterized by squamous plaques with reddish borders; ___ **eritematoso sistémico** / ___ erythematous, systemic, characterized by febrile episodes affecting the viscera and the nervous system; ___ **marginado** / marginal ___; ___ **vulgar** / ___ vulgaris.
luteína *f.* lutein, yellow pigment that derives from the corpus luteum.
luteo-a, luteínico-a *a.* luteal, rel. to the corpus luteum.
luteoma *f.* luteoma, tumor of the corpus luteum.
luxación *f.* dislocation, luxation; ___ **cerrada** / closed ___; ___ **cervical** / cervical ___; ___ **complicada** / complicated ___; ___ **congénita** / congenital ___; ___ **congénita de la cadera** / congenital ___ of hip; ___ **recidivante** / habitual ___ .
luz *f.* light; *v.* **dar ___** / to give birth; **adaptación a la ___** / ___ adaptation; ___ **del día** / daylight; ___ **deslumbrante** / glare.
Lyme, enfermedad de *f.* Lyme disease, multisystem inflammatory disorder caused by a deer tick; gen. occurs in the eastern part of the United States during spring and summer; the immediate recommendation is to remove the ticks from the body to avoid contagion.

m

M *abr.* **maduro** / mature; **maligno-a** / malignant; **minuto** / minute; **morfina** / morphine.

maceración *f.* maceration. 1. decomposition and softening of organs and tissues by soaking in water or other liquids; 2. fragmentation of the skin through exposure to humidity for a long period of time.

macerar *vt.* to macerate, to soften by soaking.

macho *m.* male; *a.* male; manly.

macrocefalia *f.* macrocephalia, abnormally large head.

macrocito *m.* macrocyte, large crythrocyte.

Macrodantina *f.* Macrodantin, trade name for furantoin, bactericide used in the treatment of urinary infections.

macrófago *m.* macrophage, mononuclear phagocytic cell; **migración de __ -s** / __ migration.

macroglubinemia *f.* macroglobinemia, increase of macroglobulins in the blood.

macroglosia *f.* macroglossia, enlargement of the tongue.

macromolécula *f.* macromolecule, a large molecule such as a protein.

macroscópico-a *a.* macroscopic, visible to the naked eye.

macrosomia *f.* macrosomia, abnormal large size of the body.

mácula *f.* macula, macule, speck, small discolored spot on the skin; **__ lútea** / __ lutea, small, yellowish area next to the center of the retina.

maculado-a *a.* maculate.

maculopapular *a.* maculopapular, rel. to macules and papules.

madrastra *f.* stepmother.

madre *f.* mother; **__ soltera** / unwed __.

madurez *f.* maturity; ripeness, stage of full development.

maduro-a *a.* mature, [*fruta*] ripened.

magnesio *m.* magnesium; **sulfato de __** / __ sulfate; **__ de cloruro** / __ chloride; **__ de lactasa** / __ lactate.

magnético-a *a.* magnetic, magnetical, rel. to or that has the properties of a magnet; **campo __** / __ field.

magnetoelectricidad *f.* magnetoelectricity, electricity induced by a magnet.

magulladura *f.* bruise, contusion.

majadero-a *a.* spoiled, cranky.

mal *m.* malady, illness, disease.

mal, malo-a *a.* bad; evil; **__ genio** / ill temper; *mal adv.* badly; wrongly; **de __ en peor** / from bad to worse; *v.* **hacer __** / to harm, to hurt.

malabsorción *f.* malabsorption, inadequate absorption of nutrients from the intestinal track.

malacia *f.* malacia, softening or loss of consistency of organs or tissues.

malacoplaquia *f.* malacoplakia, formation of soft patches in the mucous membrane of a hollow organ.

malar *a.* malar, rel. to the cheek or the cheekbone.

maléolo *m.* malleolus, hammerlike protuberance, such as the ones on either side of the ankle.

malestar *m.* malaise, discomfort, uneasiness.

maleta *f.* valise, suitcase.

malformación *f.* malformation, anomaly, or deformity, esp. congenital.

malhumor *m.* bad temper.

malignidad *f.* malignancy. 1. quality of being malignant; 2. cancerous tumor.

maligno-a *a.* malignant, virulent, pernicious, having a destructive effect.

malnutrición *f.* malnutrition, deficient nutrition.

malo-a *a.* bad, malignant.

maloclusión *f.* malocclusion, defective bite.

malpresentación *f.* malpresentation, abnormal presentation of the fetus at the time of delivery.

maltratar *v.* to abuse, to mistreat, to manhandle; **__ maltrato de palabra** / verbal abuse.

malunión *f.* malunion, imperfect union of a fracture.

malleus *L.* mallei malleus, one of the three ossicles of the middle ear.

mama *f.* mamma, breast, milk-secreting gland in the female; **enfermedad benigna de la __** / benign breast disease.

mamá *f.* mom, term of endearment for mother.

mamalgia *f.* mammalgia, pain in the [*breast*] mamma.

mamaplastia, mamoplastia

mamaplastia, mamoplastia *f.* mammaplasty, mammoplasty, plastic surgery of the breast; __ **de aumento** / augmentation __; __ **de reconstrucción** / reconstructive __; __ **de reducción** / reduction __ .

mamar *v.* to suckle, to draw milk from the breast; **dar de** __ / to breastfeed.

mamario-a *a.* mammary, rel. to the mamma; **glándulas** __ **-s /** __ glands.

mamectomía *f.* mammectomy, mastectomy.

mamífero *m.* mammal.

mamiliplastia *f.* mammilliaplasty, plastic surgery of the nipple.

mamilitis *f.* mammillitis, infl. of the nipple.

mamitis, mastitis *f.* mammitis, mastitis, infl. of the mammary gland.

mamograma *m.* mammogram, x-ray of the breast.

mancha *f.* spot, blemish, macula, stain.

manchado-a *a.* spotted, soiled.

manco-a *m., f.* one-handed person.

mandíbula *f.* mandible, mandibula, horseshoe-shaped bone that constitutes the lower jaw; __ **inferior** / lower __; __ **superior** / upper __ .

manerismo *m.* mannerism, a distinctive trait in dress, speech, or action.

manga *f.* sleeve.

mango *m.* mango, handle.

manguito *m.* cuff, bandlike fibrous tissue surrounding a joint; __ **rotador** / rotator __; musculotendinous; **ruptura del** __ **rotador** / rotator tear.

manía *f.* mania, emotional disorder characterized by extreme excitement, exalted emotions, rapid succession of ideas, and fluctuating moods.

maníaco-a, maniático-a *a.* maniac, maniacal, afflicted by mania; **maníacodepresivo** / manic-depressive

manicomio *m.* insane asylum, madhouse.

manifestación *f.* manifestation, revelation.

maniobra *f.* maneuver, skillful manual procedure such as executed by the obstetrician in the delivery of a baby.

manipulación *f.* manipulation, professional treatment involving the use of hands.

manipular *v.* to manipulate, to handle.

mano *f.* hand; **apoyo de la** __ / __ rest; **deformidades adquiridas de la** __ / acquired __ deformities; **hecho a** __ / handmade.

mantener *vi.* to sustain, to support; **mantenerse** *vr.* to hold or keep up; to support oneself.

mantenimiento *m.* maintenance, sustenance.

manto *m.* mantle, covering.

manutención *f.* maintenance, child care support.

manzanilla *f.* chamomile, sedative tea used to alleviate gastrointestinal discomfort.

máquina *f.* machine, apparatus.

marasmo *m.* marasmus, extreme malnutrition, emaciation, esp. in young children.

marca *f.* mark, sign, brand; __ **de la viruela** / pockmark; __ **de nacimiento** / birthmark; __ **enfresa** / strawberry __; __ **registrada** / trademark.

marcador *m.* marker, indicator.

marcapaso, marcapasos *m.* pacemaker, electronic cardiac pacer; pacer, regulator of cardiac rhythm; __ **de ritmo fijo** / fixed rate __; __ **ectópico** / ectopic __; __ **interno** / internal __; __ **temporal** / temporary __ .

marcha *f.* gait, walk; __ **anserina** / waddling __, widespread walk; __ **atáxica** / ataxic __, staggering; __ **cerebelosa** / cerebellar __; __ **espástica** / spastic __; __ **hemipléjica** / hemiplegic __, circular movement of one of the lower extremities.

mareado-a *a.* dizzy, light-headed.

mareo *m.* dizziness; motion sickness; __ **de altura** / altitude sickness.

marginación *f.* margination, accumulation and adhesion of leukocytes to the epithelial cells of the blood vessel walls at the beginning of an inflammatory process.

marginal *a.* marginal, rel. to a margin; **caso** __ / __ case.

marido *m.* husband.

mariguana, marihuana *f. Cannabis sativa*, marihuana, marijuana. cannabis.

marsupialización *f.* marsupialization, conversion of a closed cavity into an open pouch.

martillo *m.* hammer. 1. common name for maleus, small bone of the middle ear; 2. instrument used in physical examination.

más *adv.* more, to a greater degree; **a** __ **tardar** / at the latest; __ **allá** / beyond; __ **que** / more than; __ **vale** / better to; **por** __ **que** / however much.

masa *f.* mass, body formed by coherent particles.

masaje *m.* massage, process of manipulation of different parts of the body by rubbing or kneading; ___ cardíaco / cardiac ___, resuscitation.

masajista *m., f.* masseur, masseuse, person who performs massage.

mascar, masticar *vi.* to chew.

máscara *f.* mask. 1. covering of the face; 2. appearance of the face, esp. as a pathological manifestation.

masculinización *f.* masculinization.

masculino-a *a.* masculine, rel. to the male sex.

masetero *m.* masseter, principal muscle in mastication.

masivo-a *a.* massive.

masoquismo *m.* masochism, abnormal condition by which sexual gratification is obtained from self-inflicted pain or pain inflicted by others.

mastadenitis *f.* mastadenitis, mastitis.

mastectomía *f.* mastectomy, plastic surgery of the breast; ___ radical / radical ___ .

masticación *f.* mastication, the act of chewing.

mastitis *f.* mastitis, mastadenites, fibrocystic disease of the mama; ___ cística / cystic ___; ___ cística crónica / chronic cystic ___; ___ del neonato / neonatorum ___; ___ glandular / glandular ___; ___ granulomatosa / granulomatous ___; ___ láctea / lacteal ___; ___ por estasis / caked breast; ___ puerperal / puerperal ___; ___ supurativa / suppurative ___ .

mastocitoma *f.* mastocytoma, mast cells accumulation resembling a neoplasm.

mastocitosis *f.* mastocytosis, a condition in which neoplastic mast cells appear in several tissues or in a variety of organs.

mastoideo-a *a.* mastoid. 1. rel. to the mastoid process; **antro** ___ / ___ antrum; **células** ___ **-s** / ___ cells, air spaces in the mastoid process; 2. that resembles a breast or nipple.

mastoides *m.* mastoid process, rounded apophysis of the temporal bone.

mastoiditis *f.* mastoiditis, infl. of the air cells of the mastoid process.

mastopexia *f.* mastopexy, correction of a pendulous breast.

masturbación *f.* masturbation, autostimulation and manipulation of the genitals to achieve sexual pleasure.

materia *f.* matter, substance.

material *m.* material; *a.* material.

maternidad *f.* maternity; **hospital de** ___ / ___ hospital.

materno-a *a.* maternal, rel. to the mother; **línea** ___ / matrilineal, tracing descendency to the mother

matidez *f.* dullness, diminished resonance to palpation.

matriz *f.* womb.

matutino-a *a.* of the morning, rel. to the early hours of the day; **enfermedad** ___ **del embarazo** / morning sickness; **rigidez** ___ **muscular y de las articulaciones** / morning stiffness.

maxilar *a.* maxillary, rel. to the maxilla; **hueso** ___ **de la mandíbula** / jawbone.

maxilla *L.* maxilla, bone of the upper jaw.

mayor *a.* greater, [*edad*] older; **-mente** *adv.* mostly, mainly.

meatal *a.* meatal, rel. to a meatus.

meato *m.* meatus, passage or channel in the body.

mecanismo *m.* mechanism. 1. involuntary response to a stimulus; ___ de defensa / defense ___; ___ de ejecución / implementation ___; ___ de escape / escape ___; ___ del dolor / pain ___; 2. machine-like structure.

meconio *m.* meconium. 1. first feces of the newborn; greenish in color

media *f.* mean. 1. average; 2. middle coat of a blood vessel or artery.

mediador-a *m., f.* mediator, entity or person that mediates.

medial *a.* medial, rel. to or situated towards the middle.

mediante *adv.* by means of.

medias *f., pl.* socks, stockings; ___ elásticas / elastic stockings.

mediastinitis *f.* mediastinitis, infl. of the tissues of the mediastinum.

mediastino *m.* mediastinum. 1. mass of tissues and organs separating the lungs; 2. cavity between two organs.

mediastinoscopía *f.* mediastinoscopy, endoscopic examination of the mediastinum.

medicación, medicamento *f., m.* medication, medicine; **medicamento de patente** / patent medicine.

Medicaid *m.* Medicaid, U.S. government program to provide health care for the poor.

Medicare *m.* Medicare, U.S. government program that subsidizes health care esp. for the elderly and the disabled.

medicina *f.* 1. medicine, the healing arts; ___ **clínica** / clinical ___; ___ **comunal, al servicio de la comunidad** / community ___; ___ **de emergencia** / emergence ___; ___ **holística** / holistic ___; ___ **integral** / integral ___; ___ **del espacio** / aerospace ___; ___ **deportiva** / sports ___; ___ **ecológica** / environmental ___; ___ **familiar** / family practice; ___ **forense** / forensic ___; ___ **industrial** / industrial ___; ___ **interna** / internal ___; ___ **legal** / legal ___; ___ **nuclear** / nuclear ___; ___ **ocupacional** / occupational ___; ___ **preventiva** / preventive ___; ___ **socializada** / socialized ___; ___ **tropical** / tropical ___; ___ **veterinaria** / veterinary ___; 2. medication, medicine, drug; **estudiante de** ___ / medical student.

medicina alternativa *f.* alternative medicine, practice of medicine that relies on use of medicinal herbs, aromatherapy, and other unconventional means, rather than drugs or surgery to treat illnesses and injuries.

medicina holística *f.* holistic medicine, an approach to medicine that considers the human being as an integral functional unit.

medicinal *a.* medicinal, rel. to medicine or having medical properties.

médico-a *m., f.* physician, doctor; **cuerpo** ___ / medical staff; ___ **consultante, asesor** / consulting ___; ___ **de asistencia primaria** / primary ___; ___ **de cabecera o primario** / primary ___; ___ **de familia** / family ___; ___ **de guardia** / doctor on call; ___ **forense** / coroner; ___ **interno** / intern; ___ **recomendante** / referring ___; ___ **residente** / resident, physician serving a residency; *a.* medical, medicinal, rel. to medicine or that cures; **asistencia** ___ / ___ assistance; **atención** ___ / ___ care.

medicolegal *a.* medicolegal, rel. to the practice of medicine as related to law.

medida de salvación *f.* life-saving measure.

medidor de ritmo de dosis *m.* dose rate meter.

medio *m.* medium. 1. means to attain an effect; 2. substance that transmits impulses; 3. substance used in the culture of bacteria; **en** ___ **de** / in the middle of; **por** ___ **de** / by means of; **medio-a** *a.* half; in part; **línea** ___ **-a** / medial line; **punto** ___ / medium.

medioambiental *a.* environmental, rel. to the environment.

medio ambiente *m.* environment; **peligros del** ___ / environmental hazards.

medir *vi.* to measure; **cinta de** ___ / measuring tape; **taza de** ___ / measuring cup.

médula *f.* medulla, central or internal part of an organ; **fallo de la** ___ / bone marrow failure; ___ **oblongata, bulbo raquídeo, porción de la medulla localizada en la base del cráneo** / ___ oblongata; ___ **ósea** / ___ osseum, bone marrow.

médula espinal *f.* spinal cord, a column of nervous tissue that extends from the medulla oblongata to the first or second lumbar vertebrae, and from which arise all the nerves that go to the trunk of the body and to the extremities.

meduloblastoma *m.* medulloblastoma, a malignant neoplasm located in the fourth ventricle and the cerebellum, or the spinal cord that can also invade the meninges. This type of neoplasm is seen most frequently in children.

médula oblongata *f.* medulla oblongata, portion of the medulla located at the base of the brain.

médula ósea *f.* bone marrow, spongelike tissue present in the cavities of bones; **fallo de la** ___ / ___ failure; **punción y aspiración de la** ___ / ___ puncture and aspiration; **transplante de la** ___ / ___ transplant.

medular *a.* medullary, rel. to the medulla; **celularidad** ___ / ___ cellularity; **infiltración** ___ / ___ infiltration; **insuficiencia** ___ / ___ failure; **lesión** ___ / ___ injury.

megacéfalo-a *a.* megalocephalic; macrocefalia.

megacolon *m.* megacolon, abnormally large colon.

megadosis *f.* megadose, a nutrient dose that is much greater than the recommended daily allowance.

megaesófago *m.* megaesophagus, abnormally large dilation of the inferior portion of the esophagus.

megalofobia f. megalofobia, a fear of large objects.

megalomanía f. megalomania, delusions of grandeur.

megalómano-a a. megalomaniac, suffering from megalomania.

megavitamina f. megavitamin, a dose of vitamin that exceeds the daily requirement.

meiosis f. meiosis, process of cell division that results in the production of gametes.

mejilla f. cheek.

mejoramiento, mejoría m., f. improvement, amelioration.

mejorar vt. to improve; **mejorarse** vr. to get better.

mejoría f. improvement, amelioration.

melancolía f. melancholia, marked depression.

melanina f. melanin, dark pigmentation of the skin, hair, and parts of the eye.

melanocito m. melanocyte, melanine-producing cell.

melanoma m. melanoma, malignant tumor made of melanocytes that has the capacity to metastasize rapidly to another part of the skin, lymph, lungs, liver, and brain.

melanoma maligno m. malignant melanoma, pigmented neoplasm that can originate in any part of the skin, rarely found in the mucose; it has the capacity to metatazise rapidly in other parts of the lympha, lungs, liver, and brain.

melanosis f. melanosis, condition characterized by an unusual deposit of dark pigmentation in various tissues or organs.

melanuria f. melanuria, presence of dark pigmentation in the urine.

melasma gravídico m. melasma gravidarum; *pop.* pregnancy mask.

melena f. melena, abnormally dark and pasty stool containing digested blood.

mellizos-as m., f., pl. twins; gemelo-a.

membrana f. membrane, web, thin layer of tissue that covers or protects an organ or structure; __ **de la placenta** / placental __; __ **mucosa** / mucous __; __ **nuclear** / nuclear __; __ **permeable** / permeable __; __ **-s arteriopulmonares** / pulmonary arterial webs; __ **semipermeable** / semipermeable __; __ **sinovial** / synovial __; __ **timpánica** / tympanic __ .

memoria f. memory, faculty that allows the registration and recall of experiences; __ **inmediata** / short-term __ ; __ **pérdida de la** __ / __ loss; __ **visual** / visual __ .

memorizar vi. to memorize.

menarca m. menarche, first onset of menstruation.

mendelismo m. Mendelism, set of principles that explains the transmission of certain genetic traits.

meníngeo-a a. meningeal, rel. to the meninges.

meninges f. meninges, three layers of connective tissue that surround the brain and the spinal cord.

meningioma m. meningioma, a slow-growing vascular neoplasm arising from the meninges.

meningismo m. meningism, meningismus, congestive irritation of the meninges, gen. of a toxic nature, that presents symptoms similar to those of meningitis but without infl., seen esp. in children.

meningitis f. meningitis infl. of the meninges; __ **criptocóccica** / cryptococcal __; __ **viral** / viral __ .

meningocele m. meningocele, protrusion of the meninges through a defect in the skull or the vertebral column.

meningococo m. (*pl.* **meningocci**) meningococcus, microorganism that causes epidemic cerebral meningitis.

meningoencefalitis f. meningoencephalitis, cerebromeningitis, infl. of the encephalum and the meninges.

meniscectomía f. meniscectomy, excision of a meniscus.

menisco m. meniscus, crescent-shaped, cartilaginous, interarticular structure.

menometrorragia f. menometrorrhagia, abnormal bleeding during and between menstruation.

menopausia f. menopause, cessation of the fertility stage of adult women, accompanied by a decrease in hormone production.

menorragia f. menorrhagia, excessive bleeding during menstruation.

menorralgia f. menorrhalgia, painful menstruation.

menorrea f. menorrhea, normal menstrual flow.

(m)

menstruación

menstruación *f.* menstruation, periodic flow of bloody fluid from the uterus; **trastornos de la __** / menstrual disorders.

menstrual *a.* menstrual, rel. to menstruation; **ciclo __** / cycle.

menstruar *v.* to menstruate.

menstruo *m.* menses, menstruation, period.

mental *a.* mental, rel. to the mind; **actividad __** / __ activity, mentation; **deficiencia __** / __ deficiency; **edad __** / __ age; **enfermedad __** / __ illness; **higiene __** / __ hygiene; **retraso __** / __ retardation; **trastorno __** / __ disorder; **-mente** *adv.* mentally.

mentalidad *f.* mentality, mental capacity.

mente *f.* mind, intellectual power.

mentol *m.* menthol, an alcohol obtained from peppermint oil and used for its soothing effects.

mentón *m.* mentus, chin.

meñique *m.* fifth finger.

meralgia *f.* pain in the thigh; **__ parestética** / __ paresthetica.

mercurial *a.* mercurial, rel. to mercury.

mercurio *m.* mercury, volatile liquid metal.

mercurio de etileno *m.* ethyl mercury, element found in some fish that can be toxic to pregnant women and children.

mesa *f.* table; **__ de operaciones** / operating __; **__ de reconocimiento** / examination __ .

mescalina *f.* mescaline, poisonous alkaloid with hallucinatory properties.

mesectodermo *m.* mesectoderm, mass of cells that combine with others to form the meninges.

mesencéfalo *m.* mesencephalon, the midbrain of the embrionary stage.

mesénquima *m.* mesenchyme, embryonic tissue from which the connective tissue and the lymph and blood vessels arise in the adult.

mesenterio *m.* mesentery, peritoneal folds that fix parts of the intestine to the posterior abdominal wall.

mesmerismo *m.* mesmerism, therapy by hypnotism.

mesocardia *f.* mesocardia, displacement of the heart toward the center of the thorax.

mesocolon *m.* mesocolon, mesentery that fixes the colon to the posterior abdominal wall.

mesodermo *m.* mesoderm, middle germ layer of the embryo, between the ectoderm and the endoderm, from which bone, connective tissue, muscle, blood, blood vessels, and lymph tissue, as well as the membranes of the heart and abdomen, arise.

mesotelio *m.* mesothelium, cell layer of the embryonic mesoderm that forms the epithelium covering the serous membrances in the adult.

mestizo-a *m., f., a.* mestizo, half-breed; crossbred, hybrid.

meta *f.* goal, objective.

metabólico-a *a.* metabolic, rel. to metabolism; **índice __** / __ rate.

metabolismo *m.* metabolism, physiochemical changes that take place following the digestive process; **__ basal** / basal __, lowest level of energy waste; **__ de proteína** / metabolic protein, digestion of proteins as amino acids.

metabolito *m.* metabolite, substance produced during metabolism or essential to the metabolic process.

metacarpiano-a *a.* metacarpal, rel. to the metacarpus.

metacarpo *m.* metacarpus, the five small metacarpal bones of the hand.

metacrono *a.* metachronous, that has an effect at different times.

metadona *f.* methadone, highly potent habit-forming synthetic drug with narcotic action weaker than that of morphine.

metafase *f.* metaphase, one of the phases of cell division.

metáfisis *f.* metaphysis, the growing portion of a bone.

metal *m.* metal.

metamorfosis *f.* metamorphosis. 1. change of form or structure; 2. degenerative process.

metanefrina *f.* metanephrine, a catabolite of epinephrine found in the urine.

metanol *m.* methanol, methyl alcohol, wood alcohol.

metástasis *f.* metastasis, extension of a pathological process from a primary focus to another part of the body through blood or lymph vessels, as occurs in some types of cancer.

metastatizar *vt.* to metastasize, to spread by metastasis.

metatálamo *m.* metathalamus, part of the diencephalon.

mielatelia

metatarsiano-a *a.* metatarsal, rel. to the metatarsus.

metatarso *m.* metatarsus, the five small metatarsal bones located between the tarsus and the toes.

meteorismo *m.* meteorism, bloated abdomen due to gas in the stomach or the intestines.

método *m.* method, procedure, process, treatment.

metritis *f.* metritis, infl. of the walls of the uterus.

metrorragia *f.* metrorrhagia, uterine bleeding other than menstruation.

mialgia *f.* myalgia, muscle pain.

miastenia *f.* myasthenia, muscle weakness; __ **grave** / __ gravis.

miatonía *f.* myatonia, deficiency or loss of muscle tone.

micción *f.* urination.

micetoma *m.* mycetoma, severe infection caused by fungi that affects the skin, the connective tissue, and the bone.

micología *f.* mycology, the study of fungi and the diseases caused by them.

micoplasmas *m., pl.* mycoplasmas, the smallest free-living organisms, some of which produce diseases such as a type of viral pneumonia and pharyngitis.

micosis *f.* mycosis, general term used for any disease caused by fungi.

micotoxicosis *f.* mycotoxicosis, systemic toxic condition caused by toxins produced by fungi.

micrencefalia *f.* micrencephaly, abnormal smallness of the brain.

microabsceso *m.* microabscess, very small abscess.

microanatomía *f.* microanatomy, histology.

microbacterium *L.* microbacterium, gram-positive bacteria resistant to high temperatures.

microbiano-a *a.* microbic, microbial, rel. to microbes.

microbio *m.* microbe, minute living organism.

microbiología *f.* microbiology, science that studies microorganisms.

microcefalia *f.* microcephalia, microcephaly, congenital abnormally small head.

microcirugía *f.* microsurgery, surgery performed with the aid of special operating microscopes and very small precision instruments.

microcosmo *m.* microcosm, a world in miniature.

microfalo *m.* microphallus, abnormally small penis.

microgenitalia *m.* microgenitalia, underdevelopment of the external genitalia.

micrognatia *f.* micrognathia, congenital smallness of the lower jaw.

microgotero *m.* microdrip, an instrument used to administer a small, precise amount of a substance intravenously.

microinvasión *f.* microinvasion, invasion of the cellular tissue adjacent to a localized carcinoma that cannot be seen with the naked eye.

microlitiasis *f.* microlithiasis, minute concretions discharged in certain organs.

micromelia *f.* micromelia, abnormally small limbs.

micromélico-a *a.* micromelic, rel. to micromelia.

microorganismo *m.* microorganism, an organism that cannot be seen with the naked eye.

microqueiria *f.* microcheiria, disorder in which the hands are abnormally small.

microscopía *f.* microscopy, microscopic examination.

microscópico-a *a.* microscopic, rel. to microscopy.

microscopio *m.* microscope, optical instrument used to amplify objects that cannot be seen with the naked eye; __ **de luz** / light __; __ **electrónico** / electron __ .

microsomía *f.* microsomia, condition of having an abnormally small body with otherwise normal structure as in dwarfism.

microtomía *f.* microtomy, cutting thin sections of tissue.

micrótomo *m.* microtome, instrument used to prepare thin sections of tissue for microscopic study.

midriasis *f.* mydriasis, dilation of the pupil of the eye.

midriático *m.* mydriatic, agent used to dilate the pupil of the eye; **-a** *a.* causing dilation of the pupil of the eye.

miectomía *f.* myectomy, excision of a portion of a muscle.

mielatelia *f.* myelatelia, developmental defect of the spinal cord.

mielauxa *f.* myelauxe, hypertrophy of the spinal cord.

mielina *f.* myelin, the fat-like substance that forms a covering around certain nerve fibers.

mielinación, mielinización *f.* myelination, myelinization, growth of a myelin sheath around a nerve fiber.

mielinolisis *f.* myelinolysis, disease that destroys the myelin cover; __ **aguda** / acute __ .

mielitis *f.* myelitis, infl. of the spinal cord.

mieloblastemia *f.* myeloblastemia, the presence of myeloblasts in the blood.

mieloblasto *m.* myeloblast, an immature cell in the granulocyte series, generally present in bone marrow.

mielocele *m.* myelocele, hernia of the spinal cord through a defect in the vertebral column.

mielocito *m.* myelocyte, a large, granular leukocyte in the bone marrow that is present in the blood in certain diseases.

mielocitoma *m.* myelocytoma, an accumulation of myelocytes in certain tissues, present in certain illnesses.

mielodisplasia *f.* myelodysplasia, abnormal formation of the spinal cord.

mielofibrosis *f.* myelofibrosis, fibrosis of the bone marrow.

mielógeno-a *a.* myelogenic, myelogenous, produced in the bone marrow.

mielograma *m.* myelogram, x-ray of the spinal cord with the use of a contrasting medium.

mieloide *a.* myeloid, rel. to or resembling the spinal cord or the bone marrow; **médula** __ / __ tissue.

mieloleucemia *f.* myeloleukemia, a form of leukemia in which abnormal cells are derived from myelopoietic tissue.

mieloquiste *m.* myelocyst, a cyst composed of nerve cells that develops in a canal of the central nervous system.

mieloma *m.* myeloma, tumor formed by a type of cells usu. found in the bone marrow; __ **múltiple** / multiple __ .

mielomeningocele *m.* myelomeningocele, hernia of the spinal cord and its meninges through a defect in the vertebral canal.

mielopatía *f.* myelopathy, pathological condition of the spinal cord.

mieloproliferativo-a *a.* myeloproliferative, characterized by proliferation of bone marrow inside or outside of the medulla.

mielosquisis *f.* myeloschisis, spina bifida.

mielosupresión *m.* myelosuppression, decreased production of erythrocytes and platelets in the bone marrow.

miembro *m.* member. 1. organ or limb of the body; 2. person affiliated with an organization; *vr.* **hacerse** __ / to become a __ .

miestesia *f.* myesthesia, any type of sensation in a muscle.

migración *f.* migration, movement of cells from one place to another.

migraña *f.* migraine, severe headache usu. unilateral, accompanied by disturbed vision and in some cases by nausea and vomiting.

migratorio-a *a.* migratory, rel. to migration.

miiasis *f.* myasis, infection due to the presence of larvae from the diptera family.

milia neonatorum *n.*, *L.* milia neonatorum, small, non-pathogenic cysts sometimes found on newborns.

miliar *a.* miliary, characterized by the presence of small tumors.

miliaria *f.* miliaria, prickly heat, noncontagious cutaneous eruption caused by the obstruction of sweat glands and characterized by small red vesicles and papules accompanied by itching and prickling.

milieu *Fr.* milieu, environment, surroundings.

mimético-a *a.* mimetic, mimic, that imitates.

mineral *m.* mineral, inorganic element; *a.* rel. to a mineral; **agua** __ **efervescente** / carbonated __ water.

mineralización *f.* mineralization, abnormally large deposition of mineral in tissues.

mineralocorticoide *m.* mineralocorticoid, hormone released by the adrenal cortex involved in the regulation of fluids and electrolytes.

minilaparotomía *f.* minilaparotomy, a type of pelvic surgery performed for the purpose of diagnosis or sterilization by tubal ligation.

mínimo-a *a.* minimal, least, smallest; **dosis** __ / __ dose, smallest amount

minoría *f.* minority.

minucioso-a *a.* thorough, detailed; **examen __ / __** exam; **-mente** *adv.* very carefully; thoroughly.

minusvalía mental *f.* mental handicap

minusválido *m.* a handicapped person.

minuto *m.* minute, fraction of time.

miocárdico-a *a.* myocardial, myocardiac, rel. to the myocardium.

miocardio *m.* myocardium, the middle and thickest muscular layer of the heart wall; **contracción del __ /** myocardial contraction.

miocardiopatías *f., pl.* myocardial diseases.

miocarditis *f.* myocarditis, infl. of the myocardium.

miocito *m.* myocyte, cell of the muscular tissue.

mioclonus *m.*, *L.* myoclonus, a spasm of a muscle or a group of muscles, as seen in epilepsy.

miodistrofia *f.* myodystrophy, muscular dystrophy.

mioespasmo *m.* myospasm, spasmodic contractions of a muscle.

miofibrilla *f.* myofibril, myofibrilla; minute, slender fiber of the muscle tissue.

miofibroma *m.* myofibroma, benign tumor containing fibrous connective tissue and muscle cells in various parts of the tumor.

miofilamento *m.* myofilament, microscopic element that makes up myofibrils in muscles.

miogénico-a *a.* myogenic, originating in or starting from the muscle.

mioglobina *f.* myoglobin, muscle tissue pigment that participates in the transport of oxygen.

miografía *f.* myography, a recording of muscular activity.

miolisis *f.* myolysis, destruction of muscle tissue.

mioma *m.* myoma, benign tumor formed by muscular tissue; **__ previo /** previous __ .

miomectomía *f.* myomectomy. 1. excision of a portion of a muscle or of muscular tissue; 2. excision of a myoma, esp. one localized in the uterus.

miometrio *m.* myometrium, muscular wall of the uterus.

miometritis *f.* myometritis, infl. of the muscular wall of the uterus.

mionecrosis *f.* myonecrosis, necrosis of muscle tissue.

mioneural *a.* myoneural, rel. to muscles and nerves; **unión __ / __** junction, a nerve ending in a muscle.

miopatía *f.* myopathy, any disease of muscular tissues; **__ facial /** facial __; **__ ocular /** ocular __; **__ tirotóxica /** thyrotoxic __ .

miope *a.* myopic. 1. nearsighted; 2. rel. to myopia.

miopía *f.* myopia, nearsightedness, a defect in the eyeball that causes parallel rays to be focused in front of the retina.

miorrexia *f.* myorrhexis, rupture of any muscle.

miosarcoma *f.* myosarcoma, malignant tumor derived from muscular tissue.

miosina *f.* myosin, the most abundant protein in muscle tissue.

miosinógeno *m.* myosinogen, a protein present in the muscle tissue.

miosis *f.* miosis, excessive contraction of the pupil.

miositis *f.* myositis, infl. of a muscle or group of muscles.

mioterapia muscular *f.* muscular myotherapy, application of direct pressure on painful knots with fingers, feet and elbows.

miotomía *f.* myotomy, dissection of muscles.

miotonía *f.* myotonia, increased rigidity of a muscle following muscle contraction, with diminished power of relaxation.

mirar *vt.* to look, to view; **__ fijamente /** to stare; **mirarse** *vr.* to look at oneself.

miringectomía *f.* myringectomy, myringodectomy, excision of part or all of the tympanic membrane.

miringitis *f.* myringitis, infl. of the eardrum.

miringoplastia *f.* myringoplasty, plastic surgery of the tympanic membrane.

miringotomía *f.* myringotomy, incision of the tympanic membrane.

miscegenación *f.* miscegenation, sexual relations between individuals of different races.

miscible *a.* miscible, capable of mixing or dissolving.

mismo-a *a.* same; **dominio de sí __ /** self-control; **sí __ /** oneself.

misogamia

misogamia *f.* misogamy, aversion to marriage.

misoginia *f.* misogyny, hatred of women.

mitad *f.* half, each of the two equal parts in which a whole is divided; **a la __ /** in half.

mitigado-a *a.* mitigated, diminished, moderated.

mitocondrias *f., pl.* mitochondria, microscopic filaments of the cytoplasm that constitute the main source of energy in cells.

mitogenesia, mitogénesis *f.* mitogenesia, mitogenesis, the process of cell mitosis.

mitógeno *m.* mitogen, substance that induces cell mitosis.

mitosis *f.* mitosis, the somatic process of cell division that results in new cells with the same content of chromosomes and DNA.

mitral *a.* mitral, rel. to the mitral valve; **estenosis __ / __** stenosis, a narrowing of the left atrioventricular orifice; **incompetencia __ / __** insufficiency; **regurgitación __ / __** regurgitation, the flow of blood back from the left ventricle into the left atrium due to a lesion of the mitral valve; **soplo __ / __** murmur.

mittelschmerz *m.* mittelschmerz, lower abdominal pain related to ovulation and occuring midway in the menstrual cycle.

mixedema *m.* myxedema, condition caused by deficient thyroid gland function.

mixoma *m.* myxoma, a tumor of the connective tissue.

mixto-a *a.* mixed.

mixtura *f.* mixture.

mnemónica *f.* mnemonics, recall of memory through free association of ideas and other techniques.

moción *f.* motion, movement.

moco *m.* mucus, viscid matter secreted by the mucous membranes and glands.

modalidad *f.* modality, any form of therapeutic application.

moderación *f.* moderation.

moderado-a *a.* moderate, temperate; **-mente** *adv.* moderately.

modesto-a *a.* modest.

modificación *f.* modification, change.

modo *m.* mode. 1. manner, way; 2. in a series, the value that is repeated most frequently; **de cualquier __ /** in any way; **de ningún __ /** in no way.

modulación *f.* modulation, the action of adjusting or adapting, such as occurs with the inflection of the voice.

mojado-a *a.* wet.

mojar *vt.* to wet, to dampen; **mojarse** *vr.* to get wet.

molar *m.* molar, any of the twelve molar teeth.

molde *m.* 1. cast, hardened bandage made stiff; 2. template, pattern, mold; **__ para andar /** walking cast.

moldear *vt.* to cast.

molécula *f.* molecule, the smallest unit of a substance above the atomic level.

molécula gramo *m.* gram molecule, weight in grams equal to the molecular weight.

molecular *a.* molecular, rel. to molecules.

molestar *vt.* to annoy, to bother.

molestia *f.* discomfort, annoyance.

molesto-a *a.* annoyed.

momentum *L.* momentum, impetus, a force of motion.

momificación *f.* mummification, conversion into a state that resembles that of a mummy, as occurs in dry gangrene or in a dead fetus that dries up in the uterus.

monitor *m.* monitor. 1. electronic device used to monitor a function; 2. person who oversees an activity or function.

monitorear *v.* to monitor, to check systematically with an electronic device an organic function such as the heartbeat.

monitoreo, monitorización *m., f.* monitoring; **__ cardíaco /** cardiac **__**; **__ de presión arterial /** blood pressure **__**; **__ fetal /** fetal **__** .

monitoreo de Holter *m.* Holter monitoring, ambulatory electrocardiography.

monitorización glucosa *f.* glucose monitorization, close observation by periodic testing of the glucose percentage in the blood.

monoarticular *a.* monoarticular, rel. to only one joint.

monocigótico-a *a.* monozygotic, rel. to twins that have identical genetic characteristics.

monocito *m.* monocyte, large, granular, mononuclear leukocyte.

monoclonal *a.* monoclonal, rel. to a single group of cells; **anticuerpos —-es** / — antibodies.

monocromático-a *a.* monochromatic, having only one color.

monocular *a.* monocular, rel. to only one eye.

monogamia *f.* monogamy, legal marriage to or sexual relationship with only one person.

monomania *f.* monomania, mental fixation on one idea.

mononuclear *a.* mononuclear, having one nucleus; **célula —** / — cell.

mononucleosis *f.* mononucleosis, presence of an abnormally large number of monocytes in the blood; — **infecciosa** / infectious —, acute febrile infectious disease.

monosacárido *m.* monosaccharide, simple sugar.

monstruo *m.* monster.

montar *v.* to ride; — **en bicicleta** / — a bicycle; to set up; — **una consulta** / — to assemble, to fit, to adjust a doctor's office.

montón *m.* heap, pile.

morado *m.* bruise, black and blue mark; the color purple; **-a** *a.* purple.

mórbido-a, morboso-a *a.* morbid, rel. to disease.

morbilidad *f.* morbidity. 1. an illness or disorder; 2. the incidence of a disease in a given population or locality; **tasa de —** / — rate.

morbo *m.* illness.

mordedura *f.* 1. bite; 2. a wound caused by a bite.

morder *vt.* to bite.

mordida *f.* 1. bite; 2. the mark left in the skin by the teeth of an animal; 3. forced occlusion of the inferior jaw on the upper teeth; — **cruzada** / cross-bite; — **de perro** / dog bite.

mordido-a *pp.* de **morder,** bitten; *a.* bitten.

moretón *m.* bruise, black and blue mark.

morfina *f.* morphine, the main alkaloid of opium, used as a narcotic analgesic.

morfinismo *m.* morphinism, condition caused by addiction to morphine.

morgue *Fr.* morgue, place for temporarily holding dead bodies.

moribundo-a *a.* moribund, dying, on the verge of death.

morir *vi.* to die; — **con dignidad** / — with dignity.

morón, morona *m., f.* moron, a mentally retarded person with an IQ of 50 to 70.

mortal *m.* mortal, a human being; *a.* deadly, mortal; **herida —** / fatal wound; **veneno —** / — poison.

mortalidad, mortandad *f.* mortality, death rate; **índice de —** / death rate; — **fetal** / fetal —; — **infantil** / infant —; — **materna** / maternal —; — **neonatal** / neonatal —; — **perinatal** / perinatal — .

mortífero-a *a.* deadly, that can cause death.

mortinatalidad *f.* natimortality, index of still-births.

mortinato-a *m., f.* stillborn.

motor *f.* morula, solid, spheric mass of cells that results from the cell division of a fertilized ovum.

mosaicismo *f.* mosaicism, as in a mosaic, genetically multiple mutated chromosomes determining different characteristics, such as in female physiognomy.

mosaico *m.* 1. mosaic, the presence in one individual of different cell populations derived from just one cell as a result of mutation; 2. mosaic, inlaid artwork combining different small pieces forming a composition.

mosca *f.* fly.

mosquito *m.* mosquito.

mostaza *f.* mustard.

mostaza nitrogenada *f.* nitrogen mustard, HG_2, used in the treatment of leukemia and lymphatic neoplasms.

mostrar *vi.* to show, to point out.

motilidad gástrica *f.* gastric motility, the normal peristaltic movements of the stomach that facilitate the function of digestion.

motivación *f.* motivation, driving force.

motocicleta *f.* motorcycle.

motor *m.* motor, agent that causes or induces movement; **motor-a** *a.* that causes movement.

mover *vi.* to move, to put in motion; **moverse** *vr.* to move oneself.

movilidad *f.* mobility, motility.

movilización *f.* mobilization.

movimiento *m.* movement, move, motion; **alcance de —** / range of motion; — **corporal** / body — .

mucina *f.* mucin, glycoprotein that is the chief ingredient of mucus.

mucocele

mucocele *m.* mucocele, dilation of a cavity due to accumulated mucous secretion.

mucocutáneo-a *a.* mucocutaneous, rel. to the mucous membrane and the skin.

mucoide *m.* mucoid, glycoprotein similar to mucin; *a.* having the consistency of mucus.

mucomembranoso-a *a.* mucomembranous, rel. to the mucous membrane.

mucosa *f.* mucosa, mucous membrane, thin sheets of tissue cells that line openings or canals of the body that communicate to the outside; ___ **alveolar** / alveolar ___; ___ **bronquial** / bronchial ___; ___ **de la boca o bucal** / ___ oral; ___ **de la pelvis renal** / ___ of the renal pelvis; ___ **de la vagina** / vaginal ___; ___ **de la vejiga urinaria** / ___ of (*urinary*) bladder; ___ **del colon** / ___ of colon; ___ **del estómago o estomacal** / ___ of stomach; ___ **del intestino delgado** / ___ of small intestine; ___ **esofágica** / esophageal ___; ___ **faríngea** / gastric ___; ___ **gástrica** / gastric ___; ___ **laríngea** / laryngeal ___; ___ **lingual** / lingual ___; ___ **nasal** / nasal ___; ___ **olfatoria** / olfactory ___.

mucosidad *f.* mucosity.

muchacho-a *m., f.* boy; girl.

mudar *v.* to move; ___ **los dientes** / to get one's second teeth; ___ **la piel** / to shed skin.

mudo-a *m., f.* mute.

mueca *f.* grimace.

muela *f.* molar tooth, grinder; **dolor de ___ -s** / toothache; ___ **-s del juicio** / wisdom teeth.

muerte *f.* death; ___ **aparente** / apparent ___; ___ **cerebral** / brain ___; ___ **legal** / legal ___; ___ **por piedad** / mercy killing, euthanasia.

muerte de cuna *f.* crib-death; sudden infant death syndrome.

muerte súbita *m.* sudden death, occurring without having a known cause.

muerto-a *m., f.* a dead person; *a.* dead.

muestra *f.* sample; **tomar ___ -s** / sampling; **tomar ___ -s al azar** / random sampling.

muestreo *m.* sampling; ___ **al azar** / random ___.

muguet *Fr.* thrush, fungus infection of the oral mucosa, manifested by white patches on the lips, tongue, and the interior surface of the cheek.

mujer *f.* woman.

muletas *f. pl.* crutches.

multifocal *a.* multifocal, rel. to many foci.

multiforme *a.* multiform.

multípara *f.* multiparous, a woman who has given birth to more than one infant.

multiparidad *f.* multiparity. 1. condition of having borne more than one child; 2. multiple birth.

múltiple *a.* multiple, more than one; **fallo ___ de órganos** / ___ organ failure; **personalidad ___** / ___ personality.

mundo *m.* world.

muñeca *f.* 1. wrist; ___ **caída** / drop ___; carpo; 2. doll.

muñón *m.* stump.

mural *a.* mural, rel. to the walls of an organ or part.

muriático-a *a.* muriatic, derived from common salt; **ácido ___** / ___ acid.

murino-a *a.* murine, rel. to rodents, esp. mice and rats.

murmullo *m.* murmur, bruit, gen. in reference to an abnormal heart sound.

murmullo vesicular *m.* vesicular breath sound.

muscular, musculoso-a *a.* muscular, rel. to the muscles; **atrofia ___** / ___ atrophy; **contracción ___ brusca** / jerk; **desarrollo ___** / muscle building; **distensión ___** / muscle strain; **pérdida de la tonicidad ___** / loss of muscle tone; **relajador ___** / muscle relaxant; **rigidez ___** / ___ rigidity; **tonicidad ___** / muscle tone.

muscularis *L.* muscularis, muscular layer of an organ or tubule.

musculatura *f.* musculature, the total muscular system or arrangement of muscles in the body.

músculo *m.* muscle, a type of fibrous tissue that has the property to contract allowing movement of the parts and organs of the body; ___ **estriado voluntario** / striated voluntary ___; ___ **flexor** / flexor ___; ___ **visceral involuntario** / visceral involuntary ___.

musculoesquelético-a *a.* musculoskeletal, rel. to the muscles and the skeleton.

musculotendinoso-a *a.*
musculotendinous, having both muscle and tendons.

muslo *m.* thigh, the portion of the lower extremity between the hip and the knee.

mutación *f.* mutation, spontaneous or induced change in genetic structure.

mutágeno *m.* mutagen, substance or agent that causes mutation.

mutante *a.* mutant, rel. to an individual or organism with a genetic structure that has undergone mutation.

mutilación *f.* mutilation, castration.

mutilado-a *a.* mutilated.

mutismo *m.* mutism.

mutuo-a *a.* mutual, reciprocal.

muy *adv.* very.

Mycobacterium *L. Mycobacterium,* gram-positive, rod-shaped bacteria, including species that cause a variety of infections.

N

n

N *abr.* **nasal** / nasal; **nervio** / nerve; **nitrógeno** / nitrogen; **normal** / normal; **número** / number.

Naboth, quistes de *m.* nabothian cysts, small, usu. benign cysts that form in one of many small mucus-secreting glands of the neck of the uterus due to obstruction.

nacer *vi.* to be born.

nacido-a *a. pp.* de **nacer**, born; __ **vivo** / __ alive; **recién** __ / newly __ .

naciente *a.* nascent, incipient. 1. just born; 2. liberated from a chemical compound.

nacimiento *m.* birth; **certificado de** __ / __ certificate; __ **prematuro** / premature __; __ **tardío** / post-term __; __ **sin vida** / stillbirth.

nada *f.* nothing, nothingness; *indef. pron.* (after thanks) **de** __ / Don't mention it!; not at all; you are welcome.

nalgas *f., pl.* buttocks.

nanocefalia *f.* nanocephaly, abnormal smallness of the head.

narcisismo *m.* narcissism. 1. excessive love of self; 2. sexual pleasure derived from contemplation and admiration of one's own body.

narcisista *m.* narcissist.

narcoanálisis *m.* narcoanalysis, applied method of narcotherapy; originally used in cases of war psychosis, and later in the treatment of infantile trauma.

narcohipnosis *f.* narcohypnosis, hypnosis induced by the use of narcotics.

narcolepsia *f.* narcolepsy, chronic uncontrollable disposition to sleep.

narcoléptico-a *a.* narcoleptic, rel. to or that suffers from narcolepsia.

narcosis *f.* narcosis, unconsciousness caused by a narcotic. 1. lethargy and alleviation of pain by the effect of narcotics; 2. drug addiction.

narcoterapia *f.* narcotherapy, psychotherapy applied under the effect of a sedative or a narcotic.

narcótico *m.* narcotic, substance with potent analgesic effects that can

become addictive; **bloqueo** __ / __ blockade; **reversión** __ / __ reversal.

narcotismo *m.* narcotism, the stuporous state caused by narcotics.

naris *L.* naris, nostril.

nariz *f.* nose; **sangramiento por la** __ / nose-bleed; *vr.* **sonarse la** __ / to blow one's nose.

nasal *a.* nasal, rel. to the nose; **cavidad** __ / __ cavity; **congestión** __ / __ congestion; **fosa** __ / nostril; **goteo** __ / __ drip; **hemorragia** __ / __ hemorrhage; **instilación** __ / __ instillation; **meato** __ / __ meatus; **pólipo** __ / __ polyp; **secreción** __ / __ discharge; **tabique** __ / __ septum.

nasofaringe *f.* nasopharynx, portion of the pharynx that lies above the soft palate. See illustration on page 173.

nasogástrico-a *a.* nasogastric, rel. to the nose and the stomach; **tubo** __ / __ tube.

nasolabial *a.* nasolabial, rel. to the nose and the lip.

nata *f.* cream.

natilla *f.* custard.

natimortalidad *f.* natimortality, proportion of the death rate of perinatal and natal deaths as to the natality rate.

nativo-a *a.* native. 1. in its natural state; 2. indigenous.

natremia *f.* natremia, presence of sodium in the blood.

natriurético *m.* natriuretic. *See* **diuretic**.

natural *a.* natural; **derechos** __ **-es** / birth rights; *v.* **ser** __ **de** / to be from; **-mente** / *adv.* naturally.

naturaleza *f.* nature.

naturópata *m.* naturopath, practitioner of naturopathy.

naturopatía *f.* naturopathy, therapeutic treatment by natural means.

náusea *f.* nausea, nauseousness; seasickness; *v.* **dar, provocar** __ / to nauseate; **tener** __ **-s** / to be nauseated.

nauseado-a *a.* nauseated.

nauseoso-a *a.* nauseous, that causes nausea.

navicular *a.* navicular. 1. scaphoid bone; 2. boat-shaped; **abdomen** __ / __ abdomen; **fosa** __ **de la uretra** / __ fossa of the urethra; **hueso** __ / __ bone.

nébula *f.* nebula, slight opacity of the eye.

nebulización *f.* nebulization, conversion of liquid into spray or mist.

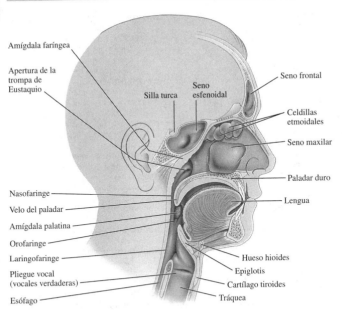

Amígdala faríngea

Apertura de la
trompa de
Eustaquio

Silla turca

Seno
esfenoidal

Seno frontal

Celdillas
etmoidales

Seno maxilar

Paladar duro

Nasofaringe

Velo del paladar

Amígdala palatina

Orofaringe

Laringofaringe

Pliegue vocal
(vocales verdaderas)

Esófago

Lengua

Hueso hioides

Epiglotis

Cartílago tiroides

Tráquea

Estructuras nasofaríngeas: sección sagital

n

nebulizador *m.* nebulizer, device used
to produce spray or mist from liquid.

nebuloso-a *a.* nebulous.

necesario-a *a.* necessary; **lo __** /
what is __; *v.* **ser __** / to be __ .

necesitado-a *a.* needy; **los __ -s** / the
needy

necesitar *vt.* to need.

necrobiosis *f.* necrobiosis, gradual
degeneration of cells and tissues as a
result of changes due to development,
aging, and use.

necrocomio *m.* morgue, place to store
dead bodies temporarily.

necrofilia *f.* necrophilia. 1. morbid
attraction to corpses; 2. sexual
intercourse with a corpse.

necrofobia *f.* necrophobia, morbid fear
of death and corpses.

necrología *f.* necrology, the study of
mortality statistics.

necropsia, necroscopia *f.*
necropsy. *See* **autopsia**.

necrosis *f.* necrosis, death of some or
all of the cells in a tissue such as occurs
in gangrene; **__ aguda de la retina** /
acute retinal __; **__ aséptica** / aseptic

__; **__ caseosa** / caseous __; **__
central** / central __; **__ cística media** /
cystic medial __; **__ de coagulación** /
coagulation __; **__ de tejidos grasos
subcutáneos del neonato** /
subcutaneous fat __ of the newborn;
__ externa progresiva de la retina /
progressive outer retinal __; **__ focal** /
focal __ ; **__ isquémica** / ischemic __;
__ laminal cortical / laminal cortical
__; **__ progresiva enfisematosa** /
progressive emphysematous __; **__
renal papilar** / renal papillary __; **__
simple** / simple __; **__ supurativa** /
suppurative __; **__ total** / total __ .

nefrectomía *f.* nephrectomy, removal
of a kidney.

nefrítico-a *a.* nephritic, rel. to or
affected by nephritis. **cólico __** / **__**
colic.

nefritis *f.* nephritis, infl. of a kidney; **__
aguda** / acute __; **__ analgésica** /
analgesic __; **__ crónica** / chronic __;
__ de complejo inmune / immune
complex __; **__ focal** / focal __; **__
glomerular** / glomerular __; **__
hemorrágica** / hemorrhagic __; **__**

173

hereditaria / hereditary __; __
intersticial / interstitial __; __
lipomatosa / lupus __; __ **sifilítica** /
syphilitic __; __ **supurativa** /
suppurative __ .

nefroesclerosis f. nephrosclerosis,
hardening of the arterial system and the
interstitial tissue of the kidney.

nefrograma m. nephrogram, kidney
x-ray.

nefrolitiasis f. nephrolithiasis,
presence of kidney stones.

nefrolitotomía f. nephrolithotomy,
incision in the kidney to remove kidney
stones.

nefrología f. nephrology, the study of
the kidney and the diseases affecting it.

nefroma m. nephroma, kidney tumor.

nefromegalia f. nephromegaly,
extreme hypertrophy of the kidney.

nefropexia f. nephropexy, fixation of a
floating kidney.

nefrosis f. nephrosis, degenerative renal
disorder associated with large amounts
of protein in the urine, low levels of
albumin in the blood, and marked
edema.

nefrostomía f. nephrostomy, creation
of a fistula in the kidney or renal
pelvis.

nefrotomía f. nephrotomy, surgical
incision into the kidney.

nefrotóxico-a a. nephrotoxic, that
destroys kidney cells.

nefrotoxina f. nephrotoxin, agent that
destroys kidney cells.

negar vt. to deny.

negativismo m. negativism, behavior
characterized by acting in a manner
opposite to the one suggested.

negativo-a a. negative; **cultivo** __ /
__ culture; **-mente** adv. negatively.

negligencia f. negligence; __
profesional / malpractice.

negro-a m., f. 1. a black person; 2. the
color black; a. black.

nematelminto m. nemathelminth,
roundworm, intestinal worm of the
phylum *Nemathelminthes*.

Nematoda Gr. Nematoda, class of
worms of the phylum
Nemathelminthes; nematode.

nematodiasis f. nematodiasis,
infection by nematode parasites.

nene-a m., f. baby.

neoartrosis f. nearthrosis,
neoarthrosis, false or artificial
joint.

neologismo m. neologism. 1. word or
phrase to which a mentally disturbed
individual attributes a meaning
unrelated to its real meaning; 2. new
word or phrase or an old one to which a
new meaning has been attributed.

neomicina f. neomycin,
broad-spectrum antibiotic.

neonatal a. neonatal, rel. to the first
four to six weeks after birth.

neonato-a a. 1. neonate, newborn;
2. infant born 37 weeks into normal
gestation.

neonatología f. neonatology, specialty
that studies the care and treatment of
newborns.

neoplasia f. neoplasia, formation of
neoplasms.

neoplasma m. neoplasm, abnormal
growth of new tissue such as a tumor.

neoplástico-a a. neoplastic, rel. to a
neoplasm.

neovascularización f.
neovascularization, abnormal
proliferation of new blood vessels as a
reaction to ischemia.

nervio m. nerve, one or more bundles of
fibers that connect the brain and spinal
cord with other parts and organs of the
body; **bloqueo del** __ / __ block;
degeneración del __ / __
degeneration; __ **pellizcado** / pinched
__; **terminación del** __ / __ ending.

nervio ciático m. sciatic nerve, nerve
that extends from the base of the spine
down to the thigh with branches
throughout the lower leg and the foot.

nerviosismo m. nervousness; pop.
jitters.

nervioso-a a. nervous, rel. to the
nerves; **crisis** __ / __ breakdown,
collapse; **fibra** __ / nerve fiber;
impulso __ / nerve impulse; **tejido** __
/ nerve tissue.

neumatización f. pneumatization,
formation of air cavities in a bone, esp.
the temporal bone.

neumatocele m. pneumatocele.
1. hernial protuberance of lung tissue;
2. a tumor or sac containing gas.

neumococal, neumocócico-a a.
pneumococcal, rel. to or caused by
pneumococci.

neumococo m. pneumococcus, one of
a group of gram-positive bacteria that
cause acute pneumonia and other
infections of the upper respiratory
tract.

neumoencefalografía *f.* pneumoencephalography, x-ray of the brain by previous injection of air or gas allowing visualization of the cerebral cortex and ventricles.

neumonía *f.* pneumonia, infectious disease of the upper respiratory tract caused by bacteria or virus that affect the lungs; ___ **doble** / double ___; ___ **estafilocócica** / staphylococcal ___; ___ **lobar** / lobar ___ .

neumonía migratoria *f.* migratory pneumonia, type of pneumonia that appears in different parts of the lung.

neumonía neumocística carinii *f.* pneumocystis pneumonia carinii, a type of acute pneumonia caused by the bacillus *Pneumocystis carinii* and one of the opportunistic diseases seen in cases of AIDS.

neumónico-a *a.* pneumonic, rel. to the lungs or to pneumonia.

neumopatía *f.* lung disease.

neumotórax *m.* pneumothorax, accumulation of gas or air in the pleural cavity that results in the collapse of the affected lung; ___ **espontáneo** / spontaneous ___; ___ **por tensión** / tension ___ .

neural *a.* neural, rel. to the nervous system; **arco** ___ / ___ arch; **cresta** ___ / ___ crest; **pliegues neurales** / ___ folds; **placa** ___ / ___ plate; **quiste** ___ / ___ cyst.

neuralgia *f.* neuralgia, pain along a nerve; ___ **facial** / facial ___; ___ **facial atípica** / atypical facial ___; ___ **glosofaríngea** / glossopharyngeal ___; ___ **halucinatoria** / hallucinatory ___; ___ **trigeminal atípica** / atypical trigeminal ___ .

neurálgico-a *a.* neuralgic, rel. to neuralgia; **puntos** ___ **-s** / tender points.

neurapraxia *f.* neurapraxia, temporary paralysis of a nerve without degeneration.

neurastenia *f.* neurasthenia, term usu. associated with increased irritability, tension, and anxiety, accompanied by physical exhaustion; ___ **angiopática** / angiopathic ___; ___ **grave** / gravis; ___ **precoz** / praecox ___; ___ **primaria** / primary ___; ___ **pulsativa** / pulsating ___ .

neurectomía *f.* neurectomy, excision or resection of a nerve.

neurilema *f.* neurilemma, thin membranous covering that encloses a nerve fiber.

neurinoma *m.* neurinoma, benign neoplasm of the sheath surrounding a nerve.

neuritis *f.* neuritis, infl. of a nerve.

neuroblasto *m.* neuroblast, the immature nerve cell.

neuroblastoma *m.* neuroblastoma, malignant tumor of the nervous system formed mostly of neuroblasts.

neurocirugía *f.* neurosurgery, the study and practice of surgery of the nervous system.

neurocirujano-a *m., f.* neurosurgeon, specialist in neurosurgery.

neurodermatitis *f.* neurodermatitis, chronic skin disease of unknown origin manifested by intense itching in localized areas.

neuroendocrinología *f.* neuroendocrinology, the study of the nervous system as it relates to hormones.

neurofarmacología *f.* neuropharmacology, the study of drugs and medications as they affect the nervous system.

neurofibroma *m.* neurofibroma, tumor of the fibrous tissue of a peripheral nerve.

neurofibromatosis *f.* neurofibromatosis, disease characterized by the presence of multiple neurofibromas along the peripheral nerves.

neurogenético-a *a.* neurogenic, neurogenetic. 1. that originates in the nervous tissue; 2. due to nervous impulses; **atrofia** ___ / ___ atrophy.

neuroglia *f.* neuroglia, connective, supportive cells that constitute the interstitial tissue of the nervous system.

neurohipófisis *f.* neurohypophysis, posterior and nervous portion of the pituitary gland.

neurolepsia *f.* neurolepsia, agitated state of consciousness due to drugs; patient shows signs of anxiety and indifference.

neuroléptico *m.* neuroleptic, tranquilizer; it belongs to the psycotropic group of drugs used in the treatment of psychosis, esp. schizophrenia; **neuroléptico-a** *a.* **anestesia** ___ / ___ anesthesia.

neurolisina

neurolisina *f.* neurolysin, injectable antibody that is obtained from a cerebral substance. *Syn.* **neurotoxina**.

neurolisis *f.* neurolysis, process of liberating a nerve from inflammatory adnexa.

neurología *f.* neurology, the study of the nervous system.

neurólogo-a *m., f.* neurologist, specialist in neurology.

neuroma *f.* neuroma, tumor composed mainly of nerve cells and fibers; ___ **acústico** / acoustic ___ .

neuromalacia *f.* neuromalacia, pathologic softening of nervous tissue.

neuromarcapaso *m.* neuropacemaker, instrument used to stimulate the spinal cord electrically.

neuromatosis *f.* neuromatosis, the presence of multiple neuromas.

neuromeníngeo-a *a.* neuromeningeal, rel. to the nervous tissues and the meninges.

neuromilitis *f.* neuromylitis, infl. of the spinal nerves.

neuromuscular *a.* neuromuscular, rel. to the nerves and the muscles; **agentes bloqueadores** ___ **-es** / ___ blocking agents; **relajador** ___ / ___ relaxant; **sistema** ___ / ___ system.

neurona *f.* neuron, nerve cell, the basic functional and structural unit of the nervous system; ___ **motor** / motor ___, carries the impulses that initiate muscle contraction.

neuro-oftalmología *f.* neuro-ophthalmology, the study of the relationship between the nervous and visual systems.

neuropatía *f.* neuropathy, a disorder or pathological change in the peripheral nerves.

neurópilo *m.* neuropil, network of nervous fibers (neurites, dendrites, and glia cells) that concentrate in different parts of the nervous system.

neurorregulador *m.* neurotransmitter, a chemical substance that affects the transmission of impulses across a synapse between nerves or between a nerve and a muscle.

neurosarcoclesis *f.* neurosarcoclesis, surgical intervention to alleviate neuralgia by resection of a wall of the osseous canal, transposing the nerve to soft tissues.

neurosicofarmacología *f.* neuropsychopharmacology, the study

of drugs as they affect the treatment of mental disorders.

neurosífilis *f.* neurosyphilis, syphilis that affects the nervous system; ___ **tabética** / tabetic ___ .

neurosis *f.* neurosis, condition manifested primarily by anxiety and the use of defense mechanisms; ___ **accidental** / accident ___; ___ **cardíaca** / cardíac ___; ___ **compulsiva** / compulsive ___; ___ **de ansiedad** / anxiety ___; ___ **de compensación** / compensation ___; ___ **de guerra** / combat ___; ___ **del carácter** / character ___; ___ **depresiva** / depressive ___; ___ **hipocondríaca** / hypochondriac ___; ___ **histérica** / hysterical ___; ___ **obsesiva** / obsessional ___; ___ **obsesiva-compulsiva** / obsessive-compulsive ___; ___ **ocupacional** / occupational ___; ___ **post-traumática** / post-traumatic ___ .

neurótico-a *a.* neurotic, rel. to or suffering from neurosis.

neurotomía *f.* neurotomy, dissection or division of a nerve.

neurotoxicidad *f.* the capacity of a substance or agent to destroy or harm the nervous tissue.

neurotóxico-a *a.* neurotoxic, that has a toxic effect on the nervous system; **agente** ___ / ___ agent

neurotoxina *f.* neurotoxin, any toxin that sets itself specifically over the nervous tissue.

neurotrasmisor *m.* neurotransmitter, chemical substance that modifies the transmission of impulses through a synapse between nerves or between a nerve and a muscle; ___ **adrenérgico** / adrenergic ___; ___ **colinérgico** / cholinergic ___ .

neurovascular *a.* neurovascular, rel. to the nervous and vascular systems.

neutral, neutro-a *a.* neutral.

neutralización *f.* neutralization, process that annuls or counteracts the action of an agent.

neutralizar *vi.* to neutralize, to counteract.

neutrofilia *f.* neutrophilia, increase in number of neutrophils in the blood.

neutrotaxis *f.* neutrotaxis, stimulation of neutrophils by a substance that either attracts or repels them.

nevar *vi.* to snow.

nevo *m.* nevus, mole, birthmark; ___ **comedónico** / comedonicus ___; ___

compuesto / compound ___; ___ **de cola de fauno** / faun tail ___; ___ **de displasia** / dysplastic ___; ___ **de Ota** / Ota's ___; ___ **de unión** / junction, junctional ___; ___ **melanocítico** / melanocytic ___; ___ **sebáceo** / sebaceous ___ .

nexo *m.* nexus, connection.

ni *conj.* neither, nor; ___ **bueno** ___ **malo** / neither good nor bad; ___ **siquiera** / not even.

niacina *f.* niacin, nicotinic acid.

nicotina *f.* nicotine, toxic alkaloid that is the main ingredient of tobacco causing ill effects on smokers.

nictalopía *f.* nyctalopia, night blindness.

nictitación *f.* nictitation, the act of winking.

nicturia, nocturia *f.* nocturia, nycturia, frequent urination during the night.

nicho *m.* niche, small defect or depression esp. in the wall of a hollow organ.

nidación *f.* nidation, implantation of the fertilized ovum into the uterine endometrium.

nido *m.* nest, small cellular mass resembling a bird's nest.

niebla *f.* fog.

nieto-a *m., f.* grandson, granddaughter.

nieve *f.* snow; *Mex.* ice cream.

nigua *f.* chigger, chigoe.

nihilismo *m.* nihilism, in psychiatry an illusory idea that nothing is real or existent.

ninfa *f.* nympha, inner lip of the vulva.

ninfectomía *f.* nymphectomy, partial or total excision of the labium.

ninfomanía *f.* nymphomania, excessive sexual desire in the female.

niña del ojo *f.* pupil of the eye.

niñez *f.* childhood.

niño-a *m., f.* child; ___ **maltratado-a** / battered ___ .

nistagmo *m.* nystagmus, involuntary spasm of the eyeball; ___ **palatino** / palatal ___ .

nistagmografía *f.* nystagmography, technique to register nystagmus.

nitrógeno *m.* nitrogen; ___ **auténtico, legítimo** / authentic, legitimate ___; ___ **ilegítimo** / illegitimate ___; ___ **monóxido** / monoxide ___; ___ **no protéico** / non protein ___; ___ **residual** / residual ___; ___ **uréico** / urea ___ .

nitroglicerina *f.* nitroglycerine, a nitrate of glycerin used in medicine as a vasodilator, esp. in angina pectoris.

nivel *m.* level.

Nocardia *f.* Nocardia, gram-positive microorganism, cause of nocardiasis.

nocardiasis *f.* nocardiasis, infection caused by the species *Nocardia* that gen. affects the lungs but can also expand to other parts of the body.

noche *f.* night; **de** ___ / at ___; **buenas** ___ **-s** / good evening, good night; **por la** ___ / in the evening.

nocivo-a *a.* noxious, harmful, pernicious.

nocturno-a *a.* nocturnal; **emisíon** ___ / ___ emission.

nodal *a.* nodal, rel. to a node.

nódulo *m.* nodule, small node; ___ **linfático** / lymphatic ___; ___ **solitario** / solitary ___; ___ **subcutáneo** / subcutaneous ___ .

noma *f.* noma, ulcer, gangrenous stomatitis usually beginning in the corner of the mouth or interior cheek, progressing to the lips; gen. following a debilitating sickness.

nombre *m.* name; ___ **genérico** / generic ___ , common name of a drug or medication that is not registered commercially; ___ **de pila** / given ___ .

nomenclatura *f.* nomenclature, terminology.

nominal *a.* nominal, rel. to the noun; **afasia** ___ / ___ aphasia, inability to name objects.

nonato-a *m., f.* 1. unborn; 2. born by Cesarean section.

non compos mentis *L.* non compos mentis, mentally incompetent.

norepinefrina *f.* norepinephrine, vasoconstrictor agent produced in the adrenal gland.

norma *f.* norm, model, standard.

normal *a.* normal.

normalización *f.* normalization, return to a normal state.

normoblasto *m.* normoblast, red blood cell, a precursor of erythrocytes in humans.

normocalcemia *f.* normocalcemia, normal level of calcium in the blood.

normoglicemia *f.* normoglycemia, normal concentration of glucose in the blood.

normopotasemia *f.* normokalemia, normal level of potassium in the blood.

normotenso-a *a.* normotensive, having a normal blood pressure.

normotermia *f.* normothermia, normal temperature.

normovolemia *f.* normovolemia, normal blood volume.

norte *m.* north; **al** ___ / to the ___ .

nosocomial *a.* nosocomial, rel. to a hospital or infirmary; **infección** ___ / ___ infection, acquired in a hospital.

nostalgia *f.* nostalgia, homesickness.

notalgia *f.* notalgia, back ache.

notar *vt.* to note; to become aware of something.

notificación *f.* notification, notice.

notocordio *m.* notochord, the axial fibrocellular cord in the embryo that is replaced by the vertebral column.

novocaína *f.* novocaine, anesthetic.

nublado-a *a.* bleary; cloudy; **vista** ___ / ___ eyed.

nuca *f.* nucha, nape, posterior part of the neck.

nucal *a.* nuchal, rel. to the nape.

nuclear *a.* nuclear. 1. rel. to the nucleus; **envoltura** ___ / ___ envelope, the two parallel membranes surrounding the nucleus, as seen under an electron microscope; 2. rel. to atomic power; **desecho** ___ / ___ waste.

núcleo *m.* nucleus, the essential part of the cell; ___ **pulposo** / ___ pulpous, central gelatinous mass within an intervertebral disk.

nucleópeto-a *a.* nucleopetal, that moves towards the nucleus.

nucleotido *m.* nucleotide, the structural unit of nucleic acid.

nudillo *m.* knuckle.

nudo *m.* node, knotlike mass of tissue; knot; ___ **de los ordeñadores** / milker's ___; ___ **del vermis** / vermis ___; **sifilítico** / syphilitic ___; ___ **vocal o de los cantantes** / vocal or singer's ___ .

nudoso-a *a.* nodose, that has nodules or protuberances.

nuevo-a *a.* new.

nuez de Adan *f.* Adam's apple.

nuligrávida *f.* nulligravida, a woman who has never conceived.

nulípara *f.* nullipara; nullipara, a woman who has never borne a living child; *a.* nulliparous, nonparous.

nulo-a *a.* null, void.

numeroso-a *a.* numerous.

nunca *adv.* never; at no time; **casi** ___ / hardly ever.

nutrición *f.* nutrition, nourishment.

nutriente *m.* nutrient, nutritious substance; *a.* nourishing.

Ñ *m.* seventeenth letter of the Spanish alphabet.

ñame *m.* yam.

ñoco-a *a. pop.* missing, **la mano-** (*le falta un dedo*), he has lost a finger in his hand.

ñoñería *f.* childishness; simplemindedness.

ñoño-a *a.* childlike; simple-minded.

O *abr.* ojo / oculus; **oral, oralmente** / oral, orally; **oxígeno** / oxygen.

o *conj.* either, or; __ **bien** __ **mal** / one way or another, anyway.

obediente *a.* obedient, compliant.

obesidad *f.* obesity, excess fat; __ **alimentaria** / alimentary __; __ **endógena** / endogenous __; __ **exógena** / exogenous __ .

obeso-a *a.* obese, excessively fat.

objetivo *m.* objective, goal; target; **-a** *a.* rel. to the perception of any happening or phenomenon as it is manifested in real life; **-mente** *adv.* objectively.

obliteración *f.* obliteration, destruction, occlusion by degeneration or by surgery.

obrar *v.* to act, to work; *Mex.* to have a bowel movement.

obscuridad, oscuridad *f.* darkness.

obscuro-a, oscuro-a *a.* dark.

observación *f.* observation; remark.

obsesión *f.* obsession, abnormal preoccupation with a single idea or emotion; *pop.* hang-up.

obsesivo-compulsivo-a *a.* obsessive-compulsive, rel. to an individual that is driven to repeat actions excessively as a relief of tension and anxiety.

obseso-a *a.* possessed, dominated by an idea or passion.

obstetra *m., f.* obstetrician.

obstetricia *f.* obstetrics, the study of the care of women during pregnancy and delivery.

obstétrico-a *a.* obstetric, rel. to obstetrics.

obstipación *f.* obstipation, severe constipation.

obstrucción *f.* obstruction, blockage; __ **crónica del pulmón** / obstructive lung disease, chronic condition caused by the physical or functional narrowing of the bronchial tree; __ **en el conducto aéreo superior** / upper airway __; __ **intestinal** / __ intestinal blockage.

obstruído-a *a.* obstructed, blocked; **no** __ / unobstructed.

obstruir *vt.* to obstruct, to block, to impede.

obtener *vt.* to obtain, to attain, to achieve.

obturación *f.* obturation, occlusion.

obturador-a *a.* obturator, that obstructs an opening.

obtuso-a *a.* obtuse. 1. lacking mental acuity; 2. [*filo*] blunt, dull.

occipital *a.* occipital, rel. to the back part of the head; **hueso** __ / __ bone; **lóbulo** __ / __ lobe.

occipitofrontal *a.* occipitofrontal, rel. to the occiput and the forehead.

occipitoparietal *a.* occipitoparietal, rel. to the occipital and parietal bones and lobes.

occipitotemporal *a.* occipitotemporal, rel. to the occipital and temporal bones.

occipucio *m.* occiput, posteroinferior part of the skull.

oclusión *f.* occlusion, obstruction; __ **coronaria** / coronary __; __ **de la pupila** / pupillar __ .

octogenario-a *m., f.* octogenarian, individual that is about eighty years old.

ocular *a.* ocular, visual, rel. to the eyes; **cuerpo extraño** __ / __ foreign body; **globo** __ / eyeball; **movimientos** __ **-es** / __ movements; **ataxia** __ / __ ataxia; **cono** __ / __ cone; __ [de un aparato óptico] / __ eyepiece; **órbita** __ / __ eyesocket; **traumatismo** __ / __ eye injury; **vértigo** __ / __ vertigo.

oculista *m., f.* oculist. oftalmólogo.

oculomotor *a.* oculomotor, rel. to the movement of the eyeball.

ocultar *vt.* to conceal, to hide.

oculto-a *a.* occult, concealed, not visible.

oculus *L.* oculus, eye.

ocupación *f.* occupation.

ocupacional *a.* occupational, rel. to an occupation; **lesiones ocupacionales** / __ injuries; **salud** __ / __ health; **terapista** __ / __ therapist.

Oddi, esfínter de *m.* Oddi's sphincter, circular contractile muscle located at the level of the angular notch of the stomach and the pancreatic ducts.

odinofobia *f.* odynophobia, morbid fear of pain.

odontectomía *f.* odontectomy, tooth extraction.

odontología *f.* odontology, the study of dentistry.

odontólogo-a

odontólogo-a *m., f.* odontologist, dentist or oral surgeon.

odontoplastia *f.* odontoplasty, surgical procedure used to improve plaque control and gingival care.

odoríforo-a *a.* odoriferous, that has a pleasant smell.

oeste *m.* west; **al ___ / to the ___.**

oficial *a.* official, authorized; **no ___ /** unofficial, rel. to medication not listed in the Pharmacopeia or standard formulary.

oficina *f.* office.

oftálmico-a *a.* ophthalmic, rel. to the eye; **nervio ___ / ___ nerve; solución ___ / ___ solution.**

oftalmología *f.* ophthalmology, the study of the eye and its disorders.

oftalmólogo-a *m., f.* ophthalmologist, oculist, specialist in eye disorders.

oftalmopatía *f.* ophthalmopathy, eye disorder.

oftalmoplastia *f.* ophthalmoplasty, plastic surgery of the eye.

oftalmoplejía *f.* ophthalmoplegia, paralysis of an eye muscle.

oftalmoscopía *f.* ophthalmoscopy, examination of the eye with an ophthalmoscope.

oftalmoscopio *m.* ophthalmoscope, instrument for viewing the interior of the eye.

oído *m.* ear. 1. hearing organ formed by the inner, middle, and external ear;

2. the sense of hearing; **dolor de ___ /** earache; **gotas para los ___ -s / ___** drops; **pliegue del lóbulo del ___ / ___** lobe crease; **___ tapado con cerumen /** ___ covered with earwax; **zumbido en los ___ -s / ringing ___ -s.** See illustration on this page.

oír *vt.* to hear.

ojeada *f.* glance; **dar una ___ / to glance.**

ojeras *f., pl.* dark circles under the eyes.

ojeroso-a *a.* haggard, referring to someone with dark circles under their eyes.

ojo *m.* eye; **banco de ___ -s / ___ bank; cuenca del ___ / ___ socket; fondo del ___ / eyeground; gotas para los ___ -s / ___ drops; ___ de vidrio / glass ___; ___ -s inyectados / bloodshot ___ -s; ___ -s llorosos / watery ___ -s; ___ -s saltones /** goggle-eyed. See illustration on page 182.

oleada *f.* tide, a space of time; rise and fall.

oler *vt.* to smell, to scent.

olfacción *f.* olfaction. 1. the act of smelling; 2. the sense of smell.

olfatear *vt.* to sniff.

olfato *m.* 1. the sense of smell; 2. odor.

olfatorio-a *a.* olfactory, rel. to smell.

oligodactilia *f.* oligodactyly, less than the normal number of toes or fingers.

oligodoncia *f.* oligodontia, hereditary condition consisting in fewer teeth than normal.

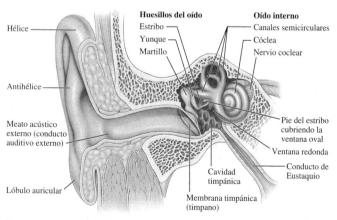

Huesillos del oído
Estribo
Yunque
Martillo

Oído interno
Canales semicirculares
Cóclea
Nervio coclear

Hélice

Antihélice

Meato acústico externo (conducto auditivo externo)

Lóbulo auricular

Pie del estribo cubriendo la ventana oval

Ventana redonda

Conducto de Eustaquio

Cavidad timpánica

Membrana timpánica (timpano)

Estructuras del oído

oligomenorrea *f.* oligomenorrhea, deficient or infrequent menstruation.

oligospermia *f.* oligospermia, diminished number of spermatozoa in the semen.

oliguria *f.* oliguria, diminished formation of urine.

oliva *f.* olive. 1. gray body behind the medulla oblongata; 2. green olive color; 3. the olive tree.

olor *m.* odor, smell, scent; __ **penetrante** / penetrating smell.

oloroso-a *a.* odorous.

olvidadizo-a *a.* forgetful.

olvidar *v.* to forget.

omalgia *f.* omalgia, pain in the shoulder.

ombligo *m.* umbilicus, navel, a depression in the center of the abdomen at the point of insertion of the uterine canal at the time of birth; *pop.* belly button.

omentectomía *f.* omentectomy, partial or total removal of the omentum.

omentum *m.* (*pl.* **omenta**) an extension of the peritoneum attached to part of the stomach, that folds organs such as the duodenum, transverse colon, and the lower intestine. *See* **epiplón.**

omisión *f.* omission.

omitir *v.* to omit.

oncogénesis *f.* oncogenesis, formation and development of tumors.

oncólisis *f.* oncolysis, destruction of tumor cells.

oncología *f.* oncology, the study of tumors.

oncótico-a *a.* oncotic, rel. to or caused by swelling.

onda *f.* wave. 1. ondulant movement or vibration that travels along a fixed direction; 2. ondulant graphic representation of an activity, such as seen in an electroencephalogram; **guía de __ -s** / waveguide; **longitud de __** / wavelength; __ **pulsátil** / pulse __; __ **Q / Q __; __ R / R __; __ -s cerebrales** / brain __ -s; __ **-s de excitación** / excitation __ -s; __ **sonora** / sound __; __ **-s ultrasónicas** / ultrasound __ -s.

onda T *f.* T wave, part of the electrocardiogram that represents the repolarization of the ventricles.

onda V *f.* V wave, positive wave that follows the T wave in an electrocardiogram.

ondulado-a *a.* ondulant, having an irregular or wavy border.

onfalitis *f.* omphalitis, infl. of the umbilicus.

onfalocele *m.* omphalocele, umbilical hernia.

onicofagia *f.* onychophagia, habit of biting the nails.

onicomalasia *f.* onychomalasia, softening of the nails.

onicopatía *f.* onicopathy, any disease of the nail.

onicosis *f.* onychosis, deformity or sickness of a nail.

oniomanía *f.* oniomania, pathological urge to spend money.

oniquectomía *f.* onychectomy, excision of a nail.

onomatonamía *f.* onomatonamia, obsessive urge to repeat words.

oocito, ovocito *m.* oocyte, female ovum before maturation.

ooforectomía *f.* oophorectomy, partial or total excision of an ovary.

ooforitis *f.* oophoritis, infl. of an ovary.

ooforocistosis *f.* oophorocystosis, formation of an ovarian cyst.

ooforopexia *f.* oophoropexy, fixation or suspension of a displaced ovary.

oogénesis, ovogénesis *f.* oogenesis, ovogenesis, formation and development of an ovum.

oospermo *m.* oosperm, a fertilized ovum.

oótide *n.* ootid, the mature ovum after the penetration of the spermatozoon and the completion of the second meiotic division.

opacidad *f.* opacity, dimness, lack of transparency.

opacificación *f.* opacification, process of rendering something opaque.

opaco-a *a.* opaque, that does not filter light.

operación *f.* operation, surgical procedure.

operar *v.* to operate, to intervene surgically.

operón *m.* operon, a system of linked genes in which the operator gene regulates the remaining structural genes.

opiáceo *m.* opiate, opium-derived drug.

opinar *v.* to express an opinion.

opinión *f.* opinion, judgment.

opio *m.* opium, *Papaver somniferum,* narcotic, analgesic, alucinogen, stimulant, addictive.

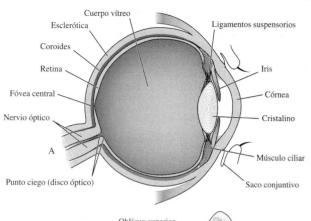

Cuerpo vítreo
Esclerótica
Coroides
Retina
Fóvea central
Nervio óptico
A
Punto ciego (disco óptico)
Ligamentos suspensorios
Iris
Córnea
Cristalino
Músculo ciliar
Saco conjuntivo

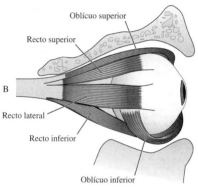

Oblícuo superior
Recto superior
B
Recto lateral
Recto inferior
Oblícuo inferior

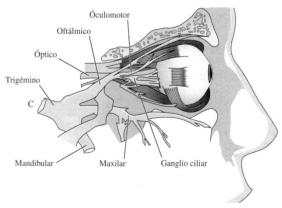

Óculomotor
Oftálmico
Óptico
Trigémino
C
Mandibular
Maxilar
Ganglio ciliar

(A) el ojo; (B) músculos extrínsecos del ojo; (C) nervios del ojo

opistótonos *m.* opisthotonos, tetanic spasm of the muscles of the back in which the heels and head bend backward and the trunk projects forward.

oponer *vt.* to oppose; *vr.* **oponerse,** to be against, to oppose.

oportunista *a.* opportunistic; opportune.

oposición *f.* opposition; objection.

opresión *f.* oppression; heaviness; __ en el pecho / an __ in the chest.

opsonina *f.* opsonin, antibody that combines with a specific antigen and makes it more susceptible to phagocytes.

óptica *f.* optics, the study of light and its relation to vision; *a.* **óptico-a,** optic, optical, rel. to vision; **disco** __ / __ disk, blind spot of the retina; **ilusión** __ / __ illusion; **nervio** __ / __ nerve.

optómetra, optometrista *m., f.* optometrist, professional who practices optometry.

optometría *f.* optometry, the practice of examining the eyes for visual acuity and prescribing corrective lenses and other optical aids.

optómetro *m.* optometer, instrument used to measure eye refraction.

oral *a.* oral, delivered or taken by mouth.

orbicular *a.* orbicular, circular; **músculo** __ / __ muscle, that surrounds a small opening such as the orbicular muscle of the mouth; __ de los labios / __ oris; __ de los párpados / __ ciliaris.

órbita *f.* orbit, bony cavity that contains the eyeball and associated structures.

orbital *a.* orbital, rel. to the orbit.

orden *m.* order, arrangement; regulation.

ordenar *vt.* to order; to arrange.

ordinario-a *a.* ordinary, usual, common.

oreja *f.* external ear; **lóbulo de la** __ / ear lobe.

orejera *f.* ear protector.

orejuela *f.* auricle, flop of tissue that partially covers the atrium.

organelo, organito *m.* organelle, minute organ of unicellular organisms.

orgánico-a *a.* organic. 1. rel. to an organ; 2. rel. to organisms of vegetable or animal origin; **enfermedad** __ / __ disease.

organismo *m.* organism, a living being.

organización *f.* organization, association.

órgano *m.* organ, part of the body with a specific function; **desplazamiento de** __ / __ displacement; **fallo de un** __ / __ failure; **terminal / end** __; **transplante de un** __ / __ transplant.

organogénesis *f.* organogenesis, growth and development of an organ.

organomegalia *f.* organomegaly, abnormal enlargement of the visceral organs. *Syn.* visceromegaly.

orgasmo *m.* orgasm, sexual climax.

orientación *f.* orientation, direction.

orientacion a la realidad *f.* reality orientation, the patient remains turned inward and in contact with his or her own environment.

orificio *m.* orifice, aperture, opening.

orín, orina *m., f.* urine, the clear fluid secreted by the kidneys, stored in the urinary bladder, and discharged by the urethra; **cultivo de** __ / __ culture; **especimen de** __ **a mitad de chorro** / midstream __ specimen; **muestra de** __ / __ sample; __ **claro-a** / clear __; __ **lechoso-a** / milky __; __ **turbio-a** / hazy __; **sedimento de** __ / __ sediment. See table on page 491.

orinal *m.* urinal, chamber pot, container or receptacle for urine.

orinar *v.* to urinate, to micturate; **ardor al** __ / burning on urination; __ **a menudo** / frequent urination; __ **con dificultad** / difficult urination; __ **con dolor** / painful urination; *vr.* **orinarse,** to wet oneself; __ **en la cama** / bedwetting.

ornitina *f.* ornithine, an amino acid not present in proteins, but an important element in the urea cycle.

orofacial *a.* orofacial, rel. to the mouth and the face.

orofaringe *m.* oropharynx, central part of the pharynx.

Oroya, fiebre de *f.* Oroya fever, Carrión disease, found in Peru, characterized by very high fever, pernicious anemia and great sensitivity of the hemopoietic tissues.

orquidectomía, orquiectomía *f.* orchidectomy, orchiectomy, removal of a testicle.

orquiditis, orquitis *f.* orchiditis, orchitis, infl. of a testicle.

orquidopexia, orquiopexia *f.* orchidopexy, orchiopexy, procedure by which an undescended testicle is lowered into the scrotum and sutured to it.

orquionco *f.* orchioncus, a tumor in the testicle.

orquiotomía *f.* orchiotomy, incision in a testicle.

ortocefálico-a *a.* orthocephalic, having a normal head with a cephalic index between 70 and 75.

ortocromático-a *a.* orthochromatic, of natural color or that accepts coloration.

ortodigita *f.* orthodigita, correction of malformations of fingers and toes.

ortodoncia *f.* orthodontics, the study of irregularities and corrective procedures of teeth.

ortodoncista *m., f.* orthodontist, specialist in orthodontics.

ortógrado-a *a.* orthograde, that walks in an erect position.

ortomixovirus *m.* orthomyxoviridae, family of viruses to which belong the three groups of influenza viruses.

ortopedia *f.* orthopedics, the study of bones, joints, muscles, ligaments, and cartilages and the preventive and corrective procedures that deal with their related disorders.

ortopédico-a, ortopedista *m., f.* orthopedist, specialist in orthopedics; *a.* **orthopedic,** rel. to orthopedia; **calzado ___ / ___ shoes.**

ortopnea *f.* orthopnea, difficulty in breathing except when in an upright position.

ortóptica *f.* orthoptics, the study and correction of disorders of binocular vision and of the movements of the eye.

ortosiquiatría *f.* orthopsychiatry, a branch of psychiatry that embraces child psychiatry, pediatrics, developmental psychology and family care and is concerned with the prevention and treatment of psychological disorders in children and adolescents.

ortostático-a *a.* orthostatic, rel. to an erect position.

ortótonos *m.* orthotonos, orthotonus, a tetanic spasm which provokes rigidity in a straight line to the neck, limbs and body.

ortotópico-a *a.* orthotopic, in the normal or correct position.

orzuelo *m.* sty, stye, infl. of the sebaceous glands of the eyelid.

oscilación *f.* oscillation, a pendulum-like motion.

oscilopsia *f.* oscillopsia, oscilating vision during the advance stage of multiple sclerosis.

óseo-a *a.* osseous, rel. to bone; **desarrollo ___ / bone development; lesiones ___ -s / bone lesions; placa ___ / bone plate.**

osículo *m.* ossicle, small bone.

osificación *f.* ossification. 1. conversion of a substance into bone; 2. bone development.

osificar *vi.* to ossify, to turn into bone.

osmolar, osmótico-a *a.* osmolar, osmotic, rel. to or of the nature of osmosis.

osmología *f.* osmology, the study of odors.

osmorreceptor *m.* osmoreceptor. 1. a group of cells in the brain that receive olfactory stimuli; 2. a group of cells in the hypothalamus that respond to changes in the osmotic pressure of the blood.

osmosis *f.* osmosis, diffusion of a solvent through a semipermeable membrane separating two solutions of different concentration.

osmótico-a *a.* osmotic, rel. to or of the nature of osmosis.

osteítis, ostitis *f.* osteitis, ostitis, infl. of a bone; **___ fibrosa quistica / ___ fibrosa cystica,** with cystic and nodular manifestations.

osteoaneurisma *m.* osteoaneurysm, aneurysm that occurs within a bone.

osteoartritis *f.* osteoarthritis, degenerative hypertrophy of the bones and joints.

osteoartropatía *f.* osteoarthropathy, disease of a joint and a bone, gen. accompanied by pain.

osteoblasto *m.* osteoblast, a cell that forms bone tissue.

osteoblastoma *m.* osteoblastoma; osteoma.

osteocarcinoma *m.* osteocarcinoma, bone cancer.

osteocartilaginoso-a *a.* osteocartilaginous, rel. to or formed by bone and cartilage.

osteocondritis *f.* osteochondritis, infl. of bone and cartilage.

osteocondroma *f.* osteochondroma, tumor of both of osseous and cartilaginous elements.

osteodistrofia *f.* osteodystrophia, osteodystrophy, defective bone formation.

otologia

osteófito *m.* osteophyte, bony outgrowth.

osteoide *a.* osteoid, rel. to or resembling bone.

osteología *f.* osteology, the study of bones.

osteoma *m.* osteoma, a tumor of bone tissue.

osteomalacia *f.* osteomalacia, softening of the bones due to loss of calcium in the bone matrix.

osteomielitis *f.* osteomyelitis, infection of bone and bone marrow.

osteonecrosis *f.* osteonecrosis, destruction and death of bone tissue.

osteópata *m., f.* osteopath, specialist in osteopathy.

osteopatía *f.* osteopathy. 1. an approach to medicine that places emphasis on a favorable environment and on normal structural relationships of the musculoskeletal system, using extensive manipulation as a corrective tool; 2. any sickness of the bones.

osteopenia *f.* osteopenia, diminished calcification of the bones.

osteoplástico-a *a.* osteoplastic. 1. rel. to bone formation; 2. plastic surgery of a bone.

osteoporosis *f.* osteoporosis, loss of bone density resulting in fragile bones that fracture easily.

osteosarcoma *m.* osteosarcoma, osseous sarcoma, the most common malignant sarcoma of the long bones.

osteosíntesis *f.* osteosynthesis, surgical fixation of a bone by mechanical means such as a plate or nail.

osteotomía *f.* osteotomy, the cutting or sawing of a bone.

ostium *L.* (*pl. ostia*) ostium, small opening.

ostium primum *n., L.* ostium primum, opening that communicates the two auricles of the fetal heart and that gradually becomes smaller and closes after birth.

ostomía *f.* ostomy, creation of an artificial opening between the bowel or intestine and the skin, as in ileostomy and colostomy.

ostra *f.* oyster.

otalgia, otodinia *f.* otalgia, otodynia, earache.

otectomía *f.* otectomy, excision of the structural contents of the middle ear.

oticodinia *f.* oticodinia, vertigo caused by an ear disorder.

otitis *f.* otitis, infl. of the external, middle, or inner ear; __ **del nadador** / swimmer's ear.

otolaringología *f.* otolaryngology, the study of the ear, nose and throat.

otolaringólogo-a *m., f.* otolaryngologist, specialist in otolaryngology.

otología *f.* otology, the study of the ear and its disorders.

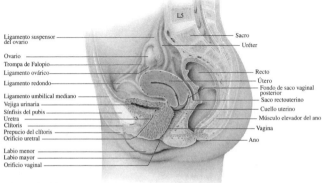

Ligamento suspensor del ovario
Ovario
Trompa de Falopio
Ligamento ovárico
Ligamento redondo
Ligamento umbilical mediano
Vejiga urinaria
Uretra
Clítoris
Prepucio del clítoris
Orificio uretral
Labio menor
Labio mayor
Orificio vaginal

L5
Sacro
Uréter
Recto
Útero
Fondo de saco vaginal posterior
Saco rectouterino
Cuello uterino
Músculo elevador del ano
Vagina
Ano

Los órganos pélvicos femeninos (sección sagital)

otoneurología

otoneurología *f.* otoneurology, the study of the inner ear as related to the nervous system.

otoplastia *f.* otoplasty, plastic surgery of the ear.

otorragia *f.* otorrhagia, bleeding from the ear.

otorrea *f.* otorrhea, purulent discharge from the ear.

otosclerosis *f.* otosclerosis, progressive deafness due to formation of spongy tissue in the labyrinth of the ear.

otoscopia *f.* otoscopy, examination of the ear with an otoscope.

otoscopio *m.* otoscope, instrument to examine the ear.

otro-a *a.* other; *pron.* another; **el ___, la ___** / the ___ one; **los ___ -s, las ___ -s** / the others.

oval *a.* oval. 1. rel. to an ovum; 2. in the shape of an egg; **ventana ___** / ___ window, membrane that separates the middle and the inner ear.

ovárico-a *a.* ovarian, rel. to the ovaries.

ovariectomía *f.* ovariectomy, ooforectomy.

ovario *m.* ovary, female reproductive organ that produces the ova. See illustration on page 185.

oviducto *m.* oviduct, uterine conduit.

ovoide *a.* ovoid, egg-shaped.

ovotestis *f.* ovotestis, hermaphroditic gland that contains both ovarian and testicular tissue.

ovulación *f.* ovulation, periodic release of the ovum from the ovary.

óvulo *m.* ovum, egg cell.

oxidación *f.* oxidation, the chemical change resulting from the combination of oxygen with another substance.

oxidado-a *a.* rusty.

oxidante *m.* oxidant, agent that causes oxidation.

oxigenación *f.* oxygenation, saturation with oxygen.

oxigenado-a *a.* oxygenated.

oxigenador *m.* oxygenator, device that oxygenates blood, gen. used during surgery.

oxígeno *m.* oxygen, free element found in the atmosphere as a colorless, tasteless, and odorless gas; **cámara de ___** / ___ tent; **distribución de ___** / ___ distribution; **falta de ___** / ___ deficiency; **tratamiento de ___** / ___ treatment.

oxigenoterapia *f.* oxygenotherapy, therapeutic use of oxygen.

oxihemoglobina *f.* oxyhemoglobin, bright red substance that forms when the red cells combine permanently with oxygen.

oxímetro *m.* oximeter, instrument used to measure the amount of oxygen in the blood.

oxitocina *f.* oxytocin, pituitary hormone that stimulates uterine contraction.

ozono *m.* ozone, O_3, powerful oxidant agent, a toxic form of oxygen.

p

P *abr.* **plasma** / plasma; **positivo-a** / positive; **posterior** / posterior; **presión** / pressure; **psiquiatría** / psychiatry; **pulso** / pulse.

paciencia *f.* patience; **con ___** / patiently.

paciente *m., f.* patient; **alta del ___** / patient's discharge; **cuidado del ___** / ___ 's care; **___ externo, no hospitalizado** / outpatient; **___ interno** / inpatient; **___ privado** / private ___; **___ solvente** / self-paying ___; *a.* patient.

padecer *vt.* to be afflicted by a sickness or injury; **___ de** / to suffer from.

padecimiento *m.* suffering; affliction.

padrastro *m.* stepfather.

padre *m.* father; **-s** / the parents, mother and father.

pagado-a *a.* paid, *pp.* of **pagar.**

palabra *f.* word.

paladar *m.* palate, the roof of the mouth; **___ blando** / soft ___; **___ duro** / hard ___; **___ hendido** / cleft ___, congenital fissure; **___ óseo** / bony ___ .

palatino-a *a.* palatine, rel. to the palate.

paliativo-a *a.* palliative, that mitigates.

palidecer *vi.* to become pale.

palidez *f.* pallor.

pálido-a *a.* pallid, pale, sallow.

paliza *f.* beating.

palma *f.* 1. palm, palm of the hand; 2. palm tree; **aceite de ___** / ___ oil.

palmacristi *f.* castor oil.

palpable *a.* palpable, that can be touched.

palpación *f.* palpation, examination with the hands.

palpar *vt.* to palpate, to feel, to touch.

palpitación *f.* palpitation, rapid pulsation or throbbing.

palpitante *a.* throbbing, that beats rapidly.

palpitar *vi.* to palpitate; to pant.

palúdico-a *a.* rel. to or afflicted by malaria.

paludismo *m.* malaria, paludism, highly infectious, febrile, and often chronic disease caused by the bite of an infected *Anopheles* mosquito.

pampiniforme *a.* pampiniform, simulating the structure of a vine.

pan *m.* bread; **___ y mantequilla** / ___ and butter.

panacea *f.* panacea, a remedy to cure all ills.

panadizo *m.* felon, painful abscess of the distal phalanx of a finger.

panartritis *f.* panarthritis. 1. infl. of some joints of the body; 2. infl. of all the tissues of a joint.

pancitopenia *f.* pancytopenia, abnormal decrease in the number of blood cells.

páncreas *m.* pancreas, gland of the digestive system that externally secretes the pancreatic juice, and internally secretes insulin and glucagon.

pancreatectomía *f.* pancreatectomy, partial or total removal of the pancreas.

pancreático-a *a.* pancreatic, rel. to the pancreas; **conducto ___** / ___ duct; **jugo ___** / ___ juice; **quiste ___** / ___ cyst.

pancreatina *f.* pancreatin, digestive enzyme obtained from the pancreas.

pancreatitis *f.* pancreatitis, infl. of the pancreas; **___ aguda** / acute ___; **___ hemorrágica aguda** / acute hemorrhagic ___ .

pancreatolitiasis *f.* pancreatolithiasis, presence of calculi in the ducts of the pancreas.

pandémico-a *a.* pandemic, that occurs over a wide geographical area.

panendoscopio *m.* panendoscope, optical instrument used to examine the urethra and the bladder.

panfleto *m.* pamphlet.

panglosia *f.* panglossia, excessive talking.

panhidrosis *f.* panhidrosis, generalized sweating.

panhipopituitarismo *m.* panhypopituitarism, deficiency of the anterior pituitary gland.

panhisterectomía *f.* panhysterectomy, total excision of the uterus.

pánico *m.* panic, excessive fear; **ataques de ___** / ___ attacks; **trastornos de ___** / ___ disorder; *v.* **tener ___** / to panic.

paniculitis *f.* paniculitis, infl. of the panniculus adiposus.

panículo *m.* panniculus, layer of tissue; **___ adiposo** / ___ adiposus; **___ carnoso** / ___ carnosus.

pannus *L.* pannus, a membrane of granulation tissue covering a normal surface.

pansinusitis *f.* pansinusitis, infl. of all the paranasal sinuses in one or both sides.

pantalla *f.* screen.

pantorrilla *f.* calf of the leg.

panza *f.* belly.

panzudo-a *a.*, *pop.* potbellied.

pañal *m.* diaper; ___ **-es desechables** / disposable ___ -s.

papá *m.* dad.

papada *f.* double chin.

Papanicolau, prueba de *f.* Papanicolau's test, Pap smear, sample of mucus from the vagina and the cervix for the purpose of early detection of cancer cells.

paperas *f.* mumps, acute, febrile, highly contagious disease characterized by swelling of the salivary glands.

papila *f.* papilla, bud, small, nipple-like eminence of the skin, esp. seen in the mouth; ___ **acústica** / acoustic ___; ___ **dérmica** / dermal ___; ___ **duodenal** / duodenal ___; ___ **filiforme** / filiform ___; ___ **gustativa** / taste bud; ___ **lagrimal** / lacrimal ___; ___ **lingual** / lingual ___ .

papilar *m.* papillary, rel. to a papilla.

papiledema *m.* papilledema, edema of the optic disk.

papilitis *f.* papillitis, infl. of the optic disk.

papiloma *m.* papilloma, benign epithelial tumor.

papilomatosis *f.* papillomatosis. 1. the development of numerous papillomas; 2. papillary projections.

papovavirus *m.* papovavirus, type of virus used in the study of cancer.

pápula *f.* papule, small, hard eminence of the skin.

papuloescamoso-a *a.* papulosquamous, rel. to papules and scales; **enfermedades cutáneas** ___ / ___ skin diseases.

paquete celular *m.* packed cells, red blood cells that have been separated from the plasma.

par *m.* pair, couple.

para *prep.* to, for; for the purpose of; in order to; ___ **siempre** / forever; ¿ ___ **qué** / what for?

paracentesis *f.* paracentesis, puncture to obtain or remove fluid from a cavity.

parado-a *a.* in a standing position.

parafimosis *f.* paraphimosis. 1. retraction or constriction of the prepuce behind the glans penis;

2. retraction of the eyelid behind the eyeball.

parafina *f.* paraffin.

parainfluenza, virus de *m.* parainfluenza virus, any of several viruses associated with some respiratory infections, esp. in children.

paralaje *m.* parallax, the apparent displacement of an object according to the position of the viewer.

parálisis *f.* palsy, paralysis, partial or total loss of function of a part of the body; ___ **alcohólica** / alcoholic ___; ___ **alterna** / alternative ___; ___ **amiotrófica** / amyotrophic ___; ___ **ascendente** / ascending ___; ___ **central** / central ___; ___ **cerebral** / cerebral ___ , partial paralysis and lack of muscular coordination due to a congenital brain lesion; ___ **cerebral atáxica infantil** / infantile cerebral ataxic ___; ___ **de acomodación** / accommodation ___; ___ **de los buzos** / diver's paralysis, decompression sickness (bends); ___ **facial** / facial ___; ___ **facial periférica** / peripheral facial ___; ___ **galopante** / rapidly progressive gen. ___; ___ **histérica** / hysterical ___; ___ **infantil** / infantile paralysis; ___ **motora** / motor ___; ___ **por enfriamiento** / cold-induced ___ .

parálisis cerebral *f.* cerebral paralysis, partial paralysis and lack of muscular coordination due to a congenital brain lesion.

paralítico-a *a.* paralytic, invalid, rel. to or suffering from paralysis; **íleo** ___ / ___ ileus, paralysis of the intestines.

paramédico-a *m.*, *f.* paramedic, individual trained and certified to offer emergency medical assistance.

parametrio *m.* parametrium, loose cellular tissue around the uterus.

paramiotonía *f.* paramyotonia, atypical myotonia, characterized by muscle spasms and abnormal muscular tonicity; ___ **atáxica** / ataxic ___; ___ **congenital** / congenital ___; ___ **sintomática** / symptomatic ___; **trastornos de** ___ / ___ disorders.

paranasal *a.* paranasal, adjacent to the nasal cavity.

paranoia *f.* paranoia, mental disorder characterized by delusions of persecution and grandeur.

paranoico-a *a.* paranoid, rel. to or afflicted with paranoia.

parto

paraplejía *f.* paraplegia, paralysis of the legs and the lower half of the body; ___ **cerebral infantil** / cerebral infantile ___; ___ **espasmódica familiar** / familiar, spasmodic ___; ___ **espasmódica, espástica** / spasmodic, spastic ___; ___ **flácida** / flaccid ___ .

parapléjico-a *a.* paraplegic, rel. to or affected with paraplegia.

parapsicología *f.* parapsychology, the study of psychic phenomena such as mental telepathy and extrasensory perception.

parar *vt.* to stop, to halt; **pararse** *vr.* to stand up; ___ **de puntillas** / to stand on tiptoe.

parasimpático-a *a.* parasympathetic, rel. to one of two branches of the autonomic nervous system.

parasístole *f.* parasystole, an irregularity in cardiac rhythm.

parásito *m.* parasite, organism that lives upon another one.

parasitología *f.* parasitology, the study of parasites.

parasomnia *f.* parasomnia, term used to designate any disorder suffered during sleep, enuresis, nightmares, sleepwalking, etc.

paratífica, fiebre *f.* paratyphoid fever, a fever that simulates typhoid fever.

paratiroidectomía *f.* parathyroidectomy, removal of one or more of the parathyroid glands.

paratiroideo-a *a.* parathyroid, located close to the thyroid gland.

paratiroides *f.* parathyroid, group of small endocrine glands situated behind the thyroid gland.

parcial *a.* partial; **-mente** *adv.* partially.

parche *m.* patch, piece of cloth or adhesive used to protect wounds; **prueba del** ___ / ___ test, for allergies.

parecido-a *a.* resembling.

paregórico *m.* paregoric, sedative derived from opium.

pareja *f.* pair, couple.

parejo-a *a.* even, equal.

parénquima *m.* parenchyma, the functional elements of an organ.

parenteral *a.* parenteral, that is introduced in the body in a way other than the gastrointestinal route.

parentesco *m.* kindred, family relationship.

paresia *f.* paresis, slight or partial paralysis.

parestesia *f.* paresthesia, sensation of pricking, tingling, or tickling, gen. associated with partial damage to a peripheral nerve.

pariente-a *m., f.* family relative; ___ **consanguíneo** / blood relation.

parietal *m.* parietal bone; *a.* parietal. 1. rel. to the parietal bone; 2. rel. to the wall of a cavity.

parir *vt.* to give birth.

Parkinson, enfermedad de *f.* Parkinson's disease, degenerative process of the brain nerves characterized by tremor, progressive muscular weakness, blurred speech, and shuffling gait.

paro *m.* standstill, arrest.

parodinia *f.* parodynia, difficult or abnormal delivery.

paroniquia *f.* paronychia, infl. of the area adjacent to a fingernail.

parótida *f.* parotid, gland that secretes saliva, situated near the ear.

parotiditis, parotitis *f.* parotiditis, parotitis. *See* **paperas**.

paroxismal, paroxístico-a *a.* paroxysmal, rel. to paroxysm.

paroxismo *m.* paroxysm. 1. attack, spasm, or convulsion; 2. recurring intensified symptoms.

parpadear *v.* to blink.

parpadeo *m.* blinking; flicker.

párpado *m.* eyelid; cilium.

parte *f.* part, portion; **por todas** ___ **-s** / everywhere.

partenogénesis *f.* parthenogenesis, unusual reproductive process in which the ovum develops without being fertilized by a spermatozoon; ___ **artificial** / artificial ___ .

partición *f.* partition, sectioning, division.

partícula *f.* particle, one of the minute parts that form matter.

parto *m.* labor, delivery, parturition; **antes del, después del** ___ / before, after delivery; **canal del** ___ / birth canal; **dolor de** ___ / ___ pains; **estar de** ___ / to be close to delivery; **etapas del** ___ / stages of ___; ___ **activo** / active ___; ___ **de un feto sin vida** / stillbirth; ___ **falso** / false ___; ___ **inducido** / induced ___; ___ **laborioso** / hard, difficult ___; ___ **natural** / natural childbirth; ___ **normal** / normal delivery; ___ **prematuro** / premature ___; ___ **prolongado, tardío** / prolonged ___; ___ **seco** / dry ___ .

parturienta *f.* parturient, a woman in the act of delivering or who has just delivered.

parturifaciente *m.* parturifacient, an agent that induces parturition.

parvovirus *m.* parvovirus, any of a group of viruses that cause diseases in animals but not in humans.

pasaje *m.* passage. 1. conduit or meatus; 2. evacuation of the bowels.

pasajero-a *a.* fleeting, that doesn't last.

pasar *v.* to pass, to pass by; to happen.

pasillo *m.* hall, hallway, corridor; covered way.

pasivo-a *a.* passive, not spontaneous or active; **ejercicio __ / __** exercise.

pasteurización *f.* pasteurization, the process of destroying microorganisms by applying regulated heat.

pasteurizar *vi.* to pasteurize, to perform pasteurization.

pastilla *f.* pill, tablet; lozenge; **__ para dormir** / sleeping **__**; **__ para el dolor** / pain **__**.

pastoso-a *a.* clammy; doughy.

patelectomía *f.* patellectomy, excision of the patella.

patella *L.* patella, kneecap.

patente *m.* 1. patent, exclusive right or privilege; **medicina de __ / __** medicine; *a.* 2. patulous; open, not obstructed; evident.

paternidad *f.* paternity; **prueba de __ / __** test.

paterno-a *a.* paternal, rel. to the father.

patético-a *a.* pathetic.

patizambo-a *a.* pigeon-toed, feet turned inward.

patofisiología *f.* pathophysiology, the study of the effects of a disease on the physiological processes.

patogénesis *f.* pathogenesis, origin and development of a sickness.

patógeno *m.* pathogen, agent that causes disease; **-a** *a.* pathogenic, that can cause a disease.

patognomónico-a *a.* pathognomonic, rel. to a sign or symptom characteristic of a given disease.

patología *f.* pathology, the study of the origin and nature of disease.

patológico-a *a.* pathologic, pathological, rel. to disease.

patrón *m.* pattern, model, type.

pausa *f.* pause, rest; interruption; **__ compensadora** / compensatory **__**, long interval of time, following a heartbeat.

paz *f.* peace; *v.* **dejar en __** / to leave alone; **en __** / at **__** .

peau d'orange *Fr.* peau d'orange, skin condition resembling that of the peel of an orange, an important sign in breast cancer.

peca *f.* freckle, spot, small discoloration of the skin.

pecho *m.* chest; **__ de paloma** / pigeon breast; *v.* **dar el __** / to breast-feed.

pecoso-a *a.* freckled.

pectina *f.* pectin, carbohydrate obtained from the peel of citrus fruits or apples.

pectus *L.* (*pl. pectora*) pectus, breast, chest.

pedazo *m.* piece, part of a whole.

pederastia *f.* pederasty, anal intercourse between males, esp. between an adult and a young boy.

pediatra *m., f.* pediatrician, specialist in pediatrics.

pediatría *f.* pediatrics, the study of the care and development of children and the treatment of diseases affecting them.

pediátrico-a *a.* pediatric, rel. to pediatrics.

pedículo *m.* pedicle, narrow, stemlike part of a tumor that connects it with its base.

pediculosis *f.* pediculosis, infestation with lice.

pedofilia *f.* pedophilia, morbid sexual attraction to children.

peinar *v.* to comb; **peinarse** *vr.* to comb one's hair.

peladura *f.* peeling, scaling, exfoliation; **__ química** / chemical **__** .

pelagra *f.* pellagra, illness caused by deficiency of niacin and characterized by dermatitis, gastrointestinal, and mental disorders.

pelar *v.* to peel; to give a haircut; **pelarse** *vr.* to get a haircut.

película *f.* 1. film, movie; 2. thin layer or membrane.

peligro *m.* danger, risk; hazard; peril; *v.* **estar en __** / to be in **__**; **poner en __** / to endanger, to jeopardize.

peligroso-a *a.* dangerous, risky, hazardous.

pellejo *m.* peel, hide; *pop.* skin.

pellizcar *vi.* to pinch.

pellizco *m.* pinch.

pelo *m.* hair; **raíz del __** / **__** root; **bola de __** / **__** ball, type of bezoar; **transplante de __** / **__** transplant.

pelota *f.* ball.

peloteo *m.* ballottement, maneuver used during examination of the abdomen and pelvis to determine the presence of tumors or enlargement of organs; ___ **renal** / renal ___ .

peludo-a *a.* hairy.

pélvico-a, pelviano-a *a.* pelvic, rel. to the pelvis.

pelvis *f.* pelvis. 1. cavity in the lower end of the trunk formed by the hip bone, the sacrum, and the coccyx; **enfermedad inflamatoria de la** ___ / pelvic inflammatory disease; 2. basin-shaped cavity.

pelvis menor, verdadera *f.* true pelvis, the inferior and contractile part of the pelvis.

pena *f.* sorrow, affliction.

pendular *a.* pendulous, oscillating or hanging.

pene *m.* penis, the external part of the male reproductive organ that contains the urethral orifice through which urine and semen pass. See illustration on this page.

peneal, peneano-a *a.* penile, rel. to the penis.

penetración *f.* penetration. 1. the act of penetrating; 2. the capacity of radiation to go through a substance.

penetrante *a.* penetrating; piercing.

penetrar *v.* to penetrate, to go through.

pénfigo *m.* pemphigus, a variety of dermatosis characterized by the presence of blisters that can become infected upon rupturing.

penicilina *f.* penicillin, antibiotic derived directly or indirectly from cultures of the fungus *Penicillium*.

pepsina *f.* pepsin, the main enzyme of the gastric juice.

péptico-a *a.* peptic, rel. to the action or the digestion of gastric juices.

pequeño-a *a.* small in size.

percepción *f.* perception. 1. the conscious mental recognition of a sensory stimulus; ___ **extrasensorial** / extrasensory ___; 2. understanding or comprehension of an idea.

percibir *vt.* to perceive, to realize.

percusión *f.* percussion, procedure that consists in tapping the surface of the body with the fingers or a small tool, in order to produce sounds or vibrations that indicate the condition of a given part of the body; ___ **auscultatoria** / auscultatory ___ .

percutáneo-a *a.* percutaneous, applied through the skin.

perder *vt.* to lose, to forfeit; ___ **sangre** / to bleed; ___ **la oportunidad** / to miss an opportunity; ___ **tiempo** / to waste time; ___ **un turno** / to miss an appointment.

pérdida *f.* loss; ___ **de sangre** / ___ of blood; ___ **del conocimiento** / ___ of consciousness; ___ **del contacto con la realidad** / ___ of contact with reality; ___ **del equilibrio** / ___ of balance; ___ **del movimiento** / ___ of motion; ___ **de la audición** / ___ of hearing; ___ **de la memoria** / ___ of memory; ___ **de la tonicidad muscular** / ___ of muscle

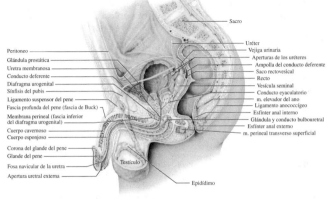

Peritoneo
Glándula prostática
Uretra membranosa
Conducto deferente
Diafragma urogenital
Sínfisis del pubis
Ligamento suspensor del pene
Fascia profunda del pene (fascia de Buck)
Membrana perineal (fascia inferior del diafragma urogenital)
Cuerpo cavernoso
Cuerpo esponjoso
Corona del glande del pene
Glande del pene
Fosa navicular de la uretra
Apertura uretral externa
Testículo

Sacro
Uréter
Vejiga urinaria
Aperturas de los uréteres
Ampolla del conducto deferente
Saco rectovesical
Recto
Vesícula seminal
Conducto eyaculatorio
m. elevador del ano
Ligamento anococcígeo
Esfínter anal interno
Glándula y conducto bulbouretral
Esfínter anal externo
m. perineal transverso superficial
Epidídimo

Los órganos pélvicos masculinos (sección sagital)

tone; __ **de la visión** / __ of vision; __ **neural de la audición** / neural hearing __ .

perecedero-a *a.* perishable, that decomposes easily.

perenne *a.* perennial, that lasts more than one year.

perfeccionismo *m.* perfectionism, excessive drive to attain perfection, regardless of the importance of the task.

perfeccionista *m., f.* perfectionist.

perfecto-a *a.* perfect; **-mente** *adv.* perfectly.

perfil *m.* profile, side view; outline; __ **bioquímico** / biochemical __; __ **físico** / physical __ .

perforación *f.* perforation, hole.

perforar *vt.* to perforate; to pierce.

perfusión *f.* perfusion, passage of a liquid through a conduit.

periamigdalino-a *a.* peritonsillar, close to the tonsils.

perianal *a.* perianal, located around the anus.

pericardial, pericárdico-a *a.* pericardiac, pericardial, rel. to the pericardium; **derrame** __ , **efusión** __ / __ effusion; **vibración** __ / __ fremitus.

pericardiectomía *f.* pericardiectomy, partial or total excision of the pericardium.

pericardio *m.* pericardium, sac-like, double-layered membrane that surrounds the heart and the origins of the large blood vessels.

pericarditis *f.* pericarditis, infl. of the pericardium; __ **constrictiva** / constrictive __; __ **localizada** / localized __; __ **reumática** / rheumatic __ .

periferia *f.* periphery, part of a body or organ away from the center.

periférico-a *a.* peripheral, rel. to or occurring in the periphery; **sistema nervioso** __ / __ nervous system, the group of nerves situated outside the central nervous system.

perilla *f.* rubber bulb.

perinatal *a.* perinatal, rel. to or occurring before, during, or right after birth.

perinatología *f.* perinatology, study of the fetus and newborn during the perinatal period.

perineo *m.* perineum, the pelvic outlet bounded anteriorly by the scrotum in the man and the vulva in the woman, and posteriorly by the anus.

periódico *a.* periodic; **-mente** *adv.* periodically.

período *m.* period. 1. interval of time, epoch; __ **de tiempo** / time span.

periodo *m.* menstruation.

periodoncia *f.* periodontics, branch of odontology dealing with areas surrounding the teeth.

periodontal *a.* periodontal, surrounding the tooth.

periostio *m.* periosteum, thick fibrous membrane that covers the entire surface of the bone except the articular surface.

peristalsis *f.* peristalsis, wavelike contractions that occur in a tubular structure such as the alimentary canal, by which the contents are forced onward.

peritoneal *a.* peritoneal, rel. to the peritoneum.

peritoneo *m.* peritoneum, serous membrane that lines the abdominopelvic walls and the viscera.

peritonitis *f.* peritonitis, infl. of the peritoneum.

periuretral *a.* periurethral, around the urethra.

perjudicial *a.* detrimental, damaging.

perleche *Fr.* perleche, disorder manifested by fissures at the corner of the mouth, seen esp. in children and gen. as a result of malnutrition.

permanente *a.* permanent, lasting; **-mente** *adv.* permanently.

permeabilidad *f.* permeability, the quality of being permeable, not obstructed; __ **capilar** / capillary __ .

permeable *a.* permeable, allowing passage through structures such as a membrane.

permiso *m.* permit; consent.

permitir *vt.* to allow, to consent, to agree.

pernicioso-a *a.* pernicious, noxious, harmful.

pero *conj.* but.

peroné *m.* perone, fibula, calf bone, the outer and thinner of the two lower leg bones.

per rectum *L.* per rectum, by the rectum.

perseveración *f.* perseveration, mental disorder manifested by the abnormal repetition of an idea or action.

persistir *vt.* to persist, to persevere.

persona *f.* person. 1. individual;

2. outward personality that conceals the real one.

personal *m.* personnel; ___ **médico** / medical ___; *a.* personal, rel. to a person.

personalidad *f.* personality, traits, characteristics, and individual behavior that distinguish one person from another; ___ **anal** / anal ___; ___ **antisocial** / antisocial ___; ___ **compulsiva** / compulsive ___; ___ **esquizoide** / schizoid, split ___; ___ **extravertida** / extroverted ___; ___ **intravertida** / introverted ___; ___ **neurótica** / neurotic ___; ___ **paranoica** / paranoid ___; ___ **psicopática** / psychopathic ___ .

perspiración *f.* perspiration, exudation.

persuasión *f.* persuasion, therapeutic treatment that tries to deal with the patient through the use of reason.

perteneciente *a.* pertaining or rel. to.

perturbación *f.* perturbation. 1. feeling of uneasiness; 2. abnormal variation from a regular state.

pertussis *L.* pertussis, whooping cough.

perversión *f.* perversion, deviation from socially accepted behavior; ___ **sexual** / sexual ___ .

pervertido-a *m., f.* pervert, individual given to sexual perversion.

pesa *f.* weighing scale.

pesadilla *f.* nightmare.

pesario *m.* pessary, a rubber cup-shaped device that is introduced into the vagina to be used as a support to the uterus.

pescuezo *m.* neck.

pesimismo *m.* pessimism, an inclination to see and judge situations in their most unfavorable light.

pesimista *m., f.* pessimist; *a.* pessimist, rel. to, or that manifests pessimism.

peso *m.* weight; **aumento de** ___ / gain; **falto de, bajo de** ___ / underweight; **pérdida de** ___ / ___ loss; ___ **al nacer** / birth ___ .

pestañas *f. pl.* eyelashes.

pestañear *v.* to blink, to wink.

pestañeo *m.* blink; blinking.

peste *f.* 1. bubonic plague, an epidemic infectious disease transmitted by the bite of infected rats or fleas; 2. plague, any epidemic contagious disease with a high rate of mortality; 3. foul smell.

peste neumónica *f.* pneumonic plague, pulmonary plague, a form of plague with symptoms of bloody sputum, chills and high fever that can be lethal.

pesticida *m.* pesticide, chemical agent that kills insects and other pests.

petequia *f.* petechiae, minute hemorrhagic spots in the skin and the mucosa that can appear in connection with some severe fevers such as typhoid.

petit mal *Fr.* petit mal, benign epileptic attack with loss of consciousness at times, but with no convulsions.

peyote *m.* peyote, plant from which the hallucinatory drug mescaline is obtained.

pezón *m.* nipple; ___ **agrietado** / cracked ___; ___ **enlechado** / engorged ___; ___ **umbilicado** / retracted ___ .

pH *m.* Potential of Hydrogen. Indicates the degree of acidity or alkalinity of a substance; ___ **cutáneo** / cutaneous ___; ___ **sanguíneo** / blood ___ .

piamadre *f.* pia mater, thin vascular membrane, the innermost of the three cerebral meninges.

pica *f.* pica, a craving for inedible substances.

picada, picadura *f.* sting, bite.

picante *a.* piquant, highly seasoned.

picar *vt.* to bite; to pierce, to prick; to itch; [*mosquito*] to sting.

picazón *f.* itching.

Pick, enfermedad de *f.* Pick's disease, type of senile dementia.

pie *m.* foot; ___ **de atleta** / athlete's ___ , dermatofitosis; ___ **en extensión** / footdrop; ___ **plano** / flatfoot; **planta del** ___ / sole; *v.* **estar de** ___ / to be standing; **ir a** ___ / to go on foot; *vr.* **ponerse de** ___ / to stand up.

pie de trinchera *m.* trench foot, infectious condition of the feet resulting from long exposure to cold.

piedra *f.* stone, calculus.

piel *f.* skin; hide, epidermis; **cáncer de la** ___ / ___ cancer; **fricción de la** ___ / skin chafing; **injerto de** ___ / ___ graft. See illustration on page 194.

pielitis *f.* pyelitis, infl. of the renal pelvis.

pielograma *m.* pyelogram, x-ray of the renal pelvis and the ureter using a contrasting medium.

pielolitotomía *f.* pyelolithotomy, incision to remove a calculus from the renal pelvis.

pielonefritis

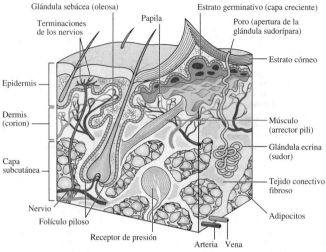

Glándula sebácea (oleosa)
Terminaciones de los nervios
Papila
Estrato germinativo (capa creciente)
Poro (apertura de la glándula sudorípara)
Estrato córneo
Epidermis
Dermis (corion)
Músculo (arrector pili)
Glándula ecrina (sudor)
Capa subcutánea
Tejido conectivo fibroso
Nervio
Adipocitos
Folículo piloso
Receptor de presión
Arteria   Vena

Corte transversal de la piel

pielonefritis *f.* pyelonephritis, infl. of the kidney and renal pelvis.

pieloplastia *f.* pyeloplasty, plastic surgery of the renal pelvis.

pielotomía *f.* pyelotomy, incision of the renal pelvis.

pierna *f.* leg, lower extremity that extends from the knee to the ankle; ___ **arqueada** / bowleg, genu varum; **traumatismo de la** ___ / ___ injury.

pigmentación *f.* pigmentation.

pigmento *m.* pigment, coloring element.

píldora *f.* pill; ___ **de control del embarazo** / birth control ___ .

piliación *f.* piliation, formation and development of hair.

pilórico-a *a.* pyloric, rel. to the pylorus.

píloro *m.* pylorus, the lower aperture of the stomach that opens into the duodenum.

piloroplastia *f.* pyloroplasty, plastic surgery to repair the pylorus.

pinchar *v.* to prick.

pinchazo *m.* prick, jab; cut.

pinna *L.* pinna, ear lap.

pinzas *f., pl.* clip, forceps, pincers, tweezers, devices used to assist in the extraction process; ___ **de secuestro** / sequestrum forceps.

piógeno-a *a.* pyogenic, that produces pus.

piojo *m.* louse, parasite that is the primary transmitter of some diseases such as typhus.

piorrea *f.* pyorrhea, periodontitis.

pipeta *f.* pipette, a narrow glass tube.

pirámide *f.* pyramid, a cone-shaped structure of the body such as the medulla oblongata.

pirético *m.* pyretic, rel. to fever.

pirexia *f.* pyrexia, high temperature; fever.

pirógeno *m.* pyrogen, agent that elevates a fever.

piscina *f.* swimming pool.

piso *m.* floor; ground.

pituitaria, glándula *f.* pituitary gland.

placa *f.* 1. plate, flat structure such as a thin layer of bone; 2. plate, thin layer of metal used to support a structure; 3. plaque, a patch on the skin or mucous membrane; 4. x-ray

placebo *m.* placebo, harmless substance of no medical value, gen. used for experimental purposes.

placenta *f.* placenta, vascular organ that develops in the wall of the uterus, through which the fetus derives its nourishment; ___ **previa** / ___ previa, placenta situated before the fetus in relation to the cervical opening, that may cause severe hemorrhaging.

placentario-a *a.* placental, rel. to the placenta; **insuficiencia** __ / __ insufficiency.

plaga *f.* plague, epidemic infectious disease.

plan *m.* plan; design.

planificación familiar *f.* family planning.

planilla *f.* [*formulario*] form.

plano *m.* plane. 1. flat surface; 2. a relatively smooth surface formed by making an imaginary or real cut through a part of the body; __ **axial** / axial __; __ **coronal** / coronal __; __ **frontal** / frontal __; __ **horizontal** / horizontal __; __ **medio** / midplane; __ **sagital** / sagittal __ .

planta *f.* plant; __ **del pie** / sole of the foot; __ **-s medicinales** [*hierbas*] / medicinal __ -s or herbs.

plantar *a.* plantar, rel. to the sole of the foot; **reflejo** __ / __ reflex, Babinski's reflex.

plaqueta *f.* platelet, thrombocyte, an element of the blood in the form of minute disks, essential to coagulation; **conteo de** __ **-s** / __ count.

plasma *f.* plasma, liquid component of the blood and lymph, made of 91 percent water and 9 percent of a combination of elements such as proteins, salts, nutrients, and vitamins.

plasticidad *f.* plasticity, the capacity to be molded.

plástico *m.* plastic; **-a** *a.* plastic.

platicar *vi.* to converse, to talk.

plétora *f.* plethora, an excess of any one of the body fluids.

pleura *f.* pleura, doublefold membrane that covers each lung; __ **parietal** / parietal __; __ **visceral** / visceral __ .

pleural *a.* pleural, rel. to the pleura; **cavidad** __ / __ cavity; **derrame** __ / __ effusion.

pleuresía *f.* pleurisy, infl. of the pleura.

pleuroscopía *f.* pleuroscopy, inspection of the pleural cavity through an incision into the thorax.

plexo *m.* plexus, an interlacing of nerves, blood, or lymphatic vessels.

pliegue *m.* fold.

plomo *m.* lead; **delantal de** __ / __ apron; **envenenamiento por** __ / __ poisoning; **sonda de** __ / __ probe.

plumbismo *m.* plumbism, chronic lead poisoning.

población *f.* population.

pobre *a.* poor.

poción *f.* draft, potion, a single dose of liquid medicine.

poco-a *a.* little, in small quantity; *adv.* little, small; **dentro de** __ / in a short while; __ **a** __ / little by little; **por** __ / almost.

poder *m.* power, strength; *vi.* to be able to; to have the power to.

podíatra *m., f.* podiatrist, specialist in podiatry.

podiatría *f.* podiatry, the diagnosis and treatment of conditions affecting the feet.

podrido-a *a.* rotten, decomposed.

polaridad *f.* polarity. 1. the quality of having two poles; 2. the quality of presenting opposite effects.

polen *m.* pollen; **conteo de** __ / __ count.

poliarticular *a.* polyarticular, affecting more than one joint.

poliartritis *f.* polyarthritis, infl. of more than one joint.

policístico-a *a.* polycystic, composed of many cysts; **enfermedad** __ **del riñón** / __ kidney disease; **síndrome** __ **ovárico** / __ ovarian síndrome.

policitemia *f.* polycythemia, excess of red blood cells; __ **primaria** / primary __ , vera; __ **rubra** / __ rubra, vera; __ **secundaria** / secondary __ , erythrocythemia; __ **vera** / __ vera, erythremia.

policlínica *f.* polyclinic, a general hospital.

polidactilia *f.* polydactylia, polydactyly, the presence of more than five fingers or toes.

polidipsia *f.* polydipsia, excessive thirst.

polígrafo *m.* polygraph, device that registers simultaneously the arterial and venous pulsations.

poli-insaturado-a *a.* polyunsaturated, denoting a fatty acid.

polimialgia *f.* polymyalgia, condition characterized by pain affecting several muscles.

polimorfonucleado-a, polimorfonuclear *a.* polymorphonuclear, having a deeply lobed nucleus; **granulocito** __ / __ granulocyte, having a nucleus with multiple lobes.

polineuropatía *f.* polyneuropathy, any disease that affects several nerves at one time.

polio, poliomielitis

polio, poliomielitis *f.* polio, poliomyelitis, contagious disease that attacks the central nervous system and causes paralysis of the muscles, esp. of the legs.

poliomiopatía *f.* polymyopathy, any disease that affects several muscles at the same time.

poliovirus *m.* poliovirus, causative agent of poliomyelitis.

polipectomía *f.* polypectomy, excision of a polyp.

pólipo *m.* polyp, tag, mass, or growth protruding from a mucous membrane.

poliposis *f.* polyposis, formation of multiple polyps.

poliquístico-a *a.* polycystic, having many cysts.

polisacárido *m.* polysaccharide, a carbohydrate capable of hydrolysis.

poliuria *f.* polyuria, excessive secretion and elimination of urine.

póliza de seguro *f.* insurance policy.

polo *m.* pole, each of the two opposite extremes of a body, organ, or part.

polución *f.* pollution.

polución de ruido *f.* noise pollution.

polvo *m.* dust; powder; **en ___ /** powdered.

pomada *f.* ointment, pomade, salve, semisolid medicinal substance for external use; **___ contraceptiva /** contraceptive jelly; **___ facial /** cold cream; **___ vaginal /** vaginal jelly.

pómulo *m.* molar bone, cheekbone.

poner *vt.* to put, to set, to lay down; **ponerse** *vr.* [*vestido*] to put on; to become; **___ viejo /** to grow or become old.

pons *L.* pons, tissue formation that connects two separate parts of an organ.

poplíteo-a *a.* popliteal, rel. to the area behind the knee.

por *prep.* for, by, through, from; **___ ahora /** for the time being; **___ atrás /** from or through the back; **___ delante /** from or through the front; **___ eso /** because of that; **___ lo tanto /** therefore.

porcino-a *a.* porcine, rel. to swine.

porción *f.* portion.

porfiria *f.* porphyria, congenital defect in metabolism manifested by the presence of great amounts of porphyrin in the blood, urine, and stools causing physical and psychiatric disorders.

poro, porus *m.* pore, porus, minute opening of the skin such as the duct of a sweat gland.

poroso-a *a.* porous, permeable.

porque *conj.* because, for the reason that; *interr.* **¿por qué? /** why?, for what reason?

porta *L.* porta, opening or entry, esp. one through which blood vessels and nerves penetrate into an organ.

porta, vena *f.* portal vein, short, thick trunk formed by branches of many veins leading from abdominal organs.

portacatéter *m.* catheter holder.

portacava *a.* portacaval, rel. to the porta and the inferior vena cava.

portador *m.* carrier, a disease causing agent that can be transmitted to other individuals; **___ de bacilos /** bacillicarrier.

portal *m.* portal, entryway; *a.* rel. to the portal system.

portal, circulación *f.* portal circulation, flow of blood into the liver via the portal vein and out via the hepatic vein.

portal, hipertensión *f.* portal hypertension, increase in pressure in the portal vein due to an obstruction in blood circulation in the liver.

portaobjeto *m.* slide, specimen holder for microscopic examination.

poseído-a *a., pp.* de **poseer**, possessed, dominated by an idea or passion.

posibilidad *f.* possibility.

posible *a.* possible; **-mente** *adv.* possibly.

posición *f.* position; **___ anatómica /** anatomic ___; **___ de litotomía /** lithotomy ___; **___ distal /** distal ___; **___ dorsal recumbente /** dorsal recumbent ___; **___ erecta /** upright ___; **___ en decúbito /** decubitus ___; **___ genucubital /** genocubital ___, knee-elbow; **___ genupectoral /** knee-chest ___; **___ inadecuada /** malposition; **___ lateral /** lateral ___; **___ prona /** prone ___, face down; **___ supina, yacente /** supine ___, face up.

positividad *f.* positivity, manifestation of a positive reaction.

positivo-a *a.* positive; certain, without doubt.

posponer *vt.* to postpone, to delay.

posterior *a.* posterior. 1. rel. to the back or the back part of a structure; 2. following in sequence.

posthipnótico-a *a.* posthypnotic, following the hypnotic state.

postictal *a.* postictal, following a seizure or attack.

postmaduro *a.* postmature, rel. to an infant born after the forty-first week of gestation.

post mortem *L.* postmortem, occurring after death; autopsy.

postnasal *a.* postnasal, behind the nose.

postparto *m.* postpartum, period of time following childbirth; **depresión del __ / __** depression; **insuficiencia pituitaria del __ / __** pituitary insufficiency; **psicosis del __ / __** psychosis.

postoperatorio-a *a.* postoperative, following surgery; **complicación __ / __** complication; **cuidado __ / __** care.

postración *f.* prostration, exhaustion, extreme fatigue.

postrado-a *a.* prostrate. 1. **__ en cama /** confined to bed; 2. exhausted, debilitated.

póstumo-a *a.* posthumous, occurring after death; **examen __ /** postmortem examination.

postura *f.* posture, position of the body.

postural *a.* postural, rel. to position or posture; **hipotensión __ / __** hypotension, decrease in blood pressure in an erect position.

potable *a.* potable, drinkable, that can be drunk without harm.

potasemia *f.* kalemia, presence of potassium in the blood.

potasio *m.* potassium, mineral which, combined with others in the body, is essential in the transmission of nerve impulses and in muscular activity.

potencia *f.* potency, strength.

potencial *m.* potential, electric pressure or tension; *a.* having a ready disposition or capacity.

potente *a.* potent, strong.

práctica *f.* practice.

practicar *vt.* to practice.

práctico-a *a.* practical.

prandial *a.* prandial, rel. to meals.

preagónico-a *a.* preagonal, rel. to a condition preceding death.

preanestésico *m.* preanesthetic, preliminary agent given to ease the administration of general anesthesia.

precanceroso-a *a.* precancerous, tending to become malignant.

precario-a *a.* precarious, uncertain.

precaución *f.* precaution.

preceder *v.* to precede.

precio *m.* price, cost.

precisión *f.* precision, exactness.

precocidad *f.* precocity, early development of physical or mental adult traits.

precoz *a.* precocious.

precursor *m.* precursor, something that precedes, such as a symptom or sign of a disease; **precursor-a** *a.* introductory, preliminary.

predisposición *f.* predisposition, propensity to develop a condition or illness, caused by environmental, genetic, or psychological factors.

predispuesto-a *a.* predisposed, prone or susceptible to develop a disease or any other condition.

predominante *a.* predominant.

preeclampsia *f.* preeclampsia, a toxic condition of late pregnancy, manifested by hypertension, albuminuria, and edema.

preferible *a.* preferable.

preferir *vt.* to prefer, to favor one thing, person, or condition over another.

pregunta *f.* question; *v.* **hacer una __ /** to ask a __ .

preguntar *vt.* to ask, to inquire.

prejuicio *m.* prejudice, bias.

preliminar *a.* preliminary.

prematuro-a *m., f.* premature baby; *a.* 1. born prior to the thirty-seventh week of gestation; 2. *pop.* preemie.

premedicación *f.* premedication.

premenstrual *a.* premenstrual; **tensión __ / __** tension.

premonitorio-a *a.* premonitory; **advertencia o señal __ / __** signal; **síntoma __ / __** symptom.

prenatal *a.* prenatal, prior to birth; **cuidado __ / __** care.

preñada *a. pop.* pregnant.

preocupación *f.* preoccupation, concern.

preocupado-a *a.* concerned, worried.

preocuparse *vr.* to worry, to be preoccupied; **no se preocupe, no te preocupes /** don't worry.

preoperativo-a *a.* preoperative; **cuidado __ / __** care.

preparación *f.* preparation. 1. the act of making something ready; 2. a medication ready for use.

preparar *v.* to prepare, to make ready.

prepubescente *a.* prepubescent, before puberty.

prepucio *m.* prepuce, foreskin, loose fold of skin that covers the glans penis.

prerrenal *a.* prerenal. 1. in front of the kidney; 2. that occurs in the circulatory system before reaching the kidney.

p

presbiopía

presbiopía *f.* presbyopia, farsightedness that occurs with increasing age due to the loss of elasticity of the lens of the eye.

prescribir *vi.* to prescribe.

prescripción *f.* prescription.

presencia *f.* presence.

presentación *f.* presentation. 1. position of the fetus in the uterus as detected upon examination; 2. position of the fetus in reference to the birth canal at the time of delivery; __ **cefálica** / cephalic __; __ **de cara** / face __; __ **de nalgas** / breech __; __ **transversa**/transverse __; 3. oral report.

presente *a.* present, manifest; *n.* [*presencia*] presence; *v.* to be present physically and psycologically assisting a patient when the patient needs it.

preservación *f.* preservation, conservation.

preservar *vt.* to preserve.

preservativo *m.* preservative. 1. agent that is added to food or medication to destroy or impede multiplication of bacteria; 2. condom.

presión *f.* pressure, stress, strain, tension; __ **arterial** / arterial __ , pressure exerted by the blood in the arteries; __ **atmosférica** / atmospheric __ , pressure exerted by the mass of air surrounding the earth; __ **central venosa** / central venous __ , blood pressure of the right atrium of the heart; __ **del pulso** / pulse __ , the difference between sistolic and diastolic pressure; __ **diastólica** / diastolic __ , lowest arterial blood pressure during diastole of the heart; __ **intracraneana** / intracranial __ , pressure exerted within the cranium; __ **osmótica** / osmotic __ ; __ **parcial** / partial __ , pressure exerted by a single gas component in a single, mixed composition; __ **sistólica** / systolic __ , arterial blood pressure during contraction of the ventricles; __ **venosa** / venous __ , pressure exerted by the blood on the walls of the veins; *v.* **hacer** __ / to exert pressure.

presión sanguínea *f.* blood pressure, pressure by the blood on the arteries, produced by the action of the left ventricle, the resistance of the arterioles and capillaries, the elasticity of the arterial walls, and the viscosity and volume of the blood expressed in relation to the atmospheric pressure; __ **alta** / high __; __ **baja** / low __; __ **normal** / normal __ .

presor *a.* pressor, that tends to raise the blood pressure.

pretender *v.* to attempt, to try.

pretérmino *m.* preterm, occurring during the period of time prior to the thirty-seventh week in a pregnancy.

prevalencia *f.* prevalence, the total number of cases of a specific disease present in a given population at a certain time.

prevención *f.* prevention.

preventivo-a *a.* preventive; **servicios de salud** __ / __ health services.

previo-a *a.* previous, prior.

previsto-a *a., pp.* de **prever**, foreseen.

priapismo *m.* priapism, painful and continued erection of the penis as a result of disease.

primario-a *a.* primary, initial; chief, principal.

primeriza *f.* primipara, a woman who has given birth to a child for the first time.

primeros auxilios *m., pl.* first aid.

primitivo-a *a.* primitive; embryonic.

primo-a *m., f.* cousin.

primogénito-a *a.* first-born.

principal *a.* main, principal, foremost; **-mente** *adv.* primarily, mainly.

principio *m.* 1. beginning, start; 2. principle, chief ingredient of a medication or chemical compound; 3. principle, rule.

principio del placer *m.* pleasure principle, behavior directed at obtaining immediate gratification and avoiding pain.

principio de la realidad *m.* reality principle, orientation to reality and self-gratification through awareness of the outside world.

prioridad *f.* priority, precedence.

privación *f.* privation, hardship; withdrawal.

privado-a *a.* private; **cuarto** __ / private room; **-mente** *adv.* privately.

privilegio *m.* privilege.

probabilidad *f.* probability.

probable *a.* probable; **-mente** *adv.* probably.

probar *vi.* [*esfuerzo*] to try; [*gusto*] to taste; [*comprobar*] to prove; to sample.

probeta *f.* pipette, glass tube.

problema *m.* problem; trouble.

proceder *v.* to proceed, to continue.

procedimiento *m.* procedure; __ **clínico** / clinical __; __ **quirúrgico** / surgical __; __ **terapéutico** / therapeutic __ .

proceso *m.* process, method, system.

procrear *v.* to procreate, to beget.

proctalgia *f.* proctalgia, pain in the rectum and anus.

proctitis *f.* proctitis, infl. of the rectum and the anus.

proctólogo-a *m., f.* proctologist, specialist in proctology.

proctoscopio *m.* proctoscope, endoscope used to examine the rectum.

prodrómico-a *a.* prodromal, rel. to the initial stages of a disease.

producir *vt.* to produce.

productivo-a *a.* productive.

producto *m.* product; result or effect.

profesión *f.* profession.

profesional *m., f.* professional; *a.* professional.

profiláctico-a *a.* prophylactic. 1. agent or method used to prevent infection; 2. condom.

profilaxis *f.* prophylaxis, preventive treatment.

profunda *L.* profunda, deep, esp. in reference to the location of some arteries.

profundo-a *a.* deep; **anillo inguinal** __ / __ inguinal ring; **arteria** __ **del brazo** / __ artery of the arm; **arteria** __ **del clítoris** / __ artery of the clitoris; **arteria** __ **del pene** / __ artery of the penis; **trombosis venenosa** __ / __ venous thrombosis; **venas cerebrales** __ / __ cerebral veins; **venas cervicales** __ / __ cervical veins; **vena facial** __ / __ facial vein.

profuso-a *a.* profuse, plentiful; **-mente** *adv.* profusely.

progesterona *f.* progesterone, steroid hormone secreted by the ovaries.

programar *vt.* to schedule; to program.

progresar *vi.* to advance; to improve; to thrive.

progresivo-a *a.* progressive, advancing.

progreso *m.* progress.

prolapso *m.* prolapse, the falling down or slipping of a body part from its usual position.

proliferación *f.* proliferation, multiplication, esp. of similar cells; __ **excesiva** / overgrowth.

prolífico-a *a.* prolific, that multiplies readily.

prolongar *vi.* to prolong, to delay.

Propiedades	Properties
abundante	abundant
alto	tall
amargo	bitter
bajo	[*estatura*] short
caliente	hot
claro	clear
dulce	sweet
espeso	thick
fresco	cool
frío	cold
fuerte	strong
grasoso	fatty
grueso, gordo	heavy, fat
húmedo	humid, moist
largo	long
ligero	light
líquido	liquid
mojado	wet
pesado	[*peso*] heavy
pobre	poor
rico	rich
seco	dry
sólido	solid
sucio	dirty
tibio	lukewarm

promedio *m.* average.

promesa *f.* promise.

prometer *v.* to promise, to give one's word.

prominencia *f.* prominence, elevation of a part; projection.

pronar *v.* to pronate, to put the body or a body part in a prone position.

prono-a *a.* prone, lying in a face down position.

pronosticar *vi.* to prognosticate, to predict.

pronóstico *m.* prognosis, evaluation of the probable course of an illness.

pronto *adv.* soon, fast, quickly; **por lo** __ / for the time being.

propagación *f.* propagation, reproduction.

propenso-a *a.* predisposed to; __ **a** / inclined to.

propiedad *f.* property. 1. possessions; 2. quality that distinguishes a person, specie, or object from another. See table on this page.

propioceptivo-a

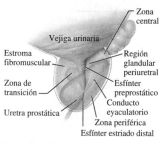

Zona central
Vejiga urinaria
Región glandular periuretral
Estroma fibromuscular
Esfínter preprostático
Zona de transición
Conducto eyaculatorio
Uretra prostática
Zona periférica
Esfínter estriado distal

La próstata

propioceptivo-a *a.* proprioceptive, capable of receiving stimulations originating within the tissues of the body.

propioceptor *m.* proprioceptor, sensory nerve ending that reacts to stimuli and gives information concerning movements and position of the body.

propósito *m.* purpose; **a __** / on purpose, by the way.

proptosis *f.* proptosis, forward displacement of a part, such as the eyeball.

prosencéfalo *m.* prosencephalon, anterior portion of the primary cerebral vesicle from which the diencephalon and the telencephalon develop.

próstata *f.* prostate, male gland that surrounds the bladder and the urethra; **hipertrofia de la __** / prostatic hypertrophy, benign enlargement of the prostate. See illustration on this page.

prostatectomía *f.* prostatectomy, partial or total excision of the prostate **__ con laser** / laser **__**; **__ perineal** / perineal **__**; **__ radical** / radical **__**; **__ trasvesical** / trasvesical **__**.

prostático-a *a.* prostatic, rel. to the prostate.

prostatismo *m.* prostatism, disorder resulting from obstruction of the bladder neck by an enlarged prostate.

prostatitis *f.* prostatitis, infl. of the prostate.

protección *f.* protection.

proteína *f.* protein, nitrogen compound essential in the development and preservation of body tissues.

proteinemia *f.* proteinemia,

concentration of proteins in the blood.

proteínico-a *a.* proteinic, rel. to protein; **balance __** / protein balance.

proteinosis *f.* proteinosis, excess protein in the tissues.

proteinuria *f.* proteinuria, the presence of protein in the urine.

prótesis *f.* prosthesis, artificial replacement of a missing part of the body, such as a limb.

protética *f.* prosthetics. 1. the art of manufacturing and adjusting artificial parts for the human body; 2. branch of surgery concerned with the replacement of parts of the body.

protocolo *m.* protocol. 1. a record taken from notes; 2. a written proposal of a procedure to be performed; **__ toxicológico** / toxicology screen.

protoplasma *m.* protoplasm, essential part of the cell that includes the cytoplasm and the nucleus.

prototipo *m.* prototype, role-model, example.

protozoario-a *a.* protozoan, rel. to protozoa.

protozoo *m.* protozoan, unicellular organism.

protracción *f.* protraction, extension of teeth or other structures of the jaw into a position anterior to their normal position.

protrombina *f.* prothrombin, one of the four major plasma proteins along with albumin, globulin, and fibrinogen.

protrusión *f.* protrusion, condition of being projected forward.

protuberancia *f.* protuberance, prominence.

provechoso-a *a.* beneficial.

proveer *vi.* to provide, to administer.

provisional *a.* provisional, temporary.

proximal *a.* proximal, closest to the point of reference.

próximo-a *a.* next to, close by.

proyección *f.* projection. 1. protuberance; 2. a mechanism by which one's own unacceptable ideas or traits are attributed to others.

prueba *f.* test, proof, trial; indication; **a __ de agua** / waterproof; **a __ de fuego** / fireproof; **__ antinuclear de anticuerpo** / antinuclear antibody **__**; **__ controlada por placebo** / placebo-controlled **__**; **__ cutánea** / skin **__**; **__ de aclaramiento de creatinina** / creatinine clearance **__**; **__ de ciego simple** / single-blind trial;

___ **de coagulación sanguínea** / blood coagulation ___; ___ **de control sin método** / random controlled trial; ___ **de doble incógnita** / double-blind trial; ___ **de esfuerzo** / stress ___ , treadmill; ___ **de función hepática** / liver function ___; ___ **de función respiratoria** / respiratory function ___; ___ **de función tiroidea** / thyroid function ___; ___ **de grasa fecal** / stool fat ___; ___ **de rasguño** / scratch ___ , allergy ___; ___ **de resistencia** / endurance ___; ___ **de tiempo limitado** / timed ___; ___ **de tipo** / type ___; ___ **de tolerancia** / tolerance ___; ___ **de tolerancia a la glucosa** / glucose tolerance ___; ___ **del embarazo** / pregnancy ___; ___ **eliminatoria** / screening ___; **hay** ___ / there is an indication; **resultado de la** ___ / results of the ___; ___ **-s sanguíneas cruzadas** / crossmatching ___ -s; ___ **serológica** / serology ___; ___ **sin pronóstico o tratamiento cierto** / double-blind technique; ___ **subsecuente, de seguimiento** / follow-up ___; ___ **visual de campimetría** / visual field ___; ___ **visual de letras** / visual ___ .

prueba del funcionamiento del páncreas *f.* pancreatic function test.

prurigo *m.* prurigo, chronic inflammatory condition of the skin characterized by small papules and severe itching.

prurito *m.* pruritus, severe itching.

pseudoaneurismo *m.* pseudoaneurysm, an aneurysm-like dilation in a vessel.

pseudoembarazo *m.* pseudopregnancy, false or imaginary pregnancy.

pseudoquiste *m.* pseudocyst, cyst-like formation.

psicoanálisis *m.* psychoanalysis, branch of psychiatry founded by Sigmund Freud that endeavors to make the patient conscious of repressed conflicts through techniques such as interpretation of dreams and free association of ideas.

psicoanalista *m., f.* psychoanalyst, one who practices psychoanalysis.

psicodélico-a *a.* psychedelic, rel. to a substance that can induce pathological states of altered perception such as hallucinations and delusions.

psicodrama *m.* psychodrama, the psychiatric method of diagnosis and therapy by which the patient acts out conflicting situations of his or her real life.

psicofarmacología *f.* psychopharmacology, the study of the effect of drugs on the mind and behavior.

psicofisiológico-a *a.* psychophysiologic, rel. to the mind's influence on bodily processes, as manifested in some disorders or diseases.

psicofisiológicos, desórdenes *m., pl.* psycho-physiologic disorders, disorders that result from the relation between psychological and physiological processes.

psicología *f.* psychology, the study of mental processes, esp. as related to the individual's environment.

psicología del desarrollo mental *f.* psychology of mental development.

psicólogo-a *m., f.* psychologist, person who practices psychology.

psicomotor-a *a.* psychomotor, rel. to motor actions that result from mental activity.

psicópata *m., f.* psychopath, sociopath, person suffering from an antisocial personality disorder.

psicopatología *f.* psychopathology, the branch of medicine that deals with the causes and nature of mental illness.

psicosis *f.* psychosis, severe mental disorder of organic or emotional origin in which the patient loses touch with reality and suffers hallucinations and mental aberrations; ___ **alcohólica** / alcoholic ___; ___ **depresiva** / depressive ___; ___ **maniacodepresiva** / manic-depressive ___; ___ **orgánica** / organic ___; ___ **por droga** / drug-related ___; ___ **senil** / senile ___; ___ **situacional** / situational ___; ___ **tóxica** / toxic ___; ___ **traumática** / traumatic ___ .

psicosocial *a.* psychosocial, rel. to both psychological and social factors.

psicosomático-a *a.* psychosomatic, rel. to both mind and body; **síntoma** ___ / ___ symptom.

psicoterapia *f.* psychotherapy, the treatment of mental or emotional disorders through psychological means, such as psychoanalysis.

psicótico-a *a.* psychotic, rel. to or suffering from psychosis.

psicotrópicas, drogas *f.*
psychotropic drugs, drugs capable of affecting mental functions or behavior.

psique *f.* psyche, conscious and unconscious mental life.

psiquiatra *m., f.* psychiatrist, specialist in psychiatry.

psiquiatría *f.* psychiatry, the study of the psyche and its disorders.

psiquiátrico-a *a.* psychiatric, rel. to psychiatry.

psíquico-a *a.* psychic, rel. to the psyche.

psoas *Gr.* psoas, one of the two muscles of the loin.

psoriasis *f.* psoriasis, chronic dermatitis manifested chiefly by red patches covered with white scales.

ptosis *Gr.* ptosis, prolapse of an organ or part, such as the upper eyelid.

púbero-a *a.* pubescent, having reached puberty.

pubertad *f.* puberty, the period of adolescence that marks the development of the secondary sexual characteristics and the beginning of reproductive capacity.

pubescencia *f.* pubescence. 1. beginning of puberty; 2. covering of soft, fine hair, lanugo.

púbico-a *a.* pubic, rel. to the pubis; **pelo** ___ / hair.

pudendum *L.* pudendum, external sexual organs, esp. the female.

puente *m.* bridge; ___ **coronario** / coronary ___; ___ **dental** / dental ___ .

pueril *a.* puerile. 1. rel. to a child; 2. childish.

puerperal *a.* puerperal, rel. to the puerperium.

pues *conj.* therefore; then; so.

pujar *vt.* to bear down.

pulga *f.* flea, blood-sucking insect.

pulgar *m.* the thumb.

pulmón *m.* lung, respiratory organ situated inside the pleural cavity of the thorax, connected to the pharynx through the trachea and the larynx; **cáncer del** ___ / ___ cancer; **colapso del** ___ / collapse of the ___ .

pulmón de granjero *m.* farmer's lung, hypersensitivity of the pulmonary alveoli caused by exposure to fermented hay.

pulmón de hierro *m.* iron lung, machine used to produce artificial respiration.

pulmonar *a.* pulmonary, pulmonic, rel. to the lungs or to the pulmonary artery; **absceso** ___ / lung abscess; **arteria** ___ / ___ artery; **elasticidad** ___ / lung elasticity; **embolismo** ___ / ___ embolism; **enfisema** ___ / ___ emphysema; **estenosis** ___ / ___ stenosis; **hemorragia** ___ / ___ hemorrhage; **insuficiencia** ___ / ___ insufficiency; **presión diferencial de la arteria** ___ / ___ artery wedge pressure; **proteinosis alveolar** ___ / ___ alveolar proteinosis; **válvula** ___ / ___ valve; **vena** ___ / ___ vein; **volumen** ___ / lung capacity.

pulmonía *f.* pneumonia. neumonia.

pulpa *f.* pulp. 1. soft part on an organ; 2. chyme; 3. soft inner part of a tooth.

pulsación *f.* pulsation, throbbing, rhythmic beat such as the heart.

pulso *m.* pulse, rhythmic arterial dilation gen. coinciding with the heartbeat. See table on this page.

punción *f.* puncture, perforation, the act of perforating a tissue with a sharp instrument.

punto *m.* 1. stitch; 2. point, a position in time or space; *v.* **estar a ___ de** / to be on the verge of; 3. spot; ___ **ciego** / blind ___; 4. *gr.* period.

puntos de presión *m., pl.* pressure points, points in an artery where the pulse can be felt or where pressure can be exerted to control bleeding.

puntual *a.* punctual, prompt, on time.

punzada *f.* twinge; sharp, sudden pain; jab.

Pulso	Pulse
alternante	alternating
bigeminado	bigeminal
de la arteria dorsal del pie	dorsalis pedis
en martillo de agua	water hammer
femoral	femoral
filiforme	filiform
irregular	irregular
lleno	full
periférico	peripheral
radial	radial
rápido	rapid
regular	regular
saltón	bounding

punzante *a.* piercing, sharp.

puño *m.* fist; **cerrar el ___** / to make a fist.

pupila *f.* pupil, contractile opening of the iris of the eye that allows the passage of light; **___ saltona** / bounding ___; **___ fija** / fixed ___ .

pupilar *a.* pupillary, rel. to the pupil.

purga *f.* purge, cathartic medication.

purgante *m.* purgative, laxative, agent used to cause evacuation of the intestines; **___ de sal** / saline cathartic.

purgar *vt.* 1. to purge, to clean; 2. to force intestinal evacuation by means of a purgative.

purificado-a *a.* purified; **agua ___** / ___ water.

puro-a *a.* pure, uncontaminated.

púrpura *L.* purpura, condition characterized by reddish or purple spots that result from the escape of blood into tissues; **___ trombocitopénica** / thrombocytopenic ___ .

purulencia *f.* purulence, the condition of being purulent.

purulento-a *a.* purulent, containing pus, pus-like.

pus *f.* pus, thick, yellowish fluid that results from inflammation; **supuración de ___** / pus discharge.

pústula *f.* pustule, sore, small elevation of the skin filled with pus.

putrefacción *f.* putrefaction, the process of decomposing.

P

q

q *abr. L.* quaque / cada; **quaque** /
every.
quadratus *L.* quadratus. 1. four-sided
muscle; 2. four-sided figure.
quebradizo-a *a.* brittle, that breaks
easily.
Queckenstedt, signo de *m.*
Queckenstedt's sign, little or no
increase in the pressure of the
cerebrospinal fluid when there is
compression of the jugular vein; in
healthy persons the pressure rises
rapidly on compression.
queilitis *f.* cheilitis, infl. of the lip.
queiloplastia *f.* cheiloplasty, plastic
surgery of the lip.
queilosis *f.* cheilosis, disorder caused
by a deficiency of vitamin B_2 complex
(riboflavin) and marked by fissures at
the angles of the lips.
queilosquisis *f.* cheiloschisis.
See **labio leporino**.
queirología *f.* cheirology. 1. the study
of the hand; 2. sign language.
queja *f.* complaint, grievance; ___
principal / chief ___ .
quejarse *vr.* to complain; to whine.
queloide *m.* keloid, thick, reddish scar
formation following a wound or
surgical incision.
quelolisis *f.* kelolysis, destruction of
ketone bodies.
quemadura *f.* burn; ___ **de primer,
segundo, tercer grado** / first-, second-,
third-degree ___ ; ___ **de sol** / sunburn;
___ **por frío** / frostbite; ___ **por
radiación** / radiation ___ ; ___ **por
viento** / windburn.
quemazón *m.* burning; [comezón],
itching.
queratina *f.* keratin, organic, insoluble
protein component of nails, skin, and
hair.
queratinización *f.* keratinization,
process by which cells become horny
due to a deposit of keratin.
queratitis *f.* keratitis, infl. of the
cornea; ___ **intersticial** / interstitial ___ ;
___ **micótica** / mycotic ___ , caused by
fungus; ___ **trófica** / trophic ___ , caused
by the herpes virus.

queratocele *m.* keratocele, hernia of
the innermost layer of the cornea.
queratoconjuntivitis *f.*
keratoconjunctivitis, simultaneous infl.
of the cornea and the conjunctiva.
queratoderma, queratodermia *f.*
keratoderma, hypertrophy of the
corneal layer of the skin, esp. in the
palms of the hands and the soles of the
feet.
queratólisis *f.* keratolysis. 1.
exfoliation of the skin; 2. congenital
anomaly that causes the skin to shed
periodically; ___ **neonatal** / ___
neonatorum.
queratomalacia *f.* keratomalacia,
degeneration of the cornea due to a
deficiency of vitamin A.
queratoplastia *f.* keratoplasty, plastic
surgery of the cornea.
queratorrexis *f.* keratorrhexis, rupture
of the cornea caused by a perforating
ulcer or trauma.
queratosis *f.* keratosis, horny condition
of the skin; ___ **actínica** / actinic ___ ,
precancerous lesion; ___ **blenorrágica** /
___ , blenorrhagica, manifested by a
scaly rash, esp. on the palms or the
soles of the feet.
queratotomía *f.* keratotomy, surgical
incision of the cornea.
querido-a *a.* dear, beloved.
quetoacidosis *f.* ketoacidosis,
acidosis caused by an increase in the
ketone bodies.
quetonuria *f.* ketonuria, presence of
ketone bodies in the urine.
quiasma *m.* chiasm, chiasma, the
crossing of two elements or structures.
quieto-a *a.* quiet, still; *v.* **estar** ___ / to
be still.
quijada *f.* jaw, osseous structure of the
mouth.
quilo *m.* chyle, milky fluid that results in
the absorption and emulsification of
fats in the small intestine.
quiluria *f.* chyluria, passage of chyle
into the urine.
química *f.* chemistry, the science that
studies the composition, structure, and
properties of matter, and the
transformations that they may undergo.
quimiocirugía *f.* chemosurgery,
removal of diseased tissue through the
use of chemicals.
quimiocoagulación *f.*
chemocoagulation, coagulation that
results from the use of chemicals.

quimionucleolisis *f.*
chemonucleolysis, dissolution of the nucleus pulposus of a hernia by injection of a proteolytic enzyme.

quimioprofilaxis *f.*
chemoprophylaxis, drug used as a preventive agent.

quimiorreceptor *m.* chemoreceptor, a cell or a receptor that can be excited by chemical change.

quimiotaxis *m.* chemotaxis, movement by a cell or an organism as a reaction to a chemical stimulus.

quimioterapia *f.* chemotherapy, treatment of a disease by chemical agents.

quimo *m.* chyme, semiliquid substance that results from the gastric digestion of food.

quimotripsina *f.* chymotrypsin, pancreatic enzyme.

quinidina *f.* quinidine, alkaloid derived from the bark of the cinchona tree, used in the treatment of cardiac arrhythmia.

quinina *f.* quinine, the most important alkaloid obtained from the cortex of the cinchona, used as an antipyretic in the treatment of malaria and typhoid fever.

quíntuple *m., f.* quintuplet, any of a set of five children born at one birth.

quiropráctica *f.* chiropractic, therapeutic treatment that consists of manipulation and adjustment of body structures, esp. of the spinal column in relation to the nervous system.

quirúrgico-a *a.* surgical, rel. to surgery; **colgajo** __ / __ flap; **equipo** __ / __ equipment; **instrumento** __ / __ instrument; **malla** __ / __ mesh.

quiste *m.* cyst, sac, or pouch containing a fluid or semifluid substance; __ **pilonidal** / pilonidal __ , containing hair and gen. occurring in the dermis of the sacrococcygeal area; __ **sebáceo** / sebaceous __ , gen. localized on the scalp.

quizás *adv.* perhaps.

q

r

R *abr.* **radioactivo-a** / radioactive;
resistencia / resistance; **respiración** /
respiration; **respuesta, reacción** /
response.

rabadilla *f.* coccyx, the extremity of the
backbone.

rabdomiosarcoma *m.*
rhabdomyosarcoma, malignant tumor
of striated muscle fibers affecting
primarily the skeletal muscles.

rabia *f.* rabies. 1. hydrophobia;
2. rage, anger; *v.* **tener ___** / to be
enraged.

rabioso-a *a.* rabid. 1. rel. to or afflicted
by rabies; 2. enraged.

racial *a.* racial, ethnic, rel. to race;
inmunidad ___ / ___ immunity, natural
immunity of the members of a race;
prejuicio ___ / ___ prejudice.

ración *f.* ration, food portion.

racionalización *f.* rationalization,
defense mechanism by which behavior
or actions are justified by explanations
that may seem reasonable but are not
necessarily based on reality.

rad *L.* rad. 1. unit of absorbed radiation;
2. *abr.* radix, root.

radiación *f.* radiation. 1. emission of
particles of radioactive material;
2. propagation of energy; 3. emission
of rays from a common center;
enfermedad por ___ / ___ sickness,
radiation syndrome, illness caused by
overexposure to x-rays or radioactive
materials; **___ electromagnética** /
electromagnetic **___**; **___ ionizante** /
ionizing **___**; **___ por rayos infrarrojos**
/ infrared **___**; **___ por rayos**
ultravioletas / ultraviolet **___** .

radiación oncológica *n.* 1. the use
of radiation for the treatment of
neoplasms; 2. radiation therapy.

radiactividad, radioactividad *f.*
radioactivity, property of some
elements to produce radiation.

radical *a.* radical. 1. aimed at
eradicating the root of a disease or all
the diseased tissue; 2. rel. to the root;
-mente *adv.* **___ mente** / radically.

radicular *a.* radicular, rel. to the root or
source.

radiculitis *f.* radiculitis, infl. of a nerve
root.

radiculoneuritis *f.* radiculoneuritis,
Guillain-Barré syndrome, infl. of the
roots of a spinal nerve.

radiculopatía *f.* radiculopathy, disease
of the roots of the spinal nerves.

radio *m.* 1. radium, metallic, radioactive,
fluorescent element used in some of its
variations in the treatment of malignant
tumors; **agujas de ___ / ___** needles,
needle-shaped, radium-containing
device used in radiotherapy; 2. radius,
the outer bone of the forearm.

radiocirugía *f.* radiosurgery,
procedure done through ionizing
radiation.

radiodensidad *f.* radiodensity, the
capacity of a substance to absorb
x-rays.

radiofármaco *m.* radiopharmaceutical,
radioactive drug used for diagnosis and
treatment of diseases.

radiografía *f.* radiography.

radioinmunoensayo *m.*
radioimmunoassay, test to determine
the concentration of protein serum as a
reaction to an injection of radioactive
substance.

radioisótopo *m.* radioisotope,
radioactive isotope.

radiología *f.* radiology, the study of
x-rays and rays emanating from
radioactive substances, esp. for medical
use.

radiólogo-a *m., f.* radiologist, specialist
in radiology.

radiolúcido-a *a.* radiolucent,
that allows the passage of most
x-rays.

radionecrosis *f.* radionecrosis,
disintegration of tissue by means of
radiation.

radiopaco-a *a.* radioopaque, that does
not allow the passage of x-rays or any
other form of radiation; **colorante ___ /**
___ dye.

radiorresistente *a.* radioresistant,
having the quality of being resistant to
the effects of radiation.

radiosensitivo-a *a.* radiosensitive,
that is affected by or responds to
radiation treatment.

radioterapia *f.* radiotherapy, radiation
therapy.

radón *m.* radon, colorless, gaseous
radioactive element.

raíz *f.* root.

ramificación *f.* ramification, separation into branches.

ránula *f.* ranula, cystic tumor under the tongue caused by an obstruction of a gland duct.

ranura *f.* groove, slit.

rápido-a *a.* quick, fast; swift; **-mente** *adv.* quickly; **movimiento ___ de los ojos /** ___ movement of the eyes.

raptus *L.* raptus, sudden, violent attack such as of a maniacal or nervous nature.

raquis *m.* rachis, the vertebral column, backbone.

raquítico-a *a.* rachitic. 1. rel. to rachitism; 2. stunted, feeble.

raquitismo *m.* rachitism, rachitis, a deficiency disease that affects skeletal growth in the young, usu. caused by lack of calcium, phosphorus, and vitamin D; *pop.* rickets.

rascar *vi.* to scratch; **rascarse** *vr.* to scratch oneself.

rasgo *m.* trait, feature, strain; ___ **adquirido /** acquired ___; ___ **heredado /** inherited ___ .

rasguño, rascuño *m.* scratch.

raspado *m.* curettage, scraping of the interior of a cavity; ___ **uterino /** ___ dilation and curettage.

raspadura, rasponazo *f., m.* scrape.

rastrear *v.* to scan, trace, and record with a sensitive detecting device.

rastreo *m.* scan, escán.

ratio *L.* ratio, quantity of one substance in relation to another.

rato *m.* while, a short time.

Rauwolfia serpentina *f.* Rauwolfia serpentina, a plant species that is the source of reserpine, an extract used in the treatment of hypertension and some mental disorders.

Raynaud, enfermedad de *f.* Raynaud's disease. acrocianosis.

Raynaud, fenómeno de *m.* Raynaud's phenomenon, the symptoms associated with Raynaud's disease.

rayo *m.* ray. ___ **láser /** laser beam; ___ **alfa /** alpha ___; ___ **infrarrojo /** infrared ___; ___ **ultravioleta /** ultraviolet ___ .

rayos gamma *m., pl.* gamma rays, high-energy rays emitted by radioactive substances.

rayos-x *m., pl.* 1. x-rays, high-energy electromagnetic short waves used to penetrate tissues and record densities on film; 2. films obtained through the use of x-rays.

raza *f.* race, a distinctive ethnic group with common inherited characteristics.

razón *f.* the faculty of reason; **a ___ de /** at the rate of; ___ **de ingreso /** ___ for admission; *v.* **tener /** to be right; ___ **de ser /** *raison d'etre.*

razonable *a.* reasonable.

razonar *vt., vi.* to reason, argue.

reacción *f.* reaction, response; ___ **alérgica /** allergic ___; ___ **anafiláctica /** anaphylactic ___; ___ **de ansiedad /** anxiety ___; ___ **de conversión /** conversion ___; ___ **depresiva psicótica /** psychotic depressive ___; ___ **en cadena /** chain ___; ___ **de formación /** formation ___; ___ **inmune /** immune ___; ___ **de tiempo /** time ___ .

reactivo *m.* reagent, agent that stimulates a reaction; **-a** *a.* reactive, that has the property of reacting or causing a reaction.

reagina *f.* reagin, antibody used in the treatment of allergies that causes the production of histamine.

realidad *f.* reality.

realimentación, retroalimentación *f.* feedback, regeneration of energy, action of taking the energy or the effects of the process back to its original source.

rebajar *vt.* to lower, to reduce, [*a liquid*] to dilute.

reblandecimiento *m.* ripening, softening, dilation, such as of the cervix during childbirth.

rebote *m.* rebound, a return to a previous condition after the removal of a stimulus; **fenómeno de ___ /** ___ phenomenon, intensified onward movement of a part when the initial resistance is removed.

recado *m.* message.

recaída *f.* relapse, setback, the recurrence of a disease after a period of recovery.

receptor *m.* 1. recipient of an organ; 2. receptor, a nerve end that receives a nervous stimulus and passes it on to other nerves; ___ **auditivo /** auditory ___; ___ **de contacto /** contact ___; ___ **de estiramiento /** stretch ___; ___ **de temperature /** temperature ___; ___ **gustativo /** taste ___; ___ **propioceptivo /** proprioceptive ___; ___ **sensorial /** sensory ___ .

recesivo-a *a.* recessive. 1. tending to withdraw; 2. in genetics, rel. to nondominant genes; **caractrísticas** ___ / ___ characteristics.

recetar *v.* to prescribe medication, to medicate.

recetario *m.* 1. prescription pad.

rechazo *m.* rejection. 1. immune reaction of incompatibility to transplanted tissue cells; ___ **agudo** / acute ___; ___ **crónico** / chronic ___; ___ **hiperagudo** / hyperacute ___; 2. denial, refusal.

recidiva *f.* recidivation, recidivism, the recurrence of a disease or symptom.

recién nacido-a *m., f.* newborn; **sala de** ___ **-s** / nursery.

reciente *a.* recent; **-mente** *adv.* recently.

recipiente *m.* 1. recipient, individual who receives blood, or an implant of tissue or organ from a donor; 2. container.

recipiente universal *m.* universal recipient, person belonging to blood group AB.

reclinado-a *a.* reclined, reclining, recumbent.

recluido-a *a.* confined.

recobrar *vt.* to regain; ___ **el conocimiento** / ___ consciousness; to regain; to retrieve.

recomendable *a.* advisable.

recomendación *f.* recommendation; referral.

recomendar *vt.* to recommend, to advise.

reconocimiento *m.* 1. physical examination; 2. recognition.

reconstitución *f.* reconstitution, restitution of tissue to its initial form.

reconstituyente *m.* tonic.

récord *m.* record, chart.

recordar *vt.* to recall; to recollect; to remind.

recordarse *vr.* to remember.

recostado-a *a.* lying down, recumbent.

recostarse *vr., vi.* to lie down.

recrudescencia *f.* recrudescence, relapse, return of symptoms.

rectal *a.* rectal, rel. to the rectum; **absceso** ___ / ___ abscess; **biopsia** ___ / ___ biopsy; **inflamación** ___ / ___ inflammation; proctitis **protuberancia, bulto** ___ / ___ lump; **prolapso** ___ / ___ prolapse.

recto *m.* rectum, the distal portion of the long intestine that connects the sigmoid and the anus; **-a** *a.* straight.

rectocele *m.* rectocele, herniation of part of the rectum into the vagina.

rectosigmoidectomía *f.* rectosigmoidectomy, surgical removal of the rectum and the sigmoid colon.

rectovaginal *a.* rectovaginal, rel. to the rectum and the vagina.

rectovesical *a.* rectovesical, rel. to the rectum and the bladder.

rectus *L.* rectus. 1. straight; 2. rel. to any of a group of straight muscles such as the ones in the eye and the abdominal wall.

recuento sanguíneo completo *m.* complete blood count.

recumbente *a.* recumbent, lying down position.

recuperación *f.* recuperation, recovery, restoration to health.

recuperar *vt.* to recover; ___ **el conocimiento** / to regain consciousness; **recuperarse** *vr.* to get well, *pop.* to pull through, to recoup.

recurrencia *f.* recurrence. 1. the return of symptoms after a period of remission; 2. relapse; repetition.

recurrente *a.* recurrent, that reappears temporarily; **cistitis** ___ / ___ cystitis; **dolor** ___ / ___ pain; **enfermedad** ___ / ___ illness.

recurso *m.* recourse; resource; ___ **-s económicos** / source of income.

red *f.* web, network, netlike arrangement of nerve fibers and blood vessels; ___ **de membranas arteriopulmonares** / pulmonary arterial ___ .

redondo-a *a.* round, circular.

reducción *f.* reduction, lowering of, diminishing.

reducción del seno *f.* reduction mammaplasty, plastic surgery that reduces the breast and improves its position and appearance.

reducir *vt.* to reduce, to cut down. 1. to restore to its normal position, such as a fragmented or dislocated bone; 2. to weaken the potency of a compound by adding hydrogen or suppressing oxygen; 3. to lose weight.

reemplazar *vt.* to replace, to substitute; to supplant.

reemplazo *m.* replacement, substitution.

referencia *f.* reference; referral; **valores de** ___ / ___ values.

reflejo *m.* reflex, a conscious or unconscious motor response to a stimulus; ___ **adquirido** / behavior ___;

__ **condicionado** / __ conditioned; __ **de estiramiento** / stretch __; __ **del tendón de Aquiles** / Achilles tendon __; __ **en cadena** / chain __; __ **instinctivo** / instinctive __; __ **no condicionado, natural** / unconditioned __; __ **patelar o rotuliano** / patellar __; __ **radial** / radial __; __ **rectal** / rectal __ .

reflejo hepatoyugular *a.* hepatojugular reflex, ingurgitation of the jugular veins, produced by pressure on the liver in cases of right cardiac failure.

reflexión *f.* reflection. 1. the throwing off or bending back of light or another form of radiant energy from a surface; 2. turning or bending back, as of a membrane lining a body wall, that passes over the surface of an organ and returns to the body wall; 3. introspection.

reflujo *m.* reflux, backflow of a fluid substance; __ **abdominoyugular** / abdominojugular __; __ **esofágico** / esophageal __; __ **hepatoyugular** / hepatojugular __; __ **intrarenal** / intrarenal __; __ **ureterorenal** / ureterorenal __ .

reflujo gastroesofágico *m.* gastroesophageal reflux, reflux concerning the stomach and the esophagus.

reforzar *vt.* to reinforce, to strengthen.

refracción *f.* refraction, the act of refracting; __ **ocular** / ocular __ .

refractar *vt.* to refract. 1. to change the direction from a straight path, such as of a ray of light when it passes from one medium to another of different density; 2. to detect abnormalities of refraction in the eyes and correct them.

refractario-a *a.* refractory. 1. resistant to treatment; 2. nonresponsive to a stimulus.

refrigerante *m.* refrigerant; antipyretic.

refugiar *vt.* to shelter; **refugiarse** *vr.* to seek refuge, to seek shelter.

refugio *m.* shelter, refuge; asylum.

regalo *m.* present, gift.

regeneración *f.* regeneration, restoration, renewal; feedback.

régimen *m.* regimen, structured plan, such as a regulated diet.

región *f.* region, a part of the body with more or less definite boundaries.

registro *m.* register, recording.

regla *f.* 1. menstruation; 2. rule; 3. ruler, device for measuring.

reglamento *m.* set of rules, policy.

regresar *v.* to return to a place.

regresión *f.* regression. 1. return to an earlier condition; 2. abatement of the symptoms or process of a disease.

regurgitación *f.* regurgitation. 1. the act of expelling swallowed food; 2. the backflow of blood through a defective valve of the heart; __ **de la válvula aórtica** __ / aortic valve __; __ **de la válvula mitral** / mitral valve __; __ **valvular** / valvular __ .

rehabilitar *vt.* to rehabilitate, to help regain normal functions through therapy.

rehidratación *f.* rehydration, establishment of normal liquid balance in the body.

rehuir *vi.* to evade, to shun.

rehusar *vt.* to refuse, deny; __ **la medicina** / __ taking the medication.

reimplantación *f.* reimplantation. 1. restoration of a tissue or part; 2. restitution into the uterus of an ovum removed from the body and fertilized *in vitro*.

reinfección *f.* reinfection, subsequent infection caused by the same microorganism.

reírse *vr., vi.* to laugh.

rejuvenecer *vi.* to rejuvenate; **rejuvenecerse** *vr.* to become rejuvenated.

relacionado-a *a.* rel. to, related.

relajación *f.* relaxation, act of relaxing or becoming relaxed.

relajado-a *a.* relaxed.

relajante *m.* relaxant, agent that reduces tension.

relativo-a *a.* relative; **-mente** *adv.* relatively.

rellenar *vt.* to refill.

reloj *m.* watch; clock.

remediar *vt.* to remedy, to help, to alleviate.

remedio *m.* remedy, relief.

remineralización *f.* remineralization, replacement of lost minerals from the body.

remisión *f.* remission. 1. diminution or cessation of the symptoms of a disease; 2. period of time during which the symptoms of a disease diminish.

remitente *a.* remittent, occurring at intervals.

r

renal *a.* renal, rel. to or resembling the kidney; **aclaración ___ , aclaramiento ___ / ___** clearance; **fallo ___ / ___** failure; **hipertensión de origen ___ / ___** hypertension; **intervención ___ / ___** intervention; **pelvis ___ / ___** pelvis; **prueba de aclaramiento o depuración ___ / ___** clearance test; **prueba funcional ___ / ___** function test; **diálisis, terapia de reemplazo ___ / ___** dialisis, replacement therapy.

rendido-a *a.* tired out, exhausted.

rendimiento *m.* output, yield; **fallo en el ___ / ___** failure.

renina *f.* renin, an enzyme released by the kidney that is a factor in the regulation of blood pressure.

renografía *f.* renography, x-ray of the kidney.

renuente *a.* reluctant.

reparación *f.* repair, restoration.

repaso *m.* review; **___ del caso / case ___**; **___ por sistemas, aparatos / ___** of systems.

repentino-a *a.* sudden; **-mente** *adv.* suddenly.

repetir *vt.* to repeat, to reiterate.

repliegue *m.* replication, reproduction, duplication.

reporte *m.* report, account.

reposo *m.* rest, repose; **cura de ___ / ___** cure; **en ___ / ___** resting.

represión *f.* repression. 1. inhibition of an action; 2. exclusion from consciousness of unacceptable desires or impulses.

reproducción *f.* reproduction.

reproducir *vt.* to reproduce.

reproductivo-a *a.* reproductive, rel. to reproduction; **sistema ___ / ___** system.

reprovisión *f.* feedback. 1. [*información*] regeneration of information; 2. regeneration of energy.

requerimiento *m.* requirement.

resbaladizo-a, resbaloso-a *a.* slippery.

resbalar *vi.* to slip; to slide.

rescatar *vt.* to rescue, to save.

resección *f.* resection, the act of cutting a portion of tissue or organ; **___ en cuña / wedge ___**; **___ gástrica / gastric ___**; **___ transuretral / transuretral ___**.

resectoscopía *f.* resectoscopy, resection of the prostate with a resectoscope.

resectoscopio *m.* resectoscope, instrument provided with a cutting electrode used in surgery within cavities, such as the one used for the resection of the prostate through the urethra.

reserpina *f.* reserpine, derivative of *Rauwolfia serpentina* used primarily in the treatment of hypertension and emotional disorders.

resfriado *m.* a cold.

resfriarse *vr.* to catch a cold.

residente *m.* resident, physician completing a residency.

residual *a.* residual, remainder; **función ___ / ___** function; **orina ___ / ___** urine.

residuo *m.* residue; **dieta de bajo ___ / low- ___ diet; dieta de ___ alto / high- ___ diet.**

resiliente *a.* resilient, elastic.

resina *f.* resin, resina, organic substance of vegetable origin, insoluble in water but readily soluble in alcohol and ether, that has a variety of uses in medicine and dentistry.

resistencia *f.* resistance, endurance, capacity of an organism to resist harmful effects; **___ adquirida / acquired ___**; **___ a un colorante / fast resistant**; **___ inicial / initial ___**; **___ periférica / peripheral ___**.

resistente *a.* resistant; **___ a la insulina / insulin ___**.

resolución *f.* resolution. 1. termination of an inflammatory process; 2. the ability to distinguish fine and subtle details as through a microscope.

resolver *vt.* to resolve. 1. to cause resolution; 2. to become separated into components.

resonancia *f.* resonance, capacity to increase the intensity of a sound; **___ normal / normal ___**; **___ vesicular / vesicular ___**; **___ vocal / vocal ___**.

resorcinol *m.* resorcinol, agent used in the treatment of acne and other forms of dermatosis.

resorción *f.* resorption, partial or total loss of a process, tissue, or exudate by means of biochemical reactions such as lysis and absorption.

respiración *f.* breathing, respiration; **aguantar o sostener la ___ / to hold one's breath; ___ abdominal / abdominal ___; ___ acelerada / accelerated ___; ___ aeróbica / aerobic ___; ___ anaeróbica / anaerobic ___; ___ diafragmática / diaphragmatic ___; ___ gruesa / coarse ___; ___ laboriosa / labored ___; ___ profunda / deep ___.**

retinitis

respiración sibilante *f.* wheezing.
respirador *m.* respirator, breather,
device used to purify the air reaching
the lungs or to administer artificial
respiration; __ **torácico** / chest __ .
respirar *v.* to breathe; __ **por la boca** /
__ through the mouth; __ **por la nariz**
/ __ through the nose.
respiratorio-a *a.* respiratory, rel. to
respiration; **alkalosis** __ / __
alkalosis; **aparato** __ **superior** / upper
__ tract; **arritmia** __ / __ arrhythmia;
ataxia __ / __ ataxia; **bronquíolos** __
-s / __ bronchioles; **capacidad** __ /
__ capacity; **cociente** __ / __ quotient;
conducto, pasaje __ / airway;
ejercicios __ -s / breathing exercises;
enzima __ / __ enzyme; **índice** __ /
__ rate; **infección del tracto** __
superior / upper __ tract infection;
**infecciones y enfermedades de las
vías** __ -s / __ tract infections and
diseases; **inhibidor** __ / __ inhibitor;
insuficiencia o fallo __ / __ failure,
insufficiency; **lóbulo** __ / __ lobule;
metabolismo __ / __ metabolism;
mucosa __ / __ mucosa; **pruebas de
función** __ / __ function tests; **paro**
__ / __ arrest; **ruidos** __ / __ sounds;
unidad de cuidado __ / __ care unit.
respiratorio, centro *m.* respiratory
center, region in the medulla oblongata
that regulates respiratory movements.
responsable *a.* responsible; **persona**
__ / responsible party.
respuesta *f.* response; answer.
1. reaction of an organ or tissue to a
stimulus; 2. reaction of a patient to a
treatment; __ **evocada** / evoked __ ,
sensorial test; __ **no condicionada** /
unconditioned __ , nonrestricted
reaction.
restablecer *vt.* to restore;
restablecerse *vr.* to recover.
restablecido-a *a.* [*de una
enfermedad*] recovered.
restaurar *vt.* to restore.
restricción *f.* restraint, confinement;
__ **de movimiento** / limitation of
motion; __ **en cama** / bed confinement.
restringido-a *a.* restricted.
resucitación *f.* resuscitation. 1. return
to life; 2. artificial respiration; __
cardiaca / cardiac __ .
resucitador *m.* resuscitator, an
apparatus to provide artificial
respiration; __ **cardiaco** / cardiac __.
resucitar *vt.* to resuscitate, to revive.

resultado *m.* result, outcome.
resumen *m.* summary.
resurgencia *f.* resurgence.
retardado-a *a.* retarded.
retención *f.* retention; **enema de** __ /
__ enema; __ **de líquido** / fluid __; __
gástrica / gastric __; __ **urinaria** /
urinary __ .
retener *vt.* to retain; to keep.
reticulación *f.* reticulation, reticular
formation.
reticular, retiforme *a.* reticular,
resembling a network.
retículo *m.* reticulum, a network, esp. of
nerve fibers and blood vessels.
reticulocito *m.* reticulocyte, an
immature red blood cell with a network
of threasds and granules that appears
primarily during blood regeneration.
reticulocitopenia *f.*
reticulocytopenia, an abnormal
decrease in the number of reticulocytes
in the blood.
reticulocitosis, reticulosis *f.*
reticulocytosis, abnormal increase in
the number of reticulocytes in the
bloodstream, as a result of active blood
regeneration by means of bone marrow
stimulation, or as a symptom of anemia.
reticuloendotelial, sistema *m.*
reticuloendothelial system, network of
phagocytic cells (except circulating
leukocytes) throughout the body,
involving processes such as blood cell
formation, elimination of worn-out
cells, and immune responses to
infection.
reticuloendotelioma *m.*
reticuloendothelioma, tumor of the
reticuloendothelial system.
reticuloendoteliosis *f.*
reticuloendotheliosis, increased growth
and proliferation of the cells of the
reticuloendothelial system.
retina *f.* retina, the innermost layer of the
eyeball that receives images and
transmits visual impulses to the brain;
conmoción de la __ / commotio
retinae, traumatic condition of the
retina that produces temporary
blindness; **desprendimiento de la** __ /
retinal detachment, separation of all or
part of the retina from the choroid;
deterioración de la __ / retinal
degeneration.
retiniano-a *a.* retinal, rel. to the retina;
perforación __ / __ perforation.
retinitis *f.* retinitis, infl. of the retina.

211

retinoblastoma *m.* retinoblastoma, gen. inherited malignant tumor of the retina genetic in origin.

retinol *m.* retinol, vitamin A1.

retinopatía *f.* retinopathy, any abnormal condition of the retina. __ **diabética** / diabetic __ .

retinoscopía *f.* retinoscopy, method of determination and evaluation of refractive errors of the eye.

retortijón *m.* brief and acute intestinal cramp.

retracción *f.* retraction, the act of drawing or pulling back; __ **del coágulo** / clot __ .

retractable, retráctil *a.* retractile, capable of being retracted.

retractar *vt.* to retract, to draw back, to withdraw.

retractor *m.* retractor. 1. instrument for holding back the edges of a wound; 2. retractile muscle.

retraído-a *a.* withdrawn, introverted, that keeps to himself or herself.

retrasado-a, retardado-a *a.* retarded; __ **mental** / mentally __ .

retraso *m.* retardation, abnormal slowness of a motor or a mental process.

retraso en el desarrollo *m.* failure to thrive, as in children that do not have a normal development.

retroauricular *a.* retroauricular, rel. to or situated behind the ear.

retrocecal *a.* retrocecal, rel. to or situated behind the cecum.

retroceder *vi.* [water] recede, diminish; to go back.

retroflexión *f.* retroflexion, the flexing back of an organ.

retrógrado-a *a.* retrograde, that moves backward or returns to the past; **amnesia** __ / __ amnesia; **aortografía** __ / __ aortography; **pielografía** __ / __ pyelography.

retrogresión *f.* 1. retrogression, return to a simpler level of development; 2. flashback, sudden vivid memory of images from the past.

retrolental *a.* retrolental, rel. to or situated behind the lens of the eye; **fibroplasia** __ / __ fibroplasia.

retroperitoneal *a.* retroperitoneal, rel. to or situated behind the peritoneum.

retroprovisión *f.* feedback.

retroversión *f.* retroversion, turning backward, such as an organ.

retroversión uterina *f.* retroversion of the uterus, condition of the uterus in which it is tipped backward.

retrovirus *m.* retrovirus, a virus belonging to a group of RNA viruses, some of which are oncogenic; __ **endógeno humano** / human endogenous __ .

reuma *f.* rheum. 1. aqueous secretion; 2. rheumatism.

reumático-a *a.* rheumatic, rel. to or afflicted by rheumatism.

reumatide *f.* rheumatid, any dermatosis associated with rheumatic fever.

reumatismo *m.* rheumatism, painful chronic or acute disease marked by infl. and pain in the joints.

reumatoide *a.* rheumatoid, rel. to or resembling rheumatism; **artritis** __ / __ arthritis.

reunión *f.* meeting; attachment. 1. meeting parts such as those of a fractured bone on the edge of a wound; 2. meeting of a group of persons.

revacunación *f.* booster shot.

revascularización *f.* revascularization. 1. restoration of blood supply to a part following a lesion or a bypass; 2. bypass.

reventar *vi.* to burst; **reventarse** *vr.* to burst open.

reversión *f.* reversal, reversion, restitution to a previously existing condition.

revisar *vt.* to review; to revise.

revivir *vt.* to revive, to bring back to life.

revólver *m.* revolver, handgun.

revulsión *f.* revulsion; contrairritación.

Reye, síndrome de *m.* Reye's syndrome, acute disease in children and adolescents manifested by severe edema that can affect the brain and other major organs of the body such as the liver.

rezar *vi.* to pray.

riboflavina *f.* riboflavin, component of vitamin B_2 complex, essential to nutrition.

ribonucleasa *f.* ribonuclease, enzyme that catalyzes the hydrolysis of ribonucleic acid.

ribonucleoproteína *f.* ribonucleoprotein, a substance containing both protein and ribonucleic acid.

ricino *m.* castor oil plant; **aceite de** __ / castor oil.

rickettsia *f.* rickettsia, any of the gram-negative microorganisms of the group *Rickettsiaceae* that multiply only in host cells of fleas, lice, ticks, and mice, and are transmitted to humans via the bite of these vectors.

riego *m.* flow; ___ **sanguíneo** / blood ___ .

riesgo *m.* risk; hazard; **grupos de alto ___ / high ___ groups ___; **posible ___** / potential ___; **___ de contaminación / ___** of contamination; **___ de infección / ___** of infection; **___ de una lesión / ___** of injury; **___ de violencia / ___** of violence; **___ -s / ___** factors.

riesgoso-a *a.* risky.

rigidez *f.* rigidity, stiffness, inflexibility; ___ **cadavérica** / cadaveric ___ , rigor mortis.

rígido-a *a.* rigid, stiff.

rigor *m.* rigor. 1. inflexibility of a muscle; 2. chill with high temperature; ___ **mortis** / ___ mortis.

rinal *a.* rhinal, rel. to the nose.

rinitis *f.* rhinitis, infl. of the nasal mucosa.

rinofaringitis *f.* rhinopharyngitis, infl. of the nasopharynx.

rinofima *f.* rhinophyma, severe form of acne rosacea in the area of the nose.

rinolaringitis *f.* rhinolaryngitis, simultaneous infl. of the mucous membranes of the nose and the larynx.

rinoplastia *f.* rhinoplasty, plastic surgery of the nose.

rinorrea *f.* rhinorrhea, liquid mucous discharge from the nose.

rinoscopia *f.* rhinoscopy, examination of the nasal cavities.

riñón *m.* kidney, organ situated in the back of each side of the abdominal cavity; **fallo del ___ / ___** failure; **necrosis papilar del ___ / renal papillary necrosis; **piedras en el ___ / ___** stones; **___ artificial** / hemodyalizer; **___ poliquístico** / polycystic ___; **transplante del ___ / renal transplant. See illustration on page 214.

risa *f.* laugh, laughter; ___ **histerica** / hysteric ___; ___ **sardónica** / sardonic ___ , contraction of facial muscles that gives the appearance of a smile.

risorio *m.* risorius, muscle inserted at the corners of the mouth.

risueño-a *a.* smiling, affable.

Ritalin, clorhidrato de *m.* Ritalin hydrochloride, stimulant and antidepressant.

ritidectomía *f.* rhytidectomy, face-lift, removal of wrinkles through plastic surgery.

ritidosis *f.* rytidosis, contraction of the cornea before death.

ritmo *m.* rhythm, regularity in the action or function of an organ of the body such as the heart; ___ **acoplado** / coupled ___; ___ **alfa** / alpha ___; **atrioventricular** / atrioventricular ___; ___ **bigeminal** / bigeminal ___; **circadiano** / circadian ___; ___ **de galope** / gallop ___; ___ **de tic-tac** / tic-tac ___; ___ **ectópico** / ectopic ___; ___ **idioventricular** / idioventricular ___; ___ **nodal** / nodal ___; ___ **pendular** / pendulum ___; ___ **sinusal** / sinus ___ .

ritmo circadiano *m.* circadian rhythm, rhythmic biological variations in a 24-hour cycle.

rizotomia *f.* rhizotomy, transection of the root of a nerve.

robustecer *vi.* to strengthen.

rociar *vt.* to spray.

rodar *vt.* to roll; to wheel.

rodeado-a *a.* surrounded.

rodilla *f.* knee; **dislocación de la ___ / ___** dislocation.

rodillera *f.* knee protector.

rodopsina *f.* rhodopsin, purple-red pigment found in the retinal rods that enhances vision in dim light.

roedor *m.* rodent.

roentgen *m.* roentgen, the international unit of x- or gamma radiation; **rayos de ___ / ___** rays, x-rays.

rojizo-a *a.* reddish.

rojo-a *a.* red; ___ **Congo** / Congo ___; ___ **escarlata** / scarlet ___ .

Romberg, signo de *m.* Romberg's sign, swaying of the body when in an erect position with eyes closed and feet close together as a sign of an inability to maintain balance.

romper *vt.* to break; **romperse** *vr.* to break into pieces.

roncar *vi.* to snore.

roncha *f.* blotch; wheal; hives.

ronco-a *a.* hoarse, with a husky voice.

ronquera *f.* hoarseness.

ronquido *m.* snore.

ropa *f.* clothing; ___ **de cama** / bed clothes, bed linens; ___ **interior** / underclothing.

Rorschach, prueba de *f.* Rorschach test, psychological test by which personality traits are revealed through

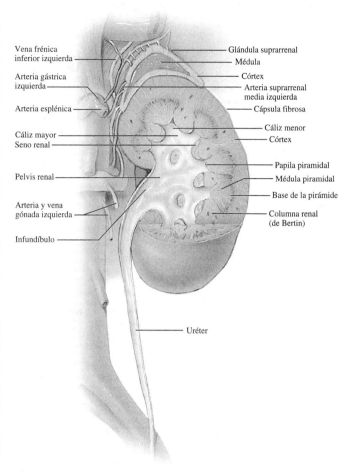

Vena frénica inferior izquierda

Arteria gástrica izquierda

Arteria esplénica

Cáliz mayor
Seno renal

Pelvis renal

Arteria y vena gónada izquierda

Infundíbulo

Glándula suprarrenal
Médula
Córtex
Arteria suprarrenal media izquierda
Cápsula fibrosa
Cáliz menor
Córtex
Papila piramidal
Médula piramidal
Base de la pirámide
Columna renal (de Bertin)

Uréter

Riñón izquierdo y glándula suprarrenal

the subject's interpretation of a series of ink blots.

rosáceo-a *a.* pinkish, rosy.

rosario *m.* rosary, structure that resembles a string of beads.

rosbif *m.* roast beef.

roséola *f.* roséola, rose-colored skin eruption.

rosette *Fr.* rosette, a rose-shaped cluster ofcells.

rostral *a.* rostral, rel. to or resembling a rostrum.

rostro *m.* rostrum. 1. human face; 2. beak or projection.

rotación *f.* rotation.

roto-a *a., pp.* de **romper,** broken.

rótula *f.* patella, kneecap; ball-and-socket joint.

rotura *f.* breakage; fracture.

rubefaciente *a.* rubefacient, that causes redness of the skin.

rubeola *f.* rubella, German measles, highly contagious benign viral infection manifested by fever, rose-colored eruption, and sore throat. It can have serious effects on the development of the fetus if acquired by the mother during early pregnancy.

rubor *m.* rubor, redness of the skin; blush.

ruborizado-a *a.* rubescent, that blushes.

ruborizarse *vr.* to blush.

rudimento *m.* rudiment. 1. a partially developed organ; 2. an organ or part with a partial or total loss of function.

rueda de andar *f.* [*acondicionamiento físico*] treadmill.

ruido *m.* noise, sound; [*corazón*] bruit, murmur; __ **sordo** / rumble.

ruptura *f.* rupture.

rutina *f.* routine.

rutinario-a *a.* routine, done habitually.

r

S

S *abr.* **sulfuro** / sulphur.

s *abr.* **sacral** / sacral; **sección** / section; **segundo** / second.

sábana *f.* sheet.

sabañón *m.* chilblain, a hand or foot sore produced by cold.

saber *vi.* to know; **hacer __** / to make known; **__ cómo** / **__** how; **__ de** / of, about.

Sabin, vacuna de *f.* Sabin vaccine, oral poliomyelitis vaccine.

sabor *m.* taste; flavor, aftertaste; *v.* **tener __ a, __ de** / to taste like.

sacar *vt.* to take out; to draw out.

sacárido *m.* saccharide, chemical compound, one of a series of carbohydrates that includes sugars.

sacarina *f.* saccharin, crystalline substance used as an artificial sweetener.

saciar *v.* to quench; to satiate; **__ la sed** / **__** the thirst.

saco *m.* sac, pocket, pouchlike structure; jacket.

sacral *a.* sacral, rel. to or near the sacrum; **nervios __ -es** / **__** nerves; **plexo __** / **__** plexus.

sacralización *f.* sacralization, fusion of the fifth lumbar vertebra and the sacrum.

sacro *m.* sacrum, the large triangular bone formed by five fused vertebrae that lies at the base of the spine between the two hip bones.

sacroilitis *f.* sacroilitis, infl. of the sacroiliac joint.

sacrolumbar *a.* sacrolumbar, rel. to the sacral and the lumbar regions.

sacudir *vt.* to shake; to jerk.

sáculo *m.* saccule, small sac.

sádico-a *a.* sadistic, rel. to sadism.

sadismo *m.* sadism, perverted sexual pleasure derived from inflicting physical or psychological pain on others.

sadomasoquismo *m.* sadomasochism, perverted sexual pleasure derived from inflicting pain on oneself or on others.

sadomasoquista *m., f.* sadomasochist, person who practices sadomasochism; *a.* sadomasochistic, rel. to the practice of sadomasochism.

safeno-a *a.* saphenous, rel. to or associated with the saphenous veins or nerves; **venas __ -s** / **__** veins, the veins of the leg.

sagital *a.* sagittal, resembling an arrow; **plano __** / **__** plane, parallel to the long axis of the body.

sal *f.* salt, sodium chloride; **__ -es aromáticas** / smelling **__ -s**; **__ corriente** / noniodized **__**; **__ yodada** / iodized **__**; *v.* **echar o poner __** / to salt or add salt; **sin __** / unsalted.

sala *f.* room; living room; [*hospital*] ward; **__ de aislamiento** / isolation ward; **__ de cuidado cardíaco** / cardiac care unit; **__ de cuidados intensivos** / intensive care unit; **__ de emergencia** / emergency **__**; **__ de espera** / waiting **__**; **__ de operaciones** / operating **__**; **__ de parto** / delivery **__**; **__ de recuperación** / recovery **__** .

salado-a *a.* salty.

salicilato *m.* salicylate, any salt of salicylic acid.

salino-a *a.* saline; **solución __** / **__** solution, distilled water and salt.

saliva *f.* saliva, spit, secretion of the salivary glands that moistens and softens foods in the mouth.

salivación *f.* salivation, excessive discharge of saliva.

salival *a.* salivary, rel. to saliva.

Salk, vacuna de *f.* Salk vaccine, poliomyelitis vaccine.

Salmonela *f.* Salmonella, a genus of gram-negative bacteria of the *Enterobacteriaceae* family that causes enteric fever, gastrointestinal disorders, and septicemia.

salmonelosis *f.* salmonellosis, infectious condition caused by ingestion of food contaminated by bacteria of the genus *Salmonella*.

salpingectomía *f.* salpingectomy, removal of one or both fallopian tubes.

salpingitis *f.* salpingitis, infl. of a fallopian tube.

salpingo-oforectomía *f.* salpingo-oophorectomy, removal of a fallopian tube and an ovary.

salpingoplastia *f.* salpingoplasty, plastic surgery of the fallopian tubes.

salpinx *Gr.* (*pl.* **salpinges**) salpinx, a tube, such as the fallopian tube.

salpullido, sarpullido *m.* heat rash.
saltar *vt., vi.* to jump; to skip; __ **un turno** / to skip an appointment or turn.
salto *m.* jump; skip; omission, [*del corazón*] palpitation.
salubre *a.* salubrious, healthy.
salubridad *f.* the state of public health.
salud *f.* health **atención a la __** / care; **centros de __** / __ care facilities; **certificado de __** / __ certificate; **cuidado de la __** / __ care; **cuidado de __ en el hogar** / home __ care; __ **de las personas de mayor edad** / senior __; **estado de __** / __ status; **instituciones de __ pública** / public __ facilities; __ **mental** / mental __; __ **precaria** / uncertain __; **profesional de atención de la __** / __ care provider; **servicios de __** / __ services; **servicios de __ para los ancianos** / __ services for the aged; __ **pública** / public __; __ **rural** / rural __; __ **urbana** / urban __ .
saludable *a.* healthy; **conducta __** / __ behavior __ .
salvado *m.* bran, a by-product of the milling of grain.
salvar *vt.* to save.
salvia *f.* sage.
sanar *v.* to cure, to heal.
sanatorio *m.* sanatorium, sanitarium, health establishment for physical and mental rehabilitation.
saneamiento *m.* sanitation.
sangrado, sangramiento *m.* bleeding; __ **por la nariz** / nosebleed.
sangrar *vi., vt.* to bleed.
sangre *f.* blood; __ **autóloga** / autologous __; **coágulo de __** / __ clot; **conteo de __** / __ count; **donante de __** / __ donor; __ **periférica** / peripheral __; **prueba selecta de __** / __ screening; **transfusión de __** / __ transfusion; __ **vital** / lifeblood; **a __ fría** / in cold __; **banco de __** / __ bank.
sangre oculta *f.* occult blood, blood that is present in such a minute amount that it cannot be seen with the naked eye.
sangría *f.* bloodletting.
sangriento-a *a.* bloody.
sanguíneo-a *a.* 1. sanguineous, rel. to blood or that contains it; **derivados __ -s, hemoderivados** / blood derivatives; **determinación de grupos __ -s** / blood grouping; **gases __ -s** / blood gases; **plasma __** / blood plasma;

producto __ / blood product; **proteína __** / blood protein; **sustitutos __ -s** / blood substitutes; **tipo __** / blood group; **tiempo de coagulación __** / blood coagulation time; 2. sanguine, of a cheerful nature.
sanguinolento-a *a.* sanguinolent, containing blood; **esputo __** / bloody sputum.
sanitario-a *m., f.* sanitarian, person trained in matters of sanitation and public health; *a.* sanitary, hygienic; **toalla, servilleta __** / __ napkin.
sano-a *a.* healthy; sound; wholesome.
saprófito *m.* saprophyte, vegetable organism that lives on decaying or dead organic matter.
sarampión *m.* measles, highly contagious disease esp. in school age children, caused by the rubeola virus; **suero de globulina preventivo al __** / __ immune serum globulin administered within five days after exposure to the disease.
sarcoidosis *f.* sarcoidosis. *See* **Schaumann, enfermedad de**.
sarcoma *m.* sarcoma, malignant neoplasm of the connective tissue. **condroblástico** / chondroblastic __; __ **de tejido blando** / soft tissue __; __ **fibroblástico** / fibropastic __; __ **gástrico** / gastric __; __ **linfático** / lymphatic __; __ **medular** / medullary __; __ **mielógeno** / myelogenic __; __ **óseo** / osteogenic __; __ **prostático** / prostatic __; __ **pulmonar** / pulmonary __; __ **renal** / renal __ .
satisfecho-a *a., pp.* de **satisfacer,** satisfied.
saturación *f.* saturation.
saturado-a *a.* saturated, unable to absorb or receive any given substance beyond a given limit; **no __** / unsaturated.
savia *f.* sap, natural juice.
Schaumann, enfermedad de *f.* Schaumann's disease, chronic disease of unknown cause manifested by the presence of small tubercles, esp. in the lymph nodes, lungs, bones, and skin.
Schilling, prueba de *f.* Schilling test, use of radioactive Vitamin B_{12} for the purpose of diagnosing primary pernicious anemia.
sebáceo-a *a.* sebaceous, rel. to or containing sebum; **glándulas __ -s** / __ glands, glands of the skin; **quiste __** / __ cyst.

sebo

sebo *m.* sebum, fatty thick substance secreted by the sebaceous glands.

seborrea *f.* seborrhea, malfunction of the sebaceous glands characterized by an excessive discharge of sebum from the glands.

seborréico-a *a.* seborrheic, rel to seborrhea; **blefaritis __ / __** blepharitis; **dermatitis __ / __** dermatitis; **queratosis __ / __** keratosis.

secar *vt.* to dry; **secarse** *vr.* to dry oneself.

sección *f.* section, portion, part; **__ media** / midsection.

seco-a *a.* dry.

secreción *f.* secretion. 1. the production of a given substance as a result of glandular activity; 2. substance produced by secretion; **__ apocrina** / apocrine __; **__ externa** / external __; **__ interna** / internal __; **__ purulenta** / purulent __ .

secretagogo *m.* secretagogue, secretogogue, agent that stimulates glandular secretion.

secretar *vt.* to secrete.

secretor-a *a.* secretory, that has the property of secreting; **capilares __ -es** / __ capillaries; **carcinoma __ / __** carcinoma; **fibra __ / __** fiber; **nervio __ / __** nerve.

secuela *f.* sequela, aftereffects, condition following or resulting from a disease or treatment.

secuestración *f.* sequestration. 1. the act of isolating; 2. the formation of sequestrum.

secuestro *m.* sequestrum, fragment of dead bone that has become separated from adjoining bone.

secundario-a *a.* secondary.

secundinas *f., pl.* afterbirth, placenta and membranes expelled at the time of delivery.

sed *f.* thirst; *v.* **tener __** / to be thirsty.

sedación *f.* sedation, the act and effect of inducing calm through medication.

sedante, sedativo *m.* sedative, agent with a quieting and tranquilizing effect.

sedentario-a *a.* sedentary. 1. having little or no physical activity; 2. rel. to a sitting position.

sediento-a *a.* thirsty.

sedimentación *f.* sedimentation, the process of depositing sediment; **índice de __ / __** rate.

sedimento *m.* sediment, matter that settles at the bottom of a solution.

segmentación *f.* segmentation, the act of dividing into parts.

segmento *m.* segment, section or part.

seguido-a *a.* continuous, unbroken; following.

seguimiento *m.* follow-up.

Seguin, síntoma de *m.* Seguin's signal symptom, involuntary contraction of the muscles before an epileptic seizure.

seguir *vt.* to follow; to continue.

según *prep.* according to; in accordance with.

segundo *m.* second, unit of time; **-a** *a.* [*ordinal number*] second, ordinal form of the number two.

seguridad *f.* safety, security; assurance; **medidas de __ / __** measures.

seguro *m.* insurance; **__ de incapacidad** / disability __; **__ de vida** / life __; **__ médico** / health __; **__ social** / social security; **seguro-a** *a.* safe; certain; **-mente** *adv.* surely.

selenio *m.* selenium, a nonmetallic chemical element resembling sulfur, used in electronic devices.

semana *f.* week; **la __ pasada** / last __; **la __ próxima, la __ que viene** / next __ .

semanal *a.* weekly; **-mente** *adv.* weekly.

semblante *m.* appearance of the face.

semejante *a.* resembling, similar.

semen *m.* semen, sperm, thick whitish secretion of the male reproductive organs.

semicoma *m.* semicoma, slight comatose state.

seminal *a.* seminal, concerning the semen or seed; **conducto __ / __** duct; **emision __ / __** emission.

seminífero-a *a.* seminiferous, that produces or bears seeds or semen; **conductos __ -s /__** tubules.

seminoma *m.* seminoma, a tumor of the testis.

seminuria *f.* seminuria, presence of semen in the urine.

semiótica *f.* semiotics, the branch of medicine concerned with signs and symptoms of diseases.

semiótico-a *a.* semiotic, rel. to the signs and symptoms of a disease.

sencillo-a *a.* simple, plain.

senescencia *f.* senescence, the process of becoming old.

senil *a.* senile, rel. to old age esp. as it affects mental and physical functions.

senilidad *f.* senility, the state of being senile.

seno *m.* breast, bust, bosom; **autoexamen de los __ -s / __** self-examination.

senos paranasales *m., pl.* paranasal sinuses, any of the air cavities in the adjacent bones of the nasal cavity.

sensación *f.* sensation, feeling, perception through the senses.

sensato-a *a.* sensible, reasonable.

sensibilidad *f.* sensitivity, the condition of being sensitive to touch or palpation; tenderness; __ **cruzada** / cross __; **entrenamiento de la __ /** training; __ **profunda** / deep __; __ **táctil** / touch sensation; __ **térmica** / thermal __ .

sensibilización *f.* sensitization, the act of making sensible.

sensible *a.* sensitive, sensible; wise, prudent.

sensífero-a *a.* sensiferous, that causes, transmits, or conducts sensations.

sensitivo-a *a.* 1. sensorial, that is perceived through the senses; 2. tender, sensitive to touch or palpation.

sensitivomotor *a.* sensorimotor, rel. to sensory and motor activities of the body.

sensorial, sensorio-a *a.* sensory, rel. to sensation or to the senses; **afasia __ /** aphasia; **epilepsia __ / __** epilepsy; **ganglio __ / __** ganglion; **imagen __ / __** image; **integración __ / __** integration; **nervio __ / __** nerve; **nivel de agudeza __ / __** acuity level; **privación __ / __** deprivation; **procesamiento __ / __** processing; **sobrecarga __ / __** overload; **umbral __ / __** threshold.

sensual *a.* sensual, sensuous; carnal.

sentado-a *a.* seated.

sentarse *vr., vi.* to sit down.

sentido *m.* sense; a perception or impression received through the senses; __ **de la vista /** __ of sight; __ **del oído /** __ of hearing; __ **del olfato /** __ of smell; __ **del sabor /** __ of taste; __ **del tacto /** __ of touch; __ **común /** common __; __ **del humor /** __ of humor.

sentimiento *m.* feeling; sentiment.

sentir *vt.* to feel, to perceive through the senses; **sentirse** *vr.* [*estado corporal*] to feel, general state of the body or mind; __ **bien /** to __ good; __ **mal /** to __ sick.

señal *f.* sign, indication.

señalado-a *a.* conspicuous, pronounced.

señalar *vt.* to point out, to indicate; to mark.

señor *m.* mister; *abr.* Mr.

señora *f.* married woman; *abr.* Mrs.

señorita *f.* miss, young lady; *abr.* Miss.

separación *f.* separation; in obstetrics, disengagement.

separado-a *a.* separate; **-mente** *adv.* separately.

sepsis *f.* sepsis, toxic condition caused by bacterial contamination.

septal *a.* septal, rel. to a septum; **desviación __ / __** deviation.

septectomía *f.* septectomy, partial or total excision of the septum.

septicemia *f.* septicemia, blood poisoning, invasion of the blood by virulent microorganisms.

séptico-a *a.* septic, rel. to sepsis; **choque __ / __** shock.

septum *L.* septum, (*pl. septa*) partition between two cavities.

sequedad *f.* dryness.

ser *vi.* to be.

serie *f.* distribution, set, succession; series, a group of specimens or types arranged in sequence; **en __ /** serial; __ **selectiva bioquímica /** biochemical screening.

serio-a *a.* serious; [*caso médico*] complicated; **en __ /** seriously; **-mente** *adv.* seriously.

seroconversión *f.* seroconversion, development of antibodies as a response to an infection or to the administration of a vaccine.

serológico-a *a.* serologic, serological, rel. to serum.

seroma *m.* seroma, accumulation of blood serum that produces a tumorlike swelling, gen. subcutaneous.

seronegativo-a *a.* seronegative, presenting a negative reaction in serological tests.

seropositivo-a *a.* seropositive, presenting a positive reaction in serological tests.

serosa *f.* serosa, serous membrane.

serosanguíneo-a *a.* serosanguineous, of the nature of serum and blood.

serositis *f.* serositis, infl. of a serous membrane, an important sign in diseases of the connective tissue such as systemic erythematous lupus.

seroso-a *a.* serous. 1. of the nature of serum; 2. producing or containing serum.

serotipo *m.* serotype, type of microorganism determined by the class and combination of antigens present in the cell; **determinación del __ /** serotyping.

serpiente *f.* snake, serpent; **__ de cascabel /** rattlesnake; **mordida de __ / __ bite; __ venenosa /** poisonous __ .

servicio *m.* service; **__ -s de cuidado exterior /** extended care facility; **__ -s de emergencia /** emergency __ ; **__ -s de salud preventiva /** preventive health __ .

sesamoideo-a *a.* sesamoid, rel. to or resembling a small mass in a joint or cartilage.

sésil *a.* sessile, attached by a broad base with no peduncle.

sesión *f.* session.

seso *m.* brain.

seudogota *f.* pseudogout, recurrent arthritic condition with symptoms similar to gout.

severo-a *a.* severe; **síndrome respiratorio __ / __** acute respiratory syndrome; **inmunodeficiencia combinada __ / __** combined immunodeficiency.

sexo *m.* sex; **__ sin riesgo / __** without risk; **relacionado con el __ / __** -linked, transmitted by genes located in the sex chromosome.

sexual *a.* sexual, rel. to sex; **agresión __ / __** assault; **características __ -es / __** characteristics; **conducta __ / __** behavior; **desarrollo __ / __** development; **educación __ / __** education; **madurez __ / __** maturity; **relaciones __ -es / __** intercourse; **salud __ / __** health; **trastorno __ / __** disorder; **vida __ / __** life; **-mente** *adv.* sexually; **enfermedad __ transmitida, enfermedad venéree / __** transmitted disease. See table on page 458.

sexualidad *f.* sexuality, collective characteristics of each sex.

Shiatsu *m.* Shiatsu, Oriental technique of applying finger pressure to specific points in the body to liberate energy.

shigelosis *f.* shigellosis, bacillary dysentery.

shock *m.* shock, abnormal state generated by insufficient blood circulation that can cause disorders such as low blood pressure, rapid pulse, pallor, abnormally low body temperature, and general weakness; **anafiláctico /** anaphylactic __ ; **endotóxico /** endotoxic __ ; **insulínico /** insulin __ ; **séptico /** septic __ .

Shy-Drager, síndrome de *m.* Shy-Drager syndrome, neurodegenerative disease of middle-aged or older persons that affects the autonomic nervous system and is characterized by chronic orthostatic hypotension and cardiac arrhythmia.

sialadenitis *f.* sialadenitis, sialoadenitis, infl. of a salivary gland.

sialoadenectomía *f.* sialoadenectomy incision and drainage of a salivary gland.

sialograma *m.* sialogram, x-ray of the salivary tract.

SIDA *abr.* AIDS, acquired immunodeficiency syndrome, characterized by immunodeficiency, infections (such as pneumonia, tuberculosis, and chronic diarrhea), and tumors esp. lymphoma and Kaposi's sarcoma.

sien *f.* temple, the flattened lateral region on either side of the head.

sietemesino-a *a.* born at seven months' gestation.

sífilis *f.* syphilis, contagious venereal disease usu. transmitted by direct contact and manifested by structural and cutaneous lesions; **__ terciaria /** tertiary __ , the third and most advanced stage of syphilis.

sifilítico-a *m., f.* syphilitic, person infected with syphilis; *a.* rel. to or caused by syphilis; **mácula __ / __** macule.

sigmoide, sigmoideo-a *a.* sigmoid. 1. shaped like the letter *s*; 2. rel. to the sigmoid colon.

sigmoidoscopía *f.* sigmoidoscopy, examination of the sigmoid flexure with a sigmoidoscope.

significado *m.* meaning, significance.

signo *m.* sign; mark, objective manifestation of a disease; **__ -s vitales /** vital __ -s.

siguiente *a.* following, next.

silencio *m.* silence.

silicosis *f.* silicosis, dust inhalation; a pathological condition of the lungs resulting from long term inhalation of silica dust.

Silvio, acueducto de *m.* aqueduct of Silvius, narrow channel connecting the third and fourth ventricles of the brain.

silla *f.* chair; ___ **de ruedas** / wheelchair.

silla turca *f.* sella turcica, depression on the superior surface of the sphenoid bone that contains the hypophysis.

simbiosis *f.* symbiosis, close association of two dissimilar organisms.

simbolismo *m.* symbolism. 1. mental abnormality by which the patient conceives occurrences as symbols of his or her own thoughts; 2. in psychoanalysis, symbolic representation of repressed thoughts and emotions.

símbolo *m.* symbol.

simetría *f.* symmetry, perfect correspondence of parts situated on opposite sides of an axis or plane of a body.

simétrico-a *a.* symmetrical.

similar *a.* similar.

simpatectomía *f.* sympathectomy, interruption of the sympathetic nerve pathways.

simpatía *f.* sympathy, relationship, affinity. 1. affinity between mind and body whereby one is affected by the other; 2. relationship between two organs in which an anomaly in one affects the other.

simpático-a *a.* sympathetic, rel. to the sympathetic nervous system.

simpatolítico-a *a.* sympatholytic, resistant to the activity produced by the stimulation of the sympathetic nervous system.

simpatomimético-a *a.* sympathomimetic, having the capacity to cause physiological changes similar to those produced by the action of the sympathetic nervous system.

simple *a.* simple; **-mente** *adv.* merely.

simplificar *vt.* to simplify.

simulación *f.* simulation, imitation; feigning an illness or symptom.

sin *prep.* without; ___ **embargo** / nevertheless.

sinapsis *f.* 1. synapse, the point of contact between two neurons, where the impulse traveling through the first neuron originates an impulse in the second one; 2. synapsis, the pairing of homologous chromosomes at the start of meiosis.

sinartrosis *f.* synarthrosis, an immovable joint in which the bony elements are fused.

sincondrosis *f.* synchondrosis, an immovable joint in which the surfaces are joined by cartilaginous tissue.

sincopal *a.* syncopal, rel. to a syncope.

síncope *m.* syncope, temporary loss of consciousness due to inadequate supply of blood to the brain; ___ **anginoso** / anginal ___; ___ **de deglución** / deglutition ___; ___ **cardíaco** / cardiac ___; ___ **convulsivo** / convulsive ___; ___ **histérico** / hysterical ___; ___ **laríngeo** / laryngeal ___ .

sincrónico-a *a.* synchronous, occurring at the same time.

sindactilia *f.* syndactylism, syndactyly, congenital anomaly consisting of the fusion of two or more fingers or toes.

síndrome *m.* syndrome, the totality of the symptoms and signs of a disease; ___ **adiposo** / adipose ___; ___ **de choque tóxico** / toxic shock ___ , blood poisoning due to *Staphylococci*; ___ **de dificultad respiratoria** / respiratory distress ___; ___ **de escaladadura** / scalded skin ___ , burns of the epidermis that gen. do not harm the underlying dermis; ___ **de intestino irritado** / irritable bowel ___; ___ **de malabsorción** / malabsorption ___ , gastro-intestinal disorder caused by poor absorption of food; ___ **de niños maltratados** / battered children ___; ___ **de privación** / withdrawal ___ , resulting from discontinued use of alcohol or a drug; ___ **de transfusión múltiple** / multiple transfusion ___ ; ___ **de vaciamiento gástrico rápido** / dumping ___ , rapid dumping of the stomach contents into the small intestine; ___ **del túnel del carpo** / carpal tunnel ___ ; ___ **del lóbulo medio del pulmón** / middle lobe ___ of the lung; ___ **del secuestro subclavicular** / subclavian steal ___; ___ **nefrótico** / nephrotic ___ , excessive loss of protein; ___ **premenstrual** / premenstrual ___; ___ **suprarrenogenital** / adrenogenital ___ .

síndrome de inmunodeficiencia adquirida (SIDA) *m.* acquired immunodeficiency syndrome. *See* **SIDA**.

S

síndrome de muerte infantil súbita (SMIS) m. sudden infant death syndrome, sudden unexplained death of an apparently healthy infant during sleep the cause of which remains unknown.

síndrome neuroléptico maligno m. neuroleptic malignant syndrome, caused by the use of neuroleptic agents and characterized by symptoms of hyperthermia, loss of consciousness, and serious reactions related to the central nervous system that could be fatal.

sinequia f. synechia, union or abnormal adherence of tissue or organs, esp. in reference to the iris, the lens, and the cornea.

sinérgico-a a. synergistic, synergic, the capacity to act together.

sinergismo m. synergism, correlated or harmonious action between two or more structures or drugs.

sínfisis f. symphysis, a joint in which adjacent bony surfaces are united by fibrocartilage.

sinoauricular o sinusal, nódulo m. sinoauricular, sinoatrial node located at the meeting point of the vena cava and the right cardiac atrium, point of origin of the impulses that stimulate the heartbeat.

sinostosis f. synostosis, osseous joining of two adjacent bones; __ senil / senile __; __ tribacilar / tribacilar __.

sinovia f. synovia, synovial fluid, transparent and viscid liquid secreted by synovial membranes that lubricates joints and connective tissue.

sinovial a. synovial, rel. to or producing synovia; **bursa, saco** __ / __ bursa; **membrana** __ / __ membrane; **quiste** __ / __ cyst.

sinovioma m. synovioma, tumor that originates in the synovial membrane.

sinovitis f. synovitis, an infl. of the synovial membrane; __ **purulenta** / purulent __; __ **seca** / dry __; __ **serosa** / serous __ .

sinquisis f. synchysis, state of fluidity of the vitreous humor.

síntesis f. synthesis, the composition of a whole by union of the parts.

sintético-a a. synthetic, rel. to or produced by synthesis.

sintetizar vi. to synthesize, to produce synthesis.

síntoma m. symptom, any manifestation of a disease as perceived by the patient; __ **constitucional** / constitutional __; __ **demorado** / delayed __; __ **de supresión** / withdrawal __; __ **objetivo** / objective __ ; __ **patognomónico** / pathognomonic __; __ **presente** / presenting __; __ **prodrómico** / prodromal __; __ **premonitorios** / warning __ -s.

sintomático-a a. symptomatic; -mente adv. symptomatically.

sintomatología f. symptomatology, symptoms pertaining to a given condition or case.

sintónico-a m., f. syntonic, a type of personality that responds and adjusts normally to his or her environment.

sinus L. sinus, cavity or hollow passage.

sinusitis f. sinusitis, infl. of a sinus, esp. a paranasal sinus.

sinusoide m. sinusoid, a minute passage that carries blood to the tissues of an organ, such as the liver; a. resembling a sinus.

siringocele m. syringocele. 1. the central canal of the spinal cord; 2. a meningomyelocele containing a cavity in the ectopic spinal cord.

siringomielia f. syringomyelia, chronic, progressive disease of the spinal cord manifested by formation of liquid-filled cavities, gen. in the cervical region and sometimes extending into the medulla oblongata.

sistáltico-a a. systaltic, that alternates dilations and contractions.

sistema m. system, a group of correlated parts or organs constituting a whole that performs one or more vital functions; __ **cardiovascular** / cardiovascular __; __ **digestivo** / digestive __; __ **endocrino** / endocrine __; __ **genitourinario** / genitourinary __; __ **hematopoyético** / hematopoietic; __ **inmunológico** / immune __; __ **linfático** / lymphatic __; __ **nervioso** / nervous __; __ **óseo** / osseous __; __ **portal** / portal __; __ **reproductivo** / reproductive __; __ **respiratorio** / respiratory __; __ **reticuloendotelial** / reticuloendothelial __.

sistema de circulación cardiopulmonar m. application of a heart-lung machine.

sistema sensorio nervioso m. sensory nervous system.

sistemático-a *a.* systematic, that follows a system; **-mente** *adv.* systematically.

sistémico-a *a.* systemic, that affects the body as a whole; **circulación** __ / __ circulation.

sístole *f.* systole, the contractive cycle of the heartbeat, esp. of the ventricles; __ **auricular** / atrial __; __ **prematura** / premature __; __ **ventricular** / ventricular __ .

sistólico-a *a.* systolic, rel. to the systole; **murmullo** __ / __ murmur; **presión** __ / __ pressure.

situación *f.* situation.

situado-a *a.* situated, placed, located.

situs *L.* situs, position or place.

Sjogren, síndrome de *m.* Sjogren's syndrome, autoimmune disorder that results in diminished salivary and lacrimal secretion, causing dryness of the eyes and the lips.

Snellen, prueba de ojo de *f.* Snellen's eye test, a chart of black letters that gradually diminish in size, used in testing visual acuity.

sobra *f.* excess, surplus; **hay de** __ / there is more than enough.

sobre *prep.* above, over; __ **todo** / above all.

sobrealimentación *f.* hyperalimentation; __ **intravenosa** / parenteral __ .

sobrecierre *m.* overclosure, condition caused when the mandible closes before the upper and lower teeth meet.

sobrecompensación *f.* overcompensation; an exaggerated attempt to conceal feelings of guilt or inferiority.

sobredosis *f.* overdose, excessive dose of a drug.

sobrellevar *vt.* to endure.

sobremordida *f.* overbite.

sobrenombre *m.* surname, family name.

sobrepeso *m.* overweight.

sobreponerse *vr.* to overcome.

sobrerrespuesta *f.* overresponse, excessive reaction to a stimulus.

sobresalir *vi.* to protrude; to be conspicuous.

sobresaltado-a *a.* frightened, startled.

sobrevivir *vt.* to survive.

sobrino-a *m., f.* nephew; niece.

sobrio-a *a.* sober.

social *a.* social; **seguro** __ / __ security; **asistencia** __ / __ work; **trabajador-a** __ / __ worker.

socialización *f.* socialization, social adaptation.

socializado-a *a.* socialized; **medicina** __ / __ medicine.

sociedad *f.* society; corporation; fellowship.

sociópata *m., f.* sociopath, an individual that manifests antisocial behavior.

socorrer *vt.* to help, to assist, to aid.

soda *f.* soda, sodium carbonate.

sodio *m.* sodium, soft alkaline metallic element found in the fluids of the body; **bicarbonato de** __ / baking soda; **carbonato de** __ / soda.

sodomía *f.* sodomy, term used in reference to dual intercourse most often between males.

sodomita *m., f.* sodomite, one who commits sodomy.

sofisticación *f.* sophistication; the adulteration of a substance.

sofocación *f.* suffocation, asphyxia, shortness of breath.

sofoco *m.* hot flash; suffocation.

sol *m.* sun; **baño de** __ / sunbathing; **bloqueador del** __ / sunscreen; **estar expuesto al** __ / exposure; **mancha del** __ / sunspot; **quemadura de** __ / sunburn; **tomar el** __ / to sunbathe.

solar *a.* solar, rel. to the sun; **bloqueador** __ / sunscreen; **energía** __ / __ energy.

sólido-a *a.* solid; firm; sound.

solo-a *a.* alone, only; **-mente** *adv.* only.

soltar *vt.* to release; to loosen.

soltero-a *a.* single, unmarried.

soluble *a.* soluble.

solución *f.* solution; __ **ocular** / eyewash.

solvente *m.* solvent, liquid that dissolves or is capable of producing a solution; thinner.

somático-a *a.* somatic, rel. to the body.

somatización *f.* somatization; the process of converting mental experiences into bodily manifestations.

sombra *f.* shadow; opacity; shade; **a la** __ / in the shade.

someter *vt.* to submit; **someterse** *vr.* to undergo; to submit oneself.

somnífero *m.* sleeping pill.

somniloquia *f.* somniloquism, the act of talking while asleep.

somnolencia *f.* sleepiness, drowsiness.

sonambulismo *m.* somnambulance, somnambulism, sleepwalking.

sonámbulo-a *m., f.* somnambule, person who walks in his or her sleep.

sonar *vt.* to sound, to ring.

sonda *f.* probe, thin, smooth, and flexible instrument used to explore cavities and body passages or to measure the depth and direction of a wound; ___ **acanalada** / hollow ___; ___ **intestinal** / intestinal decompression tube; ___ **uretral** / urethral catheter.

sonido *m.* sound.

sonografía *f.* sonography. *See* ultrasonografía.

sonograma *m.* sonogram, image obtained by ultrasonography.

sonoro-a *a.* sonorous, resonant, having a deep or full sound.

sonreír *vi.* to smile.

sonrisa *f.* smile.

soñar *vi.* to dream; ___ **despierto -a** / to daydream.

soplar *vt.* to blow.

soplo *m.* murmur, bruit, flutter; short, raspy, or fluttering sound, esp. an abnormal beat of the heart; ___ **aórtico, regurgitante** / aortic, regurgitant in value; ___ **cardíaco** / cardiac ___; ___ **continuo** / continuous ___; ___ **creciente, en crescendo** / crescendo ___; ___ **diastólico** / diastolic ___; ___ **endocardial** / endocardial ___; ___ **en vaivén** / to-and-fro ___; ___ **exocardial** / exocardial ___; ___ **funcional** / functional ___; ___ **inocente** / innocent ___; ___ **mitral** / mitral ___; ___ **pansistólico** / pansystolic ___; ___ **presistólico** / presystolic ___; ___ **sistólico** / systolic ___ .

sopor *m.* drowsiness, sleepiness.

soporífero, soporífico *m.* soporific, agent that produces sleep.

soportable *a.* bearable, tolerable.

soportar *vt.* to endure, to bear, to sustain.

soporte *m.* support.

sorber *vt.* to sip; to suck; to absorb.

sorbo *m.* sip.

sordera *f.* deafness.

sordo-a *m., f.* a deaf person; *a.* deaf.

sordomudo-a *m., f.* deaf-mute person.

sostén *m.* support, backing; buttress; brassiere.

sostener *vt.* to sustain; to maintain.

Still, enfermedad de *f.* Still's disease, juvenile rheumatoid arthritis.

Streptococcus *Gr.* Streptococcus, a genus of gram-positive bacteria of the tribe *Streptococceae* that occur in pairs or chains, many of which are causal agents of serious infection.

suavizar *vt.* to soften.

subacromial *a.* subacromial, below the acromion.

subaracnoideo-a *a.* subarachnoid, situated or occurring below the arachnoid membrane; **espacio** ___ / ___ space.

subclavicular *a.* subclavian, subclavicular, located beneath the clavicle; **arteria** ___ / ___ artery; **vena** ___ / ___ vein.

subclínico-a *a.* subclinical, without clinical manifestations.

subconsciencia, subconsciente *f., m.* subconscious, state during which mental processes affecting thought, feeling, and behavior occur without the individual's awareness.

subconsciente *a.* subconscious, rel. to the part of the mind of which one is not fully aware.

subcultivo *m.* subculture, a culture of bacteria derived from another culture.

subcutáneo-a *a.* subcutaneous, under the skin.

subdesarrollado-a *a.* underdeveloped.

subdesarrollo *m.* underdevelopment.

subdural *a.* subdural, under the dura mater; **espacio** ___ / ___ space.

subependimario-a *a.* subependymal, situated under the ependyma.

subfrénico-a *a,* subphrenic, situated below the diaphragm; **absceso** ___ / ___ abscess.

subinvolución *f.* subinvolution, incomplete involution; ___ **del útero** / ___ of the uterus.

subir *v.* to go up; to lift up; to climb; ___ **las escaleras** / to climb the stairs.

súbito-a *a.* sudden; **muerte** ___ / ___ death; **-mente** *adv.* suddenly.

subjetivo-a *a.* subjective; **síntomas** ___**-s** / ___ symptoms.

sublimación *f.* sublimation. 1. the change from a solid state to vapor; 2. a Freudian term indicating a process by which instinctual drives and impulses are modified into socially acceptable behavior.

sublingual *a.* sublingual, under the tongue; **glandula** ___ / ___ gland.

subluxación *f.* subluxation, an incomplete dislocation.

submandibular *a.* submandibular, under the mandible.

submucosa *f.* submucosa, layer of cellular tissue situated under a mucous membrane.

subrogado-a *a.* surrogate, that takes the place of someone or something.

subscripción *f.* subscription, part of the prescription that contains instructions for its preparation.

substantivo, sustantivo *m., gr.* substantive, noun.

subungueal *a.* subungual, beneath a nail.

succión *f.* suction; **dispositivo de __** / __ device.

suceder *v.* to happen.

sucesivo-a *a.* successive, consecutive.

suceso *m.* happening, event.

sucio-a *a.* dirty, filthy.

sucrosa *f.* sucrose, natural saccharose obtained mostly from sugarcane and sugar beets.

sudado-a *a.* sweaty, moist with perspiration; perspiring.

sudamina *f.* sudamina, non-inflammatory cutaneous eruption that presents whitish vesicles filled with aqueous liquid and that gen. occurs after profuse sweating or accompanying some febrile disorder.

sudar *vt.* to sweat, to perspire.

sudatorio, sudorífico *m.* sudorific, an agent promoting sweat.

sudor *m.* sweat, perspiration, secretion of the sweat glands; **__ -es nocturnos** / night __-s.

sudores fríos *m., pl.* cold sweat.

sudores nocturnos *m., pl.* night sweats.

sudorífico-a *a.* sudorific, that produces sweat.

sudoroso-a *a.* perspiring, sweaty.

suegro-a *m., f.* father-in-law; mother-in-law.

suelo *m.* ground; floor.

sueño *m.* sleep; dream; **ciclos del __** / __ cycles; **__ crepuscular** / twilight __ ; **estadíos del __** / __ stages; **__ profundo** / deep __ ; **__ reparador** / balmy __ ; **trastornos del __** / sleep disorders; *v.* **tener __** / to be sleepy.

sueño, enfermedad del *f.* sleeping sickness, endemic, acute disease of Africa caused by a protozoon transmitted by the tsetse fly and characterized by a state of lethargy, chills, loss of weight, and general weakness.

suero *m.* serum. 1. clear, watery portion of the plasma that remains fluid after clotting of blood; 2. any serous fluid; 3. immune serum of an animal that is inoculated to produce passive immunization; **__ antitóxico** / immune __; **__ de globulina** / globulin __; **__ de la verdad** / truth __ .

suficiente *a.* sufficient, enough; **-mente** *adv.* sufficiently.

sufrimiento *m.* suffering.

sufrir *vt.* to suffer; [*herida*] to sustain; [*operación*] to undergo.

sufusión *f.* suffusion, infiltration of a bodily fluid into the surrounding tissues.

sugerencia, sugestión *f.* suggestion, intimation, indication.

sugestivo-a *a.* suggestive, rel. to suggestion or that suggests.

suicida *a.* suicidal, prone to commit suicide.

suicidarse *vr.* to commit suicide.

suicidio *m.* suicide; **intento de __** / attempted __ .

sujeto *m.* subject. 1. term used in reference to the patient; 2. topic; 3. *gr.* subject of the verb.

sulfa, medicamentos de *m., pl.* sulfa drugs, *sulfonamides,* antibacterial drugs of the sulfonamide group.

sulfato *m.* sulfate, a salt of sulfuric acid.

sulfonamidas *f. pl.* sulfonamides, a group of bacteriostatic sulfur organic compounds.

sulfúrico-a *a.* sulfuric, rel. to sulfur.

sulfuro *m.* sulphur.

sumamente *adv.* extremely, very.

sumar *vt.* to add.

sumario *m.* summary, clinical history of the patient.

sumergir *vt.* to submerge, to immerse.

superfecundación *f.* superfecundation, successive fertilization of two or more ova from the same menstrual cycle in two separate instances of sexual intercourse.

superfetación *f.* superfetation, fecundation of two ova in the same uterus corresponding to two different menstrual cycles but occurring within a short period of time from each other.

superficial *a.* superficial, rel. to a surface; **tensión __** / surface tension;

shallow; **-mente** *adv.* superficially, shallowly.

superficie *f.* surface, outer portion or limit of a structure.

superinfección *f.* superinfection, new infection that occurs while a previous one is still present, gen. caused by a different organism.

superior *a.* superior; upper; higher; greater.

superolateral *a.* superolateral, situated above and to the side.

supersaturado-a *a.* supersaturated, beyond saturation.

supersaturar *v.* to supersaturate, to add a substance in an amount greater than that which can be dissolved normally by a liquid.

superyó *m.* superego, in psychoanalysis the part of the psyche concerned with social standards, ethics, and conscience.

supinación *f.* supination, turning the hand with the palm facing forward and upward.

supino-a *a.* supine, rel. to the position of lying on the back, face up, with palms of the hands turned upward.

suplemento *m.* supplement, supply.

suponer *vi.* to suppose, to surmise.

supositorio *m.* suppository, a semisolid, soluble, medicated mass that is introduced in a body passage such as the vagina or the rectum.

suprapúbico-a *a.* suprapubic, above the pubis; **catéter** __ / __ catheter; **cistotomia** __ / __ cystotomy.

suprarrenal *a.* suprarenal, above the kidney; **glandula** __ / __ gland.

supresión *f.* suppression; withdrawal; 1. arrest in the production of a secretion, excretion, or any normal discharge; 2. in psychoanalysis, inhibition of an idea or desire.

supuración *f.* suppuration, formation or discharge of pus.

supurar *v.* to suppurate, to fester, to ooze.

supurativo-a *a.* suppurative, rel. to suppuration.

surco *m.* furrow, line, wrinkle; groove, track; __ **atrioventricular** /

atrioventricular __; **bicipital** / bicipital __; __ **costal** / costal __; __ **digital** / digital __; __ **glúteo** / gluteal __ .

surfactante *m.* surfactant, active agent that modifies the surface tension of a liquid.

susceptible *a.* susceptible.

suscitar *v.* to rouse, to stir up.

suspender *vt.* to suspend, to cancel, to halt.

suspenso-a *a.* pending.

suspensorio-a *a.* suspensory, sustaining or providing support; **ligamento** __ / __ ligament.

sustancia *f.* substance, matter; __ **blanca** / white matter, neural tissue formed mainly by myelinated fibers that constitute the conducting portion of the brain and the spinal cord; __ **fundamental** / ground __ , gelatinous matter of connective tissue, cartilage, and bone that fills the space between cells and fibers.

sustantivo *m., gr.* substantive, noun.

sustento *m.* sustenance.

sustitución *f.* substitution, the act of replacing one thing for another; **terapéutica por** __ / __ therapy.

sustituir *vt.* to substitute.

sustituto *m.* substitute.

susto *m.* fright, sudden fear.

sutura *f.* suture, line of union; __ **absorbible** / absorbable __; __ **compuesta** / bolster __; __ **continua, de peletero** / continuous, uninterrupted __; __ **de aposición y aproximación** / near and far __; __ **de catgut** / catgut __; __ **de colchonero** / vertical mattress __; __ **de herida** / wound __; __ **de seda** / silk __; __ **en bolsa de tabaco** / pursestring __; __ **facial** / fascial __; __ **implantada** / implanted __; __ **interrumpida** / interrupted __; __ **no absorbible** / nonabsorbable __; __ **plana** / flat __ .

Swan-Ganz, catéter de *m.* Swan-Ganz catheter, soft, flexible catheter with a balloon near the tip used to measure the blood pressure in the pulmonary artery.

t

T *abr.* **temperatura absoluta** / absolute temperature; **T+, tensión aumentada** / T+, increased tension; **T+, tensión disminuída** / T+, diminished tension.

tabaco *m.* 1. tobacco, the dried and prepared leaves of *Nicotiana tabacum* that contain nicotine; 2. cigar; **contaminación por humo de __** / __ smoke pollution.

tabardillo *m.*, *pop.* name given to typhus or typhoid fever in certain regions of Mexico and Latin America.

tabes *L.* tabes, progressive deterioration of the body or any part of it caused by a chronic illness.

tabicado-a *a.* septate, that has a dividing wall.

tabique *m.* thin wall; **__ cellular** / cell wall; **__ nasal, o de la nariz** / nose ridge.

tabla *f.* table. 1. a flat osseous plate or lamina; 2. an arranged collection of many particulars that have a common standard.

tableta *f.* tablet, a solid dosage of medication; **__ de capa entérica** / enteric-coated __ .

tabular *a.* tabular, resembling a table or square; *v.* to tabulate, to make lists or tables.

tacón *m.* heel of a shoe.

táctil *a.* tactile, rel. to touch or to the sense of touch; **discriminación __** / __ discrimination; **sistema __** / __ system.

tacto *m.* the sense of touch.

taenia *L.* taenia. tenia.

talámico-a *a.* thalamic, rel. to the thalamus.

tálamo *m.* thalamus, one of the two large, oval-shaped masses of gray matter situated at the base of the cerebrum that are the main relay centers of sensory impulses to the cerebral cortex.

talasemia *f.* thalassemia, group of different types of hereditary hemolytic anemia found in populations of the Mediterranean region and Southeast Asia; **__ mayor** / major __; **__ menor** / minor __ .

talasofobia *f.* thalassophobia, morbid fear of the sea.

talasoterapia *f.* thalassotherapy, the treatment of disease by sea bathing or by exposure to the sea.

talidomida *f.* thalidomide, hypnotic sedative known to cause severe malformation in developing fetuses.

talipes *m.* talipes, congenital deformity in children consisting in a fixed foot.

talitoxicosis *f.* thallitoxicosis, incidental poisoning by ingestion of thallium sulfate even in pesticides.

talla *f.* size, height or length of the body taken from head to toe.

talle de la cintura *m.* waistline.

talón *m.* talus, astragalus, heel, ankle bone.

talotibial *a.* talotibial, rel. to the talus and the tibia.

tambalearse *vr.* to stagger, to waver.

tanatología *f.* thanatology, branch of medicine that deals with death in all its aspects.

tanatomania *f.* thanatomania, suicidal or homicidal mania.

tanatómetro *m.* thanatometer, instrument used to determine when a death took place by taking an internal measurement of the temperature of the body.

tapado-a *a.* plugged (*Mex.*) **oído __** / __ ear; **nariz __** / __ nose.

taponamiento *m.* tamponade, packing. 1. the process of filling a cavity with cotton, gauze or some other material; 2. wrapping.

taponamiento cardíaco *m.* cardiac tamponade, acute compression of the heart due to excess fluid in the pericardium.

taquiarritmia *f.* tachyarrhythmia, arrhythmia combined with a rapid pulse.

taquiarritmia paroxística *f.* paroxismal taquicardia, palpitation episodes that begin and end abruptly or may last hours or days and can be recurrent.

taquicardia *n.* tachycardia, acceleration of the heart activity, gen. at a frequency of more than one hundred beats per minute in adults; **__ auricular** / atrial __; **__ auricular paroxística** / paroxysmal atrial __; **__ ectópica** / ectopic __; **__ en salves** / __ en salves; **__ exoftálmica** / __ exophthalmica; **__ fetal** / fetal __;

paroximal / paroxysmal ___; ___
refleja / reflex ___; ___ **sinusal** / sinus
___; ___ **supraventricular** /
supraventricular ___; ___ **ventricular** /
ventricular ___ .

taquifagia *f.* tachyphagia, an acquired
habit of eating too fast.

taquifasia *f.* tachyphasia, characteristic
of rapid speech. *Syn.* taquifrasia.

taquipnea *f.* tachypnea, rapid
breathing.

tara *f.* 1. weight of a container deducted
from the total weight of a load;
2. physical or mental inherited
disorder of importance; 3. defect or
imperfection that devalues an
object.

tarado-a *a.* defective, damaged;
[*person*] handicapped; idiot; nitwit.

tarántula *f.* tarantula, large, black,
venomous spider.

tardar *v.* to delay; to take time; **a más ___**
/ at the latest; **¿cuánto tarda la
operación?** / how long does the
operation take?; **tarda menos de una
hora** / It takes less than an hour; *fam.*
no tardes mucho / do not be long ___;
tardarse *vr.* to be delayed.

tarde *f.* afternoon; *adv.* late; **más ___ o
más temprano** / sooner or later.

tardive *Fr.* tardive, late in appearing.

tarjeta *f.* card; ___ **de crédito** / credit
___; ___ **de visita** / calling ___ .

tarsal, tarsiano-a *a.* tarsal, rel. to the
connective tissue that supports the
eyelid or the tarsus.

tarso *m.* tarsus, posterior part of the foot
located between the bones of the lower
leg and the metatarsus; **huesos del ___ /**
tarsal bones.

tarsometatarsiano-a *a.*
tarsometatarsal, rel. to the tarsus and
the metatarsus.

tartamudo-a *m., f.* stutter, a person that
stutters.

tartamudeo, tartamudez *m., f.*
stammering, stuttering.

taxis *L.* taxis. 1. manipulation or
reduction of a part or an organ to restore
it to its normal position; 2. directional
reaction of an organism to a stimulus.

taza *f.* cup.

tebaína *f.* thebaine, toxic alkaloid
obtained from opium.

teca *f.* theca, covering or sheath of an
organ.

tecnecio 99m *m.* technetium 99m, a
radioisotope that emits gamma rays and

that is the most frequently used
radioisotope in nuclear medicine.

técnica *f.* technic, technique, method, or
procedure.

técnico-a *m., f.* technician, an
individual who has the necessary
knowledge and skill to carry out
specialized procedures and treatments,
gen. under the supervision of a health
care professional; ___ **dental** / dental
___; ___ **de rayos-x** / x-ray ___; ___ **de
terapia respiratoria** / respiratory
therapy ___ .

tecnología *f.* technology, the science of
applying technical knowledge for
practical purposes.

tecnológico-a *a.* technological.

tecnólogo-a *m., f.* technologist, an
expert in technology.

tecoma *m.* thecoma, tumor of an ovary,
gen. benign.

tectorium *L.* tectorium, membrane that
covers Corti's organ.

tegumento *m.* tegument, the skin.

tejido *m.* tissue, a group of similar cells
and their intercellular substance that act
together in the performance of a
particular function; ___ **adiposo** /
adipose ___; ___ **cartilaginoso** /
cartilaginous ___; ___ **cicatrizante** / scar
___; ___ **conectivo** / connective ___; ___
de granulación / granulation ___; ___
elástico / elastic ___; ___ **endotelial** /
endothelial ___; ___ **epitelial** /
epithelial; ___ **eréctil** / erectile ___; ___
fibroso / fibrous ___; ___ **glandular** /
glandular ___; ___ **intersticial** /
fluid; ___ **linfático** / lymphatic ___; ___
mesenquimatoso / mesenchymal ___;
___ **mucoso** / mucous ___; ___
muscular / muscular ___; ___ **nervioso** /
nerve, nervous ___; ___ **óseo** / bony,
bone ___; ___ **subcutáneo** /
subcutaneous ___ .

telangiectasia *f.* telangiectasia,
telangiectasis, condition caused by an
abnormal dilation of the capillary
vessels and arterioles that sometimes
can produce angioma.

telecardiófono *m.* telecardiophone,
an instrument that allows to hear the
heart sounds.

telediagnóstico *m.* telediagnosis,
diagnosis or progress by electronic
means by remote transmission between
medical institutions.

teléfono *m.* telephone; **llamar por ___ ,
telefonear** / to telephone.

telemetría *f.* telemetry, electronically transmitted data.

telencéfalo *m.* telencephalon, anterior portion of the prosencephalon.

teleopsia *f.* teleopsy, visual disorder by which close objects seem farther than they really are.

telepatia *f.* telepathy, apparent communication of thought by extrasensory means.

telerradiografía *f.* teleradiography, x-ray taken with the radiation source at a distance of about two meters or more from the subject to minimize distortion.

temblor *m.* tremor, an involuntary quivering or trembling; ___ **alcohólico** / alcoholic ___; **continuo** / continuous ___; ___ **de aleteo** / flapping ___; ___ **de reposo** / resting ___; ___ **de variaciones rápidas** / fine ___; ___ **esencial** / essential ___; ___ **fisiológico** / physiologic ___; ___ **intencional** / intentional ___; ___ **intermitente** / intermittent ___; ___ **lento y acentuado** / coarse ___; ___ **muscular** / muscular ___.

temblores *m., pl. pop.* the shakes.

temer *v.* to fear, to dread.

temperamento *m.* temperament, the combined physical, emotional, and mental constitution of an individual that distinguishes him or her from others.

temperatura *f.* temperature. 1. degree of heat or cold as measured on a specific scale; ___ **absoluta** / absolute ___; ___ **ambiente** / room ___; ___ **axilar** / axillary ___; ___ **crítica** / critical ___; ___ **del cuerpo** / body ___; ___ **máxima** / maximum ___; ___ **mínima** / minimum ___; ___ **normal** / normal ___; ___ **oral** / oral ___; ___ **rectal** / rectal ___; ___ **subnormal** / subnormal ___; 2. the natural degree of heat of a living body.

temple *m.* temper; character.

temporal *a.* 1. temporal, rel. to the temple; **huesos** ___ **-es** / ___ bones; **lóbulo** ___ / ___ lobe; **músculo** ___ / ___ muscle; 2. temporary, limited in time.

temporomandibular *a.* temporomandibular, rel. to or affecting the joint between the temporal bone and the mandible; **articulaciones** ___ **-es** / ___ joints.

tenáculo *m.* tenaculum, type of hook used in surg. to grasp or hold a part.

tenar *a.* thenar, rel. to the palm of the hand; **eminencia** ___ / ___ eminence; **músculos** ___ **-es** / ___ muscles.

tendinitis *f.* tendinitis, tendonitis, infl. of a tendon.

tendinoso-a *a.* tendinous, rel. to or resembling a tendon; **reflejo** ___ / tendon reflex; **reflejo** ___ **profundo** / deep tendon reflex; **tirón** ___ / tendon jerk.

tendón *m.* tendon, sinew, highly resistant, fibrous tissue that attaches the muscles to the bones or to other parts; ___ **-es de la corva** / hamstring; ___ **de Aquiles** / Achilles ___.

tener *vt.* to have, to possess; ___ **diez años** / to be ten years old; ___ **dolor** / to be in pain; ___ **ganas de** / to want to; ___ **hambre** / to be hungry; ___ **miedo** / to be afraid; ___ **que** / to have to; ___ **razón** / to be right; ___ **sed** / to be thirsty.

tenesmo *m.* tenesmus, continuously painful, ineffectual, and straining efforts to urinate or defecate.

tenia *f.* flatworm of the class *Cestoda* that in the adult stage lives in the intestines of vertebrates; *pop.* tapeworm.

teniasis *f.* taeniasis, infestation by taenia.

tenosinovitis *f.* tenosynovitis, infl. of a tendon sheath.

tensión *f.* tension, tenseness. 1. the act or effect of stretching or being extended; 2. the degree of stretching; 3. physical, emotional, or mental stress; ___ **premenstrual** / premenstrual ___; ___ **superficial** / surface ___; 4. the expansive pressure of a gas or vapor.

tensor *a.* tensor, term applied to any muscle that stretches or produces tension.

teoría *f.* theory. 1. an exposition of the principles of any science; 2. hypothesis that lacks scientific proof.

terapeuta, terapista *m., f.* therapist, person skilled in giving or applying therapy; ___ **físico** / physical ___; ___ **patólogo-a del habla y del lenguage** / speech ___.

terapéutica *f.* therapeutics, the branch of medicine that deals with treatments and remedies; ___ **electroconvulsiva** / electroconvulsive ___; ___ **endocrina** / endocrine ___; ___ **específica** / specific ___; ___ **experimental** / experimental ___; ___ **farmacológica** / pharmacological ___; ___ **hidrológica** / hydrologic ___; ___ **ocupacional** / occupational ___; ___ **química** / chemical ___; ___ **quirúrgica** / surgical ___; ___ **sustitutiva** / substitution ___.

terapia, terapéutica

terapia, terapéutica *f.* therapy, the treatment of a disease or a condition; ___ **anticoagulante** / anticoagulant ___; ___ **biológica** / biological ___; ___ **de conducta** / behavioral ___; ___ **de grupo** / group ___; ___ **de oxígeno** / oxygen ___; ___ **diatérmica** / diathermic ___; ___ **inespecífica** / nonspecific ___; ___ **inmunosupresiva** / immunosuppressive ___; ___ **ocupacional** / occupational ___; ___ **por choque** / shock ___; ___ **por inhalación** / inhalation ___; ___ **por radiación** / radiation ___; ___ **por sugestión** / suggestion ___; ___ **respiratoria** / respiratory ___; ___ **sustitutiva** / substitutive ___.

terapia de megavitaminas *f.* megavitamin therapy, a theory that advocates the ingestion of large doses of vitamins as prevention to many health disorders.

terapia genética *f.* genetic therapy, therapy that tries to correct a genetic disorder.

terapéutica por realidad *f.* reality therapy, method by which the patient is confronted with his or her real-life situation and helped to accept it as such.

terapéutico-a *a.* therapeutic. 1. rel. to therapy; **indicaciones** ___ **-s** / therapeutic ___-s; 2. that has healing properties.

teratogénesis *f.* teratogenesis, the production of gross fetal abnormalities.

teratógeno *m.* teratogen, agent that causes teratogenesis.

teratología *f.* teratology, the study of malformations in fetuses.

teratoma *m.* teratoma, neoplasm derived from more than one embryonic layer and therefore constituted by different types of tissues.

terciano-a *a.* tertian, that repeats itself every three days; **fiebre** ___ / ___ fever.

teres *L.* teres, term applied to describe some elongated, cylindrical muscles and ligaments.

termal *a.* thermal, thermic, rel. to heat or produced by it.

terminal *a.* terminal, final.

término *m.* term. 1. a definite period of time or its completion, such as a pregnancy; 2. word.

terminología *f.* terminology, nomenclature.

termocauterización *f.* thermocauterization, use of electric current or another heat medium to destroy tissue.

termocoagulación *f.* thermocoagulation, coagulation of tissue with high-frequency currents.

termodinámica *f.* thermodynamics, the science that studies the relationship between heat and other forms of energy.

termoesterilización *f.* thermosterilization, sterilization by heat.

termografía *f.* thermography, recording obtained by the use of a thermograph.

termógrafo *m.* thermograph, infrared detector that registers variations in temperature by reaction to the blood flow.

termómetro *m.* thermometer; device that measures heat or cold; ___ **clínico** / clinical ___; ___ **de Celsius** / Celsius ___ , centigrade; ___ **de Fahrenheit** / Fahrenheit ___; ___ **de registro automático** / self-recording ___; ___ **rectal** / rectal ___.

termorregulación *f.* thermoregulation, regulation by heat and temperature.

termotaxis *f.* thermotaxis. 1. regulation of the temperature of the body; 2. the reaction of an organism to heat.

termoterapia *f.* thermotherapy, therapeutic use of heat.

Terramicina *f.* Terramycin, trade name for a tetracycline antibiotic.

testicular *m.* testicular, rel. to a testicle; **tumores** ___ **-es** / ___ tumors.

testículo *m.* testicle, the male gonad, one of the two male reproductive glands that produce spermatozoa and the hormone testosterone; ___ **ectópico** / ectopic ___ ; ___ **no descendido** / undescended testis.

testificar *vi.* to testify.

testigo *m.*, *f.* to witness; ___ **experto especializado** / expert witness.

testosterona *f.* testosterone, male hormone produced chiefly by the testicle and responsible for the development of male secondary characteristics such as facial hair and a deep voice; **implante de** ___ / ___ implant.

teta *f.* teat. 1. mammary gland; 2. nipple.

tetania *f.* tetany, a neuromuscular affliction associated with parathyroid deficiencies and diminished mineral balance, esp. calcium, and manifested by intermittent tonic spasms of the voluntary muscles.

tetánico-a *a.* tetanic, rel. to tetanus; **antitoxina** ___ / tetanus antitoxin; **convulsión** ___ / ___ convulsion; **toxoide** ___ / ___ toxoid.

tétano *m.* tetanus, an acute infectious disease caused by the toxin of the tetanus bacillus, gen. introduced in the body through a wound, manifested by muscular spasms and rigidity of the jaw, neck, and abdomen; *pop.* lockjaw; **globulina inmune para el** ___ / ___ immune globulin.

tetilla *f.* male nipple.

tetraciclina *f.* tetracycline, a type of broad-spectrum antibiotic effective against gram-positive and gram-negative bacteria, rickettsia, and a variety of viruses.

tetraplejía *f.* tetraplegia, paralysis of the four extremities.

tetraploide *a.* tetraploid, having four sets of chromosomes.

tetravalente *m.* tetravalent, element that has a chemical valance of four.

textura *f.* texture, the composition of a tissue or structure.

tez *f.* [*cutis*] complexion.

thrill *m.* thrill, a vibration felt on palpation; ___ **aneurismal** / aneurysmal ___; ___ **aórtico** / aortic ___; ___ **arterial** / arterial ___; ___ **diastólico** / diastolic ___ .

tibia *f.* tibia, the inner and larger bone of the leg below the knee.

tic *Fr.* tic, spasmodic, involuntary movement or twitching of a muscle; ___ **convulsivo** / convulsive ___; ___ **coordinado** / coordinated ___; ___ **doloroso** / ___ douleureux; ___ **facial** / facial ___ .

tiempo *m.* 1. time, the duration of an event; **a** ___ / in ___; **a su debido** ___ / in due ___; **¿cuánto** ___ **?** / how long?; **espacio de** ___ / ___ frame; **medir el** ___ / to ___ , to set the ___; **pérdida de** ___ / waste of ___; **por algún** ___ / for some ___; **regulador de** ___ / timer; ___ **de coagulación** / coagulation ___; ___ **de exposición** / exposure ___; ___ **de latencia** / ___ lag; ___ **de percepción** / perception ___; ___ **de protrombina** / prothrombin ___; ___ **de sangramiento** / bleeding ___; ___ **limitado** / a limited ___; ___ **medido** / timed; ___ **suplementario** / overtime; 2. weather; **hace buen** ___ / the ___ is good; **hace**

mal ___ / the ___ is bad; **pronóstico del** ___ / ___ forecasting.

tiempo de trombina *m.* thrombin time, necessary length of time to form a fibrin clot after adding thrombin to the citrated plasma.

tienda *f.* tent, a cover or shelter made of fabric, gen. used to enclose the patient within a given area; ___ **de oxígeno** / oxygen ___ .

tífico-a *a.* typhoid, rel. to typhus.

tiflitis *f.* typhlitis, infl. of the cecum.

tifoidea, fiebre *f.* typhoid fever, acute intestinal infection caused by a bacterium of the genus *Salmonella*, characterized by fever, prostration, headache, and abdominal pain.

tifus *m.* typhus, acute infectious disease caused by *rickettsia* with manifestations of high fever, delirium, prostration, and severe headache, gen. transmitted by lice, fleas, ticks, and mites.

timectomía *f.* thymectomy, excision of the thymus.

timo *m.* thymus, glandular organ situated in the inferior portion of the neck and the antero-superior portion of the thoracic cavity. It plays an important part in the immunological process of the body.

timoma *m.* thymoma, tumor derived from the thymus.

timpanectomía *f.* tympanectomy, excision of the tympanic membrane.

timpánico-a *a.* tympanic, pertaining to a structure that has the quality of resonance when struck or that resonated on percussion by transmitting sound vibrations as occurs in the middle ear or a drumlike sound that resounds in other part of the body; **membrana** ___ / ___ membrane; **nervio** ___ / ___ nerve.

timpanismo *m.* tympanites, distension of the abdomen caused by accumulation of gas in the intestine.

timpanítico-a *a.* tympanitic, rel. to or affected with tympanites; **resonancia** ___ / ___ resonance.

timpanitis *f.* tympanitis, infl. of the middle ear.

tímpano *m.* tympanum, the eardrum, middle ear.

timpanoplastia *f.* tympanoplasty, surgical correction of a damaged middle ear.

timpanotomía *f.* tympanotomy, incision of the tympanic membrane.

tinea

tinea *L.* tinea, cutaneous fungal infection in the form of a ring; __ **capitis** / __ capitis; __ **corporis** / __ corporis; __ **pedis** / __ pedis, athlete's foot; __ **versicolor** __ / versicolor.

tinnitus *L.* tinnitus, buzzing or ringing sound in the ears.

tinte *m.* dye.

tiña *f.* tinea, ringworm. tinea.

tío-a *m., f.* uncle; aunt.

típico-a *a.* typical; characteristic.

tipificación *f.* typing, determination by types; __ **de tejido** / tissue __; __ **inmunológica** / immunotyping.

tipo *m.* type; kind, the general character of a given entity.

tirante *a.* tense, extended; pulling; stretched; [*relación*] strained.

tiritar *v.* to shiver.

tiroadenitis *f.* thyroadenitis, inf. of the thyroid gland.

tiroglobulina *f.* thyroglobulin. 1. a glycoprotein secreted by the thyroid gland; 2. a substance obtained by the fractioning of the thyroid gland of the hog, used in the treatment of hyperthyroidism.

tirogloso-a *a.* thyroglossal, rel. to the thyroid and the tongue; **conducto** __ / __ duct.

tiroidea *a.* thyroid related; **hormona estimulante** __ / thyroid stimulating hormone.

tiroidectomía *f.* thyroidectomy, excision of the thyroid gland.

tiroideo-a *a.* thyroid, rel. to the thyroid gland; **cartílago** __ / __ cartilage; **crisis** __ / __ storm; **hormonas** __ -s / __ hormones.

tiroides, glándula *f.* thyroid gland, one of the endocrine glands situated in the front part of the trachea and made up of two lateral lobules that connect in the middle; **prueba del funcionamiento de la** __ / thyroid function test.

tiroiditis *f.* thyroiditis, infl. of the thyroid gland.

tiromegalia *f.* thyromegaly, enlargement of the thyroid gland.

tiroparatiroidectomía *f.* thyroparathyroidectomy, excision of the thyroid and parathyroid glands.

tirotóxico-a *a.* thyrotoxic, rel. to or affected by toxic activity of the thyroid gland.

tirotoxicosis *f.* thyrotoxicosis, disorder caused by hyperthyroidism and marked by an enlargement of the thyroid gland, increased metabolic rate, tachycardia, rapid pulse, and hypertension.

tirotropina *f.* thyrotropin, thyroid-stimulating hormone produced in the anterior lobe of the pituitary gland; **hormona estimulante de la** __ / __ -releasing hormone.

tiroxina *f.* thyroxine, iodine containing hormone produced by the thyroid gland, also obtained synthetically for use in the treatment of hypothyroidism.

tobillera *f.* ankle brace.

tobillo *m.* ankle.

tocar *vi.* to touch, to palpate.

tocino *m.* bacon.

tocógrafo *m.* tocograph, device used to estimate and record the force of uterine contractions.

todo-a *a.* all, entire; **ante** __ / above all; __ **el día** / the whole day; __ **-s los días** / every day; __ **-s los meses** / every month.

tofáceo-a *a.* tophaceous, rel. to a tophus or of a gritty nature.

tofo *m.* tophus. 1. deposits of urates in tissues as seen in gout; 2. dental calculus.

toilette *Fr.* toilette, cleansing, as related to a medical procedure.

tolerancia *f.* tolerance, the ability to endure the use of a medication or performance of a given amount of physical activity without ill effects.

tomar *vt.* to take; to eat or drink; __ **una decisión** / to make a decision.

tomografía *f.* tomography, scan, diagnostic technique by which a series of x-ray pictures taken at different depths of an organ are obtained; __ **axial computada** / computed __; __ **axial computarizada (TAC)** / computerized axial __ (CAT); __ **computada** / computed __; __ **computada de alta resolución** / high-resolution computed __; __ **computada dinámica auricular** / atrial bolus dynamic computerized __; __ **con rayos de electrón** / electron beam __; __ **convencional** / conventional __; __ **de emisión de positron** / positron emission __; __ **dinámica computada** / dynamic computed __; __ **magnética nuclear de resonancia** / nuclear magnetic resonance __ .

tomógrafo *m.* tomograph, x-ray machine used in tomography.

tonicidad *f.* tonicity, normal quality of tone or tension.

tónico *m.* tonic, medication for restoring tone and vitality; **-a** *a.* 1. that restores the normal tone; 2. characterized by continuous tension.

tono *m.* tone; pitch. 1. the quality of the body with its organs and parts in a normal and balanced state; ___ **muscular** / muscle ___; 2. a particular quality of sound or voice.

tonometría *f.* tonometry, the measurement of tension or pressure.

tonómetro *m.* tonometer, instrument that measures tone, esp. intraocular tension.

tonsila *f.* tonsil; ___ **cerebelosa** / cerebellar ___; ___ **faríngea** / pharyngeal ___; ___ **lingual** / lingual ___; ___ **palatina** / palatine ___ .

tonsilar *a.* tonsillar, rel. to a tonsil; **cripta** ___ **o amigdalina** / ___ crypt; **fosa** ___ / ___ fossa.

tonsilectomía *f.* tonsillectomy. amigdalotomía.

tonsilitis *f.* tonsillitis. amigdalitis.

tonsiloadenoidectomía *f.* tonsilloadenoidectomy, excision of the tonsils and adenoids.

tópico-a *a.* topical, rel. to a specific area.

toracentesis *f.* thoracentesis, surgical puncture and drainage of the thoracic cavity.

torácico-a *a.* thoracic, rel. to the thorax; **cavidad** ___ / ___ cavity; **conducto** ___ / ___ duct; **pared** ___ / ___ cage, chest wall, osseous structure enclosing the thorax; **traumatismos** ___ -s / ___ injuries.

toracicoabdominal *a.* thoracicoabdominal, rel. to the thorax and the abdomen.

Toracina *f.* Thorazine, antiemetic sedative.

toracolumbar *a.* thoracolumbar, rel. to the thoracic and lumbar vertebrae.

toracoplastia *f.* thoracoplasty, plastic surgery of the thorax that consists in removing a portion of the ribs to allow the collapse of a diseased lung.

toracostomía *f.* thoracostomy, incision of the chest wall to allow for drainage.

toracotomía *f.* thoracotomy, incision of the thoracic wall.

tórax *m.* thorax, the chest; ___ **inestable** / flail chest, condition of the wall of the thorax caused by multiple fracture of the ribs.

tórax en embudo *m.* funnel thorax, depression of the sternum.

torcedura *f.* strain, sprain, warp, twisting of a joint with distension and laceration of its ligaments, usu. accompanied by pain and swelling.

torcido-a *a.* twisted, sprained.

tormenta *f.* storm, abrupt and temporary intensification of the symptoms of a disease.

torniquete *m.* tourniquet, tourniquette, device used to apply pressure over an artery to stop the flow of blood.

tórpido-a *a.* torpid, sluggish, slow.

torpor *m.* sluggishness, cloudiness; ___ **mental** / clouding of consciousness.

torsión *f.* torsion, twisting or rotating of a part on its long axis; ___ **ovárica** / ovarian ___; ___ **testicular** / testicular ___ .

torso *m.* torso, trunk of the body.

tortícolis *f.* torticollis, toniclonic spasm of the muscles of the neck that causes cervical torsion and immobility of the head.

tos *f.* cough; **ataque de** ___ / coughing spell; **calmante para la** ___ / ___ suppressant; **jarabe para la** ___ / ___ syrup; **pastillas para la** ___ / lozenges; ___ **metálica, bronca** / brassy ___; ___ **seca recurrente** / hacking ___ .

tos ferina *f.* pertussis, whooping cough, infectious children's disease that gen. begins with a cold followed by a persistent dry cough.

toser *v.* to cough.

tostado-a *a.* toasted; **pan** ___ / toast.

total *a.* total, whole; **mente** *adv.* totally.

totipotencia *f.* totipotency, ability of a cell to regenerate or develop into another type of cell.

toxemia *f.* toxemia, generalized intoxication due to absorption of toxins formed at a local source of infection.

toxicidad *f.* toxicity, the quality of being poisonous.

tóxico-a *a.* toxic, rel. to a poison or of a poisonous nature.

toxicología *f.* toxicology, the study of poisons and their effects and treatment.

toxicólogo-a *m., f.* toxicologist, a specialist in toxicology.

toxicosis *f.* toxicosis, morbid state caused by a poison.

toxina *f.* toxin, a noxious substance produced by a plant or animal microorganism; ___ **bacteriana** / bacterial ___ .

toxina antitoxina *f.* toxin-antitoxin, a nearly neutral mixture of a toxin and its antitoxin used for immunization against the specific disease caused by the toxin.

toxoide *m.* toxoid, a toxin void of toxicity that causes antibody formation and produces immunity to the specific disease caused by the toxin; ___ **diftérico** / diphtheria ___; ___ **tetánico** / tetanus ___ .

Toxoplasma *m. Toxoplasma*, a genus of parasitic protozoa; **anticuerpo del** ___ / ___ antibody; ___ **serológico** / serologic ___ .

toxoplasmosis *f.* toxoplasmosis, infection with organisms of the genus *Toxoplasma* that can cause minimal symptoms of malaise or swelling of the lymph glands, or serious damage to the central nervous system.

trabajador-a *m., f.* worker; ___ **social** / social ___ .

trabajar *v.* to work, to labor.

trabajo *m.* work, job, occupation; ___ **de beneficencia social** / welfare ___; ___ **de casa** / housework; ___ **excesivo** / overwork.

trabajoso-a *a.* laborious, hard.

tracción *f.* traction. 1. the action of drawing or pulling; 2. a pulling force; ___ **cervical** / cervical ___; ___ **lumbar** / lumbar ___ .

tracoma *f.* trachoma, a viral contagious disease of the conjunctiva and the cornea, manifested by photophobia, pain, tearing, and, in severe cases, blindness.

tracto *m.* tract, an elongated system of tissue or organs that acts to carry out a common function; ___ **alimenticio** / alimentary ___; ___ **dorsolateral** / dorsolateral ___; ___ **genitourinario** / genitourinary ___; ___ **intestinal** / intestinal ___; ___ **respiratorio** / respiratory ___ .

tragar *vi.* to swallow; ___ **apresuradamente** / to gulp down.

trago *m.* tragus, triangular cartilaginous eminence in the outer part of the ear.

trance *m.* trance, hypnotic-like state characterized by detachment from the surroundings and diminished motor activity.

tranquilizante *m.* tranquilizer, sedative.

tranquilo-a *a.* tranquil, calm, restful.

transabdominal *a.* transabdominal, through or across the abdominal wall.

transaminasa glutámica oxalacética *f.* glutamic-oxaloacetic transaminase, enzyme present in several tissues, such as the heart, liver, and brain, that presents a high concentration of serum when there is cardiac or hepatic damage.

transaminasa glutámica pirúvica *f.* glutamicpyruvic transaminase, enzyme that presents an elevated serum content when there is an injury or acute damage to liver cells.

transcutáneo-a *a.* transcutaneous, through the skin; **neuroestimulación eléctrica** ___ / ___ electrical nerve stimulation.

transección *f.* transection, cross section, cutting across the long axis of an organ.

transexual *a.* transexual. 1. individual with a psychological urge to be of the opposite sex; 2. person who has undergone a ical sex change.

transferencia *f.* transfer, transference. 1. in psychoanalysis, shifting feelings and behavior towards a new object, gen. the psychoanalyst; 2. transmission of symptoms from one part of the body to another.

transferrina *f.* transferrin, a type of beta globulin in blood plasma that fixes and transports iron.

transfixión *f.* transfixion, the act of cutting through soft tissues from the inside outwards, such as in amputations and excision of tumors.

transformación *f.* transformation, change of form or appearance.

transfusión *f.* transfusion, the process of transferring fluid into a vein or artery; ___ **directa** / direct ___; ___ **indirecta** / indirect ___; ___ **de sangre** / blood ___ .

transición *f.* transition.

transicional *a.* transitional, rel. to or subject to change; **carcinoma** ___ **celular** / ___ cellular carcinoma.

transiluminación *f.* transillumination, passage of light through a body part.

transitorio-a *a.* transitory, of a temporal nature.

translocación f. translocation, displacement of all or part of a chromosome to another chromosome.

translúcido-a a. translucent.

transmigración f. transmigration, the passing from one place to another such as of blood cells in diapedesis.

transmisible a. transmissible, that can be transmitted.

transmisión f. transmission, the act of transmitting, such as an infectious disease or a hereditary condition; ___ **patógena** / pathogen ___; ___ **placentaria** / placental ___; ___ **por contacto** / ___ by contact; ___ **por instilación** / droplet ___ .

transmisor m. transmitter.

transmitir vt. transmit, the act of transfering a genetic disease, a hereditary trait or infection from a person to another.

transmutación f. transmutation. 1. transformation, evolutionary change; 2. change of one chemical into another.

transorbitorio-a a. transorbital, occurring or passing through the orbit of the eye.

transparente a. transparent, pertaining to the clear quality of an object allowing the light to go through and show images on the opposite side.

transplacentario-a a. transplacental, occurring through the placenta.

transposición f. transposition. 1. displacement of an organ to the opposite side; 2. displacement of genetic material from one chromosome to another resulting at times in congenital defects.

transposición de los grandes vasos f. transposition of the great vessels, congenital defect by which the aorta rises from the right ventricle and the pulmonary artery from the left ventricle.

transuretral a. transurethral, occurring or administered through the urethra.

transvaginal a. transvaginal, occurring or done through the vagina.

transversal a. transverse, across; **plano** ___ / ___ plane.

transverso-a a. transverse; **colon** ___ / ___ colon.

transvestido-a, transvestita m., f. transvestite, person who practices transvestism.

transvestismo m. transvestism, adoption of modalities of the opposite sex, esp. dress; cross-dressing.

trapecio m. trapezius, flat, triangular muscle essential in the rotation of the scapula.

tráquea f. trachea, respiratory conduit between the inferior extremity of the larynx and the beginning of the bronchi; pop. windpipe.

traqueal a. tracheal, rel. to the trachea.

traqueítis f. tracheitis, infl. of the trachea.

traqueobronquitis f. tracheobronchitis, infl. of both the trachea and the bronchi.

traqueoesofágico-a a. tracheoesophageal, rel. to the trachea and the esophagus; **fistula** ___ / ___ fistula.

traqueomalacia f. tracheomalacia, softening of the cartilages of the trachea.

traqueostenosis f. tracheostenosis, narrowing of the trachea.

traqueostomía f. tracheostomy, incision into the trachea through the neck to allow the passage of air in cases of obstruction.

traqueotomía f. tracheotomy, incision into the trachea through the skin and muscles of the neck.

trasero m. pop. buttocks, rear.

trasplantación f. transplantation, the act of transplanting; ___ **autoplástica** / autoplastic ___; ___ **heteroplastíca** / heteroplastic ___; ___ **homotópica** / homotopic ___ .

trasplantar v. to transplant.

trasplante m. transplant, the transfer of an organ or tissue from a donor to a recipient, or from one part of the body to another in order to replace a diseased organ or to restitute impaired function.

trasplante de médula ósea m. bone marrow transplantation, grafting of bone marrow tissue to cancer patients after an extenuating degree of chemotherapy, or to patients suffering from aplastic anemia or severe leukemia.

trasplante de órgano m. organ transplantation.

trasplante cardíaco m. heart transplantation; ___ **de corazón** / heart ___ .

trasplante hepático m. liver transplantation

trastornado-a

Trastornos de la personalidad ejemplos	Personality disorders examples
trastorno de:	**disorder:**
__ ansiedad depresión aguda	anxiety __ acute depression
__ dependencia de adicción: dependencia en las drogas	addiction dependency__ drug dependence
__ de ajuste personalidad antisocial	adjustment__ antisocial personality
__ ciclotímico de cambios emocionales cíclicos	cyclothymic__ cyclic mood swings
__ de deglución bulimia, deglución excesiva	eating __ bulimia, binge eating
__de fobias miedo a las alturas	phobias __ fear of heights
__de cambios emocionales ataques de llanto	mood change __ crying attacks
__ de pánico miedo anormal a la oscuridad	panic__ abnormal fear of darkness
__ de falta de atención impulsividad, falta de concentración	attention deficit __ impulsivity, lack of concentration

trastornado-a *a.* deranged, mentally disturbed.

trastorno *m.* disturbance, disorder, derangement; ___ **del procesor metabólico** / deranged metabolic process; ___ **mental** / mental disorder; ___ **afectivo estacional** / seasonal affective disorder; ___ **alimenticio** / eating disorder; ___ **de ajuste** / adjustment disorder.

trastornos de la personalidad *m., pl.* personality disorders; ___ **de adicción a las drogas** / drug addiction; ___ **de ansiedad** / anxiety disorder; ___ **ciclotímico** / cyclothymic ___; ___ **de ajuste** / adjustment ___; ___ **de cambios emocionales** / mood change ___; ___ **de deglución** / eating ___; ___ **de falta de atención** / attention deficit disorder; ___ **de fobias** / phobic disorders ; ___ **de pánico** / panic ___. See table on this page.

trastornos sexuales *m., pl.* sexual disorders; **erotomanía** / erotomania; **exhibicionismo** / exhibitionism; **fetichismo** / fetishism; **fetichismo trasvestido** / transvestic fetishism; **froterismo** / frotteurism; **masoquismo** / masochism; **ninfomanía** / nymphomania; **parafilia** / paraphilia; **pedofilia** / pedophilia; **sadismo** / sadism; **satiromanía** / satyromania; **voyeurismo, mironismo** / voyeurism.

trasudado *m.* transudate, fluid that has passed through a membrane or that has been forced out from a tissue as a result of infl.

tratado-a *a.* treated; **no** ___ / untreated

tratamiento *m.* treatment, method, or procedure used in curing illnesses, lesions, or malformations; **método o plan de** ___ / ___ plan; **sujeto a** ___ / under ___; ___ **de desintoxicación** / withdrawal ___ .

tratar *v.* [*a un paciente*] to treat; to try.

trato *m.* care; treatment; **buen** ___ / good ___; **mal** ___ / bad ___ .

trauma, traumatismo *m.* 1. trauma, a psychological state; **Una muerte en la familia es un trauma familiar.** / A death in the family is a trauma; 2. traumatismo, refering to a physiological condition; **Un golpe en la cabeza es un traumatismo cerebral** ___ / A blow to the head is cerebral trauma.

traumatizado-a *a.* traumatized.

traumatología *f.* traumatology, the branch of surg. that deals with injuries and wounds and their treatment.

travestido *m.* transvestite.

trazador *m.* tracer, a radioisotope that when introduced into the body leaves a trace that can be detected and followed.

triquinosis

trazo *m.* tracing, the graphic record of movement or change made by an instrument.

trefinación *f.* trephination, the act of removing a circular disk of bone, gen. from the skull, or of removing tissue from the cornea or sclera.

Trematoda *Gr. Trematoda,* a class of parasitic worms that includes the flatworms and the flukes, both pathogenic to humans.

tremor *m.* tremor, trembling.

trémulo-a *a.* tremulous, rel. to or affected by a tremor.

trepanación *f.* trepanation, perforation of the skull with a special instrument to relieve increased pressure caused by fracture or accumulation of intracranial blood or pus.

trepanar *v.* to trepan, to perforate with a trepan.

trépano *m.* trepan, bur, burr, type of drill used for trepanation.

Treponema *Gr. Treponema,* microorganisms of the genus Spirochaetales, some of which are pathogenic to humans and other animals; __ **pallidum** / __ pallidum, causing agent of syphilis.

treponema *m.* treponema, any organism of the genus Treponema.

treponemiasis *f.* treponemiasis, infection with organisms of the genus Treponema.

tríada *f.* triad, a group of three related elements, objects, or symptoms.

triage *Fr.* triage, screening and classification of injured persons during a battle or disaster for the purpose of establishing priority of treatment in order to maximize the number who will survive.

tríceps *m.* triceps, a three-headed muscle; **reflejo del** __ / __ reflex.

Trichinella *Gr. Trichinella* a genus of nematode worms parasitic in carnivorous mammals.

Trichomonas *Gr. tricomonas m. Trichomonas,* a genus of parasitic protozoa that lodge in the alimentary and genitourinary tracts of vertebrates; __ **vaginal** / __ vaginalis.

tricobezoar *m.* trichobezoar, concretion or bezoar of hair found in the intestine or stomach.

tricomicosis *f.* trichomycosis, hair disease caused by a fungus.

tricomoniasis *f.* trichomoniasis, infestation with *Trichomonas;* __ **vaginal** / vaginal __ .

tricromático-a *a.* trichromatic, rel. to or consisting of three colors.

tricúspide *a.* tricuspid. 1. having three points; 2. rel. to the tricuspid valve of the heart; **atresia** __ / __ atresia; **soplo** __ / __ murmur; **válvula** __ / __ valve.

trifocal *a.* trifocal.

trigémino-a *a.* trigeminal, rel. to the trigeminus nerve; **neuralgia** __ / __ neuralgia.

trigeminus *L.* trigeminus, trigeminus nerve. See **craneales, nervios**.

triglicéridos *m. triglycerides* combination resulting from one molecule of glycerol and three molecules of fatty acids; elevated triglycerides are considered an important factor in heart disease.

trigonitis *f.* trigonitis, infl. of the trigone of the urinary bladder.

trigueño-a *a.* dark-complexioned, brunet, brunette.

trimestre *m.* trimester, three-month period, one of the consecutive months in which the gestation time is divided.

trinchera *f.* trench, ditch, moat; **fiebre de** __ / __ fever; **pie de** __ / __ foot, infection caused by exposure to severe cold

tripa *f.* tripe, gut.

tripanosomiasis *f.* trypanosomiasis, infection caused by a flagellated organism of the genus Trypanosoma.

triplopia *f.* triplopia, eye disorder in which three images of the same object are seen at one time.

tripsina *f.* trypsin, an enzyme present in the pancreatic juice formed by trypsinogen.

tripsinógeno *m.* trypsinogen, inactive substance released by the pancreas into the duodenum to form trypsin.

triptófano *m.* tryptophan, crystalline amino acid present in proteins essential to animal life.

triquina *f.* trichina, a worm that lives as a parasite in the muscles in the larval stage, and in the intestines when mature.

triquinosis *f.* trichinosis, disease acquired by ingestion of raw or inadequately cooked meat, esp. pork, that contains the larvae of Trichinella spiralis.

triquitis *f.* trichitis, infl. of hair bulbs.

trismo *m.* trismus, a spasm of the mastication muscles.

trisomía *f.* trisomy, genetic disorder in which there are three homologous chromosomes per cell instead of the usual two (diploid), causing severe fetal malformation.

trituración *f.* trituration; pulverization.

trocánter *m.* trochanter, each of the two outer prominences below the neck of the femur; __ **mayor** / major __; __ **menor** / lesser __ .

tróclea *f.* trochlea, structure that functions as a pulley.

trombectomía *f.* thrombectomy, removal of a thrombus.

trombina *f.* thrombin, an enzyme present in extravasated blood which catalyzes the conversion of fibrinogen to fibrin.

trombo *m.* thrombus, a blood clot that causes a total or partial vascular obstruction; __ **blanco** / white __ , pale; __ **estratificado** / stratified __ , layered; __ **mural** / mural __ , attached to the wall of the endocardium; __ **oclusivo** / occluding __ , that closes the vessel completely.

tromboangiítis *f.* thromboangiitis, thrombosis of a blood vessel.

trombocito *m.* thrombocyte, platelet.

trombocitopenia *f.* thrombocytopenia, abnormal decrease in the number of blood platelets.

trombocitosis *f.* thrombocytosis, abnormal increase in the number of blood platelets.

tromboembolia *f.* thromboembolism, obstruction of a blood vessel by a blood clot that has broken away from its site of origin.

tromboflebitis *f.* thrombophlebitis, dilation of a vein wall associated with thrombosis.

tromboflebitis migratoria *f.* thrombophlebitis migrans, slowly progressing thrombophlebitis moving from one vein to another.

trombogénesis *f.* thrombogenesis, formation of blood clots.

trombólisis *f.* thrombolysis, dissolution of a thrombus.

trombosado-a *a.* thrombosed, rel. to a blood vessel containing a thrombus.

trombosis *f.* thrombosis, formation, development, or presence of a thrombus; __ **biliar** / biliary __; __

cardíaca / cardiac __; __ **coronaria** / coronary __; __ **embólica** / embolic __; __ **traumática** / traumatic __; __ **venosa** / venous __ .

trompa *f.* tube, conduit; **ligadura de las** __ -s / tubal ligation.

troncal *a.* truncal, rel. to the trunk of the body.

tronco *m.* trunk, the human body exclusive of the head and the extremities.

tropezar *vi.* to bump or stumble into something or somebody.

tropical *a.* tropical, rel. to the tropics.

tropismo *m.* tropism, the reaction of a cell or living organism toward or away from the source of an external stimulus.

truncus *L.* truncus, trunk.

Trypanosoma *m.* *Trypanosoma*, a genus of parasitic protozoa found in the blood of many vertebrates, transmitted to them by insect vectors.

tsetsé *m.* tsetse fly, bloodsucking fly of southern Africa that transmits sleeping sickness.

tuba *L.* tuba, tube; __ **acústica** / eustachian tube.

tubárico-a *a.* tubal, rel. to a tube; **embarazo** __ / __ pregnancy occurring in the fallopian tube.

tubercular *a.* tubercular, rel. to or marked by tubercles.

tuberculicida *a.* tuberculocidal, that destroys the tubercle bacilli.

tuberculina *f.* tuberculin, compound prepared from the tubercle bacillus and used in the diagnosis of tuberculosis infection; **prueba de la** __ / __ test.

tubérculo *m.* tubercle. 1. small nodule; 2. small knobby prominence of a bone; 3. the characteristic lesion produced by the tuberculosis bacilli.

tuberculosis *f.* tuberculosis, an acute or chronic bacterial infection caused by the germ *Mycobacterium tuberculosis* that gen. affects the lungs, although it can affect other organs as well; __ **espinal** / spinal __; __ **infantil** / childhood __; __ **meníngea** / meningeal __; __ **pulmonar** / pulmonary __; __ **urogenital** / urogenital __ .

tuberculosis miliar *f.* miliary tuberculosis, disease that invades the organism through the bloodstream and is characterized by the formation of minute tubercles in the different organs affected by it.

tuberosidad *f.* tuber, a swelling or enlargement.

tubo *m.* tube, elongated, cylindrical, hollow structure; __ **colector** / collecting tubule; __ **contorneado del riñón** / convoluted tubule of the kidney; __ **de drenaje** / drainage __; __ **de ensayo** / test __; __ **de inhalación** / inhalation __; __ **de toracostomía** / thoracostomy __; __ **de traqueotomía** / tracheotomy __; __ **endotraqueal** / endotracheal __; __ **en T** / T- __; __ **nasogástrico** / nasogastric __; __ **urinífero** / uriniferous tubule.

tubo-ovaritis *f.* tubo-ovaritis, infl. of the ovary and the Fallopian tube.

tuboovárico-a *a.* tubo-ovarian, rel. to the fallopian tube and the ovary; **absceso** __ / __ abscess.

tuboplastia *f.* tuboplasty, plastic surgery of a tube, esp. the fallopian tube.

túbulo *m.* tubule, a small anatomical tube; __ **colector** / collecting __; __ **renal** / renal __ .

tuerto-a *a.* one-eyed or blind in one eye.

tularemia *f.* tularemia, rabbit fever, infection transmitted to humans by the bite of a vector insect or by handling of infected meat.

tumefacción, tumescencia *f.* tumefaction, the process of swelling.

tumor *m.* tumor, swelling, new spontaneous growth of mass or tissue of no physiological use; __ **desdiferenciado** / undifferentiated __; __ **difundido o difuso** / diffuse __; __ **escirroso** / scirrhous __; __ **inflamatorio** / inflammatory __; __ **medular** / medullary __; __ **necrótico** / necrotic __; __ **no solido** / nonsolid __; __ **radiocurable** / radiocurable __; __ **radiorresistente** / radioresistant __; __ **radiosensitivo** / radiosensitive __; __ **sin diferenciación** / undifferentiated __ .

tumoral *a.* tumorous, rel. to a tumor.

tumorectomía *f.* lumpectomy, excision of a breast tumor excluding lymph nodes and adjacent tissue.

tumoricida *a.* tumoricidal, that destroys tumorous cells.

tumorigénesis *f.* tumorigenesis, production of tumors.

túnel *m.* tunnel, a bodily channel; __ **del carpo** / carpal __; __ **flexor** / flexor __; __ **torsal, tarsiano** / torsal __ .

túnica *L.* tunica, tunic, protective membrane; __ **adventicia** / __ adventitia; __ **albugínea** / __ albuginea; __ **dartos** / __ dartos; __ **mucosa** / __ mucosa; __ **muscular** / __ muscularis; __ **serosa** / __ serosa; __ **vaginal** / __ vaginalis.

túnica *f.* tunic, covering, outer layer of an organ or part.

tupido-a *a.* plugged, obstructed; **oídos** __ / __ ears.

turbio-a *a.* turbid, cloudy, not translucent.

turgido-a *a.* turgid, distended, swollen.

turgor *m.* turgor. 1. swelling, distension; 2. normal cellular tension.

Turner, sindrome de *m.* Turner's syndrome, congenital endocrine abnormality manifested by amenorrhea, failure of sexual maturation, short stature and neck, and the presence of only forty-five chromosomes.

tussis *L.* tussis, cough.

tympanum *L.* tympanum, the middle ear. *See* **tímpano**.

u

U *abr.* unidad / unit; **uranio** / uranium; **urología** / urology.

u *conj.* or, used instead of *o* before words beginning with *o* or *ho*.

úlcera *f.* ulcer, sore, or lesion of the skin or mucous membrane with gradual disintegration of tissue; **chancroide** / chancroidal; ___ **crónica** / chronic ___; ___ **duodenal** / duodenal ___; ___ **fagedénica** / phagedenic ___; ___ **gástrica** / gastric ___; ___ **hemorrágica** / hemorrhagic ___; ___ **indolente** / indolent ___; ___ **marginal** / marginal ___; ___ **micótica** / mycotic ___; ___ **péptica** / peptic ___ ; ___ **perforante** / perforating ___; ___ **por decúbito** / decubitus ___ , bedsore; ___ **roedora** / rodent ___ , that destroys gradually; ___ **sifilítica** / syphilitic ___; ___ **varicosa crónica de la pierna** / chronic varicose leg ___; ___ **vesical** / vesical ___ . See table on page 487.

úlcera péptica *f.* peptic ulcer, ulceration of the mucous membranes of the esophagus, stomach, or duodenum caused by excessive acidity of the gastric juice, gen. produced by acute or chronic stress.

ulceración *f.* ulceration, the formation process of an ulcer; **-es genitales** / genital ___ -s.

ulcerado-a *a.* ulcerated, rel. to or of the nature of an ulcer.

ulcerativo *a.* ulcerative, rel. to or causing an ulcer.

uleritema *m.* ulerythema, erythematous dermatitis characterized by formation of scars.

ulnar *a.* ulnar, rel. to the ulna or to the arteries and nerves related to it; **disfunción del nervio** ___ / ___ nerve dysfunction.

ulocarcinoma *m.* ulocarcinoma, cancer of the gums.

ultracentrífuga *f.* ultracentrifuge, machine with a centrifugal force capable of separating and sedimenting the molecules of a substance.

ultrafiltración *f.* ultrafiltration, a filtration process that allows the passage of small molecules, holding back larger ones.

ultramicroscopio *m.* ultramicroscope, a microscope that makes visible objects that cannot be seen under a common light microscope.

ultrasónico-a *a.* ultrasonic.

ultrasonido *m.* ultrasound, a sound wave with a frequency above the range of human hearing used in ultrasonography for diagnostic and therapeutic purposes; **diagnóstico por** ___ / ultrasonic diagnosis; ___ **abdominal** / abdominal ___; ___ **de la mama** / breast ___; ___ **de la tiroides** / thyroid ___; ___ **del embarazo** / pregnancy ___ .

ultrasonografía *f.* ultrasonography, diagnostic technique that uses ultrasound waves to develop the image of a body structure or tissue.

ultrasonograma *m.* ultrasonogram, the image produced by ultrasonography.

ultravioleta *a.* ultraviolet, beyond the visible, violet end of the spectrum; **rayos** ___ / ___ rays; **terapia de radiación** ___ / ___ therapy.

umbilical *a.* umbilical, rel. to the umbilicus.

umbral *m.* threshold, the minimum degree of stimulus needed to produce an effect or response; ___ **absoluto** / absolute ___; ___ **auditivo** / auditory ___; ___ **de la conciencia** / ___ of consciousness; ___ **renal** / renal ___; ___ **sensorio** / sensory ___ .

unánime *a.* unanimous.

ungueal *a.* ungual, rel. to the nails.

ungüento *m.* unguent, liniment, salve, medicated preparation for external use.

uniarticular *a.* uniarticular, rel. to a single joint.

unibásico-a *a.* unibasal, rel. to a single base.

unicelular *a.* unicellular, having only one cell.

único-a *a.* only, sole; **-mente** *adv.* only, solely.

unidad *f.* unit. 1. one of a kind; ___ **motora** / motor ___ , that provides motor activity; 2. standard of measurement; 3. unity.

unidad de cuidado cardíaco intensivo *f.* intensive unit of cardiac care.

unidad de cuidado intensivo *f.* intensive care unit.

ureterouereterostomía

unidad internacional *f.* international unit, standard measurement of a given substance as adopted by the International Conference for Unification of Formulae.

unido-a *a.* joined; close.

uniforme *m.* uniform; *a.* uniform, even.

unigrávida *f.* unigravida, woman who is pregnant for the first time.

unión *f.* union. 1. the action or effect of joining two things into one; 2. the growing together of severed parts of a bone or of the lips of a wound.

unípara *f.* uniparous, woman who gives birth to only one child.

unipolar *a.* unipolar, having one pole, such as the nerve cells.

universal *a.* universal, general.

Unna, bota de pasta de *f.* Unna's paste boot, compression dressing applied to the lower part of the leg in the treatment of varicose ulcers consisting of layers of gauze applied with and covered with Unna's paste.

unsinaria *f.* hookworm, intestinal parasite; **enfermedad de la __ / __** disease.

untadura *f.* application; ointment.

untar *vt.* to apply ointment; to rub, to smear.

uña *f.* nail; **__ del dedo del pie** / toenail; **__ encarnada** / ingrown __; *vr.* **comerse las __ -s** / to bite one's __ -s.

uñero *m.* ingrown nail.

uránico-a *a.* uranic, rel. to uremia.

uranio *m.* uranium, heavy metallic element.

urato *m.* urate, uric acid salt.

urea *f.* urea, crystalline substance found in the blood, lymph, and urine that is the final product of the metabolism of proteins and is excreted through the urine as nitrogen.

urelcosis *f.* urelcosis, formation of ulcers in the urinary tract.

uremia *f.* uremia, toxic condition caused by renal insufficiency that produces retention of nitrogen substances, phosphates, and sulfates in the blood; **__ eclámptica** / eclamptic __ .

urémico-a *a.* uremic, rel. to or affected by uremia.

uréter *m.* ureter, one of the ducts by which urine passes from the kidney to the urinary bladder.

ureteral, uretérico-a *a.* ureteral, rel. to a ureter; **lesión __ / __** injury; **obstrucción __ / __** obstruction; **reflejo __ / __** reflex.

ureterectasis *f.* ureterectasis, abnormal dilation of the ureter.

ureterectomía *f.* ureterectomy, partial or total excision of the ureter.

ureteritis *f.* ureteritis, infl. of the ureter.

ureterocele *m.* ureterocele, cystic dilation of the distal intravesical portion of the ureter due to stenosis of the ureteral orifice.

ureterocistostomía *f.* ureterocystostomy, surgical communication made between the cervix and the bladder. *See* **ureteroneocistostomía**.

ureterografía *f.* ureterography, x-ray of the ureter with the use of a radiopaque substance.

ureteroheminefrectomía *f.* ureteroheminephrectomy, resection of a portion of the kidney and its ureter in cases of duplication of the upper urinary tract.

ureterohidronefrosis *f.* ureterohydronephrosis, distension of the ureter and the kidney due to obstruction.

ureterolitiasis *f.* ureterolithiasis, formation of a ureteral calculus.

ureterolitotomía *f.* ureterolithotomy, incision into a ureter for removal of a calculus.

ureteronefrectomía *f.* ureteronephrectomy, excision of the kidney and its ureter.

ureteroneocistostomía *f.* ureteroneocystostomy, reimplantation of the ureter into the bladder.

ureteropélvico-a *a.* ureteropelvic, rel. to the ureter and the pelvis.

ureteropieloplastia *f.* ureteropyeloplasty, plastic surgery of a ureter and the renal pelvis.

ureteroplastia *f.* ureteroplasty, plastic surgery of the ureter.

ureterosigmoidostomía *f.* ureterosigmoidostomy, implantation of a ureter in the sigmoid colon.

ureterostomía *f.* ureterostomy, formation of a permanent fistula for drainage of a ureter.

ureterotomía *f.* ureterotomy, incision into a ureter.

ureteroureterostomía *f.* ureteroureterostomy, anastomosis of two ureters or of extreme parts of the same ureter.

ureterovesical *a.* ureterovesical, rel. to the ureter and the urinary bladder.

urético-a *a.* uretic, rel. to the urine.

uretra *f.* urethra, urinary canal.

uretral *a.* urethral, rel. to the urethra; **catéter __ / __** catheter; **obstrucción __ / __** obstruction; **procedimiento __ / __** process; **secreción __ / __** discharge; **síndrome __ / __** syndrome; **suspensión __ / __** suspension.

uretralgia *f.* urethralgia, pain in the urethra.

uretrectomía *f.* urethrectomy, partial or total excision of the urethra.

uretritis *f.* urethritis, chronic or acute infl. of the urethra.

uretrografía *f.* urethrography, x-ray of the urethra after injection of a radiopaque substance.

uretroscopio *m.* urethroscope, instrument for viewing the interior of the urethra.

uretrotomía *f.* urethrotomy, incision of the urethra, usu. to alleviate a stricture.

uretrótomo *m.* urethrotome, instrument used in urethrotomy.

urgente *a.* urgent, pressing; **-mente** *adv.* urgently.

uricemia *f.* uricemia, excess uric acid in the blood.

úrico-a *a.* uric, rel. to the urine.

uricosuria *f.* uricosuria, presence of an excessive amount of uric acid in the urine.

urinación *f.* urination, the act of urinating.

urinálisis *m.* urinalysis, analysis of the urine.

urinario-a *a.* urinary, rel. to the urine; **infección __ / __** infection; **órganos __ -s / __** organs; **sedimento __ / __** sediment.

urinario, sistema *m.* urinary system, the group of organs and conduits that participate in the production and excretion of urine.

urinífero-a *a.* uriniferous, containing or carrying urine.

urinogenital, urogenital *a.* urinogenital, urogenital, rel. to the urinary and the genital tracts.

urinoma *m.* urinoma, a cyst containing urine.

urobilinógeno *m.* urobilinogen, pigment derived from the reduction of bilirubin by action of intestinal bacteria.

urocinasa *f.* urokinase, enzyme present in human urine used to dissolve blood clots.

urodinámica *f.* urodynamics, the study of the active process and pathophysiology of urination.

urodinia *f.* urodynia, painful urination.

urogenital *a.* urogenital, rel. to the urinary and the genital tracts; **diafragma __ / __** diaphragm.

urografía *f.* urography, x-ray of a part of the urinary tract by injection of a radiopaque substance; **__ descendente o excretora** / descending or excretory **__**; **__ retrógrada** / retrograde **__** .

urograma *m.* urogram, x-ray record of a urography.

urohematonefrosis *f.* urohematonephrosis, pathological condition of the kidney by which the pelvis distends with blood and urine.

urolitiasis *f.* urolithiasis, formation of urinary calculi and disorders associated with their presence.

urolítico-a *a.* urolithic, rel. to urinary calculi.

urología *f.* urology, the branch of medicine that studies the diagnosis and treatment of diseases of the genitourinary tract in men and the urinary tract in women.

urológico-a *a.* urologic, rel. to urology.

urólogo-a *m., f.* urologist, specialist in urology.

uropatía *f.* uropathy, any disease that affects the urinary tract.

urosquesis *f.* uroschesis, suspension or retention of urine.

urticaria *f.* urticaria, hives, eruptive skin disease characterized by pink patches accompanied by intense itching, gen. allergic in nature and caused by an internal or external agent; **__ papulosa** / papular **__**; **__ pigmentosa / __** pigmentosa; **__ térmica** / heat rash.

usado-a *a.* used.

usar *vt.* to use; [*ropa*] to wear.

uso *m.* use; function; usage; **de poco __** / under **__**; **__ no aprobado /** off-label **__** .

usual *a.* usual, customary; **-mente** *adv.* usually.

uterino-a *a.* uterine, rel. to the uterus; **prolapso __ / __** prolapse; **ruptura**

___ / ___ rupture; **sangramiento** ___ / ___ bleeding unrelated to menstruation.

útero _m._ uterus, womb, hollow, muscular organ of the female reproductive system that contains and nourishes the embryo and fetus during the period of gestation; **cáncer del** ___ **o de la matriz** / uterine cancer; ___ **didelfo** / didelphys ___ , double uterus.

uterosalpingografía _f._ uterosalpingography, x-ray examination of the uterus and the fallopian tubes following injection of a radiopaque substance.

uterovaginal _a._ uterovaginal, rel. to the uterus and the vagina.

uterovesical _a._ uterovesical, rel. to the uterus and the urinary bladder.

útil _a._ useful, practical.

utrículo _m._ utriculus, small bag; ___ **del oído o del vestíbulo** / ___ of the ear or of vestibule; ___ **prostático o uretral** / ___ prostaticus or urethral.

uva _f._ grape.

uvea _f._ uvea, the vascular layer of the eye formed by the iris and the ciliary body together with the choroid coat.

uveitis _f._ uveitis, infl. of the uvea.

úvula _f._ uvula, small, fleshy structure hanging in the middle of the posterior border of the soft palate; ___ **hundida** / cleft ___; ___ **vesical** / vesical ___ .

uvulitis _f._ uvulitis, infl. of the uvula.

uvulotomía _f._ uvulotomy, partial or total cutting of the uvula.

u

V

V _abr._ **válvula** / valve; **vena** / vein; **visión** / vision; **volumen** / volume.

vaccinia _L._ vaccinia, cowpox, a virus that causes disease in cattle and when inoculated in humans gives a degree of immunity against smallpox.

vaciar _vt._ to empty; to flush out, to void; **vaciarse** _vr._ to become empty.

vacilante _a._ vacillating, fluctuating; shaky.

vacío-a _a._ empty; **envasado al __ /** vacuum packed.

vacuna _f._ vaccine, a preparation of attenuated or killed microorganisms that when introduced in the body establishes immunity to the specific disease caused by such microorganisms; **reacción a la __ / __** reaction; **__ antipolio oral, trivalente atenuada de Sabin** / poliovirus, live oral trivalent __ , Sabin; **__ antirrábica** / rabies __; **__ antisarampión de virus, vivo** / measles virus __ , live; **__ antisarampión, inactivada** / measles virus __ , inactivated; **__ antitífica** / typhoid fever __; **__ antivariólica, antivariolosa** / smallpox __; **__ contra la tuberculosis** / BCG __ against tuberculosis; **__ contra el tétano** / tetanus __; **__ contra la hepatitis A** / hepatitis A __; **__ contra la hepatitis B** / hepatitis B __; **__ contra la influenza** / influenza __; **__ contra la varicela** / chickenpox __; **__ de Salk, contra la poliomielitis** / Salk __ , antipolio; **__ de virus vivo contra la rubéola** / rubella virus __ , live; **__ neumocócica polisacárida** / pneumovax __; **__ neumocócica polivalente** / pneumococcal polyvalent virus __; **__ triple contra la difteria, el tétano y la tos ferina / __** , against diphtheria, pertussis, and tetanus.

vacunación _f._ vaccination, inoculation of vaccine.

vacunar _vt._ to vaccinate.

vacuola _f._ vacuole, small cavity or space filled with fluid or air in the cellular protoplasm.

vacuolización _f._ vacuolization, formation of vacuoles.

vacuum _L._ vacuum, emptiness, a space devoid of air or matter.

vagal _a._ vagal, rel. to the pneumogastric or vagus nerve.

vagar _vi._ to wander.

vagina _f._ vagina. 1. female canal extending from the uterus to the vulva; 2. structure resembling a sheath.

vaginal _a._ vaginal, rel. to the vagina or to a sheathlike structure; **candidiasis __ / __** candidiasis; **cultivo __ / __** culture; **flujo __ / __** discharge; **hemorragia, sangrado __ / __** bleeding; **picazón __ / __** itching; **quistes __ / __** cysts; **reparación de la pared __ / __** wall repair; **tratamiento de secamiento __ / __** drying treatment; **tumor __ / __** tumor.

vaginismus _L._ vaginismus, sudden and painful spasm of the vagina.

vaginitis _f._ vaginitis, infl. of the vagina; **__ bacteriana** / bacterial __ .

vaginoplastia _f._ vaginoplasty, plastic surgery of the vagina.

vaginosis _f._ vaginosis, infl. of the vagina.

vago, nervio _m._ vagus nerve. _See_ **nervios craneales**.

vagolisis _f._ vagolysis, surgical destruction of the vagus nerve.

vagolítico-a _a._ vagolytic, inhibiting the function of the vagus nerve.

vagotomía _f._ vagotomy, interruption of the vagus nerve.

vaina _f._ sheath, a protective covering structure.

valer _vi._ to cost; to be worth; to be valid, good, or acceptable; **valerse** _vr._ __ **por sí mismo** / to be self-sufficient.

valgus _L._ valgus, bent or twisted outward.

válido-a _a._ valid, acceptable.

Valsalva, maniobra de _f._ Valsalva's maneuver, procedure to test the patency of the eustachian tubes or to adjust the pressure of the middle ear by forcibly exhaling while holding the nostrils and mouth closed.

válvula _f._ valve, a membranous structure in a canal or orifice that closes temporarily to prevent the backward flow of the contents passing through it; **__ aórtica** / aortic __ , between the left ventricle and the aorta; **__ atrioventricular derecha, tricúspide** / atrioventricular __ right, tricuspid; __

atrioventricular izquierda, bicúspide, mitral / atrioventricular __ left, bicuspid, mitral; __ **ileocecal** / ileocecal __ ; __ **pilórica** / pyloric __ ; __ **pulmonar** / pulmonary __ .

válvula mitral f. mitral valve, the left atrioventricular valve of the heart; **insuficiencia de la** __ / insufficiency of the __ ; **prolapso de la** __ / prolapse of the __ .

valvular a. valvular, rel. to a valve or of its nature; **estenosis pulmonar** __ / pulmonary stenosis.

válvulas conniventes f., pl. valvulae conniventes, circular membranous folds found in the small intestine that slow the passage of food along the bowels.

valvulitis f. valvulitis, infl. of a valve, esp. the cardiac valve.

valvuloplastia f. valvuloplasty, plastic surgery of a heart valve.

valvulótomo m. valvulotome, instrument to incise a valve.

vapor m. vapor, gas, fume.

vaporización f. vaporization. 1. action and effect of vaporizing; 2. therapeutic use of vapors.

vaporizador m. vaporizer, device used to convert a substance into a vapor for therapeutic purposes.

variable f. variable, a changing factor; a. that can change.

variante f. variant, that which is essentially the same as another but different in form; a. different, changing.

várice, variz f. varix, an enlarged and tortuous vein, artery or lymphatic vessel.

varicella L. varicella, chicken pox, viral contagious disease, gen. manifested during childhood, characterized by an eruption that evolves into small vesicles.

varicocele m. varicocele, varicose condition of the veins of the spermatic cord that produces a soft mass in the scrotum.

varicocelectomía f. varicocelectomy, surgical removal of part of the scrotal sac.

varicoso-a a. varicose, resembling or related to varices; **venas** __ -s / __ veins.

varicotomía f. varicotomy, excision of a varicose vein.

varilla f. thin, short rod; wand; __ **de aceite** / dipstick.

variola L. variola. viruela.

variólico-a, varioloso-a a. variolous, rel. to smallpox or affected by it.

varios-as a. several.

varón m. male.

varonil a. manly.

varus L. varus, twisted or turned inward.

vas deferens L. vas deferens, the excretory duct of the spermatozoa.

vascular a. vascular, rel. to the blood vessels; **cambio cutáneo** __ / __ skin change; **ectasia** __ **del colon** / __ ectasia of the colon; **espasmo** __ / __ spasm; **púrpura** __ / __ purpura; **sistema** __ / __ system, all the vessels of the body, esp. the blood vessels; **túnica** __ / __ tunic.

vascularización f. vascularization, formation of new blood vessels.

vascularizar vi. to vascularize, to develop new blood vessels.

vasculatura f. vasculature, arrangement of blood vessels in an organ or part.

vasculitis f. vasculitis. angiitis.

vasculopatía f. vasculopathy, any disease of a blood vessel.

vasectomía f. vasectomy, partial excision and ligation of the vas deferens to prevent the passage of spermatozoa into the semen, usu. done as a means of birth control.

vaselina f. vaseline, petroleum jelly.

vasija f. receptacle, vessel.

vaso m. vessel; conduit. 1. any channel or tube that carries fluid such as blood or lymph; **grandes** __ -s / great __ -s; __ **colateral** / collateral __ ; __ **linfático** / lymphatic __ ; __ **sanguíneo** / blood __ ; 2. a drinking glass.

vasoactivo m. vasoactive, agent that affects the blood vessels.

vasoconstricción f. vasoconstriction, decrease in the caliber of the blood vessels.

vasoconstrictor m. vasoconstrictor, that which causes vasoconstriction; **vasoconstrictor-a** a. vasoconstrictive, rel. to constriction of the blood vessels.

vasodepresión f. vasodepression, increase in the diameter of a blood vessel.

vasodilatación f. vasodilation, increase in the caliber of the blood vessels.

vasodilatador m. vasodilator, that which causes vasodilation;

vasodilatador-a *a.* that causes vasodilation.

vasoespasmo *m.* vasospasm. angioespasmo; ___ **coronario** / coronary ___ .

vasomotor *m.* vasomotor, that which regulates the contraction and dilation of blood vessels; **centro** ___ / ___ center; **epilepsy** ___ / ___ epilepsy; **paralysis** ___ / ___ paralysis; **reflejo** ___ / ___ reflex; **rinitis** ___ / ___ rhinitis; **sistema** ___ / ___ system; **-a** *a.* rel. to dilation or contraction of blood vessels.

vasopresina *f.* vasopressin, hormone secreted by the posterior pituitary gland that increases the reabsorption of water by the kidneys, raising the blood pressure.

vasopresor *m.* vasopressor, that which has a vasoconstrictive effect; **-a** *a.* having a vasoconstrictive effect.

vasovagal *a.* vasovagal, rel. to the vessels and the vagus nerve; **síncope** ___ / ___ syncope, brief fainting spell caused by vascular and vagal disturbances.

Vater, ámpula de *f.* Vater's ampulla or papilla, the point where the biliary and pancreatic excretory systems enter the duodenum.

vector *m.* vector, a carrier that transmits infectious agents.

vegetación *f.* vegetation, a wartlike, abnormal growth on a body part as seen in endocarditis.

vegetarianismo *m.* vegetarianism, the practice of eating only vegetables and fruits. Dairy products may not be excluded.

vegetariano-a *m., f.* vegetarian, individual that eliminates any kind of food containing animal meat in his or her diet.

vegetativo-a *a.* vegetative. 1. rel. to functions of growth and nutrition; 2. rel. to involuntary or unconscious bodily movements; 3. pertaining to plants.

vehículo *m.* vehicle. 1. agent without therapeutic action that carries the active ingredient of a medication; 2. an agent of transmission.

vejez *f.* old age.

vejiga *f.* bladder; **cálculos de la** ___ / ___ calculi; ___ **hiperactiva** / hyperactive ___; **irrigación de la** ___ / ___ irrigation; ___ **llena de aire** / air ___; ___ **neurogénica** / neurogenic ___ .

vejiga urinaria *f.* urinary bladder, sac-shaped organ that serves as a receptacle to urine secreted by the kidneys.

velar *v.* to watch over, to take care of someone.

velo *m.* veil. 1. thin membrane or covering of a body part; 2. a piece of amniotic sac seen sometimes covering the face of a newborn; 3. slight alteration in the voice.

vello *m.* body hair; ___ **axilar** / axillary ___ ; ___ **púbico** / pubic hair.

vellosidad *f.* villus, short, filiform projection from a membranous surface; ___ **aracnoidea** / arachnoid ___; ___ **coriónica** / chorionic ___; ___ **-es intestinales** / intestinal ___; ___ **-es sinoviales** / synovial ___ .

vena *f.* vein, fibromuscular vessel that carries blood from the capillaries toward the heart; ___**-s varicosas** / ___ veins, *pop.* spider ___ .

vena cava *f.* vena cava, either of two large veins returning deoxygenated blood to the right atrium of the heart; ___ **inferior** / inferior ___; ___ **superior** / superior ___ .

vencimiento *m.* expiration; **fecha de** ___ / ___ date.

venda *f.* bandage; ___ **para los ojos** / eyeband.

vendaje *m.* bandage, dressing, curative, protective covering; ___ **abdominal** / abdominal binder; ___ **de yeso** / plaster cast; ___ **protector** / surgical dressing.

vendar *vt.* to bandage.

veneno *m.* poison, venom, toxic substance; **centro de control de** ___ **-s** / ___ control center.

venenoso-a *a.* poisonous, venomous, toxic; **hiedra** ___ / poison ivy.

venéreo-a *a.* venereal, resulting from or transmitted by sexual intercourse; **enfermedad** ___ / ___ disease; **verruga** ___ / ___ wart.

venina *f.* venin, toxic substance present in snake venom.

veninantivenina *f.* venin-antivenin, vaccine to counteract the effect of snake poison.

venipuntura *a.* venepuncture, venipuncture, surgical puncture of a vein.

venoclusivo-a *a.* veno-occlusive, rel. to the obstruction of veins.

venoconstricción *f.*
venoconstriction, constriction of the
muscular walls of the veins.

venograma *m.* venogram, x-ray of a
vein with the use of a contrasting
medium; ___ **renal** / renal ___ .

venoso-a *a.* venous, rel. to the veins;
congestión ___ / ___ congestion;
insuficiencia ___ / ___ insufficiency;
retorno ___ / ___ return; **sangre** ___ / ___
blood; **seno** ___ / ___ sinus;
tromboembolismo ___ / ___
thrombo-embolism; **trombosis** ___ / ___
thrombosis.

vent *Fr.* vent, opening.

ventaja *f.* advantage.

ventilación *f.* ventilation; ___
pulmonar / pulmonary / ___ 1. the act
of circulating fresh air in a given area;
2. oxygenation of blood; 3. open
discussion and airing of grievances.

ventilador *m.* ventilator, artificial
respirator; fan.

ventolera *f.* strong gust of wind.

ventral *a.* ventral, abdominal, rel. to the
belly or to the front side of the body;
hernia ___ / ___ hernia.

ventricular *a.* ventricular, rel. to a
ventricle; **defecto del tabique** ___ / ___
septal defect; **defecto septal** ___ / ___
septal defect; **fibrilación** ___ / ___
fibrillation; **punción** ___ / ___ puncture;
taquicardia ___ / ___ tachycardia.

ventriculitis *f.* ventriculitis, infl. of a
ventricle.

ventrículo *m.* ventricle, a small cavity,
esp. in reference to such structures as
seen in the heart, the brain, or the
larynx; **cuarto** ___ **del cerebro** / fourth
___ of the brain; **tercer** ___ **del cerebro**
/ third ___ of the brain; ___ **de la laringe**
/ ___ of the larynx; ___ **derecho del
corazón** / right ___ of the heart; ___
izquierdo del corazón / left ___ of the
heart; ___ **lateral del cerebro** / lateral
___ of the brain.

venticulograma *m.* venticulogram,
radionuclide test done during
catherization that evaluates the main
pumping chamber of the left ventricle
with each heartbeat.

ventriculotomía *f.* ventriculotomy,
incision of a ventricle.

vénula *f.* venule, minute vein that
connects the capillaries with larger
veins.

ver *vi.* to see; **está por** ___ / it remains
to be seen; **tener que** ___ **con** / to have

to do with; **verse** *vr.* to see oneself; to
see each other.

verano *m.* summer.

verdad *f.* truth; **decir la** ___ / to tell the
___; **de** ___ / truly, really; **¿no es** ___ **?** /
isn't it so?

verdadero-a *a.* true, real; **pelvis** ___ /
___ pelvis; **-mente** *adv.* truly.

verdugón *m.* welt.

verdura *f.* [*vegetales*] greens.

vergonzoso-a *a.* shameful.

vergüenza *f.* shame; bashfulness;
v. **tener** ___ / to be ashamed.

verificar *vi.* to verify, to prove true.

vermicida, vermífugo *m.*
vermicide, agent that destroys worms.

vermis *L.* vermis. 1. parasitic worm;
2. wormlike structure.

vernix *L.* vernix, varnish; ___ **caseosa** /
___ caseosa, sebaceous secretion
protecting the skin of a fetus.

verruca *L.* verruca, (*pl. verrucae*) wart;
___ **filiformis** / ___ filiformis; ___
plantaris / ___ plantaris; ___ **vulgaris** /
___ vulgaris.

verruga *f.* verruca; ___ **planas juveniles**
/ ___ planae juveniles; ___ **seborreica** /
seborrheic ___; ___ **simple** / simple ___ .

verrugoso-a *a.* verrucose, warty, or rel.
to warts.

versión *f.* version. 1. change of direction
of an organ, such as the uterus; 2.
change of position of the fetus in utero
to facilitate delivery; ___ **bimanual** /
bimanual ___ ; ___ **bipolar** / bipolar ___;
___ **cefálica** / cephalic ___; ___
combinada / combined ___; ___
externa / external ___; ___ **espontánea** /
spontaneous ___ .

vértebra *f.* vertebra, any of the
thirty-three bones of the vertebral
column; ___ **cervical** / cervical ___; ___
coccígea / coccygeal ___; ___ **lumbar** /
lumbar ___; ___ **sacra** / sacral ___; ___
torácica / thoracic ___ .

vertebral *a.* vertebral, rel. to the
vertebrae; **arteria** ___ / ___ artery;
conducto ___ / ___ canal; **costillas** ___
-es / ___ ribs.

vertebrobasilar *a.* vertebrobasilar,
rel. to the basilar and vertebral arteries;
insuficiencia ___ / ___ insufficiency;
sistema ___ / ___ system;
trastornos ___ **-es de la circulación** /
___ circulatory disorders; *n.*
vertebral-basilar, union of two arteries
localized at the base of the skull
forming the basilar artery.

V

verter

verter *vi.* to spill; to pour.

vertex *n.* (*pl.* **vértices**) vertex. 1. the highest point of a structure, such as the top of the head; 2. convergence point of the two sides of an angle.

vertical *a.* vertical. 1. upright; 2. rel. to the vertex.

vértice *m.* vertex.

vértigo *m.* vertigo, sensation of whirling motion either of oneself (subjective vertigo), or of surrounding objects (objective vertigo) gen. caused by a disease of the inner ear or by gastric or cardiac disorders; ___ **laberíntico** / labyrinthine ___ .

verumontanitis *f.* verumontanitis, infl. of the verumontanum.

verumontanum *L.* verumontanum, an elevation in the urethra at the point of entry of the seminal ducts.

vesicación *f.* vesication. 1. the formation of blisters; 2. a blister.

vesical *a.* vesical, rel. to or resembling a bladder.

vesicouretral *a.* vesicoureteral, rel. to the urinary bladder and the ureters.

vesicovaginal *a.* vesicovaginal, rel. to the urinary bladder and the vagina.

vesícula *f.* vesicle, vesicula, small sac or elevation of the skin containing serous fluid.

vesícula biliar *f.* gallbladder, pear-shaped receptacle on the lower part of the liver that stores bile.

vesiculación *f.* vesiculation, formation of vesicles.

vesicular *a.* vesicular, rel. to a vesicle.

vesiculitis *f.* vesiculitis, infl. of a vesicle.

vesiculoso-a *a.* vesiculate, of the nature of a vesicle.

vestibular *a.* vestibular, rel. to a vestibule; **bulbo** ___ / ___ bulb; **nervio** ___ / ___ nerve.

vestíbulo *m.* vestibule. 1. space or cavity that gives access to a duct or canal; 2. lobby, waiting room.

vestigial *a.* vestigial, rudimentary, rel. to a vestige.

vestigio *m.* vestige, remains of a structure that was fully developed in a previous stage of the species or of the individual.

veterinaria *f.* veterinary medicine, the science that deals with prevention and cure of animal diseases, esp. domestic animals.

veterinario-a *m., f.* veterinarian, specialist in veterinary medicine; *a.* rel. to veterinary medicine.

vez *f.* time, occasion; **a la** ___ / at the same ___; **alguna** ___ / sometime; **cada** ___ / each ___; **de una** ___ / all at once; **de** ___ **en cuando** / once in a while; **en** ___ **de** / instead of; **otra** ___ / again; **rara** ___ / rarely; **tal** ___ / perhaps; **una** ___ / once.

vía *f.* tract, via, passage, conduit; ___ **olfatoria** / olfactory ___; ___ **piramidal** / pyramidal ___; ___ **-s biliares** / biliary ___; ___ **-s digestivas** / gastrointestinal ___; ___ **-s respiratorias** / respiratory ___; ___ **-s urinarias** / urinary ___ .

vías descendientes *f., pl.* descending tracts, tracts of nerves in the dorsal spine that carry impulses from the brain to the rest of the body.

viable *a.* viable, capable of surviving, gen. in reference to a newborn; **no** ___ / nonviable.

vibración *f.* vibration, oscillation.

vibratorio-a *a.* vibratory, vibratile, vibrating or producing vibration; **sentido** ___ / ___ sense.

víctima *f.* victim; ___ **de accidente** / casualty.

vida *f.* life; vitality; **medidas para el sostenimiento de la** ___ / ___ saving measures; **promedio de duración de** ___ / ___ expectancy; **que pone la** ___ **en peligro** / ___-threatening; ___ **cotidiana** / daily ___ .

vida media *f.* half-life. 1. the time required for half the nuclei of a radioactive substance to disintegrate; 2. the time required for half the amount of a substance taken in by the body to dissolve by natural means.

video *m.* video.

videocinta *f.* videotape.

viejo-a *a.* old, aged; stale.

vientre *m.* belly; abdomen.

vigente *a.* in force, in effect.

vigilar *vt.* to watch, to guard; to survey.

vigilia *f.* vigil. 1. the state of being consciously responsive to a stimulus; 2. insomnia.

vigor *m.* vigor, strength; fortitude; stamina.

vigoroso-a *a.* vigorous, strong; having fortitude; **-mente** *adv.* vigorously.

VIH *m.* HIV, human immunodeficiency virus-1, a retrovirus considered to be the cause of AIDS that can be transmitted by sexual relations or by blood transfusion from someone who is infected with HIV. The virus can be transmitted to children of mothers with HIV in utero, at birth, or, likely, through breast-feeding.

violación f. rape; violation; ___ **estatutaria** / statutory ___ .

violeta a. [color] violet.

viral a. viral, rel. to a virus; **artritis** ___ / ___ arthritis; **crup** ___ / ___ croup; **fiebre hemorrágica** ___ / ___ hemorrhagic fever; **gastroenteritis** ___ / ___ gastroenteritis; **hepatitis** ___ / ___ hepatitis; **infección** ___ **del sistema respiratorio superior** / ___ upper respiratory infection; **neumonía** ___ / ___ pneumonia; **replicación** ___ / ___ replication.

viremia f. viremia, the presence of virus in the blood.

virgen f. virgin. 1. uncontaminated, pure; 2. having had no sexual intercourse.

virilidad f. virility. 1. sexual potency; 2. the quality of being virile.

virilización f. virilization, the process by which secondary male characteristics develop in the female, gen. due to adrenal malfunction or to intake of hormones.

virión m. virion, mature viral particle that constitutes the extracellular, infectious form of a virus.

virolento-a a. 1. rel. to or afflicted with smallpox; 2. pockmarked.

virología f. virology, the study of viruses.

virtual a. virtual, existing in appearance and effect, but not in reality.

viruela f. smallpox, highly contagious viral disease characterized by high temperature and generalized blisters and pustules; ___ **-s locas** / chickenpox.

virulencia f. virulence. 1. the power of an organism to produce disease in the host; 2. the quality of being virulent.

virulento-a a. virulent, highly poisonous or infectious.

virus m. virus, ultramicroscopic microorganisms capable of causing infectious diseases; ___ **atenuado** / attenuated ___; **citomegálico** / cytomegalic ___; ___ **Coxsackie** / Coxsackie ___; ___ **de la parainfluenza** / parainfluenza ___; ___ **ECHO** / ECHO ___; ___ **entérico** / enteric ___; ___ **herpético** / herpes ___; ___ **oncogénico, tumoral** / tumor ___; ___ **sincitial**

respiratorio / respiratory syncytial ___; ___ **variólico** / pox ___ .

Virus del Nilo Occidental m. West Nile Virus, transmitted to humans and animals by mosquitoes that had bitten diseased birds and became infected. Children and adults with a normal immune system if bitten by an infected mosquito gen. develop mild "flu-like" symptoms. Persons with weakened immune systems who suffer from a serious disease could contract encephalitis and suffer severe damage to the central nervous system and the brain.

visceral a. visceral, rel. to viscera.

vísceras f., pl. viscera, large internal organs of the body, esp. the abdomen.

visceromegalia f. visceromegaly, abnormal enlargement of a viscus.

visceroptosis f. visceroptosis, descent of the viscera from their normal place.

viscosidad f. viscosity, the quality of being viscous, esp. the property of fluids to offer resistance due to molecular friction.

visible a. visible; evident; **-mente** adv. visibly.

visión f. vision, the sense of sight. 1. the ability to see, to perceive things through the action of light on the eyes and on related centers in the brain; ___ **acromática** / achromatic ___; ___ **a la distancia** / distance ___; ___ **binocular** / binocular ___; ___ **central** / central ___; ___ **cromática** / chromatic ___; ___ **diurna, fotoscópica** / day ___, photoscopic; ___ **doble, diplopía** / double ___, diplopia; ___ **en túnel** ___ / in tunnel field; ___ **estocópica** / stocopic ___; ___ **monocular** / monocular ___; ___ **nocturna** / night ___; 2. imaginary apparition. See table on page 497.

visión en tunel f. tunnel vision, eye anomaly manifested by a great reduction in the visual field, as if looking through a tunnel, such as occurs in cases of glaucoma.

visita f. visit; call; **horas de** ___ / visiting hours; ___ **médica** / house call.

visitar v. to visit.

vista f. sight; eyesight; view; **corto de** ___ / near-sighted; **enfermedades de la** ___ / eye diseases; ___ **cansada** / eyestrain; ___ **nublada** / bleary-eyed; **a primera** ___ / at first ___; **en** ___ **de** / in

vistazo

view of; **tener buena __** / to have good eyesight.

vistazo *m.* glance, glimpse; *v.* **dar un __** / to take a look.

visual *a.* visual, rel. to vision; **campo __** / __ field, field of vision; **contacto __** / eye contact; **memoria __** / __ memory.

visualización *f.* visualization, 1. the act of viewing an image or picture, as in the study of an x-ray, when a body part is examined in detail; 2. mental conception of health created for the purpose of aiding the healing process.

visualizar *vi.* to visualize. 1. to form a mental image; 2. to make visible, such as through x-rays.

vital *a.* vital, rel. to life or essential to maintaining it; **capacidad __** / capacity; **signos __ -es** / __ signs.

vitalidad *f.* vitality. 1. the quality of having life; 2. physical or mental vigor.

vitamina *f.* vitamin, any one of a group of organic compounds found in small amounts in foods, essential to the growth and development of the body and its functions; **pérdida de __ -s** / loss of __ -s.

vitiligo *m.* vitiligo, benign skin disease characterized by smooth white spots, gen. in exposed areas.

vitrectomía *f.* vitrectomy, partial or total extirpation of the vitreous humor of the eye; sometimes recommended in cases of advanced proliferative diabetic retinopathy.

vítreo-a *a.* vitreous, glassy, hyaline; **camara __** / __ chamber; **cuerpo __** / body; **humor __** / __ humor.

viudo-a *m., f.* widower; widow.

vivificante *a.* vivifying.

vivir *v.* to live.

vivisección *f.* vivisection, the cutting or operating upon living animals for research purposes.

vivo-a *a.* alive; living; *pop.* ingenuous.

vocación *f.* vocation, profession.

vocal *f. Gr.*, vowel; *a.* rel. to the voice or produced by it; **ligamentos __ -es** / __ ligaments.

vocalización *f.* vocalization.

volar *vi.* to fly; to travel by airplane.

volátil *a.* volatile, readily vaporized.

volición *f.* volition, will, the power to determine.

Volkmann, contractura de *f.* Volkmann contracture, ischemic contracture as a result of irreversible necrosis of the muscular tissue, gen. seen in the forearm and hands.

volumen *m.* volume, space occupied by a body or substance; **__ cardíaco** / heart __; **__ de reserva espiratoria o aire de reserva** / expiratory air reserve __; **__ de ventilación pulmonar** / tidal __; **__ residual** / residual __; **sanguíneo** / blood __; **__ sistólico** / stroke __ .

voluntad *f.* will, determination; **fuerza de __** / __ power.

voluntario-a *m., f.* volunteer; *a.* voluntary; **músculo __** / __ muscle.

vólvulo *m.* volvulus, intestinal obstruction a result of an intestinal twist usu. caused by a predisposed mesentery.

vómer *m.* vomer, the impaired flat bone that forms part of the nasal septum.

vomitar *v.* to vomit.

vomitivo *m.* vomitive, emetic.

vómito *m.* vomit, vomiting.

Von Gierke, enfermedad de *f.* Von Gierke disease, abnormal storage of glycogen.

Von Willenbrand, enfermedad de *f.* Von Willenbrand's disease, hereditary blood disorder characterized by bleeding episodes gen. from the mucous membranes.

vórtice *m.* vortex, spiral-shaped structure.

voyeurismo *m.* voyeurism, sexual perversion by which erotic gratification is derived from watching sexual organs or activity.

voz *f.* voice.

vuelo *m.* flight; trajectory.

vuelta *f.* turning; turn; rotation; **media __** / about-face; *v.* **dar una __** / to take a stroll, ride, or walk; *v.* **estar de __** / to be back.

vulnerable *a.* vulnerable, prone to injury or disease.

vulva *f.* vulva, external female organ.

vulvectomía *f.* vulvectomy, excision of the vulva.

vulvitis *f.* vulvitis, infl. of the vulva.

vulvovaginal *a.* vulvovaginal, rel. to the vulva and the vagina.

vulvovaginitis *f.* vulvovaginitis, infl. of the vulva and the vagina.

Waldenstrom, macroglobulinemia de *f.*
Waldenstrom's macroglobulinemia, sickness of elderly persons, hemorrhagic syndrome with anemia and symptoms of enlarged lymph nodes, liver and spleen, with frequent manifestations of bleeding and purpura.

Waldeyer, anillo de *m.* Waldeyer's ring, the ring of lymphatic tissue that consists of the palatine, lingual, and pharyngeal tonsils.

Waller, degeneración de *f.*
Wallerian degeneration, degeneration of nerve fibers that have been separated from their center of nutrition.

warfarina *f.* warfarin, generic name for Coumadine, anticoagulant used in the prevention of thrombosis and infarcts.

Wasserman, reacción de *f.*
Wasserman reaction, serological test for syphilis.

Waterhouse-Friderichsen, síndrome de *m.*
Waterhouse-Friderichsen syndrome, a condition caused by meningococcemia characterized by vomiting, diarrhea, cyanosis and convulsions usually manifested with meningitis and hemorrhage; children under 10 years are the most common victims.

Weneger, granulomatosis de *f.*
Weneger's granulomatosis, disease characterized by the formation of granulomas in the artery affecting the nasal cavity, the lungs, and the kidneys.

Western Blot *m.* Western Blot, immunoblot, test to confirm HIV infection in patients with evidence of exposure to HIV by a previous enzyme-linked immunosorbent assay.

Wharton, conducto de *m.*
Wharton's duct, excretory duct of the submandibular gland.

Whipple, enfermedad de *f.*
Whipple's disease, rare disease caused by deposit of lipids in the lymphatic and intestinal tissues.

Wilms, tumor de *m.* Wilms tumor, rapidly developing neoplasm of the kidney, seen esp. in children.

Wilson, enfermedad de *f.*
Wilson's disease, rare genetic disease, or copper's disease originating an accumulation of the metal in the liver which releases it to other organs such as the brain eventually producing dementia and liver cirrhosis.

X

X *abbr.* **xantina** / xanthine.

xantelasma *f.* xanthelasma, yellow plaques or spots that appear gen. around the eyelids.

xantina *f.* xanthine, one of a group of stimulants of the central nervous system and the heart, such as caffeine.

xantocromía *f.* xanthochromia, yellowish discoloration as it is seen in skin patches or in the cerebrospinal fluid.

xantoderma *m.* xanthoderma, yellowish coloration of the skin.

xantoma *m.* xanthoma, condition characterized by the presence of yellowish plaques or nodules in the skin, gen. due to deposit of lipids; ___ **diabético** / diabetic ___ ; ___ **diseminado** / disseminatum ___ ; ___ **eruptivo** / eruptive ___ ; ___ **plano** / planar ___ ; ___ **tendinoso** / tendinous ___ ; ___ **tuberoso** / tuberosum ___ .

xantosis *f.* xanthosis, yellowing of the skin due to excessive ingestion of foods such as carrots and egg yolks.

xenofobia *f.* xenophobia, morbid fear or aversion to anything foreign.

xenoinjerto *m.* xenograft; **rechazo de ___ / ___** rejection.

xenón *m.* xenon, a dense, colorless element found in small amounts in the atmosphere.

xenotransplante *m.* xenotransplant, the act of transplanting an organ, tissue, or part from one species to another.

xerodermia *f.* xeroderma, xerosis, excessively dry skin.

xeroftalma *f.* xerophthalmia, dryness of the conjunctiva due to lack of vitamin A.

xeromamografía *f.* xeromammography, xeroradiography of the breast.

xerorradiografía *f.* xeroradiography, dry process of registering electrostatic images by the use of metal plates covered with a substance such as selenium.

xerosis *f.* xerosis, abnormal dryness as seen in the skin, eyes, and mucous membranes.

xerostomía *f.* xerostomia, abnormal dryness of the mouth due to deficiency of salivary secretion.

xifoide, xifoideo-a *a.* xiphoid, shaped like a sword, as the xiphoid process.

xifoides, apéndice *m.* xiphoid process, cartilaginous, sword-shaped formation joined to the lowest portion of the sternum.

y *conj.* and.

ya *adv.* already; __ **que** / as long as.

yang *n.* a polarized form of chi which identifies positive energy.

yatrogénico-a, yatrógeno-a *a.* iatrogenic, rel. to the adverse condition of a patient resulting from an erroneous medical treatment or procedure.

yaws *m.* yaws; frambesia.

yema *f.* yolk. 1. the yolk of the egg of a bird; 2. contents of the ovum that supply the embryo.

yerbabuena, hierbabuena *f.* peppermint.

yerno *m.* son-in-law.

yersinia *f.* yersinia, genus of the species *Yersinia pestis*, parasitic bacteria in humans that does not form spores and that contains rods of ovoid, gamma negative cells.

yeso *m.* plaster, plaster cast.

yeyunal *a.* jejunal, rel. to the jejunum.

yeyunectomía *f.* jejunectomy, excision of part or all of the jejunum.

yeyunitis *f.* jejunitis, infl. of the jejunum.

yeyuno *m.* jejunum, portion of the small intestine that extends from the duodenum to the ileum.

yeyunostomía *f.* jejunostomy, permanent opening in the jejunum through the abdominal wall.

yin-yang *m.* yin-yang, Chinese philosophical concept of two opposing influences that complement each other and form the basis of all nature.

yo *m.* self, [*el yo*] the ego, Freudian term that refers to the part of the psyche that mediates between the person and reality; *gr. pron.* I.

yodismo *m.* iodism, poisoning by iodine.

yodo *m.* iodine, nonmetallic element used in medications, esp. those that stimulate the function and development of the thyroid gland and the prevention of goiter; **prueba radiactiva del** __ / radioactive __ excretion test, used for evaluating the function of the thyroid gland.

yododerma, yododermia *f.* iododerma, skin rash caused by allergy to the ingestion of iodites.

yodofilia *f.* iodophilia, affinity for iodine.

yodurar *v.* to iodize, to treat with iodine.

yoga *m.* yoga, Hindu system of beliefs and practices by which the individual tries to reach the union of self with a universal self through contemplation, meditation, and self-control.

yugular *a.* jugular, rel. to the throat; **foramen** __ / __ foramen; **fosa** __ / __ fossa; **glándula** __ / __ gland; **glomo** __ / __ glomus; **nervio** __ / __ nerve; **pulso** __ / __ pulse; **venas** __ -es / __ veins, veins that carry blood from the cranium, the face, and the neck to the heart.

yuxtaglomerular *a.* juxtaglomerular, close to a glomerulus; **aparato** __ / __ apparatus; group of cells that participate in the production of renin and in the metabolism of sodium situated around arterioles leading to a glomerulus of the kidney.

yuxtaposición *f.* juxtaposition, a position that is adjacent to or side by side to another.

Z

z *abr.* **zona** / zone.
zambo-a *a.* bandy-legged; bow-legged.
zanahoria *f.* carrot.
zapato *m.* shoe; __ortopédico /
orthopedic __ ; __ para escayola /
cast __ .
zinc, cinc *m.* zinc, crystalline metallic
chemical element with astringent
properties; **ácido de** __ / __ oxide;
peróxido de __ / __ peroxide;
pomada de __ / __ ointment; **sulfato
de** __ / __ sulfate.
Zollinger-Ellison, síndrome de
m. Zollinger-Ellison syndrome,
manifested by gastric hypersecretion
and hyperacidity and by peptic
ulceration of the stomach and small
intestine.
zona *f.* 1. zona, a specific area or layer;
2. zoster; 3. zone, a belt-like anatomical
structure; __ **de apoyo** / rest area; __
de bienestar / comfort __; __ **de**
deslizamiento / gliding __; __ **de**
equivalencia / equivalence __; __
de transición / transition __; __
radiada / radiated __; __
respiratoria / respiratory __ .
zona desencadenante *f.* trigger
zone, a sensitive area of the body
whose stimulation triggers a reaction in
a different part of the body.
zoofilia *f.* zoophilia. 1. excessive love of
animals; 2. bestiality.
zoofobia *f.* zoophobia, anxiety and
irrational fear of animals.
zoógeno-a *a.* zoogenous, acquired
from animals or derived from them.
zooinjerto *m.* zoograft, graft taken
from an animal.
zootoxina *f.* zootoxin, poisonous
substance produced from an animal
such as the snake venom.
zóster *f.* zoster; *pop.* shingles. herpes.
zoster oftálmico *m.* zoster
ophthalmicus, herpetic infection of
the eye, esp. affecting the optical
nerve.
zumbar *v.* to hum, to buzz, to ring.
zumbido *m.* hum, buzz, ring.
zurdo-a *m., f.* a left-handed person; *a.*
left-handed.

Glosario inglés-español

English-Spanish Glossary

a

a *abbr.* **absolute** / absoluto; **accommodation** / acomodación; **acidity** / acidez; **allergy** / alergia; **anterior** / anterior; **aqua** / agua; **artery** / arteria.

a *art. indef.* un, una; **a contagious disease** / una enfermedad contagiosa; **a good doctor** / un buen médico; (antes de vocal o *h* muda); **an; an abdominal pain** / un dolor abdominal; *a.* algún, alguna; **Is there a doctor on duty?** / ¿Hay algún médico de guardia? *prep.* a; **three times a day** / tres veces al (a+el) día.

abandon *v.* abandonar, dejar; desamparar.

abasia *n.* abasia, movimiento incierto.

abbreviation *n.* abreviación, abreviatura.

abdomen *n.* abdomen, vientre. *pop.* barriga, panza; **pendulous** ___ / ___ colgante, pendular; **scaphoid** ___ / ___ escafoideo. V. ilustración en la página 258.

abdominal *a.* abdominal, rel. al abdomen; ___ **bandage** / vendaje ___; ___ **breathing** / respiración ___; ___ **cavity** / cavidad ___; ___ **cramps** / retortijón, torzón; ___ **dyspnea** / disnea ___; ___ **distention** / distensión ___; ___ **fistula** / fístula ___; ___ **injuries** / traumatismos ___-es; ___ **puncture** / punción ___; ___ **rigidity** / rigidez ___; ___**tumor** / tumor ___ .

abdominocentesis *n.* abdominocentesis, punción abdominal.

abdominoplasty *n.* abdominoplastia, reparación de la pared abdominal.

abducent *a.* abducente; abductor; ___ **muscle** / músculo___; **nerve** / nervio___.

abduction *n.* abducción, separación.

aberrant *a.* aberrante, desviado del curso normal; anómalo.

aberration *n.* aberración. 1. visión defectuosa o imperfecta; **chromatic** ___ / ___ cromática 2. desviación de lo normal; 3. trastorno mental; **mental** ___ / ___ mental.

abetalipoproteinemia *n.* abetalipoproteinemia, condición hereditaria rara que se define por la ausencia o deficiencia de betalipoproteína en el metabolismo de las grasas.

ability *n.* habilidad, aptitud; talento, capacidad.

abiotrophy *n.* abiotrofia, pérdida prematura de la vitalidad.

ablatio *n.* ablación, separación, desprendimiento; ___ **placentae** / desprendimiento de la placenta; ___ **retinae** / desprendimiento de la retina.

able *a.* hábil, capaz, apto-a; *v.* **to be** ___ / [*to be or do something*] ser capaz de; poder.

abnormal *a.* anormal, anómalo-a; disforme, irregular.

abortifacient *n.* abortivo, estimulante para inducir un aborto.

abortion *n.* aborto, interrupción prematura del embarazo. V. cuadro en la página 258.

abortionist *n.* abortista, persona que interrumpe un embarazo.

about *prep.* cerca de; junto a; alrededor de; a eso de, sobre; **it is** ___ **a block from here** / está cerca de una cuadra de aquí *adv.* [*time*]; **it is** ___ **one thirty** / es alrededor de la una y media *v.* **to speak** ___ / hablar de.

above *n.* antecedente, precedente; *a.* antedicho-a, anterior; *prep.* sobre, por encima de; ___ **the heart** / encima del corazón *adv.* arriba; la parte alta; más de o más que; ___ **all** / sobre todo; **from** ___ / desde lo alto, desde arriba.

abrasion *n.* abrasión, excoriación, irritación o raspadura de las mucosas o de una superficie a causa de una fricción o de un trauma; ___ **collar** / círculo de ___ , marca circular de pólvora que deja en la piel el disparo de un arma de fuego.

abrasive *a.* abrasivo-a, irritante, raspante, rel. a una abrasión o que la causa.

abreast *adv.* de frente; en frente.

abrupt *a.* abrupto-a, precipitado-a, repentino-a.

abruptio *n. L.* abruptio, abrupción, acción violenta de separación, desprendimiento; ___ **placentae, placental abruption** / desprendimiento prematuro de la placenta.

abscess *n.* absceso, acumulación de pus gen. debido a una desintegración del tejido.

absence

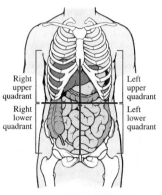

Quadrants of the abdomen:
showing the organs within each quadrant

Abortion	Aborto
accidental	accidental
afebrile	afebril
ampullar	ampollar
artificial	artifical
cervical	cervical
complete	completo
contagious	contagioso
criminal	criminal
elective	electivo
epizootic	epizoótico
incomplete	incompleto
induced	provocado o inducido
infectious	infeccioso
in progress	en curso
natural	natural
recurrent	recurrente
septic	séptico
spontaneous	espontáneo
therapeutic	terapéutico
tubal	tubárico

absence *n.* ausencia, falta; pérdida momentánea del conocimiento.
absentia epiléptica *n.* absencia epiléptica (epilepsia menor), pérdida momentánea del conocimiento en ciertos casos de ataques epilépticos.

absolute *a.* absoluto-a, incondicional; ___ **alcohol (ethyl)** / alcohol ___ (alcohol etílico).
absorb *v.* absorber, sorber, chupar.
absorbent *a.* absorbente; que puede absorber.
absorption *n.* absorción. 1. acto de ingerir o introducir líquidos u otras sustancias en el organismo; **cutaneous** ___ / ___ cutánea; **mouth** ___ / ___ bucal; **parenteral** ___ / ___ parenteral; **intestinal** ___ / ___ entérica; **stomach** ___ / ___ estomacal 2. ensimismación.
abstain *v.* abstenerse, privarse de; ___ **from sexual intercourse** / ___ de relaciones sexuales *Mex.* cuidarse.
abstinence *n.* abstinencia, privación voluntaria, templanza, moderación.
abstract *n.* extracto, cantidad pequeña; resumen; *a.* abstracto-a; *v.* separar, alejar; extractar; resumir.
abundance *n.* abundancia.
abuse *n.* abuso, uso exagerado; maltrato; ___ **of medication** / uso exagerado de medicamentos o drogas; **spouse** ___ / ___ conyugal; **verbal** ___ / ___ maltrato de palabra, insulto *v.* [*to take advantage of*] abusar de; maltratar; seducir.
acanthoma *n.* acanoma, tumor benigno de la piel.
acanthosis *n.* acantosis, enfermedad que causa una condición áspera y verrugosa en la piel.
acapnia *n.* acapnia, estado producido por una disminución de ácido carbónico en la sangre.
acariasis *n.* acariasis, infección causada por ácaros; comezón; sarna.
acarid *n.* ácaro, parásito; *a.* acárido-a.
acatalepsy *n.* deteorización de la habilidad mental
accent *n.* acento, énfasis, intensificación; *v.* acentuar, hacer énfasis; recalcar.
acceptable *a.* aceptable, permitido-a; admitido-a; ___ **daily intake** / consumo diario ___.
access *n.* 1. ataque, acceso; paroxismo; 2. [*entrance*] entrada.
accessory *a.* accesorio-a, adicional, adjunto-a; ___ **nerve** / nervio ___.
accident *n.* accidente; **by** ___ / por casualidad, sin querer; **car** ___ / ___ automovilístico; **occupational** ___ / del trabajo, ocupacional; ___ **prone** / propenso a___; **traffic** ___ / ___ de tráfico.

accommodation *n.* acomodación,
ajustamiento; [*lodging*] alojamiento;
amplitude of ___ / amplitud de ___;
histologic ___ / ___ histológica;
negative ___ / ___ negativa; **nerve** ___ /
___ del nervio; **positive** ___ / ___
positiva; **range of** ___ / jerarquía de ___.
accretion *n.* aumento,
acrecentamiento; acumulación.
accumulation *n.* acumulación,
amontonamiento; hacinamiento.
accurate *a.* exacto-a, preciso-a,
correcto-a.
accustomed *a.* acostumbrado-a; *v.* **to
be** ___ **to** / estar acostumbrado-a a.
acetabulum *n.* acetábulo, hueso
cóncavo de la cadera.
acetic *a.* acético, agrio, relacionado con
el vinagre; ___ **acid** / ácido ___ .
acetone *n.* acetona, sustancia fragante
que se usa como solvente y se observa
en cantidad excesiva en casos de
diabetes.
acetonemia *n.* acetonemia, exceso de
acetona en la sangre.
acetonuria *n.* acetonuria, exceso de
acetona en la orina, característico de la
diabetes.
acetylcholinesterase *n.*
Acetilcolinesterasa, enzima presente en
varios tejidos, células sanguíneas,
nerviosas y en músculos.
acetylsalicylic acid *n.* ácido
acetilsalicílico, aspirina.
achalasia *n.* acalasia, falta de
capacidad de relajación esp. de una
abertura o esfínter.
ache *n.* dolor constante, padecimiento,
pop. achaque.
achievement quotient *n.* cociente
de inteligencia.
Achilles tendon *n.* tendón de
Aquiles, tendón mayor que se une a los
músculos posteriores de la pierna y se
inserta en el talón del pie.
achillobursitis *n.* aquilobursitis, infl.
de la bursa situada en la parte anterior
del tendón de Aquiles.
achillodynia *n.* aquilodinia, dolor en la
región del tendón de Aquiles.
aching *a.* doloroso-a, doliente;
mortificante.
achlorhydria *n.* aclorhidria, ausencia
de ácido hipoclorhídrico en las
secreciones estomacales.
achloropsia *n.* acloropsia, inhabilidad
de distinguir el color verde.
acholia *n.* acolia, ausencia de bilis.

achondroplasia *n.* acondroplasia,
deformidad ósea de nacimiento;
enanismo.
achromasia *n.* acromasia, falta o
pérdida de la pigmentación de la piel,
característica de los albinos.
achromatic *a.* acromático-a, sin
color.
achromatopsia *n.* acromatopsia,
ceguera cromática.
achromocyte *n.* acromocito, tipo de
eritrocito con escasa hemoglobina y en
forma de semiluna.
achylia *n.* aquilia, deficiencia de jugos
estomacales.
acid *n.* ácido; **acetic** ___ / ___ acético; ___
-fast / acidorresistente; ___ **-proof** / a
prueba de ___; **aminoacetic** ___ /
aminoacético (suplemento dietético);
ascorbic ___ / ___ ascórbico; **aspartic**
___ / ___ aspártico; **boric** ___ / ___
bórico; **butyric** ___ / ___ butírico;
chlorogenic ___ / ___ clorogénico;
cholic ___ / ___ cólico o coleico; **citric**
___ / ___ cítrico; **deoxyribonucleic** ___
/ ___ desoxirribonucleico; **fatty** ___ /
___ graso; **folic** ___ / ___ fólico; **gastric**
___ / ___ gástrico; **glucuramic** ___ / ___
glucurámico; **glutamic** ___ / ___
glutámico; **glycolic** ___ / ___ glicólico;
lactic ___ / ___ láctico; **nicotinic** ___ /
___ nicotínico; **nitric** ___ / ___ nítrico;
nucleic ___ / ___ nucleico; **phenic** ___ /
___ fénico; **ribonucleic** ___ / ___
ribonucleico; **salicylic** ___ / ___
salicílico; **sulfonic** ___ / ___ sulfónico;
sulfuric ___ / ___ sulfúrico; **uric** ___ /
___ úrico.
acidemia *n.* acidemia, exceso de ácido
en la sangre.
acidity *n.* acidez, exceso de ácido,
acedia, agrura.
acidophilus milk *n.* leche con
acidófilos, leche fermentada por
lactobacillus acidophilus.
acidosis *n.* acidosis, exceso de acidez
en la sangre y los tejidos del cuerpo;
diabetic ___ / ___ diabética; **metabolic**
___ / ___ metabólica.
acknowledge *v.* reconocer, agradecer;
[*correspondence*] acusar recibo.
acne *n.* acné, condición inflamatoria de
la piel; ___ **rosacea** / ___ rosácea;
vulgaris / ___vulgar o común.
acoustic *a.* acústico-a, rel. al sonido o
la audición. ___ **neuroma** / neuroma
___; ___**radiation** / radiación ___; ___
reflex / reflejo ___ .

acoustics *n.* acústica, la ciencia de los sonidos, su producción, transmisión y efectos.

acquainted *a.* conocido-a, informado-a; **to be ___ with a case** / tener conocimiento del caso.

acquire *v.* adquirir, obtener, conseguir.

acquired *a.* adquirido-a; contraído-a.

acquired immunity *n.* inmunidad adquirida que se desarrolla desde el nacimiento.

acquired immunodeficiency syndrome (AIDS) *n.* síndrome de inmunodeficiencia adquirida, colapso del sistema inmune del organismo que lo incapacita a responder a la invasión de infecciones.

acrid *a.* amargo-a, agrio-a, acre, irritante.

acroarthritis *n.* acroartritis, infl. de las articulaciones de las extremidades.

acrocyanosis, Raynaud's disease *n.* acrocianosis, Raynaud, enfermedad de, cianosis y frialdad en las extremidades a causa de un trastorno circulatorio asociado con tensión emocional o por exposición al frío.

acrodermatitis *n.* acrodermatitis, infl. de la piel de las manos y los pies; **chronic ___** / **___ crónica** atrófica.

acromegaly *n.* acromegalia, enfermedad crónica de la edad madura manifestada por un agrandamiento progresivo de las extremidades óseas y los huesos de la cabeza debido a un malfuncionamiento de la pituitaria.

acromial *a.* acromial, rel. al acromion; **___ bone** / hueso ___; **___ process** / proceso ___; **___reflex** / reflejo ___ .

acromion *n.* acromión, parte del hueso escapular del hombro.

acrophobia *n.* acrofobia, mal de altura; temor excesivo a la altitud.

acropustulosis *n.* acropustulosis, erupciones pustulares de las manos y de los pies; forma de psoriasis; **infantile ___** / **___ infantil.**

across *adv.* a través, de una parte a otra, al otro lado de; *prep.* a través de, por, sobre, contra; *v.* **to come ___** / encontrarse con.

acrotism *n.* acrotismo, falta o deficiencia del pulso.

actine *n.* actina, proteína del tejido muscular que, unida a la miosina, hace posible la contracción muscular.

actinic *a.* actínico-a, rel. a rayos químicamente activos tal como los rayos-x, la luz ultravioleta y particularmente el sol; **___ dermatitis** / dermatitis ___; **___ granuloma** / granuloma ___; **___ keratosis** / queratosis ___ .

action *n.* acción, actuación.

activate *v.* activar.

active *a.* activo-a; diligente, hábil, enérgico-a.

active immunity *n.* inmunidad activa, inmunidad adquirida por autoproducción natural o artificial.

activities of daily living *n.* actividades de la vida diaria.

activity *n.* actividad, ejercicio, ocupación.

actual *a.* actual, real, verdadero-a; **-ly** *adv.* en realidad, actualmente; **the ___ symptom** / el síntoma verdadero.

acuity *n.* agudeza; precisión; **visual ___** / ___visual.

acupuncture *n.* acupuntura, método de cura por inserción de agujas en áreas determinadas del cuerpo con el propósito de reducir o suprimir un dolor.

acute *a.* agudo-a punzante; **___ -care-center** / centro-de-emergencia; **___ care facility** / centro de cuidado crítico; **an ___ pain** / un dolor ___ .

Adam's apple *n.* nuez de Adán.

adaptation *n.* adaptación, ajuste.

add *v.* añadir, sumar, agregar.

addict *n.* adicto-a; vicioso-a, *a.* adicto-a, entregado-a, dependiente física o psicológicamente de una sustancia esp. referente a una persona alcohólica o narcómana.

addicted *a.* enviciado-a; entregado-a, habituado-a a una sustancia, esp. alcohol o narcóticos; *v.* **to become ___** / enviciarse, entregarse a una droga.

addiction *n.* adicción, propensión, dependencia.

Addison's disease *n.* enfermedad de Addison, hipofunción de las glándulas suprarrenales.

additive *n.* aditivo, sustancia que se agrega.

address *n.* dirección, señas; *v.* [*to speak or write to*] dirigirse a; hablar con; [*to write*] escribir a; [*to speak to an audience*] hablar en público.

adduct *v.* aducir, mover hacia la línea media.

adduction *n.* aducción. 1. movimiento

hacia la línea media del cuerpo o hacia adentro de un miembro o parte del cuerpo; 2. movimiento hacia un centro común.

adductor *n.* músculo aductor, músculo que tira hacia una línea media o hacia el centro.

adenectomy *n.* adenectomía, extirpación de una glándula.

adenitis *n.* adenitis, infl. de una glándula.

adenoacanthoma *n.* adenoacantoma, cáncer en el útero que crece lentamente.

adenocarcinoma *n.* adenocarcinoma, cáncer maligno que se origina en una glándula.

adenocystoma *n.* adenocistoma, tumor benigno de una glándula formado por quistes.

adenofibroma *n.* adenofibroma, tumor benigno formado por tejido fibroso y glandular, visto en el útero y en los pechos.

adenoid *a.* adenoideo, semejante a una glándula.

adenoidectomy *n.* adenoidectomía, extirpación de la adenoide.

adenoiditis *n.* adenoiditis, infl. de la adenoide.

adenoids *n., pl.* adenoides, acumulación de tejido linfático en la nasofaringe durante la niñez.

adenoma *n.* adenoma, tumor de una consistencia parecida a la del tejido glandular; **acidophil** __ / __ acidófilo; __**of nipple** / __ de la mama; **adrenocortical** __ / __ adrenocortical; **basal cell** __ / __ de células basales; **basophil** __ / __ basófilo; **bronquial** __ / __ bronquial; **embryonal** __ / __ embriónico; **follicular** __ / __ folicular; **hepatic** __ / __ hepático; **renal cortical** __ / __ corticorenal; **sebaceous** __ / __ sebáceo; **toxic** __ / __ tóxico.

adenomyoma *n.* adenomioma, tumor benigno visto con frecuencia en el útero.

adenopathy, adenopalia *n.* adenopatía, adenopalia, enfermedad de una glándula linfática.

adenosarcoma *n.* adenosarcoma, tumor maligno.

adenosis *n.* adenosis, engrosamiento de una glándula.

adenovirus *n.* adenovirus, grupo de virus que pueden causar infecciones en el tracto respiratorioii superior.

adequate *a.* adecuado-a, proporcionado-a.

adherent lens *n.* lente de contacto.

adhesion *n.* adhesión, adherencia.

adhesive *n.* adhesivo, tela adhesiva; __ **strips** / esparadrapo.

adipocyte *n.* adipocito, célula adiposa.

adipose tissue *n.* tejido adiposo, grasa.

adjacent *a.* adyacente, contiguo, al lado de.

adjective *n.* adjetivo.

adjunct *a.* adjunto-a, unido-a, asociado-a, arrimado-a.

adjustment *n.* ajuste, adaptación; __ **disorder** / trastorno de ajuste __.

adjuvant *n.* adjutor, agente o sustancia que acentúa la potencia de un medicamento.

administer *v.* administrar, proveer, dar algo necesario.

administration *n.* administración.

admission *n.* [*to a hospital*] ingreso; internación, admisión.

admit *v.* admitir, dar entrada o ingreso a una institución.

admittance *n.* entrada, admisión.

adnexa *n., pl.* anejos, anexos, apéndices tales como las trompas de Falopio.

adolescence *n.* adolescencia, pubertad.

adolescent *n.* adolescente; pubescente.

adopt *v.* adoptar, prohijar.

adoption *n.* adopción.

adrenal *a.* suprarrenal, adrenal; __ **congenital hyperplasia** / hiperplasia __ congenital; __**crisis** / crisis __; __ **cortex hormones** / corticosteroides __-es; **gland diseases** / enfermedades de la glándula __; __ **glands** / glándulas __-es; __ **gland neoplasms** / neoplasmas de las glándulas __-es; __ **hypertension** / hipertensión __.

adrenalectomy *n.* adrenalectomía, extirpación de las glándulas suprarrenales.

adrenaline *n.* adrenalina, marca registrada de la epinefrina, hormona usada como vasoconstrictor secretada por la médula suprarrenal.

adrenalism *n.* adrenalismo, disfunción de la glándula suprarrenal que ocasiona síntomas de debilidad y decaimiento.

adrenergic blocking agents *n., pl.* agentes bloqueadores adrenérgicos. 1. tipo de drogas que copian las acciones del sistema nervioso simpático; 2. drogas que aumentan el flujo sanguíneo y reducen la tensión arterial.

adrenocorticotropin *n.* adrenocorticotropina, hormona secretada por la pituitaria, estimulante de la corteza suprarrenal.

adsorbent *a.* adsorbente.

adsorption *n.* adsorción, adherencia de un gas o líquido a una superficie sólida.

adult *n., a.* adulto-a.

adulteration adulteración, falsificación, cambiando del original.

advancement *n.* [*improvement*] mejora, mejoría, progreso; promoción, ascenso.

advantage *n.* ventaja, ganancia, beneficio; *v.* **to take** ___ / aprovecharse, valerse de.

adverb *n.* adverbio.

adverse *a.* desfavorable, adverso-a, contrario-a, opuesto-a; ___ **effects** / efectos ___; ___ **reaction** / reacción ___ .

advise *n.* advertencia, consejo; opinión, parecer; *v.* advertir; aconsejar, recomendar.

aerate *v.* airear, ventilar. 1. saturar un líquido de aire; 2. cambiar la sangre venosa en sangre arterial en los pulmones.

aerobe *n.* aerobio, organismo que requiere oxígeno para vivir.

aerobic *a.* aeróbico-a. 1. rel. a un aerobio; 2. rel. a un ejercicio coordinado como una actividad física; ___ **dance** / baile ___; ___ **exercises** / ejercicios ___-s 3. que ocurre o vive en la presencia de oxígeno.

aerobics *n.* aeróbic, técnica gimnástica que consiste en ejercicios y calistenia combinados con una rutina de baile.

aeroembolism *n.* aeroembolismo, "enfermedad de los buzos", condición causada por burbujas de nitrógeno liberadas en la sangre debido a un cambio brusco de presión atmosférica; *pop.* **the bends**.

aeroemphysema *n.* aeroenfisema, "enfermedad de los aviadores", condición causada por un ascenso súbito en el espacio sin decompresión adecuada; *pop.* **the chokes**.

aerophagia *n.* aerofagia, tragar aire en exceso.

afebrile *a.* afebril, sin fiebre, sin calentura.

affect *v.* afectar, causar un cambio en la salud; conmover, excitar.

affection *n.* [*sickness*] afección, dolencia, enfermedad; [*feeling*] expresión de cariño, afecto o afección.

affective *a.* afectivo-a; ___ **disorders** / trastornos ___ -s; ___ **symptoms** / síntomas ___ -s.

afferent *a.* aferente, que se dirige hacia el centro o hacia adentro; ___ **fibers** / fibras ___-s; ___**glomerular arteriole** / arteriola glomerular ___; ___ **lymphatic vessel** / vaso linfático ___; ___ **nerve** / nervio ___; ___**vessel** / vaso ___ .

affinity *n.* afinidad, conformidad; conexión.

affix *v.* aplicar, colocar, adaptar; ligar, unir.

affixture *n.* ligadura, adición.

afflicted *a.* afligido-a, sufrido-a.

afibrinogenemia *n.* afibrinogenemia, deficiencia de fibrinógeno en la sangre.

afraid *a.* temeroso-a, miedoso-a, intimidado-a, *v.* **to be** ___ / tener miedo.

after *prep.* después; *adv.* después, más tarde; ___ **effects** / consecuencias, secuelas; acción retardada de una droga; ___ **treatment** / tratamiento de recuperación.

afterbirth *n.* secundinas, placenta y membranas que se expelen en el parto.

aftercare *n.* convalescencia, restablecimiento; tratamiento post-operatorio.

afterimage *n.* impresión mantenida por la retina.

aftermath *n.* secuela, consecuencias de una enfermedad.

afterpains *n., pl.* entuertos, dolores siguientes al parto.

aftersound *n.* impresión auditiva que persiste después de cesar el estímulo.

aftertaste *n.* permanencia de la sensación del gusto.

afterwards *adv.* después, luego, más tarde.

again *adv.* otra vez; ___ **and** ___ / una y otra vez, muchas veces; **do it** ___ / hágalo, hazlo ___ .

against *prep.* contra, enfrente; *v.* **to be** ___ / oponerse; enfrentarse a, con.

agalorrhea *n.* agalorrea, cesación o falta de leche en los pechos.

agamic *a.* agámico-a, rel. a la reproducción sin unión sexual.

agammaglobulinemia *n.* agammaglobulinemia, deficiencia de gamma globulina en la sangre.

age *n.* edad; ___ **of consent** / mayor de

___ , mayoría de ___; **full** ___ / mayor de edad; **legal** ___ / ___ legal; **tender** ___ / infancia, primera edad.

agenesis, agenesia *n.* agénesis, agenesia. 1. defecto congénito en el desarrollo de un órgano o parte del cuerpo; 2. esterilidad; impotencia.

agent *n.* agente, factor.

Agent Orange *n.* Agente Naranja, causante de defoliación que contiene el elemento químico-tóxico dioxina.

agglomeration *n.* aglomeración, acumulación.

agglutinants *n., pl.* aglutinantes, agentes o factores que unen partes separadas en un proceso de curación.

agglutination *n.* aglutinación, acción de aglutinar o causar unión.

aggravate *v.* agravar, empeorar, irritar.

aggression *n.* agresión, actitud y acción hostil.

aggressive *a.* agresivo-a, hostil.

agile *a.* ágil, ligero-a, expedito-a.

aging *n.* envejecimiento.

agitate *v.* [*to shake*] agitar, sacudir; [*to upset*] inquietar, perturbar.

agitated *n.* agitado, perturbado, alborotado.

agnosia *n.* agnosia, desorden o incapacidad debido a una lesión cerebral por la cual una persona pierde total o parcialmente el uso de los sentidos y no reconoce a personas u objetos familiares; **visual** ___ / ___ visual.

ago *adv.* atrás; [*with time*] hace; **ten years** ___ / [*hace + length of time*] hace diez años.

agony *n.* agonía. 1. sufrimiento extremo; 2. estado que precede a la muerte.

agoraphobia *n.* agorafobia, temor excesivo a los espacios abiertos.

agranulocytosis *n.* agranulocitosis, condición aguda causada por la disminución excesiva de leucocitos en la sangre.

agraphia *n.* agrafia, pérdida de la habilidad de escribir causada por un trastorno cerebral.

agree *v.* acordar; estar de acuerdo; sentar bien, caer bien; **we** ___ / estamos de acuerdo; **coffee does not** ___ **with me** / el café no me sienta bien; el café no me cae bien.

agreement *n.* acuerdo, pacto, consolidación, ajustamiento; **to come to an** ___ / llegar a un acuerdo; acordar.

ahead *adv.* adelante, enfrente, hacia adelante; *v.* **look** ___ / mire, mira ___ .

aid *n.* ayuda, asistencia; **government** ___ / subsidio del gobierno; **nurse** ___ / enfermero, enfermera asistente.

AIDS *abbr.* acquired immunodeficiency syndrome; *n.* SIDA; síndrome de inmunodeficiencia adquirida, estado avanzado de infección por el virus VIH, caracterizado por inmunodeficiencia, infecciones (tales como neumonía, tuberculosis y diarrea crónica) y tumores (esp. linfoma y sarcoma de Kaposi).

ailing *a.* achacoso-a, enfermizo-a.

ailment *n.* dolencia, achaque, indisposición.

air *n.* aire; ___ **bladder** / vejiga llena de ___; ___ **blast injury** / lesión por una explosión; ___ **bubbles** / burbujas de ___; ___ **chamber** / cámara de ___; ___ -**conditioned** / ___ acondicionado; ___ **contamination** / ___ contaminado; ___ **dressing** / vendaje; ___ **embolism** / embolia gaseosa; ___ **hole** / respiradero; ___ **hunger** / falta de ___; ___ **mattress** / colchón neumático; ___ **passages** / conductos de ___; ___ **pocket** / bolsa de ___; ___ **pollution** / polución atmosférica; ___ **sac [lung]** / alvéolo pulmonar; **cool** ___ / ___ fresco; **tidal** ___ / ___ respiratorio; **ventilated** ___ / ___ de ventilación *v.* [*to ventilate*] airear, ventilar.

airborne *a.* en vuelo; [*transported*] llevado-a por el aire; ___ **spores** / esporas transmitidas por el aire.

airing *n.* aéreo, ventilación.

airless *a.* falto de respiración, sin aire.

airsickness *n.* mareo de altura.

airtight *a.* hermético-a.

airway *n.* 1. conducto de aire; 2. vías respiratorias; **lower** ___ / vía respiratoria inferior; **oclussive** ___ / conducto de aire; vía respiratoria oclusiva; **respiratory** ___ / vías respiratorias; **upper** ___ / vía respiratoria superior.

akin *a.* consanguíneo, de cualidades uniformes.

akinesthesia *n.* aquinestesia, falta del sentido de movimiento.

alalia *n.* pérdida del habla.

alar *a.* alar, rel. a o semejante a una ala; ___ **artery** / arteria ___; ___ **cartilage** / cartílago ___ .

alarm

alarm *n.* alarma, peligro; **fire** ___ / ___ de fuego *v.* alarmar, inquietar, impacientar; turbar.

alarming *a.* alarmante, inquietante, desesperante; sorprendente.

albinism *n.* albinismo, falta de pigmentación en la piel, el cabello y los ojos.

albino *n.* albino-a, persona afectada por albinismo.

albumin *n.* albúmina, componente proteínico.

albuminuria *n.* albuminuria, presencia de proteína en la orina, esp. albúmina o globulina.

alcohol *n.* alcohol; ___ **detoxification** / detoxificación alcohólica; ___ **withdrawal syndrome** / síndrome de privación alcohólica

alcoholic *n., a.* alcohólico-a.

alcoholism *n.* alcoholismo, uso excesivo de bebidas alcohólicas.

aldosterone *n.* aldosterona, hormona producida por la corteza suprarrenal.

aldosteronism *n.* aldosteronismo, trastorno causado por una secreción excesiva de aldosterona.

alert *a.* alerta, dispuesto-a.

alertness *n.* estado de alerta.

alexia *n.* alexia, inhabilidad de comprender la palabra escrita.

algorithm *n.* algoritmo, método aritmético y algebraico que se usa en el diagnóstico y tratamiento de una enfermedad.

alien *a.* incompatible; extranjero-a, forastero-a.

alimentary *a.* alimenticio-a, rel. a los alimentos; ___ **tract** / tubo digestivo, tracto ___ .

alimentation *n.* alimentación, nutrición; **forced** ___ / ___ forzada; **rectal** ___ / ___ por el recto.

alive *a.* vivo-a, con vida; *v.* **to be** ___ / estar ___ .

alkalemia *n.* alcalemia, exceso de alcalinidad en la sangre.

alkaloid *n.* alcaloide, grupo de sustancias orgánicas básicas de origen vegetal.

alkalosis *n.* alcalosis, trastorno patológico en el balance acidobásico del organismo.

all *n.* el todo, compuesto de partes iguales; *a.* todo-a, todos-as; [*everyone*] todo el mundo; ___ **day** / todo el día; ___ **night** / toda la noche; **at** ___ **risks** /

Allergens	Alérgenos
acarus	ácaros de polvo
alcoholic beverages	bebidas alcohólicas
aspirin	aspirina
birds (feathers, droppings)	pájaros (pluma, excremento)
cat (urine, hair)	gato (orina, pelo)
colorants (food)	colorantes (comidas)
cosmetics	cosméticos
chocolate	chocolate
detergents	detergentes
glue	pegamentos
horse (sweat, hair)	caballo (sudor, pelo)
insecticide	insecticida
medicines	medicinas
milk	leche
mushrooms	hongos
nuts	nueces
paints	pinturas
plants	plantas
pollen	polen

a todo riesgo; **before** ___ / ante todo *adv.* todo, del todo, completamente; enteramente; ___ **along** / todo el tiempo; ___ **of a sudden** / de pronto, de golpe, de repente; ___ **the better** / tanto mejor; ___ **the worse** / tanto peor; **by** ___ **means** / sin duda, por supuesto; ___ **right** / está bien.

allele *n.* alelo, alelomorfo, uno de dos o más genes de una serie que ocupa la misma posición en cromosomas homólogos y que determina características alternantes en los descendientes.

allergen *n.* alérgeno, antígeno que induce una respuesta alérgica o hipersensitiva. V. cuadro esta página.

allergens *n., pl.* alérgenos, agentes causantes de alergias.

allergic *a.* alérgico-a; ___ **reaction** / reacción alérgica; ___ **rhinitis** / rinitis ___ .

allergist *n.* alergista, especialista en alergias.

allergy *n.* alergia; **delayed** ___ / reacción alérgica retardada.

alleviate *v.* aliviar, calmar, mejorar, atenuar.

allogeneic, allogenic *a.* alogénico-a, de constitución genética distinta dentro de una misma especie; ___ **cells** / células ___ s; ___ **system** / sistema ___.

allograft *n.* aloinjerto. homograft.

allow *v.* admitir, aceptar, consentir.

Almighty *n.* Dios; **almighty** *a.* todopoderoso-a, omnipotente.

almost *adv.* casi, cerca de, alrededor de.

alone *a.* solo-a, solitario-a.

along *adv.* a lo largo de, próximo a, junto a; *v.* **come** ___ / venga; ven; **to get** ___ / llevarse bien.

alopecia *n.* alopecia, pérdida del cabello.

already *adv.* ya.

also *adv.* del mismo modo, también.

alter *v.* cambiar, variar; reformar.

alteration *n.* alteración, modificación, reforma, cambio.

alternative *n.* alternativa, opción.

alternative medicine *n.* sistema de tratamiento medicinal que proporciona diferentes selecciones y modalidades al del uso estándar de medicamentos y cirugía para tratar enfermedades y lesiones.

although *conj.* aunque, si bien, bien que.

altitude *n.* altitud, altura, elevación.

alveolar *a.* alveolar, rel. a un alvéolo.

alveolitis *n.* alveolitis. 1. infl. de los alveolos pulmonares; 2. infl. de la fosa de un diente; **allergic** ___ / ___ alérgica; **acute pulmonary** ___ / ___ pulmonar aguda; **chronic fibrotic** ___ / ___ fibrosa crónica; **cryptogenic fibrotic** ___ / ___ fibrosa criptogénica; **extrinsic allergic** ___ / ___ alérgica extrínseca.

alveolus *n.* (*pl.* **alveola**) alvéolo, cavidad.

always *adv.* siempre, para siempre.

alymphocytosis *n.* alinfocitosis, reducción anormal de linfocitos.

Alzheimer's disease *n.* enfermedad de Alzheimer, deterioración cerebral progresiva con características de demencia senil.

amastia *n.* amastia, ausencia de los pechos.

amaurosis *n.* amaurosis, ceguera sin aparente cambio en los ojos, posiblemente causada por una lesión cerebral.

amaurotic *a.* amaurótico-a, rel. a amaurosis.

amber *n.* ámbar; *a.* ambarino-a.

ambiance *n.* ambiente.

ambidextrous *a.* ambidextro-a.

ambisexual *a.* ambisexual, bisexual.

ambivalence *n.* ambivalencia.

amblyopia *n.* ambliopía, visión reducida.

ambulance *n.* ambulancia.

ambulant *a.* ambulante.

ambulatory *a.* ambulatorio-a; ambulante.

amebiasis *n.* amebiasis, amibiasis, estado infeccioso causado por amebas.

amebic *a.* amebiano-a, rel. a la ameba o causado por ésta.

amenorrhea *n.* amenorrea, ausencia del período menstrual.

American *n., a.* americano-a.

ametropia *n.* ametropía, falta de visión causada por una anomalía de los poderes refractores del ojo.

amine *n.* amina, uno de los compuestos básicos derivados del amoníaco.

amino acid *n.* aminoácido, compuesto orgánico metabólico necesario en el desarrollo y crecimiento humano esencial en la digestión e hidrólisis de proteínas.

amitosis *n.* amitosis, división nuclear directa.

ammonia *n.* amoníaco, gas alcalino que se forma por la descomposición de sustancias nitrogenadas y por aminoácidos.

ammoniuria *n.* amoniuria, excreción de orina con un alto grado de amoníaco.

amnesia *n.* amnesia, pérdida de la memoria.

amniocentesis *n.* amniocentesis, punción del útero para obtener líquido amniótico.

amnion *n.* amnios, saco membranoso que envuelve el embrión.

amnioscope *n.* amnioscopio, endoscopio que se usa para el estudio del líquido amniótico.

amnioscopy *n.* amnioscopía, visualización directa del feto y del líquido amniótico por medio de un endoscopio.

amniotic *n.* amniótico, en relación con el amnios; ___ **fluid** / fluido ___; ___ **sac** / saco ___.

amniotomy *n.* amniotomía, ruptura artificial de las membranas fetales para estimular el parto.

amoeba, ameba *n.* ameba, organismo de una sola célula.

amorphous *a.* amorfo-a, sin forma.

amphetamine

amphetamine *n.* anfetamina, tipo de droga usada como estimulante del sistema nervioso.

ampicillin *n.* ampicilina, penicilina semisintética.

amplification *n.* amplificación, ampliación, extensión.

amplify *v.* ampliar, extender, dilatar.

ampoule, ampule *n.* ámpula, ampolla, tubo de jeringuilla.

amputate *v.* amputar, desmembrar.

amputation *n.* amputación, desmembración.

Amsler Grid *n.* Amsler, gráfico de, gráfico que sirve de ayuda para revelar signos de degeneración macular aguda.

amygdala *n.* amígdala. V. tonsil.

amyloid *n.* amiloide, proteína que se asemeja a los almidones; ___ **degeneration** / degeneración ___; ___ **disease** / enfermedad ___; ___ **kidney** / riñón ___; ___ **nephrosis** / nefrosis ___ .

amyloidosis *n.* amiloidosis, acumulación de amiloide en los tejidos.

anabolic *a.* anabólico-a, rel. al anabolismo; ___ **steroid** / esteroide ___ .

anabolism *n.* anabolismo, proceso celular por el cual sustancias simples se convierten en complejas, fase constructiva del metabolismo.

anaerobe *n.* anaerobio, microorganismo que se multiplica en ausencia de aire u oxígeno.

anal *a.* anal, rel. al ano; ___ **fistula** / fístula ___ .

analgesic *n.* analgésico, calmante.

analysis *n.* análisis, prueba; **accumulation** ___ / ___ de acumulación; **amino acid** ___ / ___ de aminoácido; **bite** ___ / ___ de la mordida; **breath** ___ / ___ del aliento; **cephalometric** ___ / ___ cefalométrico; **character** ___ / ___ del carácter; **cost** ___ / ___ de costos; **data** ___ / ___ de datos; **dream** ___ / ___ de los sueños; **gastric** ___ / ___ gástrico; **hair** ___ / ___ del pelo; **qualitative** ___ / ___ cualitativo; **quantitative** ___ / ___ cuantitativo.

analyze *v.* analizar, hacer análisis.

anaphase *n.* anafase, etapa de la división celular.

anaphylactic *a.* anafiláctico-a, rel. a la anafilaxis.

anaphylaxis *n.* anafilaxis, hipersensibilidad, reacción alérgica extrema.

anaplasia *n.* anaplasia, falta de diferenciación en las células.

anasarca *n.* anasarca, edema generalizado, hidropesía.

anastomosis *n.* anastomosis, pasaje o comunicación entre dos o más órganos.

anatomic, anatomical *a.* anatómico-a, rel. a la anatomía.

anatomy *n.* anatomía, ciencia que estudia la estructura del cuerpo humano y de sus órganos; **macroscopic** ___ / ___ macroscópica, estudio de estructuras que se distinguen a simple vista; **topographic** ___ / ___ topográfica, estudio de estructuras y partes de las mismas en las distintas regiones del cuerpo.

ancestors *n., pl.* antepasados, padres o abuelos; *pop.* los mayores.

anconal *a.* anconal, referente al codo.

and *conj.* y; e (gr. used instead of y before words beginning with i or hi); **father and son** / padre *e* hijo; **two thirty** / las dos *y* media.

androgen *n.* andrógeno, hormona masculina.

androgynous *a.* androginoide, que tiene las características de ambos sexos.

anemia *n.* anemia, insuficiencia hemática o de glóbulos rojos en calidad, cantidad o en hemoglobina; **aplastic** ___ / ___ aplástica, falta anormal de producción de glóbulos rojos; **hemorrhagic, hemolytic** ___ / ___ hemorrágica, hemolítica, destrucción progresiva de glóbulos rojos; **hyperchromic** ___ / ___ hipercrómica, aumento anormal en la hemoglobina; **hypochromic microcytic** ___ / ___ hipocrómica microcítica, (células pequeñas), deficiencia de glóbulos rojos en menor cantidad que de hemoglobina; **macrocytic** ___ / ___ macrocítica, glóbulos rojos de un tamaño exagerado (anemia perniciosa); **sickle cell** ___ / ___ de glóbulos falciformes; **iron deficiency** ___ / ___ por deficiencia de hierro.

anergy *n.* anergia. 1. astenia, falta de energía; 2. reducción o falta de respuesta a un antígeno específico.

anesthesia *n.* anestesia; **endotracheal** ___ / ___ endotraquial; **epidural** ___ / ___ epidural; **general** ___ / ___ general; **general** ___ **by inhalation** / general por ___ inhalación; **general** ___ **by intubation** / general por

__ intubación; **hypnosis** __ / __ por hipnosis; **hypotensive** __ / __ con hipotensión controlada; **intercostal** __ / __ intercostal; **intravenous general** __ / __ general intravenosa; **local** __ / __ local; **regional** __ / __ regional; **saddle block** __ / __ en silla de montar; **spinal** __ / __ raquídea; **topical** __ / __ tópica; **thermal** __ / __ térmica.

anesthesiologist *n.* anestesista, anestesiólogo-a.

anesthesiology *n.* anestesiología.

anesthetic *n.* anestésico.

anesthetize *v.* anestesiar.

aneurysm *n.* aneurisma, dilatación de una porción de la pared de una arteria; **aortic** __ / __ aórtico; **berry** __ / __ cerebral saculado; **cerebral** __ / __ cerebral; **dissecting** __ / __ disecante; **false** __ / __ falso; **fusiform** __ / __ fusiforme; **true** __ / __verdadero.

aneurysmal *a.* aneurismal, rel. a un aneurisma.

aneurysmectomy *n.* aneurismectomía, extirpación de un aneurisma.

anger *n.* ira, cólera.

angina *n.* angina, sensación de dolor constrictivo o ahogo; __ **pectoris, angor pectoris** / __ de pecho, dolor en el pecho causado por insuficiencia de flujo sanguíneo al músculo cardíaco; **intestinal** __ / __ intestinal, dolor abdominal agudo debido a insuficiencia de flujo sanguíneo a los intestinos; **laryngeal** __ / __ laríngea, infl. de la garganta; **unstable** __ / __ inestable.

angiocardiography *n.* angiocardiografía, visión radiográfica de las aurículas y los ventrículos del corazón.

angiogenesis *n.* angiogénesis, desarrollo del sistema vascular.

angiogram *n.* angiograma, visualización radiográfica de un vaso sanguíneo mediante inyección de una sustancia radioopaca; **coronary** __ / __ coronario; **lymph** __ / __ linfático.

angiography *n.* angiografía, proceso de obtener una radiografía de los vasos sanguíneos haciendo resaltar su contorno.

angioma *n.* angioma, tumor vascular benigno.

angioplasty *n.* angioplastia, intervención quirúrgica para la reconstrucción de vasos sanguíneos enfermos o traumatizados; **percutaneous coronary** __ / __ coronaria percutánea; **peripheral percutaneous** __ / __ periférica percutánea.

angiosarcoma *n.* angiosarcoma, neoplasma maligno que ocurre mayormente en tejidos blandos; se cree que se origina en las células endoteliales de los vasos sanguíneos.

angiospasm *n.* angioespasmo, contracción prolongada y fuerte de un vaso sanguíneo.

angiostenosis *n.* angioestenosis, estrechamiento de un vaso, esp. un vaso sanguíneo.

angiotensin *n.* angiotensina, agente presor en los trastornos hipotensivos, estimulante de la aldosterona.

angitis *n.* angitis, infl. de un vaso linfático o de un vaso sanguíneo.

angle *n.* ángulo, abertura formada por dos líneas que salen separadamente de un mismo punto.

anhidrosis *n.* anhidrosis, deficiencia o falta de secreción sudoral.

animate *v.* animar, dar vida.

animosity *n.* animosidad, rencor, aversión, mala voluntad; *v.* **to have** __ / tener __ .

anisocoria *n.* anisocoria, condición por la cual ambas pupilas de los ojos son desiguales; **central simple** __ / __ central simple; **essential** __ / __ esencial; **physiologic** __ / __ fisiológica; **simple** __ / __ simple.

anisocytosis *n.* anisocitosis, tamaño desigual de los glóbulos rojos.

ankle *n.* tobillo; __ **bone** / hueso del __ .

ankylosis *n.* anquilosis, inflexibilidad o falta de movimiento de una articulación.

announcement *n.* anuncio, aviso, declaración pública.

annoy *v.* importunar, fastidiar, molestar.

annual *a.* anual; *-ly adv.* anualmente, cada año.

annular *a.* anular, en forma de anillo; __ **eruption** / erupción __ .

anodyne *n.* anodino, agente mitigador del dolor; *a.* insípido-a.

anomalous *a.* anómalo-a, irregular, disforme.

anomaly *n.* trastorno, anomalía, irregularidad contraída o congénita.

anorexia *n.* anorexia, trastorno causado por falta de apetito; __ **nervosa** / __ nerviosa, aversión histérica a la comida.

anosmia *n.* anosmia, falta de olfato.

another *a.* otro-a, otros-as; *pron.* el otro, la otra.

anovulation *n.* anovulación, cese de ovulación.

anovulatory drugs *n., pl.* drogas anticonceptivas, drogas para evitar la ovulación.

anoxemia *n.* anoxemia, insuficiencia de oxígeno en la sangre.

anoxia *n.* anoxia, ausencia de oxígeno en los tejidos; **altitude** __ / __ de altitud; **anemic** __ / __ anémica; **neonatorum** __ / __ del nenonato; **stagnant** __ / __ de estancamiento.

answer *n.* contestación, respuesta.

antacid *n.* antiácido, neutralizador de acidez.

antagonist *a.* antagonista, droga que neutraliza los efectos de otra.

antecubital *a.* antecubital, en posición anterior al codo.

anteflexion *n.* anteflexión, acto de doblarse hacia adelante.

antemetic *n.* antiemético, medicamento para controlar las naúseas.

antemortem *L.* antemortem, anterior a la muerte.

anterior *a.* anterior, precedente; [*body position*] anterior o ventral; [*time*] previo-a.

anteversion *n.* anteversión, vuelta hacia el frente.

anthracosis *n.* antracosis, condición pulmonar causada por la inhalación prolongada de polvo de carbón.

anthrax *n.* ántrax, infección estafilocócica causada por el *Bacillus anthracis* que da lugar a abscesos cutáneos profundos que pueden formar grandes pústulas.

anthropomorphic *a.* antropomórfico-a, de forma humana.

antiallergic *a.* antialérgico-a, rel. a los medicamentos que se usan para combatir alergias.

antiarrythmic *a.* antiarrítmico-a, que previene la arritmia cardíaca o es efectivo en tratamientos contra ésta; __ **agents** / agentes __-s.

antiarthritics *n., pl.* antiartríticos, medicamentos para combatir la artritis o aliviarla.

antibiotic *n., pl.* antibióticos, drogas antibacterianas; **antineoplastic** __ / __ antineoplástico; **bactericidal** __ / __ bactericida; **broad spectrum** __ / __ de amplio espectro; __ **sensitivity test** / prueba de sensibilidad antibiótica.

antibody *n.* anticuerpo, sustancia de proteína que actúa como respuesta a la presencia de antígenos; __ **formation** / formación de __-s; **cross-reacting** __ / __ de reacción cruzada; **monoclonal** __ / __ monoclónico, derivado de células de hibridoma.

anticancer drug, anticarcinogen *n.* anticarcinógeno, droga usada en el tratamiento del cáncer.

anticholinergic *a.* anticolinérgico-a, rel. al bloqueo de los impulsos transmitidos a través de los nervios parasimpáticos.

anticoagulant *n.* anticoagulante, medicamento usado para evitar coágulos.

anticonvulsant *n.* anticonvulsivo, medicamento usado en la prevención de convulsiones o ataques.

antidepressant *n.* antidepresivo, medicamento o proceso curativo usado para evitar estados de depresión.

antidiabetic *n.* antidiabético, medicamento usado en el tratamiento de la diabetes.

antidiarrheal *a.* antidiarreico.

antidiuretic *n.* antidiurético, sustancia que evita la emisión excesiva de orina.

antidote *n.* antídoto, contraveneno.

antiemetic *n.* antiemético, medicamento usado en el tratamiento de la náusea.

antiestrogen *n.* antiestrógeno, sustancia que detiene o modifica la acción del estrógeno.

antigen *n.* antígeno, sustancia tóxica que estimula la formación de anticuerpos; **carcinoembriogenic** __ / __ carcinoembriogénico.

antigenic *a.* antigénico-a, que tiene las propiedades de un antígeno; __ **determinant** / determinante __; __ **drift** / variaciones antigénicas menores; __ **shift** / variación mayor; __ **specificity** / especificidad __ .

antihistamine *n.* antihistamina, medicamento usado en el tratamiento de reacciones alérgicas.

antihypertensive n. antihipertensivo, medicamento para bajar la presión arterial.

anti-inflammatory agents n., pl. agentes anti-inflamatorios.

antineoplastic a. antineoplástico-a, droga que controla o mata células cancerosas.

antioncotic n. antioncótico, agente reductor de la tumefacción.

antipruritic a. antipruriginoso-a, sustancia que trata o alivia la picazón.

antipyretic n. antipirético-a, agente reductor de la fiebre.

antiseptic n. antiséptico, agente desinfectante que destruye bacterias.

antiserum anaphylaxis n. antisuero anafiláctico.

antispasmodic n. antiespasmódico, medicamento usado para aliviar o prevenir espasmos.

antitoxic n. antitóxico, neutralizador de los efectos de las toxinas.

antitoxin n. antitoxina, anticuerpo que actúa como neutralizante de la sustancia tóxica introducida por un microorganismo; **bovine** ___ / ___ bovina; **diphtheria** ___ / ___ diftérica; **scarlet fever** ___ / ___ de la escarlatina; **tetanus** ___ / ___ tetánica.

antivenum n. antiveneno. V. **antitoxin**.

antiviral a. antivirósico-a, antiviral, que detiene la acción de un virus.

antrum n. antro, cavidad o cámara casi cerrada; **auris** ___ / cavidad del oído; **cardiaum** ___ / ___ cardial; **follicular** ___ / ___ folicular; **mastoid** ___ / ___ mastoideo; **maxillary** ___ / ___ maxilar o seno maxilar; **pyloricum** ___ / ___ pilórico; **tympanic** ___ / ___ timpánico.

anuria n. anuria, escasez o ausencia de orina.

anus n. ano, orificio del recto.

anxiety n. ansiedad, angustia; estado de preocupación excesiva; aprehensión, abatimiento de ánimo, desasosiego; ___ **attack** / crisis de ___; ___ **disorders** / trastornos ___; ___ **neurosis** / neurosis de ___ .

anxious a. ansioso-a, anheloso-a, abatido-a, perturbado-a.

any a. algún, alguna, cualquier, cualquiera; **are you taking any medicine ?** / ¿toma, tomas alguna medicina?; ¿toma, tomas algún medicamento?; ___ **further** / más lejos; ___ **more** / no más; **don't go** ___ **further** / no vaya, no vayas más lejos;

don't take ___ **of those pills** / no tome, no tomes ninguna de esas pastillas; **you don't need** ___ **more pills** / no necesita, no necesitas más pastillas; [*after negation*] ningún, ninguno-a.

anybody *pron.* alguien, alguno-a; cualquiera; **did** ___ **call ?** / ¿llamó alguien?; [*negative*] nada, nadie, ninguno-a; **no one called** / no llamó nadie.

aorta n. aorta, arteria mayor que se origina en el ventrículo izquierdo del corazón; **ascending** ___ / ___ ascendiente; **arch of the** ___ / cayado de la ___; **coarctation of the** ___ / coartación o compresión de la ___; **descending** ___ / ___ descendiente, descendente.

aortic a. aórtico-a, rel. a la aorta; ___ **murmur** / soplo, ruido ___; ___ **stenosis** / estenosis o estrechamiento ___ .

aortocoronary n. aortocoronaria, rel. a las arterias aorta y coronaria.

aortogram n. aortograma, rayos-x de la aorta.

aortography n. aortografía, técnica empleada con rayos-x para ver el contorno de la aorta.

apathy n. apatía, insensibilidad.

aperture n. apertura, abertura, paso, boquete.

apex n. apex. 1. ápice, extremo superior o punta de un órgano; 2. extremidad puntiaguda de una estructura.

aphasia n. afasia, incapacidad de coordinar el pensamiento y la palabra; **amnestic** ___ / ___ amnéstica; **ataxic** ___ / ___ atáxica.

aphonia n. afonía, pérdida de la voz debido a una afección localizada en la laringe.

aphonic a. afónico-a, sin sonido, sin voz.

aphrodisiac a. afrodisíaco-a, que estimula deseos sexuales.

aphtha n. afta, úlcera pequeña que aparece como señal de infección en la mucosa oral.

aphthous stomatitis n. estomatitis aftosa, dolor de garganta acompañado de pequeñas aftas en la boca.

aplasia n. aplasia, falta de desarrollo normal en un órgano.

apnea n. apnea, falta de respiración.

aponeurosis n. aponeurosis, membrana que cubre los músculos.

apoplexy n. apoplejía, hemorragia cerebral.

apparent

apparent *a.* aparente, evidente, preciso-a; claro-a; patente; **-ly** *adv.* aparentemente, evidentemente, precisamente.

appear *v.* aparecer, parecer, responder; manifestarse.

appendage *n.* apéndice; dependencia; accesorio.

appendectomy *n.* apendectomía, extirpación del apéndice.

appendicitis *n.* apendicitis, infl. del apéndice.

appendicular *a.* apendicular, rel. al apéndice.

appendix *n.* apéndice.

appetite *n.* apetito, deseos de, ganas de comer; **altered __** / __ alterado; **excessive __** / __ excesivo; **poor __** , **loss of __** / falta de __ , pérdida del __ .

applicable *a.* aplicable, adecuado-a, apropiado-a para utilizarse.

application *n.* aplicación, solicitud; **__ blank** / formulario; [*ointment*] untadura.

applicator *n.* aplicador; **cotton __** / __ de algodón.

apply *v.* aplicar, solicitar, requerir.

appointment *n.* cita, consulta, turno; [*job related*] nombramiento, cargo.

approach *n.* [*avenue*] acceso, entrada; [*words*] las palabras acertadas; método; [*decision*] las medidas necesarias; *v.* abordar; *vr.* acercarse, aproximarse.

appropriate *a.* apropiado-a, adecuado-a, apto-a.

approve *v.* aprobar, aceptar, dar estimación.

approximate *a.* aproximado-a.

apraxia *n.* apraxia, falta de coordinación muscular en los movimientos causada por una afección cerebral.

apricot *n.* albaricoque; *Mex.* chabacano.

apron *n.* delantal.

aptitude *n.* aptitud, capacidad, destreza para hacer algo; **__ test** / prueba de __ .

aqua *n. L.* agua; **aq. abbr.** / aq. *abr.*; **__bull,** __ **bulliens** / __ hirviendo; __ **dest., __ destillata,** / __ destilada; __ **pur., __ pura** / __ pura; __ **tep., __ tepid** / __ tépida, tibia water.

aqueous *a.* acuoso-a, aguado-a; **__ humor** / humor __ .

arachnoid *n.* aracnoides, membrana media cerebral que cubre el cerebro y la médula espinal.

arch *n.* arco, estructura de forma circular o en curva; **__ like** / arqueado-a; **carotid __** / __ carotídeo; **maxillary __** / __ del paladar; **plantar __** / __ plantar.

archetype *n.* arquetipo, tipo original ideal del que se derivan versiones modificadas.

ardor *n.* ardor, sensación quemante.

areflexia *n.* arreflexia, ausencia de reflejos.

areola *n.* aréola, areola, área circular alrededor de un centro.

Argyll Robertson symptom *n.* signo de Argyll Robertson, condición de la pupila de acomodarse a una distancia, pero no a refracciones de la luz.

arm *n.* brazo, una de las extremidades superiores; **__ sling** / cabestrillo; **__ span** / de mano a mano, distancia de la mano derecha a la izquierda con los **__-s** extendidos; **open arms** / __-s abiertos.

armpit *n.* axila, *pop.* sobaco.

aroma *n.* aroma, olor agradable.

aromatic *a.* aromático-a, rel. al aroma.

around *prep.* en, cerca de; *adv.* alrededor, cerca, a la vuelta; más o menos; **__ here** / por aquí, en los alrededores *v.* **to look __** / buscar; **to turn __** / voltear, dar la vuelta; virarse.

arrest *n.* paro, arresto; detención; **cardiac __** / __ del corazón, __ cardíaco.

arrhenoblastoma *n.* arrenoblastoma, tumor ovárico.

arrhythmia *n.* arritmia, falta de ritmo, esp. latidos irregulares del corazón.

arrival *n.* arribo, llegada; **dead on __** / paciente que llega sin vida, que llega muerto-a; [*newborn*] **new __** / neonato-a, recién nacido-a.

arsenic *n.* arsénico; **__ poisoning** / envenenamiento por __ .

arterial *a.* arterial, referente a las arterias; **__ blood gases** / gases __-es ; **occlusive diseases** / enfermedades oclusivas __-es; **__ system** / sistema __ .

arteriogram *n.* arteriograma, angiograma de las arterias; **cerebral or carotid __** / cerebral o carotinoide; **mesenteric __** / __ mesentérico; **peripheral __** / __ periférico; **renal __** / __ renal.

arteriography *n.* arteriografía, proceso de obtener una radiografía de las arterias.

arteriole *n.* arteriola, arteria diminuta que termina en un capilar.

arterioplasty *n.* arterioplastia, proceso quirúrgico para reparar o reconstruir una arteria.

arteriosclerosis *n.* arterioesclerosis, endurecimiento de las paredes de las arterias.

arteriovenous *a.* arteriovenoso-a, relacionado con una arteria y una vena; ___ **fistula** / fístula ___; **malformations** / malformaciones ___-s; ___ **shunt, surgical** / anastomosis ___ quirúrgica.

arteritis *n.* arteritis, infl. de una arteria.

artery *n.* arteria, uno de los vasos mayores que llevan la sangre del corazón a otras partes del cuerpo; **innominate** ___ / ___ innominada.

arthritic *a.* artrítico-a, que padece de artritis.

arthritis *n.* artritis, infl. de una articulación o coyuntura; **acute** ___ / ___ aguda; **chronic** ___ / ___ crónica; **degenerative** ___ / ___ degenerativa; **hemophilic** ___ / ___ hemofílica; **rheumatoid** ___ / ___ reumatoidea; **juvenile rheumatoid** ___ / ___ reumatoidea juvenil; **rheumatoid coronary** ___ / ___ coronaria reumatoide; **septic** ___ / ___ séptica; **traumatic** ___ / ___ traumática.

arthrodesis *n.* artrodesis. 1. fusión de los huesos que hacen una articulación; 2. anquilosis artificial.

arthrography *n.* artrografía, radiografía de una articulación por medio de un tinte opaco.

arthroplasty *n.* artroplastia, reparación quirúrgica plástica de una articulación.

arthroscopy *n.* artroscopia, examen del interior de una articulación.

arthrotomy *n.* artrotomía, incisión en una articulación con fines terapéuticos.

articulation *n.* articulación. 1. unión de dos o más huesos; 2. pronunciación clara y distinta de los sonidos de las palabras; ___ **disorders** / trastornos de la ___.

artificial *a.* artificial, artificioso-a; ___ **impregnation** / impregnación, fecundación ___; ___ **insemination** / inseminación ___; ___ **limb** /

extremidad o parte ___; ___ **respiration** / respiración ___.

artificial heart *n.* corazón artificial, aparato que bombea la sangre con la capacidad funcional de un corazón normal.

as *conj.* como, del mismo modo; ___ **a child** / de niño *comp.* ___ **much** / tanto ___; **as much** ___ **possible** / lo más posible; ___ **soon** ___ **you can** / tan pronto como pueda, puedas; ___ **usual** / como de costumbre; ___ **you please** / como Ud. quiera, como tú quieras; **not** ___ **yet** / todavía no.

asbestos *n.* asbesto, amianto.

asbestosis *n.* asbestosis, infección crónica de los pulmones causada por el polvo del asbesto.

ascariasis *n.* ascariasis, infección causada por parásitos del género *Ascaris.*

ascaris *n. Ascaris,* género de parásitos que se aloja en el intestino de animales vertebrados.

ascendent *a.* ascendiente, ascendente.

ascites *n.* ascitis, acumulación de líquido en la cavidad abdominal.

ascorbic acid *n.* ácido ascórbico, vitamina C.

asepsia *n.* asepsia, ausencia total de gérmenes.

aseptic *a.* aséptico-a, estéril.

asexual *a.* asexual, sin género; ___ **reproduction** / reproducción sin unión sexual.

Asiatic flu *n.* gripe asiática.

ask *v.* preguntar, interrogar, hacer preguntas; [*about someone*] preguntar por; **to** ___ **for** / [*to request*] pedir.

asleep *a.* dormido-a; *v.* **to fall** ___ / dormirse, quedarse ___ .

aspartame *n.* aspartamo, dulcificante artificial de baja caloría.

aspartate transaminasa *n.* aspartato transaminasa, agente diagnóstico en casos de hepatitis viral e infarto de miocardio.

Asperger's disorder *n.* Asperger, síndrome de, trastorno de la personalidad que en casos extremos se caracteriza por retraimiento social, falta de habilidad ocupacional, habla de estilo pedante y excesivo interés en asuntos banales.

aspergillosis *n.* aspergilosis, infección producida por el hongo *Aspergillus* que suele afectar el oído; **acute invasive**

___ / ___ invasiva aguda; **disseminated**
___ / ___ diseminada.

asphyxia *n.* asfixia, sofocación, falta de respiración; ___ **fetalis** / ___ del feto.

asphyxiate *v.* asfixiarse.

aspirate *v.* aspirar.

aspiration *n.* aspiración, inhalación, succión, extracción de un líquido sin dejar entrar el aire; ___ **biopsy** / biopsia con aguja.

aspirin *n.* aspirina, ácido acetilsalicílico.

assay *n.* ensayo; análisis.

assessment *n.* evaluación; **clinical** ___ / ___ clínica; **health** ___ / ___ del estado de salud.

assimilation *n.* asimilación, transformación y absorción por el organismo de los alimentos digeridos.

assist *v.* ayudar, asistir, socorrer.

assistance *n.* asistencia, ayuda.

assistant *n., a.* asistente, ayudante.

associate *a.* asociado-a, socio-a.

asthenia *n.* astenia, pérdida de vigor.

asthma *n.* asma, condición alégica con ataques de coriza y falta de respiración a causa de la infl. de las membranas mucosas; **cardiac** ___ / ___ cardíaca.

asthmatic *a.* asmático-a, rel. al asma.

astigmatism *n.* astigmatismo, defecto de la visión a causa de una irregularidad en la curvatura del ojo.

astragalus *n.* astrágalo, calus, hueso del tobillo.

astringent *a.* astringente, agente con poder de constricción de los tejidos y las membranas mucosas.

astrocytoma *n.* astrocitoma, tumor cerebral.

asymmetry *n.* asimetría, falta de simetría.

asymptomatic *a.* asintomático-a, sin síntoma alguno.

asynclitism *n.* asinclitismo, presentación del neonato y de los planos pélvicos en el parto.

asynergy *n.* asinergia, falta de coordinación entre órganos gen. armónicos.

asystole, asystolia *n.* asístole, asistolia, paro del corazón, ausencia de contracciones cardíacas.

ataraxia *n.* ataraxia; impasividad.

atavism *n.* atavismo, reproducción de rasgos y características ancestrales.

ataxia *n.* ataxia, deficiencia de coordinación muscular.

atelectasis *n.* atelectasis, colapso parcial o total de un pulmón.

atheroma *n.* ateroma, depósito graso o lípido en la capa íntima de una arteria que causa endurecimiento de la misma.

atherosclerosis *n.* aterosclerosis, condición causada por la deposición de grasa en las capas interiores de las arterias y fibrosis de las mismas.

athetosis *n.* atetosis, condición con síntomas de contracciones involuntarias en las manos y los dedos y movimientos sin coordinación de las extremidades, esp. los brazos.

athlete's foot *n.* pie de atleta. V. **dermatophytosis.**

atmosphere *n.* atmósfera.

atmospheric *a.* atmosférico-a.

atom *n.* átomo.

atomic *a.* atómico-a.

atomizer *n.* atomizador.

atonia, atony *n.* atonía, falta de tono, esp. en los músculos.

atopy *n.* atopía, tipo de alergia considerada de carácter hereditario.

atresia *n.* atresia, cierre congénito anormal de una abertura o conducto del cuerpo.

atrial *a.* auricular, atrial, rel. al atrio o la aurícula; ___ **septal defect** / defecto septal ___ .

atrioventricular *a.* atrioventricular, rel. a la aurícula y ventrículo del corazón; ___ **node** / nudo aurículoventricular; ___ **orifice** / orificio ___ .

atrium *n.* (*pl.* **atria**) atrio-a. 1. cavidad que tiene comunicación con otra estructura; 2. cavidad superior del corazón.

atrophy *n.* atrofia, deteriorización de las células, tejidos y órganos del cuerpo; **acute yellow** ___ **of the liver** / ___ amarilla hepática aguda; **alveolar** ___ / ___ alveolar; **arthritic** ___ / ___ artrítica; **artificial** ___ / ___ artificial; **cerebellar** ___ / ___ cerebelosa; **epileptic absence** ___ / ___ por ausencia epiléptica; **infantile progressive spinal muscular** ___ / ___ músculo-espinal infantil progresiva; **ischemic muscular** ___ / ___ isquémica muscular; **juvenile muscular** ___ / ___ muscular juvenil; **macular** ___ / ___ macular; **multiple system** ___ / ___ de sistema múltiple;

neurogenic __ / __ neurogénica;
nutritional type cerebellar __ / __
cerebelar de tipo nutricional; **ocular** __
/ __ ocular; **periodontal** __ / __
periodontal; **postmenopausal** __ / __
postmenopausia; **primary macular** __
of the skin / __ macular primaria de la
piel; **primary vascular** __ **of the skin**
/ __ primaria vascular de la piel;
progressive cerebral __ / __
progresiva cerebral.

atropine sulfate n. atropina, agente
usado como relajador muscular, esp.
aplicado para dilatar la pupila y
paralizar el músculo ciliar durante un
examen de la vista.

attach v. añadir, juntar, pegar, unir.

attached a., pp., añadido-a, pegado-a,
unido-a.

attack n. ataque, acceso; **heart** __ /
ataque al corazón v. atacar, combatir.

attend v. atender, asistir, cuidar, tener
cuidado; **to __ the sick** / asistir, cuidar
a los enfermos.

attendant n. auxiliar, asistente.

attending physician n. médico-a de
cabecera.

attention n. atención, cuidado; **lack of**
__ / falta de __; v. **to pay __** /
atender, prestar atención.

attenuation n. atenuación, acto de
disminución, esp. de una virulencia.

attitude n. actitud; __ **of health**
personnel / __ del personal de salud;
__ **toward death** / __ frente a la
muerte.

attraction n. atracción.

atypical a. atípico-a, que no es común;
fuera de lo corriente.

audiogram n. audiograma, instrumento
para anotar la agudeza de la audición.

auditory a. auditivo-a, rel. a la audición;
__ **canal** / conducto __; **nerve** /
nervio __ .

augment n. aumento, crecimiento; v.
aumentar, crecer; agrandarse.

aunt n. tía.

aura n. aura, síntoma premonitorio de un
ataque epiléptico.

aural, auricular a. aural, auricular. 1.
rel. al sentido del oído; 2. rel. a una
aurícula del corazón.

auricle, auricula n. aurícula. 1.
oreja, la parte externa del oído; 2. cada
una de las dos cavidades superiores del
corazón; 3. orejuela.

auscultate v. auscultar, examinar,
detectar sonidos de órganos tales como
el corazón y los pulmones con el
propósito de hacer un diagnóstico.

auscultation n. auscultación, acto de
auscultar, detección de sonidos en un
examen directo o por medio del
estetoscopio.

authorization n. autorización.

autism n. autismo, trastorno de la
conducta que se manifiesta en un
egocentrismo extremo; **infantile** __ /
__ infantil.

autistic a. autístico-a, rel. al autismo o
que padece de éste.

autoclave n. autoclave, aparato de
esterilización al vapor.

autodigestion n. autodigestión,
digestión de tejidos por las mismas
sustancias que los producen.

autogenous n. autógeno-a, que se
produce en el mismo organismo.

autogenous vaccine n. vacuna
autógena, inoculación que proviene del
cultivo de bacterias del mismo paciente
y se hace para crear anticuerpos.

autograft n. autoinjerto, injerto que se
transfiere de una parte a otra del cuerpo
del mismo paciente.

autoimmunization n.
autoinmunización, inmunidad
producida por una sustancia
desarrollada dentro del organismo de la
persona afectada.

autoinfection n. autoinfección,
infección causada por un agente del
propio organismo.

autoinoculable a. autoinoculable,
suceptible a organismos que provienen
del propio cuerpo.

autologous a. autólogo-a, que indica
algo que proviene del propio individuo.

automatic a. automático, de
movimiento propio.

automatism n. automatismo, conducta
que no está bajo control voluntario.

autonomic, autonomous a.
autonómico-a, autónomo-a, que
funciona independientemente; __
division of nervous system / división
__ del sistema nervioso; __
dysreflexia / disrreflexia __; __
hyperreflexia / hiperreflexia __; __
imbalance / desequilibrio __; __
nervous system / sistema nervioso __;
__ **neurogenic bladder** / vejiga
neurogénica __; __ **plexus** / plexo __;
__ **seizure** / convulsión __; __
visceral motor nuclei / núcleos
viscerales motores autonómicos.

autoplasty *n.* autoplastia, cirugía plástica con el uso de un injerto que se obtiene de la misma persona que lo recibe.

autopsy *n.* autopsia, examen de un cadáver.

autosuggestion *n.* autosugestión, acto de sugestionarse.

autotransfusion *n.* autotranfusión, transfusión de la propia sangre del individuo.

autotransplant *n.* autotransplante, autoinjerto, autograft.

auxiliary *a.* auxiliar; ayudante.

available *a.* disponible, servicial; a la mano; **to be __** / estar a la disposición, estar __ .

average *n.* promedio, término medio; de mediana proporción.

aversion *n.* aversión, aborrecimiento, odio.

avitaminosis *n.* avitaminosis, trastorno o enfermedad causada por una deficiencia vitamínica.

avoid *v.* evitar.

avulsion *n.* avulsión, extracción o remoción de una estructura o parte de ésta.

awake *a.* despierto-a.

aware *a.* enterado-a; conocedor-a; *v.* **to be __** / estar al tanto.

away *adv.* lejos; *a.* distante, ausente; *v.* **to go __** / irse, ausentarse *interj.* **get __** ! / quítese, quítate; váyase, vete.

awhile *adv.* por un rato, por algún tiempo.

axial *a.* axil, axial, rel. al axis o a un eje.

axilla *n.* (*pl.* **axillae**) axila, *pop.* sobaco.

axillary *a.* axilar, rel. a la axila.

axis *n.* axis, eje, línea central imaginaria que pasa a través del cuerpo o de un órgano.

axon *n.* axon, fibra nerviosa, proyección que va desde el cuerpo celular de una neurona y transporta impulsos nerviosos lejos de ésta.

Ayerza's syndrome *n.* síndrome de Ayersa, síndrome caracterizado por múltiples síntomas, esp. dispnea y cianosis, gen. como resultado de insuficiencia pulmonar.

azoospermia *n.* azoospermia, falta de espermatozoos en el esperma.

azotemia *n.* azotemia, exceso de urea en la sangre.

azure *n.* azul celeste.

b

b *abbr.* **bacillus** / bacilo; **behavior** / conducta; **buccal** / bucal.

Babinski's sign *n.* reflejo de Babinski, dorsiflexión del dedo gordo al estimularse la planta del pie.

baby, babe *n.* bebé, *dim.* bebito-a; nene, nena.

bacillar, bacillary *a.* bacilar, rel. a un bacilo.

bacillemia *n.* bacilemia, presencia de bacilos en la sangre.

bacillicarrier *n.* portador de bacilos.

bacilluria *n.* baciluria, presencia de bacilos en la orina.

bacillus *n.* (*pl.* **bacilli**) bacilo, microbio, bacteria en forma de bastoncillo; **Calmette-Guérin, bacille bilié** ___ / ___ de Calmette Guérin, bacille bilié; **Koch's** ___ , **Mycobacterium tuberculosis** / ___ de Koch, micobacteria de la tuberculosis; **typhoid** ___ , **Salmonella typhi** / ___ de la fiebre tifoidea, Salmonela tifoidea.

bacitracin *n.* bacitracin, antibiótico efectivo en contra de ciertos estafilococos.

back *n.* espalda; ___ **tooth** / muela; **low** ___ **pain** / lumbalgia, *adv.* atrás, detrás.

backache *n.* dolor de espalda.

backbone *n.* columna vertebral, espina dorsal.

backlash *n.* contragolpe.

backward *a.* atrasado-a, tardío-a, lento-a, retraído-a; *adv.* atrás, hacia atrás, al revés; [*direction*] en sentido contrario.

bacteria *n., pl.* bacterias, gérmenes.

bacterial *a.* bacteriano-a; ___ **infections** / infecciones ___-s; ___ **endocarditis** / endocarditis ___; ___ **sensitivity tests** / pruebas de sensibilidad ___ .

bactericidal *n.* bactericida, exterminador de bacterias.

bacteriogenic *a.* bacteriogénico-a. 1. de origen bacteriano; 2. que produce bacterias.

bacteriological *a.* bacteriológico-a, rel. a las bacterias.

bacteriologist *n.* bacteriólogo-a, especialista en bacteriología.

bacteriology *n.* bacteriología, ciencia que estudia las bacterias.

bacteriolysin *n.* bacteriolisina, anticuerpo antibacteriano que destruye bacterias.

bacteriolysis *n.* bacteriolisis, destrucción de bacterias.

bacteriostasis *n.* condición en la que existe retardo en el crecimiento de bacterias.

bacterium *n.* (*pl.* **bacteria**) bacteria, germen.

bacteriuria *n.* bacteriuria, presencia de bacterias en la orina.

bad *a.* malo-a mal, nocivo-a, [*harmful*] dañino-a; ___ **from** ___ **to worse** / de mal en peor; **it is** ___ **for your health** / es dañino a la salud; ___ **breath** / mal aliento; ___ **looking** / mal parecido; ___ **mood** / mal humor; ___ **taste in the mouth** / mal sabor en la boca; *slang* ___ **trip** / mala experiencia con una droga; **to look** ___ / tener mal aspecto, tener mala cara *adv.* mal; *v.* **to feel** ___ / ___ sentirse mal -ly *adv.* mal, malamente; **to need** ___ / necesitar con urgencia.

bag *n.* bolsa, bolso; saco; ___ **of waters** / saco amniótico, *pop.* de aguas; **colostomy** ___ / bolso de colostomía; **ice** ___ / ___ de hielo.

balance *n.* balance. 1. pesa, balanza, instrumento para medir pesos; **acid-base** ___ / ___ acidobásico; **fluid** ___ / ___ hídrico 2. balance, estado de las cantidades y concentraciones de las partes y fluidos que en forma normal constituyen el cuerpo humano; 3. estado normal del equilibrio físico o emocional.

balanced *a.* balanceado-a; en control; ___ **diet** / dieta ___ .

balanitis *n.* balanitis, infl. del glande gen. acompañada de infl. del prepucio.

balanoposthitis *n.* balanopostitis, infl. del glande y del prepucio.

bald *a.* calvo-a, sin pelo; franco-a, espontáneo-a, escueto-a.

baldness *n.* calvicie.

ball *n.* bola; asiento del pie; ___ **forceps** / pinzas sacabalas; ___ **of the foot** / antepié.

ball-and-socket joint *n.* enartrosis, articulación multiaxial sinovial en la cual la cabeza del hueso hace cabida dentro de la cavidad redondeada del otro hueso, *p. ej.* la articulación de la cadera.

balloon *n.* globo, balón; slang [*heroin*] globo; **angioplasty** __ / __ de angioplastia; **detachable** __ / __ desmontable; **intraaortic** __ / __ para uso intraaórtico.

ballottement *n., Fr.* peloteo, movimiento manual de rebote por palpación usado en el examen abdominal y pélvico para determinar la presencia de un tumor o el agrandamiento de un órgano.

Band-Aid *n. pop.* curita; parche.

bandage *n.* venda, vendaje, faja; *v.* vendar, ligar, atar.

bang *n.* golpe; detonación.

bank *n.* banco; **blood** __ / __ de sangre.

B antigens *n.* antígenos B, proteínas presentes en las membranas de los eritrocitos que pueden causar una reacción seria en una transfusión.

barbiturate *n.* barbitúrico, hipnótico, sedante.

bare *a.* desnudo-a, descubierto-a; __ -legged / sin medias -ly; *adv.* apenas.

barefoot *a.* descalzo-a, sin zapatos.

barium *n.* bario, metal alcalino de número atómico 56; __ **enema** / enema de __; __ **swallow** / trago de __ .

barium sulfate *n.* sulfato de bario, suspensión lechosa de sulfato de bario que se da a los pacientes como medio de contraste antes de hacer una radiografía del tubo digestivo.

barometer *n.* barómetro, instrumento para medir la presión atmosférica.

baroreceptor *n.* barorreceptor, terminación nerviosa sensorial que reacciona a los cambios de presión.

barren *a.* estéril, infecundo-a.

bartholinitis *n.* bartolinitis, infl. de la glándula de Bartolino o glándula vulvovaginal.

basal, basilar *a.* basal, basilar, rel. a una base; __ **ganglia diseases** / enfermedades de los ganglios __ -es; __ **metabolic rate** / índice del metabolismo __ .

basal ganglia *n.* ganglios basales, masas grises localizadas debajo de la corteza cerebral que toman parte en la coordinación muscular.

base, basis *n.* base, fundación.

basic *a.* básico-a, fundamental.

basilar *a.* basilar, rel. a la base o parte basal.

basin *n.* 1. vasija redonda tal como una palangana; 2. cavidad de la pelvis.

bastard *n.* bastardo-a; hijo o hija ilegítimo-a.

bath *n.* baño; **alcohol** __ / fricción de alcohol; **antipyretic** __ / __ antipirético, para reducir la fiebre; **aromatic** __ / __ aromático; **cold** __ / __ de agua fría; **hot** __ / __ caliente; **full** __ / __ completo; **kinetotherapeutic** __ / __ cinetoterapéutico; **immersion** __ / __ con inmersión; **oil** __ / __ aceitado; **Sitz** __ / __ de asiento caliente; **sponge** __ / __ con esponja; **warm** __ / __ tibio.

bathe *v.* bañar, lavar; bañarse, lavarse.

bathrobe *n.* bata de baño.

bathroom *n.* baño, cuarto de baño.

battered *a.* abatido-a, maltratado-a.

battle *n.* batalla, lucha; *v.* batallar, combatir, luchar.

B cell receptor *n., pl.* receptor de células tipo B.

B cells *n., pl.* células tipo B, linfocitos que proceden de la médula ósea y producen anticuerpos, por lo que representan una ayuda importante en la respuesta inmune.

be *vi.* ser, estar; **there is, there are** / hay; **there was** / hubo, había; **there will be** / será, estará, habrá [*pp.*] **been** / sido, estado [*pp.*] **being** / siendo, estando; **to __ afraid** / tener miedo; **to __ at a loss** / estar confundido-a; **to __ calm** / calmarse; **to __ careful** / tener cuidado; **to __ cold** / tener frío; **to __ hot** / tener calor; **to __ hungry** / tener hambre; **to __ quiet** / callarse; estar tranquilo-a; **to __ right** / tener razón; **to __ all right** / estar bien; **to __** . . . **years old** / tener . . . años; **to __ sick** / estar enfermo-a; **to __ sleepy** / tener sueño; **to __ successful** / tener éxito; **to __ thirsty** / tener sed; **to __ warm** [*with a temperature*] / tener fiebre, tener calentura; tener calor; **to want to __** / querer ser; **to want to __** [*somewhere*] / querer estar.

bear *vi.* soportar; aguantar; __ **down** / pujar, empujar hacia afuera con fuerza.

beard *n.* barba.

bearded *a.* barbudo.

bearer *n.* soporte, apoyo.

bearing *n.* gestación; conexión; [*in obstetrics*]; __ **down** / [*second stage of labor*] pujo, expulsión hacia afuera.

beat *n.* [*heart*] latido, pulsación; **heart**

___ / ___ del corazón vi. pulsar; [*heart*] palpitar; pegar, golpear.

beaten a. pp. de to beat, maltratado-a; golpeado-a; vencido-a, derrotado-a.

become vi. hacerse, convertirse; ___ a / convertirse en; ___ accustomed / acostumbrarse; ___ a doctor / hacerse médico-a; [*conversion*] ; ___ crazy / volverse loco-a; ___ frightened / asustarse; ___ ill / ponerse enfermo-a; enfermarse; ___ inflamed / inflamarse; ___ swollen / hincharse.

bed n. cama, lecho; ___ occupancy / ocupación de ___ -s; ___ rest / reclusión en ___ .

bedding n. ropa de cama; colchón y almohada.

bedfast a. recluido-a en cama.

bedpan n. bacín, chata, cuña.

bedridden a. postrado-a en cama.

bedsore n. úlcera por decúbito.

bedtime n. hora de acostarse.

bed-wetting n. enuresis; orinarse en la cama, mojar la cama.

bee n. abeja; ___ venom / veneno de ___ .

before adv. delante; enfrente de; antes de; anterior a; conj. antes que; antes de que.

beforehand adv. con anterioridad, con anticipación; de antemano.

begin vi. comenzar, empezar, principiar.

beginner n. principiante, novicio-a; autor-a, iniciador-a.

behavior n. conducta, comportamiento; ___ reflex / reflejo adquirido; ___ therapy / terapia de la ___; high-risk ___ / comportamiento arriesgado.

behind adv., prep., detras, trás, atrás, hacia atrás.

belladonna n. belladona, yerba medicinal cuyas hojas y raíces contienen atropina y alcaloides.

Bell's palsy n. parálisis de Bell, parálisis de un lado de la cara causada por una afección del nervio facial.

belly n. abdomen, barriga, vientre, pop. panza; ___ button / ombligo; ___ worm / lombriz intestinal.

bellyache n. dolor de estómago, de barriga.

below prep. después de, debajo de; adv. abajo, bajo, debajo; down ___ / en la parte baja; más abajo.

belt n. cinturón, cinto.

bend vi. doblarse, inclinarse; ___ back / ___ hacia atrás; ___ forward / ___ hacia adelante.

beneath prep., adv. abajo, debajo, bajo.

Benedict test n. prueba de Benedict, análisis químico para encontrar la presencia de azúcar en la orina.

beneficial a. beneficioso-a, favorable, provechoso-a.

beneficiary n., a. beneficiado-a, favorecido-a.

benefit n. beneficio, favor; servicio, provecho; allocation of ___ -s / asignación de ___ -s.

benign a. benigno-a, que no es de naturaleza maligna.

bent n. inclinación, curvatura; a. encorvado-a; inclinado-a.

beriberi n. beriberi, tipo de neuritis múltiple causada por deficiencia de vitamina B1 (tiamina).

beside adv. además, prep. al lado de, cerca de, junto a; ___ oneself / fuera de sí, loco-a.

best a., sup. mejor, superior, óptimo; v. to do one's ___ / hacer lo ___ posible.

bestiality n. bestialidad, relaciones sexuales con animales.

beta blocker n. beta bloqueador, agente que bloquea la acción de la epinefrina.

better a. comp. mejor, superior; [*better than*] mejor que; so much the ___ / tanto mejor. to be ___ / estar mejor, ponerse mejor; to be ___ than / ser mejor que; to be ___ than before / estar, ser mejor que antes; to change for the ___ / recuperarse, restablecerse; to like ___ / preferir; to make ___ / mejorar, aliviar.

beverage n. bebida; alcoholic ___ -s / bebidas alcoholicas; nonalcoholic ___ / ___ no alcoholica.

beware of vi. cuidarse de; estar al tanto de.

bezoar n. bezoar, concreción formada de distintas materias como fibras vegetales y pelo, presente en el estómago y en el intestino humano así como en el de los animales.

bibliography n. bibliografía.

bicarbonate n. bicarbonato, sal de ácido carbónico.

biceps n. músculo bíceps.

bicipital a. bicipital. 1. rel. al músculo bíceps; 2. bicípite, que tiene dos cabezas.

bicycle n. bicicleta; stationary ___ / ___ estacionaria.

bifocal a. bifocal, referente a dos focos o enfoques.

bifurcation

bifurcation *n.* bifurcación, división en dos ramas o derecciones.

big *a.* grande, enorme; mayor; __ bellied / barrigón-a, panzudo-a; __ head / cabezón-a; __ sister, brother / hermana mayor, hermano mayor; __ toe / dedo gordo; __ with child / encinta, en estado.

bigeminal *a.* bigeminal, que tiene pulsación duplicada en sucesión rápida.

bigger *a. comp.* mayor, más grande.

bile *n.* bilis, hiel, producto de la secreción del hígado; __ acids and salts / ácidos y sales biliares; __ ducts / conductos biliares; __ pigments / pigmentos biliares.

biliary *a.* biliar, rel. a la bilis, los conductos biliares o la vesícula; __ duct obstruction / obstrucción del conducto __; __ stasis / colestasis; __ tract diseases / enfermedades de las vías __-es; __ tract hemorrhage / hemobilia.

bilingual *a.* bilingüe.

bilious *a.* bilioso-a, con exceso de bilis.

bilirubin *n.* bilirrubina, pigmento rojo de la bilis.

bilirubinemia *n.* bilirrubinemia, presencia de bilirrubina en la sangre.

bilirubinuria *n.* bilirubinuria, presencia de bilirrubina en la orina.

binary *a.* binario, doble.

bind *vi.* unir, ligar, vendar.

binding *n.* enlace; ligazón; venda; vendaje.

bioassay *n.* bioensayo, prueba de determinación de la potencia de una droga en animales.

biochemical *a.* bioquímico-a, rel. a la bioquímica.

biochemistry *n.* bioquímica, ciencia que estudia los organismos vivos.

biologic, biological *a.* biológico-a, rel. a la biología; __ assay / análisis __; __ control / control __; __ evolution / evolución __; __ half-life / semivida __; __ immunotherapy / inmunoterapia __; __ indicator / indicador __; __ psychiatry / siquiatría __; __ warfare / guerra __ .

biologist *n.* biólogo-a.

biology *n.* biología, ciencia que estudia los organismos vivos; **cellular** __ / __ celular; **molecular** __ / __ molecular.

biopsy *n.* biopsia, proceso para obtener un espécimen de tejido con fines de diagnóstico; **aspiration** __ / por aspiración; __ by ablation / __ por ablación; __ by frozen section / __ en frío; __ of the bone marrow / __ de la medula ósea; __ of the breast / __ de la mama, del seno; __ of the cervix / __ del cuello uterino; __ of the lymph nodes / __ de los ganglios linfáticos; **brush** __ / __ con cepillo; **endoscopic** __ / __ endoscópica; **excision** __ / __ por excisión; **fine needle** __ / __ de aguja fina; **incision** __ / __por incisión; **muscle** __ / __ muscular; **needle** __ / __ por aspiración; **sentinel** __ / __ del ganglio vigilante; **specimen wedge** __ / __ de espécimen cuneiforme; **temporal artery** __ / __ de la arteria temporal.

biosynthesis *n.* biosíntesis, formación de sustancias químicas en los procesos fisiológicos de los organismos.

bioterrorism *n.* terrorismo biológico, bioterrorismo.

birth *n.* nacimiento, parto, alumbramiento; __ canal / canal del parto; __ certificate / certificado de __; __ control / control de la natalidad, planeamiento familiar; __ -death ratio / índice de mortalidad; __ rate / natalidad; __ right / derechos naturales; __ weight / peso al nacer; **post-term** __ / __ tardío; **premature** __ / __ prematuro *v.* **to give** __ / dar a luz, estar de parto.

birth date *n.* fecha de nacimiento.

birthday *n.* cumpleaños, natalicio.

birthplace *n.* lugar de nacimiento.

bisexual *a.* bisexual, con gónadas de los dos sexos.

bite *n.* mordida, picadura; [*snake*] mordida de serpiente; [*insect*] picadura; __ block / bloque de __; __ rim / reborde de la __; __ testing / análisis de la __ *v.* morder, picar.

biting *a.* (*pain*) penetrante, picante.

Bitot spots *n., pl.* Bitot, manchas de, pequeñas manchas grises triangulares que aparecen en la conjuntiva y se asocian a la deficiencia de vitamina A.

bitter *a.* agrio-a, amargo-a; [*person*] amargado-a.

black *a.* negro-a; __ and blue / amoratado-a; __eye / ojo amoratado; __ death / peste bubónica; __ urine / melanuria.

blackhead *n.* barro, espinilla, comedón.

blackout *n.* desmayo, vértigo, condición caracterizada por la falta de visión y pérdida momentánea del conocimiento.

bladder *n.* vejiga; saco musculomembranoso situado en la cavidad pélvica; ___ **calculi** / cálculos, piedras de la ___; ___ **infection** / infección de la ___; ___ **irrigation** / irrigación de la ___; ___ , **neurogenic** / ___ neurogénica.

Blalock-Tausig operation *n.* Blalock-Tausig, operación de, cirugía para reparar una malformación congénita del corazón.

blame *n.* culpa; *v.* **to blame** / echar la culpa; **to blame someone** / echarle la culpa a alguien.

bland *a.* blando-a, suave; ___ **diet** / dieta

blanket *n.* manta, frazada, cobija.

blastomycosis *n.* blastomicosis, infección causada por hongos que se inicia gen. en los pulmones.

bleariness *n.* lagaña, secreción pegajosa del ojo; vista nublada.

bleary-eyed *a.* [*eye*] legañosos; [*sight*] vista nublada; vista cansada.

bleed *vi.* sangrar, derramar, perder sangre; [*profusely*] desangrarse.

bleeding *n.* sangrado, hemorragia; ___ **disorders** / trastornos hemorrágicos; ___ **from an artery** / hemorragia arterial; ___ **from the vagina** / ___ vaginal; ___ **from the nose** / ___ por la nariz, epistaxis; ___ **piles** / hemorroides ; ___ **tendency** / diátesis hemorrágica; ___ **rectal** / rectorrhagia; **life threatening** ___ / hemorragia con peligro mortal.

blemish *n.* mancha, imperfección, defecto.

blepharitis *n.* blefaritis, infl. de los párpados.

blepharochalasis *n.* blefarocalasis, relajación o caída del párpado superior por pérdida de elasticidad del tejido intersticial.

blepharoplasty *n.* blefaroplastia, operación plástica de los párpados.

blepharoplegia *n.* blefaroplejía, parálisis del párpado.

blind *a.* ciego, sin vista, ofuscado-a; *v.* cegar, deslumbrar; ___ **in one eye** / tuerto-a; ___ **spot** / punto ___ .

blindness *n.* ceguera; **color** ___ / acromatopsia, ___ al color; **night** ___ / nictalopía, ___ nocturna; **red** ___ / roja; **total** ___ / pérdida completa de la visión.

blister *n.* ampolla, vesícula, flictena.

bloated *a.* aventado-a, hinchado-a, inflado-a.

block *n.* bloqueo, obstrucción; *v.* obstruir, bloquear.

blocked *a.* bloqueado-a, obstruído-a; ___ **bowel** / obstrucción intestinal; ___ **ureter** / obstrucción ureteral.

blocker *n.* bloqueador; **calcium channel** ___ / del canal cálcico.

blood *n.* sangre; **autologous** ___ / ___ autóloga; ___ **alcohol concentration** / concentración de alcohol en la ___; ___ **alcohol test** / prueba de alcoholemia; ___ **bank** / banco de ___; ___ **cell count** / conteo globular, conteo de células sanguíneas; ___ **clotting ability** / propiedad de coagulación; ___ **count** / conteo sanguíneo; ___ **culture** / hemocultivo; ___ **clot** / coágulo de ___; ___ **coagulation time** / tiempo de coagulación sanguínea; ___ **derivatives** / derivados sanguíneos, hemoderivados; ___ **donor** / donante de ___; ___ **gases** / gases sanguíneos; ___ **groups** / grupos sanguíneos; ___ **grouping** / determinación de grupos sanguíneos; ___ **oxygen analysis** / análisis del oxígeno contenido en la ___; ___ **plasma** / plasma sanguíneo; ___ **pressure** / presión arterial; ___ **products** / productos sanguíneos; ___ **proteins** / proteínas sanguíneas; ___ **relation** / consanguíneo-a; ___ **screening** / prueba selecta de ___; ___ **sputum** / esputo sanguinolento; ___ **substitutes** / substitutos sanguíneos; ___ **sugar** / glucemia; ___ **transfusion** / transfusión sanguínea; ___ **type** / grupo sanguíneo; ___ **typing** / determinación del grupo sanguíneo; ___ **vessel** / vaso sanguíneo; **packed** ___ **cells** / células paquete, células sanguíneas compactadas; **peripheral** ___ / ___ periférica.

blood pressure *n.* presión sanguínea, tensión de la sangre en las arterias producida por la contracción del ventrículo izquierdo, la resistencia de las arteriolas y capilares, la elasticidad de las paredes arteriales y la viscosidad y volumen de la sangre; **high** ___ / ___ alta; **low** ___ / ___ baja; **normal** ___ / ___ normal.

bloodshot *a.* [*eye*] inyectado de sangre.

bloody *a.* ensangrentado-a, con sangre, sanguinolento-a, cruento.

bloody sputum *n.* expectoración sanguínea; expectoración hemorrágica.

blotch

blotch *n.* marca, roncha.

blow *n.* golpe; *vi.* soplar, **to __ one's nose** / soplarse, sonarse la nariz; **to give a __** / golpear.

blue *n.* color azul; *a.* triste, malancólico-a; **__ baby syndrome** / cianosis congénita, *pop.* mal azul.

blunt *a.* despuntado-a; embotado-a; **__ injuries** / heridas contusas.

blurred *a., pp.* de **to blur**, borroso-a, nublado-a, empañado-a.

body *n.* cuerpo; [*dead*] cadáver; tronco; materia, sustancia; **__ fluid** / líquido corporal; **__ height** / estatura; **__ temperature** / temperatura corporal; **__ weight** / peso corporal; **__ wall** / tronco. V. ilustración esta página.

body-building *n.* esculturismo, restauración del cuerpo con ejercicios.

boil *n.* forúnculo.

boiled *a.* hervido-a; **__ water** / agua __.

boiling point *n.* punto de ebullición.

bolster *n.* cabezal; sostén, refuerzo; **__ suture** / sutura compuesta.

bolus *n.* bolo. 1. cantidad de una sustancia que se administra en determinado tiempo por vía oral o intravenosa para obtener una respuesta inmediata; 2. masa de consistencia suave lista para ser ingerida; **alimentary __** / __alimenticio.

bone *n.* 1. hueso. 2. [*fish*] espina; **__ cell** / osteoblasto; **__ chips** / astillas de __; **__ density** / densidad ósea; **__ development** / desarrollo óseo; **__ fracture** / fractura, **__** quebrado; **__ fragility** / fragilidad ósea; **__ graft** / injerto óseo; **__ hook** / gancho óseo; **__ lesions** / lesiones en los __ -s; **__loss** / osteopenia; **__ marrow** / médula ósea, *pop.* tuétano; **__ marrow failure** / fallo de la médula ósea; **__ plate** / placa ósea; **__ splinter** / esquirla, astilla ósea; **hard __** / **__** compacto; **he swallowed a fish __** / se tragó una espina de __; **__ spongy __** / __ esponjoso *v.* **to make no __ -s about it** / hablar sin rodeos; **skin and __ -s** / piel y __-s, muy delgado *pop.* estar en el hueso *v.* deshuesar / sacar los __ -s.

bonelet *n. dim.* huesecillo.

book *n.* libro.

booster shot *n.* búster, 1. inyección de refuerzo; 2. dosis suplementaria; 3. reactivación de una vacuna o agente inmunizador.

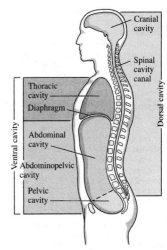

Body cavities: side view

booze *n.* bebida alcohólica.

borax *n.* bórax, borato de sodio.

border *n.* borde, margen; frontera.

bordering *a.* cercano-a, fronterizo-a, adyacente.

border-line case *n.* caso indeciso, precario, difícil de pronosticar.

bored *a.* aburrido-a.

boric acid *n.* ácido bórico.

born *a.* nacido-a; **__ alive** / __ vivo; **new __** / recién nacido-a *v.* **to be __** / nacer.

bosom *n.* seno, pecho.

both *a., pron.* ambos, los dos.

botox *n.* bótox, proteína purificada por la bacteria de botulismo *clostridium* que se emplea en aplicaciones cosméticas.

bottle *n.* botella, frasco, [*infant*] biberón, mamadera; *Mex.* pote, tele; **__ feeding** / alimentación por biberón; **__ propping** / suplemento con biberón.

bottom *n.* fondo, parte inferior; asiento; *pop.* posaderas, asentaderas; *Cuba* fondillo.

botulin *n.* botulina, toxina causante del botulismo.

botulism *n.* botulismo, intoxicación ocasionada por la ingestión de alimentos contaminados por

Clostridium botulinum que se desarrolla en alimentos que no han sido propiamente conservados.

bounding pulse *n.* pulso saltón.

bounding pupil *n.* pupila saltona

bout *n.* acceso, ataque, episodio.

bowel *n.* intestino. __ **movement** / evacuación, deposición; __ **obstruction** / obstrucción intestinal.

bowels *n., pl.* intestinos.

bowleg *n. V.* **genu varum.**

boy *n.* niño, muchacho.

boyfriend *n.* amigo, novio.

brace *n.* braguero, corsée, vendaje; abrazadera; **ankle** __ / tobillera; **neck** __ / __ de cuello; abrazadera *n., pl.* [*dentristy*] ganchos, aros.

brachial *a.* braquial, rel. al brazo; __ **artery** / arteria braquial; __ **plexus** / plexo __; __ **veins** / venas __ -es o del brazo.

brachiocephalic *a.* braquiocefálico, rel. a la cabeza y al brazo.

bradycardia *n.* bradicardia, espanocardia, lentitud anormal en los latidos del corazón.

bradypnea *n.* bradipnea, movimientos respiratorios lentos.

Braille, reading system *n.* Braille, sistema de lectura, método de escritura e impreso de puntos alzados que identifican letras, números y puntuación y permite a los ciegos leer por medio del tacto.

brain *n.* cerebro, parte del sistema nervioso central que se localiza en el cráneo y actúa como regulador principal de las funciones del cuerpo; **blood** __ **barrier** / barrera hematoencefálica; __ **abscess** / asbceso cerebral; __ **center** / centro cerebral; __ **death** / muerte cerebral; __ **edema** / edema cerebral; __ **injuries** / traumatismo cerebral; __ **or cerebral concussion** / concusión o conmoción cerebral; __ **puncture** / punción cerebral; __ **scan** / escán del __; __ **tumor** / tumor cerebral. V. ilustración en la página 282.

brain stem *n.* cuello encefálico, parte que conecta el encéfalo con la espina dorsal.

brain stimulator surgery *n.* cirugía estimuladora del cerebro, tipo nuevo de cirugía cerebral que ayuda a controlar los temblores en los pacientes de Parkinson.

brainwashing *n.* lavado de cerebro.

brainy *a.* inteligente, listo-a, talentoso-a.

branch *n.* rama, bifurcación; sección, dependencia.

brassy cough *n.* tos metálica, tos bronca.

BRCA 1 and BRCA 2 *n.* acrónimo del gene del cáncer de la mama y del cáncer uterino, son genes heredados que al presentar mutaciones pueden originar un alto riesgo canceroso. Se aconseja que mujeres con historia médica familiar de cáncer de la mama y del ovario se sometan a las pruebas llamadas BRACAnálisis con el propósito de detectar las mutaciones que pueden originar el cáncer de la mama antes de los cincuenta años y más tarde con más alto riesgo a los setenta años de edad. Igualmente las mutaciones presentan alto riesgo en desarrollar el cáncer uterino antes de los setenta años.

break *n.* fractura, rotura; quebradura; *v.* romper, quebrar, fracturar; *v.* fracturarse, romperse, quebrarse; **to __ down** / [*health*] perder la salud; **to __ in** / forzar, abrir; **to __ loose** / separarse, desprenderse; **to __ through** / avanzar; **to __ up** / fraccionar.

breakable *a.* frágil, quebradizo.

breakdown *n.* distribución detallada; descomposición; colapso; **nervous __** / crisis nerviosa.

breakout *n.* erupción.

breast *n.* pecho, seno, busto, mama; *slang* teta; **benign __ disease** / enfermedad benigna de la mama; **caked __** / mastitis por estasis*v.* to __ -**feed** / dar el pecho, dar de mamar, dar la teta, *Mex. A.* criar con pecho; __ **pump** / sacaleche, mamadera; __ **self-examination** / autoexamen de los senos.

breastbone *n.* esternón.

breastfeeding *n.* lactancia materna.

breath *n.* respiración, aliento, soplo; *pop.* resuello; __ **sounds** / ruidos respiratorios; **coarse __** / __ gruesa; **short of __** / corto de __, falto de aliento; **out of __** / falto de __, sin aliento *v.* **to be out of __** / faltar la __, estar sofacado-a; **to gasp for __** / jadear; **to take a deep __** / respirar profundamente; **to hold one's __** / sostener, aguantar la __.

breathanalyzer *n.* instrumento que

breathe

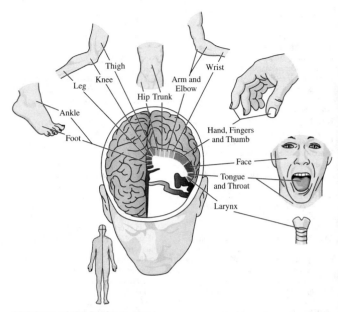

Divisions of the brain: frontal lobe

analiza el aliento de una persona para indicar el grado de consunción de alcohol.

breathe *v.* respirar; [*to exhale*] exhalar; [*to inhale*] aspirar; **to __ through the mouth** / __ por la boca; **to __ through the nose** / __ por la nariz.

breather *n.* respirador; tregua, reposo.

breathing *n.* respiración, aliento, respiro; inhalación, aspiración; __ **exercises** / ejercicios respiratorios; __ **space,** __ **time** / descanso, parada, reposo.

breathless *a.* sofocado-a, sin aliento; falto de respiración.

breech *n.* trasero, posaderas, nalgas; [*in obstetrics*] __ **birth** / presentación de nalgas, presentación trasera.

breeze *n.* brisa, aire suave.

bregma *n. Gr.* bregma, intersección de las suturas coronal y sagital del cráneo.

Bright's disease *n.* enfermedad de Bright. glomerulonephritis.

brim *n.* borde.

brittle bone disease *n.* osteogenesis imperfecta, trastorno del tejido conjuntivo que resulta en fragilidad ósea.

brittle diabetes *n.* niveles inestables de glucose en la sangre debido a falta de control.

broken *a. pp.* of **to break,** [*bone*] fracturado-a, quebrado-a; **broken arm** / brazo fracturado, quebrado; [*home, person*] **broken home** / hogar deshecho, destrozado; **broken hearted** / descorazonado.

bromhidrosis *n.* bromhidrosis, perspiración fétida; sudor fétido.

bromide *n.* bromuro, bromo, elemento no metálico, miembro del grupo de halógenos, muy irritante a las membranas mucosas. Se emplea como oxidante y antiséptico.

bronchial *a.* bronquial, rel. a los bronquios; __ **adenoma** / adenoma __; __ **arch** / arco __; __ **asthma** / asma __; __ **blockade** / bloqueo __; __ **breathing** / murmullo vesicular; __ **cleft** / fisura __; __ **glands** / glándulas bronquiales; __ **plexus injury** / lesión del plexo __; __

spasm / espasmo ___; ___ **stenosis** / estenosis ___; ___ **tree** / árbol ___; ___ **veins** / venas bronquiales; ___ **washing** / lavado ___ .

bronchiectasis *n.* bronquiectasia, dilatación crónica de los bronquios debida a una obstrucción o a una condición inflamatoria.

bronchiocele *n.* bronquiocele, dilatación localizada de un bronquiolo.

bronchiole *n.* bronquiolo, una de las ramas menores del árbol bronquial.

bronchiolitis *n.* bronquiolitis, infl. de los bronquiolos.

bronchitis *n.* bronquitis, infl. de los tubos bronquiales.

bronchoconstriction *n.* broncoconstricción, reducción de calibre bronquial.

bronchodilation *n.* broncodilatación, dilatación bronquial.

bronchodilator *n.* broncodilatador, medicamento que dilata el calibre de un bronquio; ___ **agents** / agentes ___ -es.

bronchogenic *a.* broncogénico-a, broncógeno-a, que se origina en los bronquios; ___ **carcinoma** / carcinoma ___; ___ **cyst** / quiste ___ .

bronchography *n.* broncografía, radiografía del árbol bronquial usando un medio de contraste.

broncholith *n.* broncolito, cálculo bronquial.

bronchopneumonia *n.* bronconeumonía, infl. aguda de los bronquios y de los lóbulos pulmonares que afecta gen. ambos pulmones.

bronchopulmonary *a.* broncopulmonar, rel. a los bronquios y los pulmones; ___ **lavage** / lavado ___; ___ **lymph nodes** / ganglios linfáticos ___ -es.

bronchoscopy *n.* broncoscopia, examen del árbol bronquial por medio del broncoscopio.

bronchospasm *n.* broncoespasmo, contracción espasmódica de los bronquios y los bronquiolos.

bronchospirometry *n.* broncoespirometría, proceso de medir la función de ventilación de cada pulmón separadamente por medio de un broncoespirómetro.

bronchostomy *n.* broncostomía, incisión de un bronquio.

bronchotomogram *n.* broncotomograma, escán o barrido de imágenes tomadas del sistema respiratorio superior, comprendiendo desde la tráquea a los bronquios inferiores.

bronchovesicular *a.* broncovesicular, rel. a los bronquios y alvéolos pulmonares esp. durante la auscultación. *Syn.* **broncoalveolar**.

bronchus *n.* (*pl.* **bronchia**) bronquio, uno de los tubos por los cuales el aire pasa a los pulmones; **eparterial** ___ / ___ superior a una arteria; **intermediate** ___ / ___ intermedio; **left main** ___ / ___ principal izquierdo; **lobar bronchi** / broncolobares; **main** ___ / ___ principal; **mucoid impaction of** ___ / impacto mucoso del ___; **right main** ___ / ___ principal derecho.

brother *n.* hermano; ___ **-in-law** / cuñado; **half-** ___ / medio ___ .

brow *n.* ceño; frente.

Brown-Séquard syndrome *n.* síndrome de Brown Séquard, hemisección de la médula espinal que causa hiperestesia en el lado lesionado y pérdida de la sensibilidad en el lado opuesto.

brow presentation *n.* [*delivery*] presentación frontal del feto.

brucellosis *n.* brucelosis, fiebre ondulante o fiebre mediterránea, condición infecciosa bacteriana que se contrae por contacto con ganado vacuno o sus productos.

bruise *n.* magulladura, *Lat. Am.* magullón, cardenal; *vr.* magullarse, hacerse una magulladura, un morado o cardenal.

bubonic plague *n.* peste bubónica.

bucca *n.* boca.

buccal *a.* bucal.

buccolabial *a.* bucolabial, rel. a los labios y las mejillas.

build *vi.* construir; ___ **-up phase** / fase de ascenso; **to** ___ **up one's health** / reconstituir la salud.

bulb *n.* bulbo, pera; bombillo; 1. [*syringe*] pera de goma; 2. expansión oval o circular de un conducto o cilindro.

bulbourethral *a.* bulbouretral, uretrobulbar, rel. al bulbo del pene y la uretra.

bulge *n.* hinchazón, protuberancia.

bulging

bulging *n.* protuberancia; ___ **abdomen** / abdomen prominente, vientre abombado; ___ **eyes** / ojos saltones.

bulimia *n.* bulimia, apetito exagerado.

bulla *n.* ampolla.

bullet *n.* bala; ___ **wound** / balazo, herida de ___ .

bump *n.* golpe, [*on the head*] chichón; *v.* tropezar; golpearse, darse un golpe.

bundle *n.* manojo, haz; bulto; ___ -**branch block** / bloque de rama.

bunion *n.* bunio, juanete, infl. de la bursa en la primera coyuntura del dedo pulgar del pie. V. **Hallux valgus**.

burial *n.* entierro.

burn *n.* quemadura; ___ , **dry heat** / ___ por calor seco; ___ -**s, chemical** / ___ -s por sustancias químicas; **first-, second-, and third-degree** ___ -**s** / ___ -s de primer, segundo y tercer grado; **minor** ___ / ___ leve; **sun** ___ / insolación, eritema solar; **thermal** ___ / ___ térmica; *v.* arder, quemar, incendiar.

burning *n.* ardor, quemadura; irritación; **a** ___ **feeling** / sensación de ___ , quemazón; ___ **on urination** / ___ al orinar.

burnt-out *a.* [*persona*]. extenuado-a. quemado-a; [*worn-out*] *a.* extenuado-a.

burp *n.* eructo, eructación; *v.* eructar, sacar el aire.

bursa *n.*, *L.* bursa, bolsa o saco en forma de cavidad que contiene líquido sinovial en áreas de los tejidos donde puede ocurrir una fricción.

bursitis *n.* bursitis, infl. de una bursa.

burst *n.* [*a sudden outbreak*] reventón; *v.* reventar, reventarse, abrirse; ___ **into laughter** / echarse a reír; ___ **into tears** / deshacerse en lágrimas; **to** ___ **out** / brotar, reventar; **to** ___ **open** / abrirse, reventarse; echarse a llorar.

buttocks *n.*, *pl.* nalgas, *pop. Mex.* asentaderas, *Cuba* fondillo.

button *n.* botón.

buzz *n.* murmullo, zumbido.

by *prep.* por, cerca de, al lado de, según; ___ **day** / de día, por el día; ___ **night** / de noche, por la noche.

bypass *n. pop.* baipás, derivación. 1. conducto auxiliar, comunicación, derivación; *v.* 2. cambiar el curso de fluidos de un órgano o parte a otro a través de una nueva vía quirúrgica; **aortocoronary** ___ / ___ aortocoronario o derivación aortocoronaria; **aortoiliac** ___ / ___ aortoilíaco; ___ **aortorenal** / ___ aortorenal; **cardiopulmonary** ___ / cardiopulmonar ___; **coronary** ___ / derivación coronaria; **extracraneal-intracraneal** ___ / ___ extracranial-intracranial; **internal mammary artery** ___ / derivación de la arteria mamaria interna.

by-product *n.* subproducto.

C *abbr.* **carbon** / carbono; **celsius** / Celsius; **centigrade** / centígrado; **Kilocalorie** / kilocaloría.

c *abbr.* **calorie** / caloría; **cobalt** / cobalto; **cocaine** / cocaína; **contraction** / contracción.

cachexia *n.* caquexia, condición grave que se caracteriza por pérdida excesiva de peso y debilidad general progresiva.

cadaver *n.* cadáver.

caffeine *n.* cafeína, alcaloide presente esp. en el café y el té, estimulante y diurético.

calamine *n.* calamina, antiséptico astringente secante que se usa en afecciones de la piel.

calcaneus *n.* calcáneo, hueso del talón; *pop.* calcañal, calcañar.

calcareous *n.* calcáreo, que contiene calcio o cal.

calcemia *n.* calcemia, presencia de calcio en la sangre.

calciferol *n.* calciferol, producto derivado de ergosterol, vitamina D2.

calcification *n.* calcificación, endurecimiento de tejidos orgánicos por depósitos de sales de calcio.

calcinosis *n.* calcinosis, presencia de sales cálcicas en la piel, los tejidos subcutáneos y los órganos.

calcitonin *n.* calcitonina, hormona segregada por la tiroides que estimula el transporte del calcio de la sangre a los huesos.

calcium *n.* calcio, sustancia mineral necesaria en el desarrollo de los huesos y tejidos.

calciuria *n.* calciuria, presencia de calcio en la orina.

calculus *n.* (*pl.* **calculi**) cálculo, concreción o pequeña piedra que puede formarse en las secreciones y fluidos del organismo; **biliary** ___ / ___ biliar; **calcium oxalate** ___ / ___ de oxalato de calcio; **cystine** ___ / ___ de cistina; **fibrin** ___ / ___ de fibrina; **urinary** ___ / ___ urinario.

calendar *n.* calendario, almanaque.

calf *n.* pantorrilla; [*animal*] ternero-a.

caliber *n.* calibre, diámetro de un conducto o canal.

call *n.* llamada; *v.* llamar; **to be on** ___ / estar de guardia; *v.* **to** ___ **for** / pedir.

callosity *n.* callosidad.

callous *a.* calloso-a.

callus *n.* callo, callosidad.

calm *n.* calma, serenidad; *v.* calmar, tranquilizar; calmarse, serenarse, tranquilizarse.

calmodulin *n.* calmodulina, proteína que se fija o se une a los iones de calcio e interviene en procesos celulares.

calorie *n.* caloría, unidad de calor a la que se refiere al evaluar la energía alimenticia; **kilocalorie, large** ___ / gran ___; **small** ___ / pequeña ___ .

calvaria, skullcap *n.* calvaria, bóveda craneal.

camera *n.* cámara. 1. espacio abierto o ventrículo; 2. cámara fotográfica.

camphor *n.* alcanfor; ___ **julep** / aqua alcanforada.

canal *n.* canal, pasaje, estructura tubular; **birth** ___ / ___ del parto; **femoral** ___ / ___ femoral; **inguinalis** ___ / ___ inguinal; **root** ___ / ___ radicular.

canaliculus *n.* canalículo, canal o pasaje diminuto; **biliary** ___ / ___ biliar, entre las células del hígado; **lacrimal** ___ / ___ lacrimal, lagrimal.

cancel *v.* cancelar, suprimir.

cancellous *a.* canceloso-a, esponjoso-a, reticulado-a; ___ **bone** / hueso ___ .

cancer *n.* cáncer, tumor maligno; **breast** ___ / ___ de la mama; ___ **grading** / determinacíon del grado patológico del ___; ___ **staging** / estado o extensión del tumor canceroso; ___ **survivors** / supervivientes de cáncer; **chemoprevention of** ___ / prevención química de ___; **early** ___ / ___ incipiente.

cancerophobia *n.* cancerofobia, fobia a contraer cáncer.

cancerous *a.* canceroso-a.

candida albicans susceptibility *n.* susceptibilidad a candida albicans.

candidiasis *n.* candidiasis, infección de la piel producida por un hongo semejante a la levadura.

cane *n.* bastón; caña; ___ **sugar** / azúcar de caña, sucrosa, sacarosa.

canker *n.* ulceración de la boca o los labios; ___ **sore** / afta, llaga ulcerosa.

cannabis, marijuana *n.* canabis, marijuana, mariguana, marihuana, planta de hojas que producen un efecto narcótico y halucinógeno al fumarse; *slang;* **to blast, to blow weed** / fumar marijuana.

cannula *n.* (*pl.* **cannulae**) cánula, sonda, tubo que insertado en el cuerpo conduce o saca líquidos.

cannulation *n.* canulación, acto de introducir una cánula a través de un vaso o conducto; **aortic __** / __ aórtica.

canthus *n.* 1. canto, borde; 2. ángulo formado por el párpado externo y el interno al unirse en ambas partes del ojo.

capacity *n.* 1. habilidad para contener difusión de los pulmones; **memory storage __** / __ de memoria; **reserve __** / reserva de __; **carrying __** / __ de sustención; **oxygen __ of blood** / __ oxigenadora de la sangre; **vital __** / __ vital. 2. calificación, competencia.

capillary *n.* capilar; vaso capilar; *a.* semejante a un cabello; **arterial __** / __ arterial; **lymph __** / __ linfático; **venous __** / __ venoso.

capitellum *n.* capitelum. 1. bulbo de un pelo; 2. parte del húmero.

capsula, capsule *n.* cápsula. 1. envoltura membranosa; 2. pastilla; **articular __** / __ articular, que envuelve una articulación sinovial; **enclosed in a __** / encapsulado.

car *n.* automóvil, carro; *Sp.* coche; **__ accident** / accidente automovilístico.

carbohydrate *n.* carbohidrato, grupo de compuestos de carbono, hidrógeno y oxígeno entre los que se encuentran los almidones, azúcares y celulosas.

carbon *n.* carbono; **__ dioxide** / dióxido de __; **__ monoxide** / monóxido de __ .

carbonated *a.* carbonatado-a.

carboxyhemoglobin *n.* carboxihemoglobina, combinación de monóxido de carbono y hemoglobina que desplaza el oxígeno e interrumpe la función oxidante de la sangre.

carbuncle *n.* carbunco, furúnculo, infl. con pus, *pop.* avispero.

carcinogen *n.* carcinógeno, cualquier sustancia que puede producir cáncer.

carcinogenesis *n.* carcinogénesis, origen del cáncer.

carcinogenic *n.* carcinógeno-a, de origen canceroso.

carcinoma *n.* carcinoma, tumor canceroso maligno formado por células epitelial pequeña que invadir tejidos adyacentes y tienden a metastatizar con rapidez. V. cuadro en la página 287.

carcinoma in situ *n.* carcinoma in situ, células tumorales localizadas en estado de desarrollo quo no han invadido aún estructuras adyacentes.

carcinomatosis *n.* carcinomatosis, invasión de cáncer diseminado en varias partes del cuerpo.

carcinosarcoma *n.* carcinosarcoma, neoplasma maligno formado por células carcinogénicas y de sarcoma. Este tipo de neoplasma se observa en la tiroides, la garganta y los ovarios.

cardiac *a.* cardíaco-a, referente al corazón. **__ arrest, standstill** / paro __; **__ asthma** / asma __; **__ catherization** / caterización __; **__ chambers** / cavidades __; **__ depressants** / agents antiarritmicos __; **__ edema** / edema __; **examination __** / **auscultación**; **__ failure** / insuficiencia __; **__ masage** / masaje __; **output __** / gasto, rendimiento __; **__ pacing, articifial** / estimulación artificial; **__ sounds** / ruidos __; **__ tamponade** / taponamiento __.

cardiac ultrasonography *n.* V. echocardiography.

cardias *n.* cardias, desembocadura del esófago en el estómago.

cardiectomy *n.* cardiectomía, extirpación de la región superior extrema del estómago.

cardioangiogram *n.* cardioangiograma, imagen por rayos-x de los vasos sanguíneos y las cámaras del corazón usando un medio de contraste.

cardiogram *n.* cardiograma, trazado que representa los impulsos del corazón.

cardiography *n.* cardiografía, uso del cardiógrafo para registrar los movimientos del corazón.

cardiologist *n.* cardiólogo-a, especialista del corazón.

cardiology *n.* cardiología, ciencia que estudia el corazón, sus funciones y enfermedades.

cardiomegaly *n.* cardiomegalia, hipertrofia cardíaca.

cardiomyopathy *n.* cardiomiopatía, alteración del músculo del corazón; **alcoholic __** / __ alcohólica; **congestive __** / __ congestiva; **dilated __** / __ dilatada; **familial**

Carcinoma	Carcinoma
adenocystic	adenoquístico
adenosquamous	adenoescamoso
adrenocortical	corticosuprarrenal
alveolar cells of the lung	de células alveolares del pulmón
apocrine	de apocrinocitos
basal cells of the face	de células basales de la cara
basal squamous cells	de células basales escamosas
borderline	de límite
bronchogenic	broncógeno, de broncocitos
bronchial	bronquiolar
colloid	coloide
cuboidal	cuboide
cutaneous	cutáneo
cylindromatous	cilindromatoso
cystic	quístico
duodenal	duodenal
ductal	ductal, de conducto
early cancer	precoz
embryonal	embrional
endometrial	endometrial
follicular	folicular
giant cell	de célula gigante
glandular	glandular
in situ	localizado
latent	latente
lipomatous	lipomatoso
liver cell	de hepatocitos
lobular non invasive	lobular no invasivo
medullary	medular
metastatic	metastásico
occult	escondido
of anaplastic cells	de células anaplásticas
of cervix	del cuello uterino
of salivary glands	de glándulas salivares
of the bladder	de la vejiga
of the breast	de la mama
ovarian	ovárico
papillar	papilar
pharyngeal	faríngeo
prostatic	de la próstata
uterine	del útero
verrugous	verrugoso

hypertrophic ___ / ___ hipertrófica familiar; **hypertrophic** ___ / ___ hipertrófica; **idiopathic** ___ / ___ idiopática; **puerperal** ___ / ___ puerperal.

cardiopathy n. cardiopatía, enfermedad cardíaca.

cardiopulmonary a. cardiopulmonar, rel. al corazón y los pulmones; ___ **bypass** / puente ___; ___ **resuscitation** / resucitación ___; ___ **resuscitator** / resucitador, reanimador ___.

cardiospasm n. cardiospasmo, espasmo o contracción del cardias.

cardiovascular a. cardiovascular, rel. al corazón y los vasos sanguíneos; ___ **failure** / insuficiencia ___.

cardioversion n. cardioversión, restauración del ritmo sinusal normal del corazón por medio de una corriente directa.

carditis n. carditis, infl. del pericardio, miocardio y endocardio; **rheumatic** ___ / ___ reumática.

care n. cuidado, asistencia, atención; **cardiac** ___ **unit** / sala de ___ cardíaco; **comprehensive medical** ___ / médico-comprensiva; **delivery** ___ / asistencia obstétrica; **end-of-life** ___ / ___ terminal; **free of** ___ / libre de ___; **health** ___ **system** / sistema de asistencia sanitaria; **inpatient** ___ / asistencia hospitalaria; **intensive** ___ **unit** / sala de ___ intensivo; **managed** ___ / atención administrativa; **postnatal** ___ / ___ después del parto; **prenatal** ___ / ___ y atención prenatal; **primary** ___ / ___ primario; **proper** ___ / ___ apropiado; **quality** ___ / calidad asistencial; **refusal of** ___ / negación de ___; **self-care** / atención o cuidado personal; v. **to be under the** ___ **of** / estar bajo el ___ de.

careful a. cuidadoso-a; esmerado-a; atento-a.

caregiver n. asistente de salud, facilitador de atención sanitaria.

careless a. descuidado-a; desatento-a.

caries n., pl. caries. 1. destrucción progresiva de tejido óseo; 2. caries dentales, pop. dientes picados; **dental carie** / ___ dental; **distal** ___ / ___ distal; **fissure** ___ / ___ de fisura.

carnivorous a. carnívoro-a.

carnosity n. carnosidad, excrecencia carnosa.

carotene

carotene *n.* caroteno, pigmento amarillo rojizo presente en vegetales que se convierte en vitamina A en el cuerpo.

carotid *n.* carótida, arteria principal del cuello; __ **arteries** / arterias __ -s; __ **sinus** / seno de la __; __ **sinus syncope** / síncope del seno de la __ .

carotodynia *n.* carotodinia, dolor causado por presión de la arteria carótida.

carotid sinus *n.* sinus (seno) de la carótida, pequeña dilatación de la arteria carótida y su bifurcación; __ **sinus syncope** / síncope del seno de la carótida.

carpal tunnel syndrome *n.* síndrome de estrechamiento carpiano.

carpus *n.* (*pl.* **carpi**) carpo, muñeca de la mano, porción de la extremidad superior situada entre el antebrazo y la mano.

carrier *n.* portador, agente transmisor. 1. una persona o animal que lleva oculto temporalmente un agente patógeno específico al que es inmune, y se convierte en un foco potencial de esa infección a otros; 2. un agente genético que puede convertirse en un foco de infección; __ **state** / estado portador; **latent** __ / __ latente; **manifesting** / __ manifestado; **passive** __ / __ pasivo.

carrying capacity *n.* capacidad de sustención; __ **fatality rate** / índice de letalidad; __ **management** / administración de casos.

cartilage *n.* cartílago, tejido semiduro que cubre los huesos.

caruncle *n.* carúncula, pequeña irritación de la piel; **urethral** __ / uretral.

cascara sagrada *n.* cáscara sagrada, corteza de la planta *Rhamnus purshiana*, comúnmente usada como medicamento en casos de estreñimiento crónico.

case *n.* caso; __ **fatality rate** / índice de mortalidad por __-s; __ **history** / historia clínica; __ **reporting** / presentación de __; __ **control study** / estudio comparativo de __ -s.

casein *n.* caseína, proteína principal de la leche.

caseous *a.* caseoso, de queso o parecido al queso.

cash *n.* dinero al contado; __ **payment** /

__, pago al contado; *v.* **to pay** __ / pagar al contado.

casket *n.* ataúd, caja.

cast *n.* 1. molde, vaciado; **bronchial** __ / __ bronquial 2. escayola; **plaster** __ / __ de yeso 3. cilindro; **blood** __ / cilindro hemático *v.* **to put in a** __ / enyesar, moldear; **to** __ **aside** / desechar. V. **granular cast.**

castor oil *n.* aceite de ricino, palmacristi.

casualty *n.* víctima de accidente, herido, muerto; [*war*] bajas. [*wounded*] herido-a; __ **list** / lista de accidentados.

casualty report *n.* informe de urgencias.

cat *n.* gato-a.

catabolism *n.* catabolismo, proceso por el cual sustancias complejas se reducen a compuestos más simples.

catalepsy *n.* catalepsia, condición caracterizada por la pérdida de la capacidad de movimiento muscular voluntario y disminución acentuada de la habilidad de reaccionar a estímulos, gen. asociada con transtornos psicológicos.

catalyst, catalytic *a.* catalítico-a, agente estimulante de una reacción química sin afectarla.

cataplexy *n.* cataplejía, pérdida repentina del tono muscular causada por un estado emocional intenso.

cataract *n.* catarata, opacidad del cristalino; **anular** __ / __ anular; **black** __ / __ negra; **blue** __ / __ cerúlea; **complete** __ / __ completa; **congenital** __ / __ congénita; **green** __ / __ verde; **mature** __ / __ madura; **senile** __ / __ senil; **soft** __ / __ blanda.

catarrh *n.* catarro, resfriado, constipado.

catatonia *n.* catatonía, esquizofrenia caracterizada por mutismo, postura rígida y resistencia a cooperar para activar los movimientos o el habla. Los mismos síntomas se asocian con otras enfermedades mentales.

catch *vi.* contraer; agarrar; coger; __ **an illness** / __ una enfermedad.

catecholamines *n., pl.* catecolaminas, aminas de acción simpatomimética producidas en las glándulas suprarrenales (incluyen la dopamina, la epinefrina y la norepinefrina).

category *n.* categoría, clase.

catgut *n.* catgut, tipo de ligadura que se hace con la tripa del intestino de algunos animales.

catharsis *n.* catarsis. 1. acción purgativa; 2. análisis con el fin terapéutico de liberar al paciente de un estado de ansiedad.

cathartic *n.* catártico, medicamento con efectos laxativos o purgativos; *a.* catártico-a, rel. a la catarsis.

catheter *n.* catéter, sonda, tubo usado para drenar o introducir líquidos; ___ **holder** / portacatéter.

catheterization *n.* cateterización, inserción de un catéter.

catheterize *v.* cateterizar, insertar un catéter.

cat-scratch disease *n.* enfermedad causada por rasguño de gato.

causal *a.* causal.

causalgia *n.* causalgia, dolor con ardor en la piel.

cause *n.* causa, lo que produce un efecto o condición, un cambio mórbido o enfermedad; **constitutional** ___ / ___ constitucional; **existing** ___ / ___ actual, presente; **necessary** ___ / ___ necesaria; **precipitating** ___ / factor desencadenante; **predisposing** ___ / factor predisponente; **proximate** ___ / ___ inmediata; **specific** ___ / ___ específica; **without** ___ / sin ___; *v.* causar, ocasionar.

cauterization *n.* cauterización, quemadura producida por medio de un agente cauterizante tal como el calor, la corriente eléctrica, o un cáustico.

cauterize *v.* cauterizar, quemar por medio de un agente cauterizante.

caution *n.* advertencia, precaución, cautela.

cautious *a.* precavido-a, prudente; **to make a ___ decision** / hacer una decisión precavida.

cava *n., pl.* de cavum, cavidad, hueco. V. **vein, cava**.

cavern *n.* caverna, cavidad patológica.

cavernous *a.* cavernoso-a, que contiene espacios huecos.

cavity *n.* cavidad, lugar hueco; **abdominal** ___ / ___ abdominal; **cranial** ___ / ___ craneal; **pelvic** ___ / ___ pelviana; **thoracic** ___ / ___ torácica.

cease *v.* cesar, parar, detener.

cecostomy *n.* cecostomía, creación de una apertura artificial en el ciego.

cecum *n.* ciego, bolsa que forma la primera parte del intestino grueso.

celiac *a.* celíaco, abdominal, rel. al abdomen.

celiotomy *n.* celiotomía. V. **laparotomy**.

cell *n.* célula, unidad estructural de todo organismo viviente. V. ilustración y cuadro en la página 290.

cellular *a.* celular, de naturaleza semejante o referente a la célula; ___ **compartmentation** / compartimiento ___ -es; ___ **counting device** / cuenta células; ___ **growth** / crecimiento ___; ___ **-like** / en forma ___; ___ **tissue** / tejido ___; ___ **water** / agua ___ .

cellulitis *n.* celulitis, infl. del tejido conectivo celular.

center *n.* 1. centro; 2. núcleo.

Center for Disease Control *n.* Centro para Control de Enfermedades.

centigrade *n.* centígrado.

central *a.* central; céntrico-a; ___ **nervous system** / sistema nervioso ___ .

central deafness *n.* sordera central.

centrifugal *a.* centrífugo-a, rel. al movimiento de repulsión, del centro hacia afuera.

centripetal *a.* centrípeto-a, con movimiento de atracción hacia el centro.

cephalalgia *n.* cefalalgia, dolor de cabeza, *pop.* jaqueca.

cephalic *a.* cefálico-a, rel. a la cabeza.

cephalosporin *n.* cefalosporina, antibiótico de espectro amplio.

cerebellum *n.* cerebelo, parte posterior del cerebro, centro de coordinación de los movimientos musculares voluntarios.

cerebral *a.* cerebral, rel. al cerebro; ___ **cortex** / corteza ___; ___ **cortex areas** / áreas de la corteza; ___ **edema** / edema ___; ___ **embolism and thrombosis** / embolia y trombosis ___; ___ **hemorrhage** / hemorragia ___; ___ **palsy** / parálisis ___; ___ **tumor** / tumor ___ .

cerebral paralysis *n.* parálisis cerebral, falta de coordinación muscular debido a una lesión cerebral congénita.

cerebrospinal *a.* cefalorraquídeo, cerebroespinal; ___ **axis** / eje ___; ___ **fluid** / líquido ___; ___ **meningitis** / meningitis ___; ___ **pressure** / presión ___ .

cerebrovascular

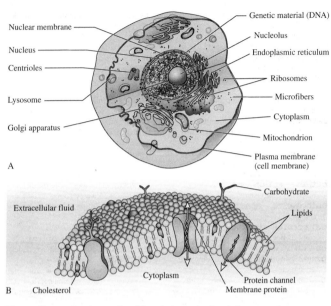

The cell: (A) cell and organelles; (B) typical animal cell and plasma membrane

Cell	Célula
adipose	adiposa
anaplastic	anaplástica
accesory	accesoria
acoustic	acústica
B lymphocyte	linfocito B, tipo de
basal	basal
columnar	columnar
giant	gigante
goblet	calciforme
ependymal	ependimaria
epidermal	epidérmica
interstitial	intersticial
mononuclear	mononuclear
phagocyte	fagocitaria
pyramidal	piramidal
red blood	sanguíneas
reproductive	reproductiva
scavenger	basurera
sickle	falciforme

cerebrovascular *a.* cerebrovascular; ___ **accident** / apoplegía, hemorragia cerebral.

cerebrum *n.* cerebro, encéfalo, centro de coordinación de actividades sensoriales e intelectuales.

certain *a.* cierto-a; seguro-a; *v.* **to be** ___ / estar seguro-a; **-ly** *adv.* ciertamente, seguramente.

certainty *n.* certeza.

certificate *n.* certificado; **death** ___ / ___ de defunción.

cerumen *n.* cerumen, segregación cerosa que lubrica y protege el óido.

cervical *a.* cervical. 1. referente al área del cuello; 2. rel. al cuello uterino; ___ **dilator** / dilatador ___; ___ **dysplasia** / displasia ___; ___ **incompetence** / incompetencia del cuello uterino; ___ **erosion** / erosión ___; ___ **polyp** / pólipo ___.

cervical cap *n.* capa o cubierta del cuello uterino.

cervical disc syndrome *n.* sindrome del disco cervical, condición causada por compresión de nervios en la región del cuello que produce dolor en el hombro.

cervical dystonia n. distonia cervical, trastorno de tonicidad en los tejidos de la nuca que resulta en incapacitación de movimiento voluntario del cuello.

cervical range of motion n. alcance del movimiento cervical.

cervical traction vest n. chaleco de tracción cervical.

cervicovesical a. cervicovesical, rel. al cuello uterino y a la vejiga.

cervix n. cuello uterino, parte baja del útero en forma de cuello; **dilation of the ___** / dilatación del ___.

cesarean n. cesárea; **___ section** / cirugía de parto.

cesium n. cesio, elemento metálico perteneciente al grupo de metales alcalinos.

chain n. cadena; **___ reaction** / reacción en ___; **___ suture** / sutura en ___.

chair n. silla.

chalazion n. chalazión, quiste del párpado, quiste meiboniano.

chalk n. yeso.

chamber n. cámara, cavidad; **anterior ___** / ___ anterior, situada entre la córnea y el iris; **aqueous ___** / ___ acuosa; **___-s of the eye** / ___-s oculares; **___-s of the heart** / cavidades del corazón: aurículas y ventrículos del corazón; **hyperbaric ___** / ___ hiperbárica.

chamomile n. manzanilla, té, sedante gastrointestinal.

chancre n. chancro; lesión primaria de la sífilis.

chancroid n. chancroide, úlcera venérea no sifilítica.

change n. cambio, alteración; **___ of life** / menopausia; v. cambiar, mudar.

channel n. canal; estructura tubular; **birth ___** / ___ del parto.

chapped a. agrietado-a, cuarteado-a; rajado-a; **___ hands** / manos ___-s; **___ lips** / labios ___-s.

character n. 1. carácter; 2. calidad, naturaleza; 3. [actor, actress in a play or movie] personaje.

characteristic n. característica, peculiaridad; a. característico-a; peculiar; **it is a symptom ___ of this illness** / es un síntoma ___ de esta enfermedad.

charity n. caridad; beneficencia.

charity institution n. institución benéfica.

charlatan n. charlatán-a; dícese de una persona que pretende tener cualidades o conocimientos para curar enfermedades.

charley horse n. dolor y sensibilidad en un músculo; pop. calambre.

chart n. plano, gráfico; **medical ___** / hoja clínica.

chat n. charla, plática; v. charlar, platicar.

cheap a. barato-a.

check n. 1. control; 2. [bank] cheque; v. controlar; chequear, verificar.

checkup n. Am. chequeo, examen físico completo.

cheek n. mejilla.

cheekbone n. carrillo, pómulo, hueso malar.

cheilectomy n. queilectomía, excisión parcial del labio.

cheilitis, chilitis n. queilitis, infl. de los labios.

cheiloplasty n. queiloplastia, reparación del labio.

cheiloschisis n. queilosquisis V. harelip.

cheilosis n. queilosis, manifestación con marcas y fisuras en la comisura de los labios debida a deficiencia de vitamina B_2 (riboflavina).

cheirology n. quirología. 1. estudio de la mano; 2. uso del lenguaje por señas como medio de comunicación con los sordomudos.

chemical a. químico-a; **___ peel** / peladura ___ .

chemist n. químico-a; farmacéutico-a, boticario-a.

chemistry n. química, ciencia que estudia los elementos, estructura y propiedades de las sustancias y las transformaciones que éstas sufren.

chemocoagulation n. quimiocoagulación, co-agulación por medio de agentes químicos.

chemonucleolysis n. quimionucleólisis, disolución por inyección de una enzima proteolítica del núcleo pulposo de una hernia.

chemoprophylaxis n. quimioprofi-laxis, uso de una droga o de una sustancia química que contiene preventivos.

chemoreceptor n. quimiorreceptor-a, célula suceptible a cambios químicos o que puede ser afectada por éstos.

chemosurgery n. quimiocirugía,

extirpación o remoción de tejidos por medio de sustancias químicas.

chemotaxis *n.* quimiotaxis, movimiento de un organismo o célula como reacción a un estímulo químico.

chemotherapy *n.* quimioterapia, tratamiento de una enfermedad por medio de agentes químicos.

chest *n.* tórax, pecho; ___ **cold** / catarro bronquial; *pop.* catarro al pecho; ___ **respirator** / respirador torácico; ___ **surgery** / cirugía torácica; ___ **wall** / pared torácica.

chew *v.* masticar, mascar.

Cheyne-Stokes respiration syndrome *n.* síndrome de respiración de Cheyne-Stokes, respiración cíclica con períodos de apnea y aumento rápido y profundo de la respiración gen. asociada con trastornos del centro neurológico respiratorio.

chiasm, chiasma *n.* quiasma. 1. cruzamiento de dos vías o conductos; 2. punto de cruzamiento de las fibras de los nervios ópticos.

chicken *n.* pollo; ___ **breast** / pechuga.

chickenpox, varicella *n.* varicela, enfermedad viral contagiosa que se manifiesta gen. en la infancia y se caracteriza por una erupción que se convierte en pequeñas vesículas; *pop.* viruelas locas.

chief *n.* jefe-a; ___ **complaint** / queja principal.

chilblain *n.* sabañón, eritema debido a frío intenso que gen. se manifiesta en las manos y los pies.

child *n.* niño-a; ___ **nurse** / niñera; ___ **nursery** / guardería infantil, jardín de la infancia; ___ **support** / manutención, pensión alimenticia; ___ **welfare** / asistencia social a la infancia.

childbearing *n.* gestación, embarazo.

childbirth *n.* parto, nacimiento, alumbramiento.

childhood *n.* infancia, niñez.

chill *n.* enfriamiento, escalofrío.

chin *n.* barba, mentón, barbilla.

chiropodist *n.* quiropodista. V. **podiatrist.**

chiropractic *n.* quiropráctica, sistema terapéutico que recurre a la manipulación y ajustamiento de las estructuras del cuerpo esp. la columna vertebral en relación con el sistema nervioso.

chloasma *n.* cloasma, hiperpigmentación facial que puede ocurrir en algunas mujeres durante el embarazo.

chlorambucil *n.* clorambucil, forma de mostaza nitrogenada usada para combatir algunas formas de cáncer.

chloramphenicol, chloromycetin *n.* cloranfenicol, cloromicetina, antibiótico esp. efectivo en el tratamiento de la fiebre tifoidea.

chlorhydria *n.* clorhidria, exceso de ácido clorhídrico en el estómago.

chloride *n.* cloruro.

chlorine *n.* cloro, agente desinfectante y blanqueador.

chlorophyll *n.* clorofila, pigmento verde de las plantas esencial en la producción de carbohidratos por fotosíntesis.

chloroquine *n.* cloroquina, compuesto usado en el tratamiento de la malaria.

chlorosis *n.* clorosis, tipo de anemia vista esp. en la mujer y usu. relacionada con deficiencia de hierro.

chlorpromazine *n.* cloropromacina, antiemético y tranquilizante.

chocolate *n.* chocolate.

choice *n.* opción, alternative; elección.

choke *v.* ahogar, sofocar, estrangular; [*choke on something*] atragantarse.

cholangiectasis *n.* colangiectasis, dilatación de los conductos biliares.

cholangiography *n.* colangiografía, rayos-x de las vías biliares.

cholangitis *n.* colangitis, infl. de los conductos biliares.

cholecystectomy *n.* colecistectomía, extirpación de la vesícula biliar.

cholecystitis *n.* colecistitis, infl. de la vesícula biliar.

cholecystoduodenostomy *n.* colecistoduodenostomía, anastomosis de la vesícula y el duodeno.

cholecystogastrostomy *n.* colecistogastrostomía, anastomosis de la vesícula y el estómago.

cholecystography *n.* colecistografía, rayos-x de la vesícula biliar usando un medio radioopaco.

choledochojejunostomy *n.* coledocoyeyunostomía, anastomosis del colédoco y el yeyuno.

choledochus *n.* colédoco, conducto biliar formado por la unión de los conductos hepático y cístico.

cirrhosis

cholelithiasis *n.* colelitiasis, litiasis biliar, presencia de cálculos en la vesícula biliar o en un conducto biliar.

cholemia *n.* colemia, presencia de bilis en la sangre.

cholera *n.* cólera, enfermedad infecciosa grave caracterizada por diarrea severa y vómitos; ___ **fulminans** / ___ fulminante.

choleric *a.* colérico-a.

cholestasis *n.* colestasis, estasis biliar.

cholesteatoma *n.* colesteatoma, tumor que contiene colesterol, situado comúnmente en el oído medio.

cholesterol *n.* colesterol, lípido precursor de las hormonas sexuales y corticoides adrenales, componente de las grasas y aceites animales, del tejido nervioso y de la sangre; ___ **reducer** / reductor de ___; **high** ___ / ___ alto.

choluria *n.* coluria, presencia de bilis en la orina.

chondritis *n.* condritis, infl. de un cartílago.

chondromalacia *n.* condromalacia, reblandecimiento anormal de los cartílagos.

chondrosarcoma *n.* condrosarcoma, tumor maligno de un cartílago.

choose *vi.* escoger, elegir.

chord *n.* cuerda; **vocal** ___ / ___ vocal.

chorea, Huntington's disease *n.* corea; enfermedad de Huntington, padecimiento nervioso que se manifiesta en movimientos abruptos coordinados aunque involuntarios de las extremidades y los músculos faciales; *pop.* baile se San Vito.

choriocarcinoma *n.* coriocarcinoma, tumor maligno visto gen. en el útero y en los testículos.

chorion *n.* corión, una de las dos membranas que rodean al feto.

chorionic *a.* coriónico-a, rel. al corión.

choroid *n.* coroides, membrana situada en el ojo entre la retina y la esclerótica.

choroiditis *n.* coroiditis, infl. de la coroides.

chromatic *a.* cromático-a, rel. al color.

chromatin *n.* cromatina, parte del núcleo de la célula más propensa a absorber color.

chromocyte *n.* cromocito, célula pigmentada.

chromosomal *a.* cromosómico-a, rel. al cromosoma; ___ **aberrations** / aberraciones ___ -s.

chromosome *n.* cromosoma, la parte dentro del núcleo de la célula que contiene los genes.

chronic *a.* crónico-a, de larga duración, de efecto prolongado; ___ **obstructive pulmonary disease** / enfermedad ___ de obstrucción pulmonary.

chronological *a.* cronológico-a, rel. a la secuencia del tiempo.

chubby *a.* regordete-a, macizo-a.

chyle *n.* quilo, sustancia lechosa que resulta de la absorción y emulsión de las grasas, presente en el intestino delgado.

chylous *a.* quiloso-a, que contiene quilo o de la naturaleza de éste; ___ **ascitis** / ascitis ___.

chyluria *n.* quiluria. V. **galacturia.**

chyme *n.* quimo, sustancia o materia semilíquida que proviene de la digestión gástrica.

chymotrypsin *n.* quimotripsina, tripsina, enzima de la secreción pancreática.

cicatrix *n.* (*pl.* **cicatrices**) *L.* cicatriz.

cicatrizant *n.* cicatrizante, agente que contribuye a la cicatrización.

cicatrization *n.* cicatrización.

ciliary *a.* ciliar, rel. a las pestañas o al párpado.

cilium *n.* (*pl.* **cilia**) *L.* párpado.

cineangiocardiography *n.* cineangiocardiografía, película de una sustancia radioopaca pasando através de vasos sanguíneos.

cineradiography *n.* cinerradiografía, película radiográfica de un órgano en movimiento.

circadian rhythm *n.* ritmo circadiano, ref. a variaciones rítmicas biológicas en un ciclo de 24 horas.

circle *n.* círculo, circunferencia.

circuit *n.* circuito, vuelta, rotación.

circulation *n.* circulación; ___ **rate** / volumen circulatorio por minuto; **peripheral** ___ / ___ periférica; **poor** ___ / mala ___.

circulatory *a.* circulatorio-a.

circumcise *v.* circuncidar.

circumcision *n.* circuncisión, excisión del prepucio.

circumference *n.* circunferencia; círculo.

cirrhosis *n.* cirrosis, enfermedad asociada con infl. intersticial, fallo en la función de hepatocitos y trastornos en la circulación de la sangre en el hígado; **alcoholic** ___ / ___ alcohólica; **biliary** ___ / ___ biliar.

cistern

cistern *n.* cisterna, receptáculo de agua, aljibe.

citizen *n.* ciudadano-a.

citizenship *n.* ciudadanía.

citric, citrous *a.* cítrico-a; ___ **acid** / ácido ___ .

claim *n.* reclamación; petición; ___ **review procedure** / proceso para revisión de peticiones (reclamaciones); *v.* reclamar, demandar.

clammy *a.* frío y húmedo.

clamp *n.* pinza; presilla.

clap *n. pop.* gonorrea, blenorragia; [*hand*] palmada.

clarification *n.* aclaración, clarificación.

clarify *v.* aclarar, clarificar.

clarity *n.* claridad.

class *n.* clase; tipo.

classification *n.* clasificación; distribución.

classify *v.* clasificar, distribuir.

claudication *n.* claudicación; **intermittent** ___ / ___ intermitente.

claustrophobia *n.* claustrofobia, miedo o fobia a espacios cerrados.

clavicle *n.* clavícula, hueso de la faja pectoral que conecta al esternón con la escápula.

clavicular *a.* clavicular, rel. a las clavículas.

claw *n.* garra; ___ **foot** / pie en ___; ___ **hand** / mano en ___ .

clean *a.* limpio-a, aseado-a; *v.* limpiar, asear.

clear *a.* claro-a.

clearance *n.* aclaramiento, eliminación renal de una sustancia en el plasma sanguíneo.

cleft *n.* fisura, abertura alargada.

cleft lip *n.* labio leporino. V. **harelip.**

cleft palate *n.* paladar hendido, defecto congénito del velo del paladar por falta de fusión en la línea media.

climacteric *a.* climatérico-a.

climate *n.* clima.

climax *n., L.* climax. 1. crisis de una enfermedad; 2. orgasmo sexual.

climb *v.* subir; trepar; subirse, treparse.

clinic *n.* clínica; **small** ___ / dispensario.

clinical *a.* clínico-a. 1. rel. a una clínica; 2. rel. a la observacíon directa de pacientes; ___ **history** / historia ___ , expediente; ___ **picture** / cuadro ___; ___ **procedure** / procedimiento ___; ___ **trials** / ensayos ___ -s.

clip *n.* pinza; *v.* sujetar con pinzas.

clitoridectomy *n.* clitoridectomía, excisión del clítoris.

clitoris *n.* clítoris, pequeña protuberancia situada en la parte anterior de la vulva.

cloaca *n.* cloaca, abertura común del intestino y de las vías urinarias en la fase de desarrollo primario del embrión.

clock *n.* reloj; **around the** ___ / durante las veinticuatro horas, de día y de noche.

clone *n.* clon, reproducción o copia idéntica.

cloning *n.* clonación.

clonus *n. Gr.* clono, serie de contracciones rápidas y rítmicas de un músculo.

close *v.* cerrar.

closed *a.* cerrado-a; ___ **-circuit television** / televisión en circuito ___; ___ **ecological system** / sistema ecológico ___ .

closure *n.* acto de cerrar o sellar; encierro.

clot *n.* cóagulo, cuajo, grumo, *pop.* cuajarón.

clothes, clothing *n.* ropa.

clotting *n.* coagulación; ___ **factor** / factor de ___; ___ **time** / tiempo de ___ .

cloudiness *n.* nebulosidad, enturbamiento.

cloudy *a.* turbio-a, nebuloso-a, oscuro-a.

clubbing *n.* dedo en palillo de tambor.

club foot *n.* pie torcido, *pop.* patizambo, *slang* chueco.

club hand *n.* mano zamba, *pop.* mano de gancho.

cluster *n.* racimo, grupo.

cluster headache, Horton's syndrome *n.* cefalalgia de Horton, dolor de cabeza producido por histaminas.

clysis *n.* clisis, administración de líquidos por cualquier vía excepto la oral.

coagglutination *n.* coagglutinación, aglutinación de grupos.

coagglutinine *n.* coaglutinina, aglutinante que afecta a dos o más organismos.

coagulant *n.* coagulante, agente que causa o acelera la coagulación. *Syn.* **coagulative.**

coagulate *v.* coagular, coagularse.

coagulation *n.* coagulación, coágulo; **disseminated intravascular** ___ / ___ intravascular diseminada.

coagulopathy *n.* coagulopatía, enfermedad o condición que afecta el mecanismo de la coagulación de la sangre.

coal miners' disease *n.* enfermedad de los mineros. V. **anthracosis**.

coarctation *n.* coartación, estrechez.

coarse *a.* grueso-a; rudo-a, tosco-a, burdo-a, ordinario-a.

coat *n.* membrana, cubierta; [*clothing*] abrigo.

coated *a.* cubierto-a, pintado-a; ___ with adhesive tape / ___ con esparadrapo.

coca *n.* coca, planta de cuyas hojas se extrae la cocaína.

cocaine *n.* cocaína, narcótico alcaloide adictivo complejo obtenido de las hojas de coca; *slang* nieve.

coccidioidomycosis, valley fever *n.* coccidioidomicosis, fiebre del valle, infección respiratoria endémica en el suroeste de los Estados Unidos, México y algunas partes de América del Sur.

coccus *n. L.* (*pl.* **cocci**) coco, bacteria de forma esférica.

coccygeal *a.* coccígeo, rel. al cóccix.

coccygodynia *n.* coccigodinia, dolor en la región coccígea.

coccyx *n.* cóccix; último hueso de la columna vertebral; *pop.* rabadilla.

cochlea *n.* cóclea, parte del oído interior en forma de caracol.

cochleare *n.*, *L.* cucharada; ___ magnum / ___ de sopa; ___ medium / ___ de postre; ___ parvum / cucharita de café.

cockroach *n.* cucaracha.

codeine *n.* codeína, narcótico analgésico.

coefficient *n.* coeficiente, indicación de cambios físicos o químicos producidos por variantes de ciertos factores.

coenzyme *n.* coenzima, sustancia que activa la acción de una enzima.

coffee *n.* café.

coffin *n.* ataúd, caja.

cognate *n.* cognado, palabra que proviene del mismo tronco o raíz; *a.* cognado-a, de la misma naturaleza o calidad.

cognition *n.* cognición, conocimiento, acción y efecto de conocer.

cognitive *a.* cognitivo-a. 1. rel. al conocimiento; 2. rel. al proceso mental de comprensión.

cognitive development *n.* desarrollo cognitivo, cambio en el desarrollo infantil de las funciones intelectuales.

cohabit *v.* cohabitar, vivir en unión sin matrimonio legal.

coherence *n.* 1. coherencia, cohesión; 2. coherencia, referencia a cualquier grupo designado, seguido o copiado por un período de tiempo, tal como en un estudio epidemiológico.

coherent *a.* coherente.

cohesion *n.* cohesión, unión, fuerza que une a las moléculas.

coil *n.* espiral, serpentina, dispositivo intrauterino.

coincidence *n.* coincidencia; **by** ___ / por casualidad.

coitus *n. L.* coito, acto sexual.

cold *n.* catarro; resfriado; [*weather*] frío; *a* [*temperature*] frío-a; ___ -**blooded** / de sangre fría o de temperatura muy baja; ___ **cream** / crema, pomada facial; ___ **pack** / compresa fría; ___ **sore** / úlcera de herpes simple; ___ **sweat** / sudor frío;*v.* **to be** ___ / tener frío; **it is** ___ / hace frío.

coldness *n.* frialdad.

colectomy *n.* colectomía, extirpación de una parte o de todo el colon.

colic *n.* cólico, dolor espasmódico abdominal agudo.

colicky *a.* rel. al cólico.

colitis *n.* colitis, infl. del colon; **chronic** ___ / ___ crónica; **pseudomembranous** ___ / ___ mucomembranosa; **spasmodic** ___ / ___ espasmódica; **ulcerative** ___ / ___ ulcerativa.

collaborate *v.* colaborar, cooperar.

collagen *n.* colágeno, principal proteína de sostén del tejido conectivo de la piel, huesos, tendones y cartílagos.

collapse *n.* colapso; postración; desplome; **circulatory** ___ / ___ circulatorio; ___ **therapy** / terapia de ___; *v.* **to collapse** / sufrir un ___.

collar *n.* cuello.

collarbone *n.* clavícula.

collateral *n.* colateral. 1. indirecto, subsidiario o accesorio a la cuestión principal; 2. una rama subsidiaria del axon de un nervio o vaso sanguíneo; *a.* accesorio-a; *adv.* al lado.

collateral vessel *n.* vaso colateral. 1. rama de una arteria que sigue el

collect

curso paralela al tronco protector; 2. un vaso que sigue su curso paralelo a otro vaso, nervio u otra estructura mayor. *Syn.* **vas collaterale.**

collect *v.* coleccionar, recoger, juntar; acumular.

collodion *n.* colodión, sustancia usada para proteger heridas en la piel.

colloid *n.* coloide, sustancia gelatinosa producida por ciertas formas de degeneración de los tejidos.

collyrium *n.* colirio, medicamento aplicado a los ojos.

coloboma *n.* coloboma, defecto congénito, patológico, o artificial especialmente manifestado en el ojo debido a un cierre incompleto de la fisura óptica; **___ iridis** / **___** del iris; **___ lentis** / **___** del lente; **___ of choroid** / **___** de la coroides; **___ of optic nerve** / **___** del nervio óptico; **___ of vitreous** / **___** del vítreo; **macular ___** / **___** macular.

colon *n.* colon, porción del intestino grueso entre el ciego y el recto; **ascending ___** / **___** ascendente; **descending ___** / **___** descendente.

colonic *a.* colónico, referente al colon; **___ neoplasms** / neoplasmas del colon.

colonoscopy *n.* colonoscopía, examen de la superficie interna del colon a través del colonoscopio.

colony *n.* colonia, cultivo de bacterias derivadas del mismo organismo.

color *n.* color; **___ index** / guía colorimétrica; *v.* colorar; teñir o dar color; **___ confusion** / confusión de colores; **___ perception** / percepción del **___**; **complementary colors** / colores complementarios; **extrinsic colors** / colores extrínsecos; **intrinsic colors** / colores intrínsecos; **primary colors** / colores primarios; **pure ___** / **___** puro; **reflected ___** / **___** reflejado; **saturated ___** / **___** saturado; **simple ___** / **___** simple; **structural ___** / **___** estructural; **tone ___** / tono de **___** . V. cuadro en la página 75.

colorectal cancer *n.* cáncer colorectal, carcinoma colónico rectal.

colostomy *n.* colostomía, creación de un ano artificial.

colostrum *n.* colostro, secreción de la glándula mamaria anterior a la leche.

colpitis *n.* colpitis, vaginitis, infl. de la vagina.

colporrhaphy *n.* colporrafia, sutura de la vagina.

colposcopy *n.* colposcopía, examen de la vagina y del cuello uterino a través de un colposcopio.

column *n.* columna.

coma *n.* coma, en estado de coma; sueño profundo o estado inconsciente.

comatose *a.* comatoso-a; **in a ___ state** / en estado de coma.

combat *n.* combate, lucha; *v.* combatir.

combine *v.* combinar, unir.

come *vi* venir; **___ in!** / pase, pasa; entre, entra; **to ___ to terms** / ponerse de acuerdo.

comfort *n.* comodidad, alivio, bienestar; *v.* confortar, alentar.

comfortable *a.* cómodo-a; a gusto.

command *n.* orden, mandato.

commensal *n.* comensal, organismo que vive a expensas de otro sin beneficiarlo ni perjudicarlo.

comminuted *a.* conminuto-a, roto-a en fragmentos tal como en una fractura.

commiserate *v.* tener compasión, tener lástima; apiadarse, compadecerse; tenerse lástima.

commissure *n.* comisura, punto de unión de estructuras tal como la unión de los labios.

commisurotomy *n.* comisurotomía, incisión de las bandas fibrosas de una comisura tal como la de los labios o la de los bordes de válvulas cardíacas.

commitment *n.* obligación, compromiso.

common *a.* común, corriente; **___ name** / nombre **___**; **___ place** / lugar **___**; **___ sense** / sentido **___** .

commotio retinae *n.*, *L.* conmoción retinal, condición traumática que produce ceguera momentánea.

communicable *a.* contagioso-a; comunicable; **___ disease control** / control de enfermedades **___** s.

communicate *v.* comunicar; [*to get in touch*] comunicarse.

communication *n.* comunicación; acceso; entrada.

community *n.* comunidad, sociedad, barrio; **___ health center** / centro de servicio de la salud; **___ medicine** / medicina comunitaria.

companion *n.* compañero-a; acompañante; **___ disease** / enfermedad concomitante.

comparative *a.* comparativo-a.

compare *v.* comparar.

compassion *n.* compasión, lástima.

compatible *a.* compatible.

compensate v. compensar, recompensar.

compensation n. compensación.
1. cualidad de compensar o equilibrar un defecto; 2. mecanismo de defensa; 3. remuneración.

competent a. competente, capaz.

complain v. quejarse, lamentarse.

complainer a. persona que se queja en exceso.

complaint n. queja, síntoma; trastorno, molestia; **chief** ___ / ___ principal.

complement n. complemento, sustancia proteínica presente en el plasma que destruye las bacterias y las células con que se pone en contacto.

complex n. complejo, serie de procesos mentales interrelacionados que afectan la conducta y la personalidad; **castration** ___ / ___ de castración; **guilt** ___ / ___ de culpa; **inferiority** ___ / ___ de inferioridad; **Electra's** ___ / ___ de Electra; **Oedipus** ___ / ___ de Edipo; a. complejo-a; complicado-a.

complexion n. cutis, complexión, tez.

compliance n. adaptabilidad, conformidad, grado de elasticidad de un órgano para distenderse o de una estructura para perder la forma; ___ **with standards** / ___ a las normas.

complication n. complicación.

component n. componente.

composition n. composición, mezcla, compuesto.

compound n. compuesto.

comprehension n. comprensión.

compress n. compresa, apósito; **cold** ___ / ___ fría; **hot** ___ / fomento; v. comprimir, apretar.

compromise v. comprometerse, obligarse.

compulsion n. compulsión.

compulsive a. compulsorio-a, compulsivo-a; obsesivo-a.

computer diagnosis n. diagnóstico computado.

concave a. cóncavo-a.

conceive v. concebir.

concentrate v. concentrar.

concentration n. concentración.

concept n. concepto, opinión, noción, idea.

conception n. concepción, acto de concebir.

concern n. preocupación, cuidado.

concise a. conciso-a; definido-a.

conclusion n. conclusión.

concoction n. cocimiento, mezcla, concocción.

concrete a. concreto-a; definido-a.

concretio cordis n., L. *concretio cordis*, obliteración parcial o total de la cavidad del pericardio debido a una pericarditis constrictiva.

concretion n. concreción, bezoar o masa inorgánica que se acumula en partes del cuerpo.

concubitus n., L. concúbito.

concussion n. concusión, conmoción, traumatismo esp. del cerebro causado por una lesión en la cabeza que puede presentar síntomas de náusea y mareos; **cerebral** ___ / ___ cerebral.

condense v. condensar, hacer más denso o compacto.

condition n. condición, cualidad; **guarded** ___ / en estado de gravedad; **preexisting** ___ / ___ preexistente; **undiagnosed** ___ / ___ sin diagnosticar.

conditioning n. acondicionamiento, condicionamiento.

condolence n. condolencia, pésame.

condom n. condón, contraceptivo masculino.

conduct v. dirigir, conducir.

conduit n. conducto; **airway** ___ / ___ para aire; **tear** ___ / ___ lagrimal.

condyle n. cóndilo, porción redondeada de un hueso, usu. en la articulación.

condyloma n. condiloma, tipo de verruga vista alrededor de los genitales y el perineo.

cone n. cono, uno de los órganos sensoriales que, con los bastoncillos de la retina, facilitan la visión del color; ___ **cells** / ___ -s de la retina.

confer v. consultar; conferencia r.

conference n. conferencia.

confidential a. confidencial; en secreto.

confidentiality n. confidencialidad.

confine v. recluir, internar, confinar; **to** ___ **in bed** / ___ en la cama.

confined a. recluido-a, confinado-a.

confirm v. confirmar.

conflict n. conflicto, problema.

confluence n. confluencia, punto de reunión de varios canales.

confront v. confrontar.

confuse v. confundir, trastornar, aturdir.

confused a. confuso-a, confundido-a, distraído-a; v. **to be** ___ / estar ___ , confundirse.

confusion

confusion *n.* confusión; atolondramiento; aturdimiento.

congenital *a.* congénito-a; engendrado-a, rel. a una característica que se hereda y existe desde el nacimiento.

congenital cataract *n.* catarata congénita, no común, usualmente bilateral, producida a causa de una infección intrauterina, a toxicidad, a una lesión, o a trastornos metabólicos o cromosomáticos.

congested *a.* congestionado-a; en estado de congestión.

congestion *n.* congestión, aglomeración; acumulación excesiva de sangre en un órgano; **active** ___ / ___ activa; **functional** ___ / ___ funcional; **passive** ___ / ___ pasiva; **venous** ___ / ___ venosa.

congestive *a.* congestivo-a, rel. a la congestión; ___ **heart failure** / insuficiencia cardíaca ___ .

conical, conic *a.* cónico-a, semejante a un cono.

conization *n.* conización, extirpación de tejido que tiene forma cónica, semejante al de la mucosa del cuello uterino.

conjunctiva *n.* conjuntiva, membrana mucosa protectora del ojo; **bulbar** ___ / ___ bulbar; **palpebral** ___ / ___ palpebral.

conjunctival *a.* conjuntivo-a, rel. a la conjuntiva; ___ **diseases** / enfermedades de la conjuntiva.

conjunctivitis *n.* conjuntivitis, infl. de la conjuntiva; **allergic** ___ / ___ alérgica; **catarrhal** ___ / ___ catarral; **chronic** ___ / ___ crónica; ___ **acute, contagious** ___ / ___ aguda contagiosa; **epidemic** ___ / ___ epidémica; **follicular** ___ / ___ folicular; **hemorrhagic** ___ / ___ hemorrágica; **infantile purulent** ___ / ___ infantil purulenta; **vernal** ___ / ___ vernal; **viral** ___ / ___ viral.

consanguineous *a.* consanguíneo-a, de la misma sangre u origen.

conscious *a.* consciente, en posesión de las facultades mentales.

consciousness *n.* consciencia, conocimiento, sentido; estado consciente; **clouding of** ___ / torpor, confusión, entorpecimiento mental; *v.* **to lose** ___ / perder el conocimiento; perder el sentido.

consensus *n.* consenso.

consent *n.* consentimiento, autorización; *v.* permitir, consentir; **informed** ___ / ___ autorizado.

consequences *n., pl.* consecuencias, secuelas.

conservation *n.* conservación, preservación.

conservative *a.* conservador-a; preservativo-a.

consider *v.* considerar, ponderar.

considerate *a.* considerado-a; moderado-a.

consideration *n.* consideración.

consistency *n.* consistencia; solidez.

consistent *a.* consistente, firme, estable.

console *v.* consolar, confortar; dar aliento.

constant *a.* constante, persistente.

constipate *v.* estreñir, constipar.

constipated *a.* estreñido-a; constipado-a; *v.* **to be** ___ / estar ___ .

constipation *n.* estreñimiento, trastorno intestinal caracterizado por la imposibilidad de evacuar con facilidad.

constitute *v.* constituir, componer, formar.

constitution *n.* constitución, fortaleza.

constrain *v.* restringir; impedir.

consult *v.* consultar.

consultant *n.* consultor-a, consejero-a.

consultation *n.* consulta.

consulting room *n.* consultorio médico.

consume *v.* consumir.

consumption *n.* consunción; desgaste progresivo; tisis, tuberculosis.

contact *n.* contacto; **close** ___ / ___ íntimo; ___ **lenses** / lentes de ___; **initial** ___ / ___ inicial.

contagion *n.* contagio, transmisión de una enfermedad por contacto.

contagious *a.* contagioso-a; infeccioso-a; que se comunica por contagio.

contain *v.* contener; reprimir.

container *n.* recipiente, envase.

contaminate *v.* contaminar, infectar.

contamination *n.* contaminación; infección.

content *n.* contenido.

contented *a.* satisfecho-a.

continence *n.* continencia, control o automoderación en relación con actividades sexuales o físicas.

continue *v.* continuar.

contraception *n.* contracepción, anticoncepción.

contraceptive *n.* contraceptivo, anticonceptivo, agente o método para impedir la concepción; __ **agents** / agentes anticonceptivos; __ **implant** / implante de __; __ **methods** / métodos __ -s, métodos anticonceptivos; **oral** __ / __ oral.

contract *v.* [*a disease*] contraer.

contracted *n.* contraído-a; retenido-a.

contractile *a.* contráctil, que tiene la capacidad de contraerse.

contraction *n.* contracción; **after** __ / __ ulterior; **deep** __ / __ de fondo; **hunger** __ / __ de hambre; **muscular** __ / __ muscular; **spasmodic** __ / __ espasmódica.

contracture *n.* contractura, contracción prolongada involuntaria.

contraindicated *a.* contraindicado-a.

contraindication *n.* contraindicación.

contrary *a.* contrario-a, adverso-a, opuesto-a.

contrast *n.* contraste; __ **medium** / medio de __; *v.* contrastar, resaltar.

contribute *v.* contribuir.

control *n.* control, regulación; *v.* controlar, regular, dominar; **to** __ **oneself** / controlarse, dominarse.

contuse *v.* magullar.

contusion *n.* contusión, magulladura.

convalesce *v.* convalecer, reponerse.

convalescence *n.* convalecencia, proceso de restablecimiento, estado de recuperación.

convalescent *a.* convaleciente.

convalescent carrier *n.* portador convaleciente, aún capaz de transmitir un agente infeccioso.

conversion *n.* conversión. 1. cambio, transformación; 2. transformación de una emoción en una manifestación física; __ **disorder** / enajenamiento.

convex *a.* convexo-a.

convulsion *n.* convulsión, contracción involuntaria de un músculo; **febrile** __ / febril; **Jacksonian** __ / __ Jacksoniana; **tonic-clonic** __ / __ tonicoclónica.

convulsive, convulsant *a.* convulsivo-a, rel. a la convulsión; __ **activity** / actividad __ .

cool *a.* fresco-a; refrescado-a; __ **headed** / sereno-a, calmado-a; [*weather*] **it is** __ / hace fresco; [*body temperature*] **he, she, it is** __ / está fresco-a.

cooler *n.* refrigerante, refresco.

coolness *n.* frialdad; serenidad.

cooperate *v.* cooperar, ayudar.

coordinate *v.* coordinar.

coordination *n.* coordinación; **lack of** __ / falta de __ .

copayment *n.* pago compartido.

copious *a.* abundante, copioso-a.

coprolith *n.* coprolito, pequeña masa fecal de consistencia dura.

copulation *n.* copulación, relaciones sexuales.

copy *n.* copia; imitación; *v.* copiar; imitar.

cor *n., L.* cor, corazón.

coracoid *n.* coracoides, apófisis del omóplato.

Coramine *n.* Coramina, nombre comercial de la niquetamida.

cord *n.* cordón, cuerda, cordel; **umbilical** __ / __ umbilical.

cordectomy *n.* cordectomía, excisión de una cuerda vocal o parte de ésta.

core *n.* centro, corazón, núcleo.

corium *n., L.* corion, dermis o piel.

corn *n.* callo, callosidad; [*grain*] maíz.

cornea *n.* córnea, parte anterior transparente del globo del ojo.

corneal grafting *n.* injerto de la córnea.

corneous *a.* córneo, rel. a la córnea; calloso-a.

coronary *a.* coronario-a, que circunda tal como una corona; __ **artery** / arteria __; __ **bypass** / desviación __; __ **care unit** / unidad de cuidado __; __ **thrombosis** / trombosis __; __ **vasospasm** / vasoespasmo __ .

coronary angiography *n.* angiografía coronaria, imágenes tomadas por medio de un medio de contraste de la circulación del miocardio, hecha gen. por caterización selectiva de cada una de las arterias coronarias.

coronary artery aneurysm *n.* aneurisma de la arteria coronaria, gen. debido a aterosclerosis, a procesos inflamatorios o a una fístula coronaria.

coronary artery bypass *n.* conducto o derivación aortocoronaria, intervención usualmente con uso de una vena como injerto, o de una arteria mamaria interna interpuesta entre la aorta y una rama de la arteria coronaria, y puesta como derivación sanguínea mas allá de la obstrucción formada. *Syn.* **aortocoronary bypass.**

coronary atherectomy

coronary atherectomy *n.* aterectomía coronaria, excisión de obstrucciones en la arteria coronaria con un instrumento cortante que se inserta usando un catéter coronario.

coronary care unit *n.* unidad de atención coronaria; sala de hospital reservada para el cuidado de pacientes que requieren atención relacionada con infarto coronario.

coronary collaterization *n.* colaterización coronaria, desarrollo espontáneo de nuevos vasos sanguíneos alrededor de las regiones cardíacas bajo un restringido fluido sanguíneo.

coronary failure *n.* insuficiencia coronaria aguda.

coronary insufficiency *n.* insuficiencia coronaria, deficiencia en la circulación coronaria con riesgo de sufrir un dolor provocado por angina, trombosis o ateroma, que puede dar como resultado un infarto del miocardio. *Syn.* **coronarism.**

coronary occlusion *n.* oclusión coronaria, bloqueo de un vaso coronario.

coronary-prone behavior *n.* conducta hostil que puede ocasionar el padecimiento de una enfermedad cardíaca.

coronary thrombosis *n.* trombosis coronaria debido a formación de un trombo, gen. como resultado de cambios ateromatosos en la pared de la arteria, posible causa de infarto de miocardio.

coroner *n.* médico-a forense.

corpse *n.* cadáver, muerto-a.

corpus *n.* (*pl.* **corpora**), *L. corpus*, el cuerpo humano.

corpus callosum *n.*, *L. corpus callosum*, comisura mayor del cerebro.

corpuscle *n.* corpúsculo, cuerpo diminuto.

corpuscular *a.* corpuscular, diminuto-a.

corpus luteum *n.*, *L. corpus luteum*, cuerpo lúteo, cuerpo amarillo, masa glandular amarillenta que se forma en el ovario por la ruptura de un folículo y produce progesterona.

correct *a.* correcto-a, exacto-a; *v.* corregir, enmendar.

correction *n.* corrección.

corrective *a.* correctivo-a.

corrective lenses *n.* lentes correctoras.

corrosive *n.* agente que causa corrosion en cualquier tejido vivo.

corset *n.* corsé.

cortex *n.* corteza, córtex, la capa más exterior de un órgano; **adrenal __ / __** suprarrenal; **cerebral __ / __** cerebral.

cortical *a.* cortical, rel. a la corteza.

corticoid, corticosteroid *n.* corticoide, corticoesteroide, esteroide producido por la corteza suprarrenal.

corticosteroid-binding globulin *n.* globulina de enlace corticoesteroide.

corticotropin *n.* corticotropina, sustancia hormonal de actividad adrenocorticotrópica.

cortisol *n.* cortisol, hormona secretada por la corteza suprarrenal.

cortisone *n.* cortisona, esteroide glucogénico derivado del cortisol o sintéticamente.

Corti's organ *n.* órgano de Corti, órgano terminal de la audición a través del cual se perciben directamente los sonidos.

cosmetic *n.* cosmético; *a.* cósmetico-a.

cosmetic surgery *n.* cirugía plástica con fines estéticos.

cost *n.* coste, costo, precio; *v.* costar.

costal *a.* costal, rel. a las costillas.

costalgia *n.* costalgia, neuralgia, dolor en las costillas.

costly *a.* costoso-a, caro-a; *adv.* costosamente.

costochondritis *n.* costocondritis, infl. de uno o más cartílagos costales.

costoclavicular *a.* costoclavicular, rel. a las costillas y la clavícula.

costovertebral *a.* costovertebral, rel. a las costillas y vértebras torácicas.

cotton *n.* algodón.

cough *n.* tos; **__ lozenges** / pastillas para la; **__ suppressant** / calmante para la **__**; **__ syrup** / jarabe para la **__**; **hacking __ / __** seca recurrente; *v.* toser; **coughing spell** / ataque de **__**; **to __ up phlegm** / expectorar la flema.

count *v.* contar.

counteract *v.* contrarrestar, oponerse a; contraatacar.

counterattack *n.* contraataque.

countercoup *n.* contragolpe.

counterpoison *n.* antídoto, contraveneno.

counterreaction *n.* reacción opuesta; reacción en contra de.

countershock *n.* contrachoque, corriente eléctrica aplicada al corazón para normalizar el ritmo cardíaco.

courage *n.* coraje, valor, firmeza.

courageous *a.* valiente, valeroso-a.

course *n.* curso, dirección.

cousin *n.* primo-a.

cover *n.* cobertor, manta, cobija; *v.* cubrir, proteger; tapar; abrigar.

covered *a.* cubierto-a; protegido-a.

cow *n.* vaca.

coward *a.* cobarde.

cowperitis *n.* cowperitis, infl. de las glándulas de Cowper (bulbouretrales).

Cowper's glands *n.* glándulas de Cowper (bulbouretrales), pequeñas glándulas adyacentes al bulbo de la uretra masculina en la que vacían una secreción mucosa.

cowpox *n.* vacuna, cowpox.

coxa *L.* (*pl.* **coxae**) coxa, cadera.

coxa magna *n.* coxa magna, ensanchamiento anormal de la cabeza y del cuello del fémur.

coxa valga *n.* coxa valga, deformidad de la cadera por desplazamiento lateral angular del fémur.

coxa vara *n.* coxa vara, deformidad de la cadera por desplazamiento angular interno del fémur.

coxalgia *n.* coxalgia, dolor en la cadera.

cradle *n.* cuna; ___ **cap** / costra láctea.

cramp *n.* calambre, entumecimiento; contracción dolorosa de un músculo.

cranial *a.* craneal, craneano-a, del cráneo o rel. al mismo.

cranial nerves *n. pl.* nervios craneales, cada uno de los doce pares de nervios que salen de la región inferior del cerebro; **olphatory** ___ / ___ olfatorio; **optic** ___ / ___ óptico; **oculomotor** ___ / ___ oculomotor; **trochlear** ___ / ___ patético; **trigeminal** ___ / ___ trigémino; **abducens** ___ / ___ abducente; **facial** ___ / ___ facial; **auditory** ___ / ___ auditivo; **glossopharyngeal** ___ / ___ glosofaríngeo; **vagus** ___ / ___ neumogástrico; **spinal** ___ / ___ espinal; **hypoglossal** ___ / ___ hipogloso.

craniopharingioma *n.* craneofaringioma, tipo de tumor cerebral maligno visto esp. en los niños.

craniotomy *n.* craneotomía, trepanación del cráneo.

cranium *n.* cráneo, parte ósea de la cabeza que cubre el cerebro.

cranky *a.* majadero-a; inquieto-a.

crawl *v.* gatear, andar a gatas, arrastrarse.

crazy *a.* loco-a, demente.

cream *n.* crema, nata.

create *v.* crear.

creatine *n.* creatina, componente del tejido muscular, esencial en la fase anaeróbica de la contracción muscular.

creatinine *n.* creatinina, sustancia presente en la orina que representa el producto final del metabolismo de la creatina; ___ **clearance** / depuración de ___, volumen de plasma libre de ___ .

creation *n.* creación, obra; universo.

credit *n.* crédito; *v.* acreditar, dar crédito.

cremasteric *a.* cremastérico, referente al músculo cremastérico del escroto.

cremate *v.* incinerar.

cremation *n.* incineración.

creosote *n.* creosota, líquido aceitoso gen. usado como desinfectante y como expectorante catarral.

crepitation *n.* crepitación, chasquido, crujido; **pleural** ___ / ___ pleural.

crest *n.* cresta, prominencia; copete. 1. reborde o prominencia de un hueso; 2. la elevación máxima de una línea en un gráfico.

cretin *n.* cretino-a, persona con manifestaciones de cretinismo.

cretinism *n.* cretinismo, hipotiroidismo congénito debido a una deficiencia acentuada de la hormona tiroidea.

crib *n.* cuna, camita.

crib death *n.* muerte de cuna, síndrome de muerte infantil súbita.

crime *n.* crimen, delito.

criminal *n.* criminal.

cripple *a.* lisiado-a, paralítico-a, inválido-a, tullido-a; *v.* lisiar, baldar, paralizar; tullir.

crisis *n.* crisis. 1. El punto culminante del estado severo del paciente en el curso de una enfermedad que puede resultar en el cambio a una condición favorable o drástica; 2. ataque convulsivo; **adolescent** ___ / ___ de maduración; **adrenal** ___ / ___ adrenal; **anaphylactoid** ___ / ___ anafiláctica; **febrile** ___ / ___ febril; **gastric** ___ / ___ gástrica; **hypertensive** ___ / ___ hipertensiva; **identity** ___ / ___ de identidad; **midlife** ___ / ___ de la edad

madura; **myasthenic** __ / __
miasténica; **tabetic** __ / __ tabética;
thyrotoxic __ / __ tiroidea tóxica.

critical *a.* crítico-a; __ condition /
estado __, gravedad extrema.

cross-dressed *n.* travestismo.

cross-legged *a.* patizambo-a;
cruzado-a de piernas.

cross matching *n.* pruebas
sanguíneas cruzadas que comprueban
la compatibilidad de la sangre antes de
una tranfusión.

cross-section *n.* sección transversal.

cross studies *n., pl.* estudios cruzados.

crossing-over, crossover *n.* acción
de cruzar a través.

crossed eyes, strabismus *n.*
estrabismo, *pop.* bizquera, debilidad de
los músculos que controlan la posición
del ojo impidiendo la coordinación
visual.

crotch *n.* bifurcación, horquilla.

croup *n.* crup, *pop.* garrotillo, síndrome
respiratorio visto en los niños, causado
gen. por una infección o una reacción
alérgica; **spasmodic** __ / __
espasmódico.

crown *n.* corona; **artificial** __ / __
artificial; **bell shaped** __ / __ en forma
de campana.

crowning *n.* coronamiento, coronación.
1. etapa del parto cuando la cabeza
se localiza en la salida pélvica;
2. preparación de un diente natural para
recubrirlo usando el material dental
elegido.

crucial *a.* crucial, definitivo-a.

crude *a.* rudo-a, crudo-a.

cruel *a.* cruel, inhumano-a.

crus *n., L. crus.* 1. pierna o parte
semejante a una pierna; 2. parte de la
pierna entre la rodilla y el tobillo.

crush *v.* triturar, moler, aplastar.

crust *n.* costra.

crutches *n., pl.* muletas.

cry *v.* llorar.

cryoanesthesia *n.* crioanestesia.
1. anestesia producida por aplicación
de frío localizado; 2. pérdida de la
sensibilidad al frío.

cryogenic *n.* criogénico, que produce
temperaturas bajas.

cryoglobulin *n.* crioglobulina,
globulina que se precipita del suero por
acción del frío.

cryosurgery *n.* criocirugía,
destrucción de tejidos por aplicación de
temperatura fría local o general.

cryotherapy *n.* crioterapia, tratamiento
terapéutico por aplicación de frío local
o general.

crypt *n.* cripta, pequeño receso
tubular.

cryptococcosis *n.* criptococosis,
infección que afecta distintos órganos
del cuerpo, esp. el cerebro y sus
meninges.

cryptorchism *n.* criptorquismo, falta
de descenso testicular al escroto.

crystal *n.* cristal, vidrio.

crystalline *a.* cristalino-a, transparente.

crystalline lens *n.* cristalino, lente
del ojo.

cubitus, ulna *n., L.* cubitus, cúbito,
hueso interno del antebrazo.

cuff *n.* manguito, tejido fibroso que rodea
una articulación; **rotator** __ / __
rotador, músculo tendinoso; **rotator** __
tear / ruptura del __ rotador.

cul-de-sac *n., Fr.* 1. cul-de-sac, fondo
de saco, bolsa sin boquete de salida;
2. saco rectouterino.

culdoscopy *n.* culdoscopía, examen de
la pelvis y la cavidad abdominal por
medio del culdoscopio.

cultivate *v.* cultivar; estudiar.

culture *n.* cultivo, crecimiento artificial
de microorganismos o células de tejido
vivo en el laboratorio; **blood** __ / __
de sangre; __; __ **medium** / medio de
__; **tissue** __ / __ de tejido.

cunnilingus *a.* cunnilinguo-a, rel. a la
práctica de estimulación oral del
clítoris.

cup *n.* copa; ventosa; **optic** __ / __ de
ojo, __ ocular; **measuring** __ / taza de
medir.

curable *a.* curable, sanable.

curare *n.* curare, veneno extraído de
varios tipos de plantas y usado como
relajante muscular y anestésico.

curative *n.* curativo, remedio, agente
que tiene propiedades curativas.

curd *n.* cuajo, cuajarón, coágulo
sanguíneo grande; [*milk*] leche cuajada.

curdle *v.* cuajarse, coagularse,
engrumecerse.

cure *n.* curación, remedio; *v.* curar, sanar,
remediar.

curettage *n.* curetaje, raspado de una
superficie o cavidad con uso de la
cureta.

curette *n.* cureta, instrumento
quirúrgico en forma de cuchara o pala
usado para raspar los tejidos de una
superficie o cavidad.

current *n.* corriente, trasmisión de fluido o electricidad que pasa por un conductor; *a.* corriente, actual; **-ly** *adv.* actualmente.

curvature *n.* curvatura.

curve *n.* curva; *v.* torcer, encorvar.

Cushing's syndrome *n.* síndrome de Cushing, síndrome adrenogenital asociado con una producción excesiva de cortisol, caracterizado por obesidad y debilitamiento muscular.

cushion *n.* cojinete, cojín.

cusp *n.* cúspide, punta.

custodial care *n.* cuidado bajo custodia.

custom *n.* costumbre, hábito.

cut *n.* cortada, cortadura; *v.* cortar; **to __ down** / rebajar, reducir; **to __ off** / extirpar, amputar; [*oneself*] cortarse.

cutaneous *a.* cutáneo-a; **__ absorption** / absorción __; **__ glands** / glándulas __ -s o sebáceas.

cuticle *n.* cutícula, capa exterior de la piel.

cutis *n.* cutis; piel de la cara.

cyanide *n.* cianuro, compuesto extremadamente venenoso; **__ poisoning** / envenenamiento por cianuro.

cyanocobalamin *n.* cianocobalamina, vitamina B_{12} usada en el tratamiento de la anemia perniciosa.

cyanosis *n.* cianosis, condición azulada o amoratada de la piel y las mucosas a causa de anomalías cardíacas o funcionales.

cyanotic *a.* cianótico-a, rel. a la cianosis o causado por ésta.

cybernetics *n.* cibernética, estudio del uso de medios electrónicos y mecanismos de comunicación aplicados a sistemas biológicos tales como los sistemas nervioso y cerebral.

cyclamate *n.* ciclamato, agente artificial dulcificante.

cycle *n.* ciclo, período; **pregnancy __** / __ gravídico.

cyclic *a.* cíclico-a, que ocurre en períodos o ciclos.

cyclical chemotherapy *n.* quimioterapia cíclica.

cyclitis *n.* ciclitis, infl. del músculo ciliar.

cyclophosphamide *n.* ciclofosfamida, droga antineoplástica usada también como inmunosupresor en trasplantes.

cyclophotocoagulation *n.* ciclofotocoagulación, fotocoagulación a través de la pupila con un laser, procedimiento usado en el tratamiento de glaucoma.

cyclosporine *n.* ciclosporina, agente inmunosupresivo usado en tranplantes de órganos.

cyclotomy *n.* ciclotomía, incisión a través del músculo ciliar.

cylinder *n.* cilindro. 1. émbolo de una jeringa; 2. forma geométrica semejante a una columna.

cylindrical *a.* cilíndrico-a.

cylindrical lens *n.* lente cilíndrico

cylindrical renal cast *n.* molde renal cilíndrico

cylindroma *n.* cilindroma, tumor generalmente maligno visto en la cara o en la órbita del ojo.

cylindruria *n.* cilindruria, presencia de cilindros en la orina.

cyst *n.* quiste, saco o bolsa que contiene líquido o materia semilíquida; **pilonidal __** / __ pilonidal, que contiene pelo, gen. localizado en el área sacrococcígea; **sebaceous __** / __ sebáceo, gen. localizado en el cuero cabelludo.

cystadenocarcinoma *n.* cistadenocarcinoma, carcinoma y cistadenoma combinados.

cystadenoma *n.* cistadenoma, adenoma que contiene uno o various quistes.

cystectomy *n.* cistectomía, extirpación o resección de la vejiga.

cystic *a.* cístico-a, rel. a la vesícula biliar o la vejiga urinaria; **__ duct** / conducto __ .

cystic fibrosis *n.* fibrosis cística del páncreas, fibroquiste.

cystine *n.* cistina, aminoácido producido durante la digestión de las proteínas, presente a veces en la orina.

cystinuria *n.* cistinuria, exceso de cistina en la orina.

cystitis *n.* cistitis, infl. de la vejiga urinaria caracterizada por ardor, dolor y micción frecuente.

cystocele *n.* cistocele, hernia de la vejiga.

cystofibroma *n.* cistofibroma, tipo de fibroma en el cual se han formado quistes o formaciones semejantes a quistes.

cystogram *n.* cistograma, rayos-x de la vejiga.

cystolithotomy *n.* cistolitotomía, extracción de una piedra o cálculo por medio de una incisión en la vejiga.

cystoscope *n.* cistoscopio, instrumento en forma de tubo usado para examinar y tratar trastornos de la vejiga, los uréteres y los riñones.

cystoscopy *n.* cistoscopía, examen por medio del cistoscopio.

cystostomy *n.* cistostomía, creación de un boquete o fístula en la vejiga para permitir el drenaje urinario.

cytology *n.* citología, ciencia que estudia la estructura, forma y función de las células.

cytolysis *n.* citolisis, destrucción de células vivas.

cytolytic *a.* citolítico-a, que tiene la cualidad de disolver o destruir células.

cytomegalic *a.* citomegálico-a, caracterizado-a por células agrandadas.

cytomegalovirus *n.* citomegalovirus, grupo de virus pertenecientes a la familia *Herpesviridae* que infectan humanos y otros animales, y son causantes de la enfermedad de inclusión citomegálica.

cytometer *n.* citómetro, dispositivo usado en el conteo y medida de los hematíes.

cytopenia *n.* citopenia, deficiencia de elementos celulares en la sangre.

cytoplasm *n.* citoplasma, protoplasma de una célula con exclusión del núcleo.

cytoreductive surgery *n.* cirugía citoreductiva, proceso de reducción de un tumor que no puede ser extirpado completamente.

cytotoxic agents *n., pl.* agentes citotóxicos, compuestos químicos usados en quimioterapia con el propósito de destruir células cancerosas.

cytotoxic T8 cell *n.* célula T8 citotóxica, lleva a cabo las funciones de destrucción de antígenos, ataque y eliminación de células infectadas por virus, parásitos y hongos.

cytotoxicity *n.* citotoxicidad, la capacidad de un agente de destruir ciertas células.

cytotoxin *n.* citotoxina, agente tóxico que afecta a las células de ciertos órganos.

cytula *n.* cítula, término que define al óvulo o pequeña célula impregnada.

d

d *abbr.* death / muerte; **deceased** / difunto-a; **degree** / grado; **density** / densidad; **dose** / dosis.

dacryadenitis *n.* dacriadenitis, infl. de una glándula lagrimal.

dacryoadenectomy *n.* dacrioadenectomía, extirpación de una glándula lagrimal.

dacryocyst *n.* dacriocisto, saco lacrimal interno.

dacryocystectomy *n.* dacriocistectomía, cirugía para restaurar el drenaje del saco lacrimal cuando ocurre obstrucción en el conducto nasolacrimal.

dacryocystitis *n.* dacriocistitis, infl. del saco lagrimal.

dacryorrhea *n.* excreción de pus por el conducto lacrimal.

dactyl *n.* dáctilo, dedo de la mano o del pie.

dactylography *n.* dactilografía, estudio de las huellas digitales.

dactylology *n.* dactilología, lenguaje mímico o por señas.

dad *n.* papá; **daddy** / *H.A.* papi, papacito, tata.

daily *a.* diario-a, cotidiano-a; __ **life** / vida cotidiana; *adv.* diariamente, todos los días, cada día, cotidianamente; __ **reference values** / referencia diurética diaria.

dairy products *n., pl.* productos lácteos.

daltonism *n.* daltonismo, dificultad para percibir colores.

damage *n.* daño, deterioro, lesión. *v.* dañar, perjudicar; dañarse, perjudicarse.

damaging *a.* perjudicial.

damp *a.* húmedo-a.

dampen *v.* humedecer, mojar.

danazol *n.* danazol, hormona sintética que suprime la acción de la pituitaria anterior.

dance *n.* baile; **St. Vitus'** __ / __ de San Vito chorea; *v.* bailar, danzar.

dandruff *n.* caspa.

danger *n.* peligro, riesgo; *v.* **to be in** __ / correr __ .

dangerous *a.* peligroso-a, arriesgado-a.

dark *a.* oscuro-a; __ **complexion**, __ **skin** / piel morena; __ **adaptation** / adaptación a la oscuridad; __ **field illumination** / iluminación del campo __ , iluminación lateral u oblicua.

darkness *n.* oscuridad.

Darwinian theory *n.* Darwin, teoría de, teoría de selección y evolución de las especies.

data *n., pl.* datos.

date *n.* fecha; **effective** __ / __ de vigencia; **expiration** __ / __ de vencimiento; **specimen** __ / __ del espécimen o muestra; **up-to-** __ / actualizado hasta la fecha; [*current*] al corriente.

daughter *n.* hija; __ **-in-law** / nuera.

day *n.* día, **all** __ / todo el __; **by** __ / por el __, de__; __ **after tomorrow** / pasado mañana; __ **before yesterday** / anteayer; __ **in** __ **out** / tras __; **each** __ / cada __; **every** __ / todos los __ -s; **every other** __ / un __ sí y un __ no; **three times a** __ / tres veces al __; **twice a** __ / dos veces al __ .

daydream *n.* ilusión, ensueño; *v.* **to** __ / soñar despierto-a.

daylight *n.* luz del día.

daze *n.* ofuscación, desorientación.

deacidify *v.* neutralizar un ácido.

deactivation *n.* desactivación, proceso de transformar lo activo en inactivo.

dead *a.* difunto-a; muerto-a.

deaden *v.* [*sound*] amortiguar; [*nerve*] adormecer; anestesiar.

deadly *a.* mortal, mortífero-a; que puede causar la muerte; __ **poison** / veneno __; __ **wound** / herida __ .

deaf *n. a.* sordo-a.

deaf-mute *n.* sordomudo-a.

deafness *n.* sordera.

deambulatory *a.* ambulatorio-a; móvil.

dear *a.* querido-a; estimado-a.

death *n.* muerte, fallecimiento; **apparent** __ / __ aparente; __ **certificate** / certificado de defunción; __ **instinct** / instinto mortal; __ **rate** / mortalidad; __ **rattle** / estertor agónico; **fetal** __ / __ del feto.

debilitate *v.* debilitar; debilitarse.

debilitated *a.* debilitado-a.

debilitating *a.* debilitante, rel. a una enfermedad o agente que debilita.

debulking operation

debulking operation *n.* extirpación de la mayor parte de un tumor.

decalcification *n.* descalcificación, pérdida o disminución de sales de calcio en los huesos o dientes.

decapsulation *n.* decapsulación, incisión y extirpación de una cápsula.

decay *n.* deteriorización, deterioro, descomposición gradual; [*teeth*] caries; **dental** __ / carie dental, *pop.* dientes picados; __ **rate** / índice de descomposición gradual *v.* deteriorar, descomponer, decaer, declinar; deteriorarse, descomponerse, [*teeth*] cariarse; [*wood*] carcomerse; [*matter*] podrirse, pudrirse.

decayed *a.* deteriorado-a, decaído-a; empeorado-a; [*teeth*] cariado-a; [*wood*] carcomido-a; [*matter*] podrido-a; putrefacto-a.

deceased *n.* difunto-a, persona muerta.

deceitful *a.* traicionero-a, engañador-a; __ **sickness** / enfermedad __ .

deceleration *n.* desaceleración, disminución de la velocidad tal como en la frecuencia cardíaca.

decent *a.* decente.

decentered *a.* descentrado-a, fuera del centro.

decide *v.* decidir, determinar.

decided *a.* decidido-a.

decidua *n.* decidua, tejido membranoso formado por la mucosa uterina durante la gestación y expulsado después del parto.

decidua menstrualis *n., L. decidua menstrual*, también llamada membrana caduca, es la capa mucosa del útero que se desprende durante la menstruación.

deciduous *a.* deciduo-a, de permanencia temporal; __ **dentition** / primera dentición; __ **teeth** / dientes __ -s, dientes de leche.

decimation *n.* gran mortalidad, diezma.

decipher *v.* descifrar, resolver un problema.

decision *n.* decisión, resolución.

decisive *a.* decisivo-a, terminante.

decline *n.* declinación; decadencia, decaimiento. *v.* declinar, decaer; [*invitation, offer*] declinar, rehusar, rechazar; [*health*] desmejorarse.

decompensation *n.* descompensación, inhabilidad del corazón para mantener una circulación adecuada.

decompose *v.* descomponerse, corromperse; [*food*] podrirse, pudrirse.

decomposed *a.* descompuesto-a; [*food*] podrido-a, putrefacto-a.

decompression *n.* descompresión, reducción de presión; __ **chamber** / cámara de __; __ **sickness** / condición por __; **surgical** __ / __ quirúrgica.

decongest *v.* descongestionar.

decongestant *n.* descongestionador, descongestionante.

decontamination *n.* descontaminación, proceso de librar el ambiente, objetos o personas de sustancias o agentes contaminados o nocivos tales como sustancias radioactivas.

decortication *n.* decorticación, excisión del tejido cortical de un órgano o estructura.

decrease *n.* disminución; reducción v. decrecer, disminuir, reducir; __ **saliva** / __ de saliva o reducción de saliva; __ **tears** / __ de lágrimas o reducción de lágrimas; __ **urine output** / __ o reducción del rendimiento urinario.

decreased *a., pp.* of **to decrease**, decrecido-a, disminuido-a, reducido-a.

decreasing *a.* decreciente; *pp.* disminuyendo.

decrepit *a.* decrépito-a, senil.

decrudescence *n.* decrudescencia, disminución de la gravedad de los síntomas.

decubitus *n.* decúbito, posición acostada; __ **ventral** / __ prono; **dorsal** __ / __ supino; **lateral** __ **x-ray** / radiografía __ lateral.

deduce *v.* deducir, inferir.

deep *a.* profundo-a, hondo-a; __ **artery of arm** / arteria __ del brazo; __ **artery of clitoris** / arteria __ del clítoris; __ **artery of penis** / arteria __ del pene; __ **breathing** / respiración __; __ **cerebral veins** / venas cerebrales __; __ **cervical veins** / venas cervicales __ -as; __ **contractions** / contracciones __ -s, de fondo; __ **-chested** / ancho-a de pecho; __ **dredging** / dragado; __ **facial vein** / vena facial __; __ **inguinal ring** / anillo inguinal __; __ **-rooted** / arraigado-a; __ **sensibility** / sensibilidad __; __ **sleep** / sueño __, sopor; __ **tendon reflex** / reflejos tendónicos __ -s; __ **venous**

delusion

thrombosis / trombosis venosa __; __
x-ray therapy / terapia __ .
deer fly disease *n*. V. tularemia.
defecate *v*. defecar, evacuar; *Mex.*
obrar.
defecation *n*. defecación, evacuación
intestinal.
defect *n*. defecto; insuficiencia; fallo.
defective *a*. defectuoso-a;
incompleto-a.
defense *n*. defensa; protección;
resistencia; __ **mechanism** /
mecanismo de __; [*organic*] antitoxina
autoprotección.
defensive medicine *n*. medicina
defensiva, medidas terapéuticas o de
diagnóstico que se toman con el
propósito de evitar un posible riesgo de
negligencia médica.
deferent *a*. deferente, hacia afuera.
defibrillation *n*. desfibrilación, acción
de cambiar latidos irregulares del
corazón a su ritmo normal.
defibrillator *n*. desfibrilador,
dispositivo eléctrico usado para
restaurar el ritmo normal del
corazón.
deficiency *n*. deficiencia, falta de algún
elemento esencial al organismo; __
disease / enfermedad por deficiencia;
galactokinasa __ / __ de
galactocinasa; **lactase** __ / __ de
lactasa; **mineral** __ / __ mineral ;
mental __ / __ mental; **oxygen**
__ / falta de oxígeno.
deficient *a*. deficiente, careciente.
definition *n*. definición.
definitive *a*. definitivo; determinado;
__ **diagnosis** / diagnóstico __ .
definitive host *n*. huésped definitivo,
aquél en el cual el parásito se desarrolla
hasta alcanzar la madurez sexual.
deflect *v*. desviar, apartar.
deflection, deflexion *n*. deflexión,
desviación, desvío; diversión
inconsciente de ideas.
deformed *a*. deformado-a, irregular.
deformity *n*. deformidad, irregularidad,
defecto congénito o adquirido.
degenerate *a*. degenerado-a;
anómalo-a.
degeneration *n*. degeneración,
deteriorización.
degenerative joint disease *n*.
enfermedad degenerativa de una
articulación o coyuntura.
deglutition *n*. deglución, acto de
ingerir.

degree *n*. grado. 1. unidad de medida
de la temperatura; 2. intensidad.
dehiscence *n*. dehiscencia, abertura
espontánea de una herida.
dehumidifier *n*. deshumectante,
aparato para disminuir la humedad.
dehydrate *v*. deshidratar, eliminar el
agua de una sustancia; deshidratarse,
perder líquido del cuerpo o de los
tejidos.
dehydrated *a*. deshidratado-a.
dehydrocholesterol *n*.
dehidrocolesterol, esterol presente en la
piel que se convierte en vitamina D por
la acción de rayos solares.
déjà vu *n*. *Fr. déjà vu*, impresión ilusoria
de haber experimentado antes una
situación que es totalmente nueva.
delay *n*. demora; *v*. demorar, atrasar;
postergar.
delayed *a*. tardío-a, demorado-a; __
delivery / parto __ .
delicate *a*. delicado-a.
delicious *a*. delicioso-a; exquisito-a.
delight *n*. deleite; delicia; *v*. agradar,
deleitar.
delighted *a*. encantado-a; *v*. **to**
be __ / tener mucho gusto.
delinquency *n*. delincuencia; **juvenile**
__ / __ juvenil.
delirious *a*. delirante, en estado de
delirio.
delirium *n*. delirium, estado de
confusión mental acompañado gen. de
alucinaciones y sensaciones
distorsionadas; __ **tremens** / __
tremens, tipo de psicosis alcohólica.
deliver *v*. extraer; partear; [*in*
childbirth] **to be delivered** / dar a
luz, estar de parto, *Mex. A.*
aliviarse.
delivery *n*. parto, alumbramiento; **after**
__ / __ después del __; **before** __ /
antes del __; __ **of the placenta** /
expulsión de la placenta; __ **room** /
sala de __ -s; sala de maternidad; **false**
__ / __ falso; **hard** __ / __ laborioso;
induction of __ / __ inducido; **normal**
__ / __ normal; **premature** __ / __
prematuro; **prolonged** __ / __
prolongado; **stages of** __ / etapas
del __ .
deltoid *a*. deltoideo-a. 1. en forma de
delta; 2. rel. al músculo deltoides.
delusion *n*. delirio, decepción, engaño;
creencias falsas; __ **of control** / __ de
control; __ **of grandeur** / __ de
grandeza; __ **of negation** / __ de

307

demand

negación; __ **of persecution** / __ de
persecución.
demand *n.* petición, demanda; __
feeding / alimentación por demanda.
demented *a.* demente, enajenado-a;
que sufre de demencia.
dementia *n.* demencia, locura;
declinación de las funciones mentales;
__ **paralytica** / __ paralítica; __
praecox / __ precoz, esquizofrenia;
organic __ / __ orgánica; **senile** __ /
__ senil.
demineralization *n.*
desmineralización, pérdida de sales
minerales del organismo.
demulcent *n.* emoliente, demulcente,
aceite u otro agente que suaviza y alivia
molestias de la piel.
demyelination *n.* desmielinización,
pérdida de la capa de mielina de un
nervio.
dendrite *n.* dendrita, prolongación
protoplasmática de la célula de un
nervio que recibe los impulsos
nerviosos.
denervated *a.* desnervado,
enervado, rel. a la pérdida de energía
nerviosa.
dengue fever *n.* dengue, fiebre
endémica producida por un virus,
transmitida por el mosquito *Aedes*.
denomination *n.* denominación,
nombre.
dense *a.* denso-a, espeso-a.
density *n.* densidad; **bone** __ / __
ósea; **optic** __ / __ óptica;
urinary __ / __ urinaria; **vapor** __ /
__ del vapor.
dental *a.* dental, dentario-a, rel. a los
dientes; __ **abscess** / absceso __; __
ankylosis / anquilosis __; __ **arch** /
arco __; __ **bulb** / bulbo __; __ **care** /
cuidado __; __ **caries** / caries __ -es;
__ **drill** / taladro, torno; __ **enamel** /
esmalte dentario; __ **floss** / hilo __,
hilo de seda encerada; __ **flossing
system** / sistema para aplicar hilo __;
__ **follicle** / folículo __; __ **health
services** / servicios de salud __; __
hygienist / técnico-a en profiláctica __;
__ **implants** / implantes __-es; __
impression / impresión, mordisco; __
impaction / inclusión dentaria; __
plaque / placa dentaria; __ **public
health** / salud pública __; __ **school** /
escuela de odontología; __ **surgeon** /
cirujano __; __ **tartar** / sarro __; __
technician / mecánico __ .

dentiform *a.* odontoide, dentado-a, de
proyección similar a un diente.
dentifrice *n.* dentífrico, pasta dental.
dentilabial *a.* dentilabial, rel. a los
dientes y los labios.
dentin *n.* dentina, marfil dentario, tejido
calcificado de un diente.
dentinogenesis *n.* dentinogénesis,
formación de la dentina.
dentist *n.* dentista.
dentistry *n.* arte o profesión de
dentistas.
dentition *n.* dentición, brote de los
dientes; __ **primary** / __ primaria
[*first teeth*] o dientes de leche; __ ,
secondary / __ secundaria o dientes
permanentes.
denture *n.* dentadura, prótesis;
[*artificial*] dentadura postiza; __
plates / __ parcial, *pop.* plancha
dental.
denudation *n.* denudación, privación
de la cubierta de superficie de una
manera traumática, sea por cirugía,
trauma, o por un cambio patológico.
deny *v.* negar, rehusar.
deodorant *n.* desodorante.
deodorize *v.* desodorizar, destruir
olores fétidos o desagradables.
deoxycorticosterone *n.*
desoxicorticosterona, hormona
producida en la corteza de las glándulas
suprarrenales de efecto marcado en el
metabolismo del agua y los
electrólitos.
deoxygenated *a.* desoxigenado-a.
deoxyhemoglobin *n.*
desoxihemoglobina, forma reducida de
hemoglobina que ocurre cuando la
oxihemoglobina pierde el oxígeno.
departed *a.* difunto-a; ausente.
dependence, dependency *n.*
dependencia, subordinación; __
producing drugs / drogas adictivas, de
dependencia.
dependent *n.* depediente *a.*
depediente; __ **drainage** / drenaje __;
__ **edema** / edema __; __ **personality**
/ personalidad __ .
depersonalization *n.*
despersonalización, pérdida de la
personalidad.
depigmentation *n.* despigmentación,
pérdida parcial o completa de
pigmento.
depilation *n.* depilación,
procedimiento de extirpación del
pelo y la raíz.

depilatory *n.* depilatorio.

depleted *a.* agotado-a, vaciado-a, depauperado-a.

depletion *n.* depleción. 1. acción de vaciar; 2. pérdida o remoción de los líquidos del cuerpo; ___ **of body liquids** / pérdida de líquidos del cuerpo; **fluid** ___ , **dehydration** / pérdida de fluido, deshidratación; **potassium** ___ / pérdida de potasio, hipopotasemia; **saline** ___ / pérdida salina.

depravation *n.* depravación.

depressant *n.* depresor; tranquilizante; ___ **drug** / medicamento tranquilizante

depressed *a.* deprimido-a, abatido-a; *v.* **to become** ___ / deprimirse.

depression *n.* depresión. 1. sensación de tristeza o melancolía acompañada de apatía y estados de abatimiento; 2. cavidad.

depressive *a.* depresivo-a, deprimente; ___ **disorder** / trastorno ___ .

depressor *n.* depresor. 1. agente usado para reducir un nivel establecido de una función o actividad del organismo; 2. tranquilizante que produce depresión.

depurate *v.* depurar.

depuration *n.* depuración, purificación.

deranged *a.* perturbado-a; trastornado-a; ___ **metabolic process** / trastorno del proceso metabólico.

derangement *n. Fr.* trastorno, desequilibrio, irregularidad de una función del cuerpo.

derivation *n.* derivación. 1. desviación, curso alterado o lateral que tiene lugar por anastomosis o por una característica anatómica natural; 2. descendencia.

dermabrasion *n.* dermabrasión, abrasión cutánea, proceso empleado para eliminar los nevos y cicatrices de la acné.

dermatitis *n.* dermatitis, dermitis, cualquier infl. de la piel; **atopic** ___ / ___ atópica; ___ **by contact** / ___ por contacto; ___ **medicamentosa** / ___ medicamentosa; ___ **papillaris capillitii** / ___ papillaris capillitii; **erythematic** ___ / ___ eritematosa; **gangrenous** ___ / ___ gangrenosa; **occupational** ___ / ___ ocupacional, industrial; **seborrheic** ___ / ___ seborréica.

dermatologist *n.* dermatólogo-a, especialista en dermatología.

dermatology *n.* dermatología, parte de la medicina que estudia la piel, su estructura, sus funciones y el tratamiento de la misma.

dermatolysis *n.* dermatolisis, exfoliación de la epidermis causada por una enfermedad.

dermatoma *n.* dermatoma, neoplasma de la piel.

dermatomycosis *n.* dermatomicosis, infl. de la piel producida por hongos.

dermatomyositis *n.* dermatomiositis, enfermedad del tejido conectivo con manifestaciones de dermatitis, edema e infl. de los músculos.

dermatoneurosis *n.* dermatoneurosis, erupción cutánea causada por un estímulo emocional.

dermatophytosis *n.* dermatofitosis, pie de atleta, infección fungosa producida por dermatófilos.

dermatoplasty *n.* dermatoplastia, cirugía plástica de la piel.

dermatosyphilis *n.* dermatosífilis, manifestación sifilítica en la piel.

dermic *a.* dermal, dermático-a, cutáneo-a.

dermis, derma *n.* dermis, piel.

dermoid *a.* dermoideo-a, semejante o rel. a la piel; ___ **cyst** / quiste ___, de origen congénito, gen. benigno.

descend *v.* descender, bajar; derivarse.

descendant *n.a.* descendiente.

descending *a.* descendente, descendiente; ___ **aorta** / aorta ___, parte mayor de la aorta; ___ **colon** / colon ___ .

descending tracts *n., pl.* ramas descendentes de nervios en la espina dorsal que llevan impulsos del cerebro al resto del cuerpo.

describe *v.* describir.

described *a.* descrito-a, narrado-a.

desensitize *v.* desensibilizar, reducir o eliminar una sensibilidad de origen físico o emocional.

deserve *v.* merecer.

desexualizing *n.* desexualización. 1. eliminación de un impulso sexual; 2. castración.

desiccant *a.* desecante, que tiene la propiedad de secar.

design *n.* diseño; ___ **drugs** / drogas de ___

desirable *a.* deseado-a; conveniente.

desmoid *a.* desmoide, en forma de ligamento.

despair *n.* desesperación; *v.* [*to lose hope*] perder la esperanza; desesperarse.

despondent *a.* desesperado-a, desalentado-a; *v.* **to be** __ / estar __; desilusionado-a.

desquamation *n.* descamación, exfoliación, desprendimiento de la piel en forma de escamas.

destroy *v.* destruir, aniquilar; arruinar.

detach *v.* separar, desprender, despegar; desprenderse; soltarse.

detachment *n.* desprendimiento, separación; __ of the retina / __ de la retina.

detail *n.* detalle; **in** __ / con detalle, detalladamente *v.* detallar, destacar; **to go into** __ / explicar todo detalladamente.

detain *v.* detener, parar.

detect *v.* detectar, descubrir.

detector *n.* detector, revelador, descubridor.

deteriorate *v.* deteriorar, desmejorar; deteriorarse; desmejorarse.

deterioration *n.* deterioración, deterioro, desmejoramiento.

determinant *n.* determinante, elemento que predomina o causa una determinación.

determination *n.* determinación, decisión, resolución.

determine *v.* determinar, decidir; resolver; concluir.

determined *a.* decidido-a; [*in tests*] comprobado-a.

detorsion *n.* destorsión. 1. corrección de la curvatura o malformación de una estructura; 2. corrección quirúrgica de la torsión de un testículo o del intestino.

detoxification *n.* destoxificación, reducción de las propiedades tóxicas de una sustancia.

detoxify *v.* destoxificar, desintoxicar, extraer sustancias tóxicas.

detrimental *a.* perjudicial, nocivo-a.

detritus *n., pl.* desechos.

detrusor *n.* detrusor, músculo que expulsa o echa hacia afuera.

deuteranopia *n.* deuteranopía, ceguera al color verde.

develop *v.* [*to expand, to grow*] desarrollar, crecer, progresar; evolucionar; avanzar; [*film*] revelar; [*symptom*] surgir; manifestarse.

developed *a.* desarrollado-a; revelado-a, manifestada-a.

development *n.* desarrollo; adelanto; progreso, crecimiento; [*germs*] proliferación; **child** __ / __ infantil; **physical** __ / __ físico; **psychomotor and physical** __ / __ psicomotor y físico.

developmental disability *n.* inhabilidades de desarrollo o pérdida de una función adquirida debido a causas congénitas o post natales, tales como la adquisición del lenguaje o la habilidad motora o social.

developmental psychology *n.* sicología del desarrollo mental.

deviation *n.* desviación, desvío. 1. alejamiento de una pauta establecida; 2. aberración mental; mala conducta, mal comportamiento.

device *n.* dispositivo; mecanismo.

devise *v.* idear, inventar, considerar.

devitalize *v.* devitalizar, debilitar, privar de la fuerza vital.

devolution *n.* devolución. V. **catabolism**.

dexter *a.* diestro-a; a la derecha.

dextrality *n.* dextrismo, preferencia de uso de la mano derecha.

dextrocardia *n.* dextrocardia, dislocación del corazón hacia la derecha.

dextrose *n.* dextrosa, glucosa, forma de azúcar simple, *pop.* azúcar de uva.

diabetes *n.* diabetes, enfermedad que se manifiesta por excesiva emisión de orina.

diabetes insipidus *n.* diabetes insípida nefrógena, causada por una deficiencia en el gasto de hormona antidiurética.

diabetes mellitus *n.* diabetes mellitus, diabetes causada por una deficiencia en la producción de insulina que resulta en hiperglucemia y glucosuria; __ **noninsulin-dependent** / __ sin dependencia de insulina.

diabetic *a.* diabético-a; rel. a la diabetes o que padece de ella; **brittle** __ / __ inestable; __ **angiopathies** / angiopatías __ -s; __ **coma** / coma __, por falta de insulina; __ **diet** / dieta __; __ **neuropathy** / neuropatía __; __ **retinopathy** / retinopatía __ ; __ **shock** / choque __ .

dichromic

diabetic retinitis *n.* retinopatia diabética.

diabetogenic *a.* diabetogénico-a, que produce diabetes.

diabetograph *n.* diabetógrafo, aparato para medir la proporción de glucosa en la orina.

diacetemia *n.* diacetemia, presencia de ácido diacético en la sangre.

diacetylmorphine *n.* diacetilmorfina, heroína.

diagnose *v.* diagnosticar, dar un diagnóstico, hacer un diagnóstico o diagnosis.

diagnosis *n.* diagnóstico, diagnosis, determinación de la enfermedad del paciente; **computer** __ / __ por computadora; __ **error** / errores de __; **differential** __ / __ diferencial, por comparación; **physical** __ / __ físico, por medio de un examen físico completo.

diagnostic *n.* diagnóstico; __ **chart** / ficha de __; __ **imaging** / __ de imágenes por medios radioactivos.

diagonal *a.* diagonal, sección transversal.

diagram *n.* diagrama.

dialysate *n.* dializado, líquido que pasa por la membrana separadora o dializadora.

dialysis *n.* diálisis, procedimiento para filtrar y eliminar toxinas presentes en la sangre de pacientes con insuficiencia renal; __ **machine** / aparato de __ (riñón artificial); **peritoneal** __ / __ peritoneal; **renal** __ / __ renal.

dialyze *v.* dializar, hacer una diálisis.

dialyzer *n.* dializador, instrumento usado en el proceso de diálisis.

diameter *n.* diámetro.

Diana, complex of *n.* complejo de Diana, la adopción de características y conducta masculina por parte de una mujer.

diapedesis *n.* diapédesis, paso de células sanguíneas, esp. leucocitos, a través de la pared intacta de un vaso capilar.

diaper *n.* pañal; culero; *Mex.* pavico; zapeta; __ **rash** / eritema de los pañales, erupción.

diaphoresis *n.* diaforesis, perspiración excesiva causada por una temperatura elevada del cuerpo debida a intenso ejercicio físico o exposición a un calor intenso.

diaphoretic *n.* diaforético, agente que estimula la transpiración.

diaphragm *n.* diafragma. 1. músculo que separa el tórax del abdomen; 2. anticonceptivo uterino.

diaphragmatic *a.* diafragmático-a, rel. al diafragma.

diaphysis *n.* diáfisis, porción media de un hueso largo tal como se presenta en el húmero.

diarrhea *n.* diarrea; **acute** __ / __ severa; __ **infantile** / __ infantil; __ **of the newborn** / __ epidémica del recién nacido; **dysenteric** __ / __ disentérica; **emotional** __ / __ emocional; **lienteric** __ / __ lientérica; **mucous** __ / __ mucosa; **nervous** __ / __ nerviosa; **pancreatic** __ / __ pancreática; **purulent** __ / __ purulenta; **summer** __ / __ estival o de verano; **travelers'** __ / __ del viajero.

diarrheal *a.* diarreico-a, rel. a la diarrea.

diastase *n.* diastasa, enzima que actúa en la digestión de almidones y azúcares.

diastasis *n.* diastasis. 1. separación anormal de partes unidas esp. huesos; 2. tiempo de descanso del ciclo cardíaco inmediatamente anterior a la sístole.

diastole *n.* diástole, fase de dilatación del corazón durante la cual se llenan de sangre las cavidades cardíacas.

diastolic *a.* diastólico-a, rel. a la diástole del corazón; __ **pressure** / presión __ .

diathermy *n.* diatermia, aplicación de calor a los tejidos del cuerpo por medio de una corriente eléctrica.

diathesis *n.* diátesis, propensión constitucional u orgánica a contraer ciertas enfermedades; **hemorrhagic** __ / __ hemorrágica; **rheumatic** __ / __ reumática.

diatrizoate meglumine *n.* diatrizoate de meglumina, sustancia radiopaca que se usa para hacer visibles las arterias y venas del corazón y del cerebro así como la vesícula, los riñones y la vejiga.

dichotomy, dichotomization *n.* dicotomía, dicotomización, división en dos partes; bifurcación.

dichromic *a.* dicrómico-a, rel. a dos colores.

311

didelphic *a.* didélfico-a, rel. a un útero doble.

didymitis *n.* didimitis. V. **orchitis**.

die *n.* molde, troquel; *v.* morir, fallecer, dejar de existir; morirse.

diembryony *n.* diembrionismo, producción de dos embriones de un solo óvulo.

diencephalon *n.* diencéfalo, parte del cerebro.

dienestrol *n.* dienestrol, estrógeno sintético.

diet *n.* dieta, régimen; **balanced** __ / __ balanceada, equilibrada; **bland** __ / __ blanda; **diabetic** __ / __ diabética; **gluten-free** __ / __ libre de gluten; **high fiber** __ / __ alta en fibra; **liquid** __ / __ líquida; **low in fat** __ / __ baja en grasa; **low-salt** __ / __ baja de sal; **salt-free** __ / __ sin sal; **weight reduction** __ / __ para bajar de peso.

dietary *a.* dietético-a; alimenticio-a; __ **vitamins** / vitaminas __ -s.

dietetic *a.* dietético-a, rel. a la dieta o aplicado a ésta.

dietetics *n.* dietética, ciencia que regula el régimen alimenticio para preservar o recuperar la salud.

dietitian *n.* dietista, especialista en nutrición.

different *a.* diferente, distinto-a.

differential *a.* diferencial, rel. a la diferenciación; __ **diagnosis** / diagnóstico __ .

differentiate *v.* diferenciar.

differentiation *n.* diferenciación, comparación y distinción de una sustancia, enfermedad o entidad con otra o de otra.

difficult *a.* difícil.

difficulty *n.* dificultad; penalidad; obstáculo.

diffraction *n.* difracción. 1. desviación de dirección; 2. la descomposición de un rayo de luz y sus componentes al atravesar un cristal o prisma; __ **pattern** / patrón de __ .

diffuse *v.* difundir, extender.

diffused *a.* difuso-a; __ **abscess** / absceso __; __ **cutaneous mastocystosis** / mastocitosis cutánea __; __ **injury** / lesión extensa; __ **obstructive enphysema** / enfisema obstructivo __ .

diffusion *n.* difusión. 1. proceso de difundir; 2. diálisis a través de una membrana.

diffusion respiration *n.* proceso de difusión de respiración en apnea.

digest *v.* digerir.

digestant *n.* digestivo, agente que facilita la digestión.

digestion *n.* digestión, transformación de líquidos y sólidos en sustancias más simples para ser asimiladas por el organismo; **gastric** __ / __ gástrica; **intestinal** __ / __ intestinal, del intestino; **pancreatic** __ / __ pancreática.

digestive *a.* digestivo-a; rel. a la digestión; __ **system** / sistema __ .

digit *n.* dedo.

digital *a.* digital, rel. a los dedos.

digitalis *n.* digitalis, agente cardiotónico que se obtiene de las hojas secas de la *Digitalis purpurea;* __ **intoxication** / intoxicación por __ .

digitalization *n.* digitalización, uso terapéutico de digitalis.

digital radiography *n.* radiografía de imagen digital, transmisión de una imagen directa de rayos-x por medio de una computadora (ordenador).

digitoxin *n.* digitoxina, glucósido cardiotónico obtenido de digitalis y usado en el tratamiento de la congestión pasiva del corazón.

digitus *n.* dígito, dedo; __ **malleus, mallet finger** / dedo en martillo; __ **valgus, varus** / desviación de un dedo.

digoxin *n.* digoxina, un derivado de digitalis que se emplea en el tratamiento de arritmias cardíacas.

dihydrostreptomycin *n.* dihidroestreptomicina, antibiótico derivado de la estreptomicina más usado que ésta por causar menos neurotoxicidad.

dilatation, dilation *n.* dilatación, aumento o expansión anormal de un órgano u orificio.

dilate *v.* dilatar, expandir.

dilation and curettage *n.* dilatación y curetaje; *pop.* raspado.

dilator *n.* dilatador. 1. músculo que dilata un órgano al contraerse; 2. instrumento quirúrgico para expandir o dilatar un orificio o paredes; **Hegar's** __ / __ de Hegar, instrumento usado para dilatar el canal uterino.

diluent *a.* diluente, diluyente, agente o medicamento que tiene la propiedad de diluir.

dimension *n.* dimensión, medida de un cuerpo.

dimercaprol *n.* dimercaprol, antídoto usado en el envenenamiento producido por metales tales como oro y mercurio.

dimethylsulfoxide *n.* dimetilsulfóxido, medicamento antiinflamatorio y analgésico.

dimetria *n.* dimetría, útero o matriz doble.

diminish *v.* disminuir, reducir; amortiguar.

diminutive *n.* diminutivo; *a.* diminuto-a, pequeño-a.

dimness *n.* opacidad; obscurecimiento de la vista.

dimorphism *n.* dimorfismo, caracterización de dos formas diferentes; **sexual** __ / __ sexual, hermafrodismo.

dimple *n.* hoyuelo o hendidura en la piel, esp. en la mejilla o la barbilla.

dinner *n.* cena.

dioptometer *n.* dioptómetro, instrumento usado para medir la refracción ocular.

dioptric *a.* dióptrico, referente a la refración de la luz.

dioptrics *n.* dióptrica, ciencia que trata de la formación de imágenes y lentes.

diphallus *n.* difalo, duplicación parcial o completa del pene.

diphenhydramine *n.* difenhidramina, nombre comercial Benadryl, antihistamínico.

diphonia *n.* difonía, producción de dos tonos diferentes.

diphtheria *n.* difteria, enfermedad contagiosa e infecciosa aguda, causada por el bacilo *Corynebacterium diphtheriae* (Klebs-Löffler), caracterizada por la formación de membranas falsas esp. en la garganta; __ **antitoxin** / antitoxina contra la __ .

diphtherotoxin *n.* difterotoxina, toxina derivada del cultivo de bacilos de la difteria.

diplacusis *n.* diplacusia, desorden auditivo caracterizado por la percepción de dos tonos por cada sonido producido.

diplegia *n.* diplejía, parálisis bilateral; **facial** __ / __ facial, parálisis de ambos lados de la cara; **spastic** __ / __ espástica.

diplocoria *n.* diplocoria, pupila doble.

diploe *n.* diploe, tejido esponjoso localizado entre las dos capas compactas de los huesos craneales.

diploid *a.* diploide, que posee dos combinaciones de cromosomas.

diplopagus *n.* diplópagos, mellizos unidos, cada uno de cuerpo casi completo, pero que comparten algunos órganos.

diplopia *n.* diplopía, visión doble.

dipsomania *n.* dipsomanía, tipo de alcoholismo en el cual el paciente sufre una urgencia incontrolable por consumir sustancias alcohólicas.

direct *a.* directo-a; *v.* dirigir, ordenar; instruir.

direction *n.* dirección; instrucción.

directory *n.* directorio; junta; **telephone** __ / guía telefónica.

dirty *a.* sucio-a, mugriento-a; *pop.* cochino-a.

disability *n.* incapacidad, inhabilidad; invalidez, impedimento; disminución de una capacidad física o mental.

disabled *a.* inválido-a; impedido-a; incapacitado-a.

disadvantage *n.* desventaja; alguna capacidad disminuida.

disagree *v.* no estar de acuerdo; disentir; altercar, argumentar.

disagreeable *a.* desagradable; ofensivo-a.

disappoint *v.* contrariar, desengañar.

disarticulation *n.* desarticulación, separación o amputación de dos o más huesos articulados entre sí.

disassimilation *n.* disasimilación, proceso destructivo.

disbelief *n.* incredulidad, escepticismo.

discard *n.* desecho, descarte; *v.* descartar, desechar.

discharge *n.* flujo; supuración; excreción; descarga; derrame; __ **summary** / sumario o nota de egreso *v.* [*fluid, pus*] secretar, supurar; [*from the hospital*] dar de alta; librar; soltar; [*electricity*] descargar.

discipline *n.* disciplina, comportamiento estricto.

discitis *n.* discitis, infl. de un disco.

disclose *v.* revelar, descubrir; destapar, abrir.

discogenic *a.* discogénico, rel. a un disco intervertebral.

discography *n.* discografía,

discolored

radiografía de un disco vertebral
usando un medio de contraste.

discolored *a.* descolorido-a, [*skin*]
ensombrecido-a, sin color,
empañado-a.

discomfort *n.* incomodidad, malestar,
aflicción.

discomposed *a.* descompuesto-a;
desordenado-a.

disconnect *v.* desconectar, desunir,
quitar la conexión; separar.

disconnected *a.* desconectado-a,
separado-a, sin conexión, desunido-a.

discontinue *v.* suspender, interrumpir,
descontinuar; **to __ the medication /
__ la medicina.**

discontinued *a.* suspendido-a,
interrumpido-a, descontinuado-a.

discourage *v.* desanimar, desalentar;
to __ from / disuadir.

discretion *n.* discreción, prudencia;
acuerdo.

discriminate *v.* discriminar;
mostrar prejuicio; hacer notar
diferencias.

discrimination *n.* discriminación;
diferenciación de raza o
cualidad.

discuss *v.* discutir, argumentar.

discussion *n.* discusión, debate,
argumento.

disease *n.* enfermedad, dolencia,
anomalía; indisposición; **a crippling
__ / __** que causa invalidez; **blood
__ / __** sanguínea; **bone __ / __**
ósea; **cardiac __ / __** cardíaca;
**chronic obstructive pulmonary __ /
__** pulmonar crónica obstructiva; **coal
miner's __ / __** de los mineros;
communicable __ / __ contagiosa;
communicable __ control / control
de __ -es contagiosas; **companion __
/ __** concomitante; **functional __ / __**
funcional; **gallbladder __ /**
colecistopatía; **heavy chain __ / __** de
red o de cadena; **kidney __ /**
nefropatía; **liver __ / __** hepática,
renal; **venereal __ / __** venérea *v.*
causar una enfermedad, contagiar,
enfermar, dañar, hacer daño.

disease related *n.* relacionado a una
enfermedad.

diseased *a.* enfermo-a.

disengage *v.* librar, separar, desplazar.

disengagement *n.* desencajamiento,
separación, desunión; [*in obstetrics*]
desplazamiento de la cabeza del feto de
la vulva.

disfiguration *n.* desfiguración,
desfiguramiento.

disillusion *n.* desencanto, desilusión; *v.*
perder la ilusión; desilusionarse.

disinfect *v.* desinfectar, esterilizar.

disinfectant *n.* desinfectante,
antiséptico, esterilizante.

disinfection *n.* desinfección.
1. proceso de limpieza extensa y
eliminación de organismos patógenos;
2. limpieza de control de eliminación
diaria de materiales contaminados y
destrucción de microorganismos, tal
como se hace en hospitales.

disinfestation *n.* desinfestación,
limpieza extensa y eliminación de
parásitos, rumiantes e insectos
causantes de infección.

disintegration *n.* desintegración,
descomposición, separación.

disjointed *a.* desarticulado-a,
descoyuntado-a, dislocado-a.

disk, disc *n.* disco; **herniated __ / __**
herniado; **ruptured __ / ruptura del __.**

dislike *n.* aversión, antipatía; *v.*
aborrecer, desagradar, repugnar; **I __
this medicine** / no me gusta, me
desagrada, me repugna esta medicina.

dislocate *v.* dislocar, descoyuntar,
desencajar.

dislocated *a. pp.* of **to dislocate**;
dislocado-a; **__ shoulder** / luxación
del hombro.

dislocation *n.* dislocación, luxación,
desviación, desplazamiento de una
articulación; **cervical __ /** luxación
cervical; **closed __ / __** cerrada;
complicated __ / __ complicada;
congenital __ / __ congénita;
congenital __ of the hip /
congénita de la cadera; **habitual __ /
__** recidivante.

dislocation of the lens *n.*
desplazamiento del cristalino.

disobedience *n.* desobediencia.

disobedient *a.* desobediente.

disorder *n.* desorden, desarreglo,
trastorno; **mental __ /** desarreglo
emocional, trastorno mental.

disorganized *a.* desorganizado-a.

disorient *v.* desorientar.

disorientation *n.* desorientación,
incapacidad de encontrar una dirección
o local, de reconocer a otras personas, y
de establecer una relación temporal
lógica.

disoriented *a.* desorientado-a;
confundido-a, confuso-a.

dispensary *n.* dispensario, clínica, establecimiento que proporciona asistencia médica y dispensa medicamentos.

displace *v.* desplazar; poner fuera de lugar.

displaced *a.* desplazado-a; dislocado-a; *v.* **to be** ___ / estar fuera de lugar, estar___ [*bone, joint*] estar dislocado-a.

displacement *n.* desplazamiento; dislocación; transferencia de una emoción a otra distinta de la inicial; ___ **of pelvic bone** / ___ del hueso pélvico.

display *n.* muestra, exhibición, *v.* mostrar, exhibir, extender.

displeased *a.* descontento-a; insatisfecho-a.

disposable *a.* desechable.

dispose *v.* disponer; desechar; **to** ___ **of** / deshacerse de.

disposition *n.* disposición; tendencia.

disproportion *n.* desproporción; desproporcionamiento.

disproportionate *a.* desproporcionado-a, desigual, sin simetría.

disregard *v.* ignorar; no prestar atención, descuidar.

dissecting knife *n.* escalpelo, bisturí.

disseminated *a.* diseminado-a, difundido-a; ___ **intravascular coagulation** / coagulación intravascular ___ .

dissemination *n.* diseminación, esparcimiento.

dissociation *n.* disociación. 1. acción y efecto de separar; 2. descomposición de un agregado molecular en otros más sencillos; 3. separación inconsciente de la personalidad propia de la esquizofrenia, con efectos que resultan en un trastorno de las asociaciones del pensamiento; **atrial** ___ / ___ atrial; **atrioventricular** ___ / ___ atrioventricular; **pupillary light-near** ___ / ___ pupilar por cercanía de luz; **sleep** ___ / ___ del sueño; **visual-kinetic** ___ / ___ visual quinética.

dissolve *v.* disolver, diluir, deshacer; destruir.

dissolvent *a.* disolvente, capaz de disolver.

distal *a.* distal, distante, rel. a la parte más lejana; ___ **end** / extremo ___ .

distance *n.* distancia, lejanía; **at a** ___ /

a lo lejos; *v.* **to keep at a** ___ / mantener a ___ .

distemper *n.* destemplanza, cualquier trastorno físico o mental.

distend *v.* distender, dilatar; distenderse, dilatarse.

distensibility *n.* distensibilidad, capacidad de una estructura de ser extendida, dilatada o agrandada en tamaño.

distension, distention *n.* distensión, condición de dilatación o expansión.

distinct *a.* diferente; definido-a; **-ly** *adv.* definidamente; con diferencia, con precisión.

distinguish *v.* distinguir; diferenciar, clasificar.

distinguished *a.* [*person*] distinguido-a; [*characteristics*] señalado-a, marcado-a.

distobuccal *a.* distobucal, rel. a la superficie distal y bucal de un diente.

distoclusion *n.* distoclusión, mordida irregular.

distort *v.* torcer, deformar, desfigurar.

distorted *a.* torcido-a; deformado-a; desfigurado-a.

distortion *n.* distorsión, deformación, desfiguración.

distracted *a.* distraído-a, [*madness*] trastornado-a.

distraction *n.* distracción. 1. inhabilidad para concentrarse en una experiencia determinada; 2. separación de articulaciones sin dislocación.

distraught *a.* atolondrado-a, confundido-a, desconcertado-a; [*irrational*] trastornado-a.

distress *n.* angustia, apuro, preocupación, aflicción. *v.* **to be in** ___ / estar angustiado-a, estar afligido-a.

distressed *a.* adolorido-a, angustiado-a, afligido-a.

distribute *v.* distribuir, dispensar, repartir.

distribution *n.* distribución.

distrust *n.* desconfianza, falta de confianza; *v.* desconfiar.

disturb *v.* perturbar, incomodar, molestar, inquietar.

diuresis *n.* diuresis, aumento en la secreción de orina.

diuretic *a.* diurético, rel. a agentes que provocan aumento en la secreción de orina.

diuria *n.* diuria, frecuencia de excreción de orina durante el día.

diver *n.* buzo-a; ___ 's paralysis / parálisis de los ___ -s.

divergence *n.* divergencia, separación de un centro común.

divergent *a.* divergente, movimiento en sentido opuesto; ___ **reactor** / reactor de potencia ___ .

diverticulitis *n.* diverticulosis, diverticulitis, infl. de un divertículo, esp. de pequeños sacos que se forman en el colon.

diverticulosis *n.* diverticulosis, formación de divertículos en las paredes del intestino grueso o colon; **degenerative** ___ / ___ degenerativa.

diverticulum *n.* (*pl.* diverticula) divertículo, saco o bolsa que se origina en la cavidad de un órgano o estructura.

divide *v.* dividir, repartir.

divided *a.* dividido-a, separado-a.

divorce *n.* divorcio, disolución.

dizygotic twins *n., pl.* gemelos dicigóticos, mellizos de embriones producidos por dos óvulos.

dizziness *n.* mareo, sensación de desvanecimiento, vahído.

dizzy *a.* mareado-a.

do *vi. aux.* hacer; ___ **it!** / ¡hágalo!, hazlo!; ___ **not** ___ **it!** / No lo haga!, no lo hagas!; ___ **you cough a lot?** / ¿Tose mucho?, ¿toses mucho? "Do" (Do is not translated in Spanish when used as an auxiliary verb.); **How do you** ___ **?** / ¿cómo está usted?, ¿cómo estás tú?; **that will** ___ / eso es suficiente; **to** ___ **away with** / deshacerse de; **to** ___ **harm** / hacer daño; **to** ___ **one's best** / hacer lo mejor posible; **to** ___ **someone good** / mejorar, ayudar a alguien; **to** ___ **without** / pasar sin, prescindir de; **What do you** ___ **?** / ¿Qué hace usted?, ¿qué haces tú?; **whatever you** ___ / cualquier cosa que haga, hagas.

doctor *n.* doctor-a, médico-a; ___ 's **discretion** / al criterio del ___; según opinión facultativa.

document *n.* documento.

documentation *n.* documentación.

dog *n.* perro-a; ___ **bite** / mordida de ___ .

dolichocephalic *a.* dolicocefálico-a, de cráneo alargado y estrecho.

dominant *a.* dominante, característica primordial; ___ **characteristics** / características ___ -s, con tendencia a heredarse; ___ **factor** / factor ___ .

donate *v.* donar, regalar.

donation *n.* donativo, donación.

done *a., pp.* of **to do**, hecho, terminado; ___ **for** / gastado-a, destruido-a.

donor *n.* donante, donador; persona contribuyente; ___ **card** / tarjeta de ___ .

Donovania granulomatosis, Donovan's body *n.* Donovania granulomatosis, cuerpos de Donovan, infección bacteriana que afecta la piel y las membranas mucosas de los genitales y el ano.

dopamine *n.* dopamina, neurotransmisor, sustancia sintetizada por la glándula suprarrenal que aumenta la presión arterial; gen. usada en el tratamiento de choque.

dope *n.* narcótico; ___ **addict** / drogadicto-a; ___ **fiend** / narcómano-a; *v.* dopar, estimar la potencia de la dosis de una droga.

Doppler technique *n.* Doppler, técnica de, técnica de diagnóstico basada en el hecho de que la frecuencia de las ondas ultrasónicas cambia cuando éstas se reflejan en una superficie en movimiento; ___ **echocardiography** / ecocardiografía de ___; ___ **effect** / efecto de ___; ___ **ultrasonography** / ultrasonografía de ___ .

dorsal *a.* dorsal, situado-a en la parte posterior del cuerpo o rel. a ésta; ___ **recumbent position** / posición recumbente; ___ **slit** / fisura o corte ___ .

dorsalgia *n.* dorsalgia, dolor de espalda.

dorsiflexion *n.* dorsiflexión, movimiento de doblar o de doblarse hacia atrás.

dorsocephalad *a.* dorsocefálico-a, situado-a en parte posterior de la cabeza.

dorsodynia *n.* dorsodinia, dolor en los músculos de la parte superior de la espalda.

dorsolateral *a.* dorsolateral, rel. a la espalda y un costado.

dorsolumbar *a.* dorsolumbar, lumbodorsal, rel. a la espalda y la región lumbar de la columna.

dorsospinal *a.* dorsoespinal, rel. a la espalda y la espina dorsal.

dorsum *n.* (*pl.* dorsa) dorso. 1. porción posterior, tal como el dorso de la mano o el pie; 2. espalda.

drivel

dose, dosage *n.* dosis, dosificación. 1. cantidad prescrita de medicina u otro agente terapéutico; 2. en medicina nuclear, una cantidad farmacéutica determinada; **absorbed** __ / __ de absorción; **average** __ / __ promedio, media; **bone marrow** __ / __ de la médula ósea; **booster** __ / __ de refuerzo; **cumulative** __ / __ acumulada; **curative** __ / __ curativa; **daily** __ / __ diaria; **divided** __ / __ dividida; **effective** __ / __ efectiva; **equivalent** __ / __ equivalente; **exposure** __ / __ de exposición; **initial** __ / __ inicial; **integral** __ / __ integral; **lethal** __ / __ letal; **maximal** __ / __ máxima; **maximal permissible** __ / máxima __ permitida; **maximum tolerated** __ / __ máxima tolerable; **minimal** __ / __ mínima; **minimal lethal** __ / __ letal mínina; **minimal reacting** __ / __ reactiva mínima; **optimum** __ / __ óptima; **preventive** __ / __ preventiva; **radiation** __ / __ de radiación; **reduction** __ / __ de reducción; **skin** __ / __ dermal; **therapeutic** __ / __ terapéutica; **tolerated** __ / __ tolerada; **unit** __ / __ individual; **volume** __ / __ de volumen.

dot *n.* cúmulo, mancha.
double *a.* doble; __ **-edged** / con dos bordes; __ **personality** / desdoblamiento de la personalidad; __ **uterus** / útero didelfo, útero o matriz doble; *v.* duplicar.
doubt *n.* duda, incertidumbre.
douche *n.* 1. ducha, regadera; 2. lavado vaginal; irrigación. *v.* tomar una ducha; ducharse.
Douglas cul-de-sac *n.* saco de Douglas, pliegue del peritoneo que se introduce entre el recto y el útero.
down *adv.* abajo, hacia abajo; __ **below** / más abajo; *v.* **to cut** __ / recortar; reducir; **to lie** __ / acostarse, recostarse.
downcast *a.* deprimido-a, alicaído-a, abatido-a.
downstairs *v.* **to go** __ / bajar las escaleras; *adv.* abajo.
Down syndrome *n.* síndrome de Down, anormalidad citogenética del cromosoma 21 caracterizada por retraso mental y facciones mongoloides.
doze *v.* dormitar, quedarse medio dormido.

dozen *n.* docena.
draft *n.* 1. líquido prescrito para ser tomado en una sola dosis; 2. [*air*] corriente de aire; 3. [*art design*] diseño, bosquejo.
drain *n.* desagüe, escurridor. *v.* drenar, desaguar, eliminar una secreción o pus de una parte infectada.
drainage *n.* drenaje; **open** __ / __ abierto; **continuous** __ / __ continuo; __ **tube** / tubo de __; **postural** __ / __ postural, por gravedad; **tidal** __ / __ periódico.
Dramamine, dimenhydrinate *n.* Dramamina, dimenhidrinato, anthistamínico usado en el tratamiento de náusea.
dramatism *n.* dramatismo, conducta espectacular y lenguaje dramatizado manifestados en ciertos trastornos mentales.
drape *v.* cubrir el campo operatorio con paños esterilizados.
drastic *a.* drástico-a; __ **therapy** / tratamiento __ .
draw *vi.* extraer, sacar; [*air*] aspirar; [*art*] dibujar, trazar; **to** __ **back** / retroceder; **to** __ **in** / atraer; incitar; **to** __ **near** / acercarse, arrimarse.
dream *n.* sueño, ilusión. *v.* soñar, imaginar, hacerse ilusiones.
drenched *a.* empapado-a, mojado-a.
dress *n.* vestido. *v.* [*a wound*] vendar, curar; [*a corpse*] amortajar; [*put on clothes*] vestirse.
dressing *n.* apósito o vendaje, venda de gasa u otro material para cubrir una herida; **adhesive, absorbent** __ / __ adhesivo, absorbente; **antiseptic** __ / __ antiséptico; **dry** __ / __ seco; **fixed** __ / __ fijo; **occlusive** __ / __ oclusivo; **pressured** __ / __ presionado; **removable** __ / __ desechable; **tie-over** __ / __ amarrado; **wet** __ / __ humedecido.
dribble *n.* goteo.
drink *n.* bebida, trago. *v.* beber, tomar.
drinker *a.* bebedor, tomador.
drip *n.* gota, goteo; gotera; **postnasal** __ / __ postnasal *v.* gotear.
drive *n.* paseo, vuelta; impulso; [*haste*] exigencia; [*energy*] energía, vigor; *v.* **to go for a** __ / dar un paseo; *vi.* [*vehicles*] conducir, manejar, guiar; **to** __ **someone crazy** / enloquecer, volver loco-a.
drivel *n.* baba o saliva que sale por los extremos de la boca.

dromotropic

dromotropic *a.* dromotrópico-a, que afecta la conductividad de una fibra muscular o nerviosa.

drop *n.* gota; caída; **— by—** / gota a gota; *v.* dejar caer; [*from school*] dejar la escuela; caerse.

droplet *n.* partícula, gotica; **— infection** / infección trasmitida por goticas o partículas.

dropper *n.* gotero.

dropsy *n.* hidropesía, acumulación excesiva de fluido seroso en una cavidad o tejido celular.

drowning *n.* ahogamiento, acción de ahogar o ahogarse.

drowse *v.* adormecerse, adormitarse.

drowsiness *n.* sopor, somnolencia, abotagamiento, pesadez.

drug *n.* droga, medicamento, narcótico, barbitúrico; **— abuse** / uso excesivo de una **—** por adicción; **— addict** / narcómano-a, drogadicto-a; **— -induced abnormality** / anomalía causada por el uso de **—** -s; **— interactions** / interacciones de medicamentos; **— resistance, microbial** / resistencia microbiana a las **—** -s; **long acting —** / **—** de acción prolongada.

drugged *a.* endrogado-a, drogado-a.

drunk *n.* borracho-a, ebrio-a.

dry *a.* seco-a; árido-a; *v.* secar; **— abscess** / absceso **—**; **— cough** / tos **—**; **— gangrene** / gangrena **—**; **to — out** / secarse.

dryness *n.* sequedad; aridez.

duct *n.* conducto, canal; **biliary —** / biliar; **common bile** / colédoco; **cystic —** / cístico; **deferent —** / defrente; **ejaculatory —** / eyaculatorio; **excretory —** / excretorio; **hepatic —** / hepático; **lacrimal —** / lacrimal; **lactiferous—** / lactífero; **lymphatic —** / linfático; **mullerian —** / mullerian; **nasolacrimal —** / nasolagrimal; **lacrimal —** / lacrimal; **mammary —** / mamario; **seminal —** / seminal; **seminiferous tubule —** / seminífero. V. cuadro en la página 76.

ductal *a.* rel. a un conducto o canal.

ductile *a.* dúctil, que tiene la propiedad de admitir deformaciones sin romperse.

ductule *n.* túbulo, conducto pequeño.

dues *n., pl.* deuda; obligación.

dull *a.* aburrido-a; [*pain*] dolor sordo; [*blade*] mellado-a.

dullness *n.* 1. matidez, resonancia disminuída en la palpación; 2. estado de aburrimiento, torpeza, estupidez; 3. [*instrument's edge*] melladura.

dumb *a.* mudo-a; torpe, estúpido-a.

dumping syndrome *n.* síndrome de vaciamiento gástrico demasiado rápido del contenido estomacal en el intestino delgado.

duodenal *a.* duodenal, rel. al duodeno.

duodenal ulcer *n.* úlcera duodenal.

duodenectomy *n.* duodenectomía, excisión del duodeno o una parte de éste.

duodenitis *n.* duodenitis, infl. del duodeno.

duodenoenterostomy *n.* duodenoenterostomía, anastomosis entre el duodeno y el intestino delgado.

duodenojejunostomy *n.* duodenoyeyunostomía, operación para construir un pasaje artificial entre el yeyuno y el duodeno.

duodenoplasty *n.* duodenoplastia, operación para reparar el duodeno.

duodenostomy *n.* duodenostomía, creación de una salida en el duodeno, para aliviar la estenosis del píloro.

duodenum *n.* duodeno, parte esencial del canal alimenticio y del intestino delgado situado entre el píloro y el yeyuno.

duplication *n.* doblez, pliegue; duplicación.

dura mater *n.* duramadre, membrana externa que cubre el encéfalo y la médula espinal.

durability *n.* durabilidad, duración.

durable *a.* durable, duradero-a; estable.

duration *n.* duración, continuación.

duress *n.* coerción; coacción, **under —** / bajo **—** .

during *prep.* durante; mientras, entre tanto.

dust *n.* polvo; [*mortal remains*] cenizas, restos mortales; **— count** / conteo de partículas de **—** en el aire.

dwarf *n.* enano-a, persona de estatura inferior a la normal; **achondroplastic —** / acondroplástico-a; **asexual —** / asexual; **infantile —** / infantil; **micrometic —** / micromético-a.

dwarfism *n.* enanismo, insuficiencia del desarrollo en el crecimiento de una persona.

dye *n.* tinte, color saturado; colorante.

dying *a.* moribundo-a, agonizante, mortal.

dynamic cardiomyoplastia *n.* cardiomioplastia dinámica, intervención que se lleva a cabo en pacientes clasificados bajo cardiopatía clase III que han sufrido fallo cardíaco o que padecen de isquemia cardíaca.

dynamics *n.* dinámica, estudio de órganos o partes del cuerpo en movimiento.

dysacousia, dysacusia *n.* disacusis, disacusia, trastorno o dificultad para oír.

dysaphia *n.* disafia, entorpecimiento del sentido del tacto.

dysarthria *n.* disartria, dificultad del habla a causa de una afección de la lengua u otro músculo esencial al lenguaje.

dysautonomy, dysautonomia *n.* disautonomía, trastorno del sistema nervioso autónomo.

dysbarism *n.* disbarismo, condición causada por descompresión.

dyscephalia *n.* discefalia, malformación de la cabeza y los huesos de la cara.

dyscoria *n.* discoria, pupila deformada.

dyscrasia *n.* discrasia, sinónimo de enfermedad.

dysentery *n.* disentería, condición inflamatoria del intestino grueso causada por bacilos o parásitos con síntomas de diarrea y dolor abdominal; **amebic** ___ / ___ amebiana; **bacillar** ___ / ___ bacilar.

dysesthesia *n.* disestesia, reacción excesiva de molestia a algunas sensaciones que por lo común no producen dolor.

dysfunction *n.* desorden, trastorno, malfuncionamiento de un órgano o parte.

dysgenesis *n.* disgénesis, defecto, malformación hereditaria.

dysgerminoma *n.* disgerminoma, tumor maligno del ovario.

dyshidrosis *n.* dishidrosis. 1. trastorno transpiratorio; 2. erupción recurrente de vesículas y picazón tal como en el pie de atleta.

dyskinesia *n.* discinesia, disquinesia,

inhabilidad de realizar movimientos voluntarios tal como sucede en la enfermedad de Parkinson.

dyslalia *n.* dislalia, impedimento en el habla debido a trastornos vocálicos funcionales.

dyslexia *n.* dislexia, impedimento en la lectura, dificultad que puede ser una condición hereditaria o causada por una lesión cerebral.

dysmenorrhea, dysmenorrhoea *n.* dismenorrea, menstruación difícil, acompañada de dolor y trastornos.

dysmetria *n.* dismetría, afección del cerebelo que incapacita el control de la distancia en movimientos musculares.

dysmnesia *n.* dismnesia, trastorno de la memoria.

dysmorphism *n.* dismorfismo, malformación anatómica.

dysmyotonia *n.* dismiotonía, distonía muscular con tonicidad muscular anormal.

dysosmia *n.* disosmia, malfuncionamiento de la función olfatoria.

dysostosis *n.* disostosis, desarrollo deficiente de los huesos y dientes.

dyspareunia *n.* dispareunia, relaciones sexuales dolorosas.

dyspepsia *n.* dispepsia, indigestión caracterizada por irregularidades digestivas tales como eructos, náuseas, acidez, flatulencia y pérdida del apetito.

dyspermia *n.* dispermia, dolor durante la eyaculación.

dysphagia *n.* disfagia, dificultad al tragar a causa de una obstrucción; **esophageal** ___ / ___ esofágica; **oropharyngeal** ___ / ___ orofaríngea.

dysphasia *n.* disfasia, defecto del habla causado por una lesión cerebral.

dysphonia *n.* disfonía, ronquera.

dysphoria *n.* disforia, excesiva depresión o angustia.

dyspigmentation *n.* despigmentación, decoloración anormal de la piel y del pelo.

dysplasia *n.* displasia, cambio o desarrollo anormal de los tejidos.

dysplastic *a.* displásico-a, pertaining to dysplasia.

dyspnea, dyspnoea *n.* disnea, dificultad en la respiración; **exertional** ___ / ___ por esfuerzo.

dyspneic *a.* disneico-a, rel. a o que padece de disnea.

dyspraxia

dyspraxia *n.* dispraxia, impedimento o dolor al realizar cualquier movimiento coordinado.

dysreflexia *n.* disrreflexia, condición por la cual las reacciones a estímulos son inapropiadas o fuera de orden.

dysrhythmia *n.* disritmia, sin coordinación o ritmo.

dysstasia *n.* distasia, dificultad de mantenerse en pie.

dyssynergia *n.* disinergia. V. **ataxia.**

dystocia *n.* distocia, parto difícil, laborioso.

dystonia *n.* distonía, tonicidad alterada, esp. muscular.

dystrophy *n.* distrofia. 1. anomalía causada por desnutrición; 2. desarrollo defectuoso o de malformación.

dysuria *n.* disuria, dificultad o dolor al orinar.

E *abbr.* **emmetropia** / emetropía; **enema** / enema; **enzyme** / enzima; **eye** / ojo.

ear *n.* oreja; oído, órgano de la audición formado por el oído interior, el medio, y el externo; __ **ache** / dolor de oídos, otalgia; __ **canal** / conducto auditivo; __ **cup** / audífono; __ **discharge** / otorrea; __ **drops** / gotas para los oídos; __ **infection** / infección auditiva; __ **injury** / oído lastimado, lesión auditiva; __ **lap** / pabellón de la oreja; __ **lobe** / lóbulo de la oreja; __ **lobe crease** / pliegue del lóbulo del oído; __ **plug** / tapón auditivo; __ **protector** / orejera; __ **specialist** / otólogo, audiólogo; __ **wax** / cerumen; *a.* __ **deafening** / ensordecedor-a. V. ilustración esta página.

earache *n.* dolor de oído.

eardrum *n.* tímpano del oído.

early *adv.* temprano, pronto; __ **ambulation** / ambulación temprana; **as** __ **as possible** / lo más __ posible; **at the earliest** / lo más __; __ **age** / infancia; __ **cancer** / cáncer incipiente; __ **childhood** / primera infancia; __ **death** / muerte prematura; __

detection / detención temprana; __ **morning** / madrugada; __ **pregnancy** / principio del embarazo; __ **stage of** / la primera fase de, al principio de.

earphone *n.* auricular, audífono.

earthworm *n.* lombriz de tierra; gusano.

ease *n.* alivio; descanso; facilidad; *v.* aliviar, facilitar; **to** __ **one's mind** / tranquilizarse.

easily *adv.* fácilmente, sin dificultad.

east *n.* este, oriente; **to the** __ / al __ .

easy *a.* fácil; **within** __ **reach** / al alcance de la mano.

easygoing *a.* sereno-a, tranquilo-a, de buena disposición.

eat *vi.* comer, sustentarse, ingerir alimentos; **to** __ **breakfast** / desayunarse, tomar el desayuno; **to** __ **lunch** / almorzar; tomar el almuerzo; **to** __ **supper** / cenar.

eating *n.* acto de comer; *a.* rel. a comer o para comer; __ **disorder** / trastorno alimenticio.

ebullition *n.* ebullición, acto de hervir.

eccentric *a.* excéntrico-a; extravagante.

ecchymosis *n.* equimosis, *pop.* morado, moratón. 1. cambio de color de la piel de azulado a verde debido a extravasación de sangre en el tejido subcutáneo celular; 2. hematoma.

eccrine sweat glands *n.* glándulas sudoríparas ecrinas, secretoras de la transpiración.

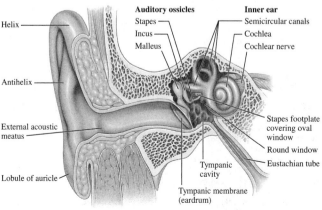

Helix

Antihelix

External acoustic meatus

Lobule of auricle

Auditory ossicles
Stapes
Incus
Malleus

Inner ear
Semicircular canals
Cochlea
Cochlear nerve

Stapes footplate covering oval window
Round window
Eustachian tube

Tympanic cavity

Tympanic membrane (eardrum)

Ear structures

echinacea *n.* equinacea, planta medicinal que reduce la inflamación.

echinococcosis *n.* equinococosis, infestación de equinococos; **hepatic** __ / __ hepática.

Echinococcus *n.* Equinococo, especie de tenia o trematodo.

echo *n.* eco, repercusión del sonido; *v.* **to** __ / hacer __.

echocardiogram *n.* ecocardiograma, gráfico producido por una ecocardiografía.

echocardiography *n.* ecocardiografía, método de diagnóstico por sonido ultrasónico para hacer visuales estructuras internas del corazón.

echoencephalography *n.* ecoencefalografía, técnica de diagnóstico por medio de ultrasonido para examinar estructuras intracraneales.

echogram *n.* ecograma, registro de una ecografía.

echolalia *n.* ecolalia, trastorno de repetición involuntaria de sonidos y palabras después de oírlas.

Echo virus *n.* Echo virus, virus presente en el tracto gastrointestinal asociado con la meningitis, enteritis e infecciones respiratorias agudas.

eclampsia *n.* eclampsia, desorden convulsivo tóxico que se presenta gen. al final del embarazo o pocos días después del parto.

ecological *a.* ecológico, __ **system** / sistema __; ecosistema.

ecology *n.* ecología, estudio de plantas y animales en relación con el ambiente.

economic *a.* económico-a; módico-a, moderado-a.

ecosystem *n.* ecosistema, microcosmo ecológico.

ecstasy *n.* 1. éxtasis, trance acompañado de un sentimiento de placer; 2. droga de diseño.

ectoderm *n.* ectodermo, la más externa de las tres capas primarias del embrión.

ectopic pregnancy *n.* embarazo ectópico, gestación fuera del útero.

ectoplasm *n.* ectoplasma, capa externa del citoplasma en una célula viva.

ectropion *n.* ectropión, anomalía de eversión congénita o adquirida, gen. vista en la comisura del párpado.

eczema *n.* eczema, infección cutánea inflamatoria no contagiosa.

edema *n.* edema, acumulación anormal de líquido en los tejidos intracelulares; **angioneurotic** __ / __ angioneurótico; **brain** __ / __ cerebral; **cardiac** __ / __ cardíaco; **dependent** __ / __ dependiente; **pitting** __ / __ de fóvea; **pulmonary** __ / __ pulmonar.

edge *n.* borde, orilla, canto; [*of cutting instruments*] filo; **on** __ / irritable, impaciente, nervioso-a.

edible *a.* comestible; edible.

educate *v.* educar, enseñar, instruir.

education *n.* educación, enseñanza; **medical** __ / __ médica.

effacement *n.* borradura, deformación de las características de un órgano tal como la del cuello uterino durante el parto.

effect *n.* efecto, impresión, resultado; *v.* **to carry into** __ / llevar a cabo; **to this** __ / en este sentido; **in** __ / en __ , en realidad; **no** __ **without results** / no __ sin resultados.

effector *n.* efector, terminación nerviosa que produce un efecto eferente en una glándula de secreción o en una célula muscular.

effeminate *a.* afeminado, *pop.* invertido-a.

efferent *a.* eferente, de fuerza centrífuga; __**arterioles** / arteriolas __; __ **nerves** / nervios __; __ **neurons** / neuronas __ -es.

effervescent *a.* efervescente, que produce efervescencia.

efficient *a.* eficiente; **-ly** *adv.* eficientemente.

effluent *a.* efluente, que tiene salida de dentro hacia afuera.

effort *n.* esfuerzo, empeño; *v.* **to make every** __ **to** / hacer todo lo posible por.

effusion *n.* efusión, derrame, escape de líquido a una cavidad o tejido; **pericardial** __ / __ pericardial; **pleural** __ / __ pleural.

egg *n.* huevo; *Mex.* blanquillos; __ **cell** / óvulo; __ **-shaped** / ovoide; __ **white** / clara de __; __ **yolk** / yema de __; **fried** __ / huevo frito; **hard-boiled** __ / huevo duro; **soft-boiled** __ / __ pasado por agua.

ego *n.* ego, el yo; la conciencia humana; término freudiano que se refiere a la parte de la psique mediadora entre la persona y la realidad.

egocentric *a.* egocéntrico-a, concentrado-a en si mismo-a.

egoism *n.* egoísmo.

elementary

egomania *n.* egomanía, concentración
excesiva en sí mismo-a.
either *a., pron.* uno-a u otro-a; *conj.* o;
adv. también; [*after negation*] tampoco.
ejaculate *v.* eyacular, expeler.
ejaculation *n.* eyaculación, expulsión
rápida y súbita tal como la emisión del
semen.
ejaculatory duct *n.* conducto
eyaculatorio.
ejection *n.* eyección, acto de expulsar
con fuerza.
elastic *n.* elástico, cinta de goma; *a.*
elástico-a, capaz de extenderse y de
volver luego a la forma inicial; __
tissue / tejido __ .
elation *n.* estado de exaltación o euforia,
caracterizado por excitación física y
mental.
elbow *n.* codo; __ **joint** / coyuntura
del __; __ **room** / espacio suficiente;
tennis __ / __ de tenista.
elder *a.* mayor, de más edad; anciano-a;
antepasados, los mayores.
elderly *adv.* de avanzada edad.
eldest *a. sup.* el mayor, la mayor.
elect *v.* elegir, escoger.
elective *a.* electivo-a, elegido-a; __
surgery / cirugía __ , planeada; __
therapy / terapia __ .
electric *a.* eléctrico-a; __ **current** /
corriente __; __ **eye** / ojo mágico,
ojo __ .
electrical *a.* eléctrico-a.
electricity *n.* electricidad.
electrocardiogram *n.*
electrocardiograma, gráfico de cambios
eléctricos que se producen durante las
contracciones del músculo cardíaco.
electrocardiograph *n.*
electrocardiógrafo, instrumento para
registrar las variaciones eléctricas del
músculo cardíaco en acción.
electrocauterization *n.*
electrocauterización, destrucción de
tejidos por medio de una corriente
eléctrica.
**electroconvulsive therapy
(ECT)** *n.* terapéutica de choque,
electrochoque, tratamiento de ciertos
desórdenes mentales con aplicación de
corriente eléctrica al cerebro.
electrode *n.* electrodo, medio entre la
corriente eléctrica y el objeto al que se
le aplica la corriente.
electrodiagnosis *n.* electrodiagnosis,
el uso de instrumentos electrónicos
para uso de diagnóstico.

electroencephalography *n.*
electroencefalografía, gráfico
descriptivo de la actividad eléctrica
desarrollada en el cerebro.
electrolysis *n.* electrolisis,
descomposición de una sustancia por
medio de una corriente eléctrica.
electrolyte *n.* electrolito, ion que
conduce una carga eléctrica.
electromagnetic *a.*
electromagnético-a; __ **spectrum** /
espectro __ .
electromyogram *n.*
electromiograma, reporte gráfico por
medio de una electromiografía.
electromyography *n.*
electromiografía. 1. grabación de la
actividad eléctrica generada en un
músculo para uso de diagnóstico;
2. estudio de laboratorio sobre
electrodiagnóstico que incluye no sólo
la electromiografía sino también
estudios sobre la conducción de los
nervios.
electronic *a.* electrónico-a; __ **fetal
monitoring** / monitoreo electrónico
fetal.
electron microscope *n.*
microscopio electrónico, microscopio
visual y fotográfico en el cual los rayos
electrónicos poseen la longitud de onda
miles de veces más corta que la luz
visible. La capacidad de resolución y
magnificación de este microscopio
permite la ampliación máxima de
objetos muy pequeños.
electrophoresis *n.* electroforesis,
movimiento de partículas coloidales en
un medio que, al someterse a una
corriente eléctrica, las separa, tal como
ocurre con la separación de proteínas
en el plasma.
electrophysiology *n.*
electrofisiología, estudio de la relación
entre procesos fisiológicos afectados
por fenómenos eléctricos.
electroretinogram *n.*
electroretinograma, registro gráfico de
la retina.
electrosurgery *n.* electrocirugía,
uso de electricidad en procesos
quirúrgicos.
electroversion *n.* electroversión,
cesación de una disrritmia cardíaca por
un medio eléctrico.
element *n.* elemento, componente.
elementary *a.* elemental;
rudimentario-a.

elephantiasis *n.* elefantiasis, enfermedad crónica caracterizada por obstrucción de los vasos linfáticos e hipertrofia de la piel y tejido celular subcutáneo que afecta gen. las extremidades inferiores y los órganos genitales externos.

elevation *n.* elevación; altura.

elevator *n.* elevador. 1. instrumento quirúrgico que se usa para levantar partes hendidas o para extirpar tejido óseo; 2. ascensor.

eligible *a.* elegible, electivo-a.

eliminate *v.* eliminar, expeler del organismo; suprimir.

elimination diet *n.* dieta de eliminación, dieta reguladora del tipo de alimentos que el paciente debe ingerir después de detectar los ingredientes que pueden producirle una reacción alérgica.

elixir *n.* elixir, licor dulce y aromático que contiene un ingrediente medicinal activo.

elongated *a.* alargado-a, estirado-a, como el sistema de las vías digestivas.

else *a.* otro-a; más; **anyone ___** / alguien más; **anything ___** / algo más; **nothing ___** / nada más; **Who ___ needs help?** / ¿Quién más necesita ayuda?

emaciated *a.* enflaquecido-a; excesivamente delgado-a; emaciado a.

emasculation *n.* emasculación; castración; mutilación.

embalming *n.* embalsamamiento, preservación del cuerpo después de la muerte por medio de sustancias químicas.

embolism *n.* embolismo, embolia, oclusión súbita de un vaso por un coágulo, placa o aire; **cerebral ___** / **___ cerebral; pulmonary ___** / **___** pulmonar.

embolus *n.* émbolo, coágulo u otro tipo de materia que, al circular a través de la corriente sanguínea, se aloja en un vaso de menor diámetro.

embryo *n.* embrión. 1. fase primitiva de desarrollo del ser humano desde la concepción hasta la séptima semana; 2. organismo en la fase primitiva de desarrollo.

embryology *n.* embriología, estudio del embrión y su desarrollo hasta el momento del nacimiento.

embryonic carcinoma *n.* carcinoma embrionario, neoplasma maligno del testículo.

emergency *n.* emergencia, urgencia; **an ___ case** / un caso de ___; **___ care** / servicio de ___; **___ childbirth** / nacimiento repentino; **___ medical identification bracelets** / brazaletes para identificación médica de ___; **___ operation** / intervención quirúrgica de urgencia; **___ room** / sala de ___; **___ tracheostomy** / traqueotomía de urgencia.

emetic *a.* emético-a, que estimula el vómito.

emigration *n.* emigración o migración, escape tal como el de leucocitos a través de las paredes de los capilares y las venas.

eminence *n.* eminencia o prominencia, forma de elevación semejante a la de la superficie de un hueso.

emission *n.* emisión, salida de líquido; derrame; **nocturnal ___** / **___ nocturna**, escape involuntario de semen durante el sueño.

emit *v.* emitir, descargar; manifestar una opinión.

emollient *a.* emoliente, que suaviza la piel o mucosas interiores.

emotion *n.* emoción, sentimiento intenso.

emotional *a.* emocional, rel. a las emociones; **___ disturbances** / síntomas afectivos; **___ life** / vida afectiva.

empathy *n.* empatía, comprensión y apreciación de los sentimientos de otra persona.

emphysema *n.* enfisema, enfermedad crónica pulmonar en la cual los alvéolos pulmonares se distienden y los tejidos localizados entre los mismos se atrofian y dificultan el proceso respiratorio.

empiric *a.* empírico-a, que se basa en observaciones prácticas.

employee *n.* empleado-a.

employment *n.* empleo, ocupación.

empty *a.* vacío-a, desocupado-a; *v.* vaciar, desocupar; **to ___ itself** / vaciarse, desocuparse.

empyema *n., L.* (*pl.* **empyemato**) empiema, acumulación de pus en una cavidad, esp. la cavidad torácica.

emulsion *n.* emulsión, mezcla de dos líquidos, uno de los cuales permanece suspendido.

enamel *n.* esmalte, sustancia dura que protege la dentina del diente.

enarthrosis *n.* enartrosis, forma ósea en la que la cabeza del hueso hace cabida dentro de la cavidad redondeada del otro hueso, como en la articulación de la cadera.

encanthis *n.* encantis, pequeño quiste en el ángulo anterior del párpado.

encephalalgia *n.* encefalalgia, dolor de cabeza intenso.

encephalic *a.* encefálico-a, rel. al encéfalo o cerebro.

encephalitis *n.* encefalitis, infl. del encéfalo; **acute hemorrhagic** __ / __ aguda hemorrágica; **acute necrotizing** __ / __ aguda necrotizante; **bacterial** __ / __ bacteriana; **epidemic** __ / __ epidémica; **experimental allergic** __ / __ experimental alérgica; **herpes** __ / __ herpética; **lethargic** __ / __ letárgica; **neonatorum** __ / __ del recién nacido; **purulent** __ / __ purulenta; **pyogenic** __ / __ piogénica; **suppurative** __ / __ supurativa.

encephalocele *n.* encefalocele, hernia del encéfalo, protrusión del encéfalo a través de una abertura congénita o traumática en el cráneo.

encephalogram *n.* encefalograma, examen radiográfico del cerebro.

encephaloma *n.* encefaloma, tumor del encéfalo.

encephalomalacia *n.* encefalomalacia, reblandecimiento del encéfalo.

encephalomyelitis *n.* encefalomielitis, infl. del encéfalo y de la médula espinal.

encephalon *n.* encéfalo, porción del sistema nervioso contenido en el cráneo.

encephalopathy *n.* encefalopatía, cualquier enfermedad cerebral.

enchondroma *n.* encondroma, tumor que se desarrolla en un hueso.

encircle *v.* rodear, circundar.

enclose *v.* encerrar, cercar; [*in a letter*] incluir, adjuntar.

enclosed *a. pp.* of **to enclose**, [*in a letter*] incluido-a, adjunto-a.

encopresis *n.* encopresis, incontinencia de heces fecales.

encourage *v.* alentar, animar.

encouragement *n.* aliento, incentivo.

encysted *a.* enquistado-a, que se encuentra envuelto en un saco o quiste.

end *n.* fin, término, extremidad; extremo; [*aim*] objetivo; **at the** __ **of** / al extremo de; [*date*] a fines de; **To what** __ **?** / ¿Con qué __ ?; *a.* terminal, final; __ **artery** / arteria terminal; __ **organ** / órgano terminal.

endanger *v.* poner en peligro. *v.* arriesgarse.

endangered *a. pp.* of **to endanger.** 1. puesto en peligro; 2. en peligro de extinción.

endarteritis *n.* endarteritis, infl. de la túnica (íntima) de una arteria.

endbrain *n.* telencéfalo, porción o parte del sistema nervioso que comprende la corteza cerebral, el cuerpo calloso, el cuerpo estriado y el rinencéfalo.

endeavor *n.* empeño, esfuerzo.

endemic *a.* endémico-a, rel. a una enfermedad que permanece por un tiempo indefinido en una comunidad o región; __ **area** / área __; __ **disease** / enfermedad __ .

endemoepidemic *n.* endemoepidemia, término que indica un aumento de casos de una enfermedad endémica.

ending *n.* final; terminación, conclusión.

endocarditis *n.* endocarditis, infl. aguda o crónica del endocardio; **acute bacterial** __ / __ aguda bacteriana; **bacterial** __ / __ bacteriana; **chronic** __ / __ crónica; **constrictive** __ / __ constrictiva; **infectious** / __ infecciosa; **malignant** __ / __ maligna; **mucomembranous** __ / __ mucomembranosa; **rheumatic** __ / __ reumática; **subacute bacterial** __ / __ subaguda bacteriana; **tuberculous** __ / __ tuberculosa; **valvular** __ / __ valvular; **vegetative** __ / __ vegetativa.

endocardium *n.* (*pl.* **endocardia**) endocardio, membrana serosa interior del corazón.

endocervicitis *n.* endocervicitis, infl. de las glándulas y epitelio del cuello uterino y el útero.

endocervix *n.* endocérvix, mucosa glandular del cuello uterino.

endocrine *a.* endocrino-a, rel. a secreciones internas y a las glándulas que las producen.

endocrine glands *n.* glándulas endocrinas, glándulas que segregan hormonas directamente en la corriente sanguínea (gónadas, pituitaria y suprarrenales).

endocrinologist *n.* endocrinólogo, especialista en endocrinología.

endocrinology

endocrinology *n.* endocrinología, estudio de las glándulas endocrinas y las hormonas segregadas por éstas.

endoderm *n.* endodermo, la más interna de las tres membranas del embrión.

endogenous *a.* endógeno-a, que ocurre debido a factores internos del organismo.

endolymphatic duct *n.* conducto endolinfático localizado en el oído.

endometrial *a.* endometrial, rel. al endometrio; ___ **biopsy** / biopsia ___ ; ___ **cyst** / quiste ___ .

endometriosis *n.* endometriosis, trastorno por el cual tejido similar al del endometrio se manifiesta en otras partes fuera del útero.

endometritis *n.* endometritis, infl. de la mucosa uterina.

endometrium *n.* endometrio, membrana mucosa interior del útero.

endomorph *a.* endomorfo-a, de torso más pronunciado que las extremidades.

endomyocarditis *n.* endomiocarditis, infl. de las capas internas del corazón, del endocardio y miocardio.

endophthalmitis, endophthalmia *n.* endoftalmitis, infl. de los tejidos interiores del globo ocular, la cual puede ser causada por una reacción alérgica, la reacción a una droga o una reacción bacteriológica. El ojo se enrojece, se infecta, y a veces tiene pus. Otros síntomas que pueden manifestarse son vómito, fiebre (calentura) y dolor de cabeza; ___ **ophthalmia nodose** / oftalmia nodular; ___ **phacoanaphylactica** / ___ facoanafiláctica; **granulomatous** ___ / ___ granulomatosa.

end organ *n.* órgano terminal.

endorphins *n., pl.* endorfinas, sustancias químicas naturales del cerebro a las que se le atribuye la propiedad de aliviar el dolor.

endoscope *n.* endoscopio, instrumento usado para examinar un órgano o una cavidad interior hueca.

endoscopy *n.* endoscopía, examen interior hecho con el endoscopio.

endosteum *n.* (*pl.* **endostea**) endostio, células localizadas en la cavidad medular central de los huesos que sirven de cobertura a la superficie interior del hueso.

endothelium *n.* (*pl.* **endothelia**) endotelio, capa celular interna que reviste los vasos sanguíneos, los canales linfáticos, el corazón y otras cavidades.

endotoxemia *n.* endotoxemia, presencia en la sangre de endotoxinas.

endotoxic shock *n.* choque endotóxico.

endotoxin *n.* endotoxina, toxina venenosa excretada después que el organismo venenoso muere; es menos potente que la exotoxina. La persona infectada puede tener síntomas de fiebre, escalofríos y choque.

endotracheal *a.* endotraqueal, dentro de la tráquea; ___ **tube, cuffed** / tubo ___ con manguito.

endotracheal anesthesia *n.* anestesia endotraqueal, el anestésico y los gases respiratorios pasan por vía bucal y nasal a través de un tubo a la tráquea.

end-stage (ESRD) *n.* fase terminal.

endurable *a.* soportable, aguantable, tolerable.

endurance *n.* resistencia; tolerancia; **beyond** ___ / más allá de lo que puede soportarse, intolerable.

endure *v.* soportar, sobrellevar, resistir, aguantar.

enema *n.* enema, lavado, lavativa; **barium** ___ / ___ de bario; **cleansing** ___ / lavativa, lavado; **double contrast** ___ / ___ de contraste doble; **retention** ___ / ___ de retención.

energetic *a.* enérgico-a, vigoroso-a, lleno-a de energía.

energy *n.* energía, la capacidad de trabajar, de moverse y hacer ejercicio con vigor; **chemical** ___ / ___ química; ___ **of activation** / ___ de activación; **free** ___ / ___ libre; **fusion** ___ / ___ de fusión; **internal** ___ / ___ interna; **kinetic** ___ / ___ cinética; **latent** ___ / ___ latente; **nuclear** ___ / ___ nuclear; **nutritional** ___ / ___ nutritiva; **potential** ___ / ___ potencial; **psychic** ___ / ___ síquica; **solar** ___ / ___ solar; **total** ___ / ___ total.

enervate *v.* 1. extirpar un nervio; 2. debilitar, enervar.

enforce *v.* [*rules, law*] hacer cumplir.

engaged *a.* encajado-a, ajustado-a, conectado-a; [*undertaken*] comprometido-a.

engagement *n.* [*birth*] encajamiento de la cabeza fetal.

English *n.* [*language*] inglés; [*native*] *a.* inglés, inglesa.

ependymoma

engorged *a.* ingurgitado-a.
1. distendido por exceso de líquidos;
2. congestionado de sangre.

engram *n.* engrama. 1. marca
permanente hecha en el protoplasma
por un estímulo pasajero; 2. vestigio o
visión imborrable producida por una
experiencia sensorial.

enhance *v.* aumentar el valor,
intensificar; [*beautify*] realzar.

enhancement *n.* aumento de un
efecto tal como el de radiaciones por
oxígeno u otro elemento químico.

enjoy *v.* disfrutar, gozar de.

enkephalins *n.*, *pl.* encefalinas,
sustancias químicas (polipéptidos)
producidas en el cerebro.

enlarge *v.* ampliar, expandir, agrandar;
ensanchar.

enlarged *pp.* dilatado, agrandado,
aumentado; ___ **liver** / hígado
agrandado; ___ **prostate** / hipertrofia
prostática.

enophthalmos *n.* enoftalmia,
hundimiento del globo ocular.

enormous *a.* enorme, muy grande.

enough *a. adv.* bastante, suficiente; **fair**
___ / de acuerdo; **large** ___ / bastante
grande; **sure** ___ / sin duda; *int.* basta!;
no más!

enriched *a.* [*added qualities*]
enriquecido-a, de valor aumentado.

enter *v.* entrar, introducir, penetrar.

enteral, enteric *a.* entérico-a, rel. al
intestino; ___ **nutrition** / nutrición.

enteric coated *n.* cubierta entérica,
revestimiento de ciertas tabletas y
cápsulas para evitar que se disuelvan
antes de llegar al intestino.

enteritis *n.* enteritis, infl. del intestino
delgado.

enteroclysis *n.* enteroclisis. 1.
irrigación del colon; 2. enema intenso.

enterococcus *n.* (*pl.* **enterococci**)
enterococo, clase de estreptococo que
se aloja en el intestino humano.

enterocolitis *n.* enterocolitis, infl. del
intestino grueso y delgado.

enteropathy *n.* enteropatía, cualquier
anomalía o enfermedad del intestino.

enterostomy *n.* enterostomía, apertura
o comunicación entre el intestino y la
piel de la pared abdominal.

enterotoxin *n.* enterotoxina, toxina
producida en el intestino.

enterovirus *n.* enterovirus, grupo
de virus que infecta el tubo
digestivo y que puede ocasionar
enfermedades respiratorias y trastornos
neurológicos.

entire *a.* entero-a, completo-a, íntegro-a;
-ly *adv.* completamente, del todo,
totalmente.

entrance *n.* [*local*] entrada;
[*acceptance*] ingreso; acceso a una
cavidad.

entropion *n.* entropión, inversión del
párpado.

entropy *n.* entropía, disminución de la
capacidad de convertir la energía en
trabajo.

entry *n.* entrada, acceso.

enucleation *n.* enucleación,
extirpación de un tumor o estructura.

enumerate *v.* enumerar, contar.

enuresis *n.* enuresis, incontinencia de
orina; **nocturnal** ___ / nocturna.

envelope *n.* sobre 1. objeto de papel de
uso postal; 2. cubierta; 3. cápsula.

envenomation *n.* 1. envenenamiento
por picadura de un miembro de la clase
Artropoda: cangrejos, langostas,
arañas, etc; 2. acto de introducir un
agente venenoso por medio de una
mordida, picazo, u otra forma
inyectable.

environment *n.* ambiente, medio
ambiente, entorno.

environmental *a.* rel. al medio
ambiente; ___ **hazards** / peligros del
medio ambiente.

enzygotic *a.* encigótico-a, que se deriva
del mismo óvulo fecundado.

enzyme *n.* enzima, proteína que actúa
como catalítico en reacciones químicas
vitales; **mucomembranous** ___ / ___
mucomenbranosa; **tuberculous** ___ /
___ tuberculosa.

eosin *n.* eosina, sustancia insoluble
usada como colorante rojo en algunos
tejidos que se estudian bajo el
microscopio.

eosinophil *n.* eosinófilo, célula
granulocítica que acepta fácilmente la
acción colorante de la eosina.

eosinophilia *n.* eosinofilia, aumento en
exceso de eosinófilos en la sangre por
unidad de volumen.

ependyma *n.* epéndimo, membrana
que cubre los ventrículos del
cerebro y el canal central de la médula
espinal.

ependymoma *n.* ependimoma, tumor
del sistema nervioso central que se
origina de inclusiones fetales
ependimarias.

ephedrine

ephedrine *n.* efedrina, alcaloide, tipo de adrenalina de efecto broncodilatador.

epicardium *n.* (*pl.* **epicardia**) epicardio, cara visceral del pericardio.

epicondyle *n.* epicóndilo, eminencia sobre el cóndilo de un hueso.

epidemic *n.* epidemia, enfermedad que se manifiesta con alta frecuencia y que afecta a un número considerable de personas en una región o comunidad; *a.* epidémico-a; __ **outbreak** / brote __ .

epidemiology *n.* epidemiología, estudio de las enfermedades epidémicas.

epidermic *a.* epidérmico-a, rel. a la epidermis; __ **growth factor** / factor __ de crecimiento.

epidermis *n.* epidermis, cubierta externa epitelial de la piel.

epidermoid *a.* epidermoide.
1. semejante a la piel; 2. rel. a un tumor que contiene células epidérmicas.

epidermolysis *n.* epidermólisis, descamación de la piel.

epididymis *n.* epidídimo, conducto situado en la parte posterior del testículo que recoge el esperma que es transportado por el conducto deferente a la vesícula seminal.

epididymitis *n.* epididimitis, infección e infl. del epidídimo.

epidural *a.* epidural, situado-a sobre o fuera de la duramadre.

epigastric *a.* epigástrico-a, rel. al epigastrio; __ **reflex** / reflejo __ .

epigastrium *n.* (*pl.* **epigastria**) epigastrio, región superior media del abdomen.

epiglottis *n.* epiglotis, cartílago que cubre la laringe e impide la entrada de alimentos en la misma durante la deglución.

epiglottitis *n.* epiglotitis, infl. de la epiglotis.

epilation *n.* epilación, depilación por medio de electrólisis.

epilepsy, grand mal *n.* epilepsia, desorden neurológico gen. crónico y con frecuencia hereditario que se manifiesta con ataques o convulsiones y a veces con pérdida del conocimiento.

epileptic *n.* epiléptico-a, persona que padece de epilepsia; *a.* epiléptico-a, rel. a la epilepsia o que sufre de ella; __ **seizure** / ataque __ , crisis __ .

epinephrine *n.* epinefrina. V. **adrenaline**.

epiphysis *n.* epífisis, extremo de un hueso largo, gen. parte más ancha que la diáfisis.

epiphysitis *n.* epifisitis, infl. de una epífisis.

epiploic foramen *n.* foramen epiploico, abertura que comunica la cavidad mayor peritoneal con la menor.

epiploon *n.* epiplón, repliegue de grasa que cubre el intestino.

episiotomy *n.* episiotomía, incisión del perineo durante el parto para evitar desgarros.

episode *n.* episodio, evento no regulado, en serie o independiente que puede formar parte de una condición física o de un estado mental, o de ambos, y se manifiestan en ciertas enfermedades tal como lo epilepsia.

epispadias *n.* epispadias, abertura congénita anormal de la uretra en la parte superior del pene.

epistaxis *n.* epistaxis, sangramiento por la nariz.

epithelial *a.* epitelial, rel. al epitelio.

epithelial cast *n.* cilindro epitelial, cilindro urinario constituido por células epiteliales renales y células redondas.

epithelialization *n.* epitelialización, crecimiento del epitelio sobre una superficie expuesta tal como en la cicatrización de una herida.

epithelioma *n.* epitelioma, carcinoma compuesto mayormente de células epiteliales.

epithelium *n., L.* (*pl.* **epitelia**) epitelio, tejido que cubre las superficies expuestas e interiores del cuerpo; **ciliated** __ / __ ciliado; **columnar** __ / __ columnar; **cuboidal** __ / __ cuboidal; **squamous** __ / __ escamoso; **stratified** __ / __ estratificado; **transitional** __ / __ de transición, transicional.

Epsom salt *n.* sal de Epsom, sal de higuera; sulfato de magnesio; medicamento usado como catártico.

Epstein-Barr virus *n.* virus de Epstein-Barr, virus del herpes que causa mononucleosis.

epulis gravidarum *n.* epúlide grávida, granuloma piogénico de la encía que puede surgir durante el embarazo.

equal *a.* igual; parejo-a; uniforme; __ **rights** / igualdad de derechos **-ly** *adv.* igualmente.

equality *n.* igualdad, uniformidad.

equalize *v.* igualar, emparejar, uniformar.

equator *n.* ecuador, línea imaginaria que divide un cuerpo en dos partes iguales.

equilibration *n.* equilibración, mantenimiento del equilibrio.

equilibrium *n.* equilibrio, balance.

equinovarus *n.* equinovaro, deformidad congénita del pie.

equipment *n.* equipo, provisión; accesorios.

equivalence *n.* equivalencia.

equivalent *a.* equivalente, del mismo valor.

equivocal *a.* equívoco-a; ___ **symptom** / síntoma equívoco.

eradicate *v.* erradicar, extirpar; desarraigar.

erase *v.* borrar; raspar.

erectile *a.* eréctil, capaz de ponerse en erección o de dilatarse; ___ **tissue** / tejido ___ .

erection *n.* erección, estado de rigidez, endurecimiento o dilatación de un tejido eréctil cuando se llena de sangre, tal como el pene.

ergonomics *n.* ergonomía, rama de la ecología que estudia la creación y diseño de maquinarias en su ambiente físico y la relación de las mismas con el bienestar humano.

ergot *n.* cornezuelo de centeno, hongo que en forma seca o en extracto se usa como medicamento para detener hemorragias o para inducir contracciones uterinas.

ergotamine *n.* ergotamina, alcaloide usado en el tratamiento de migraña.

ergotism *n.* ergotismo, intoxicación crónica producida por el uso excesivo de alcaloides del cornezuelo de centeno.

erogenous *a.* erógeno-a, que produce sensaciones eróticas; ___ **zone** / zona erótica.

erosion *n.* erosión, desgaste.

erosive *a.* erosivo-a, que causa erosión.

erotic *a.* erótico-a, rel. al erotismo o capaz de despertar impulsos sexuales.

eroticism, erotism *n.* erotismo, exaltación sexual.

erratic *a.* errático-a, que no sigue un curso o ritmo estable.

error *n.* error, falta, equivocación.

erupt *v.* brotar, salir con fuerza, hacer erupción.

eruption *n.* erupción, brote; salpullido.

erysipelas *n* erisipelas, infección de celulitis cutánea por el estreptococo β-hemolítico que se caracteriza por una erupción enrojecida, o carmelita, con tamaño definido; **ambulant** ___ / ___ ambulante; ___**internum** / ___ interna; ___ **migrans** / ___ migrante; ___ **pustulosum** / ___ pustulosa; **surgical** ___ / ___ quirúrgica.

erythema *n.* eritema, enrojecimiento de la piel debido a una congestión de los capilares.

erythroblast *n.* eritroblasto, hematíe, glóbulo rojo primitivo.

erythroblastosis *n.* eritroblastosis, número excesivo de eritoblastos en la sangre.

erythrocyte *n.* eritrocito, célula roja producida en la médula ósea que actúa como transportadora de oxígeno a los tejidos; ___ **sedimentation rate** / índice de sedimentación de ___ -s.

erythrocytopenia *n.* eritrocitopenia, deficiencia en la cantidad de glóbulos rojos circulantes.

erythrocytosis *n.* eritrocitosis, aumento de eritrocitos en la sangre.

erythroleukemia *n.* eritroleucemia, enfermedad sanguínea maligna caracterizada por el crecimiento anormal de glóbulos rojos y blancos.

erythromelia *n.* eritromelia, trastorno cutáneo de las extremidades inferiores que se manifiesta en eritema de origen desconocido y dermis atrofiada.

erythromycin *n.* eritromicina, antibiótico usado en el tratamiento de bacterias gram-positivas.

erythropoiesis *n.* eritropoyesis, producción de eritrocitos.

erythropoietic hormone *n.* hormona eritropoyética, cualquier tipo de hormona de proteína que toma parte en la formación de eritrocitos.

erythropoietin *n.* eritropoyetina, proteína no dializable que estimula la producción de eritrocitos.

erytromelalgia *n.* eritromelalgia, trastorno de las extremidades caracterizado por ataques de paroxismo con dolores severos, hinchazón, y que gen. ocurre en la edad madura.

eschar *n.* escara, costra de color oscuro que se forma en la piel después de una quemadura.

esophageal

esophageal *a.* esofágico-a, rel. al esófago; ___ **dilatation** / dilatación ___; ___ **dysphagia** / disfagia esofágica; ___ **obstruction** / obstrucción ___; ___ **scintigraphy** / cintigrafía ___; ___ **spasm** / espasmo ___ .

esophagectomy *n.* esofagectomía, excisión de una porción del esófago.

esophagitis *n.* esofagitis, infl. del esófago.

esophagodynia *n.* esofagodinia, dolor en el esófago.

esophagogastritis *n.* esofagogastritis, infl. del estómago y del esófago.

esophagogastroduodenoscopy *n.* esofagogastroduodenoscopía, examen del estómago, esófago y duodeno por medio de un endoscopio.

esophagogastroscopy *n.* esofagogastroscopía, examen del esófago y del estómago por medio de un endoscopio.

esophagus *n.* esófago, porción del tubo digestivo situado entre la faringe y el estómago.

esophoria *n.* esoforia, movimiento del ojo hacia adentro; *pop.* bizquera.

esotropia *n.* esotropia. V. **esophoria**.

essence *n.* esencia, cualidad indispensable.

essential *a.* esencial, indispensable.

establish *v.* establecer, determinar.

estate *n.* estado, condición de una persona, animal o cosa.

ester *n.* éster, compuesto formado por la combinación de un ácido orgánico con alcohol.

esterification *n.* esterificación, transformación de un ácido en un éster.

esthetics *n.* estética, rama de la filosofía que se refiere a la belleza y el arte.

estradiol *n.* estradiol, esteroide producido por los ovarios.

estrinization *n.* estrinización, cambios epiteliales de la vagina producidos por estimulación de estrógeno.

estrogen *n.* estrógeno, hormona sexual femenina producida por los ovarios; ___ **receptor** / receptor de ___ .

estrone *n.* estrona, hormona estrogénica.

eternal *a.* eterno-a.

ether *n.* éter, fluido químico cuyo vapor es usado en anestesia general.

ethics *n.* ética, normas y principios que gobiernan la conducta profesional.

ethmoid *n.* etmoides, hueso esponjoso situado en la base del cráneo.

ethmoidectomy *n.* etmoidectomía, extirpación de las células etmoideas o de parte del hueso etmoide.

ethmoid sinus *n.* seno etmoideo, cavidad aérea situada dentro del etmoide.

ethylene *n.* etileno, anestésico.

etiologic *a.* etiológico-a, rel. a la etiología.

etiology *n.* etiología, rama de la medicina que estudia la causa de las enfermedades.

eubolism *n.* eubolismo, metabolismo normal.

eucalyptus *n.* eucalipto.

eugenics *n.* eugenesia, ciencia que estudia el mejoramiento de la especie humana de acuerdo con las leyes biológicas de la herencia.

euphoria *n.* estado exagerado de sensación de bienestar.

euploidy *n.* euploidia, grupos completos de cromosomas.

Eustachian tube *n.* trompa de Eustaquio, parte del conducto auditivo.

euthanasia *n.* eutanasia, muerte infringida sin sufrimiento en casos de una enfermedad incurable.

euthyroid *a.* eutiroideo-a, rel. a la función normal de la glándula tiroides.

evacuant *a.* evacuante, catártico, estimulante de la evacuación.

evacuate *v.* evacuar, eliminar; defecar; vaciar, *Mex.* obrar.

evacuation *n.* evacuación. 1. acción de vaciar esp. los intestinos; 2. acción de hacer un vacío.

evagination *n.* evaginación, salida o protuberancia de un órgano o parte de éste de su propia localización.

evaluate *v.* evaluar, estimar.

evaluation *n.* evaluación, consideración del estado de salud mental y físico de una persona enferma o sana.

evanescent *a.* evanescente, que se desvanece, efímero-a.

evaporation *n.* evaporación, conversión de un estado líquido a vapor.

even *a.* igual, uniforme; [*same*] mismo-a, parejo-a; *adv.* ___ **so** / aún cuando; ___ **more** / aún más.

evening *n.* tardecita, anochecer, por la noche; **last** ___ / ayer por la noche; **this** ___ / esta noche.

eventration *n.* eventración, 1. protrusión de contenidos abdominales a través de una abertura en la pared abdominal; 2. una hernia.

ever *adv.* siempre; **for __ and __** / por __ jamás; **hardly __** / casi nunca; **__ since** / desde entonces, desde que.

eversion *n.* eversión, versión hacia afuera, esp. la de una mucosa que rodea un orificio natural.

every *a.* todo; cada; **__ day** / __-s los días; **__ once in a while** / a veces, de vez en cuando; **__ other day** / día por medio, cada dos días, un día sí y otro no.

everybody *pron.* todos, todo el mundo.

everything *pron.* todo.

evidence *n.* evidencia, manifestación; [*legal*] evidencia, testimonio.

evil *n.* maldad; *a.* malo-a, maligno-a.

evisceration *n.* evisceración, extirpación del contenido de una víscera o de una cavidad.

evoke *v.* evocar.

evoked response *n.* respuesta evocada.

evolution *n.* evolución, cambio gradual.

evulsion *n.* evulsión, acción de sacar hacia afuera, arranque.

exacerbation *n.* exacerbación, agravamiento de un síntoma o enfermedad.

exact *a.* exacto-a; **-ly** *adv.* exactamente.

exaggeration *n.* exageración, alarde.

exam *n.* examen, evaluación, investigación.

examination *n.* examen, exploración, reconocimiento, auscultación; **abdominal __** / exploración abdominal; **bladder __** / cistoscopia; **cardiac __** / auscultación cardíaca; **__ table** / mesa de exploración; **medical __** / reconocimiento médico; **neurological __** / exploración neurológica; **vaginal __** / examen vaginal.

examine *v.* examinar, evaluar, investigar, indagar.

example *n.* ejemplo, muestra.

exanguination *n.* pérdida severa de sangre.

exanthem, exanthema *n.* exantema, erupción cutánea secundaria a un síntoma de un virus o enfermedad cócica, por ejemplo, la escarlatina o el sarampión; **epidemic __** / __ epidémico; **__ subitum** / __ súbito; **keratoid __** / __ queratoideo.

exasperated *a.* exasperado-a.

excellent *a.* excelente, óptimo-a.

except *prep.* excepto, menos.

exception *n.* excepción; **with the __ of** / a __ de.

excess *n.* exceso, sobrante.

excessive *a.* excesivo-a.

exchange transfusion *n.* ex-sanguinotransfusión, transfusión gradual y simultánea de sangre al recipiente mientras se saca la sangre del donante.

excision *n.* excisión, extirpación, ablación.

excitation *n.* excitación, reacción a un estímulo.

excite *v.* excitar, estimular; provocar.

excited *a.* excitado-a; acalorado-a.

exclude *v.* excluir, suprimir.

exclusive *a.* exclusivo-a.

excoriation *n.* excoriación, abrasión de la epidermis.

excrement *n.* excremento, heces fecales, *pop.* [*infant's*] caca.

excrescence *n.* excrecencia, tumor saliente en la superficie de un órgano o parte.

excreta *n.* excreta, todo lo excretado por el cuerpo.

excrete *v.* excretar, eliminar desechos del cuerpo.

excretion *n.* excreción, expulsión de lo secretado.

excuse *v.* excusar, perdonar, dispensar; **__ me** / con permiso.

exercise *n.* ejercicio, esfuerzo saludable moderado con el propósito de restaurar la vitalidad máxima a los órganos y funciones del cuerpo; **active __** / __ activo; **aerobic __** / __ aeróbico; **corrective __** / __ correctivo; **deep-breathing __** / __ de respiración profunda; **electrocardiogram, stress test** / prueba de esfuerzo máximo; **__-induced amenorrea** / amenorrea inducida por __ excesivo; **__ test** / prueba de esfuerzo; **__ tolerance test** / prueba física de __ tolerado; **isometric __** / __ isométrico; **isotonic __** / __ isotónico; **passive __** / __ pasivo; **physical __** / __ físico.

exertional dyspnea *n.* disnea por esfuerzo excesivo.

exfoliation *n.* exfoliación, descamación del tejido.

exhalation *n.* exhalación, proceso de salida del aire hacia afuera.

exhale v. espirar, exhalar.

exhausted a. agotado-a, exhausto-a, extenuado-a.

exhaustion n. agotamiento, postración, fatiga extrema.

exhaustive a. completo, minucioso, extenso; **to do an __ evaluation of the case** / hacer una evaluación completa del caso.

exhibition n. exhibición, exposición.

exhibitionism n. exhibicionismo, deseo obsesivo de exhibir partes del cuerpo esp. los genitales.

exhibitionist n. exhibicionista, persona que practica el exhibicionismo.

exhumation n. exhumación, desenterramiento.

exist v. existir, ser, vivir.

existent a. existente.

exit n. salida.

exocrine a. exocrino-a, rel. a la secreción externa de una glándula.

exocrine glands n. glándulas exocrinas, glándulas que secretan hormonas a través de un conducto o tubo tal como las mamarias y las sudoríparas.

exogenous a. exógeno-a, externo-a, que se origina fuera del organismo.

exophthalmia, exophthalmos n. exoftalmia, protrusión anormal del globo del ojo.

exophthalmic a. exoftálmico-a, rel. a la exoftalmia.

exophthalmic goiter n. bocio exoftálmico.

exostosis n. exóstosis, hipertrofia ósea cartilaginosa que sobresale hacia afuera de un hueso o de la raíz de un diente.

exotoxin n. exotoxina, veneno excretado por una bacteria que es un organismo vivo, contraria a la endotoxina, que no es liberada hasta que el organismo bacteria muere.

exotropia n. exotropía, tipo de estrabismo divergente, rotación anormal de un ojo o de ambos hacia afuera por falta de balance muscular.

expand v. ensanchar, expandir, dilatar; expandirse.

expansion n. expansión, extensión.

expect v. esperar; suponer.

expectancy n. esperanza, expectativa, anhelo; (embarazo) espera; **life __ /** esperanza de vida.

expecting n. anticipación, esperanza, anhelo; **__ mother /** mujer embarazada.

expectorant n. expectorante, agente que estimula la expectoración.

expectoration n. expectoración, esputo, expulsión de mucosidades o flema de los pulmones, tráquea y bronquios.

expel v. expulsar.

experience n. experiencia, práctica.

experiment n. experimento; v. experimentar.

expert a. experto-a, perito-a.

expiration n. expiración, terminación; espiración. 1. acto de dar salida al aire aspirado por los pulmones; 2. acto de fallecer o morir.

expire v. 1. espirar, expeler el aire aspirado; 2. expirar, morir, dejar de existir.

explain v. explicar, aclarar.

explanation n. explicación, interpretación.

explanatory a. explicativo, aclaratorio; **self-explanatory /** que no necesita explicación o aclaración.

exploration n. exploración, investigación, búsqueda.

exploratory a. exploratorio-a, rel. a una exploración.

expression n. expresión, aspecto o apariencia que se registra en la cara; medio de expresar algo.

expressivity n. expresividad, apreciación de un rasgo heredado según se manifiesta en el descendiente portador del gene.

expulsion n. expulsión; **__ of the placenta /** __ de la placenta; **__ of the infant /** __ del recién nacido.

extended care facility n. centro de atención médica externa.

extended radical mastectomy n. mastectomía radical extendida.

extension n. 1. prolongación, extensión; 2. acto de enderezar un dedo o alinear un miembro o hueso dislocado.

extensor a. extensor-a, que tiene la propiedad de extender.

extenuating cases n., pl. casos atenuantes.

exterior a. exterior, externo-a; visible.

exteriorize v. exteriorizar, exponer un órgano o una parte temporalmente.

externalia n., pl. genitales externos.

extinction n. extinción; supresión; cesación.

extinguish v. extinguir, apagar.

extirpation *n.* extirpación, ablación de una parte u órgano.

extra *a.* extraordinario-a; adicional.

extracellular *a.* extracelular, fuera de la célula.

extracorporeal *a.* extracorporal, fuera del cuerpo.

extract *n.* extracto, producto concentrado; **alcoholic** __ / __ alcohólico; **allergic** __ / __ alérgico; **belladonna** __ / __ de belladona; **equivalent** __ / __ equivalente; **fluid** __ / __ líquido; **hydroalcoholic** __ / __ hidroalcohólico.

extraction *n.* extracción, proceso de extraer, separar o sacar afuera.

extradural *a.* extradural. V. **epidural**.

extraneous *a.* extraño-a, sin relación con un organismo o fuera del mismo.

extraocular *a.* extraocular, fuera del ojo.

extrasensory perception (ESP) *n.* percepción extrasensorial, percepción o conocimiento de las acciones o pensamientos de otras personas adquirido sin participación sensorial.

extrasystole *n.* extrasístole, latido arrítmico del corazón.

extravasated *a.* extravasado-a, rel. al escape de fluido de un vaso a tejidos circundantes.

extravascular *a.* extravascular, que ocurre fuera de un vaso o vasos.

extreme *a.* extremo-a, excesivo-a; último-a; **-ly** *adv.* extremadamente, excesivamente; sumamente.

extremity *n.* extremidad, la parte terminal de algo.

extrinsic *a.* extrínseco-a __ **muscle** / músculo __ .

extrovert *a.* extrovertido-a, tipo de personalidad que dirige la atención a sucesos u objetos fuera de sí mismo-a.

extrude *v.* exprimir, forzar hacia afuera.

extrusion *n.* extrusión, expulsión.

extubation *n.* extubación, extracción de un tubo.

exuberant *a.* exuberante, de proliferación excesiva.

exudate *n.* exudado, fluido inflamatorio tal como el de secreciones y supuraciones.

exudation *n.* exudación.

exude *v.* exudar, sudar, supurar a través de los tejidos.

eye *n.* ojo; **amaurotic** __ / __ amaurótico; **artificial** __ / __ postizo; **black** __ / __ amoratado, contusión ocular; **bleary** __ / __ nublado; __ legañoso; **bloodshot** __ / __ inyectado; **chemical burns in** __ / quemaduras químicas oculares; **crossed-eyed** / bizco; **cyclopian** __ / __ de cíclope; __ **bank** / banco de ojos; __ **contact** / contacto visual; __ **diseases** / enfermedades de los ojos, enfermedades de la vista; __ **drops** / gotas para los ojos; __ **injuries** / traumatismos oculares; __ **injury** / lesión ocular; __**memory** / memoria visual; __**strain** / fatiga ocular; **foreign body in the** __ / cuerpo extraño en el __; **glass** __ / __ de cristal, __ de vidrio; **lazy** __ / ambliopía; **light-adapted** __ / __ adaptado a la luz; **master** __ / __ maestro; **squinting** __ / __ estrábico; **to keep an__ on** / cuidar, vigilar; **watery** __ / __ lacrimoso. V. ilustración en la página 334.

eyeball *n.* globo del ojo, globo ocular.

eyeband *n.* venda para los ojos.

eyebrow *n.* ceja.

eyecup *n.* copita para los ojos.

eyeglasses *n. pl.* espejuelos, gafas, lentes, anteojos; **bifocal** __ / __ bifocales; **trifocal** __ / __ trifocales.

eyeground *n.* fondo del ojo.

eyelash *n.* pestaña.

eyelid *n.* párpado.

eyepiece *n.* ocular.

eyesight *n.* vista; *v.* **to have good** __ / tener buena __ .

eye socket *n.* órbita ocular; cuenca del ojo.

eye strain *n.* vista cansada.

eye wash *n.* solución ocular, colirio, solución para los ojos.

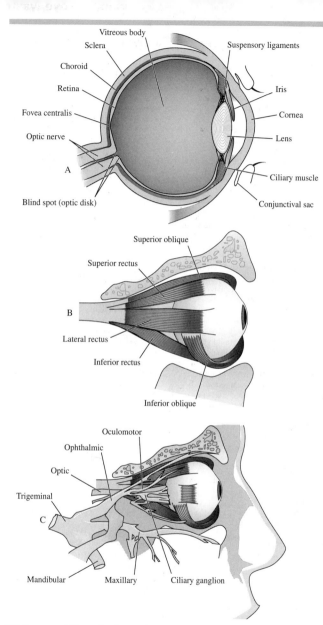

(A) the eye; (B) extrinsic muscles of the eye; (C) nerves of the eye

f

F *abbr.* **Fahrenheit** / Fahrenheit.
f *abbr.* **failure** / fallo; **feminine** / femenino; **formula** / fórmula; **function** / función.
face *n.* cara, rostro, faz; ___ **-down** / boca abajo; ___ **-lift** / estire de la cara, ritidectomía; ___ **peeling** / peladura de la ___; ___ **to face** / frente a frente; ___ **-up** / boca arriba.
facet *n.* faceta, pequeña parte lisa en la superficie de una estructura dura semejante a la de los huesos.
facetectomy *n.* extirpación de la faceta auricular.
facial *a.* facial, rel. a la cara; ___ **artery** / arteria ___; ___ **axis** / axis ___; ___ **bone defects** / defectos óseos ___ -es; ___ **bones** / huesos de la cara, huesos ___ -es; ___ **canal** / canal ___; ___ **hemiplegia** / hemiplejía ___; ___ **injuries** / traumatismos ___ -es; ___ **nerve** / nervio ___; ___ **nerves** / nervios ___ -es; ___ **palsy** / parálisis ___; ___ **paralysis** / parálisis ___; ___ **reconstruction** / reconstrucción ___; ___ **spasm** / espasmo ___; ___ **tic** / tic ___; ___ **vein** / vena ___.
facies *n. (pl.* **facies)** facies, expresión o apariencia de la cara; **leontina** ___ / ___ leontina; **masklike** ___ / ___ inexpresiva.
facilitate *v.* facilitar; proporcionar.
facility *n.* facilidad; instalación; [*conveniences*] *pl.* comodidades; servicios en general.
facioplasty *n.* facioplastia, cirugía plástica de la cara.
facioplegia *n.* facioplejía, parálisis facial.
fact *n.* de hecho, hecho, realidad; **in** ___ / en efecto, en realidad.
factor *n.* factor, elemento que contribuye a producir una acción; **antihemophilic** ___ / ___ antihemofílico; **clotting, coagulation** ___ / ___ de coagulación; **fibroblast growth** ___ / ___ de crecimiento fibroplástico; **releasing** ___ / ___ liberador; **Rh** ___ / ___ Rh [*erre ache*]; **rheumatoid** ___ / ___ reumatoideo; **tumor angiogenesis** ___ / ___ angiogenético tumoral.

factual *a.* objetivo-a, real; de hacho.
facultative *a.* facultativo-a.
1. voluntario, no obligatorio;
2. de naturaleza profesional.
faculty *n.* facultad. 1. aptitud o habilidad para llevar a cabo funciones normales;
2. cuerpo facultativo.
Faget, sign of *n.* signo de Faget, un pulso bajo en relación a la alta temperatura presente.
Fahrenheit scale *n.* escala de Fahrenheit, escala de temperatura que usa el punto de congelación a 32 y el de ebullición a 212.
failing *n.* debilidad; deterioro; flaqueza; falla, falta.
failure *n.* insuficiencia, fallo; omisión; fracaso; ___ **neurosis** / neurosis de fracaso; **gross** ___ / fiasco; **heart** ___ / ___ cardíaca, fallo cardíaco; **renal** ___ / ___ renal; **respiratory** ___ / ___ respiratoria.
failure to thrive *n.* retraso en el desarrollo visto en niños que no alcanzan un desarrollo normal.
faint *n.* desmayo, desvanecimiento, vahído; *v.* dar un vahído; desmayarse, desvanecerse; **-ly** *adv.* débilmente, lánguidamente; escasamente.
fainting *n.* desmayo; desfallecimiento; ___ **spell** / desmayo.
fair *a.* [*blonde*] rubio-a; [*light skin*] de tez blanca; [*average*] regular; ___ **complexion** / rubio-a, de tez clara; [*weather*] claro, despejado, favorable; [*decision*] imparcial, razonable, justa.
faith *n.* fe; **in good** ___ / de buena ___.
faith healer *n.* curandero-a.
faith healing *n.* cura de fe, uso de la oración para tratar enfermedades.
fake *v.* fingir; falsificar, simular.
fall *n.* caída; [*season*] otoño; *vi.* caer; caerse; **to** ___ **asleep** / quedarse dormido-a; **to** ___ **back** / echarse atrás; **to** ___ **behind** / atrasarse, quedarse atrás; **to** ___ **short** / faltar, ser deficiente.
falling *n.* caída; [*temperature*] descenso.
Fallopian tubes *n.* trompas de Falopio, conductos que se extienden del útero a los ovarios.
Fallot, tetralogy of *n.* tetralogía de Fallot, deformación cardíaca congénita que comprende cuatro defectos de los grandes vasos sanguíneos y de las paredes de las aurículas y ventrículos.

false

false *a.* falso-a, incorrecto-a. no real; ___ **anemia** / anemia ___; ___ **aneurysm** / aneurisma ___; ___ **ankylosis** / anquilosis ___; ___ **blepharoptosis** / blefaroptosis ___; ___ **diverticulum** / divertículo ___; ___ **hematuria** / hematuria ___; ___ **hermaphroditism** / hermafroditismo ___; ___ **image** / imagen ___; ___ **joint** / articulación ___; ___**lumen** / lúmen ___; ___ **membrane** / membrana ___; ___ **memory syndrome** / síndrome ___ de la memoria; ___ **negative** / ___ negativo; ___ **neuroma** / neuroma ___; ___ **positive** / ___ positivo; ___ **pregnancy** / embarazo ___; ___ **rib** / costilla ___; ___ **suture** / sutura ___; ___ **vocal chords** / cuerdas vocales ___ -s.

familial, familiar *a.* familiar, rel. a la familia; frecuente; ___ **adenomatous polyposis** / poliposis adenomatosa ___; ___ **amyloid neuropathy** / neuropatía amiloide ___; ___ **dysautonomia** / disautonomía ___; ___ **goiter** / bocio ___; ___ **hypercholesteremia** / hipercolesteremia ___; ___ **jaundice** / ictericia ___; ___ **Mediterranean fever** / fiebre ___ del Mediterráneo; ___ **periodic paralysis** / parálisis periódica ___; ___ **pseudoinflammatory macular degeneration** / degeneración macular pseudo-inflamatoria ___; ___ **screening** / escrutinio ___; ___ **tendency** / tendencia, propensión familiar.

family *n.* familia; ___ **man** / padre de familia; ___ **name** apellido; de; ___ **therapy** / terapia de familiar.

family planning *n.* planificación familiar, planeamiento de la concepción de los hijos gen. con el uso de métodos contraceptivos.

family practice *n.* medicina familiar, atención médica especial de la familia como unidad.

famished *a.* famélico-a, hambriento-a.

Fanconi's syndrome *n.* síndrome de Fanconi, anemia hipoplástica congénita.

fancy *v.* imaginar, fantasear.

fantasy, phantasy *n.* fantasía, uso de la imaginación para transformar una realidad desagradable en una experiencia satisfactoria.

far *adv.* lejos; distante; ___ **apart** / infrecuente; ___ **better** / mucho mejor; ___ **cry** / gran diferencia; ___ **off** / a lo lejos, distante; **from** ___ **away** / de lejos, a lo lejos; **so** ___ / hasta ahora, hasta aquí.

farmer's lung *n.* pulmón de granjero, hipersensibilidad de los alvéolos pulmonares causada por exposición a heno fermentado.

farsighted *a.* hiperópico-a, que sufre de hipermetropía.

farsightedness *n.* presbiopía, hiperopía, hipermetropía, defecto visual en el cual los rayos de luz hacen foco detrás de la retina y los objetos lejanos se ven mejor que los que están a corta distancia.

fascia *n.* fascia, tejido fibroso conectivo que envuelve el cuerpo bajo la piel y protege los músculos, los nervios y los vasos sanguíneos; ___ , **aponeurotic** / ___ aponeurótica, tejido fibroso que sirve de soporte a los músculos; ___ , **Buck's** / ___ de Buck, tejido fibroso que cubre el pene; ___ , **Colles'** / ___ de Colles, cubierta interna de la fascia perineal; ___ **graft** / injerto de una ___; ___ , **lata** / ___ lata, protectora de los músculos del muslo; ___ , **tranversalis** / ___ tranversal, localizada entre el peritoneo y el músculo transverso del abdomen.

fascial *a.* fascial, rel a una fascia; ___ **sheath of eye-ball** / cubierta ___ del globo del ojo.

fasciculation *n.* fasciculación. 1. formación de fascículos; 2. contracción involuntaria breve de fibras musculares.

fascietomy *n.* fascietomía, excisión parcial o total de una fascia.

fasciitis *n.* fascitis, infl. de una fascia.

fasciodesis *n.* fasciodesis, operación de adherir un tendón a una fascia.

fascioplasty *n.* fascioplastía, cirugía plástica de una fascia.

fasciotomy *n.* fasciotomía, incisión de una fascia.

fast *n.* ayuno; *a.* [*speed*] rápido-a, ligero-a; [*of a color*] que tiene resistencia a un colorante; ___ **asleep** / profundamente dormido-a; ___ **day** / día de ayuno; *v.* ayunar, estar en ayunas.

fasten *v.* sujetar; amarrar; abrochar; abotonar.

fastening *n.* amarre.

fastidious *a.* 1. fastidioso-a. 2. en bacteriología, rel. a demandas nutricionales complejas.

fasting *n.* ayuno.

fasting blood glucose *n.* glucemia en ayunas.

fastness *n.* resistencia.

fat *n.* [*grease*] grasa; *a.* gordo-a, grueso-a, obeso-a; [*greasy*] grasoso-a; **embolism** / embolia grasosa; *v.* **to get** __ / engordar.

fatal *a.* fatal.

fatality *n.* fatalidad, desgracia; muerte.

fatality rate *n.* índice de mortalidad.

father *n.* padre; papá; *pop.* tata.

father-in-law *n.* suegro.

fatigue *n.* cansancio; sensación de agotamiento; *v.* fatigarse, cansarse.

fatness *n.* gordura.

fatty *a.* adiposo-a, grasoso-a; __ **acids** / ácidos grasos; __; __ **cirrhosis** / cirrosis __; __**degeneration** / degeneración __; __ **heart** / corazón __; __ **hernia** / hernia __; __**infiltration** / infiltración __; __ **kidney** / riñón __; __ **liver** / hígado __; __ **oil** / aceite __; __ **tumor** / lipoma; __ **tissue** / tejido __.

fault *n.* falta, defecto, culpa; *v.* **to be at** __ / ser culpable.

faulty *a.* defectuoso-a, imperfecto-a.

favor *n.* favor.

fear *n.* temor, miedo, aprehensión. *v.* temer, tener miedo.

fearful *a.* temeroso-a, miedoso-a.

fearless *a.* sin temor, intrépido-a.

feature *n.* rasgo, característica.

febrile *a.* febril, calenturiento-a; __ **convulsion** / convulsión __.

fecal *a.* fecal, que contiene heces fecales; __**abscess** / absceso __; __ **examination** / examen __; __ **fistula** / fístula __.

fecalith *n.* fecalito, concreción intestinal formada alrededor de materia fecal.

fecaluria *n.* presencia de materia fecal en la orina.

feces *n., pl.* heces, excremento.

fecundity *n.* fecundidad, fertilidad.

fee *n.* honorario, cuota.

feeble *a.* débil, endeble.

feed *vi.* alimentar, dar de comer; proveer materiales o asistencia.

feedback *n.* 1. [*information*] reprovisión de material informativo distribuido; 2. retroalimentación, retorno parcial del rendimiento o efectos de un proceso a su fuente de origen o a una fase anterior; *v.* proveer de nuevo material informativo; regenerar la energía.

feeding *n.* alimentación; **breast-** __ / lactancia materna; **enteral** __ / __ enteral; __ **time** / horario de __;

forced __ / __ forzada; **intravenous** __ / __ intravenosa; **rectal** __ / __ por el recto; **tube** __ / __ por sonda.

feel *vi.* sentir, percibir, sentirse; **Do you** __ **the effects of the medication?** / ¿Siente, sientes los efectos de la medicina?; **to** __ **hungry** / tener hambre; **to** __ **the effects of** / sentir los efectos de; **to** __ **like** / tener ganas de; **to** __ **sleepy** / tener sueño; **to** __ **sorry for** / compadecerse de; tener lástima de; **to** __ **the pulse** / tomar el pulso; **to** __ **thirsty** / tener sed; **to** __ **bad** / sentirse mal; **to** __ **better** / __ mejor; **to** __ **good, fine** / __ bien; **to** __ **uncomfortable** / __ incómodo-a.

feeling *n.* sensación; [*emotion*] sentimiento, emoción, sensibilidad.

feet *n., pl.* de **foot**; pies.

feline *a.* felino-a, rel. a la familia de los gatos o con características semejantes a éstos.

felon *n.* 1. panadizo, absceso doloroso de la falange distal de un dedo; 2. felón, criminal.

female *n.* hembra; poseedora del óvulo en el proceso de procreación, y quien lleva a cabo la gestación.

feminine *a.* femenino-a; rel. al sexo femenino.

femininity *n.* feminidad; __ **complex** / complejo de __.

feminization *n.* feminización, 1. desarrollo de características femeninas. 2. características sexuales femeninas presentes en un genotipo masculino.

femoral *a.* femoral, rel. al fémur; **deep** __ **arch** / arco __ profundo; __ **artery** / arteria __; __ **canal** / canal __; __ **hernia** / hernia __; __ **nerve** / nervio __; __ **nutrient artery** / arteria nutricional __; __ **sheath** / capa __; __**triangle** / triángulo __; __ **vein** / vena __.

femorotibial *a.* femorotibial, rel. al fémur y a la tibia; __ **capillary** / capilar __; __ **membrane** / membrana __.

femur *n.* fémur, hueso del muslo.

fenestration *n.* fenestración. 1. creación de una abertura en el laberinto del oído para restaurar la audición; 2. acto de perforar.

ferment *n.* fermento. 1. sustancia o agente que activa la fermentación; 2. producto de fermentación; *v.* fermentar, hacer fermentar.

fermentation

fermentation *n.* fermentación, descomposición de sustancias complejas por la acción de enzimas o fermentos.

ferroprotein *n.* ferroproteína, proteína compuesta de un radical ferruginoso.

ferruginous *a.* ferruginoso-a, ferrugíneo-a. 1. que contiene hierro; 2. que tiene el color de hierro oxidado.

fertile *a.* fértil, fecundo-a, productivo-a.

fertility *n.* fertilidad.

fertilization *n.* fertilización, fecundación.

fertilize *v.* fecundar, hacer fértil.

fertilizer *n.* fertilizante.

fester *v.* enconarse; supurar superficialmente.

fetal *a.* fetal, rel. al feto; **___ alcohol syndrome** / síndrome alcohólico ___; **___ aspiration syndrome** / síndrome de aspiración ___; **___ circulation** / circulación ___; **___ death** / muerte ___; **___ drug syndrome** / síndrome ___ del abuso de droga; **___ dystocia** / distocia ___; **___ growth retardation** / retardo del crecimiento ___; **___ heart tone** / latido del corazón ___; **___ hydrops** / hidropesía ___; **___ maturity, chronologic** / edad gestacional; **___ medicine** / medicina ___; **___ membrane** / membrana ___; **___ monitoring** / monitorización ___; **___ placenta** / placenta ___; **___ pulse oximeter** / oxímetro de pulso ___; **___ transfusion** / transfusión de sangre *in utero*; **___ viability** / viabilidad ___; **___ wastage** / desperdicio ___.

fetid *a.* fétido-a, hediondo-a, de mal olor.

fetometry *n.* fetometría, estimación del tamaño del feto, esp. la cabeza antes del nacimiento

fetoprotein *n.* fetoproteína, antígeno presente en el feto humano.

fetoscope *n.* fetoscopio, endoscopio que se usa en la fetoscopía.

fetoscopy *n.* fetoscopía, inspección antenatal fetal transabdominal de la placenta y el feto con el propósito de diagnosticar posibles trastornos fetales.

fetus *n.* feto, embrión en desarrollo, fase de la gestación desde los tres meses hasta el parto.

fever *n.* fiebre, calentura; **enteric ___** / ___ entérica, intestinal; **___ blister** / herpes febril; **___ of unknown origin** / ___ de origen desconocido; **intermittent ___** / ___ intermitente; **rabbit ___** / ___ de conejo, tularemia; **rheumatoid ___** / ___ reumatoidea; **remittent ___** / ___ remitente; **Rocky Mountain ___** / ___ manchada de las Montañas Rocosas; **scarlet ___** / escarlatina; **yellow ___** / ___ amarilla, paludismo, malaria; **typhoid ___** / ___ tifoidea; **undulant ___** / brucelosis.

fiber *n.* fibra, filamento en forma de hilo.

fibril *n.* filamento, fibrilla, fibra pequeña.

fibrillar, fibrillary *a.* fibrilar, rel. a una fibra; **___ astrocyte** / astrocito ___; **___ contractions** / contracciones ___ -es.

fibrillation *n.* fibrilación. 1. contracción muscular involuntaria que afecta fibras musculares individuales; 2. formación de fibrillas; **atrial ___** / ___ auricular; **flutter ___** / ___ de aleteo; **ventricular ___** / ___ ventricular.

fibrin *n.* fibrina, proteína insoluble indispensable en la coagulación de la sangre.

fibrinogen *n.* fibrinógeno. 1. proteína presente en el plasma sanguíneo que se convierte en fibrina en el proceso de coagulación; 2. el Factor I.

fibrinogenemia *n.* fibrinogenemia, presencia de fibrógeno en la sangre.

fibrinogenic, fibrinogenous *a.* fibrinogénico-a, que produce fibrina.

fibrinogenolysis *n.* fibrinogenólisis, disolución o inactivación del fibrinógeno en la corriente sanguínea.

fibrinolysis *n.* fibrinólisis, disolución de fibrina por la acción de enzimas; **primary ___** / ___ primaria; **therapeutic ___** / ___ terapéutica.

fibrinous, fibrous *a.* fibrinoso-a, fibroso-a. 1. rel. a la naturaleza de una fibra; 2. semejante a un hilo; **___ bronchitis** / bronquitis ___; **___ inflammation** / inflamación ___; **___ pericarditis** / pericarditis ___; **___ pleurisy** / pleuresía ___; **___ polyp** / pólipo ___.

fibrinuria *n.* fibrinuria, presencia de fibrina en la orina.

fibroadenoma *n.* fibroadenoma, tumor benigno formado por tejido fibroso y glandular.

fibroblast *n.* fibroblasto, células de soporte de las que proviene el tejido conectivo.

fibrocartilage *n.* fibrocartílago, tipo de cartílago en el que la matriz contiene abundante tejido fibroso.

fibrochondroma n. fibrocondroma, tumor benigno compuesto por tejido conjuntivo fibroso y cartilaginoso.

fibrocyst n. fibroquiste. 1. fibroma formado por quistes; 2. neoplasma de degeneración cística.

fibrocystic a. fibrocístico-a, fibroquístico-a, de naturaleza fibrosa con degeneración cística; ___ disease of the breast / enfermedad ___ de la mama.

fibrocystoma n. fibrocistoma, tumor benigno con elementos císticos.

fibroid a. fibroide, de naturaleza fibrosa; ___adenoma / adenoma ___; ___ cataract / catarata ___.

fibroidectomy n. fibroidectomía, excisión de un tumor fibroide.

fibrolipoma n. fibrolipoma, tumor que contiene tejido fibroso y adiposo en exceso.

fibroma n. fibroma, tumor benigno compuesto de tejido fibroso.

fibromatosis n. fibromatosis, producción de fibromas múltiples en la piel o en el útero.

fibromuscular a. fibromuscular, de naturaleza muscular y fibrosa; ___ dysplasia / displasia ___.

fibromyalgia n. fibromialgia, condición crónica generalizada que resulta en dolor y rigidez en los músculos y los tejidos blandos.

fibromyoma n. fibromioma, tumor benigno formado por tejido muscular y fibroso.

fibroneuroma n. fibroneuroma, tumor del tejido conjuntivo de los nervios.

fibroplasia n. fibroplasia, producción de tejido fibroso tal como en la cicatrización de una herida.

fibrosarcoma n. fibrosarcoma, tumor maligno constituído por células fusiformes, colágeno y fibras de reticulina.

fibrosis n. fibrosis, formación anormal de tejido fibroso; **diffuse interstitial pulmonary** ___ / ___ intersticial del pulmón; **proliferative** ___ / ___ proliferativa; **retroperineal** ___ / ___ retroperineal.

fibrositis n. fibrositis, infl. de tejido blanco conjuntivo esp. en el área de las articulaciones.

fibrous a. fibroso-a. 1. rel. a la fibrina; 2. estructura en forma de hilo; ___ ankylosis / anquilosis ___; ___ cortical defect / defecto cortical ___; ___

degeneration / degeneración ___; ___ **goiter** / bocio ___; ___**joint** / articulación ___; ___ **tissue** / tejido ___; ___ **tubercule** / tubérculo ___.

fibula a. peroné, el hueso más externo y más delgado de la pierna.

fibular a. fibular, rel. al peroné; ___ **artery** / arteria ___; ___ **veins** / venas ___ .

fictitious a. ficticio-a, falso-a.

fidelity n. fidelidad, lealtad; precisión.

field n. campo. 1. área o espacio abierto; ___ **of vision** / ___ visual 2. área de especialización.

fight n. pelea, lucha; vi. pelear, combatir, luchar con.

figure n. figura; cifra, número.

filament n. filamento, fibra o hilo fino.

file n. [instrument] lima; [record] expediente, ficha; v. limar; registrar.

fill v. llenar; rellenar; llenarse.

filling n. [dental] empaste; obturación; restauración.

film n. 1. película; radiografía; 2. telilla, membrana o capa fina.

filter n. filtro; v. filtrar; **to** ___ **through** / filtrarse.

filthy a. sucio-a, mugriento-a, mugroso-a.

filtration n. filtración, colación, acción de pasar a través de un filtro.

fimbria n. (pl. **fimbriae**) fimbria, borde o canto; apéndice de ciertas bacterias; ___**hippocampi** / ___ del hipocampo; ___ **of uterine tube** / ___ del tubo uterino; ___ **ovaricae** / ___ ovárica.

final a. final, último-a; conclusivo-a; definitivo-a.

findings n., pl. hallazgos, resultados de una investigación o indagación.

fine a. fino-a, delicado-a; v. **to feel** ___ / sentirse bien.

finger n. dedo de la mano; ___ **agnosia** / agnosia del ___; ___ **nose test** / prueba de la nariz y el ___; ___ **-shaped** / digitiforme; **first** ___ / dedo índice; **little** ___ / dedo meñique; **mallet** ___ / dedo en martillo.

fingernail n. uña.

finish n. final, terminación; v. acabar, terminar.

finished a. acabado-a, terminado-a.

Finney operation n. operación de Finney, gastroduodenostomía que crea una apertura grande para asegurar el vaciamiento total del estómago.

fire n. fuego; [conflagration] incendio; ___ **alarm** / alarma de ___; ___ **department** / cuerpo de bomberos; ___

first

escape / escalera de __; v. **to catch**
__ / encenderse, prenderse; **to set** __
to / encender, quemar.

first n. primero-a; a. primero-a, primer
(before a m. singular n.) __ **degree** /
de primer grado; __ **name** / nombre de
pila.

first aid n. primeros auxilios; __ **kit** /
botiquín de __.

firstborn n. primogénito-a.

fish poisoning n. intoxicación de
pescado.

fission n. fisión. 1. división en partes;
2. división de un átomo para ser
descompuesto y desplazar energía y
neutrones.

fissure n. fisura. V. **cleft.**

fist n. puño v. **to make a** __ / cerrar
el __.

fistula n. fístula, canal o pasaje anormal
que permite el paso de secreciones de
una cavidad a otra o a la superficie
exterior; **anal** __ / __ anal;
arteriovenous __ / __ arteriovenosa;
biliary __ / __ biliar.

fistulectomy n. fistulectomía,
extirpación de una fístula.

fistulization n. fistulización, formación
de una fístula por un medio quirúrgico
o patológico súbito.

fit n. ataque súbito; convulsión; a.
[suitable] adecuado-a: vi. [glasses]
ajustar, encajar, montar.

fitness n. aptitud, vigor físico,
acondicionamiento físico; **physical** __
/ __ física.

fix v. [fasten] fijar, asegurar; **to fix up** /
arreglar, componer.

fixation n. fijación. 1. inmovilización
de una parte; 2. acción de fijar la vista
en un objeto; 3. interrupción del
desarrollo de la personalidad antes de
alcanzar la madurez.

fixed a. fijo-a; decidido-a [resolved]
resuelto; arreglado-a, determinado-a;
compuesto-a; __ **fee** / honorario __ o
definido; __ **term** / plazo __.

flabby a. blando-a, flojo-a; pop. fofo-a.

flaccid a. flácido-a; débil, flojo-a; __
paralysis / parálisis __.

flagellated a. flagelado-a, provisto de
flagelo o flagelos.

flagelliform n. flageliforme, en forma
de látigo.

flagellum n. (pl. flagella) flagelo,
prolongación o cola en la célula de
algunos protozoos.

flail chest n. tórax inestable, condición

de la pared del tórax causada por la
fractura múltiple de costillas.

flank n. flanco, parte del cuerpo entre las
costillas y el borde superior del íleo.

flap n. [sound of wings] aleteo; sonido de
alas; cubierta; colgajo.

flare n. brote, irritación rosácea o área
difundida; destello, fulgor; __ **-up** /
__ con irritación v. brotar, irritar.

flash n. fulguración, destello; **hot** __ /
fogaje, rubor.

flashback n. retrogresión; retroversión;
retrospección y actualización de
imágenes pasadas.

flatfoot n. pie plano.

flatulence n. flatulencia, distensión y
molestias abdominales por exceso de
gas en el tracto gastrointestinal.

flatus n. flato, pop. aventación, gas o aire
en los intestinos.

flatworm n. gusano plano que se aloja
en los intestinos.

flavor n. sabor, gusto.

flea n. pulga, insecto chupador de sangre;
__ **bite** / picadura de __.

flesh n. carne, tejido muscular suave del
cuerpo; __ **wound** / herida superficial.

flexibility n. flexibilidad, propiedad de
flexionar.

flexion n. flexión, acto de flexionar o de
ser flexionado.

flexor n. flexor, músculo que hace
flexionar una articulación.

flexure n. flexura, pliegue o doblez de
una estructura u órgano; **hepatic** __ /
__ hepática, ángulo derecho del colon;
sigmoid __ / sigmoidea, curvatura del
colon que antecede al recto; **splenic** __
/ __ esplénica, ángulo izquierdo del
colon.

flicker v. fluctuar, vacilar; [to quiver]
oscilar; causar una sensación visual de
contraste con interrupción de la luz.

floaters n., pl. flotadores, manchas
visuales, máculas.

floating a. flotante, libre, sin adhesión;
__ **ribs** / costillas __ -s.

flora n. flora, grupo de bacterias que se
alojan en un órgano; **intestinal** __ / __
intestinal.

flow n. flujo, salida; riego; [menstrual]
pop. pérdida; v. fluir; correr; derramar;
blood __ / riego sanguíneo; **laminar**
__ / __ laminar; **turbulent** __ / __
turbulento.

flowmeter n. medidor de flujo.

fluctuation n. fluctuación. 1. acto de
fluctuar, variación de un curso a otro;

2. sensación de movimiento ondulante producido por líquidos en el cuerpo que se percibe en un examen de palpación.

fluid *n.* líquido, fluido; secreción; **amniotic** __ / __ amniótico; **cerebroespinal** __ / __ cefalorraquídeo; **extracellular** __ / __ extracelular; **extravascular** __ / __ extravascular; **interstitial** __ / __ intersticial; **intracellular** __ / __ intracelular; **seminal** __ / __ seminal; **serous** __ / __ seroso; **synovial** __ / __ sinovial.

fluid balance *n.* balance hídrico.

fluid retention *n.* retención de líquido.

fluke *n.* duela, gusano de la orden *Trematoda;* **blood** __ / __ sanguínea; **intestinal** __ / __ intestinal; **liver** __ / __ hepática; **lung** __ / __ pulmonar.

fluorescent *a.* fluorescente, rel. a la fluorescencia; __ **antibody** / anticuerpo __; __ **troponemal antibody absorption test** / técnica del anticuerpo __.

fluoridation *n.* fluoridización, adición de fluoruro al agua.

fluoride *n.* fluoruro, combinación de flúor con un metal o metaloide.

fluoroscope *n.* fluoroscopio, instrumento que hace visibles los rayos-x en una pantalla fluorescente.

fluoroscopy *n.* fluoroscopía, uso del fluoroscopio para examinar los tejidos y otras estructuras internas del cuerpo.

fluorosis *n.* fluorosis, exceso de absorción de flúor.

flush *n.* rubor; [*cleansing*] irrigación; [*to empty out*] vaciar; irrigar; ruborizarse, sonrojarse.

flutter *n.* aleteo, acción similar al movimiento de las alas de los pájaros; **atrial** __ / __ auricular; __ **and fibrillation** / fibrilación __; **ventricular** __ / __ ventricular; *v.* aletear, sacudir; agitarse.

flux *n.* flujo excesivo proveniente de una cavidad u órgano del cuerpo.

fly *n.* mosca; *vi.* volar.

focal *a.* focal, rel. a un foco.

focus *n., L. (pl.* **foci**) foco; *v.* enfocar.

fold *n.* pliegue de un margen; **aryepiglottic** __ / __ ariepiglótico; **gastric** __ / __ gástrico; **gluteal** __ / __ glúteo.

folic acid *n.* ácido fólico, miembro del complejo de vitaminas B.

follicle *n.* folículo, saco, bolsa,

depresión o cavidad excretora; **atretic** __ / __ atrésico; **gastric** __ / __ gástrico; **hair** __ / __ piloso; **ovarian** __ / __ ovárico; **thyroid** __ / __ tiroideo.

follicular *a.* folicular, rel. a un folículo; __ **phase** / fase __.

folliculitis *n.* foliculitis, infl. de un folículo, gen. un folículo piloso.

follow *v.* seguir, continuar; __ **-up** / acción continuada, seguimiento, (estudio, procedimiento del caso); __ **-up evaluation** / evaluación del proceso evolutivo; **to __ through** / continuar el procedimiento; llevar hasta el final; continuar la observación de un caso.

fomes *n., L. (pl.* **fomites**) fomes, cualquier sustancia que puede absorber y luego transmitir agentes infecciosos.

fontanel, fontanella *n.* fontanela, *pop.* mollera, parte suave en el cráneo del recién nacido que normalmente se cierra al desarrollarse los huesos craneales.

food *n.* alimento; comida; **dietetic** __ / __ dietética; __ **additives** / aditivos alimenticios; __ **contamination** / contaminación de __ -s; __ **handling** / manipulación de __ -s; __ **poisoning** / intoxicación alimenticia; __ **requirements** / requisitos alimenticios; __ **supplements** / alimentos enriquecidos; **organic** __ / __ orgánico.

Food and Drug Administration *n.* Administración de Alimentos y Drogas, institución oficial en los Estados Unidos con regulaciones concernientes a alimentos, drogas, cosméticos y disposiciones médicas.

foot *n. (pl.* **feet**) pie; **athlete's** __ / __ de atleta; **flat** __ / __ plano.

foot and mouth disease *n.* fiebre aftosa, enfermedad viral propia de animales vacunos y equinos, y que es raramente trasmitida al ser humano, se caracteriza por la erupción de pequeñas vesículas en la lengua, la boca y los dedos de las manos y pies.

foot-drop *n.* pie caído.

footstep *n.* paso, pisada; [*print*] huella del pie.

for *prep.* [*intended for the use of*] para, **an antibiotic __ the infection** / un antibiótico __ la infección; [*in*

foramen

exchange for] por; **a thermometer __ taking the temperature** / un termómetro __ tomar la temperatura; [*for the benefit of*] para; **do it __ her** / hágalo, hazlo __ ella; **__ the time being** / __ ahora, __ el momento; **the medicine is __ the patient** / la medicina es __ el paciente; [*for the purpose of*] para; **you pay a dollar __ each pill** / paga un dólar __ cada pastilla; [*for the sake of*] por.

foramen *n.* foramen, orificio, pasaje, abertura; **intervertebral __** / __ intervertebral; **jugular __** / __ yugular; **optic __** / __ óptico; **ovale __** / __ oval; **sciatic, greater __** / __ sacrociático mayor; **sciatic, lesser __** / __ sacrociático menor

forbid *vi.* prohibir, impedir; **God __** ! / !no lo permita Dios!.

force *n.* fuerza, vigor, energía; *v.* forzar, violentar, obligar; *v.* **to __ out** / echar a la fuerza; **to __ through** / hacer penetrar a la fuerza.

forceps *n.* fórceps, pinza en forma de tenaza que se emplea para sujetar y manipular tejidos o partes del cuerpo.

forearm *n.* antebrazo.

forebrain *n.* prosencéfalo, porción anterior de la vesícula primaria cerebral de donde se desarrollan el diencéfalo y el telencéfalo.

forecast *n.* pronóstico, predicción; *v.* predecir, pronosticar.

forefinger *n.* dedo índice.

forefoot *n.* antepié, parte anterior del pie.

foregut *n.* intestino anterior, porción cefálica del tubo digestivo primitivo en el embrión.

forehead *n.* frente.

foreign bodies *n., pl.* cuerpos extraños, máculas, materia o pequeños objetos ajenos al lugar en que se alojan.

forensic *a.* forense, rel. a asuntos legales; **__ laboratory** / laboratorio __; **__ medicine** / medicina legal; **__ physician** / médico __.

foreplay *n.* estímulo erótico que precede al acto sexual.

foresight *n.* precaución, previsión.

foreskin *n.* prepucio; **prepuce.**

forever *adv.* siempre, para siempre, por siempre.

forget *vi.* olvidar; olvidarse de; **__ it** / olvídese, olvídate de eso; no se preocupe, no te preocupes.

forgetful *a.* olvidadizo-a; negligente.

form *n.* forma; [*document*] formulario; *v.* formar, dar forma; establecer.

formaldehyde *n.* formaldehído, antiséptico.

forme fruste *n. Fr.* forma frustrada, enfermedad abortada o manifestada de manera atípica.

formication *n.* formicación, sensación de hormigueo en la piel.

formula *n.* fórmula, forma prescrita o modelo a seguir.

fornix *n., L. (pl. fornices)* fornix.
1. estructura en forma de arco;
2. concavidad en forma de bóveda semejante a la vagina.

forth *adv.* [*forward*] hacia adelante; [*out, away*] afuera, hacia afuera.

forthcoming *a.* venidero-a; (*future*) próximo; (*available*) disponible

fortify *v.* fortalecer, fortificar.

fourchette *n. Fr.* horquilla, comisura posterior de la vulva.

fovea *n.* fóvea, fosa o depresión pequeña, esp. en referencia a la fosa central de la retina.

foxglove *n.* dedalera, nombre común de Digitalis purpurea.

fraction *n.* fracción, parte separable de una unidad.

fracture *n.* fractura, rotura; *pop.* quebradura. V. cuadro en la página 343.

fragility *n.* fragilidad, con disposición a romperse o quebrarse con facilidad.

frambesia, yaws *n.* frambesia, enfermedad cutánea tropical infecciosa que se manifiesta con lesiones aframbuesadas ulcerosas.

frame *n.* armazón, estructura de soporte; [*eye-glasses*] armazón. **claw type traction __** / armazón de tracción en garra; [*orthopedics*] **traction __** / armazón de tracción.

fraternal twins *n., pl.* mellizos fraternales, desarrollados de dos óvulos fecundados separadamente.

freckle *n.* peca, mácula pigmentada que se manifiesta en el exterior de la piel esp. en la cara.

free *a.* libre, suelto-a; [*of charge*] gratis; **__ association** / __ asociación; **-ly** *adv.* libremente.

freeze *n.* helada; congelación; **__ dried** / liofilizado; **__ drying** / liofilización; *vi.* congelar, helar; congelarse, helarse; **to __ to death** / morirse de frío.

freezing *n.* congelación; **__ point** / punto de __.

Fractures	Fracturas
avulsion	por avulsión
blow-out	por estallamiento
butterfly	en mariposa
closed	cerrada
comminuted	conminuta
complete	completa
complex	compleja
compressed	por compresión
depressed	con hundimiento
greenstick	de tallo verde
hairline	de raya fina
impacted	impactada
incomplete	incompleta
mallet	en martillo
open	expuesta
pathologic	patológica
perforating	perforante
rib	costal
spiral	espiral
stress	de sobrecarga
T	en T
wedge	en cuña

fremitus *n.* fremitus, frémito, vibración detectable por palpación o auscultación tal como las vibraciones del pecho al toser.

frenectomy *n.* frenectomía, excisión de un frenillo.

frenulum, frenum *n., L. (pl.* **frenulla**) frenulum, pliegue membranoso que impide los movimientos de un órgano o parte; __ **of the tongue** / frenillo de la lengua.

frequency *n.* frecuencia

frequent *a.* frecuente, habitual, regular; **-ly** *adv.* frecuentemente, con frecuencia.

fresh *a.* fresco-a, reciente.

Freudian *a.* freudiano, rel. a las doctrinas de Sigmund Freud, neurólogo vienés (1856–1939).

friction *n.* fricción, rozamiento; __ **rub** / roce de __.

frightened *a.* asustado-a, atemorizado-a.

frigidity *n.* frígidez, frialdad, esp. de la mujer incapaz de responder a estímulos sexuales.

Frohlich's syndrome *n.* síndrome de Frolich, distrofia adipogenital manifestada en infantilismo sexual con cambios en las características sexuales secundarias.

front *n.* frente; **in __ of** / en __ de, delante de.

frontal *a.* frontal, rel. a la frente; __ **bone** / hueso __; __ **muscle** / músculo __; __ **sinuses** / senos __ -es.

frostbite *n.* quemadura por frío.

froth *n.* espuma; *v.* echar espuma, espumar; **to __ at the mouth** / echar __ por la boca.

frozen *a. pp.* of **to freeze**, congelado-a; *v.* **to become __** / congelarse, helarse.

frozen section *n.* corte por congelación, espécimen de tejido fino que se toma y congela inmediatamente para ser usado en el diagnóstico de tumores.

frozen shoulder *n.* hombro rígido.

fructose *n.* fructosa, azúcar de frutas; lebulosa; __ **intolerance** / intolerancia a la __.

fructosuria *n.* fructosuria, fructosa en la orina.

fruitful *a.* productivo-a; provechoso-a.

frustrated *a.* frustrado-a.

fulguration *n.* fulgaración, uso de corriente eléctrica para destruir tejido vivo.

full *a.* completo-a; lleno-a, pleno-a; __ **answer** / respuesta __; __ **payment** / pago total; **in __** / completamente, por completo.

full-grown *a.* completamente desarrollado-a; crecido-a.

full term *n.* a término, [*in obstetrics*] embarazo a término, de 38 a 41 semanas de duración incluyendo el nacimiento.

fulminant *a.* fulminante, que aparece súbitamente con extrema intensidad tal como un dolor o enfermedad.

fumes *n., pl.* vapores o gases.

fumigation *n.* fumigación, exterminación por medio de vapores.

fuming *a.* fumante, que desprende vapores visibles.

function *n.* función; facultad; *v.* funcionar, desempeñar un trabajo.

functional disease *n.* enfermedad funcional, desorden o trastorno que no tiene una causa orgánica conocida.

fundus *n.* fondo, la parte más distante al orificio de entrada de un órgano; __ **of stomach** / __ del estómago; __ **uteri** / __ del útero.

fungal, fungous

fungal, fungous *a.* fungoso-a, rel. a hongos o causado por éstos.

fungemia *n.* fungemia, presencia de hongos en la sangre.

fungistasis *n.* fungistasis, acto de impedir o arrestar el desarrollo de hongos.

fungitoxic *a.* fungitóxico, de efecto tóxico en los hongos.

fungus *n., L. (pl.* **fungi**) hongo.

funicular *a.* funicular, rel. al cordón umbilical o espermático.

funiculitis *n.* funiculitis, infl. del cordón espermático.

funnel chest *n.* tórax en embudo.

furious *a.* furioso-a; enfurecido-a.

furosemide *n.* furosemida, diurético.

furrow *n.* surco; **atrioventricular** __ / __ atrioventricular; **digital** __ / __ digital; **gluteal** __ / __ gluteal.

furuncle *n.* furúnculo; *pop.* grano enterrado.

furunculosis *n.* furunculosis, condición que resulta por la presencia de furúnculos.

fusion *n.*fusión. 1. reacción termonuclear en la cual núcleos atómicos de luz se unen para formar átomos más potentes; 2. acto de fusionar o fundir; **nuclear** __ / __ nuclear.

future *n.* futuro, porvenir.

fuzzy *a.* 1. nublado-a, que no es claramente visible; 2. velloso-a, cubierto de pelusa.

g

g

G *abbr.* **constant of gravitation** / constante de gravitación.

g *abbr.* **gender** / género; **glucose** / glucosa; **grain** / grano.

gag *n.* abrebocas, instrumento para mantener la boca abierta durante ciertas intervenciones quirúrgicas; __ **reflex** / reflejo de arqueada.

gain *n.* ganancia, ventaja; provecho; *v.* ganar; **to __ weight** / aumentar de peso.

gait *n.* marcha, andar; **cerebellar __** / __ cerebelosa; **compensated gluteal __** / __ compensada glútea; **crutch __** / __ con muletas; **dorsiflexor __** / __ de dorsiflexión; **drag-to __** / __ de arrastre; **duck __** / __ de pato; **equine __** / __ equina; **festinating __** / __ festinante; **gastrocnemius __** / __ gemelar; **hemiplegic __** / __ hemipléjica; **petit pas __** / __ en pequeños pasos; **scissors __** / __ en tijeras; **spastic __** / __ espástica; **steppage __** / __ en estepaje; **tabetic __** / __ tabética; **three point __** / __ en tres apoyos; **Treadelenburg or gluteal __** / __ de Treadelenburg o glútea; **two point __** / __ en dos apoyos; **uncompensated gluteal __** / __ glútea descompensada; **waddling __** / __ de ánade.

galactagogue *n.* galactagogo, galactógeno, agente que promueve la secreción de leche.

galactase *n.* galactasa, enzima presente en la leche.

galactocele *n.* galactocele, quiste de la mama que contiene leche.

galactography *n.* galactografía, rayos-x de los conductos lácteos.

galactophoritis *n.* galactoforitis, infl. de los conductos lácteos.

galactophorous *a.* galactóforo-a, que conduce la leche o la lleva.

galactopoiesis *n.* galactopoyesis, producción de leche.

galactorrhea *n.* galactorrea. 1. secreción excesiva de leche; 2. continuación de secreción de leche a intervalos después que el período de lactancia ha terminado.

galactose *n.* galactosa, monosacárido derivado de la lactosa por acción de una enzima o un ácido mineral; __ **cataract** / catarata de __ .

galactosemia *n.* galactosemia, ausencia congénita de la enzima necesaria para la conversión de galactosa a glucosa o sus derivados.

galactosuria *n.* galactosuria, orina con apariencia lechosa.

galactotherapy *n.* galactoterapia. 1. tratamiento dirigido a un lactante mediante administración de medicamentos a la madre; 2. uso terapéutico de la leche en una dieta especial.

galacturia *n.* galacturia, aspecto lechoso en la orina.

gall *n.* bilis, hiel; __ **ducts** / conductos biliares.

gallbladder *n.* vesícula biliar; __ **attack** / ataque de la vesícula.

gallop *n.* galope, ritmo cardíaco que simula el galope de un caballo y que se oye cuando hay fallo del corazón.

gallop rhythm *n.* ritmo de galope, sonido anormal del corazón percibido en casos de taquicardia.

gallstone *n.* cálculo biliar; **calcium oxalate __** / __ de oxalato de calcio; **cholesterol __** / __ de colesterol; **cystine __** / __ de cistina; **fibrin __** / __ de fibrina; **pigment __** / __ de pigmento.

galvanic *a.* galvánico-a, rel. al galvanismo; __ **battery** / batería; __ **cell** / célula __; __ **current** / corriente __ .

gamete *n.* gameto, célula sexual masculina o femenina; __ **intrafallopian transfer** / transferencia de __ a los tubos de Falopio.

gametocyte *n.* gametocito, célula que al dividirse produce gametos tal como el parásito de la malaria cuando se divide y pasa al mosquito portador.

gamma globulin *n.* gamma globulina, tipo de anticuerpo producido en el tejido linfático o sintéticamente.

gamma rays *n., pl.* rayos gamma, rayos emitidos por sustancias radioactivas.

gammagraphy *n.* gammagrafía, registro de rayos gamma después de la administración de isótopos radioactivos.

gammopathy

gammopathy *n.* gammopatía, trastorno manifestado por un exceso de inmunoglobulinas como resultado de una proliferación anormal de células linfoides.

gamophobia *n.* gamofobia, temor al matrimonio.

gangliectomy *n.* gangliectomía, ganglionectomía, excisión de un ganglio.

ganglioglioma *n.* ganglioglioma, ganglioneuroma, tumor caracterizado por un gran número de células ganglionares.

ganglioma *n.* ganglioma, tumor de un ganglio, esp. linfático.

ganglion *n. (pl.* **ganglia)** ganglio. 1. masa de tejido nervioso en forma de nudo; 2. quiste en un tendón o en una aponeurosis, que se observa a veces en la muñeca, en el talón o en la rodilla; __ **-a, basal** / __ **-s basales;** __ , **carotid** / __ carotídeo; __ , **celiac** / __ celíaco.

ganglioneuroma *n.* ganglioneuroma, neuroma compuesto de células ganglionares.

ganglionitis *n.* infl. de una glándula.

gangrene *n.* gangrena, destrucción de un tejido debido a riego sanguíneo interrumpido gen. por infección bacteriana y putrefacción.

gangrenous *a.* gangrenoso, rel. a la gangrena.

gap *n.* laguna, vacío; intervalo, abertura.

Gardner's syndrome *n.* síndrome de Gardner. 1. múltiple poliposis del colon asociado con riesgo de carcinoma del colon; 2. tumor de tejido blando de la piel.

gargle *n.* gargarización; *v.* hacer gárgaras.

gargoylism *n.* gargolismo, condición hereditaria caracterizada por anormalidades físicas, en algunos casos con retraso mental.

gas *n.* gas, sustancia con propiedades de expansión indefinida; **mustard** __ / __ de mostaza; **nerve** __ / __ neurotóxico; **tear** __ / __ lacrimógeno.

gaseous *a.* gaseoso-a, rel. a o de la naturaleza del gas.

gas gangrene *n.* gangrena gaseosa.

gastradenitis *n.* gastradenitis, infl. de las glándulas del estómago.

gastralgia *n.* gastralgia, dolor de estómago.

gastrectasis, gastrectasia *n.* gastrectasia, dilatación del estómago.

gastrectomy *n.* gastrectomía, extirpación de una parte o de todo el estómago.

gastric *a.* gástrico-a, rel. o concerniente al estómago; **acid** / ácido; __ **analysis** / gastroanálisis; __ **arteries** / arterias __; __ **by-pass** / derivación __; **digestion** __ / digestión __; **emptying** / vaciamiento __; __ **feeding** / alimentación __; __ **fistula** / fístula __; __ **glands** / glándulas __; __ **juice** / jugo __ ; __ **lavage** / lavado __ ; __ **stapling** / cirugía de reducción __ para adelgazar; **ulcer** __ / úlcera __; __ **vertigo** / vértigo __ .

gastritis *n.* gastritis, infl. del estómago; **acute** __ / __ aguda; **chronic** __ / __ crónica.

gastroanalysis *n.* gastroanálisis, análisis del contenido del estómago.

gastrocele *n.* gastrocele, hernia del estómago.

gastrocnemius *n.* gastronemio, músculo mayor de la pantorrilla.

gastrocolitis *n.* gastrocolitis, infl. del estómago y del colon.

gastrocolostomy *n.* gastrocolostomía, anastomosis del estómago y el colon.

gastroduodenal *a.* gastroduodenal, rel. al estómago y el duodeno.

gastroduodenitis *n.* gastroduodenitis, infl. del estómago y el duodeno.

gastroduodenoscopy *n.* gastroduodenoscopía, uso del endoscopio para examinar visualmente el estómago y el duodeno.

gastroenteritis *n.* gastroenteritis, infl. del estómago y el intestino.

gastroenterocolitis *n.* gastroenterocolitis, infl. del estómago y el intestino delgado.

gastroesophageal *a.* gastroesofágico-a, rel. al estómago y al esófago; __ **hernia** / hernia __; __ **reflux disease** / enfermedad de reflujo __ .

gastrogavage *n.* gastrogavaje, alimentación artificial al estómago por tubo o a través de una abertura.

gastrohepatitis *n.* gastrohepatitis, infl. del estómago y del hígado.

gastroileostomy *n.* gastroileostomía, anastomosis entre el estómago y el íleo.

gastrointestinal *a.* gastrointestinal; rel. al estómago y el intestino; __ **barrier** / barrera __; __ **bleeding** / sangramiento __; __ **decompression** / descompresión __; __ **tract** / tracto __.

gastrojejunostomy *n.* gastroyeyunostomía, anastomosis del estómago y el yeyuno.

gastrolith *n.* gastrolito, concreción en el estómago.

gastrolithiasis *n.* gastrolitiasis, cálculos en el estómago.

gastromegaly *n.* gastromegalia, agrandamiento del estómago.

gastroplication *n.* gastroplicación, operación de sutura de un pliegue de la pared del estómago para reducir el tamaño del mismo. Syn. gastrorrhaphy.

gastrorrhagia *n.* gastrorragia, hemorragia estomacal.

gastrorrhaphy *n.* gastrorrafia, sutura o perforación del estómago.

gastroschisis *n.* gastrosquisis, hendidura en la pared abdominal debida a ruptura de la membrana amniótica.

gastrospasm *n.* gastroespasmo, contracciones espasmódicas de las paredes del estómago.

Gauss sign *n.* Gauss, signo de, movimiento marcado en el útero durante las primeras semanas del embarazo.

gauze *n.* gasa: **absorbable** __ / __ absorbible; **absorbent** __ / __ absorbente; **antiseptic** / antiséptica; __ **compress** / compresa de __.

gay *n.* homosexual; __ **bowel syndrome** / síndrome intestinal del __.

gender *n.* género, denominación del sexo masculino o femenino; __ **identity** / identidad de __; __ **role** / representación de __.

gene *n.* gen, gene, unidad básica de rasgos hereditarios; **dominant** __ / __ dominante; __ **frequency** / frecuencia del __; **lethal** __ / __ letal; **gene mapping** / genética cartográfica; **recessive** __ / __ recesivo; **sex-linked** __ / __ ligado al sexo.

general *a.* general; __ **appearance** / aspecto __; __ **condition** / estado __; __ **practitioners** / médicos de familia; __ **treatment** / tratamiento __.

generalization *n.* generalización.

generation *n.* generación. 1. acción de crear un nuevo organismo; 2. producción por proceso natural o artificial; 3. conjunto de personas nacidas dentro de un período de unos treinta años aproximadamente.

generic *n.* nombre común de un producto o medicamento no patentado; *a.* genérico-a, rel. al género; __ **name** / nombre genérico.

genesis *n.* génesis, acto de creación, reproducción y desarrollo.

gene therapy *n.* terapia genética, terapia con el propósito de corregir un defecto genético.

genetic *a.* genético-a, rel. a la génesis y a la genética; __ **amplification** / amplificación __; __ **association** / asociación __; __ **code** / patrón __ ; __ **counseling** / asesoramiento __; __ **determinant** / determinante __; __ **engineering** / construcción __ ; __ **epidemiology** / epidemiología __; __ **fitness** / acondicionamiento __; __ **load** / carga __; __ **marker** / marcador __ ; __ **substrate** / substrato __.

genetics *n.* genética, rama de la biología que estudia la herencia y las leyes que la gobiernan; **medical** __ / __ médica.

genicular *a.* genicular, rel. a la rodilla.

geniculate *a.* geniculado-a. 1. doblado-a, como una rodilla; 2. rel. al ganglio del nervio facial; __ **body** / cuerpo __; __ **ganglion** / ganglio __; __ **neuralgia** / neuralgia __.

genital *a.* genital, rel. a los genitales; __ **ambiguity** / ambigüedad __; __ **cord** / cordón __; __ **corpuscles** / corpúsculos __; __ **furrow** / surco __; __ **herpes** / herpes __; __ **phase** / fase __; __ **tract** / tracto __; __ **wart** / verruga __.

genitals, genitalia *n., pl.* genitales, órganos de la reproducción.

genitourinary *a.* genitourinario, rel. a los órganos reproductivos y urinarios.

genocide *n.* genocidio, exterminación sistemática de un grupo étnico.

genodermatosis *n.* genodermatosis, una condición de la piel de origen genético.

genom, genome *n.* genoma, el conjunto básico completo de cromosomas haploides en un organismo.

genomic

genomic *a.* genómico-a, rel. a un genoma; ___ **clone** / clon ___ .

genotype *n.* genotipo, constitución genética de un organismo.

gentian violet *n.* violeta de genciana, colorante para teñir tejidos y microorganismos que permiten el estudio microscópico.

genucubital *a.* genucubital, rel. a los codos, las rodillas y su posición; ___ **position** / posición ___ .

genupectoral *a.* genupectoral, rel. a las rodillas y el tórax y su posición; ___ **position** / posición ___ .

genus *n.* (*pl.* **genera**) género, categoría perteneciente a una clasificación biológica.

genu valgum, knock knee *n.* genu valgum, curvatura anormal de las rodillas hacia adentro y separación de los tobillos al caminar que comienza en la infancia a causa de una deficiencia ósea.

genu varum, bow-leg *n.* piernas arqueadas, *pop.* zambo-a, curvatura anormal de las rodillas hacia afuera.

geographic *a.* geográfico-a, que muestra señales física, natural o superficialmente; ___ **keratitis** / queratitis ___; ; ___ **retinal atrophy** / atrofia retinal ___; ___ **skull** / cráneo ___ .

geographic tongue *n.* lengua geográfica, lengua caracterizada por áreas desnudas rodeadas de epitelio grueso que simulan áreas terrestres.

geriatrics *n.* geriatría, rama de la medicina que trata de las enfermedades y de los problemas que se manifiestan en la vejez.

germ *n.* germen, microorganismo o bacteria esp. causante de enfermedades; ___ **warfare** / guerra bacteriológica.

German measles *n.* rubela, rubéola; *pop.* sarampión de tres días, infección viral benigna muy contagiosa en los niños de 3 a 10 años. Puede causar trastornos serios en el desarrollo del feto al contraerla la madre; ___ **vaccination** / vacunación antirrubeólica.

germinal *a.* germinal, rel. a o de la naturaleza de un germen o gérmenes; ___ **cell** / célula ___; ___ **disk** / disco ___; ___ **epithelium** / epitelio ___; ___ **localization** / localización ___; ___ **vesicle** / vesícula o núcleo ___ .

gestalt *n.* gestalt, teoría que mantiene que la conducta responde a la percepción íntegra de una situación y no es posible analizarla atendiendo sólo a las partes componentes de la misma.

gestation *n.* embarazo, gestación, estado de gravidez; **abdominal** ___ / ___ abdominal; **ectopic** ___ / ___ ectópica; **interstitial** ___ / ___ intersticial; **multiple** ___ / ___ múltiple; **prolonged** ___ / ___ prolongada; **secondary** ___ / ___ secundaria; **secondary abdominal** ___ / ___ abdominal secundaria; **tubal** ___ / ___ tubárica; **tubo-ovarian** ___ / ___ tubo-ovárica; **uterotubaric** ___ / ___ útero-tubárica.

gestational maturity *n.* madurez gestacional fetal.

gesticulate *v.* gesticular, expresar por medio de gestos o señas.

get *v.* obtener, adquirir, conseguir; [*communication*]; **to ___ across** / lograr comunicarse, hacer comprender; **to ___ ahead** / prosperar; **to ___ back something** / recobrar; **to ___ back** / volver; [*to swallow*] **to ___ down** / tragar; [*steps*] **to ___ down** / bajar; **to ___ into** / meterse; **to ___ it over** / acabar de una vez; **to ___** [*someone, something*] **out of the way** / sacar de, quitar de, apartar de; **to ___ sick** / enfermarse; **to ___ underway** / empezar, comenzar; **to ___ up** / levantarse; **to ___ well** / curarse, sanarse.

giant *a.* gigante, de un tamaño grande anormal; ___ **cell** / célula ___; ___ **cell tumor** / tumor de células ___ -s.

giardiasis *n.* giardiasis, infección intestinal común causada por la *Giardia lamblia* que se trasmite por contaminación de alimentos, de agua o por contacto directo.

gibbosity *n.* gibosidad, corcova, condición de joroba.

gigantism *n.* gigantismo, desarrollo en exceso del cuerpo o de una parte de éste; ___ , **acromegalic** / ___ acromegálico; ___ , **eunuchoid** / ___ eunucoide, gigantismo acompañado de características e insuficiencia sexual propias del eunuco; ___ , **normal** / ___ normal, desarrollo normal de los órganos sexuales y proporción normal de los órganos y partes del cuerpo, gen. causado por secreción excesiva de la glándula pituitaria.

Gilles de la Tourette syndrome *n.* síndrome de Gilles de la Tourette, enfermedad de la infancia que afecta más a los varones que a las hembras y que se cree ser de naturaleza neurológica; Se manifiesta en anomalías musculares y en la pubertad en la expresión involuntaria de obscenidades.

gingiva n. (pl. **gingivae**) gingiva, encía, porción de tejido que rodea el cuello de los dientes.

gingival a. gingival, rel. a la gingiva.

gingivectomy n. gingivectomía, resección de la encía.

gingivitis n. gingivitis, infl. de las encías.

girdle n. faja, cinturón; **pelvic __** / cinturón pélvico; **scapular or shoulder __** / cinturón torácico.

give vi. dar; **__ birth** / dar a luz; **to __ and take** / hacer concesiones mutuas; **to __ out** / repartir; **to __ up** / renunciar a, perder la esperanza; darse por vencido.

glad a. alegre, contento-a; v. **to be __ of** / alegrarse de; **to be __ to** / tener mucho gusto en; **-ly** adv. con mucho gusto; con satisfacción; alegremente.

gland n. glándula, órgano que segrega o secreta sustancias que realizan funciones fisiológicas específicas o que eliminan productos del organismo; **eccrine __** / __ ecrina; **endocrine __** / __ endocrina; **swollen __** / __ inflamada.

glans n. glande, masa redonda de estructura similar a una glándula situada en la extremidad del pene (glans penis) y del clítoris (glans clitorides).

glare n. resplandor, deslumbramiento, relumbrón; v. mirar con intensidad.

Glasgow coma scale n. escala de coma de Glasgow, método para evaluar el grado de un estado de coma.

glasses n., pl. lentes, espejuelos, gafas; **bifocal __** / __ bifocales; **trifocal __** / __ trifocales.

glaucoma n. glaucoma, enfermedad de los ojos producida por hipertensión del globo ocular, atrofia de la retina y ceguera; **absolutum __** / __ absoluto, etapa final del glaucoma agudo que resulta en ceguera; **chronic __** / __ crónico; **congential __** / __ congénito; **juvenile __** / __ juvenil, se manifiesta en niños mayores y jóvenes sin agrandamiento del globo ocular; **infantile __** / __ infantil, se manifiesta a partir del nacimiento o desde los tres años.

glenohumeral a. glenohumeral, rel. al húmero y la cavidad glenoide; **__ joint** / articulación __; **__ ligaments** / ligamentos __.

glenoid a. glenoideo-a, con apariencia de fosa o cuenca; **__ cavity** / cavidad __; **__ fossa** / fosa __.

glioblastoma n. glioblastoma, tipo de tumor cerebral.

gliocytoma n. gliocitoma, tumor de células de neuroglia.

glioma n. glioma, neoplasma del cerebro compuesto de células de neuroglia.

gliomyoma n. gliomioma, combinación de glioma y mioma.

glioneuroma n. glioneuroma, glioma combinado con neuroma.

gliosarcoma n. gliosarcoma, glioma con abundancia de células fusiformes.

global warming n. calentamiento global, aumento de los niveles de gases tales como el dióxido de carbono que provoca el alce de la temperatura de la tierra y que puede afectar muchos sistemas biológicos, incluyendo la salud del ser humano.

globulin n. globulina, una de las cuatro proteínas más importantes que componen el plasma; **antilymphocyte __** / __ antilinfocítica; **gamma __** / gamma __.

globulinuria n. globulinuria, presencia de globulina en la orina.

globus n. globo, esfera; **__ hystericus** / __ histérico, sensación subjetiva de tener una bola en la garganta.

glomerular a. glomerular, rel. a un glomérulo; en forma de racimo; **__ cyst** / quiste __; **__ filtration rate** / índice de filtración __; **__ nephritis** / nefritis __.

glomerulonephritis n. glomerulonefritis, enfermedad de Bright, infl. del glomérulo renal.

glomerulosclerosis n. glomeruloesclerosis, proceso degenerativo del glomérulo renal que se asocia con arteriesclerosis y diabetes.

glomerulus n., L. (pl. **glomeruli**) glomérulo, colección de capilares en forma de bola pequeña localizados en el riñón.

glomus n., L. (pl. **glomera**) glomo, bola, grupo de arteriolas conectadas directamente a las venas, ricas en inervación.

glossa n. glosa, lengua.

glossalgia

glossalgia *n.* glosalgia, dolor en la lengua.

glossectomy *n.* glosectomía, excisión parcial o completa de la lengua.

glossitis *n.* glositis, infl. de la lengua; **acute** __ / __ aguda, asociada con estomatitis.

glossodynia *n.* glosodinia, glossalgia.

glossopharyngeal *a.* glosofaríngeo, relativo a la faringe y la lengua.

glossoplasty *n.* glosoplastia, cirugía plástica de la lengua.

glossy skin *n.* liodermia, apariencia brillante de la piel, síntoma de atrofia o traumatismo de los nervios.

glottis *n.* glotis, hendidura en la parte superior de la laringe entre las cuerdas vocales verdaderas; aparato vocal de la laringe.

glucagon *n.* glucagón, una de dos hormonas producidas por los islotes de Langerhans cuya función consiste en aumentar la concentración de glucosa en la sangre y que tiene un efecto antiinflamatorio.

glucagonoma *n.* glucagonoma, tumor que secreta glucagón.

glucocorticoid *n.* glucocorticoide, grupo de hormonas segregadas por la corteza suprarrenal que intervienen en el proceso metabólico del organismo y tienen un efecto antiinflamatorio.

glucogenesis *n.* glucogénesis, proceso de desdoblamiento del glucógeno.

glucose *n.* glucosa, dextrosa, azúcar de fruta, fuente principal de energía en organismos vivos; **blood level of** __ / nivel de __ en la sangre; **tolerance test** / prueba de tolerancia a la __ .

glucose-6-phosphate dehydrogenase *n.* glucofosfato de deshidrogenasa, enzima presente en el hígado y los riñones necesaria en la conversión de glicerol a glucosa.

glucoside, glycoside *n.* glucósido, compuesto natural o sintético que al hidrolizarse libera azúcar.

glucosuria, glycosuria *n.* glucosuria, presencia excesiva de glucosa en la orina; **diabetic** __ / __ diabética; **pituitary** __ / __ pituitaria; **renal** __ / __ renal.

glucuronic acid, glycuronic acid *n.* ácido glucurónico, ácido de efecto desintoxicante en el metabolismo humano.

glutamic-oxaloacetic transaminase *n.* transaminasa glutámica oxaloacética, enzima presente en varios tejidos y líquidos del organismo cuya concentración elevada en el suero indica daño cardíaco o hepático.

glutamic-pyruvic transaminase *n.* transaminasa glutámica pirúvica, enzima cuyo aumento en la sangre es indicio de daño cardíaco o hepático.

gluteal *a.* glúteo-a, rel. a las nalgas; __ **fold** / pliegue __; __ **reflex** / reflejo __ .

gluten *n.* gluten, materia vegetal albuminoidea; __ **-free diet** / dieta libre de __ .

glycemia *n.* glicemia, glucemia, concentración de glucosa en la sangre.

glycerin *n.* glicerina, glicerol, alcohol que se encuentra en las grasas.

glychoprotein *n.* glucoproteína, compuesto de carbohidrato y proteína.

glycine *n.* glicina, ácido aminoacético, aminoácido no esencial.

glycocholic acid *n.* ácido glicocólico, combinación de glicina y ácido cólico.

glycogen *n.* glucógeno, polisacárido usu. almacenado en el hígado que se convierte en glucosa según lo necesite el organismo; __ **storage disease** / hepatina, almacenamiento de glucógeno en el hígado.

glycolic *a.* glucolítico-a, que descompone o digiere los azúcares.

glycolysis *n.* glicólisis, subdivisión de azúcar en compuestos más simples.

glycophilia *n.* glucofilia, estado en el cual una cantidad muy pequeña de dextrosa produce hiperglucemia.

glycorrhachia *n.* glucorraquia, presencia de glucosa en el líquido cefalorraquídeo.

gnathoplasty *n.* gnatoplastia, cirugía plástica de la mandíbula.

gnosia *n.* gnosia, facultad de reconocer y distinguir objetos y personas.

go *vi.* ir; irse; **to** __ **after** / seguir; **to** __ **about** / andar, caminar; [*to accompany*] **to** __ **along with** / acompañar; **to** __ **against** / ir en contra de; **to** __ **ahead** / adelantar; emprender; **to** __ **along with a decision** / aceptar, aprobar una decisión; **to** __ **bad** / echarse a perder; **to** __ **back** / volver, retroceder; **to** __ **crazy** / enloquecer; **to** __ **in or into** / entrar; **to** __ **deep into** / ahondar; **to**

__ **down with** / enfermarse, caer enfermo-a; [*distance*] **to __ far** / ir lejos; [*to succeed*] tener éxito, progresar; **to __ on** / continuar; **to __ over** / examinar, estudiar; **to __ through** / examinar o estudiar con cuidado; **to let __** / soltar, dejar; **to let oneself __** / soltarse; dejarse; relajarse.

goblet cell *n.* célula caliciforme secretora que se localiza en el epitelio del tubo digestivo y del tubo respiratorio.

godchild *n.* ahijado-a.

godfather *n.* padrino.

godmother *n.* madrina.

goggle-eyed *a.* de ojos saltones.

goiter *n.* bocio, engrosamiento de la glándula tiroides; **congenital __** / __ congénito; **endemic, colloid __** / __ endémico, coloide; **exophtalmic __** / __ exoftálmico; **toxic __** / __ tóxico (de síntomas similares a la tirotoxicosis); **wandering __** / __ móvil.

gonad *n.* gónada, glándula productora de gametos: los ovarios en la mujer y los testículos en el hombre.

gonadal *a.* gonadal, rel. a una glándula gónada; **__ dysgenesis** / disgenesia, malformación __ .

gonadectomy *n.* gonadectomía, excisión de una glándula sexual.

gonadotropin *n.* gonadotropina, hormona estimulante de las gónadas; **chorionic __** / __ coriónica, presente en la sangre y orina de la mujer durante el embarazo; base de la prueba del embarazo; **__ of the anterior pituitary** / __ hipofisaria.

gonadotropin-releasing hormone *n.* hormona que estimula la secreción de gonadotropina.

gonalgia *n.* gonalgia, dolor en la rodilla.

gonarthritis *n.* gonartritis, infl. de la articulación de la rodilla.

goniopuncture *n.* goniopuntura, tratamiento de glaucoma por punción en la cámara anterior del ojo.

goniotomy *n.* goniotomía, procedimiento para tratar el glaucoma congénito.

gonococcal *a.* gonocócico-a; rel. a los gonococos; **__ arthritis** / artritis __; **__ conjunctivitis** / conjuntivitis __ .

gonococcemia *n.* gonococcemia, presencia de gonococos en la sangre.

gonococcus *n.* (*pl.* **gonococci**)

gonococo, microorganismo de la especie *Neisseria gonorrhoeae*, causante de la gonorrea.

gonorrhea *n.* gonorrea, enfermedad infecciosa catarral contagiosa de la mucosa genital.

gonorrheal *a.* gonorreico-a, rel. a la gonorrea; **__ arthritis** / artritis __; **__ ophthalmia** / oftalmía __ .

good *a.* bueno-a; **all in __ time** / todo a su debido tiempo; **in __ time** / a buen tiempo, puntual; **very good!** / muy bien!; **__ afternoon** / buenas tardes; **__ behavior** / buena conducta, buen comportamiento; **__ -bye** / adiós; **__ cause** / causa justificada; **__ luck** / buena suerte; **__ morning** / buenos días, buen día; **__ night** / buenas noches; **in __ faith** / de__fe; **to be at** / tener talento para; **to do someone __** / hacer bien a alguien; **to put in a __ word** / recomendar.

Good Samaritan Law *n.* Ley del buen samaritano, protección legal al facultativo o a otras personas que prestan ayuda médica en casos de emergencia.

gout *n.* gota, enfermedad hereditaria causada por defecto del metabolismo de ácido úrico.

grade *n.* grado. 1. medida o evaluación estándar; 2. en la patología del cáncer, indicación de la fase de la enfermedad.

gradient *a.* gradiente, línea que indica aumento o disminución en una variable.

Graefe operation *n.* Graefe, operación de. 1. operación de la catarata por incisión de la esclerótica, distinción de la cápsula e iridectomía; 2. iridectomía para glaucoma.

Graefe's sign *n.* Graefe, signo de, fallo del párpado superior en seguir el movimiento del globo del ojo hacia abajo.

graft *n.* injerto, tejido u órgano usado en un trasplante o implante; *v.* injertar; **accordion __** / __ en acordeón; **__ allogenic __** / alogénico; **autologous __** / __ autólogo; **autoplastic __** / __ autoplástico; **bone __** / __ óseo; **choriolantoic __** / __ coriolantoideo; **corneal __** / __ de la córnea **dermal __** dérmico; **fat __** / __ adiposo; **free __** / __ libre; **heterologous __** / __ heterólogo; **heteroplastic __** / __ heteroplástico; **heterotopic __** / __ heterotópico; **homologous __** / __

351

homólogo; **homoplastic** ⸺ / ⸺ homoplástico; **isoplastic** ⸺ / isoplástico; **mucosal** ⸺ / ⸺ mucoso; **nerve** ⸺ / ⸺ de nervio; **orthotopic** ⸺ / ⸺ ortotópico; **pedicle** ⸺ / ⸺ pedicular; **sieve** ⸺ / ⸺ en criba; **skin** ⸺ / ⸺ de piel; **tendon** ⸺ / ⸺ tendinoso; **zooplastic** ⸺ / ⸺ zooplástico.

gramicidin *n.* gramicidina, antibiótico producido por *Bacillus brevis*, localmente activo contra bacterias gram-positivas.

gram-molecule *n.* molécula gramo, el peso en gramos de una sustancia igual a su peso molecular.

gram-negative *n.* gram-negativo, resultado de la aplicacion del método de Gram de decoloración de una bacteria o tejido por medio de alcohol.

gram-positive *n.* gram-positivo, retención del color o resistencia a la decoloración en la aplicación del método de Gram.

Gram's method *n.* método de Gram, proceso de coloración de bacterias para identificarlas en un análisis.

granular *a.* granuloso-a, granulado-a, hecho o formado de gránulos; ⸺ **cell tumor** / tumor celular ⸺; ⸺ **conjunctivitis** / conjuntivitis ⸺; ⸺ **corneal dystrophy** / distrofia ⸺ de la córnea; ⸺ **cortex** / corteza ⸺; ⸺ **endoplasmic reticulum** / retículo endoplásmico ⸺; ⸺ **leukocyte** / leucocito ⸺; ⸺ **ophthalmia** / oftalmia ⸺ .

granular cast *n.* cilindro granuloso, cilindro urinario visto en nefropatías degenerativas o de tipo inflamatorio.

granulation *n.* granulación, masa redonda y carnosa que se forma en la superficie de un tejido, membrana u órgano; ⸺ **tissue** / tejido de ⸺ .

granule *n.* gránulo, partícula pequeña formada de gránulos; **acidophil** ⸺ / ⸺ acidófilo, que acepta colorantes ácidos ; **basophil** ⸺ / ⸺ basófilo, que acepta colorantes básicos.

granulocyte *n.* granulocito, leucocito que contiene gránulos.

granulocytopenia *n.* granulocitopenia, deficiencia de granulocitos en la sangre.

granuloma *n.* granuloma, tumor o neoplasma de tejido granular; **foreign body** ⸺ / ⸺ de cuerpo extraño; **infectious** ⸺ / ⸺ infeccioso; **inguinal**

⸺ / ⸺ inguinal; **venereum** ⸺ / ⸺ ulcerativo de los genitales.

granulomatous *a.* granulomatoso-a, que tiene las características de un granuloma; ⸺ **colitis** / colitis ⸺; ⸺ **encephalomyelitis** / encefalomielitis ⸺; ⸺ **enteritis** / enteritis ⸺; ⸺ **inflammation** / inflamación ⸺ .

granulosa *n.* granulosa, membrana ovárica de células epiteliales que rodea el folículo ovárico.

granulosa cell tumor *n.* tumor de la granulosa.

granulosa-teca cell tumor *n.* tumor de células de la granulosa-teca, tumor ovárico de células que provienen del folículo de Graaf.

graphology *n.* grafología, estudio de la escritura como indicación de la personalidad del paciente y como ayuda en el diagnóstico de enfermedades nerviosas.

grave *a.* severo-a, serio-a, peligroso-a.

Graves' disease *n.* enfermedad de Graves, hipertiroidismo. *Syn.* **exophthalmic goiter.**

gravida *n.* mujer embarazada, encinta, en estado.

gray *n.* color gris; *a.* gris; ⸺ **cataract** / catarata ⸺; ⸺ **columns** / columnas ⸺ -es; ⸺ **degeneration** / degeneración ⸺ ; ⸺ **fibers** / fibras ⸺ -es; ⸺ **hepatization** / hepatización ⸺ ; ⸺ **induration** / induración ⸺ ; ⸺ **matter** / sustancia ⸺ .

gray matter *n.* materia o sustancia gris, tejido nervioso muy vascularizado de color gris pardo compuesto de células nerviosas y fibras nerviosas amielínicas.

green blindness *n.* ceguera al color verde.

grief *n.* pesar, aflicción.

grief reaction *n.* reacción de aflicción.

grief-stricken *a.* desconsolado-a; afligido-a; acongojado-a; lleno-a de pesar.

grinder's disease *n.* enfermedad de los pulmones producida por inhalación de polvo.

grip, grippe *n.* gripe, influenza.

griseofulvin *n.* griseofulvina, antibiótico usado en el tratamiento de algunas enfermedades de la piel.

groan *v.* gemir; quejarse.

groggy *a.* atontado-a, vacilante, tambaleante.

groin *n.* ingle.

groove *n.* surco, ranura; **bicipital __** / **__ bicipital; costal __** / **__ costal.**

gross *a.* grueso-a, denso-a; grotesco-a; **__ negligence** / imprudencia o negligencia __ seria.

gross anatomy *n.* anatomía macroscópica, estudio de los órganos y partes del cuerpo que se ven a simple vista.

ground substance *n.* sustancia fundamental que llena los espacios intercelulares de los huesos, cartílagos y tejido fibroso.

group *n.* grupo, conglomerado; **support __** / __ de soporte.

group therapy *n.* terapia de grupo.

grow *vi.* crecer, desarrollar; **to __ old** / envejecer.

growth *n.* desarrollo, crecimiento, multiplicación; proliferación.

growth hormone *n.* hormona del crecimiento, secreción de la glándula pituitaria que estimula el crecimiento.

guaiacol *n.* guayacol, antiséptico y anestésico.

guanethidine *n.* guanetidina, agente usado en el tratamiento de la hipertensión.

guard *v.* [*protect*] guardar, proteger, cuidar; guardarse, cuidarse; **to __ against** / tomar precauciones, cuidarse de, guardarse de.

guarded *a.* de cuidado; guardado-a; vigilado-a; protegido-a; **in __ condition** / de pronóstico reservado.

guardian *n.* guardián-a, custodio-a; tutor-a.

guest *n.* invitado-a, huésped, comensal; parásito.

guidance *n.* guía, consejo, dirección.

guide *n.* guía, cualquier instrumento o mecanismo que dirige a otro para conducirlo a su objetivo; *v.* guiar.

Guillain-Barré syndrome *n.* Guillan-Barré, síndrome de, enfermedad neurológica rara que se evidencia por parálisis ascendente que comienza por las extremidades y puede llegar rápidamente a los músculos respiratorios en dos o tres semanas causando fallo respiratorio.

guinea pig *n.* conejillo de Indias.

gulp down *v.* engullir, tragar apresuradamente.

gum *n.* encía. V. **gingiva;** goma; **chewing __** / goma de mascar, *pop.* chicle.

gumma *n.* (*pl.* **gummata**) goma, tumor sifilítico.

gunshot wound *n.* herida de bala.

gurney *n.* camilla.

gush *v.* salir a borbotones, derramar, verter.

gustation *n.* gustación, sentido del gusto.

gustatory *a.* gustativo-a, rel. al gusto; **__ agnosia** / agnosia __; **__ aura** / aura __; **__ hyperhidrosis** / hiperhidrosis __; **__ rhinorrhea** / rinorrea __ .

gut *n.* intestino, *pop.* tripas.

gutta-percha *n.* gutapercha, látex vegetal seco y purificado que se usa en tratamientos dentales y médicos.

guttural *a.* gutural.

gymnastics *n.* gimnasia, calistenia.

gynandroid *n.* ginandroide, persona de características hermafroditas que muestra la apariencia del sexo opuesto.

gynecologic, gynecological *a.* ginecológico-a, rel. al estudio de enfermedades del tracto reproductivo femenino.

gynecologic operative procedures *n.* procedimientos quirúrgicos ginecológicos.

gynecologist *n.* ginecólogo-a, especialista en ginecología.

gynecology *n.* ginecología, estudio de los trastornos que afectan los órganos reproductivos femeninos.

gynecomastia *n.* ginecomastia, desarrollo excesivo de las glándulas mamarias en el hombre.

gyrus *n., L.* (*pl.* **giri**) circunvolución, porción elevada de la corteza cerebral; **Broca's __** / __ de Broca, tercera, frontal inferior; **frontal, superior __** / __ frontal superior; **inferior, lateral occipital __** / __ occipital inferior lateral; **superior occipital __** / __ occipital superior.

H

h

H *abbr.* **heroin** / heroína;
hydrogen / hidrógeno;
hypermetropia / hipermetropía;
hypodermic / hipodérmico.

h *abbr.* **height** / altura; **hour** / hora;
horizontal / horizontal.

habit *n.* hábito, uso, costumbre; adicción
al uso de una droga o bebida; *v.* **to be
in the ___ of** / tener la costumbre de;
acostumbrarse a; habituarse; *pop.*
[*drugs*] to kick the ___ / dejar la
adicción; curarse.

habit training *n.* entrenamiento de
hábitos, enseñanza impartida a los
niños para realizar actividades básicas
tales como comer, dormir, vestirse,
asearse y usar el servicio sanitario.

hacking cough *n.* tos seca
recurrente.

haggard *a.* ojeroso-a; desfigurado-a;
desaliñado-a.

hair *n.* pelo, cabello, vello; **axillary ___ /
___ axilar; curly ___ / ___ rizado; gray
___ / cana; pubic ___ / vello púbico;
straight ___ / ___ lacio, liso; wavy ___ /
___ ondeado.

hairball *n.* bola de pelo, tipo de
bezoar.

hair bulb *n.* bulbo piloso.

hair follicle *n.* folículo piloso.

hairline *n.* línea fina; raya del pelo; trazo
fino; **___ fracture** / fractura de línea
fina.

hair root *n.* raíz del pelo.

hair transplantation *n.* transplante de
pelo, trasplante de epidermis que
contiene folículos pilosos de otra parte
del cuerpo.

hairy *a.* peludo-a, velludo-a; **___ tongue**
/ lengua velluda, lengua infectada de
hongos parásitos.

half *n.* mitad, medio; **___ and ___** / a
mitades, en igual proporción; **___ as
much** / la mitad; **___brother** / medio
hermano; **___ -hour** / media hora; **___
sister** / media hermana; **___ -starved** /
medio muerto de hambre; **in ___** / en
dos mitades.

half-life *n.* 1. vida media, tiempo
requerido para que la mitad de una

sustancia ingerida o inyectada en el
organismo se elimine por medios
naturales; 2. semidesintegración,
tiempo requerido por una sustancia
radioactiva para perder la mitad de su
radioactividad por desintegración.

halitosis *n.* halitosis, mal aliento.

hallucinate *v.* alucinar, desvariar.

hallucination *n.* alucinación,
alucinamiento, sensación subjetiva que
no tiene precedencia o estímulo real;
**auditory ___ , imaginary perception
of sounds** / ___ auditiva, percepción
imaginaria de sonidos; **gustatory ___ ,
imaginary sensation of taste / ___
gustativa, sensación imaginaria del
gusto; **haptic ___ , imaginary
perception of pain, temperature, or
skin sensations / ___ táctil, percepción
imaginaria de dolor, de temperatura o
de sensaciones en la piel; **motor ___ ,
imaginary movement of the body /
___ de movimiento, percepción
imaginaria de movimiento del cuerpo;
**olfactory ___ , imaginary smells / ___
olfativa, de olores imaginarios.

hallucinogen *n.* alucinógeno, droga
que produce alucinaciones o desvaríos
tal como LSD, peyote, mescalina y
otras.

hallucinosis *n.* alucinosis, delirio
alucinatorio crónico; **acute alcoholic
___ / ___ alcohólica, manifestación de
temor patológico acompañado de
alucinaciones auditivas.

hallux *n., L. (pl.* **halluces**) dedo gordo
del pie; **___ valgus / ___** valgus,
desviación del dedo gordo hacia los
otros dedos; **___varus / ___** varus,
separación del dedo gordo de los
demás dedos.

halo *n.* aureola. 1. área del seno de tono
más oscuro que rodea el pezón; 2.
círculo de luz.

ham *n.* 1. corva de la pierna, región
poplítea detrás de la rodilla; 2. jamón.

hamartoma *n.* hamartoma, nódulo de
tejido superfluo semejante a un tumor
usualmente benigno.

hammer *n.* martillo. 1. huesecillo del
oído medio; 2. instrumento empleado
en exámenes físicos; **___ finger or toe /
dedo en garra; percussion ___ / ___ de
percusión; **reflex ___ / ___** de reflejo.

hamstring *n.* 1. tendones de la corva;
2. músculos flexores y aductores de la
parte posterior del muslo.

hand n. mano; **close at __** / muy de
cerca; **give me a __** / ayúdeme,
ayúdame; **__ deformities, acquired** /
deformidades adquiridas de la __; **__
rest** / apoyo de la __; **in good __ -s** /
en buenas manos; **on the other __** /
por otra parte; **to have a free __** / tener
libertad para, tener carta blanca; **to
have one's __ -s tied** / tener atadas las
manos, sin poder hacer nada; **to keep
one's __ -s off** / no meterse; **to shake
__ -s** / dar la __; v. **to __ in a report** /
presentar un informe; **to __ out
information** / facilitar información; **to
__ out news** / facilitar noticias.

handicap n. impedimento; obstáculo,
desventaja; **handicapped person** /
persona desvalida, inválida, baldada,
impedida.

hangnail n. uñero, uña encarnada.

hang-up n. obsesión o problema que
irrita.

Hanot's disease n. enfermedad de
Hanot, cirrosis biliar, cirrosis
hipertrófica del hígado acompañada de
icteria.

Hansen's disease n. enfermedad de
Hansen. Syn. **leprosy.**

haploid n. haploide, célula sexual que
contiene en el cromosoma la mitad de
las características somáticas de la
especie.

happy a. contento-a, alegre, feliz.

hard a. duro-a, endurecido-a, sólido;
trabajoso-a, difícil; [bone] osificado;
__ of hearing / medio sordo; v. **to
grow __** / endurecerse; [parturition];
__ labor / parto laborioso **-ly** adv. a
duras penas, difícilmente,
escasamente.

hard bone n. hueso compacto.

hardbound a. estreñido-a.

hardening n. endurecimiento, solidez.

hard contact lens n. lentes de
contacto duros.

hard palate n. paladar óseo.

hard pressed a. acosado-a,
apremiado-a.

hardship n. sufrimiento, privación,
penalidad.

harelip n. labio leporino, deformidad
congénita a nivel del labio superior
causada por falta de fusión del proceso
nasal interno y el lateral maxilar; **__
suture** / sutura del __.

harelipped a. labihendido-a, que tiene
labio leporino.

harm n. daño, mal, perjuicio; v. dañar,
perjudicar.

harmful a. perjudicial, dañino-a.

harmless a. inofensivo-a, inocuo-a.

harness n. cinturón corrector.

harvest n. recolección, obtención o
separación de bacterias u otros
microorganismos de un cultivo;
cosecha.

hashish n. hachís, pop. yerba, narcótico
de efecto eufórico extraído de la
marihuana.

haustrum n., L. haustrum, cavidad o
saco, esp. el del colon.

hay fever n. fiebre del heno, asma del
heno, catarro del heno, catarro
primaveral, alergia causada por un
agente irritante externo, gen. polen.

hazard n. riesgo, peligro; **a __ to your
health** / un __ para su salud.

hazardous a. arriesgado-a, peligroso-a.

head n. 1. cabeza; 2. parte principal de
una estructura; **from __ to toe** / de la
__ a los pies; **__ birth** / presentación
cefálica; **__ drop** / caída de la __; **__
injury** / traumatismo del cráneo, golpe
en la __; **__ of the family** / __ de
familia; v. **to nod one's __** / asentir con
la __.

headache n. cefalalgia, dolor de
cabeza, jaqueca.

headrest n. apoyo para la cabeza,
cabezal.

headstrong a. voluntarioso-a,
testarudo-a.

heal v. curar, sanar, recobrar la salud; [a
wound] cicatrizar; curarse, sanarse;
recobrarse.

healing n. 1. curación, recuperación de
la salud; **__ process** / proceso de __;
2. curanderismo.

health n. salud; [government]
behavioral __ / conducta saludable;
dental __ / higiene dental;
Department of __ / Ministerio de
Salud o Salubridad; **__ and medical
assistance** / asistencia
médico-sanitaria; **__ assessment** /
evaluación del estado de __; **__
authorities** / autoridades de Sanidad;
__ care / atención o cuidado de la __;
__ care provider / profesional de
atención de la __; **__ care reform** /
reforma al sistema de __; **__ care
system** / sistema sanitario; **__ center** /
centro de __, centro de higiene
sanitaria; **__ certificate** / certificado de

___; ___ **education** / educación médica; ___ **facilities** / instituciones de ___; **food** / alimento sano; ___ **habits** / hábitos sanitarios; ___ **laws** / estatutos sanitarios; ___ **personnel** / profesionales médicos y de asistencia pública; ___ **physicist** / biofísico; ___ **planning** / planeamiento de métodos de ___; ___ **risk assessment** / evaluación de riesgo sanitario; ___ **services** / servicios o atención de la ___; ___ **services for the aged** / servicios de ___ a los ancianos; ___**statistics** / estadísticas de ___ salud mental; ___**status** / estado de ___; **home** ___ **care** / cuidado de ___ en el hogar; **mental** ___ / ___ mental; **occupational** ___ / ___ atención médica laboral; **rural** ___ / ___ rural; **uncertain** ___ / ___ precaria; **urban** ___ / ___ urbana.

healthy *a.* sano-a, saludable, fornido-a.

hear *vi.* oír, escuchar.

hearing *n.* audición, oído; ___ **acuity** / agudeza auditiva; ___ **aid** / instrumento auditivo; ___ **level** / umbral auditivo; ___ **loss** / pérdida de la audición.

heart *n.* corazón, órgano muscular cóncavo cuya función es mantener la circulación de la sangre; ruidos cardíacos; ___ **congenital** ___ **disease** / anomalías congénitas del ___; **distant** ___ **sounds** / ruidos cardíacos apagados; **enlarged** ___ / cardiomegalia; **fetal** ___ **sounds** / ruidos cardíacos fetales; ___ **atrium** / aurícula cardíaca; ___ **attack** / ataque al ___; ___ **block** / bloqueo del ___; **block, atrioventricular** / bloqueo auriculoventricular, interrupción en el nódulo A-V; ___ **block, bundle-branch** / bloqueo de rama; ___ **block, interventricular** / bloqueo interventricular; ___ **block, partial** / bloqueo parcial; **block, sinoatrial** / bloqueo senoauricular, interferencia completa o parcial del paso de impulsos del nódulo senoauricular; ___ **catherization** / cateterización o cateterismo cardíaco; ___ **disease** / cardiopatías; ___ **failure, congestive** / insuficiencia cardíaca congestiva, colapso o fallo cardíaco; ___ **failure, low output** / rendimiento bajo del ___ deficiencia en mantener un flujo sanguíneo adecuado; ___ **failure, left** / insuficiencia ventricular izquierda, deficiencia en mantener un gasto normal del ventrículo izquierdo; ___ **failure, right-sided** / insuficiencia del

ventrículo derecho; ___ **-healthy** / cardiosaludable ; ___ **hypertrophy** / hipertrofia del ___; ___ **murmur** / soplo cardíaco; ___ **output** / gasto cardíaco; ___ **pacemaker** / estimulador cardíaco, marcapasos; ___ **palpitation** / palpitación cardíaca ; ___ **pump, nuclear powered** / bomba del ___ de fuerza nuclear; ___ **rate** / frecuencia cardíaca; ___ **reflex** / reflejo cardíaco; ___ **scan** / escán cardíaco; ___ **shadow** [*as in x-ray*] / silueta cardíaca; ___ **sound** / ruido del ___; ___ **specialist** / cardiólogo; ___ **transplant** / trasplante del ___; ___ **valve** / válvula del ___; **hypertensive** ___ **disease** / cardiopatía por hipertensión; **low** ___ **output** / gasto bajo; **reduplication of** ___ **sounds** / desdoblamiento de ruidos cardíacos.

heartbeat *n.* latido del corazón, [*rapid*] palpitación; **ectopic** ___ / ___ ectópico.

heartburn *n.* acedía, acidez, *pop.* ardor en el estómago; agruras.

heart-lung machine *n.* máquina corazón-pulmón, máquina cardiopulmonar que se usa para mantener artificialmente las funciones del corazón y de los pulmones.

heat *n.* calor; **conductive** ___ / ___ de conducción; **dry** ___ / ___ seco; ___**cramps** / espasmo muscular (debido a trabajos realizados en altas temperaturas); ___ **exhaustion** / colapso por calor; ___ **loss** / pérdida de ___; ___ **prostration** / insolación con colapso; ___ **sensitive** / sensible al calor; ___ **stable** / termoestable; ___ **stroke** / insolación; ___ **unit** / caloría; ___ **therapy** / termoterapia; **to be in** ___ / estar en celo *v.* calentar; dar calor.

heating pad, electric *n.* almohadilla eléctrica.

heaviness *n.* pesadez, pesantez, peso; [*sleep*] sueño pesado, modorra; [*feelings*] abatimiento, decaimiento.

heavy *a.* pesado-a, grueso-a, fornido-a; ___ **chain disease** / enfermedad de red o cadena; ___ **drinker** / bebedor, que bebe demasiado; ___ **food** / alimento indigesto; ___ **liquid** / líquido espeso; ___ **meal** / comida fuerte; ___ **period** / hipermenorrea; ___ **sleep** / sueño profundo; ___ **traffic** / tráfico denso

hectic *a.* hético-a, febril; agitado-a; consumido-a, tísico-a.

heel *n.* talón, calcañal, parte posterior redondeada del pie.

height *n.* altura, alto; estatura.

Heimlich maneuver *n.* maniobra de Heimlich, técnica que se usa para sacar o forzar la expulsión de un cuerpo extraño que impide el paso del aire de la tráquea o la faringe.

heliotherapy *n.* helioterapia, exposición o baños de sol con propósito terapéutico

helium *n.* helio, elemento gaseoso inerte empleado en tratamientos respiratorios y en cámaras de descompresión para facilitar el aumento o disminución de la presión del aire.

helminth *n.* helminto, gusano que se localiza en el intestino humano.

helminthiasis *n.* helmintiasis, condición parasítica intestinal.

helminthicide *n.* helminticida, vermicida, medicamento que extermina parásitos.

help *n.* ayuda, asistencia, socorro, auxilio; *v.* ayudar, asistir, auxiliar; remediar.

helper *n.* ayudante, asistente, auxiliar.

helpful *a.* útil, provechoso-a.

helpless *a.* desamparado-a, indefenso-a; desvalido-a.

hemagglutination *n.* hemoaglutinación, aglutinación de células rojas sanguíneas.

hemagglutinin *n.* hemoaglutinina, anticuerpo de células rojas o hematíes que causa aglutinación.

hemangioma *n.* hemangioma, tumor benigno formado por vasos capilares en racimo que producen una marca de nacimiento de color rojo púrpura en la piel.

hemangiosarcoma *n.* hemangiosarcoma, tumor maligno del tejido vascular.

hemarthrosis *n.* hemartrosis, derrame de sangre en la cavidad de una articulación.

hematemesis *n.* hematemesis, vómito de sangre.

hematherapy, hemotherapy *n.* hematerapia, hemoterapia, uso terapéutico de la sangre.

hematic *n.* hemático, droga usada en el tratamiento de anemia; *a.* hemático-a, relacionado con la sangre.

hematochezia *n.* hematoquezia, presencia de sangre en el excremento.

hematocolpos *n.* hematocolpos, retención del flujo menstrual en la vagina debido a imperforación del himen.

hematocrit *n.* hematócrito. 1. aparato centrifugador que se usa en la separación de células y partículas del plasma; 2. promedio de eritrocitos en la sangre.

hematocyst *n.* hematoquiste. 1. quiste sanguinolento; 2. hemorragia dentro de un quiste.

hematogenesis *n.* hematogénesis. V. hematopoiesis.

hematologic, hematological *a.* hematológico-a, rel. a la sangre; ___ studies / estudios ___ -s; ___ values / valores ___.

hematologic values *n.* valores hematológicos; **bleeding time** / tiempo de sangramiento; **coagulation time** / tiempo de coagulación; **erythrocyte sedimentation** / sedimentación de eritrocitos; **hematocrit** / promedio de eritrocitos; **hemoglobin** / hemoglobina; **partial thromboplastin time** / tiempo parcial de tromboplastina; **arterial blood pH** / pH de las sangre arterial; **prothrombin time** / tiempo de protrombina

hematologist *n.* 1. hematólogo-a especialista en hematología; 2. especialista en diagnóstico de pruebas sanguínea y tratamiento de enfermedades de las sangre.

hematology *n.* hematología, ciencia que estudia la sangre y los órganos que intervienen en la formación de ésta.

hematoma *n.* hematoma, hinchazón por sangre coleccionada fuera de un vaso; *pop.* chichón; **pelvic** ___ / ___ pélvico; **subdural** ___ / derrame subdural.

hematopoiesis, hemopoiesis *n.* hematopoyesis, hemopoyesis, formación de sangre.

hemianalgesia *n.* hemianalgesia, insensibilidad al dolor en un lado del cuerpo.

hemianopia, hemianopsia *n.* hemianopia, hemianopsia, pérdida de la visión en la mitad del campo visual de uno o ambos ojos.

hemiatrophy *n.* hemiatrofia, atrofia de la mitad de un órgano o de la mitad del cuerpo.

hemicolectomy *n.* hemicolectomía, extirpación de una mitad del colon.

hemihypertrophy

hemihypertrophy *n.* hemihipertrofia unilateral con desarrollo excesivo de la mitad del cuerpo.

hemilaminectomy *n.* hemilaminectomía, extirpación de un lado de la lámina vertebral.

hemiparalysis *n.* hemiparálisis, parálisis de un lado del cuerpo.

hemiparesis *n.* hemiparesis, debilidad muscular que afecta un lado del cuerpo.

hemiparetic *a.* hemiparético-a, rel. a la hemiparesis o de la naturaleza de la misma.

hemiplegia *n.* hemiplejía, parálisis gen. ocasionada por una lesión cerebral que afecta la parte del cuerpo opuesta al hemisferio cerebral afectado. **alternating** ___ / ___ alternante; **cerebral** ___ / ___ cerebral; **crossed** ___ / ___ cruzada; **double** ___ / ___ doble; **facial** ___ / ___ facial; **spastic** ___ / ___ espástica.

hemiplegic *a.* hemipléjico-a, que sufre de hemiplejía.

hemisphere *n.* hemisferio, mitad de una estructura u órgano de forma esférica.

hemithyroidectomy *n.* hemitiroidectomía excisión de un lóbulo de la tiroides.

hemobilia *n.* hemobilia, sangramiento en los conductos biliares.

hemochromatosis, iron storage disease *n.* hemocromatosis, trastorno del metabolismo férrico acompañado por exceso de depósitos de hierro en los tejidos que causa anomalías de pigmentación de la piel, cirrosis hepática y diabetes.

hemoclasis, hemoclasia *n.* rotura, desgarro, [*hemolysis*] disolución u otro tipo de destrucción de eritrocitos.

hemoconcentration *n.* hemoconcentración, concentración de hematíes a causa de una disminución del volumen líquido sanguíneo.

hemodialysis *n.* hemodiálisis, proceso de diálisis usado para eliminar sustancias tóxicas de la sangre.

hemodialyzer *n.* hemodializador, riñón artificial, aparato que se usa en el proceso de diálisis.

hemodilution *n.* hemodilución, aumento del plasma sanguíneo en relación al de los glóbulos rojos.

hemodynamics *n.* hemodinamia, el estudio de la dinámica de la circulación de la sangre.

hemoglobin *n.* hemoglobina, la proteína de mayor importancia en la sangre a la que da color y por la que se transporta el oxígeno.

hemoglobinemia *n.* hemoglobinemia, presencia de hemoglobina libre en el plasma sanguíneo.

hemoglobinuria *n.* hemoglobinuria, presencia de hemoglobina en la orina; **epidemic** ___ / ___ epidémica; **intermittent** ___ / ___ intermitente; **malarial** ___ / ___ en malaria; **paroxysmal cold** ___ / ___ paroxística fría; **paroxysmal nocturnal** ___ / ___ paroxística nocturna; **postparturient** ___ / ___ de la posparturienta; **toxic** ___ / ___ tóxica.

hemogram *n.* hemograma, representación gráfica de un conteo sanguíneo diferencial.

hemolith *n.* hemolito, concreción en un vaso sanguíneo.

hemolysis *n.* hemólisis, ruptura de eritrocitos con liberación de hemoglobina en el plasma; **immune** ___ / ___ inmune; **venom** ___ / ___ venenosa.

hemolytic *a.* hemolítico-a, rel. a hemólisis o que la produce; **disorder** / trastorno ___.

hemolytic anemia *n.* anemia hemolítica, anemia congénita causada por agentes tóxicos de eritrocitos frágiles de forma esferoidal.

hemolytic disease of the newborn *n.* hemólisis en el recién nacido, trastorno gen. causado por la incompatibilidad del factor Rh. **Rh factor**.

hemolytic uremic syndrome *n.* síndrome hemolítico urémico, con anemia hemolítica y trombocitopenia, presentando un cuadro con fallo renal agudo; en la infancia se presenta con síntomas de sangrado gastrointestinal, hematuria, oliguria, y de anemia hemolítica.

hemophilia *n.* hemofilia, condición hereditaria caracterizada por deficiencia de coagulación y tendencia a sangrar.

hemophiliac *a.* hemofílico-a, persona afectada por hemofilia.

hemophobia *n.* hemofobia, temor patológico a la sangre.

hemopneumothorax *n.* hemoneumotórax, acumulación de sangre y de aire en la cavidad pleural.

hemoptysis *n.* hemoptisis, expectoración sanguinolenta de color rojo vivo.

hemorrhage *n.* hemorragia, derrame profuso de sangre; **cerebral** __ / __ cerebral, accidente cerebrovascular; **concealed** __ / __ oculta; **internal** __ / __ interna; **intracranial** __ / __ intracraneana; **intraventricular** __ / __ intraventricular; **nasal** __ / __ nasal; **petechial** __ / __ petequial; **postpartum** __ / __ puerperal.

hemorrhagic *a.* hemorrágico-a.

hemorrhoid *n.* hemorroide, *pop.* almorrana, masa de venas dilatadas en la pared rectal; **external** __ / __ -s externas, fuera del esfínter anal; **internal** __ / __ interna; **prolapsed** __ / __ de prolapso, protrusión de almorranas internas por el ano.

hemorrhoidectomy *n.* hemorroidectomía, extirpación de hemorroides.

hemosalpinx *n.* hemosálpinx, acumulación de sangre en las trompas de Falopio.

hemosiderin *n.* hemosiderina, compuesto insoluble de hierro derivado de la hemoglobina que se almacena para ser usado en la formación de hemoglobina en el momento necesario.

hemosiderosis *n.* hemosiderosis, depósitos de hemosiderina en el hígado y el vaso.

hemospermia *n.* hemospermia, presencia de sangre en el semen.

hemostasis *n.* hemostasis, hemostasia, detención o contención (artificial o natural) de sangramiento.

hemostat *n.* hemóstato, instrumento o medicamento que se emplea para contener un sangramiento.

hemothorax *n.* hemotorax, sangre localizada en la cavidad pleural.

heparin *n.* heparina, sustancia que actúa como anticoagulante.

heparinize *n.* heparinizar, evitar la coagulación por medio del uso de heparina.

hepatectomy *n.* hepatectomía, extirpación de una parte o de todo el hígado.

hepatic *a.* hepático-a, rel. al hígado; __ **coma** / coma __; __ **duct** / ducto __;

__ **lobes** / lóbulos o subdivisiones __ -s; __ **veins** / venas __.

hepatitis *n.* hepatitis, infl. del hígado; **amebic** __ / __ amébica; **active chronic** __ / __ crónica activa; **cholestatic** __ / __ colestática; **drug-induced** __ / __ inducida por drogas; **epidemic** __ / __ epidémica; **fulminating** __ / __ fulminante; **fulminating chronic** __ / __ fulminante crónica; **fulminant** __ / __ aguda fulminante; __ **A** / __ A, viral, afecta primordialmente a los niños; __ **B** / __ B, causada por un virus y trasmitida en líquidos del organismo; saliva, lágrimas, semen; **infectious** __ / __ infecciosa o viral; **non-A, non-B** __ / __ no A, no B, asociada con transfusiones de sangre; **serum** __ / __ sérica; **persistent chronic** __ / __ persistente crónica.

hepatojugular reflex *n.* reflejo hepatoyugular, ingurgitación de las venas yugulares producida por el hígado en casos de insuficiencia cardíaca derecha.

hepatologist *n.* hepatólogo-a, especialista en trastornos hepáticos.

hepatorenal *a.* hepatorrenal, rel. a los riñones y el hígado.

hepatosplenomegaly *n.* hepatosplenomegalia, agrandamiento del hígado y del bazo.

hepatotoxicity *n.* hepatotoxicidad, la tendencia de un fármaco o producto tóxico a dañar el hígado.

hepatotoxin *n.* hepatotoxina, toxina destructora de células hepáticas.

herb *n.* yerba, hierba, planta clasificada como medicinal o usada como condimento; __ **tea** / infusión.

hereditary *a.* hereditario-a; que se trasmite por herencia.

heredity *n.* herencia, trasmisión de características o rasgos genéticos de padres a hijos.

hermaphrodite *n.* hermafrodita, persona cuyo cuerpo presenta los tejidos ovárico y testicular combinados en un mismo órgano o separadamente.

hermetic *a.* hermético-a, que no deja pasar el aire.

hernia *n.* hernia, protrusión anormal de un órgano o víscera a través de la cavidad que la contiene; **cystic** __ / __ cística; **femoral** __ / femoral, que se protrude dentro del canal femoral; **hiatus** __ / __ hiatal, a través del hiato

hernial, herniated

esofágico del diafragma; **incarcerated**
___ / ___ incarcerada, gen. causada por
adherencias; **inguinal** ___ / ___ inguinal,
de una víscera con protrusión en la
ingle o el escroto; **lumbar** ___ / ___
lumbar, protrusión en la región lumbar;
reducible ___ / ___ reducible, que puede
tratarse por manipulación; **scrotal** ___ /
___ escrotal; **sliding** ___ / ___ por
deslizamiento, de una víscera intestinal;
strangulated ___ / ___ estrangulada,
que obstruye los intestinos; **umbilical**
___ / ___ umbilical; **ventral** ___ / ___
ventral, protrusión a través de la pared
abdominal.

hernial, herniated *a.* herniado-a, rel.
a una hernia o que padece de ella; ___
disk / disco herniado; ___ **sac** / saco de
la hernia, bolsa peritoneal en la cual
desciende la hernia.

herniation *n.* herniación, desarrollo de
una hernia; ___ **of nucleus pulposus** /
___ del núcleo pulposo, prolapso o
ruptura del disco intervertebral.

hernioplasty *n.* hernioplastia,
reparación quirúrgica de una hernia.

herniorrhaphy *n.* herniorrafia,
reconstrucción o reparación quirúrgica
de una hernia.

heroin, diacetylomorphine *n.*
heroína, diacetilomorfina, narcótico
adictivo derivado de la morfina; ___
addict / heroinómano-a.

herpangina *n.* herpangina, enfermedad
infecciosa, epidémica que ocurre en el
verano y que afecta las membranas
mucosas de la garganta.

herpes *n.* herpes, enfermedad
inflamatoria viral dolorosa de la piel
que se manifiesta con erupción y
ampollas; ___ **genitales** / ___ de los
genitales; ___ **ocular** / ___ ocular; ___
simplex / ___ simple, de simples
vesículas que recurren una y otra vez
en la misma área de la piel; ___ **zoster,**
pop. **shingles** / ___ zóster, erupción
dolorosa a lo largo de un nervio, *pop.*
culebrilla.

herpetic *a.* herpético-a, rel. al herpes o
de naturaleza similar; ___
gingivostomatitis / gingivostomatitis
___, infl. de la boca y las encías causada
por herpes simple.

heterogeneous *a.* heterogéneo-a, de
naturaleza diferente.

heterograft *n.* heteroinjerto, injerto de
un donante de especie o tipo diferente
al del receptor.

heterologous *a.* heterólogo-a;
derivado de un organismo o especie
diferente.

heteroplasia *n.* heteroplasia, presencia
anormal de tejido en un área diferente a
la que le corresponde según su origen.

heteroplastia *n.* heteroplastia,
trasplante de tejido obtenido de un
donante que pertenece a una especie
diferente.

heterosexual *n.* heterosexual,
inclinación sexual hacia el sexo
opuesto.

heterosexuality *n.* heterosexualidad.

heterotopia *n.* heterotopía,
desplazamiento de un órgano o parte de
la posición normal.

hiatus *n.* hiatus, abertura, orificio,
fisura.

hibernoma *n.* hibernoma, tumor
benigno localizado en la cadera o en la
espalda.

hiccough, hiccups *n.* hipo,
contracción involuntaria del diafragma
y la glotis.

hidradenitis *n.* hidradenitis, infl. de las
glándulas sudoríparas.

hidrosis *n.* hidrosis, sudor excesivo.

high *a.* alto-a, elevado-a; ___ **blood**
pressure / presión alta; ___ **-calorie**
diet / dieta rica en calorías; ___
cholesterol / ___ nivel de colesterol; ___
color / de color subido; ___ **nuclear**
waste / desechos nucleares de alta
radioactividad; ___ **-residue diet** / dieta
___ en residuos (fibras, celulosas); ___
-risk / ___ peligro o riesgo; ___ **-risk**
behavior / conducta o actividades de
___ riesgo; **-ly** *adv.* altamente,
sumamente, excesivamente.

high altitude sickness *n.*
enfermedad de la altura, trastorno por
altura excesiva manifestado en
dificultades respiratorias por
imposibilidad de adaptarse a la
disminución de la presión del oxígeno.

high-risk groups *n. pl.* pacientes o
personas con alto riesgo de contraer
una determinada enfermedad debido a
factores genéticos o conductales; ___
in HIV / personas de actividades
sexuales múltiples sin adecuada
protección; drogadictos que
intercambian agujas y jeringuillas; feto
in utero o infante lactante de madre
drogadicta o infectada por el virus.

hike *n.* caminata; *v.* **to go on a** ___ / ir a
caminar, ir andando.

hilum, hilus *n., L.* (*pl.* **hila**) hilio, depresión o apertura en un órgano que sirve de entrada o salida a nervios, vasos y conductos.

hinge *n.* bisagra; __ **joint** / coyuntura; __ **movement** / movimiento de bisagra; __ **position** / posición de gozne.

hip *n.* cadera, región lateral de la pelvis; __ **dislocation** / dislocación de la __; __ **dislocation, congenital** / dislocación congénita de la __; __ **joint** / articulación de la __; **snapping** __ / __ de resorte; **total** __ **replacement** / restitución total de la __.

hip-joint disease *n.* trastorno de la articulación de la cadera, coxartropatía.

hippocampus *n.* (*pl.* **hippocampi**) hipocampo, circunvolución de materia gris que forma la mayor parte de la corteza cerebral olfatoria.

hippocratic facies *n.* facies hipocrática, máscara facial que precede a la muerte.

hippocratic oath *n.* juramento hipocrático, juramento ético de la medicina.

hirsute *a.* hirsuto-a, peludo-a.

hirsutism *n.* hirsutismo, desarrollo excesivo de pelo en áreas no comunes, esp. en la mujer.

histamine *n.* histamina, sustancia que produce efecto dilatador en los vasos capilares y estimula la secreción gástrica.

histidine *n.* histidina, aminoácido esencial en el crecimiento y en la restauración de los tejidos.

histocompatibility *n.* histocompatibilidad, estado en el cual los tejidos de un donante son aceptados por el receptor; **major** __ **complex** / complejo de __ mayor.

histoplasmin *n.* histoplasmina, sustancia que se usa en la prueba cutánea de histoplasmosis.

histoplasmosis *n.* histoplasmosis, enfermedad de las vías respiratorias causada por el hongo *Histoplasma capsulatum*.

HIV *n.* **human immunodeficiency virus**,VIH, virus de inmunodeficiencia humano, retrovirus del SIDA. Se transmite sexualmente o por intercambio de agujas y jeringuillas con una persona infectada. Puede transmitirse también a través de una transfusión de sangre obtenida de donantes infectados. El virus puede ser transmitido igualmente al feto *in utero*, durante el parto o al recién nacido en la lactancia a través de la leche materna de una madre afectada.

hives *n., pl.* ronchas, erupción alérgica.

hoarse *a.* ronco-a; áspero-a.

hoarseness *n.* ronquera, manifestación en la voz de una afección de la laringe.

Hodgkin's disease *n.* enfermedad de Hodgkin, presencia de tumores malignos en los nódulos linfáticos y el bazo.

holistic *a.* holístico-a, rel. a un todo o unidad.

holistic medicine *n.* medicina holística, sistema médico que considera al ser humano integrado como una unidad funcional.

hollow *a.* hueco-a, cóncavo-a.

hollow back *n.* lordosis.

holocrine *a.* holocrino-a, rel. a las glándulas secretorias.

holodiastolic *a.* holodiastólico-a, rel. a una diástole completa.

holography *n.* holografía, figura tridimensional de un objeto por medio de una imagen fotográfica.

Holter monitoring *n.* monitoreo de Holter (de funda al hombro), electrocardiografía ambulatoria.

homeopathy *n.* homeopatía, curación por medio de medicamentos diluidos en cantidades ínfimas que producen efectos semejantes a los síntomas producidos por la enfermedad.

homogeneous *a.* homogéneo-a, semejante, de la misma naturaleza.

homograft *n.* homoinjerto, transplante tomado de la misma especie o tipo.

homologous *a.* homólogo-a, similar en estructura y origen pero no en funcionamiento.

homophobia *n.* homofobia, temor o repulsión a los homosexuales.

homophobic *a.* homofóbico-a, que tiene repulsión o temor a homosexuales.

homosexual *n.* homosexual, invertido-a, atracción sexual por las personas del mismo sexo.

homozygote *n.* homocigoto-a, que presenta alelos idénticos en una característica o en varias.

homozygous *a.* homocigótico-a, rel. a un homocigoto.

homunculus

homunculus *n.* homúnculo-a, enano-a sin deformidades y proporcionado-a en todas las partes del cuerpo.

hookworm *n.* uncinaria, lombriz de gancho, nematodo del intestino; __ **disease** / enfermedad de la __.

hope *n.* esperanza; *v.* esperar, tener esperanzas.

horizontal *n. a.* horizontal; __ **position** / posición acostada.

hormonal *a.* hormonal, rel. a una hormona o que actúa como tal.

hormone *n.* hormona, sustancia química natural del cuerpo que produce o estimula la actividad de un órgano; **growth** __ / __ del crecimiento; **therapy** / terapia hormonal; __ **receptor** / receptor hormonal.

hornet *n.* avispa, avispón.

hospice *n.* hospicio.

hospital *n.* hospital.

hospitalization *n.* hospitalización.

hospitalize *v.* hospitalizar, ingresar en un hospital; dar ingreso en un hospital.

host *n.* [*parasite*] huésped, organismo que sostiene o alberga a otro llamado parásito; __ **defenses** / defensas del __.

hostile *a.* hostil.

hot *a.* caliente, de temperatura alta; contaminado-a por material radioactivo; __ **flashes** / fogaje, sofoco; rubores, bochorno.

hour *n.* hora; **by the** __ / por hora **-ly** *adv.* a cada hora

house *n.* casa, vivienda, domicilio; __ **call** / visita médica.

housewife *n.* ama de casa, madre de familia.

housework *n.* tareas domésticas, trabajo de la casa.

how *adv.* cómo, cuánto; __ **are you?** / ¿Cómo está?, ¿Cómo estás?; __ **late?** / ¿Hasta qué hora?; __ **many?** / ¿Cuántos-as?; __ **often?** / ¿Cuántas veces?, ¿Con qué frecuencia?

however *adv.* sin embargo, no obstante.

hum *n.* susurro; tarareo; zumbido; *v.* [*music*] tararear; zumbar; susurrar.

human *a.* humano-a, rel. a la humanidad.

human immunodeficiency virus *n.* virus de inmunodeficiencia humana, retrovirus del SIDA.

humeral *a.* humeral, rel. al húmero.

humerus *n., L.* (*pl.* **humeri**) húmero, hueso largo del brazo.

humid *a.* húmedo-a, que contiene humedad.

humidifier *n.* humectante, humedecedor, aparato que controla y mantiene la humedad en el aire de una habitación.

humor *n.* humor. 1. cualquier forma líquida en el cuerpo; **aqueous** __ / __ acuoso, líquido claro en las cámaras del ojo; **crystalline** __ / __ cristalino, sustancia que forma el cristalino; **vitreus** __ / __ vítreo, sustancia transparente semilíquida localizada entre el cristalino y la retina; 2. secreción; 3. disposición de carácter; *v.* **to be in bad** __ / estar de mal __; **to be in good** __ / estar de buen __.

hump *n.* joroba, corcova, jiba.

hunchback *n.* corcova, joroba, deformación con curvatura de la espina dorsal.

hunger *n.* hambre.

hungry *a.* hambriento-a; **to be** __ / tener hambre; **to go** __ / pasar hambre.

Huntington's chorea *n.* corea de Huntington, *Syn.* **chorea**.

husband *n.* esposo, marido.

hyaline *a.* hialino-a, vítreo-a o casi transparente; __ **cast** / cilindro __, que se observa en la orina; __ **membrane disease** / enfermedad de la membrana __, trastorno repiratorio que se manifiesta en recién nacidos.

hyalinization *n.* hialinización, conversión a una sustancia semejante al vidrio.

hyalinosis *n.* hialinosis, degeneración hialina.

hyalitis *n.* hialitis, infl. del humor vítreo.

hyaluronic acid *n.* ácido hialurónico, presente en la sustancia del tejido conjuntivo, actúa como lubricante y agente conector.

hybrid *a.* híbrido-a, rel. al producto de un cruzamiento de diferentes especies en animales y plantas.

hybridoma *n.* hibridoma, célula somática híbrida capaz de producir anticuerpos.

hydatid *n.* hidátide, quiste que se manifiesta en los tejidos esp. en el hígado; *a.* hidatídico, rel. a un tumor enquistado; __ **disease** / equinococcosis; __ **mole** / quiste __ en el útero que produce hemorragia.

hydramnion *n.* hidramnios, exceso de líquido amniótico.

hydrarthrosis *n.* hidrartrosis acumulación de fluido seroso en la cavidad de una articulación indicando inflamación.

hydrate *v.* hidratar, combinar un cuerpo con el agua.

hydrated *a.* hidratado-a, que contiene agua o está húmedo.

hydrocele *n.* hidrocele, acumulación de líquido esp. en la túnica vaginal del testículo.

hydrocelectomy *n.* hidrocelectomía, extirpación de un hidrocele.

hydrocephalus *n.* hidrocéfalo, acumulación de líquido cefalorraquídeo en los ventrículos del cerebro.

hydrochloric acid *n.* ácido clorhídrico o hidroclórico, constituyente del jugo gástrico.

hydrocortisone *n.* hidrocortisona, hormona corticosteroide producida por la corteza suprarrenal.

hydrogen *n.* hidrógeno; ___ **concentration** / concentración de ___.

hydrogen peroxide *n.* peróxido de hidrógeno, agua oxigenada, limpiador y desinfectante.

hydrolysis *n.* hidrólisis, disolución química de un compuesto por acción del agua.

hydromyelia *n.* hidromielia, aumento de líquido cefalorraquídeo en el canal central de la médula espinal.

hydronephrosis *n.* hidronefrosis, distensión en la pelvis renal y cálices a causa de una obstrucción.

hydrophobia *n.* hidrofobia. 1. temor excesivo al agua; 2. *pop.* rabia.

hydropic *a.* hidrópico-a, rel. a la hidropesía.

hydrops, hydropsy *n.* hidropesía, hidropsia o edema.

hydrosalpinx *n.* hidrosálpinx, acumulación de fluido seroso en la trompa de Falopio.

hydrotherapy *n.* hidroterapia, uso terapéutico del agua con aplicaciones externas en el tratamiento de enfermedades.

hydrothorax *n.* hidrotórax, colección de fluido en la cavidad pleural sin producir inflamación.

hydroureter *n.* hidrouréter, distensión por obstrucción del uréter.

hygiene *n.* higiene, estudio de la salud y la conservación de un cuerpo sano; **mental** ___ / ___ mental; **oral** ___ / ___ oral; **public** ___ / ___ pública.

hygienic *a.* higiénico-a, sanitario-a, rel. a la higiene.

hygienist *n.* higienista, especialista en higiene; **dental** ___ / ___ dental, técnico en profiláctica dental.

hygroma *n.* hidroma, saco o bursa que contiene líquido.

hymen *n.* himen, repliegue membranoso que cubre parcialmente la entrada de la vagina.

hymenectomy *n.* himenectomía, excisión del himen.

hymenotomía *n.* himenotomía, incisión del himen.

hyoglossal *a.* hioglosal, rel. al hioides y la lengua.

hyoglossus *n.* hiogloso, músculo de la lengua de acción retractora y lateral.

hyoid *a.* hioideo-a, rel. al hueso hioides.

hyoid bone *n.* hioides, hueso en forma de herradura situado en la base de la lengua.

hypalgesia, hypalgia *n.* hipalgesia, hipalgia, disminución en la sensibilidad del dolor.

hyperacidity *n.* hiperacidez, acidez excesiva.

hyperactive *a.* hiperactivo-a, excesivamente activo-a.

hyperactivity *n., pl.* actividad excesiva; desorden caracterizado por actividad excesiva que se manifiesta en niños y adolescentes acompañado de irritabilidad e incapacidad de mantener la atención.

hyperacuity *n.* desarrollo anormal de uno de los sentidos esp. la vista o el olfato.

hyperacute *a.* sobreagudo-a, extremadamente agudo-a.

hyperalbuminosis *n.* hiperalbuminosis, exceso de albúmina en la sangre.

hyperalimentation *n.* hiperalimentación, sobrealimentación por vía intravenosa.

hyperapnea *n.* hiperapnea, aumento de la respiración en rapidez y profundidad.

hyperbilirubinemia *n.* hiperbilirrubinemia, exceso de bilirrubina en la sangre.

hypercalcemia *n.* hipercalcemia, cantidad excesiva de calcio en la sangre.

hypercapnia *n.* hipercapnia, cantidad excesiva de dióxido de carbono en la sangre.

hyperchloremia *n.* hipercloremia, exceso de cloruros en la sangre.

hyperchlorhydria *n.* hiperclorhidria, secreción excesiva de ácido clorhídrico por células que recubren el estómago.

hyperchromatic *a.* hipercromático-a, con exceso de colorante o pigmentación.

hypercoagulability *n.* hipercoagulabilidad, aumento anormal de la coagulabilidad.

hyperemesis *n.* hiperemesis, vómitos excesivos.

hyperemia *n.* hiperemia, exceso de sangre en un órgano, tejido o parte.

hyperesthesia *n.* hiperestesia, aumento exagerado de la sensibilidad sensorial.

hyperglycemia *n.* hiperglucemia, aumento excesivo de azúcar en la sangre.

hyperglycosuria *n.* hiperglucosuria, exceso de azúcar en la orina.

hyperhidrosis *n.* hiperhidrosis, sudor excesivo.

hyperhydration *n.* hiperhidratación, aumento excesivo del contenido de agua en el cuerpo.

hyperinsulinism *n.* hiperinsulinismo, exceso de secreción de insulina en la sangre causando hipoglicemia.

hyperkalemia *n.* hipercalemia, hiperpotasemia, aumento excesivo de potasio en la sangre.

hyperkinesia *n.* hipercinesia, aumento en exceso de actividad muscular.

hyperlipemia *n.* hiperlipemia, cantidad excesiva de grasas en la sangre.

hyperlipidemia *n.* hiperlipidemia, alta concentrauón de lípedo en li cornente sangainea.

hypermenorrhea *n.* hipermenorrea, período excesivo en cantidad y duración.

hypermotility *n.* hipermobilidad, movilidad excesiva.

hypernatremia *n.* hipernatremia, concentración excesiva de sodio en la sangre.

hypernephroma *n.* hipernefroma, tumor de Grawitz, neoplasma del parénquima renal.

hyperopia *n.* hiperopia, hipermetropía. V. **farsightedness**.

hyperorexia *n.* hiperorexia, apetito excesivo.

hyperosmia *n.* hiperosmia, sensibilidad olfativa exagerada.

hyperostosis *n.* hiperostosis, desarrollo excesivo del tejido óseo.

hyperpituitism *n.* hiperpituitarismo, actividad excesiva de la glándula pituitaria.

hyperplasia *n.* hiperplasia, proliferación excesiva de células normales en un tejido.

hyperpyrexia *n.* hiperpirexia, temperatura del cuerpo excesivamente alta.

hyperreflexia *n.* hiperreflexia, reflejos exagerados.

hypersalivation *n.* hipersalivación, excesiva secreción de las glándulas salivales.

hypersalpingo-oophorectomy *n.* histerosalpingo-ooforectomía, excison del útero, de los tubos uterinos y de los ovarios.

hypersecretion *n.* hipersecreción, secreción excesiva.

hypersensibility *n.* hipersensibilidad, sensibilidad excesiva al efecto de un antígeno o a un estímulo.

hypersensitive *a.* hipersensible, hiperestísico-a.

hypersplenism *n.* hiperesplenismo, funcionamiento exagerado del bazo.

hypertension *n.* hipertensión, presión arterial alta; **benign** __ / __ benigna; **essential** __ / __ esencial; **malignant** __ / __ maligna; **portal** __ / __ portal; **primary** __ / __ primaria; **renal** __ / __ renal.

hypertensive *a.* hipertensivo-a, hipertenso-a. 1. que causa elevación en la presión; 2. rel. a la hipertensión o que padece de ella.

hyperthyroidism *n.* hipertiroidismo, actividad excesiva de la tiroides.

hypertonic *a.* hipertónica-a, rel. a, o caracterizado por aumento de tonicidad o tensión.

hypertrophy *n.* hipertrofia, desarrollo excesivo o agrandamiento anormal de un órgano o parte; **cardiac** __ / __ cardíaca, corazón agrandado; **compensatory** __ / __ compensatoria, como resultado de un defecto físico.

hypertropia *n.* hipertropia, tipo de estrabismo.

hyperuricemia *n.* hiperuricemia, exceso de ácido úrico en la sangre.

hyperventilation *n.* hiperventilación, respiración excesivamente rápida y

profunda con expiración del aire
igualmente rápida.

hypervolimia *n.* hipervolimia,
sobreaumento en volumen de la
circulación sanguínea.

hyphema *n.* hifema. 1. ojo inyectado;
2. sangramiento en la cámara anterior
del ojo.

hypnosis *n.* hipnosis, estado sugestivo
durante el cual la persona sometida
responde a mandatos siempre que éstos
no contradigan convicciones
arraigadas.

hypnotherapy *n.* hipnoterapia,
tratamiento terapéutico con práctica de
hipnosis.

hypnotism *n.* hipnotismo, práctica de
la hipnosis.

hypnotize *v.* hipnotizar, producir
hipnosis.

hypoadrenalism *n.* hipoadrenalismo,
desorden causado por deficiencia de la
glándula suprarrenal.

hypoalbuminemia *n.*
hipoalbuminemia, deficiencia de
albúmina en la sangre.

hypocalcemia *n.* hipocalcemia, nivel
de calcio en la sangre anormalmente
bajo.

hypocapnia *n.* hipocapnia,
disminución del dióxido de carbono en
la sangre.

hypochlorhydria *n.* hipocloridria,
deficiencia en la secreción de ácido
clorhídrico en el estómago, condición
que puede indicar una fase primaria de
cáncer.

hypocholesteremia *n.*
hipocolesteremia, disminución de
colesterol en la sangre.

hypochondriac *n. a.* hipocondríaco-a,
hipocóndrico-a, que cree haber
contraído alguna enfermedad cuando
goza de salud y se preocupa por ello.

hypochondrium *n.* hipocondrio, parte
del abdomen a cada lado del epigastrio.

hypochromia *n.* hipocromía,
deficiencia de hemoglobina en la
sangre.

hypocyclosis *n.* hipociclosis,
deficiencia en la acomodación visual;
lenticular ___ / ___ por deficiencia
muscular o rigidez del cristalino.

hypodermic *a.* hipodérmico-a, que se
aplica por debajo de la piel.

hypofibrinogenemia *n.*
hipofibrinogenemia, contenido bajo de
fibrinógeno en la sangre.

hypofunction *n.* hipofunción,
deficiencia en el funcionamiento de un
órgano.

hypogammaglobulinemia *n.*
hipogammaglobulinemia, nivel
anormalmente bajo de gamma
globulina en la sangre; **acquired** ___ /
___ adquirida, que se manifiesta
después de la infancia.

hypogastrium *n.* hipogastrio, área
inferior media y anterior del abdomen.

hypoglossal *a.* hipoglosal, rel. a una
posición debajo de la lengua.

hypoglossal nerve *n.* nervio
hipogloso.

hypoglycemia *n.* hipoglicemia,
hipoglucemia, disminución anormal del
contenido de glucosa en la sangre.

hypoglycemic *a.* hipoglicémico-a,
hipoglucémico-a, que produce o tiene
relación con la hipoglicemia; ___
agents / agentes ___ -s; ___ **shock** /
choque ___.

hypoinsulism *n.* hipoinsulinismo,
deficiencia en la secreción de insulina.

hypokalemia *n.* hipocalemia,
deficiencia en el contenido de potasio
en la sangre.

hypokinesia *n.* hipocinesia,
disminución de la actividad motora.

hyponatremia *n.* hiponatremia,
deficiencia en el contenido de sodio en
la sangre.

hypopharynx *n.* hipofaringe, parte de
la faringe situada bajo el borde superior
de la epiglotis.

hypophysectomy *n.* hipofisectomía,
extirpación de la glándula pituitaria.

hypophysis *n.* hipófisis, glándula
pituitaria, cuerpo epitelial localizado en
la base de la silla turca.

hypopituitarism *n.* hipopituitarismo,
condición patológica debida a
disminución de la secreción de la
glándula pituitaria.

hypoplasia *n.* hipoplasia, desarrollo
incompleto de un órgano o parte.

hypoplastic *a.* hipoplástico-a, rel. a la
hipoplasia.

hypoprothrombinemia *n.*
hipoprotrombinemia, deficiencia en la
cantidad de protrombina en la sangre.

hyporeflexia *n.* hiporreflexia, reflejos
débiles.

hypospadias *n.* hipospadias,
anomalía congénita de la uretra
masculina que consiste en el cierre
incompleto de la cara ventral de la

uretra en distintos grados de longitud. (En la mujer la uretra tiene salida a la vagina.)

hypotension *n.* hipotensión, presión arterial baja.

hypothalamus *n.* hipotálamo, parte del diencéfalo.

hypothermia *n.* hipotermia, temperatura baja.

hypothesis *n.* (*pl.* **hypotheses**) hipótesis, suposición asumida en el desarrollo de una teoría.

hypothrombinemia *n.* hipotrombinemia, deficiciencia de trombina en la sangre que causa una tendencia a sangrar.

hypothyroid *a.* hipotiroideo-a, rel. al hipotiroidismo.

hypothyroidism *n.* hipotiroidismo, deficiencia en el funcionamiento de la tiroides.

hypotonic *a.* hipotónico-a. 1. rel. a la deficiencia en tonicidad muscular; 2. de presión osmótica más baja en comparación con otros elementos.

hypoventilation *n* hipoventilación, reducción en la entrada de aire a los pulmones.

hypovolemia *n.* hipovolemia, disminución del volumen de la sangre en el organismo.

hypoxemia *n.* hipoxemia, insuficiencia de oxígeno en la sangre.

hysterectomy *n.* histerectomía, extirpación del útero; **abdominal __ / __** abdominal, a través del abdomen; **total __ / __** total, del útero y del cuello uterino; **vaginal __ / __** vaginal, a través de la vagina.

hysteria *n.* histeria, neurosis extrema.

hysteric, hysterical *a.* histérico-a, rel. a la histeria o que padece de ella; *v.* **to get __ / ponerse __; __ laughter /** risa __; **-ly** *a.* histéricamente.

hysteroid *n.* histeroide, semejante a la histeria.

hysteromania *n.* histeromanía, ninfomanía.

hysterosalpingography *n.* histerosalpingografía, radiografía del útero y de los oviductos por medio de material de contraste.

hysterosalpingoophorectomy *n.* histerosalpingooforectomía, extirpación quirúrgica de los ovarios, el útero y oviductos.

hysteroscopy *n.* histeroscopía, examen endoscópico de la cavidad uterina.

hysterotomy *n.* histerectomía, incisión del útero.

I *abbr.* símbolo químico del iodo. *pron.* yo, primera persona del singular.

i *abbr.* **iatric** / iátrico; **immune** / inmune; **implant** / implante; **impotence** / impotencia; **incomplete** / incompleto.

iatric *a.* iátrico-a, rel. a la medicina, a la profesión médica, o a los que la ejercen.

iatrogenic *a.* yatrógeno-a, iatrogénico-a, rel. a un trastorno o lesión producido por un tratamiento o por una instrucción errónea del facultativo; __ **pneumothorax** / neumotórax __; __ **transmission** / transmisión __.

ibuprofen *n.* ibuprofén, agente antiinflamatorio, antipirético y analgésico usado en el tratamiento de artritis reumatoidea.

ice *n.* hielo; __ **cap,** __ **bag** / bolsa de __; __ **cream** / helado; __ **water** / agua helada, agua con __; __ **treatment** / aplicación de __; **My hands are like** __ / Tengo las manos heladas.

ichthyosis *n.* ictiosis, dermatosis congénita caracterizada por sequedad y peladura escamosa esp. de las extremidades.

icing *n.* aplicación de hielo.

icteric *a.* ictérico-a, rel. a la ictericia.

icterogenic *a.* icterogénico-a, causante de ictericia.

icterohepatitis *n.* icterohepatitis, hepatitis asociada con ictericia.

icterus *n.* icterus, ictericia. V. **jaundice.**

icterus gravis *n.* atrofia amarilla aguda del hígado.

icterus neonatorum *n.* ictericia del recién nacido.

ictus *n.* ictus, ataque súbito.

id *n.* id. 1. término en psicoanálisis que con el *ego* y el *superego* forma parte del inconsciente freudiano y actúa como reservorio de la energía psíquica y el libido; 2. sufijo que indica ciertas erupciones secundarias de la piel que aparecen distantes de la sede de la infección primaria.

idea *n.* idea, concepto; **fixed** __ / __ fija.

idée fixe *n., Fr.* idea fija.

identical *a.* idéntico-a, igual, mismo-a.

identical twins *n., pl.* gemelos idénticos formados por la fertilización de un solo óvulo.

identification *n.* identificación; proceso en el cual una persona adopta inconscientemente características semejantes a otra persona o grupo; __ **papers** / documento oficial de identidad.

identify *v.* identificar; reconocer.

identity *n.* identidad, reconocimiento propio; __ **crisis** / crisis de __.

idiocy *n.* idiotez, deficiencia mental.

idiopathic *a.* idiopático-a. 1. rel. a la idiopatía; 2. que tiene origen espontáneo; __ **aldosteronism** / aldosteronismo __; __ **infants hypercalcemia** / hipercalcemia __ en los niños; __ **neuralgia** / neuralgia __; __ **pulmonary fibrosis** / fibrosis pulmonar __; __ **subglottic stenosis** / estenosis subglótica __.

idiopathy *n.* idiopatía, enfermedad espontánea o de origen desconocido.

idiosyncrasy *n.* idiosincrasia. 1. características individuales; 2. reacción peculiar de cada persona a una acción, idea, medicamento, tratamiento o alimento.

idiot *a.* idiota, imbécil con un cociente de inteligencia inferior a 20.

idioventricular *a.* idioventricular, rel. a los ventrículos o que afecta exclusivamente a éstos.

ignorant *a.* ignorante.

ignore *v.* desatender, ignorar, desconocer, no hacer caso.

ileal *a.* ileal, rel. al íleon; __ **arteries** / arterias __ -es; __ **orifice** / orificio __; __ **ureter** / uréter __; __ **veins** / venas __ -es.

ileal bypass *n.* desviación quirúrgica del íleon.

ileectomy *n.* ilectomía, excisión parcial o total del íleon.

ileitis *n.* ileítis, infl. del íleon; **regional** __ / __ regional

ileocecal *a.* ileocecal, rel. al íleon y al ciego; __ **valve** / válvula __.

ileocecostomy *n.* ileocecostomía, anastomosis quirúrgica del íleon al ciego.

ileocolitis *n.* ileocolitis, infl. de la mucosa del íleon y el colon.

ileocolostomy *n.* ileocolostomía, anastomosis del íleon y el colon.

ileoproctostomy *n.* ileoproctostomía, anastomosis entre el íleon y el recto.

ileosigmoidostomy *n.* ileosigmoidostomía, anastomosis del íleon al colon sigmoide.

ileostomy *n.* ileostomía, anastomosis del íleon y la pared abdominal anterior estableciendo una fístula.

ileotransversostomy *n.* ileotransversostomía, anastomosis del íleon y el colon transverso.

ileum *n.* (*pl.* **ilea**) íleon, porción distal del intestino delgado que se extiende desde el yeyuno al ciego.

iliac *a.* ilíaco-a, rel. al ilion; __ **bone** / hueso __; __ **colon** / colon __; __ **crest** / cresta __; __ **muscle** / músculo __.

iliolumbar *a.* iliolumbar, rel. a las regiones ilíaca y lumbar; __ **artery** / arteria __; __ **vein** / vena __.

ilium *n.* (*pl.* **ilia**) ilion, porción del ilíaco.

ill *a.* enfermo-a, malo-a; *v.* **to be** __ / estar enfermo-a; **to become** __ / enfermarse; **to feel** __ / sentirse indispuesto-a; sentirse mal.

ill health *n.* mala salud; *v.* **to be in** __ / no estar bien de salud.

ill-mannered *a.* descortés.

ill-tempered *a.* de mal carácter, de mal genio.

illegible *a.* ilegible.

illness *n.* enfermedad, dolencia, mal.

illusion *n.* ilusión, interpretación imaginaria de impresiones sensoriales.

image *n.* imagen, figura; representación; **body** __ / __ del cuerpo propio; **direct** __ / __ directa; **double** __ / __ doble; **electric** __ / __ eléctrica; **inverted** __ / __ invertida; **latent** __ / __ latente; **mirror** __ / __ de espejo; **optic** __ / __ óptica; **radiographic** __ / __ radiográfica; **real** __ / __ real; **virtual** __ / __ virtual.

imaginary *a.* imaginario-a, ilusorio-a.

imaging *n.* creación de imágenes.

imbalance *n.* desequilibrio.

imbalanced *a.* desequilibrado.

imbecile *a.* imbécil.

imbricated *a.* imbricado-a, en forma de capas.

imitation *n.* imitación, copia.

immature *a.* inmaturo-a, inmaduro-a; prematuro-a; sin madurez.

immediate *a.* inmediato-a, cercano-a; **-ly** *adv.* inmediatamente, en seguida.

immerse *v.* sumergir, hundir.

immersion *n.* inmersión, sumersión de un cuerpo o materia en un líquido.

immigrant *n.* inmigrante.

imminent *a.* inminente; irremediable.

immobile *a.* inmóvil, estable, fijo-a; que no se puede mover.

immobility *n.* inmovilidad, sin movimiento.

immobilization *n.* inmovilización.

immobilize *v.* inmovilizar.

immune *a.* inmune, resistente a contraer una enfermedad; __ **adherence** / adherencia __; __ **adsorption** / adsorción __; __ **complex** / complejo __; __ **paralysis** / parálisis __; __ **reaction** / reacción __; __ **response** / respuesta __.

immune system *n.* sistema inmunológico.

immunity *n.* inmunidad. 1. condición del organismo de resistir a un determinado antígeno por activación de anticuerpos específicos; 2. resistencia creada por el organismo en contra de una enfermedad específica; **acquired** __ / __ adquirida; **active** __ / __ activa; **adoptive** __ / __ adoptiva; **antiviral** __ / __ antivírica; **artificial** __ / __ artificial; **bacteriophage** __ / __ bacteriófaga; **concomitant** __ / __ concomitante; **general** __ / general __; **group** __ / __ de grupo; **inborn** __ / __ nata; **innate** __ / __ innata; **maternal** __ / __ materna; **natural** __ / __ natural; **passive** __ / __ pasiva.

immunization *n.* inmunización, proceso para activar la producción de inmunidad en el organismo en contra de una determinada enfermedad. V. cuadro en la página 369.

immunize *v.* inmunizar, hacer inmune.

immunoassay *n.* inmunoanálisis, proceso para determinar la capacidad de una sustancia para actuar como antígeno y anticuerpo en un tejido; **enzyme** __ / __ enzimático.

immunochemotherapy *n.* inmunoquimioterapia, proceso combinado de inmunoterapia y quimioterapia aplicado en el tratamiento de ciertos tumores malignos.

immunocompetency *n.* inmunocompetencia, proceso de

immunotransfusion

Immunizations			Immunizaciones		
Age	Vaccine	Method	Edad	Vacuna	Método
2 months	DTP diphtheria tetanus pertussis OPV oral poliovirus	vaccination	2 meses	DTP difteria tetanus pertusis o tos ferina OPV oral de la polio	vacuna por vía oral
4 months	DTP	vaccination	4 meses	DTP	vacuna
6 months	OPV	by mouth	6 meses	VOP	por vía oral
15 months	MMR measles mumps rubella	vaccination	15 meses	SPR sarampión paperas rubéola	vacuna por vía oral
18 months	DTP OPV	vaccination by mouth	18 meses	DTP VOP	vacuna por vía oral
2 years	Hib haemophilus	vaccination	2 años	Hib hemófilo influenza b	vacuna
4-6 years	DTP OPV	vaccination by mouth	4-6 años	DTP VOP	vacuna por vía oral

alcanzar inmunidad después de la exposición a un antígeno.

immunocompromised *a.* inmunocomprometido-a, rel. a una persona con un sistema inmunológico deficiente.

immunodeficiency *n.* inmunodeficiencia, reacción inmune celular inadecuada que limita la habilidad de responder a estímulos antigénicos; **severe combined __ disease** / enfermedad grave de __ combinada.

immunogen *n.* inmunógeno, sustancia que produce inmunidad; **targeted __** / __ específico.

immunoglobuline *n.* inmunoglobulina. 1. proteína de origen animal que pertenece al grupo del sistema de respuesta inmune; 2. uno de los cinco tipos de gamma globulina capaz de actuar como anticuerpo.

immunologic *a.* inmunológico-a, rel. a la inmunología; **__ competence** / competencia __; **__ deficiency** / deficiencia __; **__ disease** / enfermedad __; **__ enhancement** / realce __; **__ mechanism** / mecanismo __; **__ paralysis** / parálisis __; **__ pregnancy test** / prueba __ del embarazo; **__ tolerance** / tolerancia __.

immunologist *n.* inmunólogo-a, especialista en inmunología.

immunology *n.* inmunología, rama de la medicina que estudia las reacciones del cuerpo a cualquier invasión extraña, tal como la de bacterias, virus o transplantes.

immunoprotein *n.* inmunoproteína, proteína que actúa como anticuerpo.

immunoreaction *n.* inmunoreacción, reacción de inmunidad entre antígenos y anticuerpos.

immunostimulant *n.* inmunoestimulante, agente capaz de inducir o estimular una respuesta inmune.

immunosuppression *n.* inmunosupresión, disminución o prevención de respuesta immune del organismo a materia foránea.

immunotherapy *n.* inmunoterapia, inmunización pasiva del paciente por medio de anticuerpos preformados (suero o gamma globulina).

immunotransfusion *n.* inmunotransfusión, transfusión indirecta; se inmuniza el donante inyectándole un antígeno de microorganismos extraídos del recibidor, luego, se hace la transfusión al recipiente con la sangre defrigenada del donante.

immunotyping

immunotyping *n.* tipificación inmunológica.

impact *n.* colisión, impacto; efecto; golpe; *v.* impactar, fijar, rellenar, asegurar; incrustar.

impacted tooth *n.* diente impactado.

impaction *n.* impacción. 1. condición de estar alojado o metido con firmeza en un espacio limitado; 2. impedimento de un órgano o parte.

impaired *a.* impedido-a, baldado-a; desmejorado-a, debilitado-a.

impalpable *n.* impalpable.

impartial *a.* imparcial.

impatient *a.* impaciente; *v.* to get, to become ___ / impacientarse, perder la paciencia.

impediment *n.* impedimento, obstáculo, obstrucción.

imperfection *n.* imperfección, deformidad, defecto.

imperforate *a.* imperforado-a; ___ hymen / himen ___.

imperil *v.* poner en peligro, arriesgar, hacer daño.

impermeable *a.* impermeable, impenetrable, que no deja pasar líquidos.

impetigo *n.* impétigo, infección bacteriana de la piel que se caracteriza por pústulas dolorosas de tamaño diferente que al desecarse forman costras amarillentas; ___ contagiosa / ___ contagioso; ___ neonatorum / ___ del neonato; ___ vulgaris / ___ vulgar.

implant *n.* implante, cualquier material insertado o injertado en el cuerpo; *v.* implantar, injertar, insertar.

implanted *a. pp.* of to implant, implantado-a.

implosion *n.* implosión. 1. colapso violento hacia adentro como sucede en la evacuación de un vaso; 2. método de tratamiento para el miedo debido a una fobia.

importance *n.* importancia.

important *a.* importante.

impossible *a.* imposible.

impotence *n.* impotencia, incapacidad de tener o mantener una erección.

impotent *a.* impotente.

impregnate *n.* impregnar; saturar.

impression *n.* impresión. 1. huella en una superficie; 2. el efecto producido en la mente a través de estímulos externos; 3. copia de la configuración de una parte o del total del arco dental, de dientes individuales, o para uso en una restauración de caries dentales.

improve *v.* mejorar; adelantar; mejorarse, recuperarse; restablecerse.

improved *a.* mejorado-a, recuperado-a.

improvement *n.* mejoría, restablecimiento, recuperación.

impulse *n.* impulso; fuerza súbita impulsiva; cardiac ___ / ___ cardíaco; excitatory ___ / ___ excitante; inhibitory ___ / ___ inhibitorio; nervous ___ / ___ nervioso; *v.* to act on ___ / dejarse llevar por un ___.

in *prep.* [*inside of*] dentro de; [*in time*] con; [*in the night, day, etc.*] durante, por; [*in place*] en; *adv.* dentro; adentro; ___ the care of / al cuidado de; ___ the meantime / mientras tanto.

in-dwelling catheter *n.* catéter permanente.

in-grown hair *n.* pelo que crece en ángulo anormal, revirtiendo el crecimiento hacia adentro.

in situ *a., L.* in situ. 1. en el lugar normal; 2. que no se extiende más allá del sitio en que se origina.

in utero *a., L.* in utero, dentro del útero.

in vitro *a., L.* in vitro, dentro de una vasija de vidrio, término aplicado a pruebas de laboratorio.

in vivo *a., L.* in vivo, en el cuerpo vivo.

inability *n.* inhabilidad, incapacidad.

inactive *a.* inactivo-a, pasivo-a.

inactivity *n.* inactividad; physical ___ / ___ física.

inadequate *a.* inadecuado-a, impropio-a.

inanimate *a.* inanimado-a, sin vida, falto de animación.

inanition *n.* inanición; debilidad; desnutrición.

inarticulate *a.* inarticulado-a, incapaz de articular palabras o sílabas.

inborn *a.* innato-a, cualidad congénita.

incapable *a.* incapaz.

incapacitate *v.* incapacitar, imposibilitar, inhabilitar.

incapacitated *a.* incapacitado-a.

incase *v.* encajar, encajonar.

incentive *n.* incentivo, estímulo; incitante, estimulante.

incest *n.* incesto.

incidence *n.* incidencia; frecuencia.

incipient *a.* incipiente, principiante, que comienza a existir.

incision *n.* incisión, corte, cortadura.

incisor *n.* diente incisivo.

incisura *n., L.* incisura, corte, raja.

inclination *n.* inclinación.

inclusion *n.* inclusión, acto de contener una cosa dentro de otra; ___ **bodies** / cuerpos de ___, presentes en el citoplasma de ciertas células en casos de infección.

incoherent *a.* incoherente, que no coordina las ideas.

income *n.* ingreso, entrada; ___ **tax** / impuestos.

incompatible *a.* incompatible.

incomplete *a.* incompleto-a.

incontinence *n.* incontinencia, emisión involuntaria, inhabilidad de controlar la orina o las heces fecales; **bowel** ___ / ___ intestinal; **fecal** ___ / ___ fecal; **overflow** ___ / ___ por rebozamiento; **reflex** ___ / ___ de reflejo; **urinary** ___ / ___ urinaria; **urinary stress** ___ / ___ urinaria de esfuerzo.

incontinent *a.* incontinente, rel. a la incontinencia.

incoordination *n.* falta de coordinación.

incorporate *v.* incorporar, añadir.

incorrect *a.* incorrecto-a.

increase *v.* aumentar, agrandar.

incrustation *n.* incrustación, formación de una postilla o costra.

incubation *n.* incubación. 1. período de latencia de una enfermedad antes de manifestarse; 2. mantenimiento de un ambiente especial ajustado a las necesidades de recién nacidos, esp. prematuros; ___ **period** / período de ___.

incubator *n.* incubadora, receptáculo usado para asegurar las condiciones óptimas en el cuidado de prematuros.

incudectomy *n.* incudectomía, excisión del incus.

incurable *a.* incurable, que no tiene cura.

incus *n.*, *L.* incus, huesecillo del oído medio.

indemnity *n.* indemnización, resarcimiento; ___ **benefits** / beneficios de ___; ___ **insurance** / seguro de ___.

indentation *n.* mella; (*print*) indentación.

indeterminate *a.* indeterminado-a, desconocido-a.

index *n.* índice; sumario; **abortion** ___ / ___ de aborto; **specific age** ___ / ___ de edad específica; **case fatality** ___ / ___ de fatalidad de casos; **death** ___ / ___ de mortalidad, de mortandad; **birth** ___ /

___ de natalidad; **zero population growth** ___ / ___ de crecimiento; **average flow** ___ / ___ medio.

indicated *a.* indicado-a; apropiado-a.

indicator *n.* indicador, señalador.

indigenous *a.* autóctono-a, indígena.

indigestion *n.* indigestión.

indirect *a.* indirecto-a; ___ **fracture** / fractura ___; ___ **hemagglutination test** / prueba de hemaglutinación ___; ___ **immunofluorescence** / inmunofluorescencia ___; ___ **laryngoscopy** / laringoscopía ___; ___ **nuclear division** / división nuclear ___; ___ **reacting bilirubine** / bilirubina reactiva ___; ___ **transfusion** / transfusión ___; ___ **vision** / visión ___.

indispensable *a.* indispensable, necesario-a.

indisposed *a.* maldispuesto-a; indispuesto-a; *v.* **to become** ___ / enfermarse.

individual *n.* individuo; *a.* individual.

indolent *a.* indolente, perezoso-a; inactivo-a, lento-a en desarrollarse, tal como sucede en ciertas úlceras.

induce *v.* inducir, provocar, suscitar, ocasionar.

induction *a.* inducción, acción o efecto de inducir.

induration *n.* induración, endurecimiento que puede suceder en tejidos blandos como en el tejido de las membranas mucosas.

inebriation *n.* embriaguez, intoxicación.

ineffective *a.* inefectivo-a; inútil.

inertia *n.* incercia, falta de actividad.

infancy *n.* infancia, menor de edad, primera edad, período desde el nacimiento hasta los primeros dos años.

infant *n.* infante, lactante.

infanticide *n.* infanticidio.

infantile *a.* infantil, pueril; ___ **acropustulosis** / acropustulosis ___; ___ **autism** / autismo ___; ___ **eczema** / eczema ___; ___ **hypothyroidism** / hipotiroidismo ___; ___ **osteomalacia** / osteomalacia ___; ___ **paralysis** / parálisis ___; ___ **purulent conjunctivitis** / conjuntivitis purulenta ___; ___ **scurvy** / escorbuto ___; ___ **spinal muscular atrophy** / atrofia muscular ___ de la espina dorsal.

infantilism *n.* infantilismo, manifestación de características infantiles en la edad adulta.

infarct, infarction

infarct, infarction *n.* infarto, necrosis de un área de tejido por falta de irrigación sanguínea (isquemia); **bland** ___ / ___ blando; **cardiac** ___ / ___ cardíaco; **cerebral** ___ / ___ cerebral; **hermorrhagic** ___ / ___ hemorrágico; **myocardial** ___ / ___ del miocardio; **pulmonary** ___ / ___ pulmonar.

infect *v.* infectar; infectarse.

infected *a.* infectado-a.

infection *n.* infección, invasión del cuerpo por microorganismos patógenos y la reacción y efecto que éstos provocan en los tejidos; **acute** ___ / ___ aguda; **airborne** ___ / ___ aerógena; **chronic** ___ / ___ crónica; **contagious** ___ / ___ contagiosa; **cross** ___ / ___ hospitalaria; **fungus** ___ / ___ de hongos parásitos; **hospital acquired** ___ / ___ intrahospitalaria; **initial or primary** ___ / ___ inicial o primaria; **massive** ___ / ___ masiva; **opportunistic** ___ / ___ enfermedad oportunista infecciosa; **pyogenic** ___ / ___ piogénica; **secondary** ___ / ___ secundaria; **subclinical** ___ / ___ subclínica; **systemic** ___ / ___ sistémica; **water-borne** ___ / ___ hídrica.

infectious *a.* 1. infeccioso-a, rel. a una infección; ___ **agent** / agente ___; ___ **disease** / enfermedad ___; ___ **hepatitis** / hepatitis ___; 2. causado por una infección.

infer *v.* inferir, deducir.

inferior *a.* inferior.

inferiority complex *n.* complejo de inferioridad.

infertility *n.* infertilidad, inhabilidad de concebir o procrear.

infestation *n.* infestación, invasión del organismo por parásitos.

infiltration *n.* infiltración, acumulación de sustancias extrañas en un tejido o célula.

infirmary *n.* enfermería, establecimiento de salud local donde se atiende a personas enfermas o lesionadas.

infirmity *n.* enfermedad.

inflammation *n.* inflamación, reacción de un tejido lesionado.

inflammatory *a.* inflamatorio-a, rel. a la inflamación; ___ **bowel disease** / enfermedad ___ de los intestinos.

inflation *n.* inflación, distensión.

inflection *n.* inflexión, torcimiento.

inflow *n.* flujo, afluencia, entrada.

influenza *n.* influenza, infección viral aguda del tracto respiratorio.

inform *v.* informar, comunicar, avisar.

information *n.* información; informe.

informed consent *n.* consentimiento informado.

infraclavicular *a.* infraclavicular, localizado debajo de la clavícula.

infracostal *n.* infracostal, el área debajo de la Costilla.

infraction *a.* infracción, fractura ósea incompleta sin desplazamiento.

infrared rays *n., pl.* rayos infrarrojos.

infrequent *a.* infrecuente, raro-a.

infundibulum *n.* (*pl.* **infundibula**) infundíbulo. 1. estructura en forma de embudo; 2. cada una de las divisiones de la pelvis renal; 3. prolongación corta del ventrículo derecho de donde procede la arteria pulmonar.

infusion *n.* infusión. 1. introducción lenta, por gravedad, de líquidos en una vena; 2. sumersión de una hierba en agua hervida para extraer una solución medicinal; **saline** ___ / ___ salina.

ingest *v.* ingerir.

ingestion *n.* ingestión, proceso de ingerir alimentos.

ingredient *n.* ingrediente, componente.

ingrowing *a.* rel. a una parte que crece hacia adentro y no hacia afuera, en forma opuesta a lo normal.

ingrown hair *n.* pelo que crece revirtiendo el crecimiento hacia adentro.

ingrown nail *n.* uña que crece en ángulo anormal, revirtiendo el crecimiento hacia adentro.

inguinal *a.* inguinal, rel. a la ingle; ___ **canal** / conducto, canal ___; ___ **hernia** / hernia ___; ___ **ligament** / ligamento ___; ___ **ring** / anillo ___.

inhalant *n.* inhalante, medicamento administrado por inhalación.

inhalation *n.* inhalación, aspiración de aire o vapor a los pulmones; **smoke** ___ / ___ de humo.

inhale *v.* inhalar, aspirar.

inherent *a.* inherente, rel. a una cualidad natural o innata.

inherited *a.* heredado-a, rel. a la herencia.

inhibition *n.* inhibición, interrupción o restricción de una acción o hábito.

inhibitor *n.* inhibidor, agente que causa una inhibición; **fusion** ___ / ___ de fusión.

initial *a.* inicial, primero-a.

initiate *v.* iniciar, comenzar, empezar.

inject *v.* inyectar, acto de introducir líquidos en un tejido, vaso o cavidad por medio de un inyector.

injection *n.* inyección, acción de inyectar una droga o líquido en el cuerpo; **booster shot** / ___ de refuerzo; **depot** / ___ de depósito, con medicamento de liberación lenta; **hypodermic** ___ / ___ hipodérmica; **insulin** ___ / ___ de insulina; **intraarticular** ___ / ___ intrarticular o de punción lumbar; **intradermic** ___ / ___ intradémica; **intramuscular** ___ / ___ intramuscular; **intrafecal** ___ / ___ intrafecal; **intravenous** ___ / ___ intravenosa; **selective** ___ / ___ selectiva; **sensitizing** ___ / ___ de sensibilización; **test** ___ / ___ de prueba.

injector *n.* inyector, jeringa, dispositivo que se usa para inyectar.

injured *a.* lastimado-a, dañado-a; herido-a.

injury *n.* lesión, lastimadura; herida; **degloving** ___ / herida de avulsión; ___ **-free** / ileso-a.

inlay *n.* incrustación.

inlet *n.* entrada, acceso.

innate error on metabolism *n.* error innato en el metabolismo, anormalidad en el metabolismo que resulta de un efecto heredado tal como sucede en la galactosemia y Ty-Sacs entre otras aflicciones.

innate immunity *n.* inmunidad innata, resistencia de un organismo que no ha sido sensibilizado por una infección específica.

inner *a.* interior.

innervation *n.* inervación. 1. acto de inervar; 2. distribución de nervios o de energía nerviosa en un órgano o área.

innocuous *a.* inocuo-a, que no daña.

inoculable *a.* inoculable, que puede ser transmitido por inoculación.

inoculate *v.* inocular, inmunizar, vacunar.

inoculation *n.* inoculación, vacunación, inmunización, acción de administrar sueros, vacunas u otras sustancias para producir o incrementar inmunidad a una enfermedad determinada.

inoperable *a.* inoperable, que no puede tratarse quirúrgicamente.

inorganic *a.* inorgánico-a; que no pertenece a organismos vivos.

inotropic *a.* inotrópico-a, que afecta la intensidad o energía de las contracciones musculares.

inpatient *n.* paciente interno, ingresado.

input-output chart *n.* hoja de balance.

inquest *n.* encuesta, investigación oficial.

insane *a.* loco-a, demente.

insanity *n.* locura, demencia.

insatiable *a.* insaciable, insatisfecho-a.

insect *n.* insecto.

insecticide *n.* insecticida.

insecurity *n.* inseguridad.

insemination *n.* inseminación, fertilización de un óvulo.

insensible *n.* insensible, que carece de sensibilidad.

insertion *n.* inserción. 1. acto de insertar; 2. punto de unión de un músculo y un hueso.

inside *prep.* por dentro, hacia adentro; adentro.

insider *n.* persona bien informada.

insidious *a.* insidioso-a, rel. a una enfermedad que se desarrolla gradualmente sin producir síntomas obvios.

insignificant *a.* insignificante, sin importancia.

insipid *a.* insípido-a, sin sabor; *pop.* soso-a.

insoluble *a.* insoluble, que no se disuelve.

insomnia *n.* insomnio, desvelo.

inspection *n.* inspección.

inspiratory *a.* inspiratorio-a, rel a la inspiración; ___ **capacity** / capacidad ___; ___ **reserve volume** / reserva de volumen ___; ___ **stridor** / estridor ___.

instability *n.* inestabilidad.

instep *n.* empeine, parte anterior del pie.

instillation *n.* instilación, goteo de un líquido en una cavidad o superficie.

instinct *n.* instinto.

instinctive *a.* instintivo-a.

institution *n.* institución; fundación; establecimiento; [*mental*] asilo; manicomio; [*home for the aged*] asilo de ancianos.

insufficiency *n.* insuficiencia, falta de; **adrenal** ___ / ___ suprarrenal; **cardiac** ___ / ___ cardíaca; **coronary** ___ / ___ coronaria; **hepatic** ___ / ___ hepática; **mitral** ___ / ___ mitral; **pulmonary valvular** ___ / ___ pulmonar-valvular; **renal** ___ / ___ renal; **respiratory** ___ / ___ respiratoria; **valvular** ___ / ___ valvular; **venous** ___ / ___ venosa.

insufficient *a.* insuficiente.

insufflate *v.* insuflar, soplar aire, polvo, gas o vapor; hacia el interior de una cavidad, parte u órgano; __ **pump** / bomba de __; __ **resistant** / __ resistente.

insula *n.* ínsula, lóbulo central del hemisferio cerebral.

insulin *n.* insulina. hormona secretada en el páncreas; __ **dependent** / insulinodependiente.

insuline shock *n.* choque insulínico, hipoglicemia severa que se manifiesta en forma de sudor, temblores, ansiedad, vértigo y diplopia, que puede ser seguida por delirio, convulsiones y colapso.

insulinemia *n.* insulinemia, exceso de insulina en la sangre.

insulinogenesis *n.* insulinogénesis, producción de insulina.

intake *n.* ingestión.

integration *n.* integración. 1. actividad anabólica; 2. el proceso de combinarse en un ser o entidad total.

intelligence *n.* inteligencia; (IQ) __ **quotient** / cociente de __.

intensify *v.* intensificar.

intensive *a.* intensivo-a; __ **care unit** (ICU) / unidad de cuidado intensivo (ICCI).

intention *n.* intención. 1. meta o propósito; 2. proceso natural en la curación de heridas.

interaction *n.* interacción; **drug** __ / __ de medicamentos.

intercalated *a.* intercalado-a, colocado-a entre dos partes o elementos.

intercostal *a.* intercostal, entre dos costillas; __ **membranes** / membranas __ -es; __ **nerves** / nervios __ -es; __ **space** / espacio __.

intercourse *n.* [*sexual*] coito, relaciones sexuales; intercambio, comunicación.

intercurrent *a.* intercurrente, que aparece en el curso de una enfermedad y que la modifica.

interdigitation *n.* interdigitación, entrecruzamiento de partes esp. los dedos.

interferon *n.* interferón, proteína natural liberada por células expuestas a la acción del virus que se usa en el tratamiento de infecciones y neoplasmas.

interfibrillar *a.* interfibrilar, localizado entre fibrillas.

interlobitis *n.* interlobitis, infl. de la pleura que separa dos lóbulos pulmonares.

interlobular *a.* interlobular, que occurre entre dos lóbulos de un órgano.

intermediary *a.* intermediario-a, situado entre dos cuerpos.

intermission *n.* intermedio, intervención, cualquier acción para mejorar el desarrollo de una enfermedad o cambiar el curso de ésta.

intermittent *a.* intermitente, que no es continuo; __ **positive-pressure breathing** / ventilación __ bajo presión positiva; __ **pulse** / pulso __.

intern *n.* interno-a; médico-a interno-a.

internal *a.* interno-a, dentro del cuerpo; __ **bleeding** / hemorragia __

internalization *n.* internalización, proceso inconsciente por el cual una persona adapta las creencias y valores de otra persona o de la sociedad en que vive.

International Red Cross *n.* Cruz Roja Internacional, organización mundial de asistencia médica.

International unit *n.* unidad internacional, medida de una sustancia definida aceptada por la Conferencia Internacional de Unificación de Fórmulas

interpret *v.* interpretar, traducir oralmente.

interstices *n., pl.* intersticios, intervalos o pequeños espacios.

interstitial *a.* intersticial, rel. a los espacios dentro de un órgano, órgano o célula; __ **cell stimulating hormone** / hormona __ que estimula células; __ **cystitis** / cistitis __; __ **disease** / enfermedad __; __ **emphysema** / enfisema __; __ **fluid** / fluido __; __ **gastritis** / gastritis __; __ **growth** / crecimiento __; __ **hernia** / hernia __; __ **nephritis** / nefritis __; __ **pregnancy** / embarazo __.

intertrigo *n.* intértrigo, dermatitis irritante que ocurre entre o debajo de los pliegues de la piel.

interval *n.* intervalo; espacio; período de tiempo.

intervention *n.* intervención, cualquier acción para mejorar la salud o cmbiar el curso de una enfermedad.

Intoxication-Poisoning	Intoxicación-Envenenamiento
alcali poisoning-ingestion of an alcali or ammoniac	ingestión de una sustancia alcalí-amoníaco, legía
caffeinism-excessive ingestion of products containing caffeine	cafeinismo-envenenamiento por ingestion excesiva de productos conteniendo cafeína
carbon monoxide-absorbtion of carbon monoxide causing a toxic condition that can be lethal	monóxido de carbono-envenenamiento por absorción e inhalación de monóxido de carbono que puede ser letal
cyanide poisoning-inhalation of smoke or ingestion of cyanide industrial chemicals	envenenamiento de cianuro-inhalación de humo o ingestión de sustancias químicas industriales
ergotism-ingestion of ergot-infected grain products that cause diarrhea, vomiting and even alteration of the heart rhythm	ergotismo-consumo de productos de grano infestado por ergot que pueden causar diarrea y hasta alteración del ritmo cardíaco
alcohol intoxication-excessive ingestion of alcohol, can be habit forming and cause serious physical and psychological problems	intoxicación alcohólica-ingestión excesiva de alcohol puede ser adictiva y causar serios problemas físicos y psicológicos
lead poisoning-by ingestion or inhalation of paints that contain lead, or containers of water such as water pipes and water tanks	envenenamiento por plomo-por ingestión o absorción, causado por pinturas que contienen plomo, o por contenedores de agua tal como tuberías y tanques
mercury poisoning by ingesting mercury, causing acute kidney damage, vomiting and diarrhea that could be lethal	envenenamiento por mercurio-puede causar daño severo al riñón, vómito y diarrea que puede ser letal
nicotine poisoning-inhalation and ingestion of great amounts of nicotine	envenenamiento por nicotina-inhalación e ingestión de una gran cantidad de nicotina
overdose of drugs-salicylates, neuroleptics, antidepressants, and opiates prescribed or obtained illegally	sobredosis de drogas-salicilatos, neurolépticos, antidepresivos, opiados, prescritos u obtenidos ilegalmente
contaminated shellfish	mariscos contaminados
ophidism-poisoning by snakes, bees, ants, spiders, producing an injected venom	ofidismo-envenenamiento causado por la ponzoña de una abeja, hormiga, avispa, o araña negra o el veneno de una serpiente
strong cleaning substances mixed with strong acids	sustancias limpiadoras fuertes mezcladas con ácidos

interventricular a. interventricular, localizado entre los ventrículos; ___ **optum** / tabique ___ del corazón.

intervertebral disk n. disco intervertebral.

intestinal a. intestinal, rel. a los intestinos; ___ **bypass surgery** / desviación quirúrgica ___; ___ **flora** / flora ___; ___ **juice** / jugo ___; ___ **obstruction** / obstrucción ___; ___ **perforation** / perforación ___.

intestine n. intestino, tubo digestivo que se extiende del píloro al ano; **large** ___ / ___ grueso; **small** ___ / ___ delgado.

intima n., L. (pl. **intimae**) íntima, la membrana o túnica más interna de las

capas de un órgano tal como en un vaso capilar.

intolerance n. intolerancia, incapacidad de soportar dolor o los efectos de una droga.

intorsion n. intorsión, rotación del ojo hacia adentro.

intoxication n. intoxicación, envenenamiento o estado tóxico producido por una droga o sustancia tóxica. V. cuadro esta página.

intra-abdominal a. intrabdominal, localizado dentro del abdomen.

intra-aortic a. intraórtico-a, rel. a o situado dentro de la aorta.

intra-arterial a. intra-arterial, dentro de una arteria.

intra-articular *a.* intra-articular, dentro de una articulación.

intracapsular *a.* intracapsular, dentro de una cápsula.

intracellular *a.* intracelular, dentro de una célula o células.

intracranial *a.* intracraneal, dentro del cráneo.

intrahepatic *a.* intrahepático-a, dentro del hígado; __ **cholestasis of pregnancy** / colestasis __ del embarazo.

intralobular *a.* intralobular, dentro de un lóbulo.

intraluminal *a.* intraluminal. 1. dentro de la luz o estructura lumínica; 2. semejante al lumen de un vaso arterial o venoso.

intramuscular *a.* intramuscular, dentro del músculo.

intraocular *a.* intraocular, dentro del ojo; __ **pressure** / presión; __ **implant** / implante __.

intraoperative *a.* intraoperatorio-a, que tiene lugar durante un proceso quirúrgico.

intraosseous *a.* intraóseo-a, dentro de la sustancia ósea.

intrarenal *a.* intrarrenal, que ocurre dentro del riñón; __ **failure** / insuficiencia __.

intrauterine *a.* intrauterino-a, dentro del útero; __ **device** (IUD) / dispositivo __.

intravenous *a.* intravenoso-a, dentro de una vena; __ **infusion** / infusión __; __ **injection** / inyección __; **feeding** / alimentación __.

intravenous pyelogram (IVP) *n.* pielograma intravenoso, procedimiento de diagnósticos que usa un agente de contraste por medio intravenoso y rayos-x para obtener claras imágenes del tracto urinario.

intraventricular *a.* intraventricular, dentro de un ventrículo.

intrinsic *a.* intrínseco-a, esencial, exclusivo-a. inherente.

intrinsic factor *n.* factor intrínseco, proteína normalmente presente en el jugo gástrico humano.

introducer *n.* intubador, divisa utilizada para intubar.

introitus *n., L.* introito, abertura o entrada a un canal o cavidad.

introspection *n.* introspección, análisis propio o de sí mismo-a.

introversion *n.* inversion, introversión, acto de concentración de una persona en sí misma, con disminución del interés por el mundo externo.

intubation *n.* intubación, inserción de un tubo en un conducto o cavidad del cuerpo.

intumesce *v.* intumecer, engrosar, agrandar.

intumescent *a.* engrosado-a, que se va hinchando.

intussusception *n.* intuscepción, invaginación tal como la de una porción del intestino que causa una obstrucción intestinal.

invaginate *v.* invaginar, replegar una porción de una estructura en otra parte de la misma.

invagination *n.* invaginación, proceso de inclusión de una parte dentro de otra.

invalid *a.* inválido-a; debilitado-a; incapacitado-a.

invasive *a.* invasor-a, invasivo-a; que invade tejidos adyacentes; **procedimiento** __ / __ **procedure**.

inverse, inverted *a.* inverso-a, invertido-a.

inversion *n.* inversión, proceso de volverse hacia adentro; __ **of chromosomes** / __ de cromosomas; __ **of the uterus** / __ del útero; **paracentric** __ / __ paracéntrica; **pericentric** __ / __ pericéntrica; **visceral** __ / __ visceral.

investigation *n.* investigación, indagación.

investment *n.* revestimiento, cubierta.

invisible *a.* invisible, que no puede verse a simple vista.

involuntary *a.* involuntario-a.

involution *n.* involución, cambio retrógrado.

involutional melancholia *n.* melancolía involucional, trastorno emocional depresivo que se observa en mujeres de 40 a 55 años y en hombres de 50 a 65 años.

iodine *n.* iodo, yodo. 1. elemento no metálico que pertenece al grupo halógeno usado como componente en medicamentos para contribuir al desarrollo y funcionamiento de la tiroides; 2. tintura de yodo usada como germicida y desinfectante.

iodism *n.* yodismo, envenenamiento por yodo.

iodize *v.* yodurar, tratar con yodo.

iododerma *n.* yododerma, afección cutánea.

iodophilia *n.* yodofilia, afinidad por el yodo, como se manifiesta en algunos leucocitos.

ion *n.* ion, átomo o grupo de átomos provistos de carga eléctrica.

ionization *n.* ionización, disociación de compuestos en los iones que los componen.

ionizing radiation *n.* radiación por ionización.

ipecac, syrup of *n.* jarabe de ipecacuana, emético y expectorante.

ipsilateral *a.* ipsilateral, ipsolateral, que afecta el mismo lado del cuerpo.

iridectomy *n.* iridectomía, extirpación de una parte del iris.

iridology *n.* iridología, estudio del iris y de los cambios que éste sufre en el curso de una enfermedad.

iris *n.* iris, membrana contráctil del humor acuoso del ojo situada entre el cristalino y la córnea, que regula la entrada de la luz.

iritis *n.* iritis, infl. del iris.

iron *n.* hierro; *v.* **to have an __ constitution** / tener una constitución de hierro.

iron-deficiency anemia *n.* anemia causada por deficiencia de hierro.

iron lung *n.* pulmón de hierro, máquina que se usa para producir una respiración artificial.

irradiation *n.* irradiación, uso terapéutico de radiaciones.

irrational *n.* irracional.

irreducible *a.* irreducible, que no puede reducirse.

irregular *a.* irregular.

irrigate *v.* irrigar, lavar con un chorro de agua.

irrigation *n.* irrigación, acto o proceso de irrigar.

irritable *n.* irritable, que reacciona con irritación a un estímulo; **__ bowel syndrome** / síndrome de irritación intestinal.

irritant *a.* irritante, que produce irritación.

ischemia *n.* isquemia, insuficiencia de riego sanguíneo a un tejido o parte; **silent __** / **__** silenciosa.

ischemic *a.* isquémico-a, que padece de isquemia o rel. a la misma.

ischium *n., L. (pl. ischia)* isquion, parte posterior de la pelvis.

ischuria *n.* iscuria, retención o suspensión de orina.

island *n.* isla, nombre dado a un grupo celular o a un tejido aislado.

isolate *v.* aislar, separar.

isolated *a.* aislado-a, separado-a.

isolation *n.* aislamiento. 1. proceso de aislar o separar; 2. la separación física de organismos infectados de otros con el fin de evitar la contaminación; **behavioral __** / **__ conductual;** **exclusion __** / **__ de exclusión;** **infectious __** / **__ de infección;** **__ ward** / sala de **__**.

isometric *a.* isométrico-a, de dimensiones iguales.

isometropia *n.* isometropía, la misma refracción en los dos ojos.

isoniazid *n.* isoniazida, medicamento antibacteriano usado en el tratamiento de tuberculosis.

isosthenuria *n.* isostenuria, condición de insuficiencia renal.

isotonic *a.* isotónico-a, que tiene la misma tensión que otra dada; **__ exercise** / ejercicio **__**.

isotope *n.* isótopo, elemento químico que pertenece a un grupo de elementos que presentan propiedades casi idénticas, pero que difiere de éstos en el peso atómico.

issue *n.* emisión; **__ of blood** / pérdida de sangre; **to avoid the __** / esquivar la cuestión *v.* brotar, fluir; emitir.

isthmectomy *n.* istmectomía, extirpación de la parte media de la tiroides.

isthmus *n.* istmo. 1. conducto estrecho que conecta dos cavidades o dos partes mayores; 2. constricción entre dos partes de un órgano o estructura; **aortic __** / **__ de la aorta; __ of auditory tube** / **__** del tubo auditivo; **__ of the encephalon** / **__** del encéfalo; **__ of the eustachian tube** / **__** de la trompa de Eustaquio; **__of the fauces** / **__** de las fauces; **__ of the ureter** / **__** del uréter; **pharyngeal __** / **__** de la faringe; **tubaric __** / **__** tubárico.

it *pron. neut.* they; **it is** / eso es; es; **it's** *contr.* of **it** and **is; the best of __** / lo mejor; **the worst of __** / lo peor.

itch *n.* picazón.

itching *n.* sensación de picazón.

ivy *n.* hiedra.

J

j

j *abbr.* **joint** / articulación

jacket *n.* forro; corsé, soporte del tronco y de la espina dorsal usado para corregir deformidades.

Jacksonian epilepsy *n.* epilepsia jacksoniana, epilepsia parcial sin pérdida del conocimiento.

Jaeger test types *n., pl.* Jaeger, tipos de prueba, líneas de tipos de letras de distintos tamaños para determinar la precisión visual.

jamais vu *n.*, *Fr. jamais vu*, nunca visto, percepción de una experiencia familiar o conocida como si fuera una experiencia nueva.

jaundice *n.* ictericia, derrame biliar por exceso de bilirrubina en la sangre que causa pigmentación amarillo-anaranjada de la piel y otros tejidos y fluidos del cuerpo; **hemolytic** ___ / ___ hemolítica; **hepatocellular** ___; / ___ hepatógena; **neonatal** ___ / ___ neonatal; **obstructive** ___ / ___ obstructiva, obstrucción de la bilis; icterus.

jaundiced *a.* ictérico-a, rel. a la ictericia o que padece de ella.

jaw *n.* mandíbula, quijada, maxilar inferior; ___ **reflex** / reflejo mandibular; ___ **winking** / pestañeo mandibular.

jawbone *n.* hueso maxilar de la mandíbula.

jejunal *a.* yeyunal, rel. al yeyuno.

jejunectomy *n.* yeyunectomía, excisión el yeyuno o parte del mismo.

jejunitis *n.* yeyunitis, infl. del yeyuno.

jejunoileal bypass *n.* derivación yeyunoilíaca, cirugía plástica para lograr pérdida de peso en personas excesivamente gruesas.

jejunostomy *n.* yeyunostomía, creación de una abertura permanente en el yeyuno a través de la pared abdominal.

jejunum *n.* yeyuno, porción del intestino delgado que se extiende del duodeno al íleon.

jelly *n.* jalea, sustancia gelatinosa; **contraceptive** ___ / ___ anticonceptiva; **petroleum** ___ / vaselina.

jerk *n.* sacudida, reflejo súbito, contracción muscular brusca; *a.* [*slang*] tonto-a, imbécil; *v.* sacudir, tirar de, mover bruscamente.

jet lag *n.* estado de cansancio que sufren los viajeros aéreos después de jornadas largas a través de diferentes zonas de tiempo.

jitters *n.* [*slang*] nerviosidad.

job *n.* trabajo, empleo; [*task*] tarea.

jogging *n.* acción de correr acompasadamente como medio de ejercicio.

join *v.* unir, juntar; [*as a member*] hacerse miembro, hacerse socio-a; [*meet*] encontrarse.

joint *n.* articulación, coyuntura, punto de unión entre dos huesos; **arthrodial** ___ / -artrodia, que permite un movimiento de deslizamiento; **ball-and-socket** ___ / ___ esferoidea, que permite movimientos en varias direcciones; **hip** ___ / ___ de la cadera; ___ **efussion** / derrame articular; ___ **inflammation** / arthritis; ___ **freely movable** / ___ con facilidad de movimiento, diartrosis; ___ **fluid** / líquido sinfial; ___ **pain** / artralgia; ___ **replacement** / artroplastia; **knee** ___ / ___ de la rodilla; **sacroiliac** ___ / ___ sacroilíaca; **shoulder** ___ / ___ del hombro.

joint capsule *n.* cápsula articular, cubierta en forma de bolsa que envuelve una articulación.

jolt *n.* sacudida, tirón.

jowl *n.* cachete, carrillo.

jugular *a.* yugular, rel. a las venas yugulares; ___ **foramen** / foramen ___; ___ **fossa** / fosa ___; ___ **gland** / glándula ___; ___ **glomus** / glomo ___; ___ **nerve** / nervio ___; ___ **pulse** / pulso ___; ___ **venous arch** / arco venoso ___ .

jugular veins *n.* venas yugulares, venas que llevan la sangre de la cabeza y del cuello al corazón.

juice *n.* jugo, zumo, líquido extraído o segregado; **apple** ___ / ___ de manzana; **carrot** ___ / ___ de zanahoria; **gastric** ___ / ___ gástrico; **grape** ___ / ___ de uva; **grapefruit** ___ / ___ de toronja; **intestinal** ___ / ___ intestinal; **pancreatic** ___ / ___ pancreático; **pineapple** ___ / ___ de piña; **plum** ___ / ___ de ciruela.

jump *n.* salto, brinco; *v.* saltar, brincar.

jumpy *a.* inquieto-a, intranquilo-a.

juncture *n.* juntura; coyuntura.

jurisprudence, medical *n.*
jurisprudencia médica, ciencia del
derecho judicial que se aplica a la
medicina.

Jurkat cells *n., pl.* células de Jurkat,
línea de linfocitos T cuya acción
primordial determina el mecanismo
diferencial de vulnerabilidad de los
tipos de cancer a drogas y
radiación.

juvenile *a.* juvenil, joven; ___ **arthritis**
/ artritis ___; ___ **cataract** / catarata
___; ___ **delinquency** / delincuencia
___; ___ **myoclonic epilepsy** / epilepsia
mioclónica ___; ___ **on-set diabetes** /
principio de diabetes ___; ___ **pelvis** /
pelvis ___; ___ **periodontitis** /
periodontitis ___; ___ **plantar
dermatitis** / dermatitis
plantar ___.

juvenile absence epilepsy *n.*
epilepsia juvenil de ausencia, síndrome
de epilepsia generalizado que se
presenta durante la adolescencia
caracterizida por episodios de
convulsiones con pérdida del
conocimiento y convulsiones clónicas.

juvenile rheumatoid arthritis *n.*
artritis reumatoidea juvenil.

juxtaglomerular *a.* yuxtaglomerular,
junto a un glomérulo.

juxtaglomerular apparatus *n.*
aparato yuxtaglomerular, grupo de
células localizadas alrededor de
arteriolas aferentes del riñón, que
intervienen en la producción
de renina y en el metabolismo del
sodio.

juxtaposition *n.* yuxtaposición,
aposición; posición adyacente.

K

k

K *abbr.* **kalium** / potasio.

k *abbr.* **kilogram** / kilogramo.

kala-azar *n.* kala-azar, infestación visceral por un protozoo.

kalemia *n.* potasemia, presencia de potasio en la sangre.

kaliuresis *n.* caliuresis, aumento en la excreción de potasio en la orina.

kallikrein *n.* calicreína, enzima potente de acción vasodilatadora.

Kamier's Syndrome *n. Kamier,* syndrome de, trastorno autístico en la niñez.

Kanner syndrome *n.* Kanner, síndrome de, autismo infantil.

kaolin *n.* caolín, silicato de aluminio hidratado, agente de cualidades absorbentes de uso interno y externo.

Kaposi's disease *n.* enfermedad de Kaposi, neoplasma maligno localizado en las extremidades inferiores de hombres adultos que se desarrolla rápidamente en casos de SIDA.

Karvonen method *n.* Karvonen, método de, método de calcular el espectro máximo del índice cardíaco durante pruebas de ejercicios de tolerancia.

karyocyte *n.* cariocito, célula nucleada.

karyogamy *n.* cariogamía, conjugación celular con unión de dos núcleos.

karyogenesis *n.* cariogénesis, desarrollo del núcleo de la célula.

karyolysis *n.* cariolisis, disolución del núcleo de una célula.

Katz formula *n.* Katz, fórmula de, fórmula para obtener la velocidad media de sedimentación de los eritrocitos.

Kawasaki disease *n.* Kawasaki, enfermedad de, enfermedad infantil febril aguda. Los síntomas más destacados son conjuntivitis, lesiones bucales, enrojecimiento, infl. y exfoliación de la epidermis en los dedos de las manos y los pies.

Kegel exercises *n.* Kegel, ejercicios de, ejercicios que consisten en alternar contracciones y relajamiento de los músculos perineales con el fin de controlar mejor la incontinencia.

keep *vi.* [*a record*] mantener; [*guard*] guardar; **to __ down** / limitar; **to __ from** / abstenerse de, guardarse de, evitar; **to __ off** / alejarse, apartarse; **to __ on** / continuar; **to __ quiet** / estarse quieto-a, quedarse callado-a; **to __ up** / mantener, continuar.

Kelly operation *n.* Kelly, operación de. 1. histerectomía abdominal subtotal; 2. operación para corregir la incontinencia urinaria poniendo suturas en la vagina debajo del cuello de la vejiga.

keloid *n.* queloide, cicatriz de tejido grueso rojizo que se forma en la piel después de una incisión quirúrgica o de una herida.

keloidosis *n.* queloidosis, formación de queloides.

kelolysis *n.* dstrucción de cuerpos cetónicos.

kelp *n.* cenizas de un tipo de alga marina rica en yodo.

keratectomy *n.* queratectomía, incisión de una parte de la córnea.

keratin *n.* queratina, proteína orgánica insoluble que es un elemento componente de las uñas, la piel y el cabello.

keratinization *n.* queratinización, proceso por el cual las células se vuelven callosas por depósitos de queratina.

keratitis *n.* queratitis, infl. de la córnea; **interstitial __ / __** intersticial; **mycotic __ / __** micótica, queratomicosis, infección fungal de la córnea; **trophic __ / __** trófica, causada por el virus del herpes.

keratocele *n.* queratocele, hernia de la membrana anterior de la córnea.

keratoconjunctivitis *n.* queratoconjuntivitis, infl. de la córnea y la conjuntiva.

keratoderma *n.* queratoderma, queratodermia, hipertrofia del estrato córneo de la piel, esp. en las regiones de las palmas de las manos y las plantas de los pies.

keratohemia *n.* queratohemia, presencia de sangre en la córnea.

keratolysis *n.* queratolisis. 1. exfoliación de la epidermis; 2. anomalía congénita por la cual se

muda la piel periódicamente; ___
neonatorum / ___ neonatal.

keratoma *n.* queratoma, callosidad,
tumor córneo.

keratomalacia *n.* queratomalacia,
degeneración de la córnea causada por
deficiencia de vitamina A.

keratoplasty *n.* queratoplastia,
cualquier modificación de la córnea por
medio de cirugía plástica.

keratorrhexis *n.* queratorrexis, rotura
de la córnea debido a un trauma o a una
úlcera perforante.

keratosis *n.* queratosis, condición
callosa de la piel tal como callos y
verrugas; **actinic** ___ / ___ actínica,
lesión solar precancerosa;
blenorrhagic ___ / ___ blenorrágica,
manifestada en la palma de las
manos y los pies con erupción
escamosa.

keratotomy *n.* queratotomía, incisión a
través de la córnea.

kernicterus *n.* kernícterus, forma de
ictericia del recién nacido.

ketoacidosis *n.* cetoacidosis, acidosis
causada por el aumento de cuerpos
cetónicos en la sangre.

ketoaciduria *n.* cetoaciduria, acidosis
causada por el aumento de cuerpos
cetónicos en la orina.

ketone bodies *n.* cuerpos cetónicos o
acetónicos, comúnmente llamados
acetonas, productos desintegrados
de las grasas en el catabolismo
celular.

ketonemia *n.* cetonemia, concentración
de cuerpos cetónicos en el plasma.

ketonuria *n.* cetonuria, presencia de
cuerpos cetónicos en la orina.

ketosis *n.* cetosis, producción excesiva
de cuerpos acetónicos como resultado
del metabolismo incompleto de ácidos
lípidos; acidosis.

key *n.* llave; [*clue, reference*] clave.

kick *n.* patada, puntapié *v.* patear, dar
puntapiés; [*addiction*] **to** ___ **the habit**
[to abstain] / dejar la droga.

kid *n.* [*child*] niño, niña, chiquillo,
chiquilla.

kidney *n.* riñón, órgano par situado a
cada lado de la región lumbar y que
sirve de filtro al organismo; **artificial**
___ / ___ artificial; **cancer** / cáncer
del ___; **dialysis** / dialysis del ___;
disease / enfermedad del ___;
failure / fallo renal; **stones** /
piedras o cálculos renales, *pop.* piedras

en los riñones; **polycystic** ___ / ___
poliquístico. V. ilustración en la página
382.

kill *v.* matar; [*germs*] exterminar; **to** ___
time / pasar el tiempo.

killer cell *n.* linfocito citolítico o
linfocito citocida.

kilometer *n.* kilómetro.

kindred *n.* parentesco.

kinesiology *n.* cinesiología, estudio de
los músculos y los movimientos
musculares.

kinesitherapy *n.* cinesiterapia,
tratamiento por medio de movimiento o
ejercicios.

kinesthesia *n.* cinestesia, experiencia
sensorial, sentido y percepción de un
movimiento.

kinetic *n.* cinético-a, rel. al movimiento.

kinship *n.* [*family relationship*]
parentesco.

klebsiella *n.* klebsiela, bacilo
gram-negativo asociado con
infecciones respiratorias y del tracto
urinario.

Klebs-Löffler bacillus *n.* bacilo
de Klebs-Löffler, bacilo de la
difteria.

kleptomania *n.* cleptomanía, deseo
incontrolable de robar.

knee *n.* rodilla, articulación del fémur,
la tibia y la patela; ___ **ankle foot
orthosis** / ortosis de la ___ y tobillo;
___ **dislocation** / dislocación de la ___;
___ **joint** / articulación de la ___;
protector / rodillera; ___ **reflex** /
reflejo de la ___; **locked** ___ / ___
bloqueada.

kneecap *n.* rótula.

knee jerk *n.* reflejo de la rodilla que se
produce con el toque de un martillo
de goma en el ligamento de la
patela.

knob *n.* protuberancia, bulto.

knot *n.* nudo; **surgical** ___ / ___
quirúrgico.

know *vi.* saber, [*to be acquainted*]
conocer; **to** ___ **how to** / saber + *inf*; **to**
___ **of** / tener noticias de, estar
enterado-a de.

knowledge *n.* conocimiento; **to the
best of my** ___ / a mi entender, por lo
que sé; *v.* **to have** ___ **of** / saber.

knuckle *n.* nudillo.

Koch's bacillus *n.* bacilo de Koch,
Mycobacterium tuberculosis,
causa de la tuberculosis en los
mamíferos.

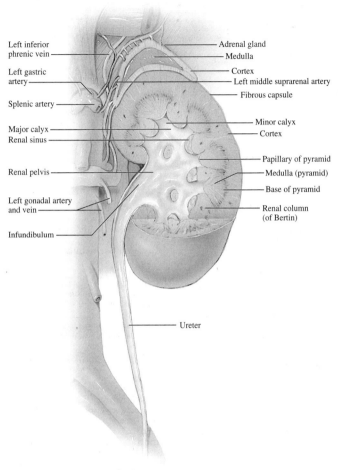

Left kidney and adrenal gland

Labels in the illustration:

Left inferior phrenic vein
Left gastric artery
Splenic artery
Major calyx
Renal sinus
Renal pelvis
Left gonadal artery and vein
Infundibulum

Adrenal gland
Medulla
Cortex
Left middle suprarenal artery
Fibrous capsule
Minor calyx
Cortex
Papillary of pyramid
Medulla (pyramid)
Base of pyramid
Renal column (of Bertin)

Ureter

kolpitis *n.* colpitis, infl. de la mucosa vaginal.

Koplic spots *n.* Koplic, manchas de, pequeños puntos blancuzcos rodeados por un anillo rojo que aparece en la parte interna de las mejillas en la fase temprana del sarampión.

kraurosis *n.* craurosis, atrofia y sequedad de la piel y de las membranes mucosas especialmente de la vulva.

Krukenberg tumor *n.* tumor de Krukenberg, tumor maligno del ovario, gen. bilateral y frecuentemente secundario a un cáncer del tracto gastrointestinal.

Kussmaul breathing *n.* respiración de Kussmaul, respiración jadeante y profunda vista en casos de acidosis diabética.

kwashiorkor *n.* Kwashiorkor, deficiencia proteínica o desnutrición durante la infancia que se manifiesta después del destete esp. en áreas tropicales y subtropicales.

kyphosis, hunchback *n.* cifosis, exageración en la curvatura posterior de la espina dorsal que da lugar a una corcova.

kyphotic *a.* cifótico-a; *pop.* corcovado-a, que sufre de una corcova; __ **pelvic** / pelvis __.

L

L *abbr.* **liter** / litro.
l *abbr.* **left** / izquierdo-a; **lethal** / letal; **light** / ligero-a; **lower** / más bajo.
labial *a.* labial, rel. a los labios; __ **branches of mental nerve** / ramas labiales del nervio mentoniano; __ **glands** / glándulas labiales; __ **hernia** / hernia __; __ **occlusion** / oclusión __; __ **splint** / férula __; __**veins** / venas labiales.
labial glands *n.* glándulas labiales, situadas entre la mucosa labial y el músculo orbicular de la boca.
labile *a.* lábil, inestable, frágil, que cambia o se altera fácilmente.
labiochorea *n.* labiocorea, espasmo crónico de los labios y trastornos del lenguaje que se derivan de esa condición.
labium *n., L.* (*pl.* **labia**) labio. 1. borde carnoso; 2. estructura semejante a un labio; **labia majora and labia minora** / __ mayor y __ menor.
labor *n.* parto; **active** __ / __ activo; **after** __ / después del __; **before** __ / antes del __; **complicated** __ / __ complicado; **contractions during** __ / contracciones durante el __; **dry** __ / __ seco; **during** __ / durante el __; **hard** __ / __ laborioso; **induction of** __ / __ inducido; __ **pains** / dolores de __; __ **room** / sala de __; **painless** __ / __ sin dolor; **stages of** __ / etapas del __; *v.* **to be in** __ / estar de parto; alumbramiento.
laboratory *n.* laboratorio; __ **findings** / resultados del análisis; __ **technician** / técnico de __.
labored *a.* laborioso-a, trabajoso-a; __ **breathing** / respiración jadeante.
labyrinth *n.* laberinto. 1. red de conductos del oído interno cuya función relaciona la audición con el equilibrio del cuerpo; 2. conductos y cavidades que forman un sistema comunicándose entre sí.
labyrinthine *a.* laberíntico-a, rel. a un laberinto; __ **artery** / arteria __; __ **fistula** / fístula __; __ **nystagmus** / nistagmo __; __**veins** / venas __; **vertigo** / vértigo __.

labyrinthitis *n.* laberintitis. 1. infl. aguda o crónica del laberinto; 2. otitis interna.
laceration *n.* laceración, desgarro.
lachrymogenous *a.* lacrimógeno-a, que produce lágrimas.
lack *n.* falta, carencia; necesidad; falta de; __ **of food** / __ de alimentos; __ **of medication** / falta de o carencia de medicina; __ **of orientation** / __ de orientación; *v.* carecer de; faltar; **they** __ **everything** / carecen de todo.
lacrimal *a.* lagrimal, rel. a las lágrimas y a los órganos y partes relacionados con éstas; __ **apparatus** / aparato __; __ **artery** / arteria __; __ **bone** / hueso __; __ **canaliculus** / canículo __; __ **duct** / conducto __; __ **fossa** / fosa __; __ **gland** / glándula __; __ **nerve** / nervio __; __**papilla** / papila; __ **punctum** / punto __; __ **sac** / saco __; __ **vein** / vena __.
lacrimotomy *n.* lacrimotomía, incisión del conducto o saco lacrimal.
lactase *n.* lactasa, enzima intestinal que hidroliza la lactosa y produce dextrosa y galactosa.
lactation *n.* lactancia, crianza; secreción de leche.
lacteal *a.* lácteo-a, rel. a la leche.
lactic acid *n.* ácido láctico.
lactiferous *a.* lactífero-a, que segrega y conduce leche; __ **ducts** / conductos __; __ **sinus** / senos __.
lacto-ovovegetarian *a.* lacto-ovovegetariano-a; que sigue una dieta de vegetales, huevos y productos lácteos.
lacto-vegetarian *a.* lactovegetariano, que sigue una dieta de vegetales y productos lácteos.
lactogen *n.* lactógeno, agente que estimula la producción o secreción de leche.
lactose, lactine *n.* lactosa, lactina, azúcar de leche; __ **deficiency** / deficiencia de __; __ **intolerance** / intolerancia a la __.
lactosuria *n.* lactosuria, presencia de lactosa en la orina.
lacuna *n., L.* (*pl.* **lacunae**) laguna, laguna, depresión pequeña tal como las cavidades del cerebro.
lag *n.* atraso, retraso; [*slow growth*] latencia; __ **time** / período de latencia.
La Leche League *n.* La Liga de la Leche, organización que promueve la lactancia materna.

Lamaze technique, Lamaze method n. método de Lamaze, procedimiento de parto natural con adiestramiento de la madre en técnicas respiratorias que facilitan el proceso del parto.

lamella n. laminilla. 1. capa fina; 2. disco que se inserta en el ojo para aplicar un medicamento.

lamina n., L. (pl. laminae) lámina, placa o capa fina; — **arcus vertebrae** / — del arco vertebral; — **basalis choroidae** / — basal de la coroide; — **limitans anterior corneae** / — elástica anterior de la córnea; — **limitans posterior corneae** / — elástica posterior de la córnea; — **multiform of cerebral cortex** / — multiforme de la corteza cerebral.

laminectomy n. aminectomía, extirpación de una o varias láminas vertebrales.

lamp n. lámpara; **infrared** — / — infrarroja; **lamplight** / luz de una —; **slit** — / — de hendidura; **sun** — / — solar.

lancet, lance n. lanceta, instrumento quirúrgico; v. abrir con una lanceta.

lancinating a. lancinante, rel. a un dolor agudo con sensación de pinchazos.

Landztainer's classification n. clasificación de Landztainer, diferenciación de grupos sanguíneos; O-A-B-AB.

language n. lenguaje; — **skills** / habilidades lingísticas.

lanolin n. lanolina, sustancia purificada que se obtiene de la lana de la oveja y se usa en pomadas.

lanugo n. lanugo, vellosidad, pelusilla suave que cubre el cuerpo del feto.

laparocele n. laparocele, hernia abdominal.

laparoscope n. laparoscopio, instrumento usado para visualizar la cavidad peritoneal.

laparoscopy n. laparoscopía, examen de la cavidad peritoneal por medio de un laparoscopio.

laparoscopy surgery n. laparoscopia, cirugía con uso de un laparoscopio.

laparotomy n. aparotomía, incisión y abertura del abdomen.

large a. grande, grueso-a, abultado-a; — **intestine** / intestino grueso.

larva n., L. (pl. **larvae**) larva, primera fase o forma de ciertos organismos tal como los insectos.

larvicide n. larvicida, agente que destruye las larvas, esp. las de los insectos.

laryngeal a. laríngeo-a; — **papillomatosis** / papilomatosis —; — **prominence** / prominencia —; — **reflex** / reflejo —, tos producida por irritación de la laringe; —**stenosis** / estenosis —; — **syncope** / síncope —; — **ventricle** / ventrículo —; — **web** / red —.

laryngectomy n. aringectomía, extirpación de la laringe.

laryngitis n. laringitis. 1. infl. de la laringe; 2. afonía, ronquera.

laryngopharyngitis n. laringofaringitis, infl. de la laringe y la faringe.

laryngopharynx n. laringofaringe, porción inferior de la faringe.

laryngoplasty n. aringoplastia, reconstrucción plástica de la laringe.

laryngoscopy n. laringoscopía, examen de la laringe; **direct** — / — directa, por medio de un laringoscopio; **indirect** — / — indirecta, por medio de un espejo.

laryngospasm n. laringoespasmo, espasmo de los músculos de la laringe.

laryngotomy n. aringotomía, incisión de la laringe.

larynx n. laringe. 1. parte del tracto respiratorio situado en la parte superior de la tráquea; 2. órgano de la voz.

laser n. láser. 1. sigla del inglés "Light Amplification by Stimulated Emission of Radiation" (amplificación de la luz por estimulación de emisión de radiación); 2. bisturí microquirúrgico usado en la cauterización de tumores; — **coagulation** / coagulación de tejido con uso de láser; — **conization** / extiración de tejido de forma cónica.

laser beams n., pl. rayos de láser, rayos de luz por efecto radioactivo de calor intenso que se usan para destruir tejidos o separar partes.

laser skin resurfacing n. renovación de la superficie de la piel a través de láser.

lassitude n. lasitud, languidez, agotamiento.

late *a.* tardío-a, último-a; *adv.* tarde; __ **auditory evoked response** / respuesta auditiva evocada __; __ **dumping syndrome** / síndrome de vaciamiento __; **luteal phase dysphoria** __ / fase luteal __ de la disforia; **to be** __ / atrasarse, retrasarse; **-ly** *adv.* últimamente, hace poco.

latency *n.* latencia, acto de permanecer latente; __ **period** / período de __.

latent *a.* latente, presente pero no activo-a; sin síntomas aparentes; sin manifestación.

later *a., comp.* of **late**. *adv.* más tarde, luego, después.

lateral *a.* lateral, rel. a un lado o costado.

lateral humeral epicondylitis *n.* epicondilitis humeral lateral, codo de tenista.

lateroflexion *n.* lateroflexión, flexión lateral o de inclinación hacia un costado.

latex *n.* látex, sustancia derivada de ciertas plantas de semillas que contienen un elemento de goma natural; en muchos casos puede causar alergia.

latter *pron.* éste, ésta; el, la más reciente, el más moderno, la más moderna.

laughter *n.* risa, carcajada; **hysteric** __ / __ histérica; **sardomic** __ / __ sardónica.

lavage *n.* lavado, irrigación de una cavidad.

lavatory *n.* [*basin*] lavatorio, lavabo, lavamanos; [*restroom*] inodoro, servicio, baño, excusado.

laxative *n.* laxante, laxativo, purgante suave.

layer *n.* capa, estrato.

laziness *n.* pereza, holgazanería, haraganería.

lazy eye *n.* ambliopía, falta de coordinación en la percepción de la profundidad visual.

lead *n.* 1. plomo; __ **apron** / delantal de __, usado como protección a radiaciones; __ **poisoning** / envenenamiento por __; 2. conductor, tal como la guía que se usa en una electrocardiografía; *v.* conducir *v.* llevar de la mano, guiar.

leakage *n.* escape, salida; **aortic** __ / __ de la aorta.

learning *n.* aprendizaje; **cognitive** __ / __ cognitivo; **incidental** __ / __ incidental; **latent** __ / __ latente; __ **disability** / impedimento en el __; **passive** __ / __ pasivo; **state**

dependent __ / __ dependiente del estado.

Leber disease *n.* enfermedad de Leber, tipo de atrofia hereditaria que causa degeneración del nervio óptico y que afecta a los hombres.

lecithin *n.* lecitina, elemento esencial en el metabolismo de las grasas presente en los tejidos de los animales, esp. el tejido nervioso.

lecture *n.* conferencia, disertación.

ledge *n.* borde.

leech *n.* sanguijuela, gusano anélido acuático chupador de sangre; **artificial** __ / ventosa.

left *a.* izquierdo-a; __ **-hand** / mano izquierda; __ **side** / lado __; **to the** __ / a la izquierda.

left-handed *a.* zurdo-a.

leg *n.* pierna, extremidad inferior que se extiende de la rodilla al tobillo; __ **injuries** / traumatismos de la __; *v.* **to pull one's** __ / tomar el pelo.

legal *a.* legal, legítimo-a, de acuerdo con la ley; __ **blindness** / ceguera __; __ **medicine, forensic medicine** / medicina __; __ **suit** / litigio, demanda, pleito.

legionnaire's disease *n.* enfermedad de los legionarios, enfermedad infecciosa grave, a veces letal, que se caracteriza por pulmonía, tos seca, dolor muscular y a veces síntomas gastrointestinales.

legislation, medical *n.* legislación médica.

leiomyoma *n.* leiomioma, tumor benigno compuesto esencialmente de tejido muscular liso.

leiomyosarcoma *n.* leiomiosarcoma, tumor formado por leiomioma y sarcoma.

Lenegre syndrome *n.* Lenegre, síndrome de, fibrosis del sistema conductivo intracardíaco que se caracteriza gen. como fibrosis idiopática del nódulo atrioventricular.

lens *n.* 1. lente; **achromatic** __ / __ acromático; **adherent** __ / __ adherido; **biconcave** __ / __ bicóncavo; **biconvex** __ / __ biconvexo; **bifocal** __ / __ bifocal; **contact** __ / __ de contacto, lentillas; **dislocation of** __ / dislocación del __; __ **implantation, intraocular** / -s intraoculares; **trifocal** __ / __ -s trifocales; 2. cristalino, lente transparente del ojo.

lentiginosis *n.* lentiginosis, presencia de un gran número de léntigos.

lentigo *n.* léntigo, mácula de la piel; **malignant** __ / __ maligno; **múltiple** __ / __ múltiple; **senile** __ / __ senil.

leper *a.* leproso-a, lazarino-a; que sufre de lepra.

leprechaunism *n.* leprecaunismo, condición hereditaria con características de enanismo acompañadas por retardo físico y mental, trastornos endocrinos y susceptibilidad a infecciones.

leprosy *n.* lepra, enfermedad infecciosa conocida también como enfermedad de Hansen causada por el bacilo *Mycobacterium leprae* caracterizada por lesiones cutáneas de pústulas y escamas.

leptomeningitis *n.* leptomeningitis, infl. de las leptomeninges.

lesbian *n.* lesbiana, mujer homosexual.

lesion *n.* lesión, herida, contusión; **degenerative** __ / __ degenerativa; **depressive** __ / __ depresiva; **diffuse** __ / __ difusa; **functional** __ / __ funcional; **gross** __ / __ grosera; **peripheral** __ / __ periférica; **precancerous** __ / __ precancerosa; **systemic** __ / __ sistemática; **toxic** __ / __ tóxica; **traumatic** __ / __ traumática; **vascular** __ / __ vascular; **whiplash** __ / __ de latigazo.

lesson *n.* lección, enseñanza, instrucción.

let *vi.* permitir, dejar, conceder; __ us go / vámonos; __ us + inf. / vamos a + *inf*; to __ be / dejar tranquilo-a; to __ blood / hacer sangrar; to __ down / dejar bajar; dejar caer; desilusionar, abandonar; to __ go / soltar; to __ in / dejar entrar, admitir; to __ out / dejar salir.

lethal *a.* letal, mortal; __ dose / dosis __; __ factor / factor __; __ gene / gene __; __ mutation / mutación __.

lethargic, lethargical *a.* letárgico-a, aletargado-a.

lethargy *n.* letargo, estupor.

leucine *n.* leucina, aminoácido esencial en el crecimiento y metabolismo.

leucinuria *n.* leucinaria, presencia de leucina en la orina.

leucocoria *n.* leucocoria, pupila de aspecto blanco producto de una catarata.

leukapheresis *n.* leucaferesis, separación de leucocitos de la sangre de un paciente con subsecuente retransfusión al mismo paciente.

leukemia *n.* leucemia, cáncer de la sangre; **acute lymphocytic** __ / __ linfoncítica aguda; **aleukemic** __ / __ aleucémica; **chronic granulocytic** __ / __ granulocítica crónica; **chronic** __ / __ crónica; **chronic myeloid** __ / __ mieloide crónica; **eosinophilic** __ / __ eosinofílica; **lymphocytic** __ / __ linfocítica; **monocytic** __ / __ monocítica.

leukemoid *n.* leucemoide, semejante a la leucemia.

leukoblast *n.* leucoblasto, leucocito inmaduro.

leukocitosis *n.* leucocitosis, aumento temporal de leucocitos en la sangre que ocurre gen. durante el acto de digerir y durante el embarazo; **absolute** __ / __ absoluta; **mononuclear** __ / __ mononuclear; **polynuclear** __ / __ polinuclear; **relative** __ / __ relativa.

leukocyte *n.* leucocito, glóbulo blanco, célula importante en la defensa y reparación del organismo; **acidophil** __ / __ acidófilo, que cambia de color con ácidos colorantes; **basophil** __ / __ basófilo, que cambia de color con colorantes básicos; **lymphoid** __ / __ linfoide, sin gránulos; **neutrophil** __ / __ neutrófilo, de afinidad con colorantes neutros; **polymorphonuclear** __ / __ polimorfonucleado, con núcleos de más de un lóbulo.

leukoencephalopathy *n.* leucoencefalopatía, cambios progresivos en la materia blanca del cerebro encontrados en niños que padecen de leucemia y que se asocian a lesiones producidas por radiación y quimioterapia.

leukopathia *n.* leucopatía, albinismo, falta de pigmentación.

leukopenia *n.* leucopenia, número anormalmente bajo de glóbulos blancos.

leukoplakia *n.* leucoplasia, áreas de color opaco en la membrana mucosa de la lengua gen. de carácter precanceroso.

leukorrhea *n.* leucorrea, flujo vaginal blancuzco.

leukosis *n.* leucosis, formación anormal de leucocitos.

leukotrichia *n.* leucotriquia, blancura del cabello.

levator *n.* 1. elevador, músculo que eleva o levanta una parte; 2. instrumento quirúrgico para levantar una depresión en una fractura del cráneo.

level *n.* nivel, plano; __ **of consciousness** / __ de conciencia *v.* nivelar, ajustar; __ **of health** / estado de salud.

levodopa *n.* levodopa, sustancia química usada en el tratamiento de la enfermedad de Parkinson.

levulose *n.* levulosa. V. **fructose**.

lewd *a.* lujurioso-a, deshonesto-a, libidinoso-a, obsceno-a.

liberation *n.* liberación.

libidinous *a.* libidinoso-a, rel. al libido.

libido *n.* libido. 1. impulso sexual, consciente o inconsciente; 2. en psicoanálisis, la fuerza o energía que determina la conducta del ser humano.

Libman-Sacks endocarditis, Libman Sacks syndrome *n.* Libman-Sacks, síndrome de, endocarditis verrugosa no bacteriana que se asocia con lupus eritematoso diseminado.

lice *n., pl.* piojos.

lichen *n.* liquen, lesiones o erupciones de la piel no contagiosas de forma papular; **atrophic sclerotic** __ / __ esclerotico atrófico; __ **scrofulosorum** / __ escrofularia; __ **planus** / __ plano; __ **urticatus** / __ de urticaria; **ulcerative** __ / __ ulcerativo.

lienal artery *n.* arteria esplénica.

lientery *n.* lientería, diarrea que muestra partículas de alimento no digerido.

life *n.* vida, modo de vivir, existencia; __ **expectancy** / expectativa de __, promedio de __; __ **insurance** / seguro de __; __ **preservers**, __ **support devices** / aparatos para prolongar la __; __ **-saving measure** / medida para prolongar o salvar la __; __ **span** / longevidad; __ **-threatening** / que puede causar la muerte.

lifetime *n.* toda la vida, curso de la vida; *a.* vitalicio-a.

lift *v.* levantar, alzar, elevar; __ **your hand** / levante, levanta la mano; **to give one a** __ / ayudar, animar, alentar.

lifting *n.* acto de levantar, levantamiento.

ligament *n.* ligamento. 1. banda de fibras de tejido conjuntivo que protege las articulaciones y evita que sufran torceduras o luxaciones; 2. banda protectora de fascias y músculos que conectan o sostienen vísceras; **acromioclavicular** __ / __ acromioclavicular; **alveolo-dental** __ / __ alveolodentario; **anococcygeal** __ / __ anococcígeo; **brachiocubital** __ / __ braquiocubital; **capsular** __ / __ capsular; **gastrocholic** __ / __ gastrocólico; **glossoepiglottic** __ / __ glosoepiglótico; **hepatoduodenal** __ / __ hepatoduodenal; **iliofemoral** __ / __ iliofemoral; __ **tear** / desgarre del __; **long plantar** __ / __ largo del plantar; **palmar** __ / __ palmar; **radiocubital** __ / __ radiocubital; **sternoclavicular** __ / __ esternoclavicular; **trapezoid** __ / __ trapezoide.

ligate *v.* ligar, aplicar una ligadura.

ligature, ligation *n.* ligadura; acción o proceso de ligar.

light *n.* luz; lumbre; __ **absorption** / absorción de la __; __ **adaptation** / adaptación de la __; __ **perception** / percepción de la __; __ **reflex** / reflejo de la __; __ **therapy** / fototerapia; *a.* ligero-a, liviano-a claro-a, pálido-a; __ **-headed** / [*dizzy*] mareado-a; **-ly** *adv.* ligeramente, levemente.

lightening *n.* [*childbirth*] aligeramiento, descenso del útero en la cavidad pélvica, gen. en la etapa final del embarazo.

like *a.* parecido-a, igual, semejante; [*to look alike*] **The boy looks** __ **the father** / El niño se parece al padre; **to look** __ / parecerse a; *v.* **I** __ **this medicine** / Me gusta esta medicina; **to** __ **someone, something** / gustar, agradar; *prep.* como; *adv.* como si, del mismo modo.

limb *n.* 1. extremidad, miembro del cuerpo; 2. porción terminal o distal de una estructura; __ **amputation** / amputación de una __; __ **rigidity** / rigidez de la __ o del miembro.

limber *a.* flojo-a, flexible.

limbic *a.* marginal.

limbic system *n.* sistema límbico, grupo de estructuras cerebrales.

limbus *n.* limbo, filo o borde de una parte; __ **corneae** / __ de la córnea.

limit *n.* límite, frontera; **assimilation** __ / __ de asimilación; __ **of perception** / umbral perceptivo; **saturation** __ / __ de saturación.

limitation *n.* limitación, restricción; __ **of motion** / __ de movimiento.

limited *a.* limitado-a, restricto-a; __

activity / actividad ___; ___ **autopsy** / autopsia parcial.

limp *n.* cojera, flojera; *v.* cojear, renquear, renguear.

line *n.* línea; rasgo; arruga; límite o guía.

linen *n.* lienzo, lino; **bed** ___ / ropa de cama.

lingering *v.* prolongación, tardanza, morosidad; *a.* prolongado-a, retardado-a, moroso-a.

lingua *n., L.* (*pl.* **linguae**) lengua o estructura semejante a la lengua.

lingual *a.* lingual, rel. a la lengua.

liniment *n.* linimento, untura de uso externo.

lining *n.* túnica, capa, forro, cubierta, revestimiento.

link *n.* eslabón, vínculo.

linkage *n.* vínculo, unión, asociación de genes.

lint *n.* 1. fibra de algodón; 2. partículas desprendidas de la ropa.

lip *n.* labio, parte externa de la boca.

lipectomy *n.* ipectomía, excisión de tejido graso; **submental** ___ / ___ submental, del cuello.

lipemia *n.* lipemia, presencia anormal de grasa en la sangre.

lipid, lipide *n.* lípido, sustancia orgánica que no se disuelve en el agua pero que es soluble en alcohol, éter o cloroformo.

lipoarthritis *n.* lipoartritis, infl. de tejidos adiposos de la rodilla.

lipodystrophy *n.* lipodistrofia, trastorno del metabolismo de las grasas; **cephalothoracic** ___ / ___ cefalotorácica; **insulin** ___ / ___ insulínica; **intestinal** ___ / ___ intestinal.

lipofuscinosis *n.* lipofuscinosis, almacenamiento anormal de cualquiera de los pigmentos adiposos.

lipogenesis *n.* lipogénesis, producción de grasa.

lipoid *n.* lipoide, sustancia que se asemeja a la grasa.

lipolysis *n.* lipólisis, descomposición de las grasas.

lipoma *n.* lipoma, tumor de tejido adiposo.

lipomatosis *n.* lipomatosis. 1. condición causada por depósito excesivo de grasa; 2. lipomas múltiples.

lipoproteins *n., pl.* lipoproteínas, proteínas combinadas con compuestos lípidos que contienen una concentración alta de colesterol.

liposarcoma *n.* liposarcoma, tumor maligno que contiene elementos grasos.

liposis *n.* obesidad, acumulación excesiva de grasa en el cuerpo.

liposoluble *a.* liposoluble, que se disuelve en sustancias grasas.

liposuction *n.* liposucción, proceso de extraer grasa por medio de alta presión al vacío.

lip reading *n.* lectura labial, interpretación del movimiento de los labios.

lipuria *n.* lipuria, presencia de lípidos en la orina.

liquid *n.* líquido, fluido; **heavy** ___ / ___ espeso; ___ **balance** / balance de ___; ___ **retention** / retención de ___.

liquor *n.* 1. licor, líquido acuoso que contiene sustancias medicinales; 2. término general aplicado a algunos líquidos del cuerpo.

lisping *n.* ceceo, sustitución de sonidos debido a un defecto en la articulación de las palabras, tal como el sonido de la *z* por la *c*, o el sonido de la *c* por la *s*.

list *n.* lista; **casualty** ___ / lista de accidentes.

listless *a.* apático-a, lánguido-a, sin ánimo; indiferente.

lithiasis *n.* litiasis, formación de cálculos, esp. biliares o del tracto urinario.

lithium *n.* litio, elemento metálico usado como tranquilizante para tratar casos severos de psicosis.

lithotomy *n.* itotomía, incisión en un órgano o conducto para extraer cálculos.

lithotripsy *n.* litotripsia, trituración de cálculos en el riñón, el uréter, la vejiga y la vesícula biliar.

lithotriptor *n.* litotriturador, aparato o mecanismo para triturar cálculos; **extracorporal shock wave** ___ / ___ extracorporal con ondas de choque.

lithuresis *n.* lituresis, arenilla en la orina.

live *v.* vivir, existir; ___ **birth** / nacimiento con vida.

livedo *n.* livedo, mancha en la piel, frecuentemente azulada o morada, similar a un morado.

lively *a.* vivo-a; vivaracho-a, animado-a.

liver *n.* hígado, glándula mayor del cuerpo que segrega bilis y sirve de estabilizador y productor de azúcar, enzimas, proteínas y colesterol además

lividity

de eliminar las sustancias tóxicas del organismo; **enlarged** __ / __ agrandado; **infantile biliary cirrhosis** / cirrosis biliar infantil; __ **circulation** / circulación hepática; __ **cirrhosis** / cirrosis hepática; __ **damage** / lesión hepática; __ **failure** / insuficiencia hepática; __ **function tests** / pruebas funcionales hepáticas; __ **spots** / manchas hepáticas.

lividity *n.* lividez, descoloración que resulta de la gravitación de sangre; **post mortem** __ / __ cadavérica.

living *n.* vida; con vida; modo de vivir; **cost of** __ / costo de __; __ **expenses** / gastos de mantenimiento; __ **under stress** / __ agitada, __ con estrés.

living will *n.* testamento hecho por una persona en completo estado de salud en el que dispone que en caso de peligro de muerte no se use ningún medio artificial para prolongarle la vida.

loading *n.* carga por administración de una sustancia en una prueba metabólica; __ **test** / prueba de carga.

loan *n.* préstamo; *v.* prestar.

lobar *a.* lobar, lobular, rel. a un lóbulo; __ **pneumonia** / pulmonía __.

lobby *n.* salón de entrada, sala de espera, vestíbulo.

lobe *n.* lóbulo, porción redondeada y más o menos delimitada de un órgano; **middle** __ **syndrome** / síndrome del __ medio del pulmón.

lobectomy *n.* lobectomía, excisión de un lóbulo; **complete** __ / __ completa; **left lower** __ / __ izquierda anterior; **partial** __ / __ parcial.

lobotomy *n.* lobotomía, incisión de un lóbulo cerebral con el fin de aliviar ciertos trastornos mentales.

lobular *a.* lobular, rel. a un lóbulo; __ **neoplasia** / neoplasia __.

lobule *n.* lobulillo, lóbulo pequeño.

local *a.* local, rel. a una parte aislada; __ **anesthesia** / anestesia __; __ **application** / aplicación __; __ **recurrence** / reaparición __.

localization *n.* localización. 1. rel. al punto de origen de una sensación; 2. determinación de la procedencia de una infección o lesión.

lochia *n.* loquios, flujo serosanguíneo del útero en las primeras semanas después del parto.

locomotion *n.* locomoción.

loculated, locular *a.* locular, rel. a un lóculo.

locus *n.* 1. lugar, sitio; 2. localización de un gene en el cromosoma.

logagraphia *n.* logagrafía, incapacidad de reconocer palabras escritas o habladas.

logamnesia *n.* logamnesia, afasia sensorial.

logical *a.* lógico-a, preciso-a, exacto-a.

logoplegia *n.* logoplejía, parálisis de los órganos del lenguaje.

loin *n.* flanco, ijar, ijada, parte inferior de la espalda y de los costados entre las costillas y la pelvis.

longevity *n.* longevidad, ancianidad, duración larga de la vida.

look *n.* [*appearance*] aspecto, apariencia, cara; mirada, ojeada. *v.* mirar; revisar; **to __ bad** / tener mal aspecto; **to __ for** / buscar; **to __ through** / examinar con cuidado; **to take a __ at** / mirar, echar una mirada.

loose *a.* suelto-a, desatado-a, libre; __ **bowels** / deposiciones blandas o aguadas; *v.* desatar, desprender, aflojar.

loose associations *n.* disociación de ideas.

lordosis *n.* lordosis, curva exagerada; aumento exagerado hacia adelante de la concavidad de la columna lumbar.

lose *vi.* perder.

loss *n.* pérdida; **at a __** / confundido-a; __ **of balance** / __ del equilibrio; __ **of blood** / __ de sangre; __ **of consciousness** / __ del conocimiento; __ **of contact with reality** / __ del contacto con la realidad; __ **of grip** / __ de la retención; __ **of hearing** / __ de la audición; __ **of memory** / __ de la memoria; __ **of motion** / __ del movimiento; __ **of muscle tone** / __ de la tonicidad muscular; __ **of vision** / __ de la visión.

lotion *n.* loción, ablución.

Lou Gehrig disease *n.* Lou Gehrig, enfermedad de, atrofia muscular progresiva.

louse *n.* (*pl.* **lice**) piojo, insecto parásito que se aloja en el pelo, trasmisor de enfermedades infecciosas tales como la fiebre tifoidea.

love *n.* amor, cariño, afecto; *v.* amar, querer; **to fall in __** / enamorarse; **to fall in __ with** / enamorarse de.

low *a.* bajo-a; [*in spirits*] abatido-a; __ **opinion** / mala opinión.

lower *a. comp.* of low, inferior; bajo-a; *v.* bajar, poner más bajo; [*in quantity, price*] reducir, disminuir; __

esophageal sphincter / esfínter esofágico ___; __ **extremity** / extremidad ___; **to __ the arm** / __ el brazo.

lozenge *n.* pastilla que se disuelve en la boca.

lubricant *n.* lubricante, agente oleaginoso que al lubricar disminuye la fricción entre dos superficies; **oil-based __** / __ oleaginoso; **waterbased __** / __ acuífero.

lucidity *n.* claridad, esp. mental.

lukewarm *a.* tibio-a, templado-a; [*feelings*] indiferente.

lumbago *n.* lumbago, dolor en la parte inferior de la espalda.

lumbar *a.* lumbar, región de la espalda entre el tórax y la pelvis; **__ nerve** / nervio ___; **__ plexus** / plexo ___; **__ puncture** / punción ___; **__ vertebrae** / vértebras __ -es.

lumen *n.* lumen. 1. unidad de flujo luminoso; 2. espacio en una cavidad, canal, conducto u órgano.

lump *n.* bulto, protuberancia, chichón; [*in the throat*] nudo en la garganta; [*of sugar*] terrón de azúcar.

lumpectomy *n.* tumorectomía, extirpación de un tumor gen. de la mama.

lunatic *a.* lunático-a, demente, loco-a.

lung *n.* pulmón, órgano par de la respiración contenido dentro de la cavidad pleural del tórax que se conecta con la faringe a través de la tráquea y la laringe; **air containing __** / __ aireado; **__ abscess** / absceso pulmonar; **__ cancer** / cáncer del __; **__ capacities** / volumen pulmonar; **__ collapse** / colapso del __; **__ diseases** / neumopatías; **__ elasticity** / elasticidad pulmonar; **__ hemorrhage** / hemorragia pulmonar; **quiet __** / __ silencioso.

lungworm *n.* gusano nematodo que infesta los pulmones.

lupus *n.* lupus, enfermedad crónica de la piel de origen desconocido que causa lesiones degenerativas locales; **anticoagulant __** / __ anticoagulante; **__ vulgaris** / __ vulgar; **marginal __** / __ marginado.

lupus erythematosus, discoid *n.* lupus eritematoso discoide, condición caracterizada por placas escamosas de bordes enrojecidos que causa irritación de la piel.

lupus erythematosus, systemic *n.* lupus eritematoso sistémico, condición caracterizada por episodios febriles que afecta las vísceras y el sistema nervioso.

luteal *a.* lúteo, rel. al cuerpo lúteo.

lutein *n.* luteína, pigmento amarillo que se deriva del cuerpo lúteo, de la yema del huevo y de las células adiposas.

luteinizing hormone *n.* hormona luteinizante producida por la pituitaria anterior que estimula la secreción de hormonas sexuales por los testículos (testosterona) y el ovario (progesterona) e interviene en la formación de esperma y óvulos.

luteoma *n.* luteoma, tumor del cuerpo lúteo.

luxation *n.* luxación, dislocación.

lycopene *n.* licopina, pigmento vegetal muy abundante en tomates y zanahorias.

lye *n.* lejía; **__ poisoning** / envenenamiento por __.

lying *a.* acostado-a; recostado-a; extendido-a.

Lyme disease *n.* Lyme, enfermedad de, trastorno inflamatorio que afecta a múltiples sistemas del cuerpo, y que es causado por una garrapata. Ocurre mayormente en el este de los Estados Unidos durante la primavera y el verano.

lymph *n.* linfa, líquido claro que se encuentra en los vasos linfáticos; **__ nodes** / ganglios linfáticos.

lymphadenectomy *n.* infadenectomía, extirpación de vasos linfáticos y ganglios.

lymphadenitis *n.* linfadenitis, infl. de los ganglios linfáticos.

lymphadenopathy *n.* linfadenopatía, enfermedad que afecta los nódulos linfáticos; **axillary __** / __ axilar; **cervical __** / __ cervical; **generalized __** / __ generalizada; **mediastinal __** / __ mediastínica; **supraclavicular __** / __ supraclavicular.

lymphangiectasis *n.* linfagiectasis, dilatación de los vasos linfáticos.

lymphangioma *n.* linfangioma, tumor simple compuesto de vasos linfáticos; **cavernous __** / __ cavernoso.

lymphangitis *n.* linfangitis, infl. de vasos linfáticos.

lymphatic *a.* linfático-a, rel. a la linfa; **__ spaces** / espacios __-s; **__ system** / sistema __.

lymphedema *n.* linfedema, edema causado por una obstrucción en los vasos linfáticos.

lymphemia *n.* linfemia, presencia en la sangre circulante de un número elevado de linfocitos extremadamente grandes, de sus precursores, o de ambos.

lymphoblast *n.* linfoblasto, forma primitiva del linfocito.

lymphoblastoma *n.* linfoblastoma, linfoma maligno formado por linfoblastos.

lymphocyte *n.* linfocito, célula linfática; __ **B cell** / __ **B**, importante en la producción de anticuerpos.

lymphocyte T *n.* linfocitos de células T, linfocitos diferenciados en el timo que dirigen la respuesta inmunológica y alertan a las células B a responder a los antígenos; **cytotoxic** __ / __ citotóxicos, ayudan a exterminar células extrañas así como en el rechazo de órganos transplantados; __ **T helper** / ayudante de __, inductores, aumentan la producción de anticuerpos de las células B; **supressor** __ / represores de __, detienen la producción de anticuerpos de las células B.

lymphocytosis *n.* linfocitosis, cantidad excesiva de linfocitos en la sangre periférica.

lymphogranulomatosis, Hodgkin's disease *n.* linfogranulomatosis, enfermedad de Hodgkin, granuloma infeccioso del sistema linfático.

lymphogranuloma venereum *n.* linfogranuloma venéreo, enfermedad viral transmitida sexualmente que puede producir elefantiasis de los genitales y estrechez rectal.

lymphoma *n.* linfoma, neoplasma del tejido linfático.

lymphopenia, lymphocytopenia *n.* linfopenia, linfocitopenia, disminución en el número de linfocitos en la sangre.

lymphosarcoma *n.* linfosarcoma, neoplasma maligno del tejido linfoide.

lysergic acid diethylamide *n.* dietilamida del ácido lisérgico.

lysin *n.* lisina, anticuerpo que disuelve o destruye células y bacterias.

lysinogen *n.* lisinógeno, agente que tiene la propiedad de producir lisinas.

lysis *n.* lisis. 1. proceso de destrucción o disolución de glóbulos rojos, bacterias o cualquier antígeno por medio de lisina; 2. desaparición gradual de los síntomas de una enfermedad.

m

m *abbr.* **male** / hombre; **malignant** / maligno; **married** / casado-a; **mature** / maduro; **melts at** / se derrite a; **minute** / minuto; **molecular weight** / peso molecular; **morphine** / morfina.

macerate *v.* macerar; suavizar una materia por medio de inmersión en un líquido.

macrocephalia *n.* macrocefalia, cabeza anormalmente grande.

macrocyte *n.* macrocito, eritrocito agrandado.

macrocytic anemia *n.* anemia macrocítica, tipo de anemia presentando un gran número de macrocitos.

macroglossia *n.* macroglosia, agrandamiento excesivo de la lengua.

macromolecule *n.* macromolécula, molécula de tamaño grande tal como la de una proteína.

macrophage, macrophagus *n.* macrófago, célula mononuclear fagocítica; ___ **migration** / migración de ___ -s.

macroscopic *a.* macroscópico-a, que se ve a simple vista, antónimo de microscópico.

macula lutea, yellow spot *n.* mácula lútea, pequeña zona amarillenta situada en el centro de la retina.

macular degeneration *n.* pérdida progresiva de la vision debida a degeneración macular.

maculopapular *a.* maculopapular, rel. a máculas y pápulas.

mad *a.* [*insane*] loco-a, demente, perturbado-a; [*moody*] enojado-a, furioso-a; *v.* **to become** ___ / enloquecer; enloquecerse, enfurecerse; volverse loco-a; enojarse.

magnesium *n.* magnesio; elemento químico cuyas sales son esenciales en la nutrición, y es necesario a la actuación de varias enzimas.

magnetic *a.* magnético-a; ___ **field** / campo ___.

magnetic resonance angiography (MRA) *n.* angiografía de resonancia magnética con aplicación de un medio de contraste.

magnetic resonance imaging (MRI) *n.* imágenes por resonancia magnética, procedimiento por imágenes basado en el análisis cualitativo de la estructura química y biológica de un tejido.

magnification *n.* magnificación, ampliación de un objeto.

magnifying glass *n.* lente de aumento; lupa.

maim *v.* mutilar; estropear; lisiar.

maintenance *n.* mantenimiento; [*feeding*] alimentación; sostén, apoyo; [*of a building*] conservación, mantenimiento; ___ **dose** / dosis de ___.

major depressive disorder *n.* trastorno mayor depresivo.

make *vi.* hacer; [*money*] ganar; [*earn*] **How much do you** ___? / ¿Cuánto gana usted?, ¿cuánto ganas tú?; **to** ___ **a prescription** / llenar, preparar una receta; **to** ___ **believe** / fingir; **to** ___ **fun of** / burlarse de; **to** ___ **known** / declarar; **to** ___ **mistakes** / hacer errores; equivocarse; **to** ___ **no difference** / no tener importancia; **to** ___ **sense** / tener sentido; **to** ___ **sure** / asegurarse; **to** ___ **up** [*time*] / recobrar el tiempo perdido; **to** ___ **up one's mind** / decidirse.

mal *n.* enfermedad, trastorno, desorden.

malabsorption syndrome *n.* síndrome de malabsorción, condición gastrointestinal con trastornos múltiples causada por absorción inadecuada de alimentos.

malacia *n.* malacia, reblandecimiento o pérdida de consistencia en órganos o tejidos.

malacoplakia *n.* malcoplaquia, formación de áreas blandas en la membrana mucosa de un órgano hueco.

maladjusted *a.* inadaptado-a, incapaz de adaptarse al medio social y de soportar tensiones.

malady *n.* enfermedad, trastorno, desorden.

malaise *n.* malestar, indisposición, molestia.

malar *a.* malar, rel. a la mejilla o a los pómulos.

malar bone *n.* pómulo, hueso en ambos lados de la cara.

malaria *n.* malaria, infección febril aguda a veces crónica causada por protozoos del género *Plasmodium* y transmitida por el mosquito *Anófeles*.

malariacidal

malariacidal *a.* malaricida, que destruye parásitos de malaria.

malassimilation *n.* malasimilación, asimilación deficiente.

maldigestion *n.* indigestión.

male *n.* varón; hombre; macho; ___ **nurse** / enfermero.

malformation *n.* deformación, anomalía o enfermedad esp. congénita.

malignancy *n.* 1. cualidad de malignidad; 2. tumor canceroso.

malignant *a.* maligno-a, pernicioso-a, de efecto destructivo.

malignant hyperthermia *n.* hipertermia maligna, brote de fiebre extremadamente alta llegando a alcanzar 106°F ó 41° + C. *Syn.* **fulminating hyperpirexia.**

malignant melanoma *n.* melanoma maligno, neoplasma maligno pigmentoso que puede originarse en cualquier parte de la piel aunque muy raramente en la mucosa. El melanoma maligno tiene la capacidad de hacer metástasis a otras partes de la piel y la linfa, los pulmones, el hígado y el cerebro. El melanoma benigno tiene la apariencia de un lunar o verruga pigmentada.

malingerer *n.* simulador-a, persona que finge o exagera los síntomas de una enfermedad.

malleolus *n.* (*pl.* **malleoli**) maléolo, protuberancia en forma de martillo tal como la que se ve a ambos lados de los tobillos.

mallet finger *n.* dedo de la mano en martillo.

mallet toe *n.* dedo del pie en martillo.

malleus *n.* (*pl.* **mallei**) malleus, uno de los huesecillos del oído medio.

malnourished *a.* desnutrido-a, malnutrido-a.

malnutrition *n.* malnutrición; mala alimentación; deficiencia nutricional.

malocclusion *n.* maloclusión, mordida defectuosa.

malposition *n.* posición inadecuada.

malpractice *n.* negligencia profesional.

malpresentation *n.* presentación anormal del feto durante el parto.

malunion *n.* malaunión, fijación imperfecta de una fractura.

mamma *n.* mama, glándula secretora de leche en la mujer localizada en la parte anterior del tórax.

mammal *n.* animal mamífero.

mammalgia *n.* mamalgia, dolor en la mama.

mammaplasty, mammoplasty *n.* mamaplastia, mamoplastia, cirugía plástica de los senos; **augmentation** ___ / ___ de aumento; **reconstructive** ___ / ___ de reconstrucción; **reduction** ___ / ___ de reducción.

mammary *a.* mamario-a, rel. a los pechos o senos; ___ **glands** / glándulas ___ -as.

mammectomy, mastectomy *n.* mamectomía, mastectomía, excisión de la mama o de una porción de la glándula mamaria.

mammilliplasty *n.* mamiliplastia, operación plástica del pezón.

mammillitis *n.* mamilitis, infl. del pezón.

mammitis, mastitis *n.* mastitis, infl. de la mama.

mammogram *n.* mamograma, rayos-x de la mama.

mammography *n.* mamografía, rayos-x de la glándula mamaria.

mammoplasty *n.* mamoplastia, operación plástica de la mama.

man *n.* (*pl.* **men**) hombre.

manageable *a.* manejable; dócil.

mandible *n.* mandíbula, hueso de la quijada en forma de herradura.

mandibular *a.* mandibular, rel. a la mandíbula.

maneuver *n.* maniobra, movimiento preciso hecho con la mano.

manhandle *v.* maltratar.

manhood *n.* virilidad; edad viril.

mania *n.* manía, trastorno emocional caracterizado por excitación excesiva, ansiedad y altas y bajas de espíritu.

maniac *a.* maníaco-a, persona afectada de manía.

manic-depressive psychosis (MDP) *n.* psicosis maníaco-depresiva cíclica, condición caracterizada por estados de depresión y manía.

manifest *v.* manifestar; expresar; revelar; manifestarse, revelarse.

manifestation *n.* manifestación; revelación.

manipulate *v.* manipular, manejar.

manipulation *n.* manipulación, tratamiento por medio del uso diestro de las manos.

manliness *n.* masculinidad, virilidad.

manly *a.* varonil.

mannerism n. manerismo, expresión peculiar en la manera de hablar, de vestir o de actuar.

mantle n. manto, capa.

many a., pron. muchos-as; tantos, tantas; **a great** __ / muchos, muchas; **as** __ **as** / tantos-as como, igual número de.

marasmus n. marasmo, emaciación debida a malnutrición, esp. en la infancia.

march n. marcha, progreso; v. marchar, poner en marcha.

marginal a. marginal; **a** __ **case** / un caso __.

margination n. marginación, acumulación y adherencia de leucocitos a las paredes de los vasos capilares en un proceso inflamatorio.

marijuana, marihuana n. mariguana. Cannabis sativa.

mark n. marca, seña, señal, signo; v. marcar; señalar.

marker n. marcador, indicador.

married a. casado-a; __ **couple** / matrimonio; __ **life** / vida conyugal, vida matrimonial.

marrow n. médula, tejido esponjoso que ocupa las cavidades medulares de los huesos; pop. tuétano; __ **aspiration** / aspiración de la __; __ **cellularity** / celularidad medular; __ **failure** / insuficiencia medular; __ **infiltration** / infiltración medular; __ **injury** / lesión medular; __ **puncture** / punción de la __ ósea; __ **transplant** / trasplante de la __.

marsupialization n. marsupialización, conversión de una cavidad cerrada a una forma de bolsa abierta.

masculation n. masculación, desarrollo de características masculinas.

masculine a. masculino-a, viril.

masculinization n. masculinización. **virilización**.

mask n. máscara. 1. cubierta de la cara; 2. aspecto de la cara, esp. como manifestación patológica; **death** __ / mascarilla; **pregnancy** __ / manchas en la cara durante el embarazo; **surgical** __ / cubreboca.

masked a. enmascarado-a; oculto-a.

masochism n. masoquismo, condición anormal de placer sexual por abuso infligido a otros o a sí mismo-a.

mass n. masa, cuerpo formado por partículas coherentes.

massage n. masaje, proceso de manipulación del cuerpo por medio de fricciones; **cardiac** __ / __ cardíaco de resucitación; v. dar masaje, sobar.

masseter n. músculo masetero, músculo principal de la masticación.

massive a. maciso-a, abultado-a.

mastadenitis n. mastadenitis, infl. de una glándula mamaria. Syn. **mastitis**.

mastadenoma n. mastadenoma, tumor de la mama, tumor del seno.

mast cell tumor n. mastocitoma, tumor compuesto de mastocitos.

mastectomy n. mastectomía. V. mammectomy.

masticate v. masticar, mascar.

mastication, chewing n. masticación.

mastitis n. mastitis **chronic cystic** __ / __ cística crónica; **glandular** __ / __ glandular; **granulomatous** __ / __ granulomatosa; **lacteal** __ / __ lacteal; **neonatorum** __ / __ del neonato; **puerperal** __ / __ puerperal; **suppurative** __ / __ supurativa.

mastitis, cystic n. mastitis cística, enfermedad fibroquística de la mama.

mastocytoma n. mastocitoma, acumulación de mastocitos con apariencia de un neoplasma.

mastocytosis n. mastocitosis, mastocitos neoplásicos que aparecen en varios tejidos como urticaria pigmentosa.

mastoid n. mastoides, apófisis del hueso temporal; a. 1. mastoideo-a, rel. a la mastoides o que ocurre en la región del proceso mastoideo; 2. semejante a una mama.

mastoid antrum n. antro mastoideo, cavidad que sirve de comunicación entre el hueso temporal, el oído medio y las células mastoideas.

mastoid cells n., pl. células mastoideas, bolsas de aire en la prominencia mastoidea del hueso temporal.

mastoiditis n. mastoiditis, infl. de las células mastoideas.

mastopexy n. mastopexia, corrección plástica del seno pendular.

masturbation n. masturbación, autoestimulación y manipulación de los genitales para obtener placer sexual.

matching n., a. semejante, igual; __ **pair** / compañero-a, pareja.

material n. materia; asunto; a. material; esencial.

maternal

maternal *a.* maternal, materno-a, rel. a la madre; __ **fetal exchange** / intercambio maternofetal; __ **welfare** / bienestar materno.
maternity *n.* maternidad; __ **hospital** / hospital de __.
mating *n.* emparejamiento de sexos opuestos esp. para la reproducción.
matrilineal *a.* de línea materna, descendiente de la madre.
matter *n.* materia, sustancia; asunto; **as a __ of fact** / en realidad; **gray __** / __ gris; **Let's take care of this __** / Vamos a hacernos cargo de este asunto; **What is the __ ?** / ¿Qué pasa?, ¿qué ocurre?
mature *a.* [*fruit*] maduro-a; sazonado-a.
maturity *n.* madurez; etapa de desarrollo completo.
maxilla *n.* maxila, hueso del maxilar superior.
may *v. aux.* poder, [*possibility*]; **it __ be** / puede ser; [*permission*] __ **I see you?** / ¿Puedo verlo-a?, ¿puedo verte?; __ **I come in?** / ¿Puedo entrar?
maze *n.* laberinto.
mean *n.* media, ídice, término medio; __ **corpuscular hemoglobin** / índice corpuscular de hemoglobina *a.* malo-a, desconsiderado-a, de mal humor.
meaning *n.* significado.
measles *n.* sarampión; *pop. Mex.* tapetillo de los niños, enfermedad sumamente contagiosa esp. en niños de edad escolar causada por el virus de la rubéola.
measles immune serum globulin *n.* suero de globulina preventivo contra el sarampión, se inyecta en uno de los cinco días siguientes a la exposición al contagio.
measles virus vaccine, live *n.* vacuna antisarampión de virus vivo, de uso en la inmunización contra el sarampión.
measure *n.* medida, dimensión, capacidad de algo; *v.* medir.
meatal *a.* meatal, concerniente al meato.
meatus *n.* meato, pasaje, abertura, apertura.
mechanical *a.* mecánico-a.
mechanism *n.* mecanismo. 1. respuesta involuntaria a un estímulo; **defense __** / __ de defensa; **implementation __** / __ de ejecución; **pain __** / __ del dolor; **escape __** / __ de escape; 2. estructura semejante a una máquina.

meconium *n.* meconio, primera fecalización del recién nacido.
medial *a.* medial, localizado-a hacia la línea media.
median *n.* mediana; __ **plane** / plano medio.
mediastinal *a.* mediastínico-a, rel. al mediastino.
mediastinitis *n.* mediastinitis, infl. del tejido del mediastino.
mediastinoscopy *n.* mediastinoscopía, examen del mediastino por medio de un endoscopio.
mediastinum *n.* mediastino. 1. cavidad entre dos órganos; 2. masa de tejidos y órganos que separa los pulmones.
mediator *a.* mediador-a; intercesor-a.
medic *n.* técnico-a entrenado para dar primeros auxilios.
Medicaid *n.* Asistencia Médica, programa del gobierno de los Estados Unidos que provee asistencia médica a los pobres.
medical *n.* médico-a; medicinal, curativo-a; __ **assistance** / asistencia __; __ **examiner** / médico forense; __ **history** / historia clínica; __ **records** / registros __ -s; [*patient's record*] expediente del paciente; __ **staff** / cuerpo médico; __ **student** / estudiante de medicina.
medical record *n.* expediente médico.
medical record linkage *n.* conexión del expediente médico. 1. cualquier información que conecte al paciente con su expediente médico; 2. colección de datos de la historia clínica de un paciente proporcionada por varias fuentes; 3. cualquier dato referente a un paciente participante en un estudio clínico que pueda revelar su identidad como sujeto participante.
medical waste *n.* deshechos de efectos médicos.
Medicare *n.* Programa de asistencia médica del gobierno de los Estados Unidos a personas desde los 65 años de edad o a adultos incapacitados para trabajar.
medicate *v.* recetar, medicinar.
medication *n.* medicina, medicamento; *pop.* remedio.
medicinal *a.* medicinal, rel. a la medicina, o con propiedades curativas.

membrane

medicine *n.* medicina. 1. ciencia que se dedica al mantenimiento de la salud por medio de tratamieno de curación y prevención de enfermedades; **alternative__** / __ alternativa; **aerospace __** / __ del espacio; **Chinese herbal __** / fitoterapia de medicina china; **clinical __** / __ clínica; **community __** / __ comunal, al servicio de la comunidad; **environmental __** / __ ecológica; **forensic __** / __ forense; **holistic medicine __** / __ psicosomática; **integrative __** / __ integrativa; **legal __** / __ legal; **chest** / botiquín; **nuclear __** / __ nuclear; **preventive __** / __ preventiva; **socialized __** / __ socializada; **sports __** / __ deportiva; **tropical __** / __ tropical; **veterinary __** / __ veterinaria; 2. una droga o medicamento.

medicine man *n.* curandero.

medicolegal *a.* médicolegal, rel. a la medicina en relación con las leyes.

mediolateral *a.* mediolateral, rel. a la parte media y a un lado del cuerpo.

medium *n.* (*pl.* media) medio. 1. intermediario-a, elemento mediante el cual se obtiene un resultado; 2. sustancia que transmite impulsos; 3. sustancia que se usa en un cultivo de bacterias.

medulla *n.* médula, *pop.* tuétano, parte interna o central de un órgano; **__ oblongata** / __ oblongata, bulbo raquídeo, porción de la médula localizada en la base del cráneo; **__ ossium, bone marrow** / __ ósea; **bone marrow failure** / fallo de la __ ósea.

medullar, medullary *a.* medular, rel. a la médula.

medulloblastoma *n.* medulloblastoma, neoplasma maligno localizado en el cuarto ventrículo y en el cerebelo, que puede invadir las meninges.

meet *n.* reunión; concurso; *vi.* encontrar; reunirse con; **I am glad to __ you** / Mucho gusto en conocerlo-a.

meeting *n.* reunión, junta. 1. partes que se unen, tales como las partes de un hueso a las márgenes de una herida; 2. reunión de un grupo de personas.

megabladder, megalocystis *n.* megalocisto, vejiga distendida.

megacephalic *a.* megacefálico-a. V. **macrocephalia.**

megacolon *n.* megacolon, colon anormalmente agrandado.

megadose *n.* megadosis, una dosis de una sustancia nutritiva que supera exageradamente la cantidad diaria recomendada.

megaesophagus *n.* megaesófago, dilatación anormal de la parte inferior del esófago.

megalomania *n.* megalomanía, delirio de grandeza.

megalophobia *n.* megalofobia, miedo a los objetos grandes.

megavitamin *n.* megavitamina, dosis de vitamina en exceso de la cantidad normal requerida diariamente.

megavitamin therapy *n.* terapia de megavitaminas, teoria que propulsa la toma de gran dosis de vitaminas como prevención de múltiples trastornos de la salud.

meibomian cyst *n.* quiste meibomiano, quiste del párpado.

meiosis *n.* meiosis, proceso de subdivisión celular que resulta en la formación de gametos.

melancholia *n.* melancolía, depresión acentuada.

melanin *n.* melanina, pigmento oscuro de la piel, el pelo y partes del ojo.

melanocyte *n.* melanocito, célula que produce melanina.

melanoma *n.* melanoma, tumor maligno compuesto de melanocitos que puede originarse en diferentes partes de la piel y tiende a hacer metástasis rapidamente en la linfa, pulmón y cerebro.

melanosis *a.* melanosis, condición que se caracteriza por la pigmentación oscura presente en varios tejidos y órganos.

melanuria *n.* melanuria, presencia de pigmentación oscura en la orina.

melena *n.* melena, masa de heces fecales negruscas y pastosas que contiene sangre digerida.

member *n.* miembro. 1. órgano o parte del cuerpo; 2. socio-a de una organización.

membrane *n.* membrana, capa fina que sirve de cubierta o protección a una cavidad, estructura u órgano; **elastic __** / __ elástica; **mucous __** / __ mucosa; **nuclear __** / __ nuclear; **permeable __** / __ permeable; **placental __** / __ de la placenta; **semipermeable __** / __

memorize

semipermeable; **synovial** __ / __ sinovial; **tympanic** __ / __ timpánica.

memorize *v.* memorizar, aprender de memoria.

memory *n.* memoria, retentiva, facultad de la mente para registrar y recordar experiencias; **bad** __ / mala __; **good** __ / buena __; **short-term** __ / __ inmediata; **visual** __ / __ visual; *v.* **Do you have a good** __ ? / ¿Tiene, tienes buena __ ?; **to have memories from** / tener recuerdos de; __ **loss** / pérdida de la __.

menace *n.* amenaza; *v.* amenazar, atemorizar.

menarche *n.* menarca, inicio de la menstruación.

mendelism *n.* mendelismo, principios que explican la trasmisión genética de ciertos rasgos.

meningeal *a.* meníngeo-a, rel. a las meninges.

meninges *n., pl.* meninges, las tres capas de tejido conjuntivo que rodean al cerebro y a la médula espinal.

meningism *n.* meningismo, irritación congestiva de las meninges gen. de naturaleza tóxica con síntomas similares a los de la meningitis pero sin inflamación.

meningitis *n.* meningitis, infl. de las meninges cerebrales o espinales; **cryptococcal** __ / __ criptocócica; **viral** __ / __ viral.

meningocele *n.* meningocele, protrusión de las meninges a través del cráneo o de la espina dorsal.

meningococcus *n.* meningococo, uno de los microorganismos causantes de la meningitis cerebral epidémica.

meningoencephalitis *n.* meningoencefalitis, cerebromeningitis, infl. del encéfalo y de las meninges.

meniscectomy *n.* meniscectomía, extirpación de un menisco.

meniscus *n.* (*pl.* **menisci**) menisco, estructura cartilaginosa de forma lunar.

menometrorrhagia *n.* menometrorragia, sangrado anormal entre menstruaciones.

menopause *n.* menopausia, cambio de vida en la mujer adulta, terminación de la etapa de reproducción y disminución de la producción hormonal.

menorrhagia *n.* menorragia, períodos o reglas muy abundantes.

menorrhalgia *n.* menorralgia, menstruación dolorosa.

menorrhea *n.* menorrea, flujo menstrual normal.

menses *n.* menses, menstruo, menstruación, período, regla.

menstrual *a.* menstrual, rel. a la menstruación; __ **cycle** / ciclo __; __ **disorder** / trastorno __.

menstruation *n.* menstruación, flujo sanguíneo periódico de la mujer.

mental *a.* mental, rel. a la mente; __ **age** / edad __; __ **disorder** / trastorno __; __ **deficiency** / retraso __; __**handicap** / minusvalía __; __ **health** / salud __; __ **hygiene** / higiene __; __ **illness** / enfermedad __; __ **retardation** / retraso __; __ **test** / examen de capacidad __.

mentality *n.* mentalidad, capacidad mental.

menthol *n.* mentol, sustancia que se obtiene del alcanfor de menta y que tiene efecto sedante.

mentum *n.* mentón, barbilla, prominencia de la barba.

meralgia *n.* meralgia, dolor en el pie que puede extenderse hasta el muslo; __ **paresthetic** / __ parestética.

mercurial *a.* mercurial, perteneciente o rel. al mercurio.

mercurochrome *n.* mercurocromo, nombre registrado de la merbromina.

mercury *n.* mercurio, metal líquido volátil; __ **poisoning** / envenenamiento por __.

mercy *n.* misericordia, compasión; __ **killing** / eutanasia.

meridian *n.* meridiano, línea imaginaria que conecta los extremos opuestos del axis en la superficie de un cuerpo esférico.

mescaline *n.* mescalina, alcaloide alucinogénico, *pop.* peyote.

mesectoderm *n.* mesectodermo, masa de células que componen las meninges.

mesencephalon *n.* mesencéfalo, el cerebro medio en la etapa embrionaria.

mesenchyme *n.* mesénquima, red de células embrionarias que forman el tejido conjuntivo y los vasos sanguíneos y linfáticos en el adulto.

mesentery *n.* mesenterio, repliegue del peritoneo que fija el intestino a la pared abdominal posterior.

mesmerism *n.* mesmerismo, uso del hipnotismo como método terapéutico.

mesocardia *n.* mesocardia, desplazamiento anormal del corazón hacia el centro del tórax.

mesocolon *n.* mesocolon, mesenterio que fija el colon a la pared abdominal posterior.

mesoderm *n.* mesodermo, capa media germinativa del embrión situada entre el ectodermo y endodermo de la cual provienen el tejido óseo, el muscular, los vasos sanguíneos y linfáticos, y las membranas del corazón y abdomen.

mesothelium *n.* mesotelio, capa celular del mesodermo embrionario que forma el epitelio que cubre las membranas serosas en el adulto.

metabolic *a.* metabólico-a, rel. al metabolismo; **___ rate** / índice **___**.

metabolism *n.* metabolismo, suma de los cambios fisicoquímicos que tienen efecto a continuación del proceso digestivo; **constructive ___** / anabolismo, asimilación; **destructive ___** / **___** destructivo, catabolismo; **basal ___** / **___** basal, el nivel más bajo del gasto de energía; **protein ___** / **___** de proteínas, digestión de proteínas y conversión de éstas en aminoácidos.

metabolite *n.* metabolito, sustancia producida durante el proceso metabólico.

metacarpal *a.* metacarpiano-a, rel. al metacarpio.

metacarpus *n.* metacarpo, la parte formada por los cinco huesecillos metacarpianos de la mano.

metachronous *a.* metacrono, que tiene efecto en tiempos diferentes.

metal *n.* metal; **___ fume fever** / fiebre por aspiración de vapores metálicos

metamorphosis *n.* metamorfosis. 1. cambio de forma o estructura; 2. cambio degenerativo patológico.

metanephrine *n.* metanefrina, catabolito de epinefrina que se encuentra en la orina.

metaphase *n.* metafase, una de las etapas de la división celular.

metaphysis *n.* metáfisis, zona de crecimiento del hueso.

metastasis *n.* metástasis, extensión de un proceso patológico de un foco primario a otra parte del cuerpo a través de los vasos sanguíneos o linfáticos como se observa en algunos tipos de cáncer.

metastasize *v.* metastatizar, esparcirse por metástasis.

metatarsial *n.* metatarsiano-a, rel. al metatarso.

metatarsophalangeal joints *n.* articulación o coyuntura del metatarso y los dedos de los pies.

metatarsus *n.* metatarso, la parte formada por los cinco huesecillos del pie situados entre el tarso y los dedos.

meteorism *n.* meteorismo, abdomen distendido causado por acumulación de gas en el estómago o los intestinos.

methadone *n.* metadona, droga sintética potente de acción narcótica menos intensa que la morfina.

methanol, wood alcohol *n.* metanol, alcohol de madera.

method *n.* método, procedimiento; proceso; tratamiento.

methylene blue *n.* azul de metileno.

methylmercury *n.* mercurio de metileno, sustancia orgánica de mercurio abundante en algunos peces de efecto tóxico en mujeres embarazadas y sobre todo a los niños.

metric *a.* métrico-a; **___ system** / sistema **___**.

metritis *n.* metritis, infl. de la pared uterina.

metroflebitis *n.* metroflebitis, infl. de las venas uterinas.

micrencephaly *n.* micrencefalia, cerebro anormalmente pequeño.

microabscess *n.* microabsceso, absceso diminuto.

microanalysis *n.* microanálisis, análisis químico de ínfimas partículas.

microanatomy *n.* microanatomía, histología.

microbe *n.* microbio, microorganismo, organismo diminuto.

microbial, microbian *a.* microbiano-a, rel. a los microbios.

microbiology *n.* microbiología, ciencia que estudia los microorganismos.

microcephaly *n.* microcefalia, cabeza anormalmente pequeña de origen congénito.

microcheiria *n.* microquiria, trastorno en el cual las manos son de un tamaño más pequeño que lo normal.

microcosmus *n.* microcosmo. 1. universo en miniatura; 2. cualquier entidad o estructura considerada en sí misma un pequeño universo.

microdrip *n.* microgotero, instrumento para administrar una cantidad precisa pequeña de una sustancia por medio intravenoso.

microfilm *n.* microfilm, microfilme, película que contiene información reducida a un tamaño mínimo.

microgenitalia

microgenitalia *n.* microgenitalia, escaso desarrollo de los genitales externos.

microglia cells *n.* células de microglia, pequeñas células intersticiales migratorias que pertenecen al sistema nervioso.

micrognathia *n.* micrognatia, mandíbula inferior anormalmente pequeña.

microinvasion *n.* microinvasión, invasión de tejido celular adyacente a un carcinoma localizado que no puede verse a simple vista.

microlithiasis *n.* microlitiasis, pequeñas concreciones excretadas en ciertos órganos.

micromelia *n.* micromelia, extremidades anormalmente pequeñas.

micromelic *a.* micromélico-a, rel. a la micromelia.

micrometer *n.* micrómetro, instrumento para medir distancias cortas.

microorganism *n.* microorganismo, organismo que no puede verse a simple vista.

microphallus *n.* microfalo, pene anormalmente pequeño.

microscope *n.* microscopio, instrumento óptico con lentes que amplifican objetos que no pueden verse a simple vista; **electron** __ / __ electrónico; **light** __ / __ con luz o lumínico.

microscopic *a.* microscópico-a, rel. al microscopio.

microscopy *n.* microscopía, examen que se realiza con un microscopio.

microsomia *n.* microsomia, cuerpo anormalmente pequeño de proporciones normales.

microsurgery *n.* microcirugía, operación efectuada con el uso de microscopios quirúrgicos e instrumentos minúsculos de precisión.

microtome *n.* micrótomo, instrumento de precisión que se usa en la preparación de secciones finas de tejido para ser examinadas bajo el microscopio.

microtomy *n.* microtomía, corte de secciones finas de tejido.

miction *n.* emisión de orina.

middle *n.* medio, centro; **in the __ of** / en el __ de.

middle age *n.* mediana edad, madurez.

middle ear *n.* oído medio, parte del oído situada más allá del tímpano.

middle finger *n.* el dedo cordial.

middle lobe syndrome *n.* síndrome del lóbulo medio del pulmón.

midget *n.* enano-a.

midgut *n.* intestino medio del embrión.

midline *n.* línea media del cuerpo.

midnight *n.* medianoche.

midplane *n.* plano medio.

midsection *n.* sección media.

midstream specimen *n.* especimen de orina que se toma después de comenzar la emisión y poco antes de terminarse.

midwife *n.* comadrona, partera, mujer que se especializa en el cuidado y atención de la salud de mujeres durante el embarazo, el parto y el postpartum.

midyear *n.* mediados de año.

migraine *n.* migraña, jaqueca, ataques severos de dolor de cabeza que gen. se manifiestan en un solo lado acompañados de visión alterada y en algunos casos de náuseas y vómitos.

migrans thrombophlebitis *n.* tromboflebitis migratoria, tromboflebitis de progreso lento de una vena a otra.

migration *n.* migración, movimiento de las células de un lugar a otro.

migratory cell *n.* célula migratoria, célula que tiene locomoción.

migratory pneumonia *n.* neumonía migratoria, tipo de neumonía que aparece en diferentes partes del pulmón.

mild *a.* [pain] leve, tolerable; moderado-a, indulgente.

mildew *n.* moho.

milia neonatorum *n.* milia neonatorum, pequeños quistes no patógenos vistos a veces en los recién nacidos.

miliary *a.* miliar, caracterizado-a por pequeños tumores o nódulos.

miliary tuberculosis *n.* tuberculosis miliar, enfermedad que invade el organismo a través de la sangre y se caracteriza por la formación de tubérculos diminutos en los órganos afectados.

milieu *n.* medio ambiente.

milk *n.* leche; **boiled __ / __** hervida; **clotted __ / __** cuajada; **condensed __ / __** condensada; **dry __ / __** en polvo; **evaporated __ / __** evaporada;

__ albumina / lactoalbúmina; __ ascites / ascites seudoquilosa; __ of magnesia / __ de magnesia / mother's __ / leche materna; skim __ / __ desnatada; sterilized __ / __ esterilizada.

milk leg *n.* flegmasia cerúlea dolorosa, trombosis de una de las venas de la pierna (gen. femoral) que manifiesta dolor agudo, infl., sianosis y edema, que puede producir un problema circulatorio severo.

mimetic, mimic *a.* mimético-a, que imita.

mind *n.* mente, entendimiento; __ -body medicine / medicina psicosomática; *v.* atender, tener en cuenta; to bear in __ / tener presente; to be out of one's __ / volverse loco-a; to make up one's __ / decidirse; to speak one's __ / dar una opinión; dar su parecer.

mineral *n.* mineral, elemento inorgánico; *a.* mineral; __ water (carbonated) / agua __ efervescente.

mineralization *n.* mineralización, depósitos de minerales en los tejidos.

mineralocorticoid *n.* mineralocorticoide, tipo de hormona liberada por la glándula suprarrenal que participa en la regulación del volumen de la sangre.

minilaparotomy *n.* minilaparotomía, un tipo de intervención pélvica para uso de diagnóstico o con el propósito de esterilización por medio de ligación de las trompas.

minimal *a. comp.* mínimo-a, más pequeño-a.

minimal dose *n.* dosis mínima, la menor dosis necesaria para producir un efecto determinado.

minimal lethal dose *n.* dosis letal mínima, la menor dosis de una sustancia que puede ocasionar la muerte.

minimize *v.* aliviar, atenuar, mitigar; reducir al mínimo; This pill is to __ the pain / Esta pastilla es para __ el dolor.

minor *n.* [*in age*] menor de edad; *a.* [*smaller, youngest*] menor, más pequeño; a __ problem / un problema sin importancia; __ burn / quemadura leve; __ surgery / cirugía menor.

minority *n.* minoría, minoridad.

minute *n.* [*time*] minuto, momento; *a.* menudo-a, mínimo-a, diminuto-a.

miosis *n.* miosis, contracción excesiva de la pupila.

miraculous *a.* milagroso-a, prodigioso-a.

misbehavior *n.* mala conducta, mal comportamiento.

miscalculate *v.* hacer un error o falta; equivocarse.

miscarriage *n.* aborto, malparto, expulsión del feto por vía natural.

miscegenation *n.* mestizaje, cruzamiento de razas o de culturas.

miscible *a.* capaz de mezclarse o disolverse.

misdiagnosis *n.* diagnóstico equivocado o erróneo.

misery *n.* sufrimiento, pena; desesperación; miseria.

misguide *v.* dirigir mal, aconsejar mal.

misguided *a.* mal aconsejado-a, mal dirigido-a.

misogamy *n.* misogamia, aversión al matrimonio.

misogyny *n.* misoginia, aversión a las mujeres.

miss *n.* señorita, jovencita; *v.* [*to fail, to overlook*] perder; to __ an appointment / perder el turno; [sentiment] to __ one's family / echar de menos a la familia; [to skip] to __ a period / faltar la regla, faltar el período.

misshaped, misshapen *a.* deforme, desfigurado-a.

missing *a.* desaparecido-a; extraviado-a.

mission *n.* misión; destino.

mistake *n.* error, equivocación, desacierto, falta; *vi.* equivocar, entender mal, confundir; *vr.* equivocarse, confundirse.

mistyping of blood *n.* error the emparejamiento de sangre; blood transfusion __ / error de emparejamiento en una transfusión sanguínea; *pop.* error de "tipaje".

mitigated *a.* mitigado-a, aliviado-a, calmado-a; disminuido-a.

mitochondria *n.* mitocondria, filamentos microscópicos del citoplasma que constituyen la fuente principal de energía de la célula.

mitogen *n.* mitógeno, sustancia que induce mitosis celular.

mitogenesis, mitogenia *n.* mitogénesis, causa de la mitosis celular.

mitosis *n.* mitosis, división celular que da lugar a nuevas células y reemplaza tejidos lesionados.

mitral

mitral *a.* mitral, rel. a la válvula mitral o
bicúspide **___ disease** / enfermedad de
la válvula **___** del corazón; **___**
incompetence / insuficiencia **___**; **___**
murmur / soplo; **___ orifice** / orificio
___; **___ valve insuficiency** /
insuficiencia de la válvula **___**; **___**
valve prolapse / prolapso de la válvula
___ , cierre defectuoso de la válvula **___**.

mitral regurgitation *n.*
regurgitación mitral, flujo sanguíneo
retrógrado del ventrículo izquierdo a la
aurícula izquierda causado por lesión
de la válvula mitral.

mitral stenosis *n.* estenosis mitral,
estrechez del orificio izquierdo
aurículo-ventricular.

mitral valve *n.* válvula mitral, válvula
aurículoventricular izquierda del
corazón.

mittelschmerz *n.* dolor en el vientre
relacionado con la ovulación que
ocurre gen. a mitad del ciclo
menstrual.

mix *v.* mezclar, juntar, asociar.

mixture *n.* mezcla, mixtura; poción.

mnemonics *n.* mnemónica,
adiestramiento de la memoria por
medio de asociación de ideas y otros
recursos.

moan *n.* quejido, gemido, queja,
lamento; *vr.* quejarse, lamentarse.

mobility *n.* movilidad.

mobilization *n.* movilización.

modality *n.* modalidad, cualquier
método de aplicación terapéutica.

mode *n.* 1. moda, manera, valor repetido
con mayor frecuencia en una serie;
2. modo.

model *n.* modelo, patrón, molde.

moderated *a.* moderado-a,
mesurado-a; [*price*] módico, [*weather*]
templado; **___ temperature** /
temperatura **___**.

moderation *n.* moderación, sobriedad.

modern *a.* moderno-a, reciente.

modest *a.* modesto-a, recatado-a.

modification *n.* modificación, cambio.

modulation *n.* modulación, acto de
ajustar o adaptar tal como ocurre en la
inflexión de la voz.

molar *n.* diente molar, muela.

molding *n.* amoldamiento de la cabeza
del feto para adaptarla a la forma y
tamaño del canal del parto.

mole *n.* mancha, lunar.

molecular *a.* molecular, rel. a una
molécula; **___ biology** / biología **___**.

molecule *n.* molécula, unidad mínima
de una sustancia.

molest *v.* dañar físicamente, vejar;
humillar; asaltar.

mollusc, mollusk *n.* (*pl.* **mollusca**)
molusco.

momentum *n.*, *L.* momentum; ímpetu;
fuerza de movimiento.

monarticular *a.* monarticular, que
concierne o afecta a una sola
articulación.

mongoloid *a.* mongoloide, rel. al
mongolismo o que sufre del mismo.

monitor *n.* monitor. 1. instrumento
electrónico usado para monitorear una
función; 2. persona que supervisa una
función o actividad; *v.* monitorear,
chequear sistemáticamente con un
instrumento electrónico una función
orgánica, tal como los latidos del
corazón.

monitoring *n.* monitoreo, acción de
monitorear; **blood pressure ___** / **___**
de la presión arterial; **cardiac ___** / **___**
cardíaco; **fetal ___** / **___** del corazón
fetal.

monochromatic *a.* monocromático-a,
de un solo color.

monoclonal *a.* monoclonal, rel. a un
solo grupo de células; **___ antibodies** /
anticuerpos **___ -es**.

monocular *a.* monocular, rel. a un solo
ojo.

monocyte *n.* monocito, glóbulo blanco
mononuclear granuloso.

monogamy *n.* monogamia, unión
matrimonial legal con una sola persona.

monomania *n.* monomania, trastorno
mental de preocupación por una sola
idea fija.

mononuclear *a.* mononuclear, que
tiene un solo núcleo; **___ cell** /
célula **___**.

mononucleosis *n.* mononucleosis,
presencia de un número anormalmente
elevado de leucocitos mononucleares
en la sangre; **infectious ___** / **___**
infecciosa, infección viral aguda.

monosaccharide *n.* monosacárido,
azúcar simple.

monozygotic twins *n.*, *pl.* gemelos
monocigóticos con características
genéticas idénticas.

monster *n.* monstruo.

mood *n.* humor, disposición, estado de
ánimo; **changeable ___ -s** / cambios de
humor, cambios de disposición; **___**
disorders / cambios de estado de

mucin

ánimo; **to be in a sad** ___ / sentirse triste; **to be in the** ___ **to** / tener ganas de.

moon *n.* luna; **moonlight** / luz de la ___.

moonface *n.* cara de luna, cara llena redonda característica de pacientes sometidos a un tratamiento prolongado de un esteroide.

moonlighter *n.* persona que tiene más de un empleo.

morality *n.* ética, rectitud, moral.

morbid *a.* mórbido, insano-a, morbosa-a, rel. a una enfermedad.

morbidity *n.* morbidez, morbosidad, enfermedad; ___ **rate** / taza de ___, número de casos de cierta enfermedad.

mordacious *a.* mordaz, satírico-a.

more *a.* más; *adv.* más; **more and more** / cada vez ___; **once** / una vez ___; [*before numeral*] ___ **than a hundred** / ___ de cien; [*before a verb*] ___ **than** / más de lo que ___; ___ **than he needs** / más de lo que necesita.

morgue *n.*, *Fr.* morgue, necrocomio, depósito temporal de cadáveres.

moribund *a.* moribundo-a, cercano-a a la muerte, agonizante.

morning *n.* mañana, madrugada; **early in the** ___ / muy de ___; **Good** ___ / buenos días, buen día; **in the** ___ / por la ___, en la ___; ___ **stiffness** / rigidez matutina muscular y de las articulaciones; **tomorrow** ___ / ___ por la ___.

morning sickness *n.* trastorno matutino de náuseas y vómitos que sufren algunas mujeres en la primera etapa del embarazo.

moron *n.* morón-a, persona con retraso mental de un cociente intelectual de 50 a 70.

morphine *n.* morfina, alcaloide que se obtiene del opio y se usa como analgésico y sedante.

morphinism *n.* morfinismo, condición morbosa ocasionada por la adicción a la morfina.

mortal *a.* mortal, mortífero-a, fatal, letal.

mortality *n.* mortalidad, mortandad. 1. estado de ser mortal; 2. índice de mortalidad.

mórula *n.* mórula, masa esférica y sólida de células que resulta de la división celular del óvulo fecundado.

mosaic *n.* mosaico, la presencia en una persona de distintos tejidos adyacentes derivados de la misma célula como resultado de mutaciones.

mosaicism *n.* mosaicismo, así como en un mosaico, los cromosomas son genéticamente mutadores diferentes que pueden establecer características distintas en humanos, tal como se muestra en la fisonomía por diferencias de sexo.

mosquito *n.* mosquito.

mother *n.* madre, mamá.

motherhood *n.* maternidad.

mother-in-law *n.* suegra.

motility *n.* movilidad.

motion *n.* movimiento; [*sign*] seña, indicación; moción; ___ **sickness** / mareo producido por movimiento.

motionless *a.* sin movimiento, inmóvil.

motivation *n.* motivación, estimulación externa.

motor *n.* motor, agente que produce o induce movimiento; *a.* motor-a, que causa movimiento.

motor development *n.* desarrollo motor.

motor neuron *n.* neurona motora, células nerviosas que conducen impulsos que inician las contracciones musculares.

mouth *n.* boca. 1. cavidad bucal; 2. abertura de cualquier cavidad; **by** ___ / por vía bucal.

mouth breathing *n.* respiración de boca a boca, método de ventilación artificial inducido por el asistente para restaurar la respiración de la víctima. Se inflan los pulmones acompasadamente seguido por repetidas fases expiratorias deteniéndose al oír que el pecho se expande al exhalar el aire.

move *n.* movimiento; paso; *v.* mover; mudar; ___ **your fingers** / Mueva, mueve los dedos; ___ **your hand** / Mueva, mueve la mano; **to** ___ **about,** **to** ___ **around** / caminar, andar, ir; **to** ___ **down** / bajar.

movement *n.* movimiento, moción, acción, maniobra; [*of the intestines*] evacuación, defecación.

much *a.* mucho-a; abundante; *adv.* excesivamente, demasiado, en gran cantidad; **as** ___ **as** / tanto como; **How** ___? / ¿Cuánto?; **not as** ___ **as before** / no tanto como antes; **How** ___ **does it hurt?** / ¿Cuánto le duele?; **too** ___ / en exceso, demasiado.

mucin *n.* mucina, glucoproteína, ingrediente esencial del mucus.

403

mucocele

mucocele *n.* mucocele, dilatación de una cavidad ósea debida a una acumulación de secreción mucosa.

mucoid *n.* mucoide, glucoproteína similar a la mucina; *a.* de consistencia mucosa.

mucomembranous *a.* mucomembranoso-a, rel. a la membrana mucosa.

mucosa *n.* mucosa, membrana mucosa. **alveolar** ___ / ___ alveolar; **bronchial** ___ / ___ bronquial; **esophageal** ___ / ___ esofágica; **gastric** ___ / ___ gástrica; **laryngeal** ___ / ___ laríngea; **lingual** ___ / ___ lingual; ___ **of colon** / ___ del colon; ___ **of mouth** / ___ de la boca or bucal; ___ **of nose** / ___ nasal o de la nariz; ___ **of pharynx** / ___ de la nariz; ___ **of renal pelvis** / ___ de la pelvis renal; ___ **of small intestine** / ___ del intestino delgado; ___ **of stomach** / ___ del estómago or estomacal; ___ **of (urinary) bladder** / ___ de la vejiga urinaria; **nasal** ___ / ___ nasal; **olfactory** ___ / ___ olfatoria; **pharyngeal** ___ / ___ faríngea; **vaginal** ___ / ___ de la vagina.

mucosal *a.* mucosal, rel. a cualquier membrana mucosa.

mucosity *n.* mucosidad.

mucous membrane *n.* membrana mucosa, láminas finas de tejido celular que cubren aberturas o canales que comunican con el exterior.

mucus *n.* moco, mucosidad, sustancia viscosa segregada por las membranas y glándulas mucosas.

multicellular *a.* multicelular, que consiste de muchas células.

multifocal *a.* multifocal, rel. a más de un foco.

multiparity *n.* multiparidad.
1. condición de una mujer que ha tenido más de un parto logrado;
2. parto múltiple.

multiparous *n.* multípara, mujer que ha parido más de una vez.

multiple *a.* múltiple, más de uno; ___ **family therapy** / terapia familiar ___; ___ **organ failure** / fallo ___ de órganos; ___ **personality disorder** / trastorno de personalidad ___.

multiple sclerosis *n.* esclerosis múltiple, enfermedad progresiva lenta del sistema nervioso central causada por pérdida de la capa de mielina que cubre las fibras nerviosas del cerebro y de la médula espinal.

mummification *n.* momificación, conversión a un estado similar al de una momia tal como en la gangrena seca o en el estado de un feto que muere y permanece en la matriz.

mumps *n.* paperas, parotiditis, enfermedad febril aguda de alta contagiosidad que se caracteriza por la infl. de las glándulas parótidas y otras glándulas salivales.

mural *a.* mural, rel. a las paredes de un órgano o parte.

murmur *n.* soplo, ruido; sonido breve raspante, esp. un sonido anormal del corazón; **aortic regurgitation** ___ / ___ regurgitación aórtica; **bronchial** ___ / ___ bronquial; **cardiac** ___ / ___ cardíaco; **continious** ___ / ___ continuo; **crescendo** ___ / ___ crescendo; **diastolic** ___ / ___ diastólico; **endocrdial** ___ / ___ endocardial; a **exocardial** ___ / ___ exocardial; **functional** ___ / ___ funcional; **mitral** ___ / ___ mitral; **pansystolic** ___ / ___ pansistólico; **systolic** ___ / ___ sistólico.

muscle *n.* músculo, tipo de tejido fibroso capaz de contraerse y que permite el movimiento de las partes y los órganos del cuerpo; **cardiac** ___ / ___ cardíaco; **flexor** ___ / ___ flexor; **involuntary, visceral** ___ / involuntario, visceral; **loss of** ___ **tone** / pérdida de la tonicidad muscular; ___ **building** / desarrollo muscular; ___ **relaxants** / relajadores musculares, medicamentos para aliviar espasmos musculares; ___ **strain** / distensión muscular; ___ **toning** / tonicidad muscular; **striated, voluntary** ___ / ___ estriado, voluntario.

muscular *a.* muscular, musculoso-a, rel. al músculo; ___ **atrophy** / atrofia ___; ___ **contractions** / contracciones ___ -es; ___ **dystrophy** / distrofia ___; ___ **rigidity** / rigidez ___.

muscularis *n.* muscularis, capa muscular de un órgano.

musculature *n.* musculatura; aparato muscular del cuerpo.

musculoskeletal *a.* musculoesquelético-a, rel. a los músculos y el esqueleto.

musculotendinous *a.* musculotendinoso-a, que está formado por músculo y tendón.

mushroom *n.* hongo, seta, champiñón; __ **poisoning** / envenenamiento por __ -s.

mutagen *n.* mutágeno, sustancia o agente que causa mutación.

mutant *a.* mutante, rel. a un organismo que ha pasado por mutaciones.

mutation *n.* mutación, alteración, cambios espontáneos o inducidos en la estructura genética.

mute *n.* mudo-a.

mutilation *n.* mutilación.

mutism *n.* mutismo, mudez.

myalgia *n.* mialgia, dolor muscular.

myasis *n.* miiasis, cualquier infección causada por la larva de insectos dípteros que infecta una cavidad cualquiera del organismo.

myasthenia *n.* miastenia, debilidad muscular; __ **gravis** / __ grave.

myatonia *n.* miatonía, deficiencia o pérdida del tono muscular.

mycetoma *n.* micetoma, infección causada por hongos parásitos que afectan a la piel, al tejido conjuntivo y a los huesos.

mycobacterium *n.*, *L.* *Mycobacterium*, especie de bacterias gram-positivas en forma de bastoncillo que incluyen las causantes de la lepra y la tuberculosis.

mycology *n.* micología, estudio de hongos y de las enfermedades que ellos producen.

mycoplasmas *n.*, *pl.* microplasmas, la más diminuta forma de organismos vivos libres a la cual pertenecen los virus que causan enfermedades como la pulmonía y la faringitis.

mycosis *n.* micosis, cualquier enfermedad causada por hongos; __ **fungoide** / __ fungosa.

mycotoxicosis *n.* micotoxicosis, condición sistémica tóxica causada por toxinas creadas por hongos.

mydriasis *n.* midriasis, dilatación prolongada de la pupila del ojo.

mydriatic *a.* midriático-a, que causa dilatación de la pupila del ojo.

myectomy *n.* miectomía, extirpación de una porción de un músculo.

myelatelia *n.* mielatelia, defecto en el desarrollo de la espina dorsal.

myelauxe *n.* mielauxa, hipertrofia de la espina dorsal.

myelin *n.* mielina, sustancia de tipo grasoso que cubre las fibras nerviosas.

myelination, myelinization *n.* mielinización, crecimiento de mielina alrededor de una fibra nerviosa.

myelinolysis *n.* mielinólisis, enfermedad que destruye la mielina alrededor de ciertas fibras nerviosas; **acute** __ / __ aguda; __ **transverse** / __ transversa.

myelitis *n.* mielitis, infl. de la espina dorsal.

myeloblast *n.* mieloblasto, una célula no madura en la serie granulocítica, generalmente presente en la médula ósea.

myeloblastemia *n.* mieloblastemia, la presencia de mieloblastos en la sangre.

myelocele *n.* mielocele, hernia de la médula espinal a través de la columna vertebral.

myelocyst *n.* mieloquiste, un quiste compuesto de células nerviosas que se desarrolla en un canal del sistema nervioso central.

myelocyte *n.* mielocito, leucocito granular de la médula ósea presente en la sangre en ciertas enfermedades.

myelocytoma *n.* mielocitoma, una acumulación de mielocitos en ciertos tejidos, presente en ciertas enfermedades.

myelodysplasia *n.* mielodisplasia, desarrollo anormal de la columna vertebral.

myelofibrosis *n.* mielofibrosis, fibrosis de la médula ósea.

myelogenic, myelogenous *a.* mielógeno-a, que se produce en la médula.

myelogenic sarcoma *n.* sarcoma que se origina en la médula ósea.

myelogram *n.* mielograma, radiografía de la médula usando un medio de contraste.

myelography *n.* mielografía, radiografía de la columna vertebral con inyección de medio de contraste en la región subaracnoidea.

myeloid *n.* mieloide; *a.* rel. a la médula espinal o similar a la médula espinal o a la médula ósea; __ **tissue** / médula roja.

myeloleukemia *n.* mieloleucemia, una forma de leucemia en la cual las células anormales provienen de tejido mielopoyético.

myeloma *n.* mieloma. 1. cualquier tumor de la médula espinal u ósea; 2. tumor formado por el tipo de células que se encuentran en la médula ósea; **multiple __ / __ múltiple.**

myelomeningocele *n.* mielomeningocele, hernia de la médula espinal y de las meninges con protrusión a través de un defecto en el canal vertebral.

myelopathy *n.* mielopatía, cualquier condición patológica de la médula espinal o de la médula ósea.

myeloproliferative *a.* mieloproliferativo-a, que se caracteriza por una proliferación de la médula ósea dentro o fuera de la médula.

myeloschisis *n.* mielosquisis, secuela de espina bífida.

myelosuppression *n.* mielosupresión, producción reducida de eritrocitos y de plaquetas en la médula ósea.

myesthesia *n.* miestesia, sensaciones en un músculo de cualquier tipo.

myocardial, myocardiac *a.* miocárdico-a, rel. al miocardio; **__ contraction** / contracción del miocardio; **__ diseases** / miocardiopatías.

myocardial infarction *n.* infarto cardíaco, necrosis de células del músculo cardíaco debido a un bloqueo del abastecimiento de sangre que lo irriga, condición usu. conocida como "ataque al corazón".

myocardial ischemia *n.* isquemia miocardial, deficiencia de abastecimiento de sangre al corazón debida a un bloqueo de una o más de una de las arterias coronarias.

myocardiography *n.* miocardiografía, trazado de los movimientos del músculo cardíaco.

myocarditis *n.* miocarditis, infl. del miocardio.

myocardium *n.* miocardio, capa media de la pared cardíaca.

myoclonus *n.* mioclonus, contracción o espasmo muscular tal como se manifiesta en la epilepsia.

myocyte *n.* miocito, célula del tejido muscular.

myodystrophy *n.* miodistrofia, distrofia muscular.

myofibril *n.* miofibrilla, fibrilla diminuta delgada del tejido muscular.

myofibroma *n.* miofibroma, tumor compuesto de elementos musculares.

myofilament *n.* miofilamento, filamentos microscópicos que constituyen las fibrillas musculares.

myogenic *a.* miogénico-a, que se origina en un músculo.

myoglobin *n.* mioglobina, pigmento del tejido muscular que participa en la distribución de oxígeno.

myography *n.* miografía, gráfico que registra la actividad muscular.

myolysis *n.* miolisis, destrucción de tejido muscular.

myoma *n.* mioma, tumor benigno compuesto de tejido muscular. **__ previum** / **__** previo.

myomectomy *n.* miomectomía. 1. excisión de una porción de un músculo o de tejido muscular; 2. extirpación de un tumor miomatoso localizado gen. en el útero.

myometrium *n.* miometrio, pared muscular del útero.

myonecrosis *n.* mionecrosis, necrosis del tejido muscular.

myoneural *a.* mioneural, rel. a una terminación nerviosa en un músculo; **__ junction** / unión **__.**

myopathy *n.* miopatía, cualquier enfermedad muscular; **ocular __** / **__** ocular.

myope *n.* miope, persona que tiene miopía.

myopia *n.* miopía, defecto del globo ocular por el cual los rayos de luz hacen foco enfrente de la retina, lo que causa dificultad para ver objetos a distancia.

myopic *a.* miope. 1. que padece de miopía; 2. rel. a la miopía.

myorrhexia *n.* miorexia, desgarro en cualquier músculo.

myosarcoma *n.* miosarcoma, tumor maligno derivado de tejido muscular.

myosin *n.* miosina, la proteína más abundante del tejido muscular.

myositis *n.* miositis, infl. de uno o de más músculos.

myotherapy *n.* mioterapia, método de terapia con ejercicios musculares ejerciendo presión sobre nudos dolorosos y articulaciones para aliviar el dolor.

myotomy *n.* miotomía, sección o disección de un músculo.

myotonia *n.* miotonía, condición muscular con aumento en rigidez y contractibilidad muscular y disminución de relajamiento.

myringectomy, myringodectomy *n.* miringectomía, extirpación de la membrana timpánica o de una parte de ésta.

myringitis *n.* miringitis, infl. del tímpano.

myringoplasty *n.* miringoplastia, cirugía plástica de la membrana del tímpano.

myxedema *n.* mixedema, condición causada por deficiencia funcional de la tiroides.

myxoma *n.* mixoma, tumor compuesto de tejido conjuntivo.

N

N *abbr.* **nasal** / nasal; **nerve** / nervio; **nitrogen** / nitrógeno; **normal** / normal; **number** / número.

Nabothian cysts *n., pl.* quistes de Naboth, quistes pequeños gen. benignos formados por obstrucción de las glándulas secretoras de mucus del cuello uterino.

nail *n.* 1. toe nail. uña de los dedos del pie; finger nail, uña de los dedos de la mano; **ingrown** ___ / uñero, encarnada; ___ **scratch** / arañazo; ___ **biting** / comerse la uñas 2. clavo.

nailbed *n.* matriz de la uña, porción de epidermis que cubre la uña.

naked *a.* desnudo-a, descubierto-a; *pop.* en cuero, en pelota; **with the** ___ **eye** / a simple vista; *v.* **to strip** ___ / desnudarse.

name *n.* nombre; [*first name and surname*] nombre completo, nombre y apellido; **What is your** ___? / ¿Cómo se llama usted?, ¿cómo te llamas tú?, ¿cuál es su, tu nombre?

nanocephaly *n.* nanocefalia, desarrollo anormal de la cabeza caracterizada por su pequeñez.

nape *n.* nuca, cerviz, parte posterior del cuello; *pop.* pescuezo, cogote.

narcissism *n.* narcisismo. 1. amor excesivo a sí mismo; 2. placer sexual derivado de la contemplación del propio cuerpo.

narcissistic *a.* narcisista.

narcoanalysis *n.* narcoanálisis, tratamiento de psicoterapia usado originalmente en casos de psicosis de guerra, y también en el tratamiento de trauma infantil. *Syn.* **narcosynthesis.**

narcohypnosis *n.* narcohipnosis, hipnosis inducida por el uso de narcóticos.

narcolepsy *n.* narcolepsia, padecimiento crónico de accesos de sueño.

narcoleptic *a.* narcoléptico-a, rel. a la narcolepsia o que padece de ella.

narcosis *n.* narcosis. 1. letargo y alivio de dolor por el efecto de narcóticos; 2. drogadicción.

narcotherapy *n.* narcoterapia, psicoterapia que se lleva a cabo bajo el efecto de un sedativo o narcótico.

narcotic *a.* narcótico-a, estupefaciente de efecto analgésico que puede producir adicción; ___ **blockade** / bloqueo ___; ___ **reversal** / reversión ___.

narcotism *n.* narcotismo. v. narcosis.

naris *n.* (*pl.* **nares**) naris, orificios o ventanas de la nariz.

narrowing *n.* estenosis, pinzamiento; **aortic** ___ / estenosis de la aorta; **mitral** ___ / **mitral** ___ or ___ de la vávula mitral.

nasal *a.* nasal, rel. a la nariz; ___ **cavity** / cavidad ___; ___ **congestion** / congestión ___; ___ **discharge** / secreción ___; ___ **drip** / goteo ___; ___ **hemorrhage** / epistaxis, hemorragia ___; ___ **instillation** / instilación ___, moquera; ___ **meatus** / meato ___; ___ **passages** / fosas nasales; ___ **polyp** / pólipo ___; ___ **septum** / tabique ___.

nascent *a.* 1. naciente, incipiente; 2. liberado de un compuesto químico.

nasogastric *a.* nasogástrico-a, rel. a la nariz y el estómago; ___ **tube** / tubo ___.

nasolabial *a.* nasolabial, rel. a la nariz y al labio.

nasolacrimal duct *n.* conducto nasolagrimal.

nasopharynx *n.* nasofaringe, parte de la faringe localizada sobre el velo del paladar. V. ilustración en la página 409.

nasty *a.* agresivo-a, de mal carácter; ___ **illness** / enfermedad grave, seria; ___ **weather** / mal tiempo.

natality *a.* natalidad, índice de nacimientos en una comunidad.

natimortality *n.* natimortalidad, índice de mortalidad de muertes perinatales y natales en proporción a la mortalidad.

native *n.* nativo-a, [*indigenous*] indígena; *a.* nativo-a, autóctono-a; ___ **born** / nacido-a en; oriundo-a de; ___ **tongue** / lengua materna.

natremia *n.* natremia, presencia de sales de sodio en la sangre.

natriuretic *n.* natriurético-a, diuretic.

natural *a.* natural; sencillo-a; ___ **childbirth** / parto ___; **-ly** *adv.* naturalmente.

natural parents *n., pl.* madre y padre biológicos.

nature *n.* naturaleza.

naturopath *n.* naturópata, persona que practica la naturopatía.

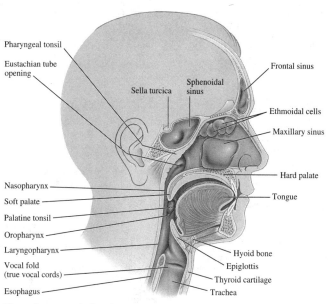

Pharyngeal tonsil

Eustachian tube opening

Sella turcica

Sphenoidal sinus

Frontal sinus

Ethmoidal cells

Maxillary sinus

Hard palate

Tongue

Nasopharynx

Soft palate

Palatine tonsil

Oropharynx

Laryngopharynx

Vocal fold (true vocal cords)

Esophagus

Hyoid bone

Epiglottis

Thyroid cartilage

Trachea

Nasopharyngeal structures: sagittal section

naturopathy *n.* naturopatía, tratamiento terapéutico por medio de recursos naturales.

nausea *n.* náusea, asco, ganas de vomitar.

nauseate *v.* dar o causar náuseas, dar asco; **to be nauseated** / tener náuseas.

nauseous *a.* nauseoso-a. 1. propenso a tener náuseas; 2. que produce náusea o asco.

navel *n.* ombligo, umbilicus.

navicular *n.* navicular, hueso escafoide; *a.* en forma de nave; ___ **abdomen** / abdomen ___; ___ **bone** / hueso ___; ___ **fossa of urethra** / fosa ___ de la uretra.

near *a.* cercano-a, próximo-a, a corta distancia; **a ___ relative** / un pariente ___; [*almost*] casi; *prep.* cerca de, junto a; [*at hand*] a la mano; [*toward*] ___ **the right** / hacia la derecha, cerca de la derecha, **-ly** *adv.* casi, por poco; **He, she ___ died** / él, ella por poco se muere.

nearsighted *a.* miope, corto-a de vista.

nearsightedness *n.* miopía, myopia.

nebula *n.* nébula, opacidad ligera de la córnea.

nebulization *n.* nebulización, atomización, conversión de un líquido a una nube de vapor.

nebulizer *n.* nebulizador, atomizador de líquido.

nebulous *a.* nebuloso-a.

necessary *n.* necesidad; *a.* necesario-a, indispensable; **It is ___** / Es necesario; **what is ___** / lo necesario; **whatever is ___** / lo que sea necesario.

neck *n.* cuello, pescuezo. 1. parte del cuerpo que une la cabeza al tronco; 2. región de un diente entre la corona y la raíz.

neck of uterus *n.* cuello uterino.

necrobiosis *n.* necrobiosis, degeneración gradual de células y tejidos como resultado de cambios debidos al desarrollo, el envejecimiento y el uso.

necrology *n.* necrología, estudio de estadísticas referentes a la mortalidad.

necrophilia *n.* necrofilia. 1. atracción mórbida por los cadáveres; 2. relación sexual con un cadáver.

necrophobia *n.* necrofobia, temor anormal a la muerte y a los cadáveres.

necropsy *n.* necropsia, autopsy.

necrosis *n.* necrosis, muerte parcial o total de las células que forman un tejido tal como ocurre en la gangrena; **acute massive liver __ / __** hepática masiva aguda; **acute retinal __ / __** aguda de la retina; **aseptic __ / __** aséptica; **caceous __ / __** caseosa; **central __ / __** central; **coagulation __ / __** de coagulación; **cystic medial __ / __** cística media; **fat __ / __** grasa; **focal __ / __** focal; **ischenic __ / __** isquémica; **laminar cortical __ / __** laminar cortical; **__of epiphysis / __** epifisaria; **progressive emphysematous __ / __** progresiva enfisematosa; **progressive outer retinal __ / __** externa progresiva de la retina; **renal papillary __ / __** renal papilar; **simple __ / __** simple; **subcutaneous fat __ of newborn / __** de tejidos grasos subcutáneos del neonato; **suppurative __ / __** supurativa; **total __ / __** total.

necrotize *v.* necrosar, causar la muerte, producir necrosis.

needle *n.* aguja; **hypodermic __ / __** hipodérmica.

needle stick puncture *n.* pinchazo accidental que pueda ocasionar la transmision de fluidos infecciosos tal como hepatitis B, C, or de otras enfermedades.

needy *n., pl.* necesitados; **the __ / los __**; *a.* necesitado-a; pobre.

negative *a.* negativo-a; **__ culture /** cultivo __; **-ly** *adv.* negativamente.

negative predictive value *n.* valor pronóstico de un diagnóstico con resultado negativo.

negative transference *n.* transferencia negativa, en el análisis psicológico, el resultado de casos de transferencia que se caracterizan por hostilidad de parte del paciente hacia el analista.

negativism *n.* negativismo, conducta caracterizada por una actuación opuesta a la sugerida.

neglect *n.* negligencia, descuido, desamparo.

negligence *n.* negligencia, descuido.

negligent *a.* negligente, descuidado-a.

neighbor *n.* vecino-a.

nemathelminth *n.* nematelminto, gusano intestinal de forma redondeada que pertenece al orden de los *Nemathelmintes.*

Nematoda *n., L. Nematoda,* clase de gusanos del orden de los *Nemathelmintes.*

nematodiasis *n.* nematodiasis, infección por parásitos nematodos.

neoarthrosis, nearthrosis *n.* neoartrosis, neartrosis, articulación artificial o falsa.

neologism *n.* neologismo. 1. vocablos a los cuales el paciente mental atribuye nuevos significados no relacionados con el verdadero; 2. vocablo al cual se le atribuye un giro nuevo.

neomycin *n.* neomicina, antibiótico de espectro amplio.

neonatal *a.* neonatal, rel. a las primeras seis semanas después del nacimiento.

neonate *n.* neonato-a, recién nacido-a, de seis semanas o menos de nacido-a.

neonatology *n.* neonatología, estudio y cuidado de los recién nacidos.

neoplasia *n.* neoplasia, formación de neoplasmas.

neoplasm *n.* neoplasma, crecimiento anormal de tejido nuevo tal como un tumor.

neoplastic *a.* neoplástico-a, rel. a un neoplasma.

neoplastic growth *n.* neoplasia o tumor.

neovascularization *n.* neovascularización, proliferación anormal de nuevos vasos sanguíneos como reacción a la isquemia.

nephew *n.* sobrino.

nephralgia *n.* nefralgia, dolor en el riñón.

nephrectomy *n.* nefrectomía, extirpación de un riñón.

nephritic *n.* nefrítico-a, rel. a la nefritis o afectado por ella.

nephritis *n.* nefritis, infl. del riñón; **acute __ / __** aguda; **analgesic __ / __** analgésica; **chronic __ / __** crónica; **focal __ / __** focal; **glomerular __ / __** glomerular; **hemorrhagic __ / __** hemorrágica; **hereditary __ / __** hereditaria; **immune complex __ / __** de complejo inmune; **interstitial __ / __** intersticial; **lupus __ / __** lipomatosa; **suppurative __ / __** supurativa; **syphilitic __ / __** sifilítica.

nephrogram *n.* nefrograma, radiografía del riñón.

nephrolithiasis *n.* nefrolitiasis, presencia de cálculos renales.

nephrolithotomy *n.* nefrolitotomía, incisión en el riñón para extraer cálculos renales.

nephrology *n.* nefrología, estudio del riñón y de las enfermedades que lo afectan.

nephroma *n.* nefroma, tumor del riñón.

nephromegaly *n.* nefromegalia, extrema hipertrofia de los riñones.

nephropexy *n.* nefropexia, fijación de un riñón flotante.

nephrosclerosis *n.* nefroesclerosis, endurecimiento del sistema arterial y del tejido intersticial del riñón.

nephrosis *n.* nefrosis, afección renal degenerativa asociada con gran cantidad de proteína en la orina, niveles bajos de albúmina en la sangre y edema pronunciado.

nephrostomy *n.* nefrostomía, formación de una fístula en el riñón o en la pelvis renal.

nephrotic syndrome *n.* síndrome nefrótico, afección del riñón caracterizada por un exceso de pérdida de proteína.

nephrotomy *n.* nefrotomía, incisión en el riñón.

nephrotoxic *a.* nefrotóxico, que destruye células renales.

nephrotoxin *n.* nefrotoxina, toxina que destruye células renales.

nerve *n.* nervio, cada una de las fibras libres o fibras en haz que conectan al cerebro y la médula espinal con otras partes y órganos del cuerpo; __ **block** / bloqueo del __; __ **cells** / neuronas; __ **degeneration** / degeneración nerviosa; __ **ending** / terminación del __; **fiber** / fibra nerviosa; __ **tissue** / tejido nervioso; **pinched** __ / __ pellizcado.

nervous *a.* nervioso-a, ansioso-a, excitable; __ **breakdown** / colapso __, crisis __; __ **debility** / fatiga __; __ **disorder** / trastorno __; __ **impulse** / impulso __; __ **system** / sistema __.

nervousness *n.* nerviosismo, nerviosidad.

nervus *n.*, *L.* (*pl.* **nervi**) nervio.

nest *n.* nido de células, masa de células en forma de nido de pájaro.

network *n.* red, encadenación; arreglo de fibras en forma de malla.

neural *a.* neural, rel. al sistema nervioso; __ **arch** / arco __; __ **crest** / cresta __; __ **cyst** / quiste __; __ **folds** / pliegues neurales; __ **plate** / placa __.

neural hearing loss *n.* pérdida neural de la audición debida a una lesión del octavo nervio craneal.

neuralgia *n.* neuralgia, dolor intenso a lo largo de un nervio; **atypical facial** __ / __ facial atípica; **atypical trigeminal** __ / __ trigeminal atípica; **facial** __ / __ facial; **glossopharyngeal** __ / __ glosofaríngea; **hallucinatory** __ / __ halucinatoria.

neuralgic *a.* neurálgico-a, rel. a la neuralgia.

neurapraxia *n.* neurapraxia, parálisis temporal de un nervio sin causar degeneración.

neurasthenia *n.* neurastenia, término asociado con un estado general de irritabilidad y agotamiento nervioso; **angiopathic** __ / __ angiopática; **gravis** __ / __ grave; **praecox** __ / __ precoz; **primary** __ / __ primaria; **pulsating** __ / __ pulsativa.

neurectomy *n.* neurectomía, corte de un segmento del nervio.

neurilemma *n.* neurilema, membrana fina que cubre una fibra nerviosa.

neurinoma *n.* neurinoma, neoplasma benigno de las capas que rodean un nervio.

neuritis *n.* neuritis, infl. de un nervio.

neuro-ophthalmology *n.* neurooftalmología, rama de la oftalmología que se especializa en la parte del sistema nervioso relacionada con la visión.

neuroblast *n.* neuroblasto, célula nerviosa primitiva.

neuroblastoma *n.* neuroblastoma, tumor maligno del sistema nervioso formado en gran parte por neuroblastos.

neurocyte *n.* neurocito. V. **neuron**.

neurocytoma *n.* neurocitoma, neoplasma, gen. intraventricular.

neurodermatitis *n.* neurodermatitis, trastorno de lesiones cutáneas blanquecinas que gen. se observan en personas nerviosas, y que suelen ser crónicas, diseminadas o localizadas.

neurofibroma *n.* neurofibroma, tumor del tejido fibroso que cubre un nervio periférico.

neurofibromatosis *n.* neurofibromatosis, condición que se caracteriza por la manifestación de múltiples neurofibromas a lo largo de los nervios periféricos.

neurogenic, neurogenetic

neurogenic, neurogenetic *a.*
neurogenético. 1. que se origina en el
sistema nervioso; 2. rel. a
neurogenesis; ___ **atrophy** / atrofia ___.

neuroglia *n.* neuroglia, células que
sirven de sostén y constituyen el tejido
intersticial del sistema nervioso.

neurohypophysis *n.* neurohipófisis,
porción nerviosa posterior de la
glándula pituitaria.

neurolepsis *n.* neurolepsia, estado
alterado de la conciencia producido por
drogas antipsicóticas; el paciente
muestra síntomas de ansiedad e
indiferencia.

neuroleptic *n.* neuroléptico, agente
tranquilizante, pertenece a la clase
psicotrópica de fármacos usada en el
tratamiento de psicosis, esp.
esquizofrenia; **anesthesia** ___ /
anestesia con el uso de un ___.

**neuroleptic malignant
syndrome** *n.* síndrome maligno de
neurolepsis causado por el uso de
agentes neurolépticos y que se
manifiesta en síntomas de hipertermia,
pérdida del conocimiento y otras
reacciones graves relacionadas con el
sistema nervioso central que pueden
ocasionar la muerte.

neurologist *n.* neurólogo-a,
especialista del sistema nervioso.

neurology *n.* neurología, rama de la
medicina que estudia el sistema
nervioso.

neurolysin *n.* neurolisina, anticuerpo
inyectable que se obtiene de una
sustancia cerebral. *Syn.* **neurotoxin.**

neurolysis *n.* neurólisis. 1. proceso de
librar un nervio de anejos inflamatorios;
2. destrucción de tejido nervioso.

neuroma *n.* neuroma, tumor constituido
principalmente por fibras y células
nerviosas; **acoustic** ___ / ___ acústico.

neuromagnetic field *n.* campo
neuromagnético.

neuromalacia *n.* neuromalacia,
reblandecimiento patológico de un
tejido nervioso.

neuromatosis *n.* neuromatosis, la
presencia de neuromas múltiples.

neuromeningeal *a.* neuromeníngeo,
rel. al tejido nervioso y las meninges.

neuromuscular *a.* neuromuscular, rel.
a nervios y músculos; ___ **blocking
agents** / agentes bloqueadores
neuromusculares; ___ **relaxant** /
relajador ___; ___ **system** / sistema ___.

neuromylitis *n.* neuromilitis, infl. de
nervios y de la espina dorsal.

neuron *n.* neurona, célula que constituye
la unidad básica funcional del sistema
nervioso.

neuropacemaker *n.*
neuromarcapasos, instrumento para
estimular eléctricamente la médula
espinal.

neuropathology *n.* neuropatología,
ciencia que estudia las enfermedades
nerviosas.

neuropathy *n.* neuropatía, trastorno o
cambio patológico en los nervios
periféricos; **autonomic** ___ / ___
autónoma; **motor** ___ / ___ motora.

neuropharmacology *n.*
neurofarmacología, estudio
farmacológico del efecto de drogas en
el sistema nervioso.

neuropil *n.* neurópilo, red de fibras
nerviosas (dendritas y neuritas) y de las
células de la glia interrumpidas por
sinapsis en partes del tejido nervioso.

neuropsychopharmacology *n.*
neurosicofarmacología, estudio de
medicamentos y del efecto que causan
en el tratamiento de trastornos
mentales.

neurosarcocleisis *n.*
neurosarcocieisis, cirugía paliativa a la
neuralgia de uno de los taabiques del
canal óseo atravezado por el nervio
traasponiendo éste a los tejidos blandos.

neurosis *n.* neurosis, condición que se
manifiesta principalmente por ansiedad
y por el uso de mecanismos de defensa;
accidental ___ / ___ accidental; **anxiety**
___ / ___ de ansiedad; **cardiac** ___ / ___
cardíaca; **character** ___ / ___ del
carácter; **combat** ___ / ___ de guerra;
compensation ___ / ___ de
compensación; **compulsive** ___ / ___
compulsive; **depressive** ___ / ___
depresiva; **hypochondriacal** ___ / ___
hipocondríaca; **hysterical** ___ / ___
histérica; **obsessional** ___ / ___
obseesiva; **obsessive-compulsive** ___ /
___ obsesiva compulsive; **occupational**
___ / ___ ocupacionaal; **post-traumatic**
___ / ___ post-traumática.

neurosurgeon *n.* neurocirujano-a,
especialista en neurocirugía.

neurosurgery *n.* neurocirugía, cirugía
del sistema nervioso.

neurosyphilis *n.* neurosífilis, sífilis
que afecta el sistema nervioso central;
tabetic ___ / ___ tabética.

neurotic *a.* neurótico-a, que sufre de neurosis.

neurotomy *n.* neurotomía, disección o división de un nervio.

neurotoxic *a.* neurotóxico-a, que ejerce un efecto tóxico sobre el sistema nervioso. __ **agent** / __ agente.

neurotoxicity *n.* neurotoxicidad. 1. la capacidad de una sustancia o agente de destruir o lesionar el tejido nervioso; 2. acción tóxica destructiva, sistema nervioso.

neurotoxin *n.* neurotoxina, cualquier toxina que se asienta específicamente sobre tejido nervioso.

neurotransmitter *n.* neurotransmisor, neurorregulador, sustancia química que modifica la transmisión de impulsos a través de una sinapsis entre nervios o entre un nervio y un músculo; **adrenergic** __ / __ adregénico; **cholinergic** __ / __ colinérgico.

neurotropic atrophy *n.* atrofia neurotrópica, sinónimo de atrofia neurogénica, anomalía de la piel, tejidos subcutáneos y huesos debida a lesiones de nervios periféricos.

neurovascular *a.* neurovascular, rel. a los sistemas nervioso y vascular.

neutral *a.* neutral.

neutralization *n.* neutralización, proceso de anular o contrarrestar la acción de un agente.

neutralize *v.* neutralizar; contrarrestar.

neutrophilia *n.* neutrofilia, aumento de neutrófilos en la sangre.

neutrotaxis *n.* neutrotaxis, estimulación de neutrófilos con una sustancia que los atrae o repele.

never *adv.* nunca, jamás; __ **fear** / pierda cuidado; __ **mind** / no importa.

nevertheless *adv.* sin embargo, no obstante.

nevus *n.* (*pl.* **nevi**) nevo, lunar, marca de nacimiento. **comedonicus** __ / __ comedónico; **compound** __ / __ compuesto; **dysplastic** __ / __ de displasia con algunas células malignas; **faun tail** __ / __ de cola de fauno; **flammeus** __ / __ flamante; **junction, junctional** __ / __ de unión; **melanocytic** __ / __ melanocítico; **sebaceous** __ / __ sebáceo.

new *a.* nuevo-a; **What is new?** / ¿Qué hay de __ ?.

newborn *n.* neonato-a, infante nacido a las 37 semanas de una gestación normal.

next *a.* próximo-a, siguiente; __ **door** / al lado; __ **of kin** / el pariente más cercano; __ **to nothing** / casi nada; **The table is** __ **to the bed** / La mesa está al lado de la cama; **Who is** __**?** / ¿Quién es el, la __?.

nexus *n.* (*pl.* **nexus**) nexo, conexión, unión.

niacin *n.* ácido nicotínico.

nice *a.* delicado-a, fino-a, bueno-a; **-ly** *adv.* finamente, delicadamente; **nicely done** / bien hecho.

niche *n.* nicho, depresión o defecto pequeño esp. en la pared de un órgano hueco.

nicotine *n.* nicotina, alcaloide tóxico, ingrediente principal del tabaco.

nictitation *n.* nictitación, acto de guiñar.

nidation *n.* nidación, fijación del óvulo fecundado en la mucosa uterina.

nidus *n.* (*pl.* **nidi**) nido.

niece *n.* sobrina.

night *n.* noche; **by** __ / de noche, por la noche; **Good** __ / Buenas noches; **last** __ / anoche; __ **before last** / anteanoche.

night-blindness *n.* ceguera nocturna. v. nyctalopia.

nightfall *n.* atardecer, anochecer.

nightmare *n.* pesadilla.

night sweats *n.* sudor excesivo durante el sueño, gen. una señal semejante a la de enfermedades tal como la tuberculosis. o de immunodefiiciente síndrome.

night vision *n.* visión nocturna. V. **scotopia**.

nihilism *n.* nihilismo, en psiquiatría una idea ilusoria en la cual nada es real o inexistente.

nipple *n.* pezón; [*of male*] tetilla; [*nursing bottle*] mamadera, tetera; **cracked** __ / __ agrietado; **engorged** __ / __ enlechado; **retracted** __ / __ retractado.

nitric acid *n.* ácido nítrico.

nitrogen *n.* nitrógeno; **authentic, legitimate** __ / __ auténtico, legítimo; **blood urea** __ / concentración plasmática de urea; **illegitimate** __ / __ ilegítimo; __ **monoxid** / monóxido de __; **residual** __ / __ residual.

nitroglycerine *n.* nitroglicerina, nitrato de glicerina usado como vasodilatador esp. en la angina de pecho.

Nocardia *n. Nocardia*, microorganismo grampositivo que causa nocardiosis.

nocardiosis *n.* nocardiosis, infección generalmente pulmonar causada por *Nocardia* que puede expandirse a varias partes del cuerpo.

nocturia, nycturia *n.* nocturia, nicturia, frecuencia aumentada de emisión de orina esp. durante la noche.

nocturnal *a.* nocturno-a, nocturnal, de noche; ___ **emission, emiction** / micciones ___ s orinarse en la cama; emisión ___ involuntaria de semen.

node *n.* nudo, nódulo, ganglio; **lymphatic** ___ / ___ linfático; **milker's** ___ / ___ de los ordeñadores; **singer's** ___ / ___ vocal o de los cantantes; **syphilis** ___ / ___ sifilítico; **vermis** ___ / ___ del vermis.

nodose *a.* nudoso-a, formado por nódulos o protuberancias.

nodule *n.* nódulo o nudo pequeño; **solitary** ___ / ___ solitario; **subcutaneous** ___ / ___ subcutáneo.

noise *n.* ruido; *v.* **to make** ___ / hacer ___.

noiseless *a.* callado-a, tranquilo-a.

noise pollution *n.* polución de ruido.

noisy *a.* ruidoso-a, turbulento-a, bullicioso-a.

noma *n.* noma, úlcera, estomatitis gangrenosa en la cara interna de la mejilla.

nomenclature *n.* nomenclatura, terminología.

nominal *a.* nominal; ___ **aphasia** / afasia ___.

non compos mentis *a., L. non compos mentis*, mentalmente incompetente.

noninvasive *a.* no invasor, que no se propaga o invade.

nonparous *a.* nulípara. V. **nulliparous.**

nonsense *n.* tontería, bobería, disparate.

nonspecific *a.* sin especificación.

nonviable *n.* que no puede sobrevivir.

norm *n.* norma, regla.

normal *a.* normal, natural, regular.

normalization *n.* normalización, regreso al estado normal.

normoblast *n.* normoblasto, célula roja precursora de los eritrocitos en los humanos.

normocalcemia *n.* normocalcemia, nivel normal de calcio en la sangre.

normoglycemia *n.* normoglucemia, concentración normal de azúcar en la sangre.

normokalemia *n.* normopotasemia, nivel normal de potasio en la sangre.

normotensive *a.* normotenso-a, de presión arterial normal.

normothermia *n.* normotermia, temperatura normal.

normotonic *a.* normotónico-a, de tono muscular normal.

normovolemia *n.* normovolemia, volumen normal de la sangre.

nose *n.* nariz; **bridge of the** ___ / tabique nasal, puente de la nariz; **running** ___ / nariz destilante; coriza.

nosebleed *n.* sangramiento por la nariz.

nosocomial *a.* nosocomial, rel. a un hospital o clínica; ___ **infection** / infección ___, enfermedad adquirida en un hospital.

nostalgia *n.* nostalgia, tristeza, añoranza.

nostril *n.* naris, fosa nasal, ventana o ala de la nariz.

notalgia *n.* notalgia, dolor en la espalda.

notice *n.* aviso, informe, nota; observación; *v.* notar, hacer caso, observar.

notification *n.* notificación, aviso, información.

notochord *n.* notocordio, sostén fibrocelular del embrión que se convierte más tarde en la columna vertebral.

noun *n.* nombre, sustantivo.

nourish *v.* alimentar, nutrir, sustentar.

nourishing *a.* alimenticio-a, nutritivo-a.

nourishment *n.* alimento, nutrición, sustento.

novocaine *n.* novocaína, anestésico.

now *adv.* ahora, ahorita, en este momento, actualmente; **from** ___ **on** / de ___ en adelante; **just** ___ / ___ mismo, hace un momento; ___ **and then** / de vez en cuando; ___ **then** / ahora bien.

nowadays *adv.* hoy en día, al presente.

no way *adv.* de ningún modo, de ninguna manera.

nowhere *adv.* en ninguna parte; ___ **else** / en ninguna otra parte.

nucha *n.* nuca, parte posterior del cuello.

nuclear *a.* nuclear. 1. rel. al núcleo de la célula; 2. rel. a la fuerza atómica.

nuclear magnetic resonance *n.* resonancia magnética nuclear.

nuclear medicine n. medicina nuclear, rama de la medicina que concierne el empleo de radionúclidos para usos de diagnóstico y servicios terapéuticos.

nucleic acid n. ácido nucleico.

nucleopetal a. nucleópeto-a, que se mueve en dirección al núcleo.

nucleotide n. nucleótido, unidad estructural de ácido nucleico.

nucleus n. (pl. **nuclei, nucleuses**) núcleo, parte esencial de una célula; ___ **pulpous** / ___ pulposo, masa gelatinosa contenida dentro de un disco intervertebral.

null a. nulo-a, sin valor, inútil; ___ **hypothesis** / hipótesis ___.

nulligravida n. nuligrávida, mujer que nunca ha concebido.

nulliparous n. nulípara, mujer que nunca ha dado a luz un feto con vida.

numb a. [extremity] entumecido-a, adormecido-a; aturdido-a; **my fingers are** ___ / mis dedos están ___ -s; **I feel** ___ / Me siento entumecido-a; me siento aturdido-a.

numb chin syndrome n. síndrome del mentón entumecido, pérdida de sensación y parestesia con calambre en un lado del mentón y el labio inferior como resultado de una condición de infiltración neoplásica del nervio mental ipsilateral obstruido por un mioloma o un carcinoma de la mama o de la próstata.

number n. número, cifra.

numbness n. [in a part] entumecimiento, adormecimiento;

[confusion] aturdimiento, entorpecimiento.

numerous a. numeroso-a.

nurse n. enfermero-a; **chief** ___, **head** ___ / jefe-a de ___ -s; **community health** ___ / ___ de salud pública; ___ **aid** / asistente de ___; ___ **anesthetist** / ___ anestesista; ___ **practitioner** / practicante de ___; **surgical** ___ / ___ de cirugía; v. [care] **to nurse** / cuidar a una persona enferma; [breast-feeding] amamantar, dar el pecho, dar de mamar.

nursery n. guardería; [in a hospital] sala de niños recién nacidos.

nursing n. 1. cuidado de los enfermos; 2. lactancia.

nutrient n. alimento, nutriente, sustancia nutritiva.

nutrition n. nutrición, mantenimiento, alimentación.

nutritious a. nutritivo-a, alimenticio-a, que proporciona nutrición.

nutritive a. nutritivo-a, sustancioso-a, alimenticio-a.

nyctalopia n. nictalopía, visión imperfecta bajo iluminación baja.

nympha n. ninfa, labio interior de la vulva.

nymphectomy n. ninfectomía, excisión parcial o total de la labia menor.

nymphomania n. ninfomanía, fuego uterino, deseo sexual mórbido en la mujer.

nystagmus n. nistagmo, espasmo involuntario del globo ocular; **palatal** ___ / ___ palatal.

O

O *abbr.* **oculus** / ojo; **oral** / oral; **orally** / oralmente, por la boca; **oxygen** / oxígeno.

oat cell carcinoma *n.* carcinoma maligno, anaplástico microcelular indeferenciado, que se manifiesta en el pulmón.

oath *n.* juramento, promesa; **Hippocratic __** / __ hipocrático; **under __** / bajo __; *v.* **to take an __** / jurar, prestar __.

obedient *a.* obediente.

obese *a.* obeso-a, excesivamente grueso-a.

obesity *n.* obesidad, grasa excesiva en el cuerpo; **alimentary __** / __ alimentaria; **endogenous __** / __ endógena; **exogenous __** / __ exógena.

obfuscation *n.* ofuscación, confusión mental.

OB/GYN abreviatura de obstetricia y ginecología.

object *n.* objeto, cosa; *v.* objetar, oponerse, tener inconveniente.

objective *n.* objetivo, propósito; *a.* objetivo-a, rel. a la percepción de fenómenos y sucesos tal como se manifiestan en la vida real; **__ sign** / señal __; **__ symptoms** / síntomas __ -s; **-ly** *adv.* objetivamente.

obligation *n.* obligación, deber, compromiso.

obliteration *n.* obliteración, destrucción; oclusión por degeneración o por cirugía.

obscure *a.* oscuro-a; oculto-a, escondido-a.

observation *n.* observación, examen, estudio.

obsession *n.* obsesión, preocupación excesiva con una idea o emoción fija.

obsessional *a.* obsesivo-a, rel. a una obsesión o causante de ésta.

obsessive-compulsive *n.* estado neurótico obsesivo-compulsivo con repetición morbosa de acciones como desahogo de tensiones y ansiedades.

obstacle *n.* obstáculo, *pop.* traba.

obstetric *a.* obstétrico-a, rel. a la obstetricia.

obstetrician *n.* obstetra, partero-a, tocólogo-a, especialista en obstetricia.

obstetrics *n.* obstetricia, rama de la medicina que se refiere al cuidado de la mujer durante el embarazo y el parto.

obstinate *a.* obstinado-a, *pop.* cabeza dura, cabeciduro-a.

obstipation *n.* obstipación, estreñimiento rebelde.

obstruct *v.* obstruir, impedir.

obstructed *a.* obstruido-a, tupido-a.

obstruction *n.* obstrucción, bloqueo, obstáculo, impedimento; **intestinal __** / __ intestinal.

obstructive lung disease, chronic (OLD) *n.* obstrucción crónica del pulmón que impide la entrada libre del aire a causa de un estrechamiento físico o funcional del árbol bronquial.

obtain *v.* obtener, adquirir, conseguir.

obturation *n.* obturación, obstrucción o bloqueo de un pasaje.

obturator *a.* obturador-a, bloqueador-a, que obstruye una abertura.

obtuse *a.* obtuso-a. 1. que le falta agudeza mental; 2. romo-a, mellado-a.

occasional *a.* infrecuente, casual, accidental; **-ly** *adv.* a veces; de vez en cuando, ocasionalmente.

occipital *a.* occipital, rel. a la parte posterior de la cabeza; **__ bone** / hueso __; **__ condyle** / cóndilo __; **__ lobe** / lóbulo __.

occipitofrontal *a.* occipitofrontal. rel. al occipucio y la frente.

occipitoparietal *a.* occipitoparietal, rel. a los huesos y lóbulos occipital y parietal.

occipitotemporal *a.* occipitotemporal, rel. a los huesos occipital y temporal.

occiput *n.* occipucio, porción postero-inferior del cráneo.

occlusion *n.* oclusión, cierre, obstrucción; **coronary __** / __ coronaria; **pupillar __** / __ de la pupila.

occult *a.* oculto-a, desconocido-a; escondido-a.

occult blood *n.* sangre oculta, presencia de sangre en cantidad tan ínfima que no puede verse a simple vista.

occupation *n.* ocupación, trabajo, profesión, oficio; **__ neurosis** / neurosis del trabajo, de la profesión.

occupational *a.* ocupacional, rel. a una ocupación; __ **health** / salud __; __ **injuries** / lesiones laborales; __ **therapist** / terapista __ ; __ **therapy** / terapia __.

occurrence *n.* ocurrencia, suceso, acontecimiento; **of frequent** __ / que sucede con frecuencia.

octogenarian *n.* octogenario-a, persona de ochenta años de edad o más; *a.* octogenario-a.

ocular *a.* ocular, visual, rel. a los ojos o a la vista. __ **foreign body** __ / cuerpo extraño; __ **movements** / movimientos ; __; **ataxia** / ataxia __; __**cone** / cono __; **vertigo** __ / vértigo __.

oculist *n.* oculista. V. **ophthalmologist.**

oculomotor *a.* oculomotor, rel. al movimiento del globo ocular.

oculus *L.* oculus, ojo, órgano de la visión.

odd *a.* extraño-a, irregular, raro-a, inexacto-a; **an** __ **case** / un caso __; __ **or even** / nones o pares; **thirty** __ **pills** / treinta píldoras más o menos, treinta y tantas píldoras; **at** __ **times** / en momentos imprevistos, a horas imprevistas.

Oddi's sphincter *n.* Oddi, esfínter de, músculo circular contráctil localizado al nivel de la incisura angular del estómago y de los conductos pancreáticos.

odontectomy *n.* odontectomía, extracción de una pieza dental.

odontologist *n.* odontólogo-a, dentista o cirujano-a dental.

odontology *n.* odontología, estudio de los dientes y del tratamiento de las enfermedades dentales.

odontoplasty *n.* odontoplastia, procedimiento quirúrgico que se usa para mejorar el control de placas y cuidado de las encías.

odoriferous *a.* odorifero, de olor agradable.

odorless *a.* sin olor, inodoro-a.

odynophobia *n.* odinofobia, temor excesivo al dolor.

Oedipus complex *n.* complejo de Edipo, amor patológico del hijo a la madre acompañado de celos y antipatía al padre.

of *prep.* de; [*possession*] __ **the** / del, de la; [*telling time*] / menos; **call at a quarter** __ **six** / Llame, llama a las seis __ cuarto.

off *adv.* fuera de aquí, lejos; __ **and on** / a veces, a intervalos; __ **the record** / confidencial; *v.* [*work*] **to be** __ / ausente, [*without work*] sin trabajo ; **the operation is** __ / se ha suspendido la operación; **to put** __ / aplazar, posponer, diferir; **to turn** __ / cerrar, apagar; *int.* ¡fuera!, ¡salga!, ¡sal!

office *n.* oficina; **doctor's** __ / consulta, consultorio; [*business*] __; **hours** / horas de __; horas de consulta.

official *a.* oficial, autorizado-a.

offspring *n.* descendencia, sucesión, hijos.

often *adv.* con frecuencia, frecuentemente, a menudo; **how** __? / ¿Cuántas veces?; **as** __ **as needed** / tantas veces como sea necesario; **not** __ / pocas veces; **too** __ / demasiadas veces.

oil *n.* aceite; **castor** __ / __ de ricino; **cod liver** __ / __ de hígado de bacalao; **mineral** __ / __ mineral; **olive** __ / __ de oliva; **salad** __ / __ para ensalada; *v.* aceitar, lubricar, engrasar, untar con aceite.

oily *a.* grasoso-a, grasiento-a, oleaginoso-a, lubricante.

ointment *n.* ungüento, pomada, unto, untura; medicamento oleaginoso semisólido de uso externo.

old *a.* viejo-a, anciano-a; antiguo-a; **an** __ **man** / un anciano, un hombre __; **an** __ **method** / un método antiguo; **How** __ **are you?** / ¿Cuántos años tiene, tienes?; **I am fifty years** __ / Tengo cincuenta años; __ **wives' tale** / cuento de __ -s.

olfaction *n.* olfacción. 1. el acto de oler; 2. el sentido del olor.

olfactory *a.* olfatorio-a, rel. al sentido del olfato.

oligodactylia *n.* oligodactilia, carencia del número normal de dedos en las manos o los pies.

oligodontia *n.* oligodoncia, condición hereditaria que resulta en un numéro menor de dientes que el normal.

oligomenorrhea *n.* oligomenorrea, deficiencia en la menstruación.

oligospermia *n.* oligospermia, disminución del número de espermatozoos en el semen.

oliguria *n.* oliguria, disminución en la formación de orina.

olive

olive *n.* oliva. 1. materia gris localizada detrás de la médula oblongata; 2. color aceitunado, verde oliva; 3. árbol del olivo; 4. aceituna.

omalgia *n.* omalgia, dolor en el hombro.

omega 3 fatty acids *n.* ácidos grasos presentes en algunos peces tales como el salmon o la tuna, de propiedad antioxidante que baja el colesterol.

omental *a.* omental, rel. a un omento o formado por él.

omentectomy *n.* omentectomía, extirpación total o parcial de un omento.

omission *n.* omisión; exclusión.

omit *v.* omitir, suprimir, excluir.

omnivorous *a.* omnívoro-a, que come alimentos de origen vegetal y animal.

omphalitis *n.* onfalitis, infl. del ombligo.

omphalocele *n.* onfalocele, hernia congénita del ombligo.

on *prep.* sobre, encima, en, hacia; [*before inf.*] después de; al; __ **an average** / por término medio; __ **the contrary** / al contrario; __ **the left foot** / en el pie izquierdo; __ **the right eye** / en el ojo derecho; __ **the table** / sobre la mesa, encima de la mesa; *adv.* __ **account of** / a causa de; __ **all sides** / por todos lados; *v.* **to be** __ **call** / estar de guardia; **caught** __ / atrapado-a en; __**later** __ / más tarde; **off and** __ / a intervalos, de vez en cuando; __ **and** __ / continuamente, sin cesar, sin parar; __ **purpose** / a propósito; [*function*] funcionando; **The machine is on** / El aparato está funcionando; *a.* [*clothing*] puesto-a; [*after a verb*]; **Go** __! / Siga, sigue!; ¡Continúe, continúa!.

once *n.* una vez; *adv.* **all at** __ / al mismo tiempo, de pronto; **at** __ / en seguida, ahora mismo; __ **in a while** / algunas veces, de vez en cuando.

oncogenesis *n.* oncogénesis, formación y desarrollo de un tumor.

oncologist *n.* oncólogo-a. especialista en oncología.

oncology *n.* oncología, rama de la medicina que estudia los neoplasmas.

oncolysis *n.* oncólisis, destrucción de las células de un tumor.

oncotic *a.* oncótico-a, rel. a una tumefacción o a una causa de ésta.

oncotomy *n.* oncotomía, incisión en un tumor, absceso o quiste.

one *n.* [*number*] uno; *a.* un, uno-a, solo, único-a; **just** __ / solamente uno; **only**
__ **form** / una sola forma; **from** __ **day to another** / de un día a otro; **he is** __ **good patient** / él es un buen paciente; *pron.* **the only** __ / el único, la única; **the** __ **I have** / el que tengo; **this** __ / éste; __ **and all** / todos; __ **of them** / __ de ellos.

one-eyed *n.* tuerto-a.

oneiric *a.* onírico-a, rel. a los sueños.

oneirism *n.* onirismo, estado de ensoñación; soñar despierto.

onicopathy *n.* onicopatía, cualquier enfermedad de la uña.

oniomania *n.* oniomanía, psicosis de urgencia de gastar dinero.

onion *n.* cebolla.

onlay *n.* injerto, esp. en la reparación de defectos óseos.

only *a.* único-a, solo-a; *adv.* sólo, solamente.

onomatomania *n.* onomatomanía, repetición obsesiva de palabras.

onychectomy *n.* oniquectomía, extirpación de una uña.

onychia *n.* oniquia, infl. de la matriz de una uña.

onychomalacia *n.* onicomalacia, reblandecimiento de las uñas.

onychophagia *n.* onicofagia, mal hábito de morderse las uñas.

onychosis *n.* onicosis, enfermedad o deformidad de las uñas.

oocyte *n.* oocito, ovocito, el óvulo antes de la madurez.

oogenesis *n.* oogénesis, formación y desarrollo del óvulo.

oophorectomy *n.* ooforectomía, excisión parcial o total de un ovario.

oophoritis *n.* ooforitis, infl. de un ovario.

oophorocystosis *n.* ooforocistosis, formación de un ovario cístico.

oophoropexy *n.* ooforopexia, fijación o suspensión de un ovario desplazado.

oosperm *n.* oospermo, óvulo fecundado.

ootid *n.* oótide, óvulo maduro después de la penetración del espermatozoide y de ocurrir la segunda division meiótica.

oozing *n.* exudado; supuración.

opacification *n.* opacificación, proceso de opacar.

opacity *n.* opacidad, falta de transparencia.

opaque *a.* opaco-a, sin brillo, que no deja pasar la luz.

open *a.* abierto-a, descubierto-a, destapado-a, libre de paso; ___ **heart surgery** / operación a corazón ___; *v.* abrir, descubrir, destapar, abrir paso; cortar, rajar.

open reduction *n.* reducción abierta, [*in fractures*] técnica de reducir fracturas con exposición de la dislocación o del hueso.

opening *n.* abertura, orificio de entrada o salida.

operate *v.* operar, intervenir, proceder.

operating room *n.* sala de operaciones, quirófano.

operation *n.* operación, intervención quirúrgica, procedimiento quirúrgico.

operon *n.* operon, sistema de genes combinados en el cual el gene operador regula los demás genes estructurales.

ophthalmic *a.* oftálmico-a, visual, rel. al ojo; ___ **nerve** / nervio ___; ___ **solutions** / soluciones ___ -s.

ophthalmologist *n.* oftalmólogo-a, médico oculista especializado en trastornos y enfermedades de la vista.

ophthalmology *n.* oftalmología, rama de la medicina que trata del estudio del ojo y trastornos de la vista.

ophthalmopathy *n.* oftalmopatía, enfermedad de los ojos.

ophthalmoplasty *n.* oftalmoplastia, cirugía plástica del ojo.

ophthalmoplegia *n.* oftalmoplegia, parálisis de un músculo ocular.

ophthalmoscope *n.* oftalmoscopio, instrumento usado para visualizar el interior del ojo.

ophthalmoscopy *n.* oftalmoscopía, examen del ojo con un oftalmoscopio.

opiate *n.* opiáceo, opiato, cualquier droga derivada del opio; ___ **abstinence syndrome** / síndrome provocado por la abstinencia de opio o sus derivados.

opinion *n.* opinión, juicio, parecer; *v.* **to have an** ___ / opinar, hacer juicio, dar el parecer; **to be of the same** ___ / estar de acuerdo, acordar.

opioids *n. pl.* drogas que no son derivadas del opio pero pueden producir efectos similares a éste.

opisthotonos *n.* opistótonos, espasmo tetánico de los músculos de la espalda por el cual los talones se viran hacia atrás y el tronco se proyecta hacia adelante.

opium *n.* opio, *Papaver somniferum*, narcótico, analgésico, estimulante venenoso y alucinógeno cuya adicción produce deteriorización física y mental.

opportune *a.* oportuno-a, conveniente.

opportunistic *a.* oportunista.

opportunistic infectious disease *n.* enfermedad oportunista infecciosa, infección parasítica oportunista, producida por un microorganismo gen. no dañino, que no causa una enfermedad severa o prolongada pero se convierte en patógeno cuando la inmunidad del organismo ha sido ya quebrantada.

opportunity *n.* oportunidad, ocasión.

oppose *v.* oponer, resistir; oponerse, resistirse.

opposition *n.* oposición, objeción.

oppression *n.* opresión, pesadez; **an** ___ **in the chest** / una ___, una sofocación en el pecho.

opsoclonus *n.* opsoclono, movimiento irregular del ojo, esp. relacionado con algunos casos de trastorno cerebral.

opsonin *n.* opsonina, anticuerpo que al combinarse con un antígeno hace que éste sea más suceptible a los fagocitos.

optic, optical *a.* óptico-a, rel. a la visión; ___ **disk** / disco ___, punto ciego de la retina; ___ **illusion** / ilusión ___; ___ **nerve** / nervio ___.

optics *n.* óptica, ciencia que estudia la luz y la relación de ésta con la visión.

optimist *a.* optimista.

option *n.* opción, alternativa.

optometer *n.* optómetro, instrumento usado para medir el poder de refracción del ojo.

optometrist *n.* optometrista, optómetra, profesional que practica la optometría.

optometry *n.* optometría, práctica de examinar los ojos para determinar la agudeza visual y para la prescripción de lentes correctivos y otros auxilios visuales.

oral *a.* oral, bucal, rel. a la boca; verbal, hablado; ___ **contraceptive** / píldora contraceptiva; ___ **diagnosis** / diagnóstico bucal; ___ **hygiene** / higiene bucal.

orbicular *a.* orbicular, circular; ___ **ciliaris** / ___ de los párpados ; ___ **muscle** / músculo ___, rodea una pequeña abertura tal como la de la boca; ___ **oris** / ___ de los labios.

orbit *n.* órbita, cavidad ósea de la cara que contiene los ojos.

orbital

orbital *a.* orbital. rel. a la órbita; ___
fractures / fracturas ___ -es.
orchidectomy *n.* orquidectomía,
orquectomía, extirpación de un
testículo.
orchiditis, orchitis *n.* orquiditis,
orquitis, infl. de los testículos.
orchioncus *n.* orquioncus, tumor
localizado en un testículo.
orchiotomy *n.* orquiotomía, incisión en
un testículo.
order *n.* orden, reglamento, disposición;
in ___ **that** / para que, a fin de que; **in**
___ **to** / para *v.* ordenar, disponer,
mandar; [*arrange*] arreglar; **to be in**
good ___ / estar en buen estado; **to get**
out of ___ / descomponerse.
orderly *n.* asistente de enfermera-o.
ordinary *a.* ordinario-a, corriente, común.
organ *n.* órgano, parte del cuerpo que
realiza una función específica; **end** ___ /
___ terminal; ___ **displacement** /
desplazamiento de un ___; ___ **failure** /
fallo de un ___; ___ **transplant** /
trasplante de un ___.
organelle *n.* organelo, organito, órgano
diminuto de los organismos
unicelulares.
organic *a.* orgánico-a. 1. rel. a un
órgano u órganos; 2. rel. a organismos
de origen vegetal o animal; ___
disease / enfermedad ___.
organism *n.* organismo, ser vivo.
organization *n.* organización;
asociación.
organogenesis *n.* organogénesis,
desarrollo y crecimiento de un
órgano.
organomegaly *n.* organomegalia,
agrandamiento de los órganos viscerales.
orgasm *n.* orgasmo, clímax sexual.
orient *n.* oriente, este.
orientation *n.* orientación, dirección.
orifice *n.* orificio, salida, boquete,
abertura.
origin *n.* origen, principio.
original *n.* original, prototipo; *a.*
original; primitivo-a.
ornithine *n.* ornitina, aminoácido que
aunque no está presente en las
proteínas desempeña un papel
importante en el ciclo de la urea.
orofacial *a.* orofacial, rel. a la boca y a
la cara.
oropharynx *n.* orofaringe, parte central
de la faringe.
orphanage *n.* orfanato, hospicio, asilo
de huérfanos.

orthocephalic *a.* ortocefálico-a, que
posee un cráneo normal proporcionado
al cuerpo, con un índice cefálico
vertical entre 70 y 75.
orthochromatic *a.* ortocromático-a,
de color normal o que acepta
coloración sin dificultad.
orthodontia *n.* ortodoncia, rama de la
odontología que trata las
irregularidades dentales por medio de
procedimientos correctivos.
orthomyxovirus *n.* ortomixovirus,
familia de virus a la cual pertenecen los
tres grupos de virus de la influenza.
orthopedia, orthopedics *n.*
ortopedia, rama de la medicina que
trata de la prevención y corrección de
trastornos en los huesos, articulaciones,
músculos, ligamentos y cartílagos.
orthopedic *a.* ortopédico-a, rel. a la
ortopedia; ___ **shoes** / calzado ___; ___
surgery / cirugía ___.
orthopedist *n.* ortopédico-a,
ortopedista, especialista en ortopedia.
orthopnea *n.* ortópnea, dificultad para
respirar excepto en posición erecta.
orthopsychiatry *n.* ortopsiquiatría,
rama de la psiquiatría que comprende
psiquiatría infantil, pediatría e higiene
mental y se dedica a la prevención y
tratamiento de trastornos psicológicos
en niños y adolescentes.
orthoptics *n.* ortóptica, el estudio y
corrección de trastornos de la visión
binocular y los movimientos oculares.
orthoscopic *a.* ortoscópico, rel. a los
instrumentos que se usan para corregir
distorsiones ópticas.
orthosis *n.* ortosis, corrección de una
deformidad o impedimento.
orthotonos, orthotonus *n.*
ortótonos, espasmo como el del tétano
que se caracteriza por una rigidez en
línea recta de la nuca, las extremidades
y el cuerpo.
orthotopic *a.* ortotópico-a, que ocurre
en una posición normal o correcta.
oscillation *n.* oscilación, movimiento
de vaivén, tal como el de un péndulo.
oscillopsia *n.* oscilopsia, visión
oscilante durante el progreso de la
esclerosis múltiple.
osmolar *a.* osmolar, de naturaleza o
propiedad osmótica.
osmology *n.* osmología. estudio de los
olores.
osmoreceptor *n.* osmorreceptor. 1.
grupo de células cerebrales que reciben

estímulos olfatorios; 2. grupo de células en el hipotálamo que responden a cambios en la presión osmótica de la sangre.

osmosis *n.* osmosis, difusión de un solvente a través de una membrana semipermeable interpuesta entre soluciones de concentración diferente.

osmotic *a.* osmótico-a, rel. a la osmosis.

osseous *a.* óseo-a, rel. a los huesos; __ tissue / tejido __.

ossicle *n.* huesillo, osículo.

ossification *n.* osificación, proceso de desarrollo óseo.

ossification, ostosis *n.* osificación. 1. conversión de una sustancia en hueso; 2. desarrollo del hueso.

ossify *v.* osificar, transformarse en hueso.

osteitis *n.* osteítis, ostitis, infl. de un hueso; __ **fibrosa cystica** / __ fibrosa cística, con degeneración fibrosa y manifestación de quistes y nódulos en el hueso.

osteoaneurysm *n.* osteoaneurisma, aneurisma que ocurre en un hueso.

osteoarthritis *n.* osteoartritis, hipertrofia degenerativa del hueso y de las articulaciones esp. en la vejez.

osteoarthropathy *n.* osteoartropatía, enfermedad gen. dolorosa que afecta las articulaciones y los huesos.

osteoblast *n.* osteoblasto, célula desarrollada aisladamente en una laguna de la sustancia ósea.

osteoblastoma *n.* osteoblastoma. V. osteoma.

osteocarcinoma *n.* osteocarcinoma, cáncer del hueso.

osteocartillaginous *a.* osteocartilaginoso-a, rel. a la formación de huesos y cartílagos.

osteochondritis *n.* osteocondritis, infl. del hueso y del cartílago.

osteochondroma *n.* osteocondroma, tumor compuesto de elementos óseos y cartilaginosos.

osteoclasia *n.* osteoclasia, destrucción de tejido óseo.

osteodystrophy *n.* osteodistrofia, hipertrofia ósea múltiple degenerativa.

osteoid *a.* osteoide, rel. o semejante a un hueso.

osteology *n.* osteología, rama de la medicina que estudia la estructura y funcionamiento de los huesos.

osteoma *n.* osteoma, tumor formado de tejido óseo.

osteomalacia *n.* osteomalacia, reblandecimiento de los huesos debido a la pérdida de calcio en la matriz del hueso.

osteomyelitis *n.* osteomielitis, infección del hueso y de la médula ósea.

osteonecrosis *n.* osteonecrosis, destrucción y muerte del tejido óseo.

osteopath *n.* osteópata, especialista en osteopatía.

osteopathy *n.* osteopatía. 1. sistema terapéutico médico con énfasis en la relación entre los órganos y el sistema muscular esquelético que hace uso de la manipulación como medio de corrección; 2. cualquier enfermedad de los huesos.

osteopenia *n.* osteopenia, disminución de la calcificación ósea.

osteophyte *n.* osteófito, prominencia ósea.

osteoplastic *a.* osteoplástico-a. 1. rel. a la formación de un hueso; 2. cirugía plástica de un hueso.

osteoporosis *n.* osteoporosis, pérdida en la densidad del hueso, resultando en continuas fracturas.

osteosarcoma *n.* osteosarcoma, sarcoma óseo maligno.

osteosynthesis *n.* osteosíntesis, fijación quirúrgica de un hueso mediante el uso de un medio mecánico tal como una placa o un clavo.

osteotomy *n.* osteotomía, cirugía empleada en cortar o serruchar un hueso.

ostium *n., L. (pl.* **ostia**) ostium, pequeña abertura.

ostium primum *L.* ostium primum, apertura que comunica las dos aurículas del corazón fetal y que se empequeñece gradualmente.

ostomy *n.* ostomía, creación de una abertura entre un órgano y la piel como medio de salida exterior, tal como se efectúa en colostomías e ileostomías.

otalgia, otodynia, otoneuralgia *n.* otalgia, otodinia, otoneuralgia, dolor de oídos.

Ota's nevus *n.* Ota, nevus de, nevus que puede desarrollarse en melanoma.

otectomy *n.* otectomía, extirpación del contenido estructural del oído medio.

other *a.* otro-a, diferente, nuevo-a; **every** __ **day** / un día sí y otro no; *pron.* **the** __ **one** / el otro, la otra; **the** __ **ones** / los otros, las otras.

otherwise

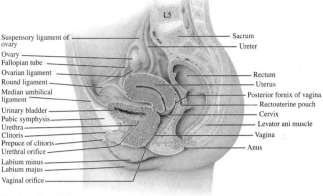

Suspensory ligament of ovary — Sacrum
Ovary — Ureter
Fallopian tube
Ovarian ligament — Rectum
Round ligament — Uterus
Median umbilical ligament — Posterior fornix of vagina
— Rectouterine pouch
Urinary bladder — Cervix
Pubic symphysis — Levator ani muscle
Urethra — Vagina
Clitoris —
Prepuce of clitoris — Anus
Urethral orifice —
Labium minus —
Labium majus —
Vaginal orifice —

The female pelvic organs (sagittal section)

otherwise *adv.* de otra manera, de otro modo, por otra parte.

oticodinia *n.* oticodinia, vértigo causado por una enfermedad del oído.

otitis *n.* otitis, infl. del oído externo, medio o interno.

otolaryngologist *n.* otolaringólogo-a, especialista en otolaringología.

otolaryngology *n.* otolaringología, estudio de la garganta, nariz y oídos.

otologist *n.* otólogo-a, especialista en enfermedades del oído.

otology *n.* otología, rama de la medicina que estudia el oído, su función y las enfermedades que lo afectan.

otoneurology *n.* otoneurología, estudio del oído interno en su relación con el sistema nervioso.

otoplasty *n.* otoplastia, cirugía plástica del oído.

otorrhagia *n.* otorragia, sangramiento por el oído.

otosclerosis *n.* otosclerosis, sordera progresiva debida a la formación de tejido esponjoso en el laberinto del oído.

otoscopy *n.* otoscopia, uso del otoscopio en un examen del oído.

ototomy *n.* ototomía, incisión en el oído.

out *adv.* afuera, fuera; [*light, appliance*] apagado-a [*unconscious*] inconsciente, sin conocimiento; __ **of** / __ de; **three** __ **of ten cases** / tres de diez casos; __ **of work** / sin trabajo, sin empleo, desempleado-a; *v.* **to be** __ / estar ausente; **to go** __ / salir; **get** __! / salga!, sal!.

outbreak *n.* erupción; [*of an epidemic*] brote epidémico.

outburst *n.* erupción; estallido; arranque; manifestación abrupta, brote.

outcome *n.* resultado, consecuencia; [*good*] éxito.

outdated *a.* anticuado-a; [*medication*] de fecha vencida.

outflow *n.* derrame, salida, flujo.

outgrow *vi.* sobrepasar, crecer más.

outgrowth *n.* excrecencia, bulto.

outlive *v.* sobrevivir, vivir más que; durar más.

outlook *n.* punto de vista, expectativa, opinión.

outpatient *n.* paciente externo, paciente de consulta externa, paciente no hospitalizado.

output *n.* rendimiento; producción; salida; __ **failure** / fallo en el __.

outroot *v.* sacar de raíz, desarraigar, extirpar.

outside *n.* exterior, apariencia; *prep.* fuera de, más allá de.

outspoken *a.* franco-a, que habla sin rodeos.

outstretch *v.* extender, alargar, expandir.

outweigh *v.* pesar más que; exceder.

oval *a.* oval; rel. al óvulo.

oval window *n.* ventana oval; abertura del oído medio.

ovarian *a.* ovárico-a, rel. a los ovarios.

ovariectomy *n.* ovariectomía. V. oophorectomy.

ovary *n.* ovario, órgano reproductor

femenino que produce el óvulo. V. ilustración en la página 422.

over *a.* acabado-a, terminado-a; *prep.* sobre, encima, por; a través de; *adv.* por encima, de un lado; a otro; al otro lado; al revés ___ **again** / otra vez; ___ **and** ___ **again** / muchas veces; *v.* [*years*] **to be** ___ / tener más de; **It is** ___ / ya se pasó, ya se acabó; **turn** ___ / vuélvase, vuélvete.

overactive bladder *n.* vejiga hiperactiva, superactiva.

overanxious *a.* demasiado inquieto-a, excitado-a, muy ansioso-a.

overbite *n.* sobremordida.

overclosure *n.* sobrecierre, cierre de la mandíbula antes de que los dientes superiores e inferiores se junten.

overcome *vi.* vencer, rendir; sobreponerse; **you must** ___ **this** / debe sobreponerse, debes sobreponerte a esto; **you must** ___ **this sickness** / debe, debes ___ a esta enfermedad.

overcompensation *n.* sobrecompensación, intento exagerado de ocultar sentimientos de inferioridad o de culpa.

Over the Counter (OTC) *n.* medicamento a la venta sin necesidad de receta médica.

overdose *n.* dosis excesiva; dosis tóxica; sobredosis.

overdue *a.* retrasado-a, tardío-a.

overeat *vi.* comer con exceso; hartarse.

overexposure *n.* superexposición; exposición excesiva.

overfeed *vi.* sobrealimentar, alimentar en exceso.

overflow *n.* rebosamiento; derramamiento; *pop.* desparramo.

overgrown *a.* demasiado crecido-a, muy grande o agrandado-a.

overgrowth *n.* proliferación excesiva.

overhear *v.* oir por casualidad; alcanzar a oir.

overnight *n.* velada, la noche completa; *adv.* durante la noche; la noche pasada.

overpowering *a.* abrumador-a; irresistible.

overreact *v.* reaccionar en exceso.

overresponse *n.* sobrerespuesta, reacción excesiva a un estímulo.

oversight *n.* descuido, equivocación, inadvertencia.

overtime *n.* tiempo suplementario; horas extras de trabajo.

overweigh *v.* pesar más que; sobrecargar.

overweight *n.* peso excesivo, sobrepeso.

overwork *n.* trabajo excesivo, trabajo en exceso.

ovicular, ovoid *a.* ovicular, en forma de huevo.

oviduct *n.* oviducto, conducto uterino; trompas de Falopio.

ovotestis *n.* ovotestis, glándula hermafrodita que contiene tejido ovárico y testicular.

ovulation *n.* ovulación, liberación periódica del óvulo o gamete por el ovario.

ovulatory *a.* ovulatorio-a, rel. al proceso de ovulación.

ovum *n.* (*pl.* **ova**) óvulo, gamete **fecundado.**

oxalic acid *n.* ácido oxálico.

oxidant *a.* oxidante, que causa oxidación o rel. a ésta.

oxidation *n.* oxidación, combinación de una sustancia con oxígeno.

oxidize *v.* oxidar, combinar con oxígeno.

oximeter *n.* oxímetro, instrumento para medir la cantidad de oxígeno en la sangre.

oxygen *n.* oxígeno, elemento o gas incoloro e inodoro no metálico que circula libremente en la atmósfera; ___ **deficiency** / falta de ___; ___ **distribution** / distribución de ___; ___ **treatment** / tratamiento de ___.

oxygen tent *n.* cámara de oxígeno, tienda de oxígeno.

oxygen therapy *n.* terapia de oxígeno, tratamiento de oxígeno por el cual se distribuye una concentración de oxígeno para aliviar la respiración del paciente por medio de un catéter nasal, tienda, cámara o máscara.

oxygenation *n.* oxigenación, saturación de oxígeno.

oxygenator *n.* oxigenador, instrumento para oxigenar la sangre gen. usado durante cirugía.

oxygenotherapy *n.* oxigenoterapia, uso terapéutico del oxígeno.

oxyhemoglobin *n.* oxihemoglobina, sustancia de color rojo brillante que se forma cuando los glóbulos rojos se combinan permanentemente con el oxígeno.

oxytocin *n.* oxitocina, ocitocina, hormona pituitaria que estimula las contracciones del útero.

oyster *n.* ostra, ostión.

ozone *n.* ozono, O_3, agente oxidante, forma tóxica de oxígeno.

P

p

P *abbr.* **part** / parte; **phosphorous** / fósforo; **plasma** / plasma; **population** / población; **positive** / positivo; **posterior** / posterior; **postpartum** / postpartum; **pressure** / presión; **psychiatry** / psiquiatría; **pulse** / pulso.

pace *n.* marcha, paso, el andar; *v.* andar, marchar.

pacemaker, pacer *n.* marcapasos, estabilizador del ritmo cardíaco; **internal** ___ / ___ interno; **temporary** ___ / ___ temporal.

pacify *v.* apaciguar, tranquilizar.

pack *n.* 1. cubierta fría o caliente en la cual se envuelve el cuerpo; 2. compresa; *v.* [*to wrap*] envolver.

packed cells *n. pl.* eritrocitos separados del plasma.

pad *n.* cojín, almohadilla; *v.* [*to fill*] rellenar.

pain *n.* [*ache*] dolor; [*suffering*] sufrimiento, pena; [*colicky*] cólico; **constant** ___ / ___ constante; **strong** ___ / ___ fuerte; **pressing** ___ / ___ oprimente; **mild** ___ / ___ leve; **localized** ___ / ___ localizado; **oppressive** ___ / ___ opresiivo; **piercing** ___ / ___ penetrante; **deep** ___ / ___ profundo; **burning** ___ / ___ quemante; **referred** ___ / ___ referido; **dull** ___ / ___ sordo; **subjective** ___ / ___ subjetivo.

painful *a.* doloroso-a, penoso-a, aflictivo-a. ___ **menstrual period** / menstruación ___; ___ **intercourse** / dispareunia, relaciones sexuales ___ -as; ___ **urination** / dolor al orinar.

painkiller *n.* calmante, sedante, remedio, pastilla para el dolor.

painless *a.* sin dolor; [*easy*] fácil.

pair *n.* par, pareja.

palatal myoclonus *n.* mioclono palatino, contracciones rítmicas del paladar, los músculos faciales y el diafragma debido a lesiones cerebrales.

palatal reflex *n.* reflejo palatino, deglución estimulada por el paladar.

palate *n.* paladar; velo del paladar; *pop.* cielo de la boca; **bony** ___ / ___ óseo;

hard ___ / ___ duro; **soft** ___ / ___ blando.

palatine *a.* palatino, rel. al paladar.

pale *a.* pálido-a, descolorido-a.

paleface *n.* rostro pálido, carapálida.

palindromic *a.* palindrómico-a, recurrente.

palliative *a.* paliativo-a, lenitivo-a, que alivia.

pallor *n.* palidez.

palm *n.* palma, parte inferior de la mano; ___ **oil** / aceite de ___ .

palmer *a.* palmer. rel a la palma de la niano.

palpable *a.* palpable.

palpate *v.* palpar, acto de palpación.

palpation *n.* palpación, acto de tocar y examinar con las manos un área del cuerpo.

palpitate *v.* palpitar, latir.

palpitation *n.* palpitación, latido; pulsación; aleteo rápido.

palsy *n.* perlesía, parálisis, pédida temporal o permanente de la sensación, de la función o control de movimiento de una parte del cuerpo; **cerebral** ___ / ___ cerebral, parálisis parcial y falta de coordinación muscular debida a una lesión cerebral congénita.

paludism *n.* paludismo, enfermedad infecciosa febril gen. crónica, transmitida por la picadura de un mosquito *Anófeles* infectado por un protozooario *Plasmodium*.

pamphlet *n.* folleto.

panacea *n.* panacea, remedio para todas las enfermedades.

panarthritis *n.* panartritis. 1. infl. de varias articulaciones del cuerpo; 2. infl. de los tejidos de una articulación.

pancreas *n.* pancreas, glándula del sistema digestivo que secreta externamente el jugo pancreático e interiormente la insulina y el glucagón; ___ **transplant** / trasplante del ___ .

pancreatalgia *n.* pancreatalgia, dolor en el páncreas.

pancreatectomy *n.* pancreatectomía, excisión parcial o total del páncreas.

pancreatic *a.* pancreático-a, rel. al páncreas; ___ **cyst** / quiste ___; ___ **duct** / conducto ___; ___ **juice** / jugo ___; ___ **neoplasms** / neoplasmas ___ -s.

pancreatic function test *n.* prueba del funcionamiento del páncreas.

pancreatin *n.* pancreatina, enzima digestiva del páncreas.

pancreatitis *n.* pancreatitis, infl. del páncreas; **acute** ___ / ___ aguda; **hemorrhagic, acute** ___ / ___ hemorrágica aguda.

pancreatolithiasis *n.* pancreatolitiasis, presencia de cálculos en los conductos del pancreas.

pancytopenia *n.* pancitopenia, disminución anormal del número de células sanguíneas.

pandemic *a.* pandémico-a, de contagiosidad epidémica en un área geográfica extensa.

panendoscope *n.* panendoscopio, instrumento óptico usado para examinar la vejiga.

pang *n.* dolor agudo penetrante.

panglossia *n.* panglosia, verborrea.

panhidrosis *n.* panhidrosis, transpiración generalizada.

panhypopituitarism *n.* panhipopituitarismo, deficiencia de la pituitaria anterior.

panhysterectomy *n.* panhisterectomía, excisión total del útero.

panic *n.* pánico, temor excesivo; ___ **attacks** / ataques de ___; *v.* tener un miedo excesivo; sobrecogerse de pánico.

panicked *a.*, *pp.* of **to panic,** sobrecogido-a de pánico; *pop.* muerto-a de miedo.

panniculitis *n.* paniculitis, infl. del panículo grasoso.

panniculus *n.* panículo, capa de tejido adiposo; ___ **adiposus** / ___ adiposo; ___ **carnosus** / ___ carnoso.

pannus *n.*, *L.* pannus, paño, membrana de tejido granulado que cubre una superficie normal.

pansinusitis *n.* pansinusitis, infl. de los senos paranasales de un lado o de ambos.

pant *v.* jadear, resollar.

panting *n.* jadeo, respiración rápida.

Papanicolaou test, Pap smear *n.* prueba de Papanicolaou (frotis, unto), recolección de mucosa de la vagina y del cuello uterino para detectar un cáncer incipiente.

papilla *n.* (*pl.* **papillae**) papila, protuberancia esp. en la lengua; **acoustic** ___ / ___ acústica; **dermal** ___ / ___ dérmica; **duodenal** ___ / ___ duodenal; **filiform** ___ / ___ filiforme; **lacrimal** ___ / ___ lagrimal; **lingual** ___ / ___ lingual.

papillary *a.* papilar, rel. a una papila.

papillary carcinoma *n.* carcinoma papilar, tumor de la tiroides caracterizado por tener varias tumoraciones en forma de dedos.

papilledema *n.* papiledema, edema del disco óptico.

papillitis *n.* papilitis, infl. del disco óptico.

papilloma *n.* papiloma, tumor epitelial benigno.

papillomatosis *n.* 1. desarrollo de numerosos papilomas; 2. proyecciones de papilares.

papovavirus *n.* papovavirus, miembro de un grupo de virus de gran importancia en el estudio del cáncer.

papular *a.* papular, rel. a una pápula.

papule *n.* pápula, protuberancia en la piel compuesta de materia sólida.

papulosquamous *a.* papuloescamoso-a, rel. a pápulas y escamas; ___ **skin diseases** / enfermedades cutáneas ___ -s.

para-aminobenzoic acid *n.* para-amino ácido benzóico, un factor en el complejo de vitamina B requerido en la síntesis de ácido fólico.

paracentesis *n.* paracentesis, punción para obtener o eliminar líquido de una cavidad.

paraffin *n.* parafina.

parainfluenza viruses *n.*, *pl.* virus de parainfluenza, virus asociados con infecciones respiratorias, esp. en los niños.

parallax *n.* paralaje, posición de desplazamiento aparente de un objeto de acuerdo con la posición del observador.

paralysis *n.* parálisis, pérdida parcial o total de movimiento o de función de una parte del cuerpo; **accomodation** ___ / ___ de acomodación; **alcoholic** ___ / ___ alcohólica; **amyotrofic** ___ / ___ amiotrófica; **ascending** ___ / ___ ascendente; **central** ___ / ___ central; **cold induced** ___ / ___ por enfriamiento; **diver's** ___, *pop.* **bends** / ___ de los buzos; **hysterical** ___ / ___ histérica; **motor** ___ / ___ motor; **peripheral fascial** ___ / ___ periférica facial; **rapidly progressive** ___ / ___ galopante.

paralytic

paralytic *a.* paralítico-a, inválido-a; impedido-a, rel. a o que sufre de parálisis; __ **ileus** / parálisis del intestino.

paralyzer *a.* paralizador, que causa parálisis.

paramedic *n.* paramédico-a, profesional con entrenamiento para ofrecer asistencia médica esp. de emergencia.

parametrium *n.* parametrio, tejido celular suelto alrededor del útero.

paramyotonia *n.* paramiotonía, miotonía atópica caracterizada por espasmos musculares y tonicidad anormal de los músculos. **ataxic** __ / __ atáxica; **congenital** __ / __ congénita; __ **disorder** / trastorno de __; **symptomatic** __ / __ sintomática.

paranasal *a.* paranasal, adyacente a la cavidad nasal.

paranasal sinuses *n., pl.* senos paranasales, cualquiera de las cavidades aéreas en los huesos adyacentes a la cavidad nasal.

paranoia *n.* paranoia, trastorno mental caracterizado por delirio de persecución o de grandeza.

paranoid *a.* paranoico-a, persona afectada por paranoia.

paraphasia *n.* parafasia, tipo de afasia que se caracteriza por el uso incoherente de palabras.

paraphimosis *n.* parafimosis. 1. constricción del prepucio detrás del glande del pene; 2. retracción del párpado por detrás del globo ocular.

paraplegia *n.* paraplejía, parálisis de la parte inferior del tronco y de las piernas. **cerebral infantile** __ / __ cerebral infantil; **familiar, spasmodic** __ / __ espasmódica, familiar; **spasmodic, spastic** __ / __ espasmódica, espástica.

paraplegic *a.* parapléjico-a, rel. a, o afectado por paraplejía.

parapsychology *n.* parapsicología, estudio de fenómenos psíquicos tales como la telepatía y la percepción extrasensorial.

parasite *n.* parásito, organismo que vive a expensas de otro.

parasitology *n.* parasitología, estudio de los parásitos.

parasomnia *n.* parasomnia, término que se refiere a cualquier trastorno sufrido durante el sueño, enuresis, pesadillas, sonambulismo, etc.

parasympathetic *a.* parasimpático, rel. a una de las dos ramas del sistema nervioso autónomo; __ **nervous system** / sistema nervioso autónomo.

parasympatholytic *a.* parasimpatolítico, que destruye o bloquea las fibras nerviosas del sistema nervioso parasimpático.

parasystole *n.* parasístole, irregularidad en el ritmo cardíaco.

parathormone *n.* hormona paratiroidea, hormona reguladora del calcio.

parathyroid *n.* paratiroides, grupo de glándulas endocrinas pequeñas situadas junto a la tiroides; __ **hormone** / hormona __, reguladora de calcio; *a.* paratiroideo-a, localizado-a cerca de la tiroides.

parathyroidectomy *n.* paratiroidectomía, extirpación de una o más de las glándulas paratiroideas.

paratyphoid *n.* paratífica, fiebre similar a la tifoidea.

paregoric *n.* paregórico, narcótico, calmante derivado del opio.

parenchyma *n.* parénquima, partes funcionales de un órgano.

parent *n.* padre o madre; *pl.* __ **-s** / padres.

parenteral *a.* parenteral, rel. a la introducción de medicamentos o sustancias en el organismo por otra vía que no sea la del canal alimenticio; __ **hyperalimentation** / sobrealimentación intravenosa.

parenthood *n.* paternidad o maternidad.

paresis *n.* paresia, parálisis parcial o leve.

paresthesia *n.* parestesia, sensación de hormigueo o de calambre que se asocia a una lesión de un nervio periférico.

parietal bone *n.* hueso parietal, uno de los dos huesos situados en la parte superior y lateral del cráneo.

Parkinson's disease *n.* enfermedad de Parkinson, atrofia o degeneración de los nervios cerebrales que se manifiesta con temblores, debilidad muscular progresiva, cambios en el habla, la manera de andar y la postura.

parodynia *n.* parodinia, parto difícil.

paronychia *n.* paroniquia, infl. del área adyacente a la uña.

parotid *n.* parótida, glándula secretora de saliva localizada cerca del oído.

parotiditis *n.* parotiditis, parotitis. V. **mumps**.

paroxysm *n.* paroxismo, ataque. 1. espasmo o convulsión; 2. síntomas que se repiten y se intensifican.

paroxysmal nocturnal dyspnea *n.* disnea paroxística nocturna, que gen. despierta al paciente inesperadamente y es causada por congestión pulmonar.

paroxysmal tachycardia *n.* taquicardia paroxística, episodios de palpitaciones que comienzan y terminan abruptamente, pero también pueden durar horas y a veces varios días y pueden ser recurrentes.

part *n.* parte, porción; [*component of an instrument*] pieza; **-ly** *adv.* parcialmente, en parte.

parthenogenesis *n.* partenogénesis, reproducción en la cual el óvulo se desarrolla sin ser fecundado por un espermatozoo; **artificial __ / __** artificial.

partial *a.* parcial; **-ly** *adv.* parcialmente.

partial lung colapse *n.* colapso parcial del pulmón.

particle *n.* partícula, porción ínfima de una materia.

parturient *a.* parturienta, mujer que acaba de dar a luz o está en el acto de dar a luz.

parturifacient *n.* parturifaciente, droga que induce el parto.

parturition *n.* parto, alumbramiento.

parvovirus *n.* parvovirus, grupo de virus patógenos que originan enfermedades en animales aunque no en personas.

pass *v.* pasar, aprobar; **to __ away /** morir, fallecer; **to __ on /** contagiar, pegar; **to __ out /** desmayarse; **to __ over /** pasar por, atravesar.

passage *n.* pasaje. 1. conducto o meato; 2. evacuación del intestino.

passing *a.* [*fleeting*] pasajero; **a __ pain /** un dolor __; [*of person*] fallecimiento.

passive *a.* pasivo-a; sumiso-a; inactivo-a, que no es espontáneo o activo; **__ exercise /** ejercicio __ .

passive movement *n.* movimiento pasivo, movimiento creado por una persona asistente que ayuda al paciente a realizar movimientos sin que el paciente tenga que hacer esfuerzo muscular alguno.

passive smoker *n.* fumador-a pasivo-a, persona que inhala el humo producido por un fumador-a próximo-a; **he smokes and his wife is a __ /** él fuma y su esposa es una __ .

pasteurization *n.* pasteurización, proceso de destrucción de microorganismos nocivos por medio de la aplicación de calor regulado.

patch *n.* placa, mancha. 1. pequeña porción de tejido que se caracteriza por pigmentación diferente a la del área que lo rodea; 2. parche, adhesivo aplicado para proteger heridas; **__ test /** prueba alérgica.

patella *n.*, *L.* patella, rótula.

patellectomy *n.* patelectomía, excisión de la patella.

patent *n.* patente, producto de marca autorizada o derecho exclusivo; **medicine /** medicina de __; *a.* patente; accesible; abierto-a.

paternal *a.* paterno, rel. al padre.

paternity *n.* paternidad.

paternity test *n.* prueba de la paternidad, comparación del tipo sanguíneo de un niño o niña con el de un hombre para comprobar si éste puede ser el padre.

path *n.* vía, curso.

pathetic *a.* patético-a.

pathogen *n.* patógeno, agente capaz de producir una enfermedad.

pathogenesis *n.* patogénesis, origen y desarrollo de una enfermedad.

pathogenic *a.* patógeno-a, que causa una enfermedad.

pathognomonic *a.* patognomónico-a, rel. a un signo o síntoma característico de una enfermedad.

pathologic, pathological *a.* patológico-a, rel. a o producido por enfermedades.

pathology *n.* patología, ciencia que estudia la naturaleza y causa de las enfermedades.

pathophysiology *n.* patofisiología, estudio de los efectos de una enfermedad en los procesos fisiológicos.

patience *n.* paciencia.

patient *n.* paciente, enfermo-a, **__ discharge /** alta, egreso del __; **__'s care /** cuidado del __; **private __ /** privado-a; **self-paying __ /** solvente; **-ly** *adv.* con paciencia, pacientemente.

patrilineal *a.* de descendencia paterna; rel. a rasgos heredados del padre.

pattern *n.* patrón, modelo, tipo.

pause

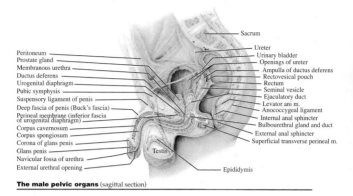

Peritoneum
Prostate gland
Membranous urethra
Ductus deferens
Urogenital diaphragm
Pubic symphysis
Suspensory ligament of penis
Deep fascia of penis (Buck's fascia)
Perineal membrane (inferior fascia of urogenital diaphragm)
Corpus cavernosum
Corpus spongiosum
Corona of glans penis
Glans penis
Navicular fossa of urethra
External urethral opening

Sacrum
Ureter
Urinary bladder
Openings of ureter
Ampulla of ductus deferens
Rectovesical pouch
Rectum
Seminal vesicle
Ejaculatory duct
Levator ani m.
Anococcygeal ligament
Internal anal sphincter
Bulbourethral gland and duct
External anal sphincter
Superficial transverse perineal m.

Testis

Epididymis

The male pelvic organs (*sagittal section*)

pause *n.* pausa, interrupción; paro; **compensatory** ___ / ___ compensatoria; *v.* **to give** ___ / dar que pensar.

peace *n.* paz; ___ **of mind** / tranquilidad de espíritu *v.* **to be at** ___ / estar en paz, tranquilizarse; **to keep, to hold one's** ___ / quedarse tranquilo-a.

peak *n.* [*sickness*] crisis, [*diagram*] cresta; cima, punta.

peau d'orange *n.*, *Fr.* piel de naranja, condición cutánea que asemeja la cáscara de naranja y que es señal importante en el cáncer de la mama.

pectin *n.* pectina, carbohidrato que se obtiene de la cáscara de frutas cítricas y de manzana.

pectoral *a.* pectoral, rel. al pecho.

pectus *n.*, *L.* pecho, tórax.

pederasty *n.* pederastia, relación homosexual anal esp. entre un hombre adulto y un muchacho.

pediatric *a.* pediátrico-a, rel. a la pediatría.

pediatrician *n.* pediatra, médico-a especialista en enfermedades de la infancia.

pediatrics *n.* pediatría, rama de la medicina relacionada con el cuidado y desarrollo de los niños y el tratamiento de las enfermedades que los afectan.

pedicle *n.* pedículo, porción estrecha que conecta un tumor o colgajo con su base.

pediculosis *n.* pediculosis, infestación de piojos.

pedophilia *n.* pedofilia, atracción mórbida sexual de un adulto hacia los niños.

peel *n.* [*fruits*] cáscara, hollejo, corteza; *v.* pelar; [*to shed skin*] despellejarse, pelarse.

peeling *n.* peladura; **chemical** ___ / química; exfoliation.

pellagra *n.* pelagra, enfermedad causada por deficiencia de niacina y caracterizada por dermatitis, trastornos gastrointestinales y finalmente mentales.

pelvic *a.* pélvico-a, pelviano-a, rel. a la pelvis.

pelvic inflammatory disease *n.* enfermedad inflamatoria de la pelvis.

pelvis *n.* pelvis. 1. cavidad en la parte inferior del tórax formada por los huesos de la cadera, el sacro y el cóccix; 2. cavidad en forma de vasija o copa.

pemphigus *n.*, *L.* pénfigo, término usado para definir una variedad de dermatosis, cuya característica común consiste en la manifestación de ampollas que se infectan y revientan.

pendulous *a.* pendular, que oscila o cuelga.

peneal, penial *a.* peneano-a, rel. al pene.

penetrate *v.* penetrar, pasar, atravesar.

penetrating *a.* [*as a pain*] penetrante, agudo-a.

penetration *n.* penetración. 1. acción de penetrar; 2. paso de radiación a través de una sustancia.

penicillin n. penicilina, antibiótico que se obtiene directa o indirectamente de un grupo de cultivos del hongo de la especie *Penicillium*.

penis n. pene, parte exterior del aparato reproductor masculino que contiene la uretra y a través de la cual pasan el semen y la orina. V. ilustración en la página 428.

people n. [*of a nation*] pueblo; [*population*] población, personas, habitantes; gente.

peppermint n. hierbabuena, yerbabuena.

pepsin n. pepsina, enzima principal del jugo gástrico.

peptic ulcer n. úlcera péptica, ulceración de las membranas mucosas del esófago, estómago o duodeno causada por acidez excesiva en el jugo gástrico y producida por tensión aguda o crónica; __ **perforation** / perforación de la __.

per *prep.* por; __ **rectum** / __ el recto, __ vía rectal.

perceive v. darse cuenta de, percibir, advertir.

perception n. percepción, acción de reconocer conscientemente un estímulo sensorial; **extrasensory** __ / __ extrasensorial.

percussion n. percusión, procedimiento de palpación de toque firme en la superficie del cuerpo para producir sensaciones vibratorias que indiquen el estado de una parte interior determinada; **auscultatory** __ / __ auscultatoria.

percutaneous a. percutáneo-a, aplicado-a a través de la piel.

percutaneous transluminal angioplasty n. angioplastia transluminal percutánea, proceso de dilatación de una arteria por medio de un balón inflado a presión.

perennial a. perenne, que perdura más de un año.

perfect a. perfecto-a, completo-a, acabado-a; **-ly** *adv.* perfectamente, completamente.

perfectionism n. perfeccionismo, tendencia al fervor exagerado en la ejecución de actividades sin distinción de importancia entre las mismas.

perfectionist a. perfeccionista.

perforate v. perforar, abrir un agujero.

perforation n. perforación, agujero.

perform v. llevar a cabo, realizar, hacer; **to __ an operation** / operar, intervenir quirúrgicamente.

perfusion n. perfusión, pasaje de un líquido o sustancia a través de un conducto.

perianal a. perianal, situado alrededor del ano.

pericardial, pericardiac a. pericárdico-a, pericardial, rel. al pericardio; __ **effusion** / derrame __; __ **window** / resección __, creación de una apertura en el pericardio.

pericardiectomy n. pericardiectomía, excisión parcial o total del pericardio.

pericarditis n. pericarditis, infl. del pericardio; **constrictive** __ / __ constrictiva; **fibrinous** __ / __ fibrinosa.

pericardium n. pericardio, membrana delicada de capa doble en forma de saco que envuelve el corazón y el inicio de los grandes vasos.

perimetrium n. perimetrio, membrana exterior del útero.

perinatal n. perinatal, rel. a o que ocurre antes, durante o inmediatamente después del nacimiento.

perinatology n. perinatología, estudio del feto y del recién nacido durante el período perinatal.

perineum n. perineo, suelo pelviano delimitado anteriormente por la raíz del escroto en el hombre y la vulva en la mujer y posteriormente por el ano.

period n. período. 1. intervalo de tiempo; época; **incubation** __ / __ de incubación; **latency** __ / __ de latencia; 2. período, menstruación, menses, regla; 3. *gr.* punto.

periodic a. periódico-a.

periodontal a. periodontal, localizado alrededor de un diente.

periodontics n. periodoncia, rama de la odontología que estudia las enfermedades que atacan las áreas que envuelven los dientes.

periosteum n. periosteo, membrana fibrosa gruesa que cubre la superficie de los huesos excepto la superficie articular.

peripheral a. periférico-a, rel. a la periferia.

peripheral nervous system n. sistema nervioso periférico, nervios situados fuera del sistema nervioso central.

periphery n. periferia, parte de un cuerpo fuera del centro.

perishable a. perecedero-a, de fácil descomposición debido al contenido orgánico.

peristalsis n. peristalsis, contracciones ondulantes de estructuras tubulares tal como el canal alimenticio, cuyo movimiento fuerza el contenido almacenado hacia afuera en dirección descendiente.

peritoneal a. peritoneal, rel. al peritoneo; **___ cavity / cavidad ___** .

peritoneal fluid n. fluido peritoneal, fluido excretado por las células del peritoneo.

peritoneum n. peritoneo, membrana que cubre la pared abdominal y las vísceras.

peritonitis n. peritonitis, infl. del peritoneo.

peritonsillar a. periamigdalino-a, que rodea o está cerca de una amígdala.

periurethral a. periuretral, alrededor de la uretra.

perlèche n., Fr. perlèche, pop. boquera, infección en la comisura de los labios y manifestaciones de infl. y fisuras, gen. causada por desnutrición.

permanent a. permanente; **-ly** adv. permanentemente.

permeability n. permeabilidad, cualidad de ser permeable; **capillary ___ / ___** capilar.

permeable a. permeable, que permite el paso de sustancias a través de una membrana u otras estructuras.

permit n. permiso, consentimiento; v. permitir, autorizar.

pernicious a. pernicioso-a, nocivo-a, destructivo-a.

peroxide, hydrogen n. peróxido de hidrógeno, agua oxigenada.

perpendicular a. perpendicular.

persecution n. persecución, acosamiento.

perseveration n. perseveración, tipo de trastorno mental que se manifiesta con repetición anormal de palabras y acciones.

persist v. persistir, perseverar, insistir.

person n. persona.

persona n. persona, personalidad adoptada que encubre la verdadera.

personal a. personal, privado-a.

personality n. personalidad, rasgos, características y conducta individual que distinguen a una persona de otras;

anal **___ / ___** anal; **antisocial ___ / ___** antisocial; **compulsive ___ / ___** compulsiva; **extroverted ___ / ___** extrovertida; **introverted ___ / ___** introvertida; **neurotic ___ / ___** neurótica; **paranoid ___ / ___** paranoica; **psychopathic ___ / ___** psicopática; **split ___ / ___** desdoblada; **schizoid ___ / ___** esquizoide.

personality disorder n. trastorno de la personalidad, término general para un grupo de trastornos de conducta caraacterizados por alteración de los patrones de percepción y cognición; **attention deficit disorder / ___** de falta de atención; **depression disorder / ___** de depresión; **addictive disorder / ___** de adicción; **adjustment disorder / ___** de ajuste; **cyclothymic disorder / ___** ciclotímico; **eating disorder / ___** de deglución; **mood disorder / ___** de cambios emocionales; **panic disorder / ___** de pánico; **phobic disorder / ___** de fobias. V. cuadro en la página 236.

personnel n. personal; **medical ___ /** equipo médico, cuerpo facultativo.

perspective n. perspectiva.

perspiration n. sudor, transpiración.

perspire v. sudar, transpirar.

persuasion n. persuasión, técnica terapéutica que consiste en un acercamiento racional al paciente para orientarle en sus actuaciones.

pertaining a. perteneciente; referente a.

perturbation n. perturbación. 1. sentimiento de inquietud; 2. variación anormal de un estado regular a otro.

pertussis, whooping cough n. pertusis, tosferina, enfermedad infantil infecciosa que se inicia con un estado catarral seguido de una tos seca persistente.

perversion n. perversión, desviación depravada, gen. de índole sexual.

pervert n. pervertido-a, persona que manifiesta alguna forma de perversión.

pessary n. pesario, dispositivo de goma en forma de copa que se inserta en la vagina y se usa como soporte del útero.

pessimism n. pesimismo, propensión a juzgar situaciones negativamente.

pessimist n. pesimista, persona que muestra pesimismo.

pest n. 1. insecto nocivo; 2. peste. V. **plague**.

pesticide n. pesticida, exterminador de insectos y roedores.

pet *n.* 1. animal doméstico favorito; 2. niño-a mimado-a.

petechia *n.* (*pl.* **petechiae**) petequia, mancha hemorrágica pequeña que se manifiesta en la piel y las mucosas en casos de estado febril esp. en la tifoidea.

petit mal *n.*, *Fr. petit mal*, ataque epiléptico benigno con pérdida del conocimiento pero sin convulsiones.

peyote *n.* peyote, planta de la que se extrae la mescalina, droga alucinatoria.

pH *n.* indica el grado de acidez o alcalinidad de una sustancia; **cutaneous** ___ / ___ cutáneo; **blood** ___ / ___ sanguíneo.

phagocyte *n.* fagocito, célula que ingiere y destruye otras células, sustancias y partículas extrañas.

phagocytosis *n.* fagocitosis, proceso de ingestión y digestión realizado por fagocitos.

phalanx *n.* (*pl.* **phalanxes, phalanges**) falange, uno de los huesos largos de los dedos de los pies o las manos.

phallic *a.* fálico, rel. al pene.

phantom *n.* fantasma, fantoma. 1. imagen mental; 2. patrón transparente del cuerpo y sus partes.

pharmaceutics *n.* preparaciones farmacéuticas.

pharmacist *n.* farmacéutico-a, boticario-a.

pharmacokinetics *n.* farmacocinética, estudio *in vivo* del metabolismo y acción de las drogas.

pharmacology *n.* farmacología, estudio de drogas, medicamentos, su naturaleza, origen, efectos y usos.

pharmacopeia *n.* farmacopea, compendio de drogas, agentes químicos y medicamentos regidos por una autoridad oficial que sirve de estándar en la preparación y dispensación de productos farmacéuticos.

pharmacy *n.* farmacia, botica.

pharyngitis *n.* faringitis, infl. de la faringe.

pharynx *n.* faringe, pasaje del aire de las fosas nasales a la laringe y de la boca al esófago en el tracto alimenticio.

phase *n.* fase, estado de desarrollo, estado transitorio.

phasic *a.* fásico-a, rel. a una fase.

phenobarbital *n.* fenobarbital, hipnótico, sedante, nombre comercial Luminal.

phenomenon *n.* (*pl.* **phenomena**) fenómeno. 1. evento o manifestación de cualquier índole; 2. síntoma objetivo de una enfermedad.

phenotype *n.* fenotipo, características visibles de un organismo como resultado de interacción entre el ambiente y los factores hereditarios.

phimosis *n.* fimosis, estrechamiento del orificio del prepucio que impide que éste pueda extenderse hacia atrás sobre el glande.

phlebitis *n.* flebitis, infl. de una vena, trastorno común esp. en las extremidades.

phlebolith *n.* flebolito, depósito calcáreo en una vena.

phlebotomy *n.* flebotomía, venotomía, incisión en una vena para sacar sangre.

phlegm *n.* flema. 1. mucus; 2. uno de los cuatro humores del cuerpo.

phlegmon *n.* flemón, infl. del tejido celular.

phobia *n.* fobia, temor exagerado e irracional.

phonation *n.* fonación, emisión de la voz.

phone *n.* teléfono; ___ **call** / llamada telefónica.

phonetic *a.* fonético-a, rel. a la voz y a los sonidos articulados.

phonetics *n.* fonética, ciencia que estudia la articulación de los sonidos y su pronunciación.

phonogram *n.* fonograma, representación gráfica de la intensidad de un sonido.

phonoscope *n.* fonoscopio, instrumento para registrar los sonidos del corazón.

phosphorus *n.* fósforo, elemento no metálico que se encuentra en alcaloides.

photochemotherapy *n.* fotoquimioterapia, tratamiento con drogas que producen una reacción a la luz de rayos ultravioleta o rayos solares.

photocoagulation *n.* fotocoagulación, proceso usado en cirugía óptica por el cual un rayo intenso de luz controlada (laser) produce una coagulación localizada.

photodermatitis *n.* fotodermatitis, reacción anormal a la exposición a los rayos solares.

phototherapy *n.* fototerapia, exposición a los rayos del sol o a una luz artificial con propósito terapéutico.

phrenetic *a.* frenético-a, maníaco-a.

physic *n.* medicamento, esp. un catártico o purgante.

physical *a.* físico-a, rel. al cuerpo y su condición; __ **examination** / examen __; __ **fitness** / acondicionamiento __; __ **therapist** / terapeuta __; __ **therapy** / terapia __.

physician *n.* médico-a; **attending** __ / __ de cabecera; **consulting** __ / __ consultante, consultor; **family** __ / __ de familia; __ **on call** / __ de guardia; **primary** __ / __ de asistencia primaria; **referring** __ / __ recomendante.

physiology *n.* fisiología, ciencia que estudia las funciones de los organismos vivos y los procesos químicos o físicos que los caracterizan.

physiotherapy *n.* fisioterapia, tratamiento por medio de agentes físicos como agua, calor o luz.

physique *n.* físico, presencia, figura.

phytobezoar *n.* fitobezoar, concreción formada por fibra vegetal que se deposita en el estómago o el intestino y no se digiere.

pia mater *n.*, *L.* piamáter, piamadre, membrana vascular fina, la más interna de las meninges.

pica *n.* pica, deseo insaciable de ingerir sustancias que no son comestibles.

Pick's disease *n.* Pick, enfermedad de, tipo de demencia senil.

picture *n.* fotografía; lámina; retrato.

piece *n.* pedazo, parte.

piercing *a.* penetrante, agudo-a.

pigeon-toed *a.* patizambo-a.

pigment *n.* pigmento, colorante.

pigmentation *n.* pigmentación, coloración.

piles *n., pl.* almorranas, hemorroides.

piliation *n.* piliación, formación y desarrollo de pelo.

pill *n.* pastilla, píldora; **birth control** __ / la píldora, píldora de control del embarazo; **pain** __ / calmante, sedativo, __ para el dolor; **sleeping** __ / sedativo, __ para dormir.

pillow *n.* almohada; [*inflatable*] almohadilla, cojín.

pimple *n.* barrillo, [*blackhead*] espinilla, grano de la cara.

pin *n.* clavo ortopédico, pieza de metal o hueso que se usa para unir partes de un hueso fracturado.

pinch *n.* pellizco; *v.* pellizcar; comprimir, apretar.

pinched nerve *n.* nervio pellizcado.

pineal gland *n.* glándula o cuerpo pineal.

pinkeye *n.* conjuntivitis catarral, oftalmia purulenta.

pinna *n.*, *L.* pinna, pabellón de la oreja.

pipet, pipette *n.* pipeta, probeta, tubo de ensayo.

pitch *n.* tono, diapasón, cualidad de un sonido de acuerdo con la frecuencia de las ondas que lo producen.

pituitary gland *n.* glándula pituitaria. hypophysis.

pity *n.* lástima, compasión; **what a** __ ! / ¡qué __ !

place *n.* lugar, sitio; **in** __ **of** / en __ de *v.* colocar; **to put in** __ / colocar en su __.

placebo *n.* placebo, sustancia anodina sin valor medicinal gen. usada en experimentos por comparación; __ **controlled trial** / prueba controlada por __.

placenta *n.* placenta, órgano vascular que se desarrolla en la pared del útero a través del cual el feto se nutre de la madre por medio del cordón umbilical; **early, previa** __ / __ previa, anterior al feto en relación con la apertura externa del cuello uterino, lo que puede causar una hemorragia grave.

placental *a.* placentario-a, de la placenta, rel. a la placenta; __ **insufficiency** / insuficiencia __.

plague *n.* peste. 1. peste bubónica, infección epidémica transmitida por la picadura de pulgas de ratas; 2. enfermedad epidémica que causa alta mortalidad.

plain *a.* común, ordinario-a.

plan *n.* plan, planificación; intento; *v.* planear.

plane *n.* plano. 1. superficie lisa y plana; 2. superficie relativamente lisa formada por un corte imaginario o un corte real a través de una parte del cuerpo; **axial** __ / __ axial; **coronal** __ / __ coronal, frontal; **sagittal** __ / __ sagital.

planned parenthood *n.* planificación familiar.

planning *n.* planeamiento, planificación; organización; **family** __ / __ familiar.

plant *a.* planta; **medicinal** __ / __, yerba medicinal.

plantar *a.* plantar, rel. a la planta del pie; __ **reflex** / reflejo plantare Babinski's sign.

plaque, placque *n.* placa; plaqueta. 1. cualquier superficie de la piel o membrana mucosa; 2. plaqueta sanguínea.

plasma *n.* plasma, componente líquido de la sangre y linfa que se compone en su mayor parte (91%) de agua; __ **proteins** / proteínas sanguíneas.

plaster *n.* yeso, emplaste, molde; __ **cast** / vendaje enyesado, tablilla de __.

plastic *n.* plástico; *a.* plástico-a

plasticity *n.* plasticidad, capacidad para moldearse.

plastic surgery *n.* cirugía plástica, proceso quirúrgico para reparar o reconstruir estructuras del cuerpo.

plate *n.* placa. 1. estructura lisa tal como una lámina ósea; 2. pieza de metal que se usa como soporte de una estructura.

platelet *n.* plaqueta, elemento celular esencial en la coagulación de la sangre.

play therapy *n.* terapia infantil aplicada en un ambiente de juguetes y juegos infantiles por medio de los cuales se estimula a los niños a revelar conflictos interiores.

please *int.* por favor; **come in** __! / ¡entre, entra por favor!; *v.* gustar, agradar, satisfacer; tener placer, tener gusto en.

pleasing *a.* agradable, placentero-a, gustoso-a.

pleasure principle *n.* principio del placer, conducta dirigida a satisfacer deseos propios y evadir el dolor.

plethora *n.* plétora, exceso de cualquiera de los líquidos del organismo.

plethysmography *n.* pletismografía, registro de las variaciones de volumen que ocurren en una parte u órgano en relación con la cantidad de sangre que pasa sobre los mismos.

pleura *n.* pleura, membrana doble que cubre los pulmones y la cavidad torácica; **parietal** __ / __ parietal; **visceral** __ / __ visceral.

pleural *a.* pleural, rel. a la pleura; __ **cavity** / cavidad __; __ **effusion** / derrame __.

pleuralgia *n.* pleuralgia, dolor en la pleura o en un costado.

pleurisy *n.* pleuresía, infl. de la pleura.

pleuroscopy *n.* pleuroscopía, examen de la cavidad pleural a través de una incisión en el tórax.

plug *n.* tapón.

plumbism *n.* plumbismo, envenenamiento crónico con plomo.

pneumatization *n.* neumatización, formación de cavidades llenas de aire en un hueso esp. en el hueso temporal.

pneumatocele *n.* neumatocele. 1. hernia de tejido pulmonar; 2. saco o tumor que contiene gas.

pneumococcal *a.* neumocócico-a, rel. a la neumonía o que la causa.

pneumococcus *n, L.* (*pl.* **pneumococci**) neumococo, microorganismo o tipo de bacteria gram-positiva que causa neumonía aguda y otras infecciones del tracto respiratorio superior.

pneumocystis carinii pneumonia *n.* neumonía neumocística carinii, tipo de pulmonía aguda intersticial causada por el bacilo *Pneumocysti carinii*, considerada una de las infecciones oportunistas comunes del SIDA.

pneumoencephalography *n.* neumoencefalografía, rayos-x del cerebro por medio de aire o gas inyectado para permitir distinguir visualmente la corteza y los ventrículos cerebrales.

pneumomediastinum *n., L.* neumomediastinum, presencia de gas o de aire en los tejidos del mediastino.

pneumonia *n.* pulmonía, neumonía, enfermedad infecciosa causada por bacterias o virus presentes en el tracto respiratorio superior; **double** __ / __ doble; __ **lobar** / __ lobar; **staphylococcal** __ / __ estafilocócica.

pneumonic *a.* neumónico-a, rel. a los pulmones o a la neumonía.

pneumonic plague *n.* peste neumónica, forma de peste con síntomas de esputos sanguíneos, escalofríos y fiebre (calentura) alta que puede ser letal.

pneumothorax *n.* neumotórax, acumulación de aire o gas en la cavidad pleural que resulta en colapso del pulmón afectado; **spontaneous** __ / __ espontáneo; **tension** __ / __ por tensión.

pocket *n.* saco, bolsa; [*clothing*] bolsillo.

pockmark *n.* marca, señal o cicatriz. 1. marca de una pústula; 2. señal que deja la viruela.

podiatrist *n.* podiatra, especialista en podiatría.

podiatry *n.* podiatría, diagnóstico y tratamiento de afecciones de los pies.

poison *n.* veneno; [*insect, reptile bite*] ponzoña; substancia tóxica; __ ivy / hiedra venenosa.

poisoning *n.* envenenamiento.

poisonous *a.* venenoso-a; tóxico-a.

polarity *n.* polaridad. 1. cualidad de poseer polos; 2. presentación de efectos opuestos en dos extremos o polos.

polarization *n.* polarización.

pole *n.* polo. 1. cada uno de los extremos opuestos de un cuerpo u órgano o de una parte esférica u oval.

policy *n.* póliza; reglamento; **insurance** __ / __ de seguros.

polio, poliomyelitis *n.* polio, poliomielitis, parálisis infantil, enfermedad contagiosa que ataca el sistema nervioso central y causa parálisis en los músculos esp. de las piernas.

poliovirus *n.* poliovirus, agente causante de la poliomielitis.

pollen *n.* polen.

pollute *v.* contaminar, corromper.

pollution *n.* polución, contaminación; **air** __ / __ del aire; **water** __ / __ del agua.

polyarthritis *n.* poliartritis, infl. de varias articulaciones.

polyarticular *a.* poliarticular, que afecta varias articulaciones.

polyclinic *n.* policlínica, hospital general.

polycystic *a.* poliquístico-a, que está formado-a por varios quistes; __ **kidney disease** / enfermedad __ del riñón; __ **ovarian syndrome** / síndrome __ ovárico.

polycythemia *n.* policitemia, aumento excesivo de glóbulos rojos; __ **rubra** / __ vera secundaria, __ vera; **primary** __ / __ primaria.

polydactyly *n.* polidactilia, condición anormal de poseer más de cinco dedos en la mano o el pie.

polydipsia *n.* polidipsia, sed insaciable.

polygraph *n.* polígrafo, instrumento para obtener diversas pulsaciones arteriales y venosas simultáneamente.

polymorphonuclear *a.* polimorfonucleado-a, que tiene un núcleo lobular complejo.

polymorphonuclear leukocyte *n.* leucocito polimorfonucleado, granulocito con núcleo de lóbulos múltiples.

polymyalgia *n.* polimialgia, condición caracterizada por dolor en distintos músculos; __ **rheumatica** / __ reumática.

polymyopathy *n.* polimiopatía, cualquier enfermedad que afecta varios músculos simultáneamente.

polyneuropathy *n.* polineuropatía, enfermedad que afecta varios nervios a la vez.

polyp *n.* pólipo, cualquier protuberancia o bulto que se desarrolla de una membrana mucosa.

polypectomy *n.* polipectomía, excisión de un pólipo.

polyposis *n.* poliposis, formación numerosa de pólipos.

polysaccharide *n.* polisacárido, carbohidrato que puede disolverse en agua.

polyunsaturated *a.* poli-nosaturado, que denota un ácido graso.

polyuria *n.* poliuria, excesiva secreción y eliminación de orina asi como en diabetes.

pomade *n.* pomada, sustancia medicinal semisólida para uso externo.

pons *n.*, *L.* pons, formación de tejido que sirve de puente entre dos partes.

pontiac fever *n.* legionnaire's disease.

poor *a.* pobre, necesitado-a; deficiente; **in** __ **condition** / en mala condición, en mal estado.

popliteal *a.* poplíteo-a, área posterior de la rodilla.

popper *n.*, *pop.* nombre atribuído a algunas drogas adictivas.

population *n.* población, habitantes de un área.

porcine *a.* porcino-a, rel. al cerdo.

pore, porus *n.* poro, abertura diminuta tal como la de una glándula sudorípara.

porosis *n.* porosis, formacion de una cavidad.

porous *a.* poroso-a, permeable.

porphyria *n.* porfiria, defecto metabólico congénito que se caracteriza por exceso de porfirina en la sangre, en la orina y en las heces fecales, causando numerosos trastornos físicos y psiquiátricos.

porta *n.*, *L.* porta, entrada, esp. la parte de un órgano por donde penetran vasos sanguíneos y nervios.

portacaval *a.* portacava, rel. a la vena porta y la vena cava inferior.

portal *a.* portal, rel. al sistema portal.

portal circulation *n.* circulación portal, curso por el cual la sangre entra al hígado por la vena porta y sale por la vena hepática.

portal hypertension *n.* hipertensión portal, aumento de la presión en la vena porta debido a una obstrucción.

portal vein *n.* vena porta, vena formada por varias ramas de venas que provienen de órganos abdominales.

portion *v.* porción.

position *n.* posición. 1. actitud o postura del cuerpo; **anatomic** ___ / ___ anatómica; **central** ___ / ___ central; **decubitus** ___ / ___ decúbito; **deep** ___ / ___ dentro de, profunda; **distal** ___ / ___ distal; **genupectoral** ___ / ___ genupectoral; **inferior** ___ / ___ inferior; **lateral** ___ / ___ lateral, de un lado; **lithotomy** ___ / ___ de litotomía; **lying down** ___ / ___ yacente, acostada; **medial** ___ / ___ media; **posterior** ___ / ___ posterior, detrás de; **prone** ___ / ___ prona, boca abajo; **superficial** ___ / ___ superficial; **superior** ___ / ___ superior, encima de; **supine** ___ / ___ supina, boca arriba; **upright** ___ / ___ erecta; 2. posición y presentación del feto.

positive *a.* positivo-a, afirmativo-a.

positivity *n.* positividad, manifestación de una reacción positiva.

possessed *a.* poseído-a, dominado-a por una idea o pasión.

possession *n.* posesión.

posterior *a.* posterior. 1. rel. a la parte dorsal o trasera de una estructura; 2. que continúa.

posthumous *a.* póstumo, que ocurre después de la muerte.

posthypnotic *a.* posthipnótico-a, que sigue al estado hipnótico.

postictal *a.* post ictal, después de un ataque o convulsión.

post mature *a.* postmaduro-a, rel. a un recién nacido después de un embarazo prolongado.

postmortem *n.*, *L.* post mortem, después de la muerte; autopsia.

postnasal *a.* postnasal, detrás de la nariz.

postnasal drip *n.* goteo postnasal.

postoperative *a.* postoperatorio-a, que ocurre después de la operación; ___ **care** / cuidado ___; ___ **complication** / complicación ___ .

postpartum *n.*, *L.* postpartum, después del parto; ___ **blues** / estado de depresión que sigue al parto; ___ **pituitary insufficiency** / insuficiencia pituitaria del ___.

postpartum period, puerperium *n.* puerperio, período de aproximadamente seis semanas después del parto durante el cual los órganos de la madre vuelven a su estado normal.

postpartum psychosis *n.* psicosis del postpartum.

postpone *v.* posponer, demorar, aplazar.

postsurgical pain treatment *n.* tratamiento de dolor posoperatorio.

postural *a.* postural, rel. a la postura del cuerpo; ___ **hypotension** / hipotensión ___, descenso de la presión arterial en posición erecta.

posture *n.* postura, posición del cuerpo.

potable *a.* potable, salubre, que puede beberse.

potassium *n.* potasio, mineral que se encuentra en el cuerpo combinado con otros, esencial en la conducción de impulsos nerviosos y actividad muscular.

potbelly *n.* panza, barriga.

potency *n.* fuerza, potencia.

potent *a.* potente, fuerte; eficaz.

potential *a.* potencial, que existe en forma de cierta capacidad o disposición.

potion *n.* poción, dosis de líquido medicinal.

pouch *n.* bolsa, saco, cavidad.

pour *v.* verter, vaciar, derramar.

poverty *n.* pobreza, carencia.

powder *n.* polvo; **powdered** *a.* en polvo.

power *n.* poder, fuerza.

pox *n.* enfermedad eruptiva de la piel caracterizada por manifestación de vesículas que se convierten en pústulas.

practical *a.* práctico-a.

practice *n.* práctica; costumbre; **private** ___ / ___ privada *v.* practicar.

prandial *a.* prandial, rel. a las comidas.

preagonal *a.* preagónico-a; moribundo-a, al borde de la muerte.

preanesthetic *n.* preanestésico, agente preliminar que se administra con anticipación a la anestesia general.

precancerous *a.* precanceroso-a, susceptible a o que puede convertirse en un cáncer.

precarious *a.* precario-a.

precaution *n.* precaución.

precede

precede *v.* preceder, anteceder.

precipitate *n.* precipitado, depósito de partes sólidas que se asientan en una solución; *a.* precipitado-a, que sucede con rapidez.

precision *n.* precisión, exactitud.

precocious *a.* precoz, de un desarrollo más avanzado que el normal para la edad; **__ child** / niño-a __ .

precocity *n.* precocidad, desarrollo de rasgos físicos o facultades mentales más avanzados que lo normal en comparación con la edad cronológica.

precursor *n.* precursor-a, predecesor-a, manifestación tal como la aparición de un síntoma o señal antes de desarrollarse una enfermedad; *a.* precursor-a, predecesor-a; preliminar.

predict *v.* predecir.

predisposed *a.* predispuesto-a, que tiene susceptibilidad o tendencia a contraer una enfermedad.

predisposition *n.* predisposición, inclinación a desarrollar una condición o enfermedad debido a factores genéticos, ambientales o psicológicos.

predominant *a.* predominante.

preeclampsia *n.* preeclampsia, condición tóxica que se ve en la última etapa del embarazo y que se manifiesta con hipertensión, albuminuria y edema.

prefer *v.* preferir, seleccionar.

preferable *a.* preferible, favorito-a.

pregnancy *n.* embarazo, gravidez, estado de gestación; **ectopic __** / __ ectópico; **extrauterine __** / __ extrauterino; **incomplete __** / __ incompleto; **interstitial __** / __ intersticial; **false __** / __ falso; **multiple __** / __ múltiple; **prolonged __** / __ prolongado; **surrogate __** / __ subrogado; **tubal __** / __ tubárico.

pregnant *a.* embarazada, encinta, en estado de gestación; grávida.

prejudice *n.* prejuicio.

preliminary *a.* preliminar.

premature *a.* [*newborn*] prematuro-a, nacido antes de llegar a término.

premedication *n.* premedicación.

premenstrual *n.* premenstrual, antes de la menstruación; **__ tension** / tensión __ .

premenstrual syndrome *n.* síndrome premenstrual, síndrome que se manifiesta días anteriores a la menstruación y que se caracteriza por irritabilidad, retención de líquidos y tensión emocional.

prenatal *a.* prenatal, anterior al nacimiento; **__ care** / cuidado __ .

preoccupation *n.* preocupación.

preoccupy *v.* preocupar; preocuparse.

preoperative care *n.* cuidado preoperatorio, cuidado preliminar a la operación.

prep *abbr.* término que se usa esp. para referirse a todo lo relacionado con el proceso preoperatorio.

preparation *n.* preparación. 1. acción de preparar algo; 2. un medicamento que se prepara para ser administrado.

prepare *v.* preparar.

prepubescent *a.* prepubescente, anterior a la pubertad.

prepuce *n.* prepucio, pliegue de piel sobre el glande del pene.

prerenal *a.* prerrenal. 1. situado frente al riñón; 2. que tiene lugar en la circulación antes de llegar al riñón.

presbiopia *n.* presbiopía, presbicia, condición de la visión que ocurre en la vejez a causa de una deficiencia en la elasticidad del cristalino.

prescribe *v.* prescribir, recetar.

prescribed *a.*, *pp.* of **to prescribe**, recetado, ordenado-a.

prescription *n.* receta; **__ tablet, pad** / formulario.

presence *n.* [*looks*] presencia, aspecto; [*attendance*] asistencia.

present *n.* [*presence*] presencia; *v.* **to be __** / asistir, estar presente física y psicológicamente asistiendo a un paciente cuando lo necesite.

presentation *n.* presentación. 1. reporte oral; 2. posición del feto en el útero según se detecta en un examen, o posición de salida en relación al canal del parto en el momento del nacimiento; **breech __** / __ de nalgas; **brow __** / __ de cejas o frente; **cephalic __** / __ de cabeza; **face __** / __ de cara; **footling __** / __ de pies; **shoulder __** / __ de hombro; **transverse __** / __ transversa.

preservation *n.* preservación, conservación.

preservative *n.* preservativo, conservador. 1. agente que se añade a un alimento o medicamento para impedir el desarrollo de bacterias; 2. profiláctico.

preserve *v.* preservar, conservar.

pressor *a.* presor, que tiende a aumentar la presión sanguínea.

pressure *n*. presión, tensión, compresión; **arterial** ___ / ___ arterial, presión o tensión de la sangre sobre las paredes de los vasos capilares; **atmospheric** ___ / ___ atmosférica, la que ejerce la masa de aire alrededor de la tierra; **central venous** ___ / ___ central venosa, presión de la sangre en la aurícula derecha del corazón; **diastolic** ___ / ___ diastólica, presión arterial durante la diástole; **intracranial** ___ / ___ intracraneana o intracraneal, presión ejercida dentro de la cavidad craneana; **intrathoracic** ___ / ___ intratorácica, presión dentro del tórax; **osmotic** ___ / ___ osmótica; osmosis; **partial** ___ / ___ parcial, la que ejerce uno de los gases de una composición mixta; **pulse** ___ / ___ de pulso; **systolic** ___ / ___ sistólica, presión arterial durante la contracción de los ventrículos; **venous** ___ / ___ venosa, la de la sangre en las venas; *v.* hacer presión, presionar.

pressure point *n*. punto de presión, área donde puede sentirse el pulso o hacer presión para contener un sangramiento.

pressure sore *n*. úlcera de decúbito.

pretend *v*. pretender, fingir, aparentar.

preterm *n*. pretérmino, lo que concierne a sucesos anteriores a completar el término de treinta y siete semanas en un embarazo.

prevalence *n*. prevalencia, número de casos en una población afectados por la misma enfermedad en un tiempo determinado.

prevent *v*. prevenir, precaver, evitar.

preventive *a*. preventivo-a; ___ **health services** / servicios de salud ___ -s.

previous *a*. previo-a, anterior.

priapism *n*. priapismo, erección prolongada y dolorosa del pene a consecuencia de una enfermedad.

price *n*. precio, valor, costo.

prick *n*. pinchazo; punzada; picadura, aguijón; *v.* picar, punzar, aguijonear, pinchar.

prickly heat *n*. salpullido, sarpullido.

primarily *adv*. primeramente; principalmente, primordialmente.

primary *a*. inicial, primario-a, rel. al contacto o atención de un caso en su principio; ___ **physician** / médico de cabecera, facultativo que atiende al paciente inicialmente, esp. un pediatra o médico de familia.

primary care *n*. atención inicial del paciente.

prime *a*. primero-a, principal; *v.* **to be in one's** ___ / estar en la flor de la vida.

primitive *a*. primitivo-a; embriónico-a.

principal *a*. principal, más importante.

principle *n*. principio. 1. ingrediente esencial de un compuesto químico; 2. regla; orden.

prior *n*. antecesor, predecesor; *a.* previo-a; ___ **to** / anterior a, antes de.

priority *n*. prioridad, preferencia, precedencia.

privacy *n*. vida privada; aislamiento.

private *a*. privado-a, particular, exclusivo-a; ___ **hospital** / clínica; ___ **practice** / consulta particular; ___ **room** / cuarto ___; **-ly** *adv*. privadamente.

privation *n*. privación, necesidad.

privilege *n*. privilegio, derecho.

privileged *a*. confidencial, privilegiado-a; reservado-a; ___ **information** / información ___ o reservada.

probability *n*. probabilidad.

probable *a*. probable, casi posible; **-ly** *adv*. probablemente.

probe *n*. sonda, instrumento flexible que se usa para explorar cavidades o conductos y para medir la penetración de una herida; **hollow** ___ / ___ acanalada.

problem *n*. problema; cuestión; trastorno; ___ **solving** / solución de ___ -s.

procedure *n*. procedimiento; **clinical** ___ / ___ clínico; **invasive** ___ / ___ invasivo; **noninvasive** ___ / ___ no invasivo; **surgical** ___ / ___ quirúrgico; **therapeutic** ___ / ___ terapéutico.

proceed *v*. proceder, continuar, seguir adelante, avanzar.

process *n*. proceso, método, sistema.

procreate *v*. engendrar, procrear, reproducir.

procreation *n*. procreación, reproducción.

proctalgia *n*. proctalgia, dolor en el recto y el ano.

proctitis *n*. proctitis, infl. de la mucosa del recto y del ano.

proctologist *n*. proctólogo-a, especialista en proctología.

proctoscope *n*. proctoscopio, espéculo rectal, tipo de endoscopio usado para examinar el recto.

prodromal *a*. prodrómico-a, rel. a la fase inicial de una enfermedad.

product

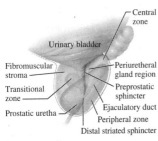

Central zone
Urinary bladder
Fibromuscular stroma
Transitional zone
Prostatic uretha
Periurethral gland region
Preprostatic sphincter
Ejaculatory duct
Peripheral zone
Distal striated sphincter

The prostate

product *n.* producto; resultado, efecto.
productive *a.* productivo-a, fecundo-a.
profession *n.* profesión, carrera, oficio.
professional *n.* profesional, facultivo-a; __ **care** / cuidado __; __ **help** / asistencia __; *a.* profesional; facultativo-a.
profile *n.* perfil, bosquejo, esbozo; **biochemical** __ / __ bioquímico); **physical** __ / __ físico.
profit *n.* beneficio, ganancia; ventaja.
profunda *a., L* (*pl.* **profunda**) muy interior, en referencia esp. a algunas arterias.
profuse *a.* profuso-a; abundante; **-ly** *adv.* profusamente; abundantemente.
progeny *n.* descendencia, prole.
progesterone *n.* progesterona, hormona esteroide segregada por los ovarios.
prognose *v.* pronosticar o predecir el desarrollo de una enfermedad.
prognosis *n.* pronóstico, evaluación del curso probable de una enfermedad.
prognosticate *v.* pronosticar.
progress *n.* progreso; *v.* **to make** __ / progresar, mejorar.
progressive *a.* progresivo-a, que avanza.
projection *n.* proyección. 1. protuberancia; 2. mecanismo por el cual el (la) paciente atribuye inconscientemente a otras personas u objetos las cualidades y sentimientos propios que rechaza.
prolapse *n.* prolapso, caída de un órgano o parte.
proliferation *n.* proliferación, multiplicación en número por reproducción esp. de células similares.
proliferous, prolific *a.* prolífero-a, que se reproduce fácilmente.
prolong *v.* prolongar, extender; retardar.

prominence *n.* prominencia, proyección; *pop.* bulto.
promise *n.* promesa; *v.* prometer, dar la palabra.
prompt *a.* puntual, a tiempo.
pronate *v.* pronar, poner el cuerpo o parte del mismo en posición prona.
prone *a.* acostado-a, postrado-a. 1. en posición acostada boca abajo; 2. con la mano virada, apoyada en el dorso; 3. propenso, susceptible a contraer una enfermedad.
pronounce *v.* pronunciar, articular sonidos de letras.
proof *n.* prueba, comprobación; *v.* probar, demostrar.
propagation *n.* propagación, reproducción.
property *n.* propiedad, cualidad, característica, atributo. V. cuadro en la página 199.
prophylactic *n.* profiláctico. 1. agente o método para evitar infecciones; 2. contraceptivo.
prophylaxis *n.* profilaxis, medidas para prevenir enfermedades o su propagación.
proprietary medicine *n.* medicamento de patente.
proprioceptive *a.* propioceptivo-a, que recibe estímulos.
proprioceptor *n.* propioceptor, terminación nerviosa receptora que responde a estímulos y transmite información de los movimientos y posiciones del cuerpo.
proptosis *n.* proptosis, desplazamiento de un órgano hacia adelante tal como el globo ocular.
prosencephalon *n.* prosencéfalo, porción anterior de la vesícula cerebral de la que se desarrollan el diencéfalo y el telencéfalo.
prostate *n.* próstata, glándula masculina que rodea el cuello de la vejiga y la uretra. V. ilustración esta página.
prostatectomy *n.* prostatectomía, excisión parcial o total de la próstata; **laser**__ / __ de láser; **perineal** __ / __ perineal; **radical** __ / __ radical; **transvesical** __ / __ transvesical.
prostatic *a.* prostático-a, rel. a la próstata; __ **hypertrophy** / hipertrofia __, agrandamiento benigno de la próstata debido a la vejez.
prostatic specific antigen (PSA) *n.* antígeno prostático específico (APE), examen sanguíneo

psychodrama

para evaluar los antígenos prostáticos específicos en la circulación.

prostatism *n.* prostatismo, trastorno debido a una obstrucción del cuello de la vejiga por agrandamiento de la próstata.

prostatitis *n.* prostatitis, infl. de la próstata.

prosthesis *n.* prótesis, reemplazo de una parte del cuerpo con un sustituto artificial.

prosthetics *n.* prostética, rama de la cirugía que se dedica al reemplazo de partes del cuerpo.

prostrate *a.* postrado-a. 1. en posición prona o supina; 2. débil, abatido-a; *v.* postrar; abatir; *vr.* postrarse; abatirse, debilitarse.

prostration *n.* postración, debilidad, abatimiento.

protean *n.* protéico, que se manifiesta en distintas formas.

protection *n.* protección, cuidado.

protective isolation *n.* aislamiento protector, estado que se recomienda en casos de pacientes de baja resistencia o inmunidad.

protein *n.* proteína, complejo compuesto nitrogenado esencial en el desarrollo y preservación de los tejidos del cuerpo;
— **balance** / balance de las — -s;
— **concentration** / — concentración de — .

proteinemia *n.* proteinemia, proteínas en la sangre.

proteinosis *n.* proteinosis, acumulación en exceso de proteínas en los tejidos.

proteinuria *n.* proteinuria, presencia de proteínas en la orina.

prothrombin *n.* protrombina, una de las cuatro proteínas principales del plasma junto a la albúmina, la globulina y el fibrinógeno.

protocol *n.* protocolo, notas oficiales de un procedimiento.

protoplasm *n.* protoplasma, parte esencial de la célula que incluye el citoplasma y el núcleo.

prototype *n.* prototipo, modelo, ejemplo.

protozoon *n.* (*pl.* **protozoa**) protozoo, organismo unicelular.

protraction *n.* protracción, tracción hacia afuera, como en la mandíbula.

protruding *a.* saliente.

protrusion *n.* protrusión, posición

saliente o impulsado hacia adelante de un estado o trastorno.

protuberance *n.* protuberancia, prominencia.

provide *v.* proveer, dar, abastecer.

providence *n.* providencia.

provisional *a.* provisional, interino; **-ly** *adv.* provisionalmente, por lo pronto.

proximal *a.* próximo, cerca del punto de referencia.

prurigo *n.* prurigo, condición cutánea crónica inflamatoria que se caracteriza por pápulas pequeñas y picazón intensa.

pruritus *n.* prurito, comezón, picazón.

pseudoaneurysm *n.* pseudoaneurisma, condición semejante a la dilatación de un aneurisma.

pseudocyst *n.* pseudoquiste, formación semejante a la de un quiste.

pseudogout *n.* seudogota, condición artrítica recurrente con síntomas similares a los de la gota.

pseudopregnancy *n.* embarazo falso o imaginario.

psoriasis *n.* psoriasis, dermatitis crónica que se manifiesta con manchas rojas cubiertas de escamas blancas.

psyche *n.* psique, proceso mental consciente o inconsciente.

psychedelic *a.* psicodélico-a, rel. a substancias o drogas que pueden inducir alteraciones perceptuales tales como alucinaciones y delirios.

psychiatric *a.* psiquiátrico-a, siquiátrico-a.

psychiatrist *n.* psiquiatra, siquiatra, especialista en psiquiatría.

psychiatry *n.* psiquiatría, rama de la medicina que estudia los trastornos mentales.

psychic *a.* psíquico-a, rel. a la mente o psique.

psychoanalysis *n.* psicoanálisis, método de análisis psicológico creado por Sigmund Freud que se vale de la interpretación de los sueños y de la libre asociación de ideas para hacer al paciente consciente de conflictos reprimidos y tratar de ajustar su conducta emocional.

psychoanalyst *n.* psicoanalista, analista.

psychodrama *n.* psicodrama, método de terapia psíquica en el cual se dramatizan situaciones conflictivas de la vida del paciente con la participación de éste.

psychologist *n.* psicólogo-a, profesional que practica la psicología.

psychology *n.* psicología, sicología, ciencia que estudia los procesos mentales y la conducta de un individuo; **mental development** ___ / psicología del desarrollo mental.

psychomotor *a.* psicomotor-a, rel. a acciones motoras como resultado de actividades mentales.

psychopath *n.* psicópata, persona que padece de trastornos mentales.

psychopathology *n.* psicopatología, rama de la medicina que trata de las causas y naturaleza de las enfermedades mentales.

psychopharmacology *n.* psicofarmacología, estudio del efecto de drogas y medicamentos en la mente y la conducta.

psychophysiological *a.* psicofisiológico-a, rel. a la influencia mental sobre procesos físicos tal como se manifiesta en algunos desórdenes y enfermedades.

psychosis *n.* psicosis, trastorno mental severo de origen orgánico o emocional en el cual el paciente pierde contacto con la realidad y sufre de alucinaciones o aberraciones mentales; **alcoholic** ___ / alcohólica; **depressive** ___ / depresiva; **drug** ___ / ___ por drogas; **manic-depressive** ___ / ___ maníaco depresiva; **organic** ___ / ___ orgánica; **senile** ___ / ___ senil; **situational** ___ / ___ situacional; **toxic** ___ / ___ tóxica; **traumatic** ___ / ___ traumática.

psychosocial *a.* psicosocial, rel. a factores psicológicos y sociales.

psychosomatic *a.* psicosomático-a, rel. al cuerpo y a la mente; ___ **symptom** / síntoma ___ .

psychotherapy *n.* psicoterapia, tratamiento de trastornos mentales o emocionales por medios psicológicos tales como el psicoanálisis.

psychotic *a.* psicótico-a, rel. a o que sufre de una psicosis.

psychotropic drugs *n.* drogas psicotrópicas, compuestos químicos que afectan la estabilidad mental.

ptosis *n.*, *Gr.* ptosis, prolapso de un órgano o parte, esp. visto en el párpado superior.

puberty *n.* pubertad, adolescencia, desarrollo de las características sexuales secundarias y comienzo de la capacidad reproductiva.

pubescense *n.* pubescencia.
1. principio de la pubertad;
2. aparición de la vellosidad.

pubic *a.* púbico-a, rel. al pubis; ___ **hair** / vello ___ .

pubis *n.* (*pl.* **pubes**) pubis, región púbica, estructura ósea frontal de la pelvis.

public health *n.* salubridad pública, rama de la medicina que se dedica a la atención social, física y mental de los miembros de una comunidad.

pudendum *n.* (*pl.* **pudenda**) pudendum, órganos genitales externos, esp. los femeninos.

puerile *a.* pueril, infantil.

puerperal *a.* puerperal, concerniente al puerperio.

pull *n.* tirón; *v.* tirar, halar, arrancar, sacar; **to** ___ **in** / tirar hacia adentro; **to** ___ **oneself together** / calmarse; **to** ___ **through** [*as in a sickness*] / recuperarse; **to** ___ **up one's knees** / levantar las rodillas.

pulmonary, pulmonic *a.* pulmonar, pulmónico-a, rel. al pulmón o a la arteria pulmonar; ___ **alveolar proteinosis** / proteinosis alveolar ___ ; ___ **artery wedge pressure** / presión diferencial de la arteria ___ ; ___ **edema** / edema ___ ; ___ **embolism** / embolia ___ ; ___ **emphysema** / enfisema ___ ; ___ **insufficiency** / insuficiencia ___ ; ___ **stenosis** / estenosis ___ ; ___ **valve** / válvula ___ ; ___ **vein** / vena ___ .

pulp *n.* pulpa. 1. parte blanda de un órgano; 2. quimo; 3. pulpa dental, parte central blanda de un diente.

pulsatile *a.* pulsátil, de pulsación rítmica.

pulsation *n.* pulsación, latido rítmico tal como el del corazón.

pulse *n.* pulso, dilatación arterial rítmica que gen. coincide con los latidos cardíacos; **alternating** ___ / alternante; **bigeminal** ___ / bigeminado; **bounding** ___ / ___ saltón; **dorsalis pedis** ___ / ___ de la arteria dorsal del pie; **femoral** ___ / femoral; **filiform** ___ / ___ filiforme; **full** ___ / ___ lleno; **irregular** ___ / ___ irregular; **peripheral** ___ / ___ periférico; ___ **pressure** / presión del pulso, diferencia entre la presión sistólica y la diastólica; **radial** ___ / ___ radial; **rapid** ___ / ___ rápido; **regular** ___ / ___ regular; **water hammer** / ___ en martillo de agua. V. cuadro en la página 202.

pump n. bomba; **intravenous** ___ / ___ intravenosa; **oxigenator** ___ / ___ oxigenadora; **stomach** ___ / ___ gástrica; v. bombear; **to** ___ **out** / ___ hacia afuera, sacar por bomba.

pumping n. bombeo; **heart** ___ / ___ del corazón; **stomach** ___ / ___ estomacal.

punch n. sacabocados, instrumento quirúrgico que se usa para perforar o cortar un disco o un segmento de tejido.

punctuate n. puntuar, acto de perforar un tejido con un instrumento afilado.

puncture n. punción, perforación; v. punzar, pinchar; agujerear.

puncture wound n. herida por perforación con un instrumento afilado.

pupil n. pupila, abertura contráctil del iris que da entrada a la luz.

pupillary a. pupilar, rel. a la pupila.

pure a. puro-a, sin contaminación.

purgative n. purgante, catártico, agente que causa evacuación intestinal; ___ **enema** / enema, lavativa, lavabo; ___ **saline** / ___ salino.

purge n. purga, medicamento o catártico; v. 1. purgar o limpiar; 2. forzar la evacuación de los intestinos por medio de un purgante.

purified a. depurado-a, purificado-a; ___ **water** / agua ___ .

purpose n. propósito, intención.

purpura n. púrpura, condición caracterizada por manchas rojizas o de color púrpura en la piel, debidas al escape de sangre a los tejidos; **thrombocytopenic** ___ / ___ trombocitopénica.

purulence n. purulencia, pus.

purulent a. purulento-a, que está supurando.

pus n. pus, excreción, fluido amarillento espeso que se forma por supuración; ___ **discharge** / supuración; ___ **-like** / purulento-a.

push n. empujón; pujo; ___ **button** / botón de llamada; v. [as to bear down] pujar.

pustule n. pústula, costra, elevación pequeña de la piel que contiene pus; pop. postilla.

put vi. poner; **to** ___ **in** / poner dentro de, echar en, meter; **to** ___ **off** / aplazar, cancelar; **to** ___ **on** [clothes] / ponerse la ropa, vestirse; **to** ___ **out** [light, fire] / apagar; **to** ___ **together** / unir, juntar; **to** ___ **up with** / aguantar, soportar, tolerar.

putrefaction n. putrefacción, condición de ser pútrido-a, corrompido-a.

pyelitis n. pielitis, infl. de la pelvis renal, con posible manifestación de orina purulenta y sanguinolenta.

pyelogram n. pielograma, radiografía de la pelvis renal y uréter usando un medio de contraste.

pyelolithotomy n. pielolitotomía, incisión para extraer un cálculo de la pelvis renal.

pyelonephritis n. pielonefritis, infl. del riñón y de la pelvis renal.

pyeloplastia n. pieloplastia, operación de reparación plástica de la pelvis renal.

pyelotomy n. pielotomía, incisión de la pelvis renal.

pyloric a. pilórico, rel. al píloro.

pyloroplasty n. piloroplastia, reparación del píloro.

pylorus n. píloro, abertura u orificio circular entre el estómago y el duodeno.

pyoderma n. pioderma, cualquier enfermedad de la piel que presenta supuración.

pyogenic a. piógeno-a, purulento-a.

pyorrhea n. piorrea, periodontitis.

pyramid n. pirámide, estructura semejante a un cono, tal como la médula oblongata.

pyrectic, pyretic a. pirético-a, rel. a la fiebre.

pyretolysis n. piretolisis. 1. reducción de fiebre; 2. proceso de curación que se acelera con la fiebre.

pyrexia n. pirexia, condición febril.

pyrogen n. pirógeno, sustancia que produce fiebre.

Q

q

q. *abbr.* **quantity** / cantidad; **quaque** / cada.

Q fever *n.* Fiebre Q, enfermedad de temperature febril aguda causada por la rickettsia *Coxiella burnetii*. La enfermedad se contrae por medio de contacto con animales infectados.

quack *n.* charlatán, persona que pretende tener cualidades o conocimientos para curar enfermedades.

quadrant *n.* cuadrante, cuarta parte de un círculo.

quadrate *a.* cuadrado, que tiene cuatro lados iguales; ___ **lobe** / lóbulo cuadrado; ___ **lobule** / lobulillo cuadrado.

quadriceps *n.* cuadríceps, músculo de cuatro cabezas, extensor de la pierna.

quadriplegia *n.* cuadriplegia, parálisis de las cuatro extremidades.

quadriplegic *a.* cuadriplégico, que sufre de parálisis en las cuatro extremidades.

quadruplet *a.* cuádruple, cada uno de los cuatro hijos nacidos en un parto múltiple.

qualified *a.* competente, capaz.

qualitative *a.* cualitativo-a, rel. a cualidad o clase.

qualitative test *n.* prueba cualitativa.

quality *n.* cualidad, propiedad.

quantitative test *n.* prueba cuantitativa.

quantity *n.* cantidad.

quarantine *n.* cuarentena, período de cuarenta días durante los cuales se restringen las actividades de personas o animales para prevenir la propagación de una enfermedad contagiosa.

queasy *a.* nauseabundo-a; ___ **stomach** / naúseas, asco.

Queckensted sign *n.* signo de Queckensted, falta de aumento en la presión del líquido cerebroespinal cuando hay compresión de las venas del cuello; en personas saludables, la presión aumenta rápidamente cuando ocurre la compresión.

queer *a.* raro-a, excéntrico-a; [*slang*] homosexual, invertido, maricón.

quench *v.* extinguir, apagar; [*thirst*] saciar.

question *n.* pregunta; cuestión, problema; *v.* interrogar, preguntar.

questionnaire *n.* cuestionario.

quick *a.* rápido-a, ligero-a, [*alert*] listo-a; ___ **-frozen** / congelado-a al instante; **-ly** *adv.* pronto, rápidamente, al instante.

quicken *v.* acelerar; animar, avivar, estimular.

quickening *n.* 1. animación; 2. percepción por la madre del primer movimiento del feto en el útero.

quiet *a.* quieto-a, sosegado-a, tranquilo-a; *v.* calmar, tranquilizar.

quinidine *n.* quinidina, alcaloide derivado de una *Cinchona* que se usa en irregularidades cardíacas.

quinine *n.* quinina, alcaloide que se obtiene de la corteza de una *Cinchona* usado como antiséptico y antipirético esp. en el tratamiento de paludismo, tifoidea y malaria.

quintuplet *a.* quíntuple, cada uno de los cinco hijos nacidos en un parto múltiple.

quit *v.* desistir, dejar, parar.

quota *n.* cuota.

quotidian *a.* cotidiano-a, de todos los días; ___ **malaria** / malaria ___.

quotient *n.* cuociente, cociente, cifra que resulta de una división; **achievement** ___ / ___ de realización; **blood** ___ / ___ sanguíneo; **growth** ___ / ___ de crecimiento; **intelligence** ___ / ___ de inteligencia.

R *abbr.* **radioactive** / radioactivo; **resistance** / resistencia; **respiration** / respiración; **response** / respuesta, reacción.

rabid *a.* rabioso-a, rel. a la rabia o afectado por ella.

rabies *n.* rabia. V. **hydrophobia.**

race *n.* raza, grupo étnico diferenciado por características comunes heredadas.

racemose *a.* racimoso-a, racimado-a, similar a un racimo de uvas.

rachis *n.* raquis, la columna vertebral.

rachitic *a.* raquítico-a. rel. al raquitismo; débil, endeble.

rachitism, rhachitis, rachitis *n.* raquitismo, enfermedad por deficiencia que afecta el desarrollo óseo en los adolescentes, causada por falta de calcio, fósforo y vitamina D.

racial *a.* racial, étnico-a, de la raza; __ **prejudice** / prejuicio __; __ **immunity** / inmunidad __, tipo de inmunidad natural de los miembros de una raza.

racial immunity *n.* inmunidad racial.

rad *n.* rad. 1. dosis de radiación absorbida; 2. rad, *abbr.* of radix, raíz.

radial *a.* radial. 1. rel. al hueso del radio; 2. que se expande en todas direcciones a partir de un centro.

radiate *v.* irradiar, expandirse.

radiation *n.* radiación. 1. emisión de materiales o partículas radioactivas; 2. propagación de energía; 3. emisión de rayos desde un centro común; __ **dosage** / dosis de __; __ **hazards** / riesgos y peligros causados por una __; __ **therapy** / radioterapia; **electromagnetic** __ / __ electromagnética; **infrared** __ / __ por rayos infrarrojos; **ionizing** __ / __ ionizante; **ultraviolet** __ / __ de rayos ultravioleta.

radiation oncology *n.* uso de radiación en el tratamiento de neoplasmas.

radiation sickness *n.* enfermedad por radiación causada por exposición a rayos-x o a materiales radioactivos.

radiation therapy *n.* terapia de radiación, tratamiento de un tumor o enfermedad por medio de radiaciones de radium o radon. *Syn.* **Radiotherapy.**

radical *a.* radical, rel. a erradicar drásticamente la raíz de una enfermedad o de todo tejido enfermo; __ **surgery** / cirugía __; __ **treatment** / tratamiento __ .

radicular *a.* radical, rel. a la raíz u origen.

radiculitis *n.* radiculitis, infl. de la raíz de un nervio.

radiculoneuritis, Guillain-Barré syndrome *n.* radiculoneuritis, síndrome de Guillain-Barré, infl. de las raíces de los nervios espinales.

radiculopathy *n.* radiculopatía, cualquier afección de las raíces de los nervios espinales.

radioactive iodine excretion test *n.* prueba radiactiva del yodo, evaluación de la función de la tiroides por medio del uso de yodo radiactivo.

radioactivity *n.* radiactividad, propiedad de ciertos elementos de producir radiaciones.

radiocardiography *n.* radiocardiografía, registro gráfico de una sustancia radioactiva durante su paso a través del corazón.

radiocontrast media *m.* medio de contraste de sustancia radioactiva usado en el proceso de efectuar varios tipos de pruebas para diagnóstico.

radiodensity *n.* radiodensidad, la habilidad de una sustancia de absorber rayos-x.

radiodiagnosis *n.* radiodiagnosis, diagnosis por medio de rayos-x.

radiography *n.* radiografía, uso de rayos-x para producir imágenes en placas o en una pantalla fluorescente.

radioimmunity *n.* radioinmunidad, disminución de la sensibilidad a las radiaciones.

radioimmunoassay (RIA) *n.* radioinmunoensayo, radioinmuno análisis método para determinar o evaluar la concentración de un antígeno o proteína en el suero.

radioisotope *n.* radioisótopo, isótopo radioactivo utilizado como medio de diagnóstico o de terapia.

radiologist *n.* radiólogo-a, especialista en radiología.

radiology *n.* radiología, ciencia que trata de los rayos-x o rayos que provienen de sustancias radioactivas, esp. para uso médico.

radiolucent *a.* radiolúcido-a, que permite el paso de la mayor parte de rayos-x.

radionecrosis *n.* radionecrosis, desintegración de tejidos por radiación.

radiopaque *a.* radioopaco-a, que no deja pasar rayos-x u otra forma de radiación; ___ **dye** / colorante ___ .

radiopharmaceutical agents *n.* radiofármacos, drogas radioactivas usadas en el tratamiento y diagnóstico de enfermedades.

radioreceptor *n.* radiorreceptor, receptor que recibe energía radiante como la de los rayos-x, de la luz o del calor.

radioresistant *a.* radiorresistente, que tiene la propiedad de resistir efectos radioactivos.

radiosensitive *a.* radiosensitivo-a, que es afectado por o que responde a un tratamiento de radiación.

radiosurgery *n.* radiocirugía, procedimiento quirúrgico de destrucción de tejido con uso de radiación ionizante.

radiotherapy *n.* radioterapia, tratamiento de una enfermedad por medio de rayos-x o por otras sustancias radioactivas.

radium *L.* radium, radio, elemento metálico radioactivo y fluorescente usado en algunas de sus variaciones en el tratamiento de tumores malignos; ___ **needle** / aguja de radio, divisa en forma de aguja que contiene radio usado en radioterapia.

radium therapy *n.* radioterapia, terapia con el uso de radio.

radius *n.* radio. 1. hueso largo del antebrazo; 2. línea recta que une el centro y cualquier punto de la circunferencia.

radon *n.* radón, elemento radiactivo gaseoso.

raise *v.* levantar; [*increase*] aumentar, subir.

rale *n.* estertor, sonido anormal originado en el pulmón que se percibe durante la auscultación; **coarse** ___ / ___ áspero; **crackling** ___ / ___ crujiente; **crepitant** ___ / ___ crepitante; **dry** ___ / ___ seco; **moist** ___ / ___ húmedo.

ramification *n.* ramificación, distribución en ramas.

range *n.* escala de diferenciación, amplitud, margen; ___ **of motion** / amplitud de movimiento; ___ **of colors** / gama de colores; ___ **of vision** / campo visual.

ranula *n.* ránula, quiste situado debajo de la lengua causado por la obstrucción de un canal glandular.

rape *n.* violación; *v.* violar, abusar sexualmente.

rapid *a.* rápido-a, veloz; ___ **eye movement** / movimientos oculares ___; **-ly** *adv.* rápidamente

rapid respiration *n.* taquipnea, respiración excesivamente rápida.

rapidly progressive sickness *n.* enfermedad rápidamente progresiva.

rapport *n.* relación armoniosa y entendimiento, congenio amistoso entre dos personas.

raptus *L.* raptus, arrebato, ataque súbito violento.

rash, rasche *n., Fr.* rasche, erupción; **diaper** ___ / eritema de los pañales; **heat** ___ / salpullido; **hemorrhagic** ___ / ___ hemorrágica; **maculopapular** ___ / ___ maculopapular; **papular** ___ / papular; **squamous** ___ / ___ escamosa.

rating *n.* evaluación; clasificación, determinación.

ratio *L.* relación, proporción, razón, expresión de la cantidad de una sustancia en relación con otra.

ration *n.* ración, porción alimenticia.

rationalization *n.* racionalización, mecanismo de defensa por el cual se justifica la conducta o actividades propias con explicaciones que aunque razonables no se ajustan a la realidad.

rattlesnake *n.* serpiente de cascabel; ___ **poison** / veneno de la ___ .

Rauwolfia serpentina *n. Rauwolfia serpentina,* planta tropical de la cual se obtiene la reserpina, extracto que se usa en el tratamiento de hipertensión y en algunos casos de trastornos mentales.

ray *n.* rayo.

Raynaud's disease *n.* síndrome de Raynaud. V. **acrocyanosis.**

Raynaud's phenomenon *n.* fenómeno de Raynaud, síntomas asociados con el síndrome de Raynaud.

razor *n.* navaja, cuchilla.

reaction *n.* reacción, respuesta; **allergic** ___ / ___ alérgica; **anaphylactic** ___ / ___ anafiláctica; **anxiety** ___ / ___ de ansiedad; **chain** ___ / ___ en cadena; **conversion** ___ / ___ de conversión; **immune** ___ / ___ inmune; **runaway** ___ / ___ de escape; **time** ___ / ___ de tiempo; **formulation** ___ / ___ de formulación.

reactive *a.* reactivo-a, que tiene la propiedad de reaccionar o de causar una reacción.

reading *n.* lectura; ___ **glasses** / anteojos, espejuelos, gafas para leer; ___ **disorders** / trastornos o impedimentos en la ___ .

ready *a.* listo-a, preparado-a; *v.* **to get** ___ / prepararse, arreglarse.

reagent *n.* reactivo, agente que produce una reacción.

reagin *n.* regina, anticuerpo usado en el tratamiento de alergias que estimula la producción de histamina.

real *a.* real, verdadero-a, cierto-a; **-ly** *adv.* realmente, verdaderamente, ciertamente.

realistic *a.* verdadero-a, realista.

reality *n.* realidad.

reality principle *n.* principio de realidad, método de orientación del paciente hacia el mundo externo para provocar el reconocimiento de objetos y actividades olvidadas, esp. dirigido a personas severamente desorientadas.

reality therapy *n.* terapéutica por realidad, método por el que se enfrenta al paciente con la realidad ayudándolo a aceptarla.

realize *v.* realizar; llevar a cabo; darse cuenta de.

rear *a.* posterior, trasero-a.

reason *n.* razón; justificación; *v.* razonar; justificar; ___ **for admission** / razón de ingreso.

reasonable *a.* razonable; justificado-a; sensato-a; ___ **care** / cuidado justificado; ___ **charge** / honorarios ___ -s; ___ **cost** / costo ___ .

reattachment *n.* acción de volver a unir, re-unión; acción de repegar; ___ **of amputated fingers** / re-unión de dedos amputados.

rebound *n.* rebote, regreso a una condición previa después que el estímulo inicial se suprime; *v.* rebotar, repercutir.

rebound phenomenon *n.* fenómeno de rebote, movimiento intensificado de una parte hacia adelante cuando se elimina la fuerza inicial contra la cual ésta hacía resistencia.

recall *v.* recordar; reclamar; hacer volver; acordarse de.

recede *v.* disminuir, [*water*] bajar, retroceder.

recent *a.* reciente; moderno; nuevo-a;

-ly *adv.* recientemente, hace poco tiempo.

receptor *n.* receptor, terminación nerviosa que recibe un estímulo y lo transmite a otros nervios; **auditory** ___ / ___ auditivo; **contact** ___ / ___ de contacto; **mechanoreceptor** / mecanoreceptor; **chemoreceptor** / quimoreceptor; **proprioceptive** ___ / ___ propioceptivo; **sensory** ___ / ___ sensorial; **taste** ___ / ___ gustativo; **temperature** ___ / ___ de temperatura.

recessive *a.* recesivo-a. 1. que tiende a retraerse; 2. en genética, rel. al gene que permanece latente; ___ **characteristics** / características ___ -s.

recidivism *n.* recidiva, reincidencia, tendencia a recaer en una condición, enfermedad o síntoma previo.

recipient *n.* 1. receptor; vasija; recipiente; 2. persona que recibe una transfusión, un implante de tejido o un órgano de un donante. 3. [*as in organ receiver*] receptor, [*mail*] destinatario-a.

reclined position *n.* posición en decúbito.

reclining *a.* recostado-a, inclinado-a.

recognition *n.* reconocimiento, estado de ser reconocido.

recollection *n.* recuerdo, memoria.

recommend *v.* recomendar; aconsejar.

recommendation *n.* recomendación.

recompense *n.* recompensa, compensación, reparación.

reconciliation *n.* reconciliación, conformidad.

reconstitution *n.* reconstitución, restitución de un tejido a la forma inicial.

reconstruction *v.* reconstrucción.

record *n.* registro; [*medical history*] historia clínica, expediente; informe; **off the** ___ / confidencialmente; **patient** ___ / ___ del paciente; **to go on** ___ / expresar públicamente; *v.* registrar, inscribir.

recording *n.* registro, [*tape*] grabación.

recoup *v.* recuperar; recobrar; recuperarse, recobrarse; restablecerse.

recourse *n.* recurso, auxilio.

recover *v.* recobrar, recuperar, restablecer; restablecerse, recobrarse, reponerse.

recovery *n.* recuperación, restablecimiento, recobro, mejoría; **past** ___ / sin remedio, sin cura; ___ **room** / sala de ___ .

recovery room *n.* sala de recuperación.

recrudescence *n.* recrudescencia, relapso, reaparición de síntomas.

rectal *a.* rectal, del recto, rel. al recto; ___ **abscess** / absceso ___; ___ **biopsy** / biopsia ___; ___ **inflammation** / inflamación ___; ___ **lump** / protuberancia, bulto ___; ___ **prolapse** / prolapso ___ .

rectify *v.* rectificar, corregir, enmendar.

rectocele *n.* rectocele, hernia del recto con protrusión en la vagina.

rectosigmoidectomy *n.* rectosigmogdoscopia, excisión del recto y del colon pelviano.

rectovaginal *a.* rectovaginal, rel. a la vagina y el recto.

rectovesical *a.* rectovesical, rel. al recto y la vejiga.

rectum *n.* recto, la porción distal del intestino grueso que se extiende de la flexura sigmoidea al ano.

rectus *L.* (*pl.* **recti**) músculo recto; ___ **muscles** / músculos ___, grupo de músculos rectos tales como los situados alrededor del ojo y en la pared abdominal.

recumbent *a.* yacente, acostado-a, recostado-a, reclinado-a, recumbente; acostado-a de espalda; ___ **position** / posición ___ .

recuperation *n.* recuperación, restablecimiento.

recur *v.* repetir, volver a ocurrir; recaer, repetirse.

recurrence *n.* recidiva. 1. reaparición de síntomas después de una remisión; 2. relapso, recaída.

recurrent *a.* recurrente, que reaparece temporalmente; repetido-a, constante; ___cystitis / cistitis ___; ___ **pain** / dolor constante; ___ **disease** / enfermedad ___.

red *n., a.* rojo; ___ **cell** / glóbulo rojo, hematíe, eritrocito; **Congo** ___ / ___ Congo; **scarlet** ___ / ___ escarlata.

redress *v.* volver a vendar; poner un nuevo vendaje; remediar.

reduce *v.* reducir, rebajar; disminuir. 1. restaurar a la situación normal, tal como un hueso fracturado o dislocado; 2. disminuir la potencia al dar hidrógeno o quitarle oxígeno a un compuesto; 3. bajar de peso.

reducing diet *n.* régimen para bajar de peso.

reducing exercises *n., pl.* ejercicios para adelgazar, ejercicios para bajar de peso.

reducing factor *n.* factor que afecta el proceso de peso.

reduction *n.* reducción, baja, disminución; rebaja.

reduction mammaplasty *n.* cirugía plástica de reducción del seno, con mejoramiento a la posición y apariencia.

reference *n.* referencia; ___ **values** / valores de ___ .

referral *n.* recomendación; remisión; ___ **and consultation** / ___ y consulta.

refill *n.* repuesto; repetición; relleno; repetición de una receta; *v.* reponer; repetir; rellenar.

reflection *n.* reflexión. 1. acomodamiento o vuelta hacia atrás tal como una membrana que después de llegar a la superficie de un órgano se repliega sobre sí misma; 2. rechazo de la luz u otra forma de energía radiante de una superficie; 3. introspección.

reflex *n.* reflejo, respuesta motora involuntaria a un estímulo; **Achilles tendon** ___ / ___ del tendón de Aquiles; ___ **action** / acto, acción ___; ___ **arch** / arco ___; **behavior** ___ / ___ adquirido; **chain** ___ / ___ en cadena; ___ **conditioned** ___ / ___ condicionado; **instinctive** ___ / ___ instintivo; **patellar** ___ / ___ patelar o rotuliano; **radial** ___ / ___ radial; **rectal** ___ / ___ rectal; **stretch** ___ / ___ de estiramiento; **unconditioned** ___ / ___ no condicionado; **vagal** ___ / ___ vagal.

reflux *n.* reflujo, flujo retrógrado; **abdominojugular** ___ / ___ abdominoyugular; **esophageal** ___ / ___ esofágico; **hepatojugular** ___ / ___ hepatoyugular; **intrarenal** ___ / ___ intrarenal; **ureterorenal** ___ / ___ ureterorenal.

refraction *n.* refracción, acto de refractar; **ocular** ___ / ___ ocular.

refractive surgery *n.* cirugía refractiva, corrección del cristalino del ojo.

refractory *a.* refractario-a. 1. resistente a un tratamiento; 2. que no responde a un estímulo.

refrigerant *a.* refrigerante; antipirético-a.

refuge *n.* refugio; asilo; *v.* **to take** ___ / refugiarse.

refusal *n.* rechazo, negación.

refuse *n.* desecho, basura; desperdicios; *v.* rehusar, rechazar, denegar; __ **the hospital food** / __ la comida del hospital; __ **to take the medication** / rehusar tomar la medicina.

regain *v.* recuperar, recobrar; **to __ consciousness** / recobrar el conocimiento.

regarding *prep.* respecto a.

regeneration *n.* regeneración, restauración, renovación.

regime *n.* régimen, regla, plan, esp. en referencia a una dieta o ejercicio físico.

region *n.* región, parte del cuerpo más o menos delimitada.

regression *n.* regresión, retrogresión. 1. vuelta a una condición anterior; 2. apaciguamiento de síntomas o de un proceso patológico.

regular *a.* regular, común, **-ly** *adv.* regularmente, con regularidad.

regurgitant *a.* regurgitante, rel. a la regurgitación.

regurgitation *n.* regurgitación. 1. acto de devolver o expulsar la comida de la boca; 2. flujo retrógrado de la sangre a través de una válvula defectuosa del corazón; **aortic __** / __ aórtica; **mitral __** / __ de la válvula mitral; **valvular __** / __ valvular.

rehabilitate *v.* rehabilitar, ayudar a recobrar funciones normales por medio de métodos terapéuticos.

rehydration *n.* rehidratación, restablecimiento del balance hídrico del cuerpo.

reimplantation *n.* reimplantación. 1. restauración de un tejido o parte; 2. restitución de un óvulo al útero después de extraerlo y fecundarlo *in vitro*.

reinfection *n.* reinfección, infección subsecuente por el mismo microorganismo.

reinfusion *n.* reinfusión, reinyección de suero sanguíneo o líquido cefalorraquídeo.

reject *n.* rechazar, rehusar.

rejection *n.* rechazo, reacción inmunológica de incompatibilidad a células de tejidos transplantados; **acute __** / __ agudo; **chronic __** / __ crónico; **hyperacute __** / __ hiperagudo.

relapse *n.* recidiva, recaída, reincidencia; *v.* recaer, volver a sufrir una enfermedad o los síntomas de ésta después de cierta mejoría.

relapsing fever *n.* fiebre recurrente.

related *a.* relacionado-a; emparentado-a.

relationship *n.* relación; parentesco, lazo familiar.

relative *n.* pariente, familiar; *a.* relativo-a; *gr.* pronombre relativo.

relaxant *n.* relajante, tranquilizante; agente que reduce la tensión; **muscle __** / __ muscular.

relaxation *n.* relajación, acto de relajar o de relajarse; reposo, descanso.

release *n.* liberación; *v.* soltar, librar, desprender; [*to inform*] informar, dar a conocer.

releasing hormone *n.* hormona estimulante.

reliable *a.* [*person*] formal, responsable; seguro-a.

relief *n.* alivio, mejoría; ayuda, auxilio; **what a __!** / ¡ay, qué __ !; *v.* **to be on __** / recibir asistencia social.

relieve *v.* [*pain*] aliviar, mejorar.

reluctant *a.* renuente; resistente; contrario-a.

rely *v.* depender, contar con, confiar en.

remain *v.* permanecer; **to __ in bed** / guardar cama.

remains *n., pl.* restos.

remark *n.* observación, nota, advertencia; *v.* observar, indicar, advertir.

remedy *n.* remedio, cura, medicamento; *v.* remediar, curar.

remember *v.* recordar, acordarse; __ **correctly!** / ¡Acuérdese, acuérdate bien!; **Don't you __?** / ¿No se acuerda?, ¿no te acuerdas? ¿no se recuerda?, ¿no te recuerdas?

remineralization *n.* remineralización, reemplazo de minerales perdidos en el cuerpo.

reminiscense *n.* memoria, recordatorio, reminiscencia.

remission *n.* remisión. 1. disminución o cesación de los síntomas de una enfermedad; 2. período de tiempo durante el cual los síntomas de una enfermedad disminuyen.

remittent *a.* remitente, que se repite a intervalos.

removal *n.* extirpación, remoción.

remove *v.* sacar; quitar, extraer; extirpar.

renal *a.* renal, rel. a o semejante al riñón; __ **cell carcinoma,** / carcinoma de células renales; __ **clearance __** / aclaración __, aclaramiento __; __ **clearance test** / prueba de aclaramiento o depuración ___; __ **colic** / cólico nefrítico, cólico renal; __ **failure** / insuficiencia renal; __ **failure, acute** / insuficiencia __ aguda; __ **function test** / prueba funcional ___; __ **gammagraphy** / gamagrafía, barrido ___; __ **hypertensión** / hipertensión de origen renal; __ **insufficiency** / insuficiencia ___; __ **involvement** / [*participation*] intervención ___; __ **papillary necrosis** / necrosis papilar ___; __ **pelvis** / pelvis ___; __ **replacement therapy** / __ diálisis, terapia de reemplazo; __ **scanning** / gammagrafía renal, barrido renal; __ **transplantation** / transplante __ .

renal ballottement *n.* peloteo renal, maniobra para mover por presión el riñón y determinar la forma, tamaño y mobilidad del riñón.

renin *n.* renina, enzima segregada por el riñón que interviene en la regulación de la presión arterial.

renogram *n.* renograma, proceso de monitoreo del índice de eliminación sanguínea a través del riñón usando una sustancia radioactiva inyectada previamente.

repair *n.* reparación, restauración; *v.* reparar, restaurar.

repeat *n.* repetir, reiterar.

repellent *a.* repelente.

replace *v.* reemplazar, reponer, substituir.

replacement *n.* reemplazo, substitución, repuesto.

replete *a.* repleto-a, lleno-a en exceso.

replication *n.* reproducción, duplicación.

repolarization *n.* repolarización, restablecimiento de la polarización de una célula o de una fibra nerviosa o muscular después de su depolarización.

report *n.* informe, reporte; *v.* informar, reportar.

repression *n.* represión. 1. inhibición de una acción; 2. mecanismo de defensa por el que se eliminan del campo de la conciencia deseos e impulsos en conflicto.

reproduce *v.* reproducir; reproducirse.

reproducer *n.* reproductor.

reproduction *n.* reproducción; **sexual** __ / __ sexual.

reproductive *a.* reproductivo-a, rel. a la reproducción ___; **system** / sistema de __ .

repudiate *v.* repudiar, repeler.

reputed *a.* reputado-a, distinguido-a, de buena fama.

request *n.* petición, encargo; solicitud; *v.* pedir, hacer una petición, [*of supplies*] encargar.

requirement *n.* requerimiento.

rescind *v.* rescindir, anular; terminar.

rescue *v.* salvar, rescatar, librar; __ **method** / método de __, de salvamento.

research *n.* investigación, indagación, pesquisa; *v.* investigar, indagar, hacer investigaciones.

resection *n.* resección, extirpación de una porción de órgano o tejido; **bloc** __ / __ en bloque; **gastric** __ / __ gástrica; **transurethral** __ / __ transuretral; **wedge** __ / __ en cuña.

resectoscope *n.* resectoscopio, instrumento quirúrgico provisto de un electrodo cortante como el que se usa para la resección de la próstata a través de la uretra.

resectoscopy *n.* resectoscopía, resección de la próstata con un resectoscopio.

resemble *v.* tener semejanza; parecerse a.

resentment *n.* resentimiento, rencor.

reserpine *n.* reserpina, derivado de la *Rauwolfia serpentina* que se usa principalmente en el tratamiento de la hipertensión y de desórdenes emocionales.

resident *n.* médico-a residente, que cursa una residencia.

residual *a.* residual, restante, remanente; __ **function** / función ___; __ **urine** / orina __ .

residue *n.* residuo; __ **diet, high** / dieta de __ alto; __ **diet, low** / dieta de __ bajo.

resilient *a.* elástico-a.

resin *a.* resina, sustancia vegetal insoluble en el agua aunque soluble en alcohol y éter que tiene una variedad de usos medicinales y dentales.

resist *v.* resistir; rechazar.

resistance *n.* resistencia, oposición; capacidad de un organismo para resistir efectos dañinos; **initial** __ / __ inicial; **acquired** __ / __ adquirida; **peripheral** __ / __ periférica; *v.* **to offer** __ / oponerse; hacer resistencia.

resistant *a.* resistente; **fast** __ / __ resistencia a un colorante; **bacterial** __ / __ bacteriana; **insulin** __ / a la insulina __.

resolution n. resolución.
1. terminación de un proceso inflamatorio; 2. habilidad de distinguir detalles pequeños y sutiles tal como se hace a través de un microscopio; 3. descomposición sin supuración.

resolve v. resolver. 1. encontrar una solución; 2. descomponer, analizar, separar en componentes.

resonance n. resonancia, capacidad de aumentar la intensidad de un sonido; **normal** __ / __ normal; **vesicular** __ / __ vesicular; **vocal** __ / __ vocal.

resorcinol n. resorcinol, agente usado en el tratamiento de acné y otras dermatosis.

resorption n. resorción, pérdida total o parcial de un proceso, tejido o exudado por resultado de reacciones bioquímicas tales como lisis y absorción.

respiration n. respiración, proceso respiratorio; **abdominal** __ / __ abdominal; **aerobic** __ / __ aeróbica; **accelerated** __ / __ acelerada; **anaerobic** __ / __ anaeróbica; **diaphragmatic** __ / __ diafragmática; **air hunger, gasping** __ / __ jadeante; **labored** __ / __ laboriosa.

respirator n. respirador, aparato para purificar el aire que se inhala o para producir respiración artificial; **chest** __ / __ torácico.

respiratory a. respiratorio-a, rel. a la respiración; __ **airway** / conducto, pasaje __; __ **alkalosis** / alkalosis __; __ **arrest** / paro __; __ **arrhythmia** / arritmia __; __ **ataxia** / ataxia __; **bronchioles** / bronquíolos __; **capacity** / capacidad; __ **care unit** / unidad de cuidado __; __ **distress syndrome** / síndrome de dificultad __; __ **enzyme** / enzima __; __ **failure, acute** / insuficiencia __ aguda; __ **failure, chronic** / insuficiencia __ crónica; __ **function tests** / pruebas de función __; __ **inhibitor** / inhibidor __; __ **lobule** / lóbulo __; __ **metabolism** / metabolismo __; __ **mucosa** / mucosa __; __ **quotient** / cociente __; __ **rate** / índice __; __ **sounds** / ruidos __; __ **system** / sistema __; __ **tract infections and diseases** / infecciones y enfermedades de las vías __ -s.

respiratory acidosis n. acidosis respiratoria, causada por retención de

dioxido de carbono debido a hipoventilación.

respiratory center n. centro respiratorio, área en la médula oblongata que regula los movimientos respiratorios.

response n. respuesta. 1. reacción o cambio de un órgano o parte a un estímulo; **immune** __ / __ inmune; 2. reacción de un paciente a un tratamiento.

responsible a. responsable.

rest n. descanso, reposo; residuo, resto; __ **cure** / cura de reposo; v. decansar, reposar.

restenosis n. reestenosis, recurrencia de estenosis después de cirugía correctiva.

restful a. tranquilo-a, quieto-a.

resting a. inactivo-a, en reposo, en estado de descanso.

restore v. restituir, restablecer.

restraint n. restricción; confinamiento; __ **in bed** / __ en cama; **mechanical** __ / __ mecánica; **medicinal** __ / __ con uso de medicamentos.

restrict v. restringir, confinar.

restricted a. limitado-a, confinado; __ **area** / área __.

restroom n. servicio, aseos, _Lat. Am._ inodoro, cuarto de baño.

result n. resultado, conclusión.

resuscitate v. resucitar; reanimar.

resuscitation n. resucitación. 1. devolver la vida; reanimar el corazón; 2. respiración artificial.

resuscitator n. resucitador, aparato automático de asistencia respiratoria.

retain v. retener, guardar; quedarse con.

retainer n. [_dentistry_] aro, freno de retención.

retardate a. retardado-a, retrasado-a, atrasado-a.

retardation n. retraso, atraso, retardo anormal de una función motora o mental; **psychomotora** __ / __ psicomotor. V. **mental retardation**.

retch n. arcada, basca, contracciones abdominales espasmódicas que preceden al vómito.

retention n. retención, conservación; **fluid** __ / __ de líquido; **gastric** __ / __ gástrica; __ **enema** / enema de __; **urinary** __ / __ urinaria.

reticular a. reticular, retiforme, en forma de red.

reticulation n. reticulación, disposición reticular.

reticulocyte *n.* reticulocito, célula roja inmadura, eritrocito en red o gránulos que aparece durante la regeneración de la sangre; __ **count** / recuento de __ .

reticulocytopenia, reticulosis *n.* reticulocitopenia, reticulosis, disminución anormal del número de reticulocitos en la sangre.

reticulocytosis *n.* reticulocitosis, sobreaumento de nuevos reticulocitos circulantes en la corriente sanguínea como regeneración activa de la sangre, estimulantes de la médula ósea después del tratamiento de anemia hemolítica genética o por adaptación ambiental.

reticuloendothelial system *n.* sistema reticuloendotelial, red de células fagocíticas (excepto leucocitos circulantes) esparcidas por todo el cuerpo que intervienen en procesos tales como la formación de células sanguíneas, destrucción de grasas, eliminación de células gastadas y restauración de tejidos participantes en el proceso inmunológico del organismo.

reticuloendothelioma *n.* reticuloendotelioma, tumor del sistema reticuloendotelial.

reticuloendotheliosis *n.* reticuloendoteliosis, crecimiento y proliferación anormal de las células del sistema reticuloendotelial.

Retin-A *n.* Retin-A, nombre comercial del ácido retinoico, medicamento usado en el tratamiento de acné.

retina *n.* retina, la capa más interna del ojo que recibe imágenes y transmite impulsos visuales al cerebro; **detachment of the** __ / desprendimiento de la __ .

retinal *a.* de la retina, retiniano-a; rel. a la retina; __ **degeneration** / deterioro retiniano, deterioración retiniana; __ **perforation** / perforación __ .

retinitis *n.* retinitis, infl. de la retina.

retinoblastoma *n.* retinoblastoma, tumor maligno de la retina gen. hereditario.

retinol *n.* retinol, vitamina A1.

retinopathy *n.* retinopatía, cualquier condición anormal de la retina.

retinoscopy *n.* retinoscopía, determinación y evaluación de errores visuales de refracción.

retiree *n.* jubilado-a; retirado-a.

retract *v.* retraer, retractar; retraerse, volverse hacia atrás.

retraction *n.* retracción, encogimiento, contracción; acto de echarse hacia atrás; **clot** __ / __ del coágulo; **uterine** __ / __ uterina

retractor *n.* retractor. 1. instrumento para separar los bordes de una herida; 2. tipo de músculo que retrae una parte u órgano.

retroauricular *a.* retroauricular, rel. a o situado detrás de la oreja o aurícula.

retrocecal *a.* retrocecal, rel. a o situado detrás del ciego.

retroflexion *n.* retroflexión, flexión de un órgano hacia atrás.

retrograde *a.* retrógrado-a, que se mueve hacia atrás o retorna al pasado; __ **amnesia** / amnesia __ ; __ **aortography** / aortografía __ ; __ **pyelography** / pielografía __ .

retrogression *n.* retrogresión, regreso a un estado más primitivo de desarrollo.

retrolental *a.* retrolental, situado detrás del cristalino; __ **fibroplasia** / fibroplasia __ .

retroperitoneal *a.* retroperitoneano-a, rel. a o situado detrás del peritoneo.

retroversion *n.* retroversión, inclinación o vuelta hacia atrás; __ **of the uterus** / desplazamiento del útero hacia atrás.

retrovirus *n.* retrovirus, virus que pertenece al grupo ácido ARN, algunos de los cuales son oncogénicos; **human endogenous** __ / __ endógeno humano.

reunion *n.* reunión, unión de partes o tejidos esp. en un hueso fracturado o en partes de una herida al cicatrizar.

revascularization *n.* revascularización, proceso de restauración de la sangre a una parte del cuerpo después de una lesión o una derivación quirúrgica.

reversal *n.* reversión, restitución a un estado anterior.

review *n.* revisión, análisis, repaso; **admission** __ / revisión de ingresos; **case** __ / __ del caso ; __ **of systems** / __ de sistemas; [*literary*] reseña; *v.* repasar, volver a ver.

revise *v.* revisar, repasar, mirar con detenimiento.

revision *n.* revisión.

revitalize *n.* revitalizar, vivificar, volver a dar fuerzas.

revive *v.* revivir.

revulsion *n.* revulsión.

Reye's syndrome *n.* síndrome de Reye, enfermedad aguda que se manifiesta en niños y adolescentes con edema agudo en órganos importantes esp. en el cerebro y el hígado.

Rh blood group *n.* grupo sanguíneo Rh.

Rh genes *n., pl.* genes Rh, determinantes de los distintos tipos sanguíneos Rh.

rhabdomyosarcoma *n.* rabdomiosarcoma, tumor maligno de fibras musculares estriadas que afecta gen. los músculos esqueléticos.

rheum, rheuma *n.* 1. reuma, secreción catarral o acuosa por la nariz; 2. reumatismo.

rheumatic *a.* reumático-a, rel. a o afectado por reumatismo.

rheumatic fever *n.* fiebre reumática, fiebre o condición acompañada de dolores en las articulaciones que puede dejar como secuela trastornos cardíacos y renales.

rheumatism *n.* reumatismo, enfermedad aguda crónica caracterizada por infl. y dolor en las articulaciones.

rheumatoid *a.* reumatoide, de naturaleza semejante al reumatismo.

rhinal *a.* rinal, rel. a la nariz.

rhinitis *n.* rinitis, infl. de la mucosa nasal.

rhinolaryngitis *n.* rinolaringitis, infl. simultánea de las mucosas nasales y laríngeas.

rhinopharyngitis *n.* rinofaringitis, infl. de la nasofaringe.

rhinophyma. *n.* rinofima, acné rosácea aguda en el área de la nariz.

rhinoplasty *n.* rinoplastia, cirugía plástica de la nariz.

rhinorrhea *n.* rinorrea, secreción mucoso-líquida por la nariz.

rhinoscopy *n.* rinoscopía, examen de los pasajes nasales a través de la nasofaringe o de los orificios nasales.

rhizotomy *n.* rizotomía, división o transección de la raíz de un nervio.

rhodopsin *n.* rodopsina, pigmento de color rojo púrpura que se encuentra en los bastoncillos de la retina y que facilita la visión en luz tenue.

rhythm *n.* ritmo, regularidad en la acción o función de un órgano u órganos del cuerpo tal como el corazón.

rhytidectomy *n.* ritidectomía, estiramiento de la piel de la cara por medio de cirugía plástica.

rib *n.* costilla, uno de los huesos de una serie de doce pares que forman la pared torácica.

riboflavin *n.* riboflavina, vitamina B2, componente del complejo vitamínico B esencial en la nutrición.

ribonucleoprotein *n.* ribonucleoproteína, sustancia que contiene proteína y ácido ribonucleico.

ridge *n.* borde, reborde, elevación prolongada.

rifampicin *n.* rifampicina, sustancia semisintética, antibacteriana que se usa en el tratamiento de la tuberculosis pulmonar.

right *n.* justicia; derecho; *a.* derecho-a, rel. a la parte derecha del cuerpo; recto-a, correcto-a; ___ -handed / diestro-a, que usa con preferencia la mano derecha; **on the** ___ **side** / al costado o lado derecho; [*health*] sano-a; **the** ___ **medication** / la medicina necesaria; **the** ___ **treatment** / el tratamiento adecuado; [*in a problem*]; **taking the** ___ **direction** / la solución indicada; **everything is all** ___ / todo está bien; ___ **or wrong** / con o sin razón; *adv.* bien, correctamente; mismo; **It is going all** ___ / Todo sigue bien; ___ **here** / aquí mismo.

right to refuse treatment *n.* derecho a rehusar tratamiento, el derecho que tiene el (la) paciente de negarse a recibir tratamiento en contra de su voluntad.

right to treatment *n.* derecho a recibir tratamiento, el derecho que tiene el (la) paciente de recibir atención médica de una institución de salud que ha asumido la responsabilidad de tratar al paciente.

rights of the patient *n., pl.* derechos del paciente.

rigid *a.* rígido-a, tieso, inmóvil.

rigidity *n.* rigidez, tesura, inmovilidad, inflexibilidad; **cadaveric** ___ / ___ cadavérica, rigor mortis.

rigor *n.* rigor. 1. escalofrío repentino con fiebre alta; 2. tesura, inflexibilidad muscular.

rigor mortis *L.* rigidez muscular inmediata sequida a la muerte.

ringing *a.* resonante, retumbante; ___ **ears** / tintineo, zumbido, ruido en los oídos.

ringworm

ringworm *n*. tiña.

ripe *a*. [*fruit*] maduro-a; [*boil, cataract*] maduro-a.

ripening *n*. reblandecimiento, dilatación tal como la del cuello uterino durante el parto.

ripping *n*. laceración, rasgadura; descosedura.

risk *n*. riesgo, peligro; ___ **of contamination** / riesgo o peligro de contaminación; ___ **factors** / factores de ___; **high- ___ groups** / grupos de alto ___; **potential ___** / ___ posible; ___ **of infection** / ___ de infección; ___ **of injury** / ___ de una lesión; ___ **of violence** / ___ de violencia; *v*. poner en peligro; arriesgarse.

risky *a*. arriesgado-a, peligroso-a.

risorious *n*. risorio, músculo que se inserta en la comisura de la boca.

Ritalin hydrochloride *n*. clorhidrato de Ritalin, estimulante y antidepresivo benigno.

roach *n*. cucaracha.

robust *a*. robusto-a, vigoroso-a.

rod *n*. bastoncillo; varilla.

rodent *n*. roedor; *a*. roedor-a; ___ **ulcer** / úlcera ___, que destruye poco a poco.

role model *n*. prototipo, modelo.

roll *n*. panecillo; *v*. rodar.

Romberg's sign *n*. signo de Romberg, oscilación del cuerpo que indica inhabilidad de mantener el equilibrio en posición erecta, con los pies juntos y los ojos cerrados.

room *n*. cuarto, sala; **bath ___** / ___ de baño; **delivery ___** / sala de partos; **operating ___** / sala de operaciones, quirófano; **the patient's ___** / ___ del paciente; **recovery ___** / sala de recuperación; ___ **temperature** / temperatura ambiente; **waiting ___** / sala de espera.

root *n*. raíz; radical.

Rorschach test *n*. prueba de Rorschach, prueba psicológica por la cual se revelan rasgos de la personalidad a través de la interpretación de una serie de borrones de tinta.

roseola *n*. roséola, condición de la piel caracterizada por manchas rosáceas de varios tamaños.

rosette *F*. rosette, células en formación semejante a una rosa.

rostral *a*. rostral, rel. o semejante a un rostro.

rot *v*. podrirse, pudrirse, echarse a perder.

rotation *n*. rotación; **fetal ___** / ___ de la cabeza del feto.

rotten *a*. podrido-a, putrefacto-a, corrompido-a; [*tooth*] cariado-a.

rough *a*. [*surface, skin*] áspero-a, escabroso-a; [*character*] rudo-a. grosero-a; *v*. **to have a ___ time** / pasarla mal.

round *a*. redondo-a, circular; ___ **-shouldered** / cargado de espaldas; **all year ___** / todo el año.

routine *n*. rutina, hábito, costumbre; *a*. rutinario-a.

rub *n*. 1. fricción, frote, frotación, masaje; 2. sonido producido por el roce de dos superficies secas que se detecta en auscultación; *v*. frotar, hacer penetrar un ungüento o pomada en la piel; friccionar; **to ___ off** / limpiar frotando, borrar; **to ___ down** / dar un masaje.

rubber *n*. goma; ___ **bulb** / perilla de ___; ___ **gloves** / guantes de ___ .

rubbing *n*. masaje.

rubbing alcohol *n*. alcohol para fricciones.

rubella *n*. rubéola, sarampión alemán; *pop. Mex.* pelusa, enfermedad infecciosa viral que se manifiesta con dolor de garganta, fiebre y una erupción rosácea y que puede ocasionar serios trastornos fetales si la madre la contrae durante los primeros tres meses del embarazo.

rubella virus vaccine, live *n*. vacuna de virus vivo contra la rubéola.

rubor *n*. rubor, enrojecimiento de la piel.

rudiment *n*. rudimento. 1. órgano parcialmente desarrollado; 2. órgano o parte que ha perdido total o parcialmente su función anterior.

rugose *a*. arrugado-a, lleno-a de arrugas.

rule *n*. régimen, regla, precepto; ___ **s and regulations** / según el reglamento; **as a ___** / por lo general *v*. gobernar, administrar; **to ___ out** / prohibir, desechar; **to be ruled by one's emotions** / dejarse llevar por las emociones.

run *n*. carrera; *vi*. correr, hacer correr; **to ___ a fever** / tener calentura, tener fiebre.

rupture *n*. [*hernia*] ruptura; [*bone*] rotura, fractura; [*boil*] reventazón; *v*. reventar, romper, fracturar; abrirse, reventarse, romperse, fracturarse.

rusty *a*. oxidado-a.

salt

S

S *abbr.* **sacral** / sacral; **section** / sección; **stimulus** / estímulo; **subject** / sujeto; **sulphur** / sulfuro, azufre.

s *abbr.* **second** / segundo; **singular** / singular.

Sabin vaccine *n.* vacuna de Sabin, vacuna oral contra la poliomielitis.

sac *n.* saco, bolsa; estructura u órgano en forma de saco o bolsa.

saccharide *n.* sacárido, compuesto químico que pertenece a una serie de carbohidratos que incluye los azúcares.

saccharine *n.* sacarina, sustancia sumamente dulce, agente dulcificante artificial, *a.* sacarino-a, azucarado-a.

saccule *n.* sáculo, saco o bolsa pequeña.

sacral *a.* sacral, rel. al sacro o situado cerca de éste; **plexus** ___ / plexo ___; ___ **nerves** / nervios ___ -es.

sacralization *n.* sacralización, fusión de la quinta vértebra lumbar con el sacro.

sacroilitis *n.* sacroilitis, infl. de la articulación sacroilíaca.

sacrolumbar *a.* sacrolumbar, rel. a las regiones sacral y lumbar.

sacrum *n.* sacro, hueso triangular formado por cinco vértebras fusionadas en la base de la espina dorsal y entre los dos huesos de la cadera.

sad *a.* triste, desconsolado-a.

saddle back *n.* espalda caída. lordosis.

sadism *n.* sadismo, perversión por la cual se obtiene placer sexual infligiendo dolor físico o psicológico a otros.

sadist *n.* sadista, persona que practica sadismo.

sadness *n.* tristeza, melancolía.

sadomasochism *n.* sadomasoquismo, derivación de placer sexual infligiendo dolor físico a sí mismo o a otros.

sadomasochist *n.* sadomasoquista, persona que practica sadomasoquismo.

safe *a.* seguro-a, sin peligro; sin riesgo; ___ **sex** / sexo sin riesgo; **-ly** *adv.* seguramente; sin peligro.

safety *n.* seguridad, protección; ___ **pin** / imperdible.

sag *v.* perder elasticidad, perder la forma; combarse; pandearse; [*to weaken*] debilitarse.

sage *n.* salvia.

sagittal *a.* sagital, semejante a una saeta; ___ **plane** / plano ___, paralelo al eje longitudinal del cuerpo.

said *a. pp.* of **to say**, dicho; dicho-a, citado-a, antes mencionado.

salicylate *n.* salicilato, cualquier sal de ácido salicílico; ___ **poisoning** / envenenamiento por aspirina.

salicylic acid *n.* ácido salicílico, ácido cristalino blanco derivado del fenol.

salient *a.* saliente, pronunciado-a.

saline *a.* salino-a; ___ **cathartic** / purgante ___; ___ **solution** / solución ___, agua destilada con sal.

saliva *n.* saliva, secreción de las glándulas salivales que envuelve y humedece el bolo alimenticio en la boca y facilita la deglución.

salivant *a.* salivoso-a, rel. a la saliva.

salivary glands *n., pl.* glándulas salivales o salivares.

salivation *n.* salivación. 1. acto de secreción de saliva; 2. secreción excesiva de saliva.

Salk vaccine *n.* vacuna de Salk, vacuna contra la poliomielitis.

salmonella *n.* Salmonela, género de bacterias gram-negativas de la familia *Enterobacteriaceae* que causan fiebres entéricas, otras infecciones gastrointestinales y septicemia.

salmonellosis *n.* salmonelosis, infección causada por ingestión de comida contaminada por bacterias del género Salmonela.

salpingectomy *n.* salpingectomía, extirpación de una o de ambas trompas de Falopio.

salpingitis *n.* salpingitis, infl. de las trompas de Falopio.

salpingo-oophorectomy *n.* salpingo-ooforectomía, extirpación de un ovario y un tubo uterino.

salpingoplasty *n.* reparación plástica de las trompas de Falopio.

salpinx *n., Gr.* (*pl.* **salpinges**) trompa, estructura similar a la trompa de Eustaquio o a la trompa de Falopio.

salt *n.* sal, cloruro de sodio; **iodized** ___ / ___ yodada; **low-** ___ **diet** / dieta hiposódica; **noniodized** ___ / ___ corriente; ___ **-free diet** / dieta libre de ___ o sin ___; ___ **shaker** / salero;

smelling __ -s / __ -es aromáticas *v.*
salar, echar sal; [*to season with*]
condimentar con sal, sazonar.

salty *a.* salado-a, salobre, salino-a.

salubrious *a.* salubre, saludable.

salve *n.* ungento, pomada.

same *a.* mismo-a, idéntico-a, igual.

sample *n.* espécimen, muestra; *v.*
probar; sacar o tomar una muestra.

sampling *n.* muestreo; hacer muestras;
selección partitiva; **random** __ / __ al
azar.

sanatorium *n.* sanatorio, institución de
rehabilitación física o mental.

sanction *n.* sanción, pena.

sand *n.* arena.

sandy *a.* arenoso-a.

sane *a.* sano-a; [*mentally*] cuerdo-a.

sanguine *a.* sanguíneo-a. 1. rel. a la
sangre; 2. de complexión rosácea, con
disposición alegre.

sanguineous *a.* sanguíneo-a, rel. a la
sangre o de abundante sangre.

sanguinolent *a.* sanguinolento-a, que
contiene sangre.

sanitarian *a.* sanitario-a, persona
entrenada en problemas de salubridad.

sanitarium *n.* sanatorio, institución de
salud de rehabilitación física o mental.

sanitary *a.* higiénico-a; __ **napkin** /
servilleta __ absorbente, toalla __ .

sanitation *n.* saneamiento, sanidad.

sanity *n.* cordura, sensatez, bienestar
mental.

sap *n.* savia, jugo natural de algunas
plantas.

saphenous *a.* safeno-a, rel. a las venas
safenas.

saphenous veins *n., pl.* venas
safenas, dos venas superficiales de la
pierna.

saprophyte *n.* saprófito, organismo
vegetal que vive en materia orgánica
pútrida.

sarcoidosis *n.* sarcoidosis. V.
Schaumann's disease.

sarcoma *n.* sarcoma, neoplasma
maligno formado por tejido conectivo;
chondroblastic __ / __
condroblástico; **fibropastic** __ / __
fibroblástico; **gastric** __ / __ gástrico;
lymphatic __ / __ linfático;
medullary __ / __ medular;
myelogenic __ / __ mielógeno;
osteogenic __ / __ óseo; **prostatic** __
/ __ prostático; **pulmonary** __ / __
pulmonar; **renal** __ / __ renal; **soft
tissue** __ / __ de tejido blando.

sardonic laugh *n.* risa sardónica,
contracción espasmódica de los
músculos risorios en forma de una
sonrisa.

satisfactory *a.* satisfactorio-a.

satisfied *a.* satisfecho-a, contento-a.

saturated *a.* saturado-a, empapado-a,
incapaz de absorber o recibir una
sustancia más allá de un límite; __ **fat** /
grasa __; __ **solution** / solución __ .

saturation *n.* saturación, acto de
saturar; __ **index** / índice de __; __
time / tiempo de __ .

save *v.* salvar, [*energy, money*] ahorrar;
[*time*] aprovechar el tiempo.

scab *n.* costra, escara.

scabies *n.* sarna, infección cutánea
parasitaria muy contagiosa que causa
picazón.

scald *n.* escaldadura, quemadura de la
piel causada por vapor o por un líquido
caliente; *v.* lavar en agua hirviendo,
quemar con un líquido caliente.

scale *n.* 1. escala, balanza; 2. escama,
costra, lámina que se desprende de la
piel seca.

scalp *n.* cuero cabelludo; __
dermatoses / dermatosis del __ .

scalpel *n.* escalpelo; bisturí,
instrumento quirúrgico.

scaly *a.* escamoso-a.

scan, scintiscan *n.* tomografía,
escán; rastreo, proceso que reproduce
la imagen de un tejido u órgano
específico usando un detector de la
sustancia radiactiva tecnecio 99 m.
inyectada como medio de contraste;
bone __ / __ de los huesos; **brain** __ /
__ del cerebro; **heart** __ / __ cardíaco;
lung __ / __ pulmonar; **thyroid** __ /
__ de la tiroide.

scanner *n.* escáner.

scanning *n.* exploración, barrido,
escrutinio y registro por medio de un
instrumento de detección de la emisión
de ondas radiactivas de una sustancia
específica que ha sido inyectada y que
se concentra en partes o tejidos en
observación.

scant *a.* escaso-a, parco-a, insuficiente.

scanty *a.* escaso-a, limitado-a, no
abundante.

scaphoid *a.* escafoide, en forma de bote
esp. en referencia al hueso del carpo y
al del tarso.

scapula *n.* escápula, hueso del hombro.

scar *n.* cicatriz, marca en la piel; *v.*
cicatrizar.

scare v. asustar, atemorizar.

scarification n. escarificación, acto de hacer punturas o raspaduras en la piel.

scarlet fever, scarlatina n. escarlatina, enfermedad contagiosa aguda caracterizada por fiebre y erupción con enrojecimiento de la piel y la lengua.

scatology n. escatología. 1. estudio de las heces fecales; 2. obsesión con el excremento y las inmundicias.

scattered a. esparcido-a, diseminado-a; desparramado-a, regado-a.

scene n. escena, escenario.

scent n. olor; aroma, perfume.

Schaumann's disease n. enfermedad de Schaumann, enfermedad crónica manifestada con pequeños tubérculos esp. en los pulmones, los nódulos linfáticos, los huesos y la piel.

schedule n. horario; v. hacer un horario; programar.

Schilling test n. prueba de Schilling, uso de vitamina B_{12} radioactiva en el diagnóstico de anemia perniciosa primaria.

Schistosoma n. Schistosoma, esquistosoma, duela, especie de trematodo cuyas larvas entran en la sangre del huésped por contacto con agua contaminada a través del tubo digestivo o la piel.

schistosomiasis n. esquistosomiasis, infestación producida por la duela.

schizoid a. esquizoide, semejante a la esquizofrenia.

schizophrenia n. esquizofrenia, desintegración mental que transforma la personalidad con varias manifestaciones psicóticas tales como alucinaciones, retraimiento y distorsión de la realidad.

schizophrenic a. esquizofrénico-a, rel. a la esquizofrenia o que padece de ella.

sciatica n. ciática, neuralgia que se irradia a lo largo del nervio ciático.

sciatic nerve n. nervio ciático, nervio que se extiende desde la base de la columna vertebral a lo largo del muslo y se ramifica en la pierna y el pie.

scintigraphy n. escintigrafía, técnica de diagnóstico que emplea radioisótopos para obtener una imagen bidimensional de la distribución de un radiofármaco en un área designada del cuerpo.

scintillation n. escintilación, centelleo, sensación visual de destellos de luz.

scirrhous a. escirroso-a, duro-a, rel. a un escirro.

scirrhus n. escirro, tumor canceroso duro.

sclera, sclerotica n. esclerótica, parte blanca del ojo compuesta de tejido fibroso.

scleritis n. escleritis, infl. de la esclerótica.

scleroderma n. escleroderma, esclerodermia, induración y casi total atrofia de la epidermis.

scleroma n. escleroma, área endurecida y circunscrita de tejido granuloso en la piel o en la membrana mucosa.

sclerosis n. esclerosis, endurecimiento progresivo de los tejidos y órganos; **Alzheimer's** ___ / ___ de Alzheimer; **amyotrophic lateral** ___ / ___ lateral amiotrófica; **arterial** ___ / ___ arterial; **multiple** ___ / ___ múltiple.

sclerotherapy n. escleroterapia, tratamiento con una solución química que se inyecta en las várices para producir esclerosis.

sclerotic a. esclerótico-a, rel. a la esclerosis o afectado por ella.

scoliosis n. escoliosis, desviación lateral pronunciada de la columna vertebral.

scorpion n., Gr. escorpión, alacrán; ___ **sting** / picadura de ___ .

scotoma n., Gr. (pl. **scotomata**) escotoma, área del campo visual en la cual existe pérdida parcial o total de la visión.

scotopia n. escotopia, visión nocturna, adaptación visual a la oscuridad.

scotopic a. escotópico-a, rel. a la escotopia; ___ **vision** / visión ___ .

scrape n. raspadura, rasponazo, raspado; v. raspar, rasguñar.

scratch n. rasguño, arañazo; v. raspar, rascar, rascarse; ___ **test** / prueba del rasguño, gen. para uso en pruebas alérgicas.

screen n. pantalla; v. examinar sistemáticamente un grupo de casos; escrutar; **toxicology** ___ / protocolo toxicológico.

screening n. escrutinio, averiguación, selección; **biochemical** ___ / serie selectiva bioquímica; **multiphasic** __ / __ múltiple; **prescriptive** __ / __ prescrito.

scribble *n.* garabato.

scrofula *n.* escrófula, tuberculosis de la glándula linfática.

scrofuloderma *n.* escrofuloderma, *pop.* lamparón, tipo de escrófula cutánea.

scrotal *a.* escrotal, rel. al escroto.

scrotum *n.* escroto, saco o bolsa que envuelve o contiene los testículos.

scrub *v.* limpiar, fregar, restregar; __ **nurse** / enfermera de cirugía.

scrubbing *n.* limpieza rigurosa de las manos y brazos antes de la cirugía.

scrutiny *n.* escrutinio.

scum *n.* espuma; escoria.

scurvy *n.* escorbuto, enfermedad causada por deficiencia de vitamina C que se manifiesta con anemia, encías sangrantes y un estado general de laxitud.

seam *n.* còstura, línea de costura.

search *n.* bùsqueda, investigación; registro; *v.* buscar, registrar; investigar.

seasickness *n.* mareo; mareo por movimiento.

season *n.* estación; temporada; *v.* [*cooking*] sazonar.

seasonal affective disorders (SAD) *n., pl.* trastornos afectivos estacionales.

seasoned *a.* sazonado-a; __ **foods** / alimentos __ -s.

sebaceous *a.* sebáceo-a, seboso-a, rel. al sebo o de la naturaleza de éste; __ **cyst** / quiste __; __ **gland** / glándula __

seborrhea *n.* seborrea, trastorno de las glándulas sebáceas, caracterizado por una secreción excesiva de sebo.

seborrheic *a.* seborréico-a, rel. to seborrhea; __ **blepharitis** / blefaritis __; __ **dermatitis** / dermatitis __; __ **keratosis** / queratosis __ .

sebum *n.* sebo, secreción espesa que segregan las glándulas sebáceas.

second *n.* segundo; *a.* segundo-a.

secondary *a.* secundario-a.

secretagogue, secretogogue *n.* secretogogo, agente que estimula la secreción glandular.

secrete *v.* secretar, segregar.

secretion *n.* secreción. 1. producción de un tejido o sustancia como resultado de una actividad glandular; **purulent** __ / __ purulenta; 2. sustancia producida por secreción.

secretory *a.* secretor-a, que tiene la propiedad de secretar; __ **capillaries** / capilares secretores; __ **carcinoma** / carcinoma __; __ **fiber** / fibra __; __ **nerve** / nervio __.

section *n.* sección, porción, parte; *v.* cortar; seccionar.

sectioning *n.* el acto de seccionar, dividir, cortar.

secure *a.* seguro-a; *v.* asegurar.

security *n.* seguridad; __ **measures** / medidas de __.

sedation *n.* sedación, acción o efecto de calmar o sedar; *v.* **to put under** __ / dar un sedante, calmante o soporífero.

sedative *n.* calmante, sedante, agente con efectos tranquilizantes.

sedentary *a.* sedentario-a. 1. de poca actividad física; 2. rel. a la posición sentada.

sediment *n.* sedimento, materia que se deposita en el fondo de un líquido.

sedimentation *n.* sedimentación, acción o proceso de depositar sedimentos; __ **rate** / índice de __.

see *vi.* ver; **I see!** / ¡Ya veo!; **Let's** __ / Vamos a ver; **to** __ **to it** / atender, ver que, hacer que.

seeing *n.* vista, visión.

segment *n.* segmento, porción, sección.

segmentation *n.* segmentación, acto de dividir en partes.

Seguin's signal symptom *n.* Seguin, síntoma de, contracción involuntaria de los músculos antes de un ataque epiléptico.

seizure *n.* ataque repentino, acceso; __ **activity** / actividad convulsiva.

seldom *adv.* rara vez, con rareza, raramente.

selection *n.* selección, elección.

self *n.* el yo; *pron.* uno-a mismo-a; *a.* sí mismo-a; mismo-a; propio-a; __ -assurance / confianza en __; __ -centered / egoísta, egocéntrico-a; __ -conscious / concentrado-a en __, cohibido-a; __ -contained / autónomo; [*personality*] reservado-a; __ -contamination / autocontaminación; __ -control / dominio de __; __ -defense / defensa propia; __ -delusion, deception / engaño a __; __ -denial / abnegación; __ -determination / autodeterminación; __ -distrust / falta de confianza en __; __ -esteem / amor propio,

reconocimiento de valores propios; ___
-identity / conciencia de la identidad
del yo; ___ **-induced** / auto-inducido-a;
___ **-medication** / automedicación; ___
-pity / compasión por ___; v. **to be** ___
-sufficient / valerse por ___ .

sella turcica n. silla turca, depresión
en la superficie superior del esfenoide
que contiene la hipófisis.

semen n. semen, esperma, secreción
espesa blanca segregada por los
órganos reproductivos masculinos.

semicoma n. semicoma, estado
comatoso leve.

seminal a. seminal, rel. a una semilla o
que consiste de una semilla.

seminiferous a. seminífero-a, que
produce semen; ___ **tubular** /
conductor ___.

seminoma n. seminoma, tumor del
testículo.

seminuria n. seminuria, presencia de
semen en la orina.

semiotic n. semiótico-a, rel. a los
síntomas o señales de una enfermedad.

semiotics n. semiótica, rama de la
medicina que trata de las señales y
síntomas de una enfermedad.

senescence n. senescencia, senectud,
proceso de envejecimiento.

senile a. senil, rel. a la vejez esp. en lo
que afecta a las funciones mentales y
físicas.

senility n. senilidad, cualidad de ser
senil.

senior citizen n. persona mayor;
jubilado-a.

sensation n. sensación, percepción de
una estimulación por un órgano
sensorial.

sense n. sentido, facultad de percibir por
medio de los órganos sensoriales;
common ___ / ___ común; ___ **of
hearing** / ___ del oído; ___ **of humor** /
___ del humor; ___ **of sight** / ___ de la
vista; ___ **of smell** / ___ del olfato; ___ **of
taste** / ___ del gusto; ___ **of touch** / ___
del tacto; v. sentir.

sensibility n sensibilidad, capacidad de
recibir sensaciones.

sensiferous a. sensífero-a, que causa,
transmite o conduce sensaciones.

sensitive a. sensitivo-a, sensible.

sensitivity n. sensibilidad,
susceptibilidad.

sensitivity training n. entrenamiento
de la sensibilidad o capacidad
sensorial.

sensitization n. sensibilización, acto
de hacer sensible ho sensorial.

sensorial a. sensorial, sensitivo-a; que
se percibe por los sentidos.

sensorimotor a. sensitivomotor, rel. a
las actividades motoras y sensitivas del
cuerpo.

sensory a. sensorial, sensorio-a, rel. a
las sensaciones o los sentidos; ___
acuity level / nivel de agudeza ___; ___
aphasia / afasia ___; ___ **depravation**
/ depravación ___; ___ **epilepsy** /
epilepsia ___; ___ **ganglion** / ganglio
___; ___ **image** / imagen ___; ___
integration / integración ___; ___
overload / sobrecarga ___; ___
processing / procesamiento ___ .

sensory nervous system n.
sistema nervioso sensorial.

sensory threshold n. umbral
sensorial.

sensual a. sensual, carnal.

sensuous a. sensual.

sentiment n. sentimiento.

sepsis n., L. sepsis, condición tóxica
producida por una contaminación
bacteriana.

septal a. septal, rel. a un septum; ___
deviation / desviación ___ .

septate a. septado-a, rel. a una
estructura dividida por un
septum.

septectomy n. septectomía, escisión
parcial o total del tabique nasal.

septic n. séptico-a, rel. a la sepsis; ___
shock / choque ___ .

septicemia, blood poisoning n.
septicemia, envenenamiento de la
sangre, invasión de la sangre por
microorganismos virulentos.

septum n., L. (pl. **septa**) septum,
tabique o membrana que divide dos
cavidades o espacios; **ventricular** ___ /
___ ventricular.

sequela n. (pl. **sequelae**) secuela,
condición que resulta de una
enfermedad, lesión o tratamiento.

sequestration n. secuestro,
aislamiento. 1. acto de aislar;
2. formación de un sequestrum.

sequestrum n. sequestrum, secuestro,
fragmento de un hueso necrosado
que se separa de un hueso sano
adyacente.

series n. serie, grupo de especímenes en
una secuencia.

serious a. serio-a; complicado-a; **-ly**
adv. seriamente.

seroconversion *n.* seroconversión, desarrollo de anticuerpos como respuesta a una infección o a la administración de una vacuna.

serologic, serological *a.* serológico-a, rel. a un suero; __ test / prueba __ .

seroma *n.* seroma, acumulación gen. subcutánea de suero sanguíneo que produce una hinchazón que se asemeja a un tumor.

seronegative *a.* seronegativo-a, que presenta una reacción negativa a pruebas serológicas.

seropositive *a.* seropositivo-a, que presenta una reacción positiva a pruebas serológicas.

serosa *n.* membrana serosa.

serosanguineous *a.* serosanguíneo-a, de naturaleza serosa y sanguínea.

serositis *n.* serositis, infl. de una membrana serosa, signo importante en enfermedades del tejido conjuntivo tal como el lupus sistémico eritematoso.

serotype *n.* serotipo, tipo de microorganismo que se determina por las clases y combinaciones de antígenos presentes en la célula.

serotyping *n.* determinación del serotipo.

serous *a.* seroso-a. 1. de la naturaleza del suero; 2. que produce o contiene suero.

serum *n.* suero, líquido seroso. 1. elemento del plasma que permanece líquido y claro después de la coagulación; 2. cualquier líquido seroso; 3. suero inmune de animales o personas que se inocula para producir inmunizaciones pasivas o temporales.

services *n.* servicios; **emergency** __ / __ de emergencia; **extended care facility** __ / __ de cuidado o atención extendida; **preventive health** __ / __ de salud preventiva.

sesamoid *a.* sesamoideo, semejante a una pequeña masa o semilla incrustada en una articulación o cartílago.

sessile *a.* sésil, insertado o fijo en una base ancha que carece de pedúnculo.

session *n.* sesión.

set *n.* conjunto, equipo; grupo; instrumentos y accesorios; [*surgical*] instrumental quirúrgico; **it is all** __ / todo está arreglado; *vi.* poner, colocar; [*a broken bone*] encasar, fijar, ajustar; __ **a fracture** / componer una fractura.

setback *n.* recaída; retraso, contrariedad.

sever *v.* cortar, romper; separar.

several *a.* varios-as, muchos-as, algunos-as.

severe *a.* grave, severo-a; __ **acute respiratory syndrome** / síndrome respiratorio agudo __ .

severe combined immunodeficiency disease *n.* enfermedad grave de inmunodeficiencia combinada, una de las enfermedades genéticas raras que se caracteriza por el desarrollo defectivo de las células que generan anticuerpos.

sex *n.* sexo; __ **determination** / determinación del __; __ **disorders** / trastornos o anomalías sexuales; __ **distribution** / distribución según el __ .

sex-linked *a.* 1. relacionado con el sexo; 2. que se refiere a cromosomas sexuales o es transmitido por ellos.

sexual *a.* sexual, rel. al sexo; __ **assault** / agresión __; __ **behavior** / conducta __; __**characteristics** / características __ -es; __**development** / desarrollo __; __ **health** / salud __; __ **intercourse** / relaciones __ -es, coito; __ **life** / vida __; __ **maturity** / madurez __; **-ly** *adv.* sexualmente; __ **transmitted disease.** / enfermedad transmitida __ . V. cuadro esta página.

sexuality *n.* sexualidad, características de cada sexo.

shadow *n.* sombra; opacidad.

shake *vi.* agitar; [*hands*] dar la mano; [*from cold*] temblar, tiritar de frío; __ **well before using** / agítese bien antes de usarse.

Sexual Disorders	Trastornos Sexuales
erotomania	erotomanía
exhibitionism	exhibicionismo
fetishism	fetichismo
frotteurism	froterismo
masochism	masoquismo
nymphomania	ninfomanía
paraphilia	parafilia
pedophilia	pedofilia
sadism	sadismo
satyromania	satiromanía
transvestic fetishism	fetichismo trasvestido
voyeurism	voyeurismo, mironismo

shakes n. pl. temblores, *pop.*
tembladera; escalofríos; fiebre
intermitente.

shaking palsy n. parálisis agitante.
Parkinson's disease.

shaman n. curandero.

shameful a. vergonzoso-a,
penoso-a.

shank n. canilla de la pierna.

shape n. forma, aspecto; condición
[*health*] **in bad __** / enfermo-a;
destruido-a; **out of __** / deformado-a,
imperfecto [*physically*] desajuste
físico; v. formar, moldear.

sharp a. [*pain*] agudo-a; [*instrument*]
afilado-a.

shave v. afeitar; afeitarse.

sheath n. cubierta, capa o membrana
protectora.

shed vi. [*blood, tears*] derramar; [*light*]
dar, esparcir; difundir; [*skin, hair*]
mudar; pelar; soltar; descamar.

sheet n. lámina, hoja de metal;
[*bedclothes*] sábana.

Shiatsu n. técnica oriental de aplicación
de terapia de puntos de presión con los
dedos, codos, rodillas y pies con
suavidad para liberar la energía.

shift n. cambio de posición, desviación;
[*work period*] turno; v. cambiar,
desviar.

shigellosis n. shigelosis, disentería
bacilar.

shinbone n. espinilla, borde anterior de
la tibia.

shingles n. *pop.* culebrilla, herpes
zóster, erupción inflamatoria de la piel
con vesículas o ampollas gen.
localizadas en el tronco.

shiver n. estremecimiento, escalofrío,
temblor; v. tener escalofríos; tiritar de
frío; estremecerse.

shock, choc n., *Fr.* shock, choque,
estado anormal generado por una
insuficiencia circulatoria sanguínea que
puede causar descenso en la presión
arterial, pulso rápido, palidez,
temperatura anormalmente baja y
debilidad; **anaphylactic __ / __**
anafiláctico; **endotoxic __ / __**
endotóxico; **septic __ / __** séptico; **__**
therapy, electric / terapia
electroconvulsiva.

shoe n. zapato, calzado; **cast __ / __** en
escayola; **orthopedic __ -s** / calzado
ortopédico.

short a. corto-a; [*time*] breve; [*height*]
bajo-a; **in a __ time** / en breve, dentro

de poco; **on __ notice** / en corto plazo;
__ of breath / falto-a de respiración.

shortage n. carencia, falta, déficit.

shortsightedness,
nearsightedness n. miopía.

shot n. (*injection*) inyección; tiro, (*bullet
wound*) balazo; tiro, disparo.

shoulder n. hombro, unión de la
clavícula, la escápula y el húmero.

shout n. grito, alarido; v. gritar.

show vi. mostrar, enseñar, manifestar;
revelar.

shower n. ducha; v. ducharse, darse una
ducha.

shrink n. *pop.* psiquiatra o alienista,
psicólogo; vi. encoger; encogerse.

shunt n. desviación, derivación, *shunt*;
low-flow __ / derivación de flujo
lento; v. desviar, derivar.

shy a. tímido-a, temeroso-a; cauteloso-a.

Shy-Drager syndrome n.
Shy-Drager, síndrome de, enfermedad
neurodegenerativa vista en personas de
edad media y mayores de edad, que
afecta el sistema nervioso autónomo y
se caracteriza por hipotensión crónica
ortostática, con pérdida del
conocimiento, impotencia,
incontinencia y arrítmia cardíaca.

sialadenitis, sialoadenitis n.
sialoadenitis, infl. de una glándula
salival.

Sialoadenectomy n.
sialoadenectomía, incision and drenaje
de una clándula salival.

sialogram n. sialograma, rayos-x del
conducto de la glándula salival.

sibling n. hermanos de los mismos
padres.

sick n. a. enfermo-a; **__ leave** / licencia
por enfermedad.

sickly a. enfermizo-a, achacoso-a,
endeble.

sickness n. enfermedad, dolencia, mal;
acute African sleeping __ / __
africana del sueño; **altitude __** / mal
de altura; **beriberi __** / de Ceylon;
bleeding __ / hemofilia; **car __** /
cinetosis, mareo; **decompression __** /
__ de los buzos; **falling __** / epilepsia;
gall __ / anaplasmosis; **green __** /
clorosis, cloroanemia; **milk __** /
brucelosis; **morning __** / trastorno de
las embarazadas; **motion __ / __** de
los viajeros; **radiation __ / __** por
radiación.

side n. lado, costado; **by the __ of** / al
__ de; **right __ / __** derecho; **left __ /**

459

__ izquierdo; __ **effect** / efecto secundario, reacción gen. adversa a un medicamento, tratamiento o droga.

sight *n.* vista; **at first** __ / a primera __ .

sigmoid *a.* sigmoide, sigmoideo. 1. que tiene forma de sigmoid; 2. rel. al colon sigmoide.

sigmoidoscopy *n.* sigmoidoscopía, uso de un sigmoidoscopio para examinar la flexura sigmoide.

sign *n.* señal, signo, indicación, manifestación objetiva de una enfermedad; **vital** __ **-s** / signos vitales.

signature *n.* 1. firma; 2. parte de una receta médica que contiene las instrucciones.

significance *a.* significado; **of no** __ / sin importancia.

significant *a.* importante, significativo-a.

sign language *n.* lenguaje mímico por señales. V. dactylology.

silent *a.* silencioso-a.

silicosis *n.* silicosis, inhalación de partículas de polvo.

silver *n.* plata; __ **nitrate** / nitrato de __ .

similar *a.* similar, semejante, parecido-a.

simple *a.* simple, sencillo-a; **-ly** *adv.* simplemente, meramente.

simplify *v.* simplificar.

simulation *n.* simulación, fingir un síntoma o enfermedad.

since *adv.* desde; __ **then, ever** __ / entonces; __ **when?** / ¿__ cuándo?

sinew *n.* tendón.

single *a.* sencillo-a, simple, solo-a; [*unmarried*] soltero-a.

sinoatrial *a.* sinoatrial, rel. a la región del seno auricular.

sinoatrial, sinoauricular node *n.* nódulo sinusal o senoauricular, localizado en la unión de la vena cava y la aurícula derecha, y que se considera el punto de origen de los impulsos que estimulan los latidos del corazón.

sinus *n., L.* sinus, seno, cavidad de abertura estrecha; __ **rhythm** / ritmo sinusal.

sinusal *a.* sinusal, rel. a un sinus.

sinusitis *n.* sinusitis, infl. de la mucosa de un seno o cavidad, esp. los senos paranasales.

sinusoid *n.* sinusoide, conducto diminuto que lleva sangre a los tejidos de un órgano; *a.* rel. a un sinus.

sip *n.* sorbo, trago; *v.* sorber.

sister *n.* hermana; __ **-in-law** / cuñada.

situated *a.* situado-a, localizado-a.

situation *n.* situación, localización.

situs *n., L.* situs, posición, sitio.

size *n.* tamaño; [*garments*] talla.

Sjogrens' Syndrome *n.* Sjogren, síndrome de, trastorno autoinmune que resulta en escasa secreción salival y lacrimal causando sequedad en la boca y los ojos.

skeleton *n.* esqueleto, armazón ósea del cuerpo.

skill *n.* destreza, habilidad.

skin *n.* piel, epidermis, cutis; *pop.* pellejo; **sagging facial** __ / cutis colgante; __ **cancer** / cáncer de la __; __ **chafing** / fricción de la __; __ **diseases** / enfermedades de la __, dermatosis; __ **graft** / injerto de la __; __ **rash** / erupción cutánea, urticaria; __**rejuvenation** / rejuvenecimiento de la __; __ **tests** / pruebas cutáneas; __ **ulcer** / úlcera cutánea. V. ilustración en la página 461.

skinny *a.* flaco-a, delgado-a, descarnado-a.

skip *v.* omitir, pasar por alto; [*jump*] saltar.

skull *n.* cráneo; calavera, estructura ósea de la cabeza; **base of the** __ / base del __; __ **fractures** / fracturas del __.

slant *n.* inclinación, plano inclinado; *v.* inclinar; [*words*] distorsionar; inclinarse.

slanted *a.* oblicuo-a, inclinado-a; sesgado-a.

sleep *n.* sueño; **balmy** __ / __ reparador; __ **apnea** / apnea intermitente que ocurre durante el sueño; __ **cycles** / ciclos del __; __ **disorders** / trastornos del __; __ **stages** / fases del __; **twilight** __ / __ crepuscular; *vi.* dormir; dormirse; **to** __ **soundly** / __ profundamente.

sleepiness *n.* somnolencia, adormecimiento.

sleeping pill *n.* soporífero, somnífero, pastilla para dormir.

sleeping sickness *n.* enfermedad del sueño, dolencia aguda endémica de África que se manifiesta con fiebre, letargo, escalofríos, pérdida de peso y debilidad general, causada por un protozoo transmitido por la picadura de la mosca tsetse.

sleepwalking *n.* sonambulismo.

sleeve *n.* manga; **Put up your** __ / Súbase, súbete la manga.

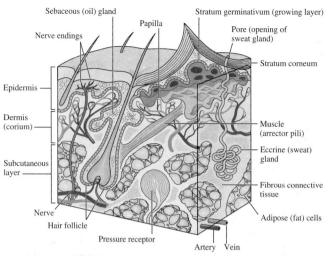

Sebaceous (oil) gland

Papilla

Stratum germinativum (growing layer)

Nerve endings

Pore (opening of sweat gland)

Stratum corneum

Epidermis

Dermis (corium)

Muscle (arrector pili)

Eccrine (sweat) gland

Subcutaneous layer

Fibrous connective tissue

Adipose (fat) cells

Nerve

Hair follicle

Pressure receptor

Artery   Vein

Cross section of the skin

---

slender *a.* esbelto-a; delgado-a.

slide *n.* diapositiva, laminilla; [*specimen holder*] portaobjeto; *v.* deslizarse.

slight *a.* ligero-a, leve; ___ **fever** / fiebrecita, fiebre ___ .

slim *a.* delgado-a; esbelto-a; insuficiente; **a ___ chance** / poco probable.

sling *n.* cabestrillo, soporte de vendaje.

slip *v.* resbalarse.

slippery *a.* resbaladizo-a, resbaloso-a.

slit *n.* incisión, hendidura, rajadura; *v.* **to make a ___** / hacer una incisión, hacer una hendidura; rajar, cortar en tiras.

slow *a.* lento-a, pausado-a, despacioso-a; [*clock*] atrasado, retrasado; *v.* **to ___ down** / ir más despacio; tener más calma; **-ly** *adv.* lentamente, pausadamente, más despacio.

sluggish *a.* flojo-a, inactivo-a, de movimiento lento.

small *a.* pequeño-a; **smaller** / *comp.* más pequeño; **smallest** / *sup.* el menor, el más pequeño.

smallpox *n.* viruela, enfermedad infecciosa viral que se manifiesta con un cuadro febril agudo y erupción de ampollas y pústulas diseminadas por todo el cuerpo.

smart *a.* inteligente, listo-a.

smear *n.* frotis, unto; *v.* untar, embarrar.

smegma *n.* esmegma, secreción producida por las glándulas sebáceas vista esp. en los órganos genitales exteriores.

smell *n.* 1. olor, aroma; **penetrating ___** / ___ penetrante; 2. sentido del olfato; *v.* oler, percibir un olor.

smile *n.* sonrisa; *v.* sonreír.

smog *n.* mezcla de niebla y humo.

smoke *n.* humo; ___ **inhalation** / inhalación de ___; ___ **screen** / cortina de ___; *v.* fumar; **Do not ___ here** / No fume, no fumes aquí.

smooth *a.* liso-a; [*cutis*] suave, terso-a, delicado-a.

snake *n.* serpiente, culebra; ___ **-bite** / mordedura de ___; **poisonous ___** / ___ venenosa.

snap *n.* chasquido, ruido cardíaco relacionado con la apertura de una válvula del corazón, gen. la válvula mitral; **opening ___** / ___ de apertura.

sneeze *n.* estornudo; *v.* estornudar.

Snellan's eye test Snellan, prueba de ojo, uadro de letras negras que gradualmente disminuyen en tamaño, usado para probar la agudeza visual.

sniff *v.* olfatear, oler; absorber por la nariz; resoplar.

sniffle *n.* catarro nasal; *v.* sorber repetidamente por la nariz.

snore n. ronquido; v. roncar.

snort v. aspirar a través de la mucosa nasal.

snow n. nieve; v. nevar.

snuff v. inhalar; resoplar hacia adentro; **to ___ up** / tomar por la nariz.

so adv. así, de este modo, de esta manera; **it is not ___** / no es ___; **not ___ much** / no tanto; **so-so** / más o menos, regular; **___ that** / de manera que.

soap n. jabón; v. enjabonar; **to ___ oneself** / enjabonarse.

sober a. sobrio-a, serio; v. **to get ___** / dejar de beber, dejar de tomar bebidas alcohólicas

social a. social, sociable; **___ behavior** / conducta o comportamiento ___; **___ security** / seguro ___; **___ work** / asistencia ___; **___ worker** / trabajador-a ___ .

socialization n. socialización, adaptación social.

socialized a. socializado-a; **___ medicine** / medicina ___ .

society n. sociedad; organización social.

sociopath n. sociópata, persona caracterizada por una conducta antisocial.

socket n. hueco, [of a bone] fosa; [electric] enchufe.

soda n. soda, carbonato de sodio; **baking ___** / bicarbonato de sodio.

sodium n. sodio, elemento metálico alcalino que se encuentra en los líquidos del cuerpo.

sodomite n. sodomita, persona que comete sodomía.

sodomy n. sodomía, término que denota relación sexual entre personas del mismo sexo; bestialidad o felación.

soft a. blando-a, suave, delicado-a; [metals] flexible, maleable; **___ diet** / dieta ___; **___ drinks** / refrescos, bebidas no alcohólicas; **-ly** adv. suavemente, blandamente.

soften v. ablandar, suavizar.

softening n. reblandecimiento, ablandamiento; suavidad.

soil n. tierra, terreno; [dirt] suciedad.

solar a. solar, rel. al sol; **___ energy** / energía ___.

sole n. suela, planta del pie.

solid a. sólido-a, macizo-a; [person] serio-a, formal.

soluble a. soluble.

solution n. solución.

solvent n. solvente, líquido que disuelve o es capaz de producir una solución.

somatic a. somático-a, rel. al cuerpo.

somatization n. somatización. proceso de conversión de experiencias mentales en manifestaciones corporales.

some a. alguno-a; algún, algo de, un poco de; unos, unos cuantos, unas, unas cuantas, algunos-as.

somebody n. alguien; **___ else** / otra persona.

somehow adv. de algún modo, de alguna manera.

something n. alguna cosa, algo; **___ else** / otra cosa.

somnambulance, somnambulism n. sonambulismo.

somnambule n. sonámbulo-a, persona que anda mientras está dormida.

somniferous n. soporífero.

somniloquism n. somniloquia, el acto de hablar dormido-a.

somnolence n. somnolencia.

son n. hijo; **___ -in-law** / yerno; **sonny** / hijito.

sonogram n. sonograma, registro de una imagen producida por ultrasonido.

sonography n. sonografía. V. **ultrasonography**.

sonorous a. sonoro-a, resonante, con un sonido vibrante.

soon adv. pronto, dentro de poco, en poco tiempo.

soothe v. calmar, aliviar, mitigar; suavizar.

sophistication n. sofisticación, adulteración de una sustancia.

soporific n. soporífico, agente que produce el sueño.

soporose, soporous a. soporosa, soporoso, en estado de sopor.

sore n. llaga, úlcera, herida; a. [feeling] adolorido-a, doloroso-a, con dolor; **___ all over** / malestar general, dolor en todo el cuerpo; **___ eyes** / malestar en los ojos, ojos adoloridos; **___ throat** / dolor de garganta; v. **to be ___** / estar adolorido-a.

sorrow n. pena, aflicción, pesar, dolor.

sorry a. apesadumbrado-a; **I am ___** / Lo siento; v. **to be ___** / arrepentirse de; **to be ___ for** [someone] / tener lástima de (alguien).

sort n. clase, especie, género; **all ___ -s of** / una variedad de; **out of ___ -s** / malhumorado-a, indispuesto-a; v. separar, clasificar, distribuir.

soul n. alma, espíritu.

sound *n.* sonido, ruido; ruido de soplo percibido por auscultación; *v.* sonar.

source *n.* origen; foco; fuente.

space *n.* área, espacio, segmento, lugar.

span *n.* lapso, instante, momento; tiempo limitado; intervalo; distancia.

Spanish *n.* [*language*] español; [*native*] español-a *a.* español-a;
Spanish-American / hispanoamericano-a.

spasm *n.* espasmo, convulsión, contracción muscular involuntaria.

spasmodic *a.* espasmódico-a.

spastic *a.* espástico-a, convulsivo-a, espasmódico-a. 1. de naturaleza espasmódica; ___ **colon** / colon espasmódico o espástico; 2. que sufre espasmos.

spasticity *n.* espasticidad, aumento en la tensión normal de un músculo que causa movimientos rígidos y dificultosos.

speak *vi.* hablar; ___ **louder** / hable, habla más alto; ___ **slowly** / hable, habla despacio.

special *a.* especial, único-a; extraordinario-a; **-ly** *adv.* especialmente.

specialist *n.* especialista.

specialty *n.* especialidad. V. cuadro en la página 108.

species *n.* especie, clasificación de organismos vivos pertenecientes a una categoría biológica.

specific *a.* específico-a; determinado-a; preciso-a; ___ **gravity**/gravedad ___.

specimen *n.* espécimen, muestra.

speck *n.* mácula, mancha.

spectacles *n., pl.* lentes, espejuelos, gafas.

spectrum *n.* (*pl.* **spectra**) espectro. 1. amplitud en la actividad de un antibiótico contra variedades de microorganismos; 2. serie de imágenes que resultan de la refracción de radiación electromagnética; 3. banda matizada de rayos solares discernibles a simple vista o con un instrumento sensitivo.

speculum *n.* espéculo, instrumento para dilatar un conducto o cavidad.

speech *n.* habla, lenguaje; **garbled** ___ / ___ enredada; ___ **defect** / defecto del ___; ___ **disorder** / trastorno del ___; ___ **therapy** / terapéutica del ___ .

spell *n.* ataque súbito; *v.* **to have a** ___ / tener un ataque o acceso de; deletrear; **to** ___ **a word** / deletrear una palabra.

spend *vi.* [*energy*] gastar, [*time*] pasar, [*money*] gastar, consumir.

sperm *n.* esperma, semen; **decreased** ___ **count** / conteo disminuido de ___; ___ **count** / espermiograma; semen; ___ **donor** / donante de ___ .

spermatic *a.* espermático, rel. al esperma; ___ **cord** / cordón ___.

spermaticidal, spermaticide *n.* espermaticida, que destruye o causa la muerte de espermatozoos.

spermatocele *n.* espermatocele, quiste del epidídimo que contiene espermatozoos.

spermatogenesis *n.* espermatogénesis, proceso de formación y desarrollo de espermatozoos.

spermatozoid, spermatozoon *n., Gr.* (*pl.* **spermatozoa**) espermatozoo, célula sexual masculina que fertiliza el óvulo.

spermaturia *n.* espermaturia, semen en la orina.

spermiogram *n.* espermiograma, evaluación de los espermatozoides en el proceso de determinación de la esterilidad.

sphenoid *n.* esfenoide, hueso situado en la base del cráneo.

sphere *n.* esfera. 1. estructura en forma de globo; 2. ambiente sociológico.

spherocyte *n.* esferocito, eritrocito de forma esférica.

spherocytosis *n.* esferocitosis, presencia de esferocitos en la sangre.

sphincter *n.* esfínter, músculo circular que abre y cierra un orificio.

sphincter of Oddi *n.* Oddi, esfínter de, músculo circular contráctil situado en la apertura intestinal de la bilis y los conductos pancreáticos.

sphincteroplasty *n.* esfinteroplastia, operación plástica de un esfínter.

sphincterotomy *n.* esfinterotomía, corte de un esfínter.

sphygmomanometer *n.* esfigmomanómetro, instrumento para determinar la presión arterial.

spica *n.* espica, tipo de vendaje.

spicule *n.* espícula, cuerpo en forma de aguja.

spider *n.* araña; **black** ___ / araña negra.

spike *n.* espiga; [*in a graphic*] cresta o elevación brusca.

spina *n.* spina, espina. 1. protuberancia en forma de espina; 2. la espina dorsal o columna vertebral.

spina bifida

spina bifida *n.* espina bífida, malformación congénita en el cierre de un conducto de la estructura ósea de la espina vertebral, con o sin protrusión de las meninges medulares, gen. a nivel lumbar; **occult** ___ / ___ oculta, sin protrusión.

spinal *a.* espinal, raquídeo-a, rel. a la médula espinal o a la espina o columna vertebral; ___ **anesthesia** / anestesia raquídea; ___ **canal** / canal raquídeo; ___ **cord** / médula ___; ___ **fluid** / líquido cefalorraquídeo; ___ **fusion** / fusión ___; ___ **muscular atrophy** / atrofia muscular ___; ___ **puncture** / punción ___; ___ **shock** / choque ___; ___ **stenosis** / estenosis ___.

spinal column *n.* columna o espina vertebral, estructura ósea formada por treinta y tres vértebras que rodean y contienen la médula espinal.

spinal cord *n.* médula espinal, columna de tejido nervioso que se extiende desde el bulbo raquídeo hasta la segunda vértebra lumbar y de la cual parten todos los nervios que van al tronco y a las extremidades; ___ **compression** / compresión de la ___.

spine *n.* columna o espina vertebral; *pop.* espinazo.

spine-shaped *a.* espinoso-a, acantoso-a.

spiral *a.* espiral, que se envuelve alrededor de un centro o axis.

spirit *n.* 1. espíritu, alma; 2. solución alcohólica de una sustancia volátil.

spiritual healing *n.* cura mental, cura espiritual.

spirochetal *a.* espiroquetósico-a, rel. a espiroquetas.

spirochete *n.* espiroqueta, microorganismo espiral de la especie *Spirochaetales* que incluye el microorganismo causante de la sífilis.

spirometer *n.* espirómetro, instrumento que se usa para medir la cantidad de aire que se inhala y la que se expele del pulmón.

spirometry *n.* espirometría, medida de la capacidad respiratoria tomada por medio de un espirómetro.

spit *n.* saliva, escupo; *vi.* escupir, expectorar.

spittle *n.* saliva; expectoración; salivazo, escupitajo.

splanchnic *a.* esplácnico-a, rel. a las vísceras o que llega a éstas; ___ **nerves** / nervios ___ -s.

spleen *n.* bazo, órgano vascular linfático, situado en la cavidad abdominal; **accesory** ___ / ___ accesorio.

splenectomy *n.* esplenectomía, excisión del bazo.

splenic *a.* esplénico-a, rel. al bazo; ___ **infart** / infarto ___.

splenitis *n.* esplenitis, inf. del bazo.

splenoportography *n.* esplenoportografía, radiografía de las venas esplénica y cava usando un medio de contraste radioopaco inyectado en el bazo.

splenorenal *a.* esplenorrenal, rel. al bazo y al riñón.

splenorenal shunt *n.* derivación esplenorrenal, anastomosis de la vena o arteria esplénica a la vena renal esp. en el tratamiento de la hipertensión portal.

splint *n.* férula, tablilla, soporte de madera, metal, plástico, vidrio de fibra o yeso usado para dar apoyo, inmovilizar un hueso fracturado o proteger una parte del cuerpo.

splinter *n.* espina; esquirla; astilla.

split *n.* división, desunión; abertura; *v.* dividir, desunir, separar; dividirse, separarse.

spoken language *n.* lenguaje hablado.

spondylitis *n.* espondilitis, infl. de una o más vértebras; **ankylosing** ___ / anquilosante, reumatoide.

spondylolisthesis *n.* espondilolistesis, desplazamiento anterior de una vértebra sobre otra, gen. la cuarta lumbar sobre la quinta o ésta sobre el sacro.

spondylolysis *n.* espondilólisis, disolución o destrucción de una vértebra.

spondylopathy *n.* espondilopatía, cualquier enfermedad que afecta las vértebras.

spondylosis *n.* espondilosis. 1. anquilosis vertebral; 2. toda lesión degenerativa de la columna vertebral.

sponge *n.* esponja; *v.* esponjar, remojar con una esponja.

spontaneous *a.* espontáneo-a.

sporadic *a.* esporádico-a, infrecuente.

spore *n.* espora, célula reproductiva unicelular.

sporicide *n.* esporicida, agente que destruye esporas.

sport *n.* deporte; ___ **-s medicine** / medicina del deporte.

spot n. mancha, marca, pápula; **blind** __ / punto ciego; **liver** __ / __ hepática; v. [*stain*] manchar; [*notice*] notar.

spotting n. manchas de flujo vaginal sanguinolento.

spouse n. esposo-a.

sprain n. torcedura, esguince, torsión de una articulación con distensión y laceración parcial de los ligamentos; v. torcer; torcerse; **to __ one's ankle** / __ el tobillo.

spray n. atomizador de líquido para rociar; v. rociar con un líquido.

spread n. extensión, diseminación, esparcimiento; a. extendido-a, esparcido-a; diseminado-a; vi. diseminar; esparcir; extender; diseminarse, esparcirse, extenderse.

sprue n. esprue, enfermedad digestiva crónica caracterizada por la inhabilidad de absorber alimentos que contienen gluten.

spur n. espolón, protuberancia esp. de un hueso; **calcaneal** __ / __ calcáneo.

sputum n. esputo, flema; **bloody** __ / __ sanguinolento.

squamous a. escamoso-a; __ **cell** / célula __ .

squat v. agacharse; sentarse en cuclillas; acuclillarse.

squeal n. chillido, alarido; v. chillar.

squeeze v. apretar, comprimir; [*cloth, fruit*] exprimir.

squint n. estrabismo; acción de encoger los ojos como protección contra una luz intensa, o para tratar de ver mejor. V. **strabismus**.

stab n. puñalada; v. apuñalar, acuchillar.

stability n. estabilidad, permanencia, seguridad.

stabilize v. estabilizar, evitar cambios o fluctuaciones.

stable a. estable, que no fluctúa.

staff n. personal de una institución.

stage n. [*sickness*] estadío, etapa o período de transición durante el desarrollo de una enfermedad; fase; **in a recuperating** __ / en una fase de recuperación.

stagger v. escalonar, saltear, distribuir con una secuencia; vacilar; tambalear; tambalearse.

staging n. estadificación, clasificación de la extensión y gravedad durante el proceso de una enfermedad.

stagnation n. estancación, estancamiento, falta de circulación en los líquidos.

stain n. 1. colorante, tinte; 2. mancha, mácula.

staining n. coloración, tintura.

stammer n. tartamudeo, balbuceo; v. tartamudear, balbucear.

stand n. sitio, puesto, situación; vi. ponerse o estar de pie; sostenerse; __ **on your toes** / pararse en la punta de los pies; **to __ back** / retroceder; **to __ still** / no moverse, estarse quieto-a.

standard n. estándar, norma, criterio, pauta a seguir; lo normal, lo usual o común; __ **deviation** / desviación __ ; __ **error** / error __ ; __ **of care** / atención o cuidado __ ; __ **procedure** / procedimiento __ , procedimiento usual establecido.

standardization n. estandarización, uniformidad; normalización.

standing n. [*position*] de pie; [*pending*] vigente; __ **orders** / órdenes o reglamento vigente.

standstill n. paro, cese de actividad.

stapedectomy n. excisión del estribo para mejorar la audición.

stapes n. estribo, el más interno de los huesecillos del oído.

staphylococcal a. estafilocócico-a, rel. a o causado por estafilococos; __ **food poisoning** / intoxicación alimenticia por estafilococos; __ **infections** / infecciones __ .

staphylococcemia n. estafilococemia, presencia de estafilococos en la sangre.

Staphylococcus n., *Gr.* estafilococo. 1. especie de bacteria gram-positiva que puede causar diferentes clases de infecciones; incluye parásitos que se alojan en la piel y las mucosas; 2. término aplicado a cualquier micrococo patológico.

staphylotoxin n. estafilotoxina, toxina producida por estafilococos.

starch n. almidón, fécula, elemento principal de los carbohidratos. v. almidonar.

starchy a. feculento-a; almidonado-a; __ **foods** / alimentos __ -s, almidones que contienen carbohidratos.

start n. comienzo, principio, inicio; v. empezar, comenzar, iniciar; hacer andar o funcionar un aparato; [*motor*] arrancar, poner en marcha.

starvation n. desnutrición, inanición, hambre, privación de alimentos.

starve v. pasar hambre, privar de alimentos.

stasis *n.* estasis, estancamiento de la circulación de un líquido tal como la sangre y la orina en una parte del cuerpo.

state *n.* estado, condición; **nutritional** __ / __ nutricional.

station *n.* estación; **nursing** __ / puesto de enfermeras.

stationary *a.* estacionario-a, estacionado-a, que permanece en una posición fija.

stature *n.* estatura, altura.

status *n.*, *L.* status, estado o condición; __ **asthmaticus** / __ **asmaticus**, condición de un ataque de asma agudo; __ **epilepticus** / __ epiléptico, serie de ataques sucesivos con pérdida del conocimiento.

stay *n.* estancia; **short** __ / __ breve; *v.* permanecer; quedarse; **to** __ **awake** / desvelarse; **to** __ **in bed** / __ en cama, guardar cama.

steam *n.* vapor.

steatorrhea *n.* esteatorrea, exceso de grasa en las heces fecales.

stem *n.* tallo, pedúnculo, estructura semejante al tallo de una planta; **brain** __ / __ encefálico; __ **cell** / célula madre.

stenosed *a.* estenosado-a, rel. a una estenosis.

stenosis *n.* estenosis, estrechamiento o contracción anormal de un pasaje; **aortic** __ / __ aórtica; **pyloric** __ / __ pilórica.

stent *n.* endoprotesis, dispositivo instalado en el organismo para sostener extructuras tubulares que se unen.

steppage *n.* estepaje, alteración en la marcha que resulta de la caída pendular del pie obligando a levantar la rodilla y flexionar el muslo sobre la pelvis.

stereotaxis *n.* estereotaxia, técnica de localización de áreas cerebrales usada en procedimientos neurológicos.

stereotype *n.* estereotipo; cliché.

sterile *a.* estéril. 1. que no es fértil; 2. aséptico-a; que no contiene ni produce microorganismos.

sterility *n.* esterilidad, incapacidad de concebir o procrear.

sterilization *n.* esterilización. 1. procedimiento que impide la reproducción; 2. destrucción completa de microorganismos; **dry heat** __ / __por calor seco; **gas** __ / __ por gas; **vapor** __ / __ por vapor.

sterilize *v.* esterilizar.

sternal *a.* esternal, rel. al esternón; __ **puncture** / punción __ .

sternocostal *a.* esternocostal, rel. al esternón y las costillas.

sternum *n.* esternón, hueso frontal en el medio del tórax.

steroid *n.* esteroide, compuesto orgánico complejo del cual se derivan varias hormonas como el estrógeno, la testosterona y la cortisona.

stersialgia *n.* estersialgia, dolor en el esternón.

stertor *n.* estertor. rale.

stethoscope *n.* estetoscopio, instrumento médico usado en la auscultación.

sticky *a.* pegajoso-a.

stiff *a.* tieso-a, rígido-a; __ **neck** / cuello __ .

stigma *n.* estigma, huella. 1. señal específica de una enfermedad; 2. marca o señal en el cuerpo.

still *a.* inmóvil, quieto-a, tranquilo-a.

stillbirth *n.* nacimiento sin vida.

stillborn *a.* mortinato-a, muerto-a al nacer.

Still's disease *n.* enfermedad de Still, artritis reumatoidea juvenil.

stimulant *n.* estimulante, agente que produce una reacción.

stimulate *v.* estimular; motivar; excitar.

stimulation *n.* estimulación; motivación.

stimulus *n.* (*pl.* stimuli) estímulo, cualquier agente o factor que produce una reacción; **conditioned** __ / __ condicionado; **subliminal** __ / __ sublimado.

sting *n.* picadura; **bee-** __ / picadura de abeja; **wasp** __ / __ de avispa.

stink *n.* olor desagradable, mal olor.

stippling *n.* punteado, condición de apariencia con manchas.

stir *n.* movimiento; excitación; *v.* revolver, agitar.

stirrup bone *n.* estribo. stapes.

stitch *n.* punto de sutura; *v.* dar puntos.

stocking *n.* medias; **elastic** __ / calceta, media elástica.

stoma *n.* estoma, abertura hecha por cirugía, esp. en la pared del abdomen.

stomach *n.* estómago, órgano en forma de saco que forma parte del tubo digestivo; **on an empty** __ / en ayunas; __ **-ache** / dolor de __; __ **pump** / bomba estomacal; __ **pumping** / lavado de __; __ **ulcer** / úlcera gástrica; *v. pop.* soportar, tolerar.

stomachal *a.* estomacal, rel. al estómago; ___ **tonic** / tónico ___ .

stomatitis *n.* estomatitis, infl. de la mucosa de la boca; **aphthous** ___ / ___ aftosa.

stone *n.* piedra, cálculo.

stool *n.* heces fecales, excremento; ___ **fat** / grasa fecal; ___ **softener** / copro-emoliente.

stop *n.* parada, alto, interrupción; *v.* detener, parar, interrumpir; **to make a** ___ / hacer alto, hacer una parada; detenerse, pararse.

stoppage *n.* bloqueo; obstrucción; taponamiento.

storm *n.* tormenta; intensificación repentina de síntomas de una enfermedad.

strabismus *n.* estrabismo, alineamiento anormal de los ojos debido a una deficiencia muscular; *pop.* bizquera.

straight *a.* derecho-a, recto-a; estirado-a, erguido-a.

straightjacket *n.* camisa de fuerza.

strain *n.* esfuerzo, torcedura, sprain; [*inherited trait*] rasgo, cepa; *v.* forzar; **to ___ a muscle** / torcer un músculo; [*filter*] colar, pasar; esforzarse demasiado; **to ___ the eyes** / forzar la vista.

strange *a.* extraño-a, raro-a; extranjero-a; no relacionado-a con un organismo o situado-a fuera del mismo.

strangulated *n.* estrangulado-a; constreñido-a; ___ **hernia** / hernia ___ .

strangulation *n.* estrangulación. 1. asfixia o sofocación gen. causada por obstrucción de las vías aéreas; 2. constricción de un órgano o estructura debida a compresión.

strap *n.* faja, banda, correa, tira; *v.* poner una faja; amarrar, atar.

stratification *n.* estratificación, formación en capas.

stratified *a.* estratificado-a, colocado-a en capas; ___ **epithelium** / epitelio ___ .

stratum *n.* estrato; capa.

strawberry *n.* fresa; ___ **mark** / marca en forma de ___ .

stream *n.* chorro, flujo, corriente.

strength *n.* fuerza, vigor, resistencia.

strep throat *n.* infección y dolor de garganta causados por un estreptococo.

streptococcal *a.* estreptocócico-a, rel. a estreptococos; ___ **infections** / infecciones ___ -s.

streptococcemia *n.* estreptococemia, infección de la sangre debida a la presencia de estreptococos.

streptococcus *n.* estreptococo, género de microorganismo de la tribu *Streptococceae*, bacterias gram-positivas que se agrupan en pares o cadenas y que causan enfermedades serias.

streptomycin *n.* estreptomicina, antibiótico que se usa contra infecciones bacterianas.

stress *n.* estrés, tensión emocional, compulsión. 1. factor químico, físico o emocional que provoca un cambio como respuesta inmediata o demorada en las funciones del cuerpo o en sus partes; ___ **test** / prueba de esfuerzo; 2. *gr.* énfasis, acento tónico.

stretch *n.* tirón, estirón, esfuerzo; *v.* extender, alargar, estirar; **to ___ forth, to ___ out** / estirarse, extenderse, alargarse; ___ **receptor** / receptor de estiramiento.

stretcher *n.* camilla, andas; dilatador, extendedor.

stretching *n.* dilatación, estiramiento.

stria *n.* lista, fibra.

striated *a.* estriado-a, enlistado-a; ___ **muscle** / músculo ___ .

stricken *a.* afectado-a súbitamente; afligido-a.

strict *a.* estricto-a; exacto-a.

stricture *n.* estrechez, estrechamiento, constricción.

stridor *n.* stridor, estridor, ruido sordo respiratorio.

strike *n.* golpe, ataque repentino; *vi.* golpear, atacar súbitamente.

stroke *n.* 1. embolia cerebral, apoplejía; ataque súbito; 2. choque, golpe.

stroking *n.* acto de frotar suavemente.

stroma *n.* estroma, armazón de tejido que sirve de soporte a un órgano.

strong *a.* fuerte, fornido-a, robusto-a; ___ **-minded** / determinado-a, decidido-a.

structure *n.* estructura; orden.

struggle *n.* lucha, esfuerzo; *v.* luchar, esforzarse.

struma *n., L.* estruma, engrosamiento de la tiroides; *pop.* bocio.

strychnine *n.* estricnina, alcaloide cristalino muy venenoso.

stubborn *a.* obstinado-a, testarudo-a, caprichoso-a; *v.* **to be ___** / obstinarse, encapricharse.

467

student

student *n.* estudiante; **medical __ / __** de medicina.

study *n.* estudio; **double-blind __ -ies / __ -s** de doble incógnita, de doble desconocimiento; *v.* estudiar.

stump *n.* muñón, parte que queda de una extremidad amputada.

stupid *n.* estúpido-a, imbécil.

stupidity *n.* estupidez.

stupor *n.* estupor, letargo.

sturdy *a.* fuerte, vigoroso-a.

stuttering *n.* tartamudeo.

sty *n.* orzuelo, condición inflamatoria de las glándulas sebáceas del párpado.

subacromial *a.* subacromial, rel. al acromión o localizado debajo de éste.

subarachnoid *a.* subaracnoideo-a, que ocurre debajo de la membrana aracnoidea o de posición inferior a ésta; **__ hemorrhage / hemorragia __ ; __ space / espacio __ .**

subclavian, subclavicular *a.* subclavicular, localizado debajo de la clavícula; **__ artery / arteria __; __ steal syndrome / síndrome del secuestro __; __ vein / vena __ .**

subclinical *a.* subclínico-a, sin manifestación clínica.

subconscious *n.* subconsciente, subconsciencia, estado durante el cual los procesos mentales que afectan el pensamiento los sentimientos y la conducta ocurren sin que la persona esté consciente de ello; *a.* rel. a. la zona mental en la que la persona no se encuentra totalmente consciente.

subcostal *a.* subcostal, debajo de las costillas.

subculture *n.* subcultivo, cultivo de bacterias que se deriva de otro.

subcutaneous *a.* subcutáneo-a, debajo de la piel.

subdural *a.* subdural, situado debajo de la dura madre; **__ hematoma / hematoma __; __ hemorrhage / hemorragia __; __ space / espacio __ .**

subinvolution *n.* subinvolución, involución incompleta; **__ of uterus / __ del útero.**

subject *n.* sujeto. 1. término usado en referencia al paciente; 2. tópico; 3. *gr.* sujeto del verbo.

subjective *a.* subjectivo-a; **__ symptoms / síntomas __ -s.**

sublethal dose *a.* dosis subletal, cantidad insuficiente de una sustancia para causar la muerte.

sublimation *n.* sublimación. 1. cambio de un estado sólido a vapor; 2. término freudiano que se refiere al proceso de transferir un impulso o deseo instintivo a una conducta aceptada socialmente.

sublingual *a.* sublingual, situado-a debajo de la lengua; **__ gland / glándula __ .**

subluxation *a.* subluxación, dislocación incompleta.

submandibular *a.* submandibular, debajo de la mandíbula.

submental *a.* submental, debajo del mentón.

submerge *v.* sumergir, colocar debajo de un líquido.

submit *v.* someter; someterse.

submucosa *n.* submucosa, capa de tejido celular situado debajo de una mucosa.

subphrenic *a.* subfrénico-a, situado-a debajo del diafragma; **__ abscess / absceso __ .**

subscription *n.* subscripción, parte de la receta médica que da instrucciones para la preparación de un medicamento.

subside *v.* menguar, apaciguar, bajar, cesar.

substance *n.* sustancia, líquido; droga; **ground __ / __ fundamental; __ abuse / abuso de drogas; __ dependence / dependencia de drogas; __ withdrawal syndrome / síndrome de abstinencia de drogas.**

substantive *n. gr.* substantivo, sustantivo, nombre.

substitute *n.* sustituto-a; reemplazo; *v.* sustituir, reemplazar.

substitution *n.* substitución; **__ therapy / terapia por __ .**

subungual *a.* subungual, debajo de una uña.

succeed *v.* tener éxito, salir bien; lograr.

success *n.* éxito, acierto, triunfo.

successful *a.* afortunado-a, de excelente resultado.

successive *a.* sucesivo-a, consecutivo-a.

such *a.* tal, semejante; **in __ manner / en __ forma.**

suck *v.* chupar, [*mother's milk*] mamar; **to __ out / chupar sacando; vaciar, extraer.**

sucrose *n.* sucrosa, sacarosa que se obtiene de la caña de azúcar o la remolacha.

suction *n.* succión, aspiración; ___ **device** / dispositivo de ___ .

sudamen *n.* sudamina, erupción cutánea no inflamatoria que presenta vesículas blanquecinas llenas de líquido acuoso y que se manifiestan después de una sudación copiosa o una enfermedad febril.

sudden *a.* súbito-a, imprevisto-a, repentino-a; ___ **death** / muerte ___ .

sudden infant death syndrome (SID) *n.* síndrome de muerte infantil súbita, muerte súbita de un bebé menor de un año de edad cuya causa permanece desconocida.

sudorific *a.* sudorífico-a, que promueve el sudor.

sudoriparous *a.* sudoríparo-a, que secreta sudor; ___ **gland** / glándula ___ .

suffer *v.* sufrir, padecer; **to** ___ **from** / padecer de.

suffering *n.* sufrimiento, padecimiento.

sufficient *a.* suficiente; **-ly** *adv.* suficientemente.

suffocate *v.* sofocar, asfixiar; faltar la respiración.

suffocation *n.* asfixia, paro de la respiración.

suffusion *n.* sufusión, infiltración de un líquido del cuerpo en los tejidos circundantes.

sugar *n.* azúcar, carbohidrato que consiste esencialmente de sucrosa; **beet** ___ , **cane** ___ / sucrosa; **fruit** ___ / fructosa; **grape** ___ / glucosa; **milk** ___ / lactosa.

suggestion *n.* sugerencia, consejo, indicación; sugestión.

suggestive *a.* sugestivo-a, rel. a la sugestión o que sugiere.

suicidal *a.* suicida, rel. al suicidio o con tendencia al mismo.

suicide *n.* suicidio; suicidarse; **attempted** ___ / tentativa o intento de ___ .

sulfa drugs *n.* sulfa, medicamentos del grupo sulfonamida, antibacterianos.

sulfacetamide *n.* sulfacetamida, sulfonamida antibacteriana.

sulfate *n.* sulfato, sal de ácido sulfúrico.

sulfonamides *n., pl.* sulfonamidas, grupo de compuestos orgánicos sulfuro-bacteriostáticos.

sulfur *n.* azufre, sulfuro.

sulfuric *a.* sulfúrico-a, rel. al sulfuro.

summary *n.* sumario, historia clínica del paciente; ___ **of hospital records** / sumario del expediente.

sun *n.* sol; ___ **-bathing** / baño de ___ ; ___ **-burn** / quemadura de ___, eritema solar; ___ **-burnt** / quemado-a, tostado-a por el sol; ___ **exposure** / estar expuesto-a al ___; *v.* **to** ___ **-bathe** / tomar el ___ .

sunscreen *n.* bloqueador de sol, sustancia que bloquea los rayos solares.

sunspot *n.* mancha de sol.

sunstroke *n.* insolación.

super ego *n.*, *L.* el yo, término freudiano que se refiere a la parte de la psique que concierne a los valores sociales, morales y éticos.

superfecundation *n.* superfecundación, fertilización sucesiva de dos óvulos que pertenecen al mismo ciclo menstrual en dos actos sexuales distintos.

superfetation *n.* superfetación, fecundación de dos óvulos en el mismo útero en un intervalo de tiempo corto aunque correspondientes a dos períodos menstruales diferentes.

superficial *a.* superficial, rel. a la superficie; **-ly** *adv.* superficialmente.

superinfection *n.* superinfección, infección subsecuente producida gen. por un microorganismo diferente que ocurre durante el curso de una infección presente.

superior *n.* superior, más alto; [*position*] hacia arriba; al exterior.

superiority complex *n.* complejo de superioridad.

supernumerary *a.* supernumerario-a, en número mayor que el normal.

superolateral *a.* superolateral, en posición superior y lateral.

supersaturate *v.* supersaturar, saturar excesivamente, añadir una sustancia en una cantidad mayor de la que puede ser disuelta normalmente por un líquido.

supersaturated *a.* supersaturado-a.

supine *a.* supino-a, de posición acostada de espalda, boca arriba y con la palma de la mano hacia arriba.

supplement *n.* suplemento; *v.* complementar.

support *n.* soporte, sostén.

suppose *v.* suponer.

suppository *n.* supositorio, medicamento semisólido que se inserta en una cavidad natural del cuerpo (vagina, recto).

suppression *n.* supresión. 1. fallo súbito del cuerpo en la producción de una excreción o secreción normal;

2. en psicoanálisis, la inhibición de una idea o deseo.

suppuration *n.* supuración, formación o salida de pus.

suprapubic *a.* suprapúbico-a, localizado-a encima del pubis; __ **catheter** / catéter __; __ **cystostomy** / cistostomía __ .

sure *a.* seguro-a, decidido-a; positivo-a.

surface *n.* superficie; porción o límite exterior de una estructura; __ **tension** / tensión superficial.

surfactant *n.* surfactante, agente tensoactivo que modifica la tensión superficial de un líquido.

surgeon *n.* cirujano-a.

surgery *n.* cirugía, rama de la medicina que comprende procesos operatorios de reparación, diagnosis de enfermedades y corrección de estructuras del cuerpo. V. cuadro esta página.

surgical *a.* quirúrgico-a; __ **dressing** / vendaje __ protector; __ **equipment** / equipo __; __ **flaps** / colgajos __ -s; __ **incision** / incisión __; __ **instruments** / instrumentos __ -s; __ **mesh** / malla __; __ **resident** / residente de cirugía.

surname *n.* apellido, nombre de familia.

surplus *n. a.* sobrante, excedente.

surrogate *a.* subrogado-a, que sustituye algo o a alguien; *v.* subrogar, sustituir.

survey *n.* encuesta; cuestionario.

survival *n.* supervivencia.

survive *v.* sobrevivir.

survivor *n.* sobreviviente.

susceptible *a.* susceptible.

suspect *a.* sospechoso-a.

suspend *v.* suspender, cancelar.

suspensory *a.* suspensorio, que sostiene y da soporte; **ligament** __ / ligamento de __.

sustain *v.* sostener, mantener; [*a wound*] sufrir una herida.

sustenance *n.* sustentación, sustento.

suture *n.* sutura; puntada; línea de unión; **absorbable surgical** __ / __ quirúrgica absorbible; **bolster** __ / __ compuesta; **catgut** __ / __ de catgut; **near and far** __ / __ de aposición o aproximación; **purse-string** __ / __ en bolsa de tabaco; **uninterrupted continuous** __ / __ continua, de peletero; **vertical mattress** __ / __ de colchonero.

swallow *n.* trago; deglución; *v.* tragar, deglutir.

Surgery	Cirugía
ambulatory	ambulatoria
arthroscopic	artroscópica
cardiothoracic	cardiotorácica
cosmetic	cosmética
cytoreductive	citorreductiva
conservative	conservadora
corrective	correctiva
endoscopic	endoscópica
excisional	de excisión
exploratory	exploratoria
major	mayor
minor	menor
orthopedic	ortopédica
oral	oral
plastic	plástica
radical	radical
reconstructive	reconstructiva
sustenance	de sustentación, sustento

swallowing *n.* deglución.

Swan-Ganz catheter *n.* catéter de Swan-Ganz, sonda flexible que contiene un balón cerca de la punta y que se emplea para medir la presión sanguínea en la arteria pulmonar.

sweat *n.* sudor, secreción de las glándulas sudoríparas; **cold** __ / __ -es fríos; **night** __ -s / __ -es nocturnos; *v.* sudar; hacer sudar.

sweat glands *n., pl.* glándulas sudoríparas.

sweating *n.* sudor, perspiración, transpiración.

sweaty *a.* sudado-a, sudoroso-a.

sweet *a.* dulce, azucarado-a; [*tempered*] dulce, agradable, gentil.

sweeten *v.* endulzar, azucarar.

sweetener *n.* dulcificante.

sweets *n., pl.* golosinas, dulces.

swelling *n.* hinchazón; tumefacción; *pop.* bulto, chichón.

swift *a.* ligero-a; fácil, sin complicación; **a** __ **operation** / una operación fácil, sin complicaciones.

swim *vi.* nadar.

swimmer *n.* nadador-a; __ **'s ear** / otitis del __ .

switch *n.* [*instrumento*] cambio; conector eléctrico; *v.* cambiar; **to** __ **off** / desconectar; cambiar; **to** __ **on** / conectar.

syndrome

swollen *a., pp.* of **to swell**, hinchado-a.
Sydenham's chorea *n.* Sydenham, corea de; tipo de corea menor o reumática, gen. vista en la infancia causada por una infección estreptococa, y que en su comienzo se manifiesta con contracciones musculares de la cara y brazos.
Sylvian aqueduct *n.* acueducto de Silvius, conducto estrecho que conecta los ventrículos cerebrales tercero y cuarto.
symbiosis *n.* simbiosis, unión estrecha de dos organismos que pertenecen a especies diferentes.
symbol *n.* símbolo, representación o señal que sustituye o representa en la práctica otra cosa o idea.
symbolism *n.* simbolismo. 1. uso de símbolos en la práctica para dar una representación a las cosas; 2. anormalidad mental por la cual el paciente percibe todos los sucesos y cosas como reflejos de sus propios pensamientos.
symmetrical *a.* simétrico-a.
symmetry *n.* simetría, correspondencia perfecta entre partes de un cuerpo colocadas en posición opuesta a un centro o axis.
sympathectomy *n.* simpatectomía, extirpación de una porción del simpático.
sympathetic *a.* simpático-a, rel. al sistema nervioso simpático.
sympathetic nervous system *n.* sistema nervioso simpático, abastecedor de los músculos involuntarios, formado por nervios motores y sensoriales.
sympatholytic *a.* simpatolítico-a, que ofrece resistencia a la actividad producida por la estimulación del sistema nervioso simpático.
sympathomimetic *a.* simpatomimético-a, que puede causar cambios fisiológicos similares a los causados por el sistema nervioso simpático.
sympathy *n.* simpatía, asociación, relación. 1. afinidad; 2. relación entre dos órganos afines por la cual una anomalía en uno afecta al otro; 3. afinidad entre la mente y el cuerpo que causa que se afecten entre sí.
symphysis *n.* sínfisis, articulación en la cual las superficies óseas adyacentes se

unen por un fibrocartílago; **pubic** ___ / ___ púbica.
symptom *n.* síntoma, manifestación o indicio de una enfermedad según se percibe por el paciente; **constitutional** ___ / ___ constitucional ___ / ___ demorado; **objective** ___ / ___ objetivo; **pathognomic** ___ / ___ patognómico; **presenting** ___ / ___ presente; **prodromal** ___ / ___ prodrómico; **withdrawal** ___ / ___ de supresión.
symptomatic *a.* sintomático-a, de la naturaleza de un síntoma o rel. a éste.
symptomatology *n.* sintomatología, conjunto de síntomas que se refieren a una enfermedad o a un caso determinado.
symptom complex *n.* complejo de síntomas concurrentes que caracterizan una enfermedad.
synapse *n.* sinapsis, punto de contacto entre dos neuronas donde el impulso que pasa por la primera neurona origina un impulso en la segunda.
synapsis *n.* sinapsis, apareamiento de cromosomas homólogos al comienzo de la meiosis.
synarthrosis *n.* sinartrosis, articulación inmóvil en la cual los elementos óseos están fusionados.
synchondrosis *n.* sincondrosis, articulación inmóvil de superficies unidas por tejido cartilaginoso.
synchysis *n.* sinquisis, estado de fluidez del humor vítreo; ___ **scintillans** / ___ centelleante.
synclonus *n.* sinclono, espasmo o temblor de varios músculos a la vez.
syncopal *a.* sincopal, rel. a un síncope.
syncope *n.* síncope, desmayo o pérdida temporal del conocimiento; **anginal** ___ / ___ anginoso; **deglutition** ___ / ___ de deglución; **cardiac** ___ / ___ cardíaco; **convulsive** ___ / ___ convulsivo; **hysterical** ___ / ___ histérico; **laryngeal** ___ / ___ laríngeo.
syndactylism *n.* sindactilia, anomalía congénita que consiste en la fusión de dos o más dedos de la mano o los pies.
syndrome *n.* síndrome, síntomas y señales que caracterizan una enfermedad; **acquired immune deficiency** ___ / ___ de inmunodeficiencia adquirida; **adipose** ___ / ___ adiposo; **adrenogenital** ___ / ___ suprarrenogenital; **battered children** ___ / ___ de niños

maltratados; **congenital rubella** __ /
__ congénito de rubéola; **dumping**
/ __ de vaciamiento gástrico rápido;
hepatorenal __ / __ hepatorrenal;
irritable bowel __ / __ de intestino
irritado, irritable; **malabsorption** __ /
__ de malabsorción gastrointestinal;
middle lobe __ / __ del lóbulo
medio del pulmón; **nephrotic** __ /
nefrótico; **respiratory stress** __ /
de dificultad respiratoria; **scalded skin**
__ / __ de escaldadura, quemadura
de la epidermis; **sick sinus** __ / __
del seno carotídeo; **subclavian steal** __
/ __ del secuestro subclavicular;
sudden death __ / __ de muerte
súbita; **multiple transfusion** __ / __
de transfusión múltiple; **premenstrual**
__ / __ premenstrual; **toxic shock** __
/ __ de choque tóxico, envenenamiento
de la sangre causado por estafilococos;
withdrawal __ / __ de privación.
synechia n. sinequia, unión o
adherencia anormal de tejidos u
órganos esp. referente al iris, al
cristalino y a la córnea.
synergic n. sinérgico-a, que posee la
propiedad de actuar en cooperación.
synergism n. sinergismo, correlación o
unión armoniosa entre dos o más
estructuras o sustancias.
synostosis n. sinostosis, union ósea
entre dos huesos adyacentes; **senile** __
/ __ senil; **tribacillary** __ / __
tribacilar.
synovia n. sinovia, líquido que lubrica
las articulaciones y los tendones.
synovial a. sinovial, rel. a la membrana
sinovial; __ **bursa** / bursa __; __ **cyst**
/ quiste __ .
synovial fluid n. líquido sinovial,
líquido viscoso transparente.
synovioma n. sinovioma, tumor que se
origina en una membrana sinovial.
synovitis n. sinovitis, infl. de la
membrana sinovial; **dry** __ / __ seca;
purulent __ / __ purulenta; **serous** __
/ __ serosa.
synthesis n. síntesis, composición de
un todo por la unión de las partes.
synthesize v. sintetizar, producir
síntesis.
synthetic a. sintético-a, rel. a una
síntesis o producido por ésta.
syntonic a. sintónico-a, rel. a un tipo de
personalidad estable que se adapta
normalmente al ambiente.
syphilis n. sífilis, enfermedad venérea

contagiosa que se manifiesta en
lesiones cutáneas. usu. transmitida
sexualmente por contacto
directo.
syphilitic n. a. sifilítico-a, rel. a la sífilis
o causado por ella; __ **macula** /
mácula __ .
syphiloma n. tumor sifilítico.
syringe n. jeringa, jeringuilla;
disposable __ / __ desechable; **glass
cylinder** __ / __ con tubo de cristal;
hypodermic __ / __
hipodérmica.
syringocele n. siringocele.
1. conducto central de la médula
espinal; 2. meningomielocele que
contiene una cavidad en la médula
espinal ectópica.
syringomyelia n. siringomielia,
enfermedad crónica progresiva de la
columna vertebral caracterizada por
cavidades llenas de líquido en la región
cervical y que a veces se extiende a la
médula oblongata.
systaltic a. sistáltico-a, que alterna
contracciones y dilataciones.
system n. sistema, grupo de partes u
órganos combinados que constituyen
un conjunto que desempeña una o más
funciones vitales en el organismo;
cardiovascular __ / __ cardiovascular;
digestive __ / __ digestivo; **endocrine**
__ / __ endocrino; **genitourinary** __ /
__ genitourinario; **hematopoietic** __ /
__ hematopoyético; **integumentary**
__ / __ tegumentario; **immune** __ /
__ de inmunidad; **lymphatic** __ / __
linfático; **muscular** __ / __ muscular;
nervous __ / __ nervioso; **osseous** __
/ __ óseo; **portal** __ / __ portal;
reproductive __ / __ reproductís;
respiratory __ / __ respiratorio;
reticuloendothelial __ / __
reticuloendotelial.
systematic a. sistemático-a,
que se ajusta a un régimen o sistema.
systemic a. sistémico-a; que afecta el
cuerpo en general; __ **circulation** /
circulación __; __ **disease** /
enfermedad diseminada.
systole n. sístole, contracción del
corazón esp. de los ventrículos; **atrial**
__ / __ auricular; **premature** __ / __
prematura; **ventricular** __ / __
ventricular
systolic a. sistólico-a, rel. a la sístole;
__ **murmur** / soplo __; __ **pressure** /
presión __ .

t

T *abbr.* absolute temperature / temperatura absoluta; **T+, increased tension** / tensión aumentada; **T–, diminished tension** / tensión disminuida.

tabardillo *n. pop.* nombre dado al tifus y la fiebre tifoidea en México y otros países de América Latina.

tabes *n.* tabes, deterioro progresivo del organismo o de una parte del mismo debido a una enfermedad crónica.

table *n.* tabla. 1. capa o lámina ósea; 2. mesa; **examination __ /__** de reconocimiento; **operating __ /__** de operaciones; 3. tabla, colección de datos o de referencia con una variante determinada.

tablet *n.* tableta, comprimido, dosis en un compuesto sólido; **enteric-coated __ /__** de capa entérica.

tabular *a.* tabular, dispuesto en forma de tabla o cuadro.

tachyarrhythmia *n.* taquiarritmia, forma de arritmia acompañada de pulso rápido.

tachycardia *n.* taquicardia, aceleración de la actividad cardíaca, gen. a una frecuencia de más de 100 por minuto en una persona adulta; **atrial __ /__** auricular; **ectopic __ /__** ectópica; **en salves __ /__** en salves; **exophthalmic __ /__** exoftálmica; **fetal __ /__** fetal; **paroxysmal atrial __ /__** auricular paroxística; **reflex /__** refleja; **sinus __ /__** sinusal; **supraventricular __ /__** supraventricular; **ventricular __ /__** ventricular.

tachyphagia *n.* taquifagia, hábito de comer muy rápido.

tachypnea *n.* taquipnea, respiración rápida.

tact *n.* tacto; diplomacia, discreción.

tactile *a.* táctil, palpable; rel. al sentido del tacto; **__ discrimination** / discriminación __; **system /** sistema __ .

taenia, tenia *n.* tenia, parásito de la clase *Cestoda* que en la etapa adulta vive en el intestino de los vertebrados.

taint *n.* [*stain*] mancha, mácula; *v.* manchar, podrirse o causar putrefacción; corromperse.

take *vi.* [*to get*] tomar; [*to seize*] coger, agarrar; [*to carry something, to take someone*] llevar; [*to remove*] quitar; **to be taken ill** / enfermarse; **to __ notes /** anotar; **to __ a trip /** viajar; **to __ a walk /** dar un paseo.

talipes *n.* talipes, pie fijo, deformidad congénita del pie.

talon *n.* parte posterior de un diente molar.

talotibial *a.* talotibial, rel. al talón y la tibia.

talus *n.* (*pl.* **tali**) talón, astrágalo, tubillo.

tambour *n.* tambor. 1. tímpano del oído medio; 2. instrumento de precisión que se usa para registrar y transmitir movimientos ligeros tales como las contracciones peristálticas.

tampon *n.* tapón, gasa o algodón prensado que se aplica o inserta en la vagina u otra cavidad para absorber secreciones.

tamponade *n., Fr.* taponamiento, aplicación de tapones a una herida o cavidad para detener una hemorragia o absorber secreciones; **balloon __ /__** por balón insuflable; **cardiac __ /__** cardíaco, compresión aguda del corazón causada por un exceso de sangre acumulada en el pericardio.

tangle *n.* enredo, confusión; *v.* enredarse; confundirse.

tangy *a.* [*smell*] fuerte, penetrante.

tap *n.* punción, perforación; acto de perforar un tejido con un instrumento afilado; **bloody __ /__** lumbar hemática; **spinal __ /__** lumbar; *v.* tocar ligeramente; punzar, perforar, hacer una punción; **__ water /** agua corriente.

tapeworm *n.* tenia, solitaria. taenia, tenia.

tapping *n.* 1. percusión; 2. extracción de fluido.

tarantula *n.* tarántula, araña negra venenosa.

target *n.* 1. [*area*] blanco; 2. objetivo de una investigación; 3. célula "en diana" u órgano afectado por un agente definido (droga u hormona).

tarsal *a.* tarsal, tarsiano-a. 1. rel. al tarso; 2. rel. al tejido conectivo que soporta el párpado del ojo.

tarsal bones *n., pl.* huesos del tarso.

tarsometatarsal *a.* tarsometatarsiano-a, rel. al tarso y al metatarso.

tarsus *n.* tarso, parte posterior del pie situada entre los huesos de la pierna y los huesos metatarsianos.

taste *n.* gusto; **in good __ / de buen __; __ buds** / papilas gustativas; *v.* probar, saborear.

taxis *n., L.* taxis. 1. manipulación o reducción de una parte u órgano para llevarlo a la posición normal; 2. reflejo direccional del movimiento de un organismo en respuesta a un estímulo.

T cell regulator *n.* célula T reguladora, dirige otras células del sistema inmune a hacer otras funciones especiales, incluso ataque al SIDA.

T cells *n., pl.* linfocitos T, linfocitos diferenciados en el timo que dirigen la respuesta inmunológica y que asisten a los linfocitos B a responder a antígenos; **helper __ / __** inductores, ayudantes, estimulantes de la producción de anticuerpos formados por células que se derivan del linfocito B; **cytotoxic __ / __** citotóxicos, destructores de células extrañas al cuerpo (como en el caso de órganos transplantados); **suppressor __ / __** supresores de la producción de anticuerpos formados por células que se derivan del linfocito B.

T8-suppressor cell *n.* célula T8 supresora, grupo de células cuya función es de inhibir la respuesta inmune.

teamwork *n.* esfuerzo coordinado; trabajo en coordinación.

tear *n.* lágrima; desgarramiento, desgarro; **__ gas** / gas lacrimógeno; *v.* rasgar, desgarrar, romper; **to shed __-s** / lagrimear, llorar; **to __ off** / arrancar.

tear duct *n.* conducto lacrimal.

tearful *a.* lagrimoso-a.

tearing *n.* lagrimeo.

teat *n.* tetilla. 1. glándula mamaria; 2. pezón.

technetium 99m *n.* technecio 99m, radioisótopo que emite rayos gamma, de uso frecuente en medicina nuclear.

technician *n.* técnico-a, persona entrenada en la administración de tratamientos o pruebas de laboratorio y que gen. actúa bajo la supervisión de un facultativo; **dental __ / __** dental; **electrocardiographic __ / __** electrocardiógrafo-a; **emergency medical __ / __** de emergencia; **medical laboratory __ / __** laboratorista; **radiologic __ / __** radiólogo-a; **respiratory therapy __ / __** de terapia respiratoria.

technique *n.* técnica, método o procedimiento.

technologist *n.* tecnólogo-a, persona experta en tecnología.

technology *n.* tecnología, ciencia que trata de la aplicación de procedimientos técnicos.

tectorium *L.* tectorium, membrana que cubre el órgano de Corti.

teenage *a.*, adolescente.

teenager *n.* jovencito-a de trece a diecinueve años de edad.

teeth *n., pl.* dientes; **deciduous __ / __** de leche o primera dentición; **permanent __ / __** permanentes; **secondary __ / __** secundarios; **wisdom __ / __** cordales; *pop.* muelas del juicio.

teething *n.* dentición.

tegument *n.* tegumento, la piel.

telangiectasia *n.* telangiectasia, telangiectasis, condición causada por dilatación de los vasos capilares y arteriolas que puede formar un angioma.

telecardiophone *n.* telecardiófono, instrumento que permite escuchar los latidos del corazón.

telediagnosis *n.* telediagnóstico, diagnóstico o pronóstico dado por medios electrónicos de transmision remota entre instituciones médicas.

telemedicine *n.* telemedicina, uso de la televisión como medio de asistencia en el cuidado de la salud.

telemetry *n.* telemetría, información transmitida electrónicamente a distancia.

telencephalon *n.* telencéfalo, porción anterior del encéfalo.

teleopsy *n.* teleopsia, desorden visual por el cual los objetos parecen estar más lejos de lo que están en realidad.

telepathy *n.* telepatía, comunicación aparente de pensamientos de una persona a otra por medios extrasensoriales.

teleradiography *n.* telerradiografía, rayos-x tomados a dos o más metros de distancia del objectivo para disminuir distorsiones.

temper *n.* carácter, disposición; temple, humor; genio; *v.* **to have a bad __ /**

tener mal ___; **to have a good** ___ / tener buen ___ .

temperament *n.* temperamento, combinación de la constitución física, mental y emocional de una persona que la distingue de otras.

temperate *a.* moderado-a; sobrio-a, abstemio-a.

temperature *n.* temperatura. 1. grado de calor o frío según se mide en una escala específica; 2. calor natural de un cuerpo vivo; 3. fiebre o calentura; **absolute** ___ / ___ absoluta; **ambient** ___ / ___ ambiental; **axillary** ___ / ___ axilar; **body** ___ / ___ del cuerpo; **critical** ___ / ___ crítica; **maximum** ___ / ___ máxima; **minimum** ___ / ___ mínima; **normal** ___ / ___ normal; **oral** ___ / ___ oral; **rectal** ___ / ___ rectal; **subnormal** ___ / ___ subnormal.

template *n.* patrón, molde.

temple *n.* sien, superficie lisa a cada lado de la parte lateral de la cabeza.

temporal *a.* temporal. 1. rel. a la sien; ___ **bone** / hueso ___; ___ **lobe** / lóbulo ___; 2. rel. al tiempo.

temporary *a.* temporal; pasajero-a; [*transition period*] interino-a; transitorio-a.

temporomandibular joint *n.* articulación temporomaxilar, rel. a la articulación entre la mandíbula y el hueso temporal.

tender *a.* sensitivo-a al tacto o la palpación; ___ **points** / puntos neurálgicos; [*soft*] blando-a, tierno-a

tenderness *n.* blandura; delicadeza. 1. sensibilidad, condición sensible al tacto o palpación; 2. ternura.

tendinitis, tendonitis *n.* tendinitis, tendonitis, infl. de un tendón.

tendinous *a.* tendinoso-a, rel. a o semejante a un tendón.

tendon *n.* tendón, tejido fibroso que sirve de unión a los músculos y los huesos y a otras partes; **deep** ___ **reflexes** / reflejos profundos de los ___ -es; ___ **jerk** / tirón tendinoso; ___ **reflex** / reflejo tendinoso.

tenesmus *n.* tenesmo, condición dolorosa e ineficaz al orinar o defecar.

tennis elbow *n.* codo de tenista.

tenosynovitis *n.* tenosinovitis, infl. de la vaina que cubre un tendón.

tense *a.* tenso-a, rígido-a, tirante, en estado de tensión.

tension *n.* tensión. 1. acto o efecto de estirarse o ser extendido; 2. grado de estiramiento; 3. sobreesfuerzo mental, emocional o físico; **premenstrual** ___ / ___ premenstrual; 4. expansión de un gas o vapor; **surface** ___ / ___ superficial.

tension headache *n.* dolor de cabeza causado por una tensión nerviosa mental.

tensor *n.* tensor, músculo que estira o hace tensión.

tent *n.* tienda, cámara esp. para cubrir un espacio en el cual se incluye al paciente; **oxygen** ___ / ___ o cámara de oxígeno.

teratogen *n.* teratógeno, agente que causa teratogénesis.

teratogenesis *a.* teratogénesis, producción de anomalías severas en el feto.

teratoid *a.* teratoide. 1. semejante a un monstruo; 2. que proviene de un embrión malformado; ___ **tumor** / tumor ___ .

teratology *n.* teratología, estudio de malformaciones en el feto.

teratoma *n.* teratoma, neoplasma que deriva de más de una capa embrionaria y por lo tanto se compone de tejidos de distintas clases.

teres *a., L.* teres, término empleado para describir ciertos tipos de músculos o ligamentos alargados y cilíndricos.

term *n.* término. 1. período de tiempo de duración efectiva o limitada tal como en el embarazo; 2. vocablo.

terminal *a.* terminal, final.

terminal illness *n.* enfermedad maligna que causa la muerte.

terminology *n.* terminología, nomenclatura.

ternary *a.* ternario-a, que se compone de tres elementos.

tertian *a.* terciano-a, que se repite cada tercer día; ___ **fever** / fiebre ___ .

tertiary syphilis *n.* sífilis terciaria, el estado más avanzado de la sífilis.

test *n.* prueba; examen; análisis; **antinuclear antibody** ___ / ___ antinuclear de anticuerpo; **creatinine clearance** ___ / ___ de aclaramiento de creatinina; **endurance** ___ / ___ de resistencia; **fat stool** ___ / ___ de grasa fecal; **follow-up** ___ / ___ subsecuente; **glucose tolerance** ___ / ___ de tolerancia a la glucosa; **liver function** ___ / ___ de función hepática; **outcome of** ___ / resultado de la ___; **pregnancy** ___ / ___ del embarazo; **random** ___ /

___ de control sin método; **respiratory function** ___ / ___ de función respiratoria; **skin** ___ / ___ cutánea; **scratch** ___ / ___ de rasguño, ___ de alergia; **screening** ___ / ___ eliminatoria; **single-blind** ___ / ___ de ciego simple; **stress** ___ / ___ de esfuerzo; **double-blind** / ___ de doble incógnita; ___ **tube** / tubo de ensayo; ___ **type** / ___ de tipo, prueba visual de letras; **thyroid function** ___ / ___ de función tiroidea; **timed** ___ / ___ de tiempo limitado o medido; **treadmill** ___ / ___ de esfuerzo; **visual** ___ / ___visual; **visual field** ___ / ___ visual de campimetría.

testicle n. testículo, una de las dos glándulas reproductivas masculinas que produce espermatozoos y la hormona testosterona; **ectopic** ___ / ___ ectópico; **undescended** ___ / ___ no descendido.

testicular a. testicular, rel. al testículo; ___ **examination** / examen ___; ___ **tumors** / tumores ___ -es.

testosterone n. testosterona, hormona producida en el testis estimulante del desarrollo de algunas características masculinas secundarias tales como el vello facial y la voz grave; ___ **implant** / implante de ___ .

test-tube baby n. fertilización *in vitro*, embarazo en probeta o que resulta de un óvulo fecundado fuera de la madre en el laboratorio y reimplantado en el útero.

tetanic a. tetánico-a, rel. al tétano; ___ **antitoxin** / antitoxina ___; ___ **convulsion** / convulsión ___; ___ **toxoid** / toxoide ___ .

tetanus, lockjaw n. tétano, enfermedad infecciosa aguda causada por el bacilo del tétano gen. introducido a través de una lesión y que se manifiesta con espasmos musculares y rigidez gradual de la mandíbula, el cuello y el abdomen.

tetany n. tetania, afección neuromuscular que se manifiesta con espasmos intermitentes de los músculos voluntarios asociada con deficiencia paratiroidea y disminución del balance de calcio.

tetracycline n. tetraciclina, antibiótico de espectro amplio usado para combatir microorganismos gram-positivos y gram-negativos, ricketsia y cierta variedad de virus.

tetraplegia n. tetraplejía, parálisis de las cuatro extremidades.

tetraploid n. tetraploide, que posee cuatro grupos de cromosomas.

tetravalent n. tetravalente, que posee una valencia química igual a cuatro.

texture n. textura, composición de la estructura de un tejido.

thalamic a. talámico-a, rel. al tálamo.

thalamus n. tálamo, una de las dos estructuras formadas por masas de materia gris que se encuentran en la base del cerebro y que constituyen el centro principal por donde los impulsos sensoriales pasan a la corteza cerebral.

thalassemia n. talasemia, grupo de diferentes tipos de anemia hemolítica hereditaria encontrada en poblaciones de la región mediterránea y sureste de Asia; **major** ___ / ___ mayor; **minor** ___ / ___ menor.

thalassophobia n. talasofobia, miedo mórbido al mar.

thalassotherapy n. talasoterapia, tratamiento de una enfermedad por medio de baños de mar o exposición al aire marino.

thalidomide n. talidomida, sedativo e hipnótico, causante probado de malformaciones en niños de madres que tomaron la droga durante el embarazo.

thallitoxicosis n. talitoxicosis, envenenamiento incidental de ingestión de sulfato de talio usado en pesticidas.

thanatology n. tanatología, rama de la medicina que trata de la muerte en todos sus aspectos.

thanatomania n. tanatomanía, manía suicida o de asesinato.

thanatometer n. tanatómetro, instrumento usado para determinar cuando una muerte ocurrió midiendo la temperatura interna del cuerpo.

theca n. teca, envoltura o capa que actúa esp. como protectora de un órgano.

thecoma n. tecoma, tumor ovárico gen. benigno.

thenar a. tenar, rel. a la palma de la mano; ___ **eminence** / eminencia ___; ___ **muscles** / músculos ___ -es.

theory n. teoría. 1. conocimientos relacionados con un tema sin verificación práctica de los mismos; 2. especulación u opinión que no ha sido probada científicamente.

therapeutic *a.* terapéutico-a. 1. que tiene propiedades curativas; 2. rel. a la terapéutica; __ **indications** / indicaciones __ -s; __ **plasma exchange** / intercambio __ de plasma.

therapeutics *n.* terapéutica, rama de la medicina que estudia tratamientos y curaciones.

therapist *n.* terapeuta, persona experta en una o más áreas de aplicación de tratamientos en el campo de la salud; **physical** __ / __ físico; **speech** __ / finiatra, logopeda.

therapy *n.* terapia, terapéutica, tratamiento de una enfermedad; **adjuvant** __ / __ adjunta; **anticoagulant** __ / __ anticoagulante; **behavioral** __ / __ de conducta; **biological** __ / __ biológica; __ **by substitution** __ / __ substitutiva; **diathermic** __ / __ diatérmica; **electroshock** __ / electrochoque; **group** __ / __ de grupo; **inhalation** __ / __ por inhalación; **immune suppressive** __ / __ inmunosupresiva; **non-specific** __ / __ inespecífica; **occupational** __ / __ ocupacional; **oxygen** __ / __ de oxígeno; **radiation** __ / __ por radiación; **respiratory** / __ respiratoria; **supportive** __ / __ de apoyo; **systemic** __ / __ sistémica.

thermal, thermic *a.* termal, térmico-a, rel. al calor o producido por éste.

thermocautery *n.* termocauterización, uso de corriente eléctrica o de otro medio de calor para destruir un tejido.

thermocoagulation *n.* termocoagulación, coagulación de tejidos por medio de corrientes de alta frecuencia.

thermodynamics *n.* termodinámica, ciencia que trata de la relación entre el calor y otras formas de energía.

thermograph *n.* termógrafo, detector infrarrojo que registra variaciones de la temperatura corporal según reacciona a los cambios de la circulación sanguínea.

thermography *n.* termografía, registro obtenido con un termógrafo.

thermometer *n.* termómetro, instrumento usado para medir el grado de calor o frío; **Celsius** __ / __ de Celsius o centígrado; **clinical** __ / __ clínico; **Fahrenheit** __ / __ de Fahrenheit; **rectal** __ / __ rectal;

self-recording __ / __ de registro automático.

thermoregulation *n.* termorregulación, regulación del calor o de la temperatura; termotaxis.

thermosterilization *n.* termoesterilización, esterilización por medio del calor.

thermotaxis *n.* termotaxis. 1. mantenimiento de la temperatura del cuerpo; 2. reacción de un organismo al estímulo del calor.

thermotheraphy *n.* termoterapia, uso terapéutico del calor.

thicken *v.* engrosar, espesar; condensar.

thigh *n.* muslo, porción de la extremidad inferior entre la cadera y la rodilla; **bone** / fémur.

think *vi.* pensar; [*believe*] creer; **to __ it over** / pensarlo bien; **to __ nothing of** / tener en poco; **to __ through** / considerar; **to __ well of** / tener buena opinión de.

thinner *n.* solvente, diluyente; líquido que es capaz de disolverse o puede producir una solución.

third degree burn *n.* quemadura de tercer grado.

thirst *n.* sed.

thirsty *a.* sediento-a; *v.* **to be** __ / tener sed.

thoracentesis *n.* toracentesis, punción y drenaje quirúrgicos de la cavidad torácica.

thoracic *a.* torácico-a, rel. al tórax; __ **cage** / caja o pared __; __ **cavity** / cavidad __; __ **duct** / conducto __; __ **injuries** / traumatismos __ -s; __ **neoplasms** / neoplasmas __ -s.

thoracicoabdominal *a.* toracicoabdominal, rel. al tórax y al abdomen.

thoracolumbar *a.* toracolumbar, rel. a las vértebras torácicas y lumbares.

thoracoplasty *n.* toracoplastia, cirugía plástica del tórax por medio de excisión de costillas para provocar la caída de un pulmón afectado.

thoracostomy *n.* toracostomía, incisión en la pared del tórax usando la abertura como drenaje.

thoracotomy *n.* toracotomía, incisión de la pared torácica.

thorax *n.* tórax, el pecho.

thorough *a.* completo-a, minucioso-a, acabado-a; **-ly** *adv.* completamente, minuciosamente, a fondo.

thought *n.* pensamiento, concepto, idea; *a. pp.* of to think, pensado.

thoughtful *n.* atento, solícito-a, esmerado-a.

thread *n.* hilo; fibra, filamento; línea fina. 1. material de sutura; 2. cualquier filamento fino semejante a un hilo; *v.* enhebrar, ensartar; **___ -like** / hiliforme, fibroso-a, filamentoso-a.

threatened abortion *n.* amenaza de aborto.

threshold *n.* umbral. 1. grado mínimo necesario de un estímulo para producir un efecto; 2. dosis mínima que puede producir un efecto; **absolute ___** / **___** absoluto; **auditory ___** / **___** auditivo; **renal ___** / **___** renal; **sensory ___** / **___** sensorio; **___dose** / dosis mínima; **___ of consciousness** / **___** de la consciencia.

thrill *n.* "thrill", estremecimiento, vibración o ruido especial que se siente por palpación; **aneurysmal ___** / **___** aneurismal; **aortic ___** / **___** aórtico; **arterial ___** / **___** arterial; **diastolic ___** / **___** diastólico; **presystolic ___** / **___** presistólico; **systolic ___** / **___** sistólico; *v.* emocionar, excitar; *v.* emocionarse, excitarse.

throat *n.* garganta, área que incluye la faringe y la laringe; **___ swab** / muestra faríngea.

throat culture *n.* muestra de cultivo del mucus extraído de la garganta y detección en el laboratorio de la presencia o no de agentes infecciosos en el mismo.

throb *n.* latido, pulsación; *v.* latir, palpitar, pulsar.

throbbing *a.* pulsátil, palpitante

thrombectomy *n.* trombectomía, extracción de un trombo.

thrombin *n.* trombina, enzima presente en la sangre extravasada que cataliza en la conversión de fibrinógeno en fibrina.

thrombin time *n.* tiempo de trombina, espacio de tiempo necesario para que se forme un coágulo de fibrina después de añadirle trombina al plasma citrado.

thromboangiitis *n.* tromboangiitis, infl. de un vaso sanguíneo con trombosis; trombosis de un vaso sanguíneo.

thrombocyte *n.* trombocito, plaqueta.

thrombocytopenia *n.* trombocitopenia, disminución anormal del número de las plaquetas sanguíneas.

thrombocytosis *n.* trombocitosis, aumento excesivo de plaquetas en la sangre.

thromboembolism *n.* tromboembolia, obstrucción de un vaso sanguíneo por un coágulo desprendido del lugar de origen.

thrombogenesis *n.* trombogénesis, formación de cóagulos o trombos.

thrombolysis *n.* trombólisis, lisis o disolución de un coágulo.

thrombophlebitis *n.* tromboflebitis, dilatación de la pared de una vena asociada con trombosis.

thrombophlebitis migrans *n.* tromboflebitis migratoria, tromboflebitis de progreso lento de una vena a otra.

thrombosed *a.* trombosado-a, rel. a un vaso sanguíneo que contiene un trombo.

thrombosis *n.* trombosis, formación, desarrollo y presencia de un trombo; **biliary ___** / **___** biliar; **cardiac ___** / **___** cardíaca; **coronary ___** / **___** coronaria; **embolic ___** / **___** embólica; **traumatic ___** / **___** traumática; **venous ___** / **___** venosa.

thrombus *n.* (*pl.* **thrombi**) (trombo, coágulo que causa una obstrucción vascular parcial o total.

thrush *n.* muguet, afta, infección fungosa de la mucosa oral que se manifiesta con placas blancas en la cavidad bucal y la garganta.

thumb *n.* dedo pulgar; **___ sucking** / chuparse el dedo gordo.

thumbnail *n.* uña del pulgar.

thymectomy *n.* timectomía, extirpación del timo.

thymoma *n.* timoma, tumor que se origina en el timo.

thymus *n.* timo, glándula situada en la parte inferior del cuello y anterosuperior de la cavidad torácica que desempeña un papel de importancia en la función inmunológica.

thyroglobulin *n.* tiroglobulina. 1. iodina que contiene glicoproteína secretada por la tiroides; 2. sustancia que se obtiene de tiroides porcinas y se administra como suplemento en el tratamiento de hipertiroidismo.

thyroglossal *a.* tirogloso-a, rel. a la tiroides y a la lengua.

thyroid *n.* glándula tiroides, una de las glándulas endocrinas situadas delante de la tráquea y constituída por dos lóbulos laterales conectados en el centro; __ **function tests** / pruebas del funcionamiento de la __; *a.* tiroideo-a, rel. a la tiroides; __ **cartilage** / cartílago __; __ **hormones** / hormonas __ -as; __ **storm** / tormenta __, crisis __ .

thyroidectomy *n.* tiroidectomía, extirpación de la tiroides.

thyroidism *n.* tiroidismo, condición por exceso de secreción tiroidea.

thyroiditis *n.* tiroiditis, infl. de la tiroides.

thyroid-stimulating hormone *n.* hormona estimulante de la secreción tiroidea. V. thyrotropin.

thyromegaly *n.* tiromegalia, agrandamiento de la tiroides.

thyroparathyroidectomy *n.* tiroparatiroidectomía, excisión de la tiroides y la paratiroides.

thyrotoxicosis *n.* tirotoxicosis, trastorno causado por hipertiroidismo que se manifiesta con agrandamiento de la tiroides, aumento en el metabolismo, taquicardia, pulso rápido e hipertensión.

thyrotropin *n.* tirotropina, hormona estimulante de la tiroides secretada por el lóbulo anterior de la pituitaria; __ **releasing factor** / factor liberador de la __; __ **releasing hormone** / hormona estimulante de __ .

thyroxine *n.* tiroxina, hormona producida por la tiroides que contiene yodo; se obtiene sintéticamente de la tiroides de animales y se usa en el tratamiento de hipotiroidismo.

tibia *n.,* tibia, hueso triangular anterior de la pierna situado debajo de la rodilla.

tic *n., Fr.* tic, espasmo súbito o involuntario de un músculo que ocurre esp. en la cara; **convulsive** __ / __ convulsivo; **coordinated** __ / __ coordinado; **douloureux** __ / __ doloroso; **facial** __ / __ facial.

tick *n.* garrapata, ácarido chupador de sangre transmisor de enfermedades; __ **bite** / picadura de __ .

tickling *n.* cosquilleo.

tidal *a.* rel. al volumen de inspiración y expiración.

tight *a.* [*fitted*] apretado-a, ajustado-a; [*airtight*] hermético-a; tirante; **a** __ **situation** / una situación grave; __ **squeeze** / *pop.* aprieto; *v.* **to hold on** __ / agarrarse bien.

tighten *v.* apretar, ajustar.

time *n.* tiempo, medida de duración; **a limited** __ / __ limitado; **at the same** __ / a la vez; **at** __ **s** / a veces; **At what** __? / ¿A qué hora?; **behind** __ / atrasado-a; **bleeding** __ / __ de sangramiento; **coagulation** __ / __ de coagulación; **for some** __ / por algún __; **for the** __ **being** / por el momento, por ahora; **from** __ **to** __ / de vez en cuando; **in due** __ / a su debido __; **on** __ / a tiempo; **perception** __ / __ de percepción; **prothrombin** __ / __ de protrombina; __ **exposure** / __ de exposición; __ **frame** / espacio de __; __ **lag** / __ de latencia; **What** __ **is it?** / ¿Qué hora es?; *v.* marcar, medir el tiempo; **to set the** __ / regular el tiempo.

tinea *n., L.* tinea, tiña, infección cutánea fungosa; __ **capital** / __ capitis; __ **pedis** / __ pedis; *pop.* pie de atleta; __ **versicolor** / __ versicolor.

tingle *n.* hormigueo, comezón, sensación de picazón.

tinnitus *n.* zumbido, chasquido, sonido que se siente en el oído.

tint *n.* tinte, colorante; *v.* teñir, colorar, dar color.

tireless *a.* incansable, infatigable.

tiresome *a.* pesado-a, tedioso-a.

tiring *a.* agotador-a, que cansa o fatiga.

tissue *n.* tejido, grupo de células similares de función determinada unidas por una sustancia intercelular que actúan conjuntamente; **adipose** __ / __ adiposo; **bone, bony** __ / __ óseo; **cartilaginous** __ / __ cartilaginoso; **connective** __ / __ conectivo; **endothelial** __ / __ endothelial; **epithelial** __ / __ epithelial; **erectile** __ / __ eréctil; **fibrous** __ / __ fibroso; **glandular** __ / __ glandular; **lymphatic** __ / __ linfático; **mesenchymal** __ / __ mesenquimatoso; **muscular** __ / __ muscular; **scar** __ / __ cicatrizante; **subcutaneous** __ / __ subcutáneo.

tissue typing *n.* tipificación, clasificación por tipo; tipificación de tejido.

titer, titre *n.* título, la cantidad de una sustancia que se requiere para producir una reacción con un volumen determinado de otra sustancia.

tobacco *n.* tabacco, planta americana de la *Nicotiana tabacum* cuyas hojas preparadas contienen nicotina, sustancia tóxica perjudicial a la salud; __ **smoke pollution** / contaminación por humo de __; __ **use disorder** / trastorno por uso de __ .

tocograph *n.* tocógrafo, instrumento para estimar la fuerza de las contracciones uterinas.

toddler *n.* niño-a que comienza a caminar.

toe *n.* dedo del pie.

toe drop *n.* caída de los dedos del pie.

toe nail *n.* uña de un dedo del pie.

toilet *n.* 1. servicio, inodoro; 2. limpieza relacionada con un procedimiento médico o quirúrgico; __ **paper** / papel higiénico.

toilet training *n.* entrenamiento de los niños para controlar el acto de orinar y de defecar.

tolerance *n.* tolerancia, capacidad de soportar una sustancia o un ejercicio físico sin sufrir efectos dañinos, tal como el uso de una droga o una actividad física prolongada.

tomograph *n.* tomógrafo, máquina radiográfica que se usa para hacer una tomografía.

tomography *n.* tomografía, técnica de diagnóstico por la cual se hacen radiografías de un órgano por secciones del mismo a profundidades distintas; **computed** __ / __ computada; **computerized axial** __ (CAT) / __ axial computarizada (TAC); **conventional** __ / __ convencional; **dynamic computed** __ / __ dinámica computada; **electron beam** __ / __ con rayos de electrón; **high-resolution computed** __ / __ computada de alta resolución; **nuclear magnetic resonance** __ / __ de resonancia magnética nuclear; **positron emission** __ / __ de emisión por positrón.

tone *n.* tono. 1. grado normal de vigor y tensión en el funcionamiento de los órganos y músculos de un cuerpo sano; **muscular** __ / __ muscular; 2. cualidad definida de un sonido o voz.

tongue *n.* lengua; **black hairy** __ / __ negra velluda, lengua infectada de hongos parásitos; **dry** __ / __ seca; **geographic** __ / __ geográfica; **red** __ / __ roja o enrojecida; **sticky** __ / __ pegajosa; __ **depressor** / depresor de __ .

tonic *n.* tónico, reconstituyente que restaura la vitalidad del organismo *a.* tónico-a. 1. que restaura el tono

normal; 2. caracterizado-a por una tensión continua.

tonicity *a.* tonicidad, cualidad normal de tono o tensión.

tonometer *n.* tonómetro, instrumento usado para medir la tensión o presión esp. intraocular.

tonometry *n.* tonometría, medida de la presión o tensión.

tonsil *n.* amígdala, tonsila; **cerebellar** __ / __ cerebelosa; **lingual** __ / __ lingual; **palatine** __ / __ palatina; **pharyngeal** __ / __ faríngea.

tonsillar *a.* tonsilar, rel. a una tonsila; __ **crypt** / cripta __ o amigdalina; __ **fossa** / fosa amigdalina.

tonsillectomy *n.* amigdalectomía, extirpación de las amígdalas.

tonsillitis *n.* amigdalitis, infl. de las amígdalas.

tonsiloadenoidectomy *n.* tonsiloadenoidectomía, extirpación de las adenoides y las amígdalas.

tooth *n.* (*pl.* **teeth**) diente; **impacted** __ / __ impactado; __ **unerupted** / __ no erupcionado.

toothache *n.* dolor de muelas.

tophus *n.* tofo. 1. depósito de sal de ácido úrico en los tejidos, gen. visto en casos de gota; 2. cálculo dental.

topical *a.* tópico-a, rel. a un área localizada.

topographic anatomy *n.* anatomía topográfica, descripción de las partes del cuerpo humano.

torpid *a.* tórpido-a, torpe en los movimientos.

torpor *n.* embotamiento; estancamiento; inactividad física.

torsion *n.* torsión, rotación de una parte sobre su propio eje longitudinal; **ovarian** __ / __ ovárica; **testicular** __ / __ testicular.

torso *n.* torso, el tronco humano.

torticollis *n.* tortícolis, espasmo tonicoclónico de los músculos del cuello que causa torsión cervical e inmovilidad de la cabeza.

total *a.* total; completo-a.

totipotency *n.* totipotencia, habilidad de una célula de regenerarse o desarrollarse en otro tipo de célula.

touch *n.* 1. sentido del tacto, percepción a través de la piel o de las membranas mucosas; 2. [*act of touching*] toque; *v.* tocar, palpar.

tourniquet *n.* torniquete, dispositivo usado para aplicar presión sobre una arteria y contener la salida de la sangre.

toxemia *n.* toxemia, condición tóxica provocada por la absorción de toxinas que provienen de un foco infeccioso.

toxic *a.* tóxico-a, venenoso-a, rel. a un veneno o de naturaleza venenosa.

toxicity *n.* toxicidad, cualidad de ser venenoso.

toxicologist *n.* toxicólogo-a, especialista en toxicología.

toxicology *n.* toxicología, estudio de los venenos o sustancias tóxicas, los efectos que causan en el organismo y su tratamiento; __ **screen** / protocolo toxicológico.

toxicosis *n.* toxicosis, estado morboso debido a un veneno.

toxin *n.* toxina, veneno, sustancia nociva de origen animal o vegetal; **bacterial** __ / __ bacteriana.

toxin-antitoxin *n.* toxina antitoxina, mezcla casi neutra de toxina diftérica y antitoxina que se usa en inmunizaciones contra la difteria.

toxoid *n.* toxoide, toxina desprovista de toxicidad que al introducirse en el organismo causa la formación de anticuerpos; *a.* toxoide, de naturaleza tóxica o venenosa; **diphtheria** __ / __ diftérico; **tetanus** __ / __ tetánico.

Toxoplasma *n. Toxoplasma*, género de parásito protozoario.

toxoplasmosis *n.* toxoplasmosis, infección causada por un microorganismo de la familia *Toxoplasma* que invade los tejidos, con síntomas leves de malestar o posible infl. de las glándulas linfáticas; puede ocasionar daños a la vista y al sistema nervioso central.

tracer *n.* trazador, radioisótopo que al introducirse en el cuerpo crea un rastro que puede detectarse.

trachea *n.* tráquea, conducto respiratorio entre la parte extrema inferior de la laringe y el comienzo de los bronquios.

tracheitis *n.* traqueítis, infl. de la tráquea.

tracheoesophageal *a.* traqueoesofágico-a, rel. a la tráquea y al esófago; __ **fistula** / fístula __.

tracheomalasia *n.* traqueomalasia. reblandecimiento de los cartílagos traqueales.

tracheostenosis *n.* traqueostenosis, estrechez de la tráquea.

tracheostomy *n.* traqueostomía, incisión en la tráquea para permitir el paso de aire en caso de obstrucción.

tracheotomy *n.* traqueotomía, incisión en la tráquea a través de la piel y los músculos del cuello.

trachoma *n.* tracoma, infección viral contagiosa de la conjuntiva y la córnea que se manifiesta con fotofobia, dolor, lagrimeo y, en casos severos, ceguera total.

tracing *n.* trazo, gráfica descriptiva que hace un instrumento al registrar un movimiento.

tract *n.* tracto, tubo, vía, vías, sistema alargado compuesto de tejidos y órganos que actúan coordinadamente para desempeñar una función; **alimentary** __ / __ alimenticio; **ascending** __ / __ ascendiente; **biliary** __ / __ biliar; **digestive** __ / __ digestivo; **genitourinary** __ / __ genitourinario; **olfactory** __ / vía olfatoria; **pyramidal** __ / __ piramidal; **respiratory** __ / __ o vía respiratoria

traction *n.* tracción. 1. acto de tirar o halar; 2. fuerza que tira con tensión; **cervical** __ / __ cervical; **lumbar** __ / __ lumbar.

tragus *n.* (*pl.* **tragi**) trago, protuberancia triangular en la parte externa del oído.

trained nurse *n.* enfermero-a graduado-a.

training *n.* entrenamiento; capacitación; adiestramiento.

trait *n.* rasgo o característica; **acquired** __ / __ adquirido; **inherited** __ / __ heredado.

trance *n.* trance, condición semejante a un estado hipnótico que se caracteriza por la disminución de la actividad motora.

tranquil *a.* apacible, tranquilo-a, calmado-a.

tranquility *n.* tranquilidad, descanso.

tranquilizer *n.* tranquilizante, calmante.

transabdominal *a.* transabdominal, a través del abdomen o de la pared abdominal.

transcutaneous *a.* transcutáneo-a, a través de la piel; __ **electrical nerve stimulation** / estimulación eléctrica __ de un nervio.

transection

transection *n.* corte transversal a través del eje largo de un órgano.

transfer, transference *n.* transferencia. 1. reorientación que hace el paciente de sentimientos negativos o positivos (esp. reprimidos inconscientemente) hacia otra persona, esp. el psicoanalista; 2. transmisión de síntomas o fluidos de una parte a otra del cuerpo.

transferrin *n.* transferrina, globulina beta en el plasma de la sangre que fija y transporta el hierro.

transfixion *n.* transfixión, acto de atravesar y cortar al mismo tiempo los tejidos blandos de dentro hacia afuera como en la extirpación de tumores o en amputaciones.

transformation *n.* transformación, cambio de forma o apariencia.

transfusion *n.* transfusión, acto de transferir un fluido a una vena o arteria; **blood** ___ / ___ de sangre; **direct** ___ / ___ directa; **exchange** ___ / exsanguino-transfusión; **indirect** ___ / ___ indirecta; ___ **reaction** / reacción a la ___.

transitional *a.* transitorio-a, rel. a transición o cambio.

transitional cell carcinoma *n.* carcinoma maligno de células de transición, localizado gen. en la vejiga, uréter o en la pelvis renal.

transitory *a.* transitorio-a, pasajero-a.

translocation *n.* translocación, desplazamiento de un cromosoma o parte del mismo hacia otro cromosoma.

transmigration *n.* transmigración, paso de un lugar a otro tal como las células sanguíneas en diapédesis.

transmissible *a.* transmisible, trasmisible, que puede transmitirse.

transmission *n.* transmisión, acto de transmitir o transferir tal como una enfermedad contagiosa o hereditaria; **droplet** ___ / ___ por instilación; **pathogen** ___ / ___ patógena; **placental** ___ / ___ placentaria; ___ **by contact** / ___ por contacto.

transmission electron microscope *n.* microscopio electrónico de transmisión, instrumento usado para visualizar las células con una capacidad superior de un millón más de visualización que el microscopio común.

transmit *v.* transmitir, el acto de transferir una condición hereditaria, enfermedad genética o infección de una persona a otra.

transmutation *n.* transmutación. 1. transformación, cambio evolutivo; 2. cambio de una sustancia en otra.

transocular *a.* transocular, que pasa a través de la órbita ocular.

transonance *n.* transonancia, resonancia transmitida.

transparency *n.* transparencia; [*slide*] diapositiva.

transparent *a.* transparente, rel. a la cualidad de claridad de un objeto que permite el paso de la luz mostrando imágenes situadas en el lado opuesto.

transpiration *n.* transpiración, perspiración.

transplacental *a.* transplacental, a través de la placenta.

transplant *n.* trasplante. 1. acto de transferir un órgano o tejido de un donante a un recipiente, o de una parte del cuerpo a otra para sustituir una parte enferma o restituir un órgano a su función normal; 2. parte artificial o natural que se usa como reemplazo; *v.* trasplantar.

transplant of the bone marrow *n.* trasplante de la medula ósea, injerto de tejido de la medula. 1. a pacientes de cáncer después de un tratamiento de quimioterpia; 2. a pacientes que sufren de anemia plástica, o en casos severo de leucemia.

transplantation *n.* transplantación, trasplantación, acto de hacer un trasplante; **autoplastic** ___ / ___ autoplástica; **heteroplastic** ___ / ___ heteroplástica; **heterotopic** ___ / ___ heterotópica; **homotopic** ___ / ___ homotópica.

transposition *n.* transposición. 1. desplazamiento de un órgano o parte a una posición opuesta; 2. cambio genético de un cromosoma a otro que resulta a veces en defectos genéticos.

transposition of great vessels *n.* transposición de los grandes vasos, anomalía congénita en la cual la aorta sale del ventrículo derecho mientras que el tronco pulmonar sale del ventrículo izquierdo.

transrectal ultrasound *n.* ultrasonido transrectal, procedimiento que se usa para examinar la próstata por medio de ultrasonido. Se introduce un instrumento por el recto para captar distintas imágenes de la próstata que se proyectan por medio de ondas sonoras emitidas por ecos reproducidos por una computadora (ordenador); ___ **resection prostate** / resección ___ de la próstata.

transsexual *a.* transexual. 1. persona que tiene una urgencia psicológica de pertenecer al sexo opuesto; 2. persona que ha cambiado de sexo sometiéndose a una operación quirúgica.

transudate *n.* transudado, fluido que ha pasado a través de una membrana o ha sido expulsado como resultado de una inflamación.

transurethral *a.* transuretral, que ocurre o se administra a través de la uretra; ___ **resection prostate** / resección ___ de la próstata.

transvaginal *a.* transvaginal, a través de la vagina.

transversal *a.* transversal ___ **plane** / plano ___.

transverse *a.* transversal, atravesado-a; ___ **colon** / colon ___ ; ___ **plain** / plano ___ .

transvestism *n.* trasvestismo, adopción de modales del sexo opuesto, esp. la manera de vestir.

transvestite *n.* transvestido-a, transvestita, persona que practica el transvestismo.

trapezius *n.* trapecio, músculo triangular plano esencial en la rotación de la escápula.

trauma *n.* 1. trauma, estado psicológico; 2. traumatismo, si se refiere a una condición física.

traumatism *n.* traumatismo.

traumatized *a.* traumatizado.

traumatology *n.* traumatología, rama de la cirugía que trata del cuidado de lesiones y heridas.

treadmill *n.* [*physical fitness*] rueda de andar; tapiz rodante.

treatment *n.* tratamiento, método o procedimiento que se usa en la cura de enfermedades, lesiones y deformaciones; **preventive** ___ / ___ preventivo; **symptomatic** ___ / ___ sintomático; ___ **plan** / plan o método de ___ .

tree *n.* 1. árbol; 2. estructura anatómica semejante a un árbol.

Trematoda *n. Trematoda*, clase de gusanos parásitos de la especie de los *Platyhelminthes* que incluye la duela y los gusanos planos que infectan el organismo humano.

trematode *n.* trematodo, gusano parásito de la clase *Trematoda*.

tremble *n.* temblor, estremecimiento, movimiento involuntario oscilatorio; *v.* temblar; estremecerse.

tremor *n.* temblor, estremecimiento; **alcoholic** ___ / ___ alcohólico; **coarse** ___ / ___ lento y acentuado; **continuous** ___ / ___ continuo; **essential** ___ / ___ esencial; **fine** ___ / ___ de variaciones rápidas; **flapping** ___ / ___ de aleteo; **intention** ___ / ___ intencional; **intermittent** ___ / ___ intermitente; **muscular** ___ / ___ muscular; **physiological** ___ / ___ fisiológico; **resting** ___ / ___ de reposo.

tremulous *a.* trémulo-a, afectado-a por un estremecimiento o que posee las características de un temblor.

trench *n.* trinchera, zanja, foso; ___ **back** / rigidez y dolor de espalda; ___ **fever** / fiebre de ___, fiebre remitente transmitida por piojos; ___ **foot** / pie de ___, infección en los pies por exposición al frío; ___ **-mouth** / infección con ulceración de las mucosas de la boca y la faringe.

trepan *n.* trépano, instrumento usado en la trepanación; *v.* trepanar, perforar el cráneo con un trépano.

trepanation *n.* trepanación, perforación del cráneo con un instrumento especial para reducir el aumento de la presión intracraneal causada por fractura, acumulación de sangre o pus.

trephination *n.* trefinación, acto de cortar un tejido o un hueso dando un corte circular o de disco, operación gen. efectuada en el cráneo.

treponema *n.* treponema, parásito de la orden *Spirochaetales* que invade a humanos y animales; ___ **pallidum** / ___ pallidum, parásito causante de la sífilis.

treponemiasis *n.* treponemiasis, infección causada por espiroquetas del género *Treponema*.

triage *n., Fr.* triage, triada, clasificación y evaluación de víctimas en acontecimientos catastróficos para establecer prioridades según la urgencia del tratamiento y aumentar el número de sobrevivientes.

trial *n.* prueba, ensayo.

triceps *n., L.* tríceps, músculo de tres porciones o cabezas; ___ **reflex** / reflejo del ___ .

Trichinella *n.* *Trichinella*, género de gusanos nematodos, parásitos de animales carnívoros.

trichinosis *n.* triquinosis, enfermedad adquirida por la ingestión de carne cruda o mal cocinada, esp. de cerdo, que contiene larvas enquistadas de *Trichinella spiralis*.

trichitis *n.* triquitis, infl. de los bulbos pilosos.

trichobezoar *n.* tricobezoar, concreción o bezoar formado de pelo que se aloja en el intestino o el estómago.

Trichomonas *n.* *Trichomonas*, parásitos protozoarios que se alojan en el tubo digestivo y en el tracto genitourinario de vertebrados; ___ **vaginalis** / ___ vaginalis, agente causante de la vaginitis.

trichomoniasis *n.* trichomoniasis, infestación por *Trichomonas*.

trichomycosis *n.* tricomicosis, enfermedad del cabello causada por hongos.

tricuspid *a.* tricúspide. 1. que posee tres puntas o cúspides; 2. rel. a la válvula tricúspide del corazón; ___ **atresia** / atresia ___ ; ___ **murmur** / soplo ___ .

trifocal *a.* trifocal; ___ **lenses** / lentes ___ -es.

trigeminal *a.* trigeminal, rel. al nervio trigémino; ___ **cough** / tos ___ ; ___ **neuralgia** / neuralgia ___ ; ___ **pulse** / pulso ___ .

trigeminal nerve *n.* nervio trigémino.

trigger *n.* desencadenamiento; impulso o reacción que inicia otros eventos; ___ **finger** / dedo en resorte ___ ; ___ **points** / puntos de ___ ; *v.* desencadenar, iniciar.

trigger zone *n.* área de resorte, area sensitiva que al recibir un estímulo ocasiona una reacción en otra parte del cuerpo.

triglycerides *n., pl.* triglicéridos, combinación que resulta de una molécula de glicerol con tres moléculas de ácidos grasos diferentes; la presencia elevada de triglicéridos es un factor importante en el desarrollo de enfermedades cardiovasculares.

trigonitis *n.* trigonitis, infl. del trígono de la vejiga urinaria.

trimester *n.* trimestre, tres meses, periodo de tres consecutivas etapas en que se divide el embarazo hasta terminar en el parto.

triplopia *n.* triplopia, trastorno visual por el cual se producen tres imágenes del mismo objeto.

trismus *n., Gr.* trismus, espasmo de los músculos de la masticación debido a una condición patológica.

trisomy *n.* trisomía, trastorno genético por el cual una persona posee tres cromosomas homólogos por célula en lugar de dos (diploide), lo cual causa deformaciones fetales serias.

trochanter *n.* trocánter, una de las dos prominencias exteriores localizadas bajo el cuello del fémur; **greater** ___ / ___ mayor; **lesser** ___ / ___ menor.

trochlea *n.* tróclea, estructura que sirve de polea.

trochlear nerve *n.* nervio troclear. cranial nerves.

tropical *a.* tropical; ___ **diseases** / enfermedades ___ -es; ___ **medicine** / medicina ___ .

tropism *n.* tropismo, tendencia de una célula u organismo a reaccionar de una forma definida (positiva o negativa) en respuesta a estímulos externos.

trouble *n.* aflicción, calamidad, problema; **What is the trouble?** / ¿qué sucede? ¿qué pasa?; *v.* **to be in** ___ / estar en un apuro; **to be worth the** ___ / valer la pena.

true pelvis *n.* pelvis verdadera o menor, parte inferior contráctil de la pelvis.

truncal *a.* troncal, truncado-a, rel. al tronco.

trunk *n.* tronco, torso, la parte anatómica excluyendp la cabeza y las extremidades.

truss *n.* braguero, faja para mantener una hernia reducida en su lugar; *v.* ligar, amarrar.

truthful *a.* veraz, verdadero-a; **-ly** *adv.* verdaderamente, realmente.

try *n.* prueba, ensayo; *v.* probar, ensayar, hacer una prueba; intentar; **to** ___ **out** / probar, someter a prueba; **to** ___ **on** / probarse.

Trypanosoma *n.* *Tripanosoma*, género de parásito protozoario que se aloja en la sangre y es transmitido a los vertebrados por insectos vectores.

trypanosomiasis *n.* tripanosomiasis, cualquier infección causada por un parásito flagelado del género *Tripanosoma*.

trypsin *n.* tripsina, enzima formada por el tripsinógeno presente en el jugo pancreático.

trypsinogen *n.* tripsinógeno, sustancia inactiva segregada por el páncreas en el duodeno para formar tripsina.

tryptophan *n.* triptófano, aminoácido cristalino presente en las proteínas, esencial a la vida animal.

tsetse fly *n.* mosca tsetsé, insecto del sur de Africa, transmisor de la enfermedad del sueño.

tubal *a.* tubárico-a; **__ pregnancy /** embarazo ectópico en una trompa de Falopio; **__ ligation /** ligadura o ligazón de las trompas.

tube *n.* tubo, conducto, trompa; **drainage __ / __** de drenaje; **endotracheal __ / __** endotraqueal; **inhalation __ / __** de inhalación; **intestinal decompression __ /** sonda intestinal; **nasogastric __ / __** nasogástrico; **tracheotomy __ / __** de traqueotomía; **thoracostomy __ / __** de toracostomía.

tubercle *n.* tubérculo. 1. nódulo pequeño; 2. pequeña prominencia de un hueso; 3. lesión producida por el bacilo de la tuberculosis.

tubercular *a.* tubercular, caracterizado por lesiones tubcrosas.

tuberculin *n.* tuberculina, compuesto preparado del bacilo de la tuberculosis usado en las pruebas de diagnóstico de infecciones de la tuberculosis.

tuberculin test *n.* prueba de la tuberculina.

tuberculocidal *a.* tuberculocida, que destruye el bacilo de la tuberculosis.

tuberculosis (TB) *n.* tuberculosis, infección bacteriana aguda o crónica causada por el germen *Mycobacterium tuberculosis* que gen. afecta los pulmones pero que también puede afectar otros órganos; **meningeal __ /** __ meníngea; **pulmonary __ /** __ pulmonar; **spinal __ / __** espinal; **__ in childhood / __** infantil; **urogenital __ / __** urogenital.

tuberosity *n.* tuberosidad, elevación o protuberancia.

tuberous sclerosis *n.* esclerosis tuberosa, enfermedad familiar marcada por ataques convulsivos, deficiencia mental progresiva y formación de múltiples tumores cerebrales cutáneos.

tuboabdominal pregnancy *n.* embarazo tuboabdominal.

tubo-ovarian *a.* tuboovárico-a, rel. a la trompa de Falopio y el ovario; **__ abscess /** absceso __ .

tubo-ovaritis *n.* tubo-ovaritis, infl. del ovario y la trompa de Falopio.

tuboplasty *n.* tuboplastia, reparación plástica de un conducto esp. de una trompa de Falopio.

tubule *n.* túbulo, conducto o canal pequeño; **collecting __ / __** colector; **renal __ / __** renal; **seminiferous __ /** conduto seminífero.

tularemia *n.* tularemia, fiebre de conejo, infeción transmitida a las personas por la picadura de un insecto vector o contraída en la manipulación de carne infectada.

tumefaction *n.* tumefacción, tumescencia, proceso de hinchazón.

tumor *n.* tumor. 1. bulto o hinchazón; 2. crecimiento espontáneo de tejido nuevo en masa sin propósito fisiológico alguno; **diffuse __ / __** difuso; **inflammatory __ / __** inflamatorio; **medullary __ / __** medular; **necrotic __ / __** necrótico; **nonsolid __ / __** no sólido; **radioresistant __ / __** radiorresistente; **radiosensitive __ / __** radiosensivo; **scirrhous __ / __** escirroso; **undifferentiated __ / __** no diferenciado.

tumor makers, serum *n., pl.* sustancias en el plasma sanguíneo indicativas de la posible presencia de un tumor maligno.

tumor virus *n.* virus tumoroso, capaz de producir cáncer.

tumoricidal *a.* tumoricida, que destruye células tumorales.

tumorigenesis *n.* tumorigénesis, formación de tumores.

tunic *n.* túnica, membrana protectora; **__ adventitia / __** adventicia; **__ albuginea /** cápsula albugínea; **externa / __** externa; **__ interna /** interna; **__ media / __** media; **__ mucosa / __** mucosa; **__ muscularis /** __ muscular; **__ serosa / __** serosa; **__ vaginalis / __** vaginal.

tunnel *n.* túnel, canal o conducto estrecho; **carpal __ / __** del carpo; **flexor __ / __** flexor; **tarsal __ / __** tarsiano.

tunnel vision *n.* visión en túnel, trastorno frecuente en casos de glaucoma avanzado que produce al paciente una disminución visual considerable tal como si mirara a través de un túnel.

turbid *a.* turbio-a, túrbido-a; nebuloso-a.

turgid *a.* túrgido-a; hinchado-a, distendido-a.

turgor *n.* turgor. 1. distensión; 2. tensión celular normal.

turn *n.* vuelta, giro; turno; *v.* voltear, virar, dar vuelta, torcer; **to ___ back** / volver, regresar, retroceder; **to ___ down** / doblar; desaprobar, rechazar; [*when referring to one's body*] volverse, darse vuelta, virarse; **to ___ into** / volverse, convertirse en, transformarse; **to ___ out** / resultar; **to ___ pale** / palidecer; **to ___ red** / enrojecerse.

Turner's syndrome *n.* síndrome de Turner, trastorno endocrino congénito que se manifiesta con deficiencia ovárica, amenorrea, estatura baja y la presencia de cromosomas X solamente.

turning *n.* 1. versión, término obstétrico referente a la manipulación del feto en el útero para facilitar el parto; 2. vuelta; *a.* giratorio-a; **the ___ point** / la crisis, el momento decisivo.

turnover *n.* cambio; *a.* cambiado-a de posición; *v.* voltear, cambiar de posición; transferir.

T wave *n.* onda T, parte del electrocardiograma que representa la repolarización de los ventrículos.

twilight *n.* crepúsculo; **___ sleep** / sueño crepuscular; **___ state** / estado de somnolencia.

twinge *n.* punzada, dolor agudo.

twins *n., pl.* gemelos, mellizos, jimaguas, uno de dos hijos nacidos de un mismo embarazo; **dizygotic ___** / **___** dicigóticos; **identical ___** / **___** idénticos; **monozygotic ___** / **___** monocigotos; **Siamese ___** / **___** siameses; **true ___** / **___** verdaderos.

twist *n.* torsión, torcedura; sacudida, contorsión; peculiaridad; *v.* [*an ankle*] torcer, virar, doblar.

twitch *n.* tic nervioso espasmódico; sacudida.

tympanectomy *n.* timpanectomía, excisión de la membrana timpánica.

tympanic *a.* timpánico-a, que se refiere a una estructura con cualidad de resonancia cuando es tocada, o que resuena en percusión transmitiendo vibraciones de sonido tal como en el oído medio o sonido de tambor en otra parte del cuerpo; **___ membrane** / membrana ___; **___ nerve** / nervio ___; **resonance** / resonancia ___; **nerve** / nervío ___.

tympanites *n.* timpanitis, distensión del abdomen causada por acumulación de gas en los intestinos.

tympanoplasty *n.* timpanoplastia, reconstrucción del oído medio.

tympanotomy *n.* timpanotomía, incisión de la membrana timpánica.

tympanum *n.* tímpano, oído medio.

type *n.* tipo, género, clase, modelo o ejemplar distintivo.

typhlitis *n.* tiflitis, infl. del ciego.

typhoid *a.* tifoideo-a, rel. al tifus o semejante a éste.

typhoid fever *n.* fiebre tifoidea, infección abdominal aguda que es causada por una bacteria de la clase *Salmonella* y que se manifiesta con infl. abdominal, postración, fiebre alta y dolor de cabeza.

typhus *n.* tifus, infección aguda causada por una *Rickettsia* que se manifiesta con fiebre alta, intensos dolores de cabeza y delirio.

typhus vaccine *n.* vacuna tífica.

typical *a.* típico-a, conforme a un tipo.

typing *n.* tipificación de tejidos, determinación por tipos; **blood ___** / determinación del grupo sanguíneo.

u

ulcer *n.* úlcera, llaga o lesión en la piel o en la membrana mucosa con desintegración gradual de los tejidos. V. cuadro esta página.

ulcerated *a.* ulcerado-a, de la naturaleza de una úlcera o afectado por ella.

ulceration *n.* ulceración, supuración; proceso de formación de una úlcera.

ulcerative *a.* ulcerativo-a, rel. a una úlcera o caracterizado-a por una condición ulcerosa; ___ **colitis** / colitis ___ .

ulerythema *n.* uleritema, dermatitis eritematosa caracterizada por la formación de cicatrices; ___ **ophryogenes** / ___ ofriógeno; ___ **sycosiforme** / ___ sicosiforme.

ulnar *n.* ulnar, rel. al cúbito o a los nervios y arterias relacionados con éste; ___ **nerve dysfunction** / disfunción del nervio ___ .

ulocarcinoma, ulocarcinomata *n.* ulocarcinoma, ulocarcinomata, cáncer de las encías.

Ulcer	Úlcera
chancroidal	chancroide
chronic	crónica
chronic leg varicose	varicosa crónica de la pierna
decubitus	por decúbito
duodenal	duodenal
gastric	gástrica
hemorrhagic	homorrágica
indolent	indolente
marginal	marginal
mycotic	micótica
peptic	péptica
perforating	perforante
phagedenic	fagedénica
rodent	roedora
syphilitic	sifilítica
vesical	vesical

ultracentrifuge *n.* ultracentrífuga, aparato de fuerza centrífuga que separa y sedimenta las moléculas de una sustancia.

ultrafiltration *n.* ultrafiltración, proceso de filtración que deja pasar pequeñas moléculas pero impide el paso de moléculas mayores.

ultramicroscope *n.* ultramicroscopio, microscopio de campo oscuro capaz de hacer visibles objetos que no se distinguen en un microscopio de luz común.

ultrasonic *a.* ultrasónico-a, supersónico-a; ___ **diagnosis** / diagnóstico por ultrasonido.

ultrasonogram *n.* ultrasonograma, imagen producida por medio de ultrasonografía.

ultrasonography *n.* ultrasonografía, técnica de diagnóstico que emplea ultrasonido para producir imágenes de una estructura o de tejidos del cuerpo.

ultrasound *n.* ultrasonido, ondas de frecuencia superior a las del oído humano que se usan en ultrasonografía en procedimientos terapéuticos y de diagnóstico; **abdominal** ___ / ___ abdominal; **breast** ___ / ___ de la mama; **pregnancy** ___ / ___ del embarazo; **thyroid** ___ / ___ de la tiroides.

ultrasound imaging *n.* imágenes por ultrasonido, captación de imágenes de órganos o tejidos del cuerpo por medio de ultrasonido empleando técnicas de reflejo (ecograma).

ultraviolet *a.* ultravioleta, que se extiende más allá de la zona violeta del espectro; ___ **rays** / rayos ___; ___ **therapy** / terapia de radiación ___ .

umbilical *a.* umbilical, rel. al ombligo; ___ **notch** / ligamento ___; ___ **hernia** / hernia ___ .

umbilical cord *n.* cordón umbilical, estructura que sirve de conexión entre el feto y la placenta durante la gestación.

umbilicus, navel *n.* ombligo, depresión en el centro del abdomen que marca el punto de inserción del cordón umbilical.

unacceptable *a.* inaceptable, no aprobado-a.

unaccustomed *a.* no usual, no acostumbrado-a, desacostumbrado-a.

unadulterated *a.* natural, puro-a, sin mezcla, no adulterado-a.

unaffected *a.* no afectado-a.

unanswered

unanswered *a.* por contestar, no contestado-a.

unassisted *a.* sin ayuda, sin auxilio, desamparado-a.

unattached *a.* suelto-a, sin conexión.

unattended *a.* desatendido-a.

unaware *a.* sin conocimiento de causa; que ignora.

unbearable *a.* insoportable, intolerable, insufrible, imposible de soportar.

unbiased *a.* imparcial, sin prejuicios.

uncomfortable *a.* incómodo-a, molesto-a, desagradable.

uncommon *a.* poco común, raro-a, extraño-a.

unconditioned reflex *n.* reflejo no condicionado o natural.

unconditioned response *n.* respuesta no condicionada o reacción no restringida.

unconscious *a.* inconsciente. 1. que ha perdido el conocimiento; 2. que no responde a estímulos sensoriales.

unconsciousness *n.* inconsciencia, pérdida del conocimiento.

unction *n.* unción, aplicación de un ungüento o aceite.

undecided *a.* indeciso-a, indeterminado-a.

under *a.* inferior; *prep. adv.* debajo, menos, menos que; bajo; ___ **observation** / bajo observación; ___ **treatment** / bajo tratamiento.

underage *a.* menor de edad.

underdeveloped *a.* subdesarrollado-a; en desarrollo.

underdevelopment *n.* subdesarrollo.

underestimate *v.* subestimar; menospreciar.

undergo *vi.* someterse a; sufrir, padecer, soportar; **to ___ surgery** / someterse a una operación.

undernourished *a.* desnutrido-a; malnutrido-a.

understand *vi.* comprender, entender.

underway *n.* en camino; bajo estudio.

underweight *n.* falta de peso, peso deficiente; bajo de peso; de peso insuficiente.

undetected *a.* no detectado-a, no descubierto-a, inadvertido-a.

undeveloped *a.* no desarrollado-a, sin manifestación.

undifferentiation *n.* indiferenciación. V. **anaplasia**.

undiluted *a.* no diluido-a, sin diluirse, concentrado-a.

undisclosed *a.* no revelado-a, no dado-a a conocer.

undo *vi.* deshacer, desatar; desabrochar.

undress *v.* desvestirse; quitarse la ropa.

undulated *a.* ondulado-a, de borde ondulado o irregular.

uneasy *a.* inquieto-a.

unequal *a.* desigual; desproporcionado-a.

unexpected *a.* inesperado-a, imprevisto-a.

unfinished *a.* incompleto-a, sin terminar.

unfit *a.* inepto-a, inhábil, incapaz.

unforeseen *a.* inesperado-a, imprevisto-a.

unfortunate *a.* infeliz, desafortunado-a, desgraciado-a.

unfriendly *a.* poco amistoso-a, poco amigable.

ungual *a.* ungueal, rel. a una uña.

unguent *n.* ungüento, medicamento preparado para uso externo.

unhappy *a.* infeliz, desgraciado-a.

unharmed, unhurt *a.* ileso-a; *pop.* sano-a y salvo-a.

unhealthy *a.* [*environment*] insalubre, malsano-a; [*person*] enfermizo-a, achacoso-a.

uniarticular *a.* uniarticular, rel. a una sola articulación.

unicellular *a.* unicelular, de una sola célula.

uniform *n.* [*garment*] uniforme; *a.* uniforme; invariable.

unigravida *a.* unigrávida, mujer embarazada por primera vez.

union *n.* unión. 1. acción de unir dos cosas en una; 2. juntura de dos partes cortadas (amputadas) de un hueso o de los bordes de una herida.

uniparous *a.* unípara, mujer que tiene un parto simple.

unipolar *a.* unipolar, de un solo polo, tal como las células nerviosas.

unique *a.* único-a; solo-a; que se distingue de otros.

unit *n.* unidad. 1. estándar de medida; 2. unidad internacional / **international** ___; 3. unidad fisiológica, la más mínima división de un órgano capaz de realizar una función; **motor** ___ / ___ motora.

united *a.* unido-a.

universal *a.* universal, general; ___ **antidote** / antídoto ___ .

488

universal donor *n.* donante universal, persona que pertenece al grupo de sangre tipo O, de factor RH negativo, cuya sangre puede ser dada a personas con sangre tipo ABO con poco riesgo de complicaciones.

universal recipient *n.* recipiente universal, persona que pertenece al grupo de sangre AB.

unlicensed *a.* no acreditado-a, sin licencia o sin permiso.

unlucky *a.* desafortunado-a.

Unna's paste boot *n.* bota de pasta de Unna, compresión que se usa en el tratamiento de úlceras varicosas en la pierna, con vendajes en espiral aplicados y cubiertos con la pasta medicinal de Unna.

unnecessary *a.* innecesario-a.

unobstructed *a.* abierto-a, suelto-a; libre; no obstruido.

unorganized *a.* desorganizado-a; no estructurado; sin orden.

unreasonable *a.* irrazonable, intransigente.

unrest *n.* desasosiego, inquietud; intranquilidad.

unsalted *a.* sin sal, que le falta sal.

unsanitary *a.* insalubre, malsano.

unsaturated *a.* no saturado-a.

unstable *a.* inestable; __ **angina** / angina __; __ **bladder** / vejiga __ .

untreated *a.* no tratado-a.

unwanted *a.* no deseado-a.

update *v.* [*to improve*] modernizar; [*documents*] poner al día; arreglar.

upgrowth *n.* crecimiento, desarrollo, maduración.

upper *n. pop.* droga estimulante, esp. una anfetamina; *a. comp.* superior, más alto-a.

upper airway obstruction *n.* obstrucción en el conducto aéreo superior.

upper GI *n.* examen radiográfico del estómago y duodeno con ingestión de una sustancia que sirve de medio de contraste.

upper jaw *n.* mandíbula superior.

upper respiratory infection *n.* infección del tracto respiratorio superior.

upper respiratory tract *n.* aparato respiratorio superior compuesto de la nariz, los conductos nasales y la nasofaringe.

upset *a.* indipuesto-a; nervioso-a; disgustado-a; *v.* trastornar; enfadar.

uptake *n.* absorción, fijación o incorporación de alguna sustancia a un organismo vivo; __ **and storage** / toma y almacenamiento.

uranic *a.* uránico-a, rel. a la uremia.

uranium *n.* uranio, elemento metálico pesado.

urate *n.* urato, sal de ácido úrico.

urea *n.* urea, producto del metabolismo de las proteínas, forma en la cual el nitrógeno se excreta por la orina; **hereditary** __ **cycle abnormality** / ciclo ureico hereditario anormal.

urelcosis *n.* urelcosis, ulceración de las vías urinarias.

uremia *n.* uremia, condición tóxica causada por insuficiencia renal que produce retención en la sangre de sustancias nitrogenadas, fosfatos y sulfatos.

ureter *n.* uréter, uno de los conductos que llevan la orina del riñón a la vejiga.

ureteral *a.* ureteral, uretérico-a, rel. o concerniente al uréter; __ **injury** / lesión __; __ **reflex** / reflejo __ .

ureterectasis *n.* ureterectasis, dilatación anormal del uréter.

ureterectomy *n.* ureterectomía, extirpación parcial o total del uréter.

ureteritis *n.* ureteritis, infl. del uréter.

ureterocele *n.* ureterocele, dilatación quística de la porción distal intravesical del uréter debida a una estenosis del orificio ureteral.

ureterocystostomy *n.* ureterocistostomía, trasplantación de un uréter a otra parte de la vejiga.

ureterography *n.* ureterografía, radiografía del uréter usando un medio radioopaco.

ureteroheminephrectomy *n.* ureteroheminefrectomía, resección de la porción de un riñón y el uréter en ciertos casos de duplicación del tracto urinario superior.

ureterohydronephrosis *n.* ureterohidronefrosis, distensión del uréter y del riñón debida a una obstrucción.

ureterolithiasis *n.* ureterolitiasis, desarrollo de un cálculo ureteral.

ureterolithotomy *n.* ureterolitotomía, incisión del uréter para extraer un cálculo.

ureteroneocystostomy *n.* ureteroneocistostomía. V. **ureterocystoneostomy**.

ureteronephrectomy

ureteronephrectomy *n.* ureteronefrectomía, excisión del riñón y su uréter.

ureteropelvic *a.* ureteropélvico-a, rel. al uréter y a la pelvis; __ junction obstruction / obstrucción de la unión __ .

ureteroplasty *n.* ureteroplastia, cirugía plástica del uréter.

ureteropyeloplasty *n.* ureteropieloplastia, cirugía plástica del uréter y la pelvis renal.

ureterosigmoidostomy *n.* ureterosigmoidostomía, implantación del uréter en el colon sigmoideo.

ureterostomy *n.* ureterostomía, formación de una fístula permanente para drenar un uréter.

ureterotomy *n.* ureterotomía, incisión de un uréter.

ureteroureterostomy *n.* ureteroureterostomía, anastomosis de dos uréteres o de dos extremos del mismo uréter.

urethra *n.* uretra, canal o conducto urinario.

urethral *a.* uretral, rel. a la uretra; __ catheter / catéter __; __ obstruction / obstrucción __; __ procedure / procedimiento __ ; __ stricture / estrechez __ ; __ suspension / suspensión __; __ syndrome / síndrome __ .

urethralgia *n.* uretralgia, dolor en la uretra.

urethrectomy *n.* uretrectomía, excisión parcial o total de la uretra.

urethritis *n.* uretritis, infl. aguda o crónica de la uretra.

urethrography *n.* uretrografía, rayos-x de la uretra usando una sustancia radioopaca inyectada.

urethroscope *n.* uretroscopio, instrumento para visualizar el interior de la uretra.

urethrotome *n.* uretrótomo, instrumento quirúrgico empleado en una uretrotomía.

urethrotomy *n.* uretrotomía, incisión efectuada para aliviar una estrechez uretral.

urgent *a.* urgente; __ care / cuidado de urgencia.

uric acid *n.* ácido úrico, producto del metabolismo de las proteínas presente en la sangre y excretado en la orina.

uricemia *n.* uricemia, exceso de ácido úrico en la sangre.

uricosuria *n.* uricosuria, presencia excesiva de ácido úrico en la orina.

urinal *n.* orinal, vasija en que se recoge la orina; *pop.* taza, pato.

urinalysis *n.* urinálisis, examen de orina.

urinary *a.* urinario-a, rel. o concerniente a la orina. __ calculi / cálculos __ -s; __ infection / infección renal o __; __ sediments / sedimentos __ -s.

urinary bladder *n.* vejiga urinaria, órgano muscular en forma de saco que recoge la orina que secretan los riñones.

urinary system *n.* sistema urinario, órganos y conductos que participan en la producción y excreción de la orina.

urinary tract *n.* vías urinarias. __ infections / infecciones de las __ .

urinate *n.* orinar, mear.

urination *n.* orina, acto de emisión de la orina; **frequent** __ / orinar con frecuencia, micción frecuente *Mex. A. pop.* meadera; **difficult** __ / orinar con dificultad, micción difícil; **painful** __ / orinar con dolor, micción dolorosa.

urine *n.* orina, orín, *pop.* aguas menores, líquido ambarino secretado por los riñones que se almacena en la vejiga y se elimina en la uretra. V. cuadro en la página 491.

uriniferous *a.* urinífero-a, que contiene o conduce orina.

urinogenital *a.* urinogenital. V. **urogenital**.

urinoma *n.* urinoma, tumor o quiste que contiene orina.

urobilinogen *n.* urobilinógeno, pigmento derivado de la reducción de bilirrubina por acción de bacterias intestinales.

urodynamics *n.* urodinámica, estudio del proceso activo patofisiológico de la micción.

urodynia *n.* urodinia, micción dolorosa.

urogenital *a.* urogenital, rel. a la vía urinaria o al tracto urinario y genital; __ diaphragm / diafragma __ .

urogram *n.* urograma, rayos-x hechos por urografía.

urography *n.* urografía, rayos-x de una parte de las vías urinarias con el uso de una sustancia radioopaca inyectada; **excretory or descending** __ / __ excretora o descendiente; **retrograde** __ / __ retrógrada.

Urine, anomalies	Orina, anomalías
acute retention (inability to urinate)	retención aguda (incapacidad de orinar)
abnormal color	color anormal
abnormal odor	olor anormal
blood in urine	sangre en la orina
midstream changes	cambios a mitad de chorro
frequent urination	micción frecuente
involuntary urine leak	escape o goteo involuntario de orina
little or no urination	escasa o ninguna cantidad de orina
painful urination	micción dolorosa
urge incontinence	micción imperiosa

urohematonephrosis *n.* urohematonefrosis, condición patológica del riñón en la cual la pelvis se distiende con sangre y orina.

urokinase *n.* urocinasa, enzima presente en la orina que se emplea en la disolución de coágulos.

urolithiasis *n.* urolitiasis, formación de cálculos urinarios y trastornos asociados con su presencia.

urologist *n.* urólogo-a, especialista en urología.

urology *n.* urología, estudio y tratamiento de las enfermedades del aparato genitourinario en el hombre y del tracto urinario en la mujer.

uropathy *n.* uropatía, enfermedades de las vías urinarias.

uropyourether *n.* uropiouréter, acumulación de orina y pus en la pelvis renal.

uroschesis *n.* urosquesis, supresión o retención de orina.

urticaria *n.* urticaria, erupción cutánea gen. alérgica que se manifiesta con ronchas rosáceas, se acompaña de picazón intensa y puede producirse por un factor interno o externo; ___ **pigment** / ___ pigmentosa.

usage *n.* uso, costumbre.

use *n.* uso, utilidad, provecho; *v.* usar, emplear; **off-label** ___ / ___ no aprobado.

useful *a.* útil, provechoso-a, práctico-a.

usual *a.* usual, de costumbre; **-ly** *adv.* usualmente, generalmente.

uterine *a.* uterino-a, rel. al útero o matriz; ___ **bleeding** / sangramiento ___, sangramiento no relacionado con la menstruación; ___ **cancer** / cáncer del útero o de la matriz; ___ **prolapse** / prolapso ___; ___ **rupture** / rotura ___ .

uterosalpingography *n.* uterosalpingografía, examen de rayos-x de la matriz y la trompa de Falopio usando una sustancia radioopaca inyectada.

uterovaginal *a.* uterovaginal, rel. al útero y a la vagina.

uterovesical *a.* uterovesical, rel. al útero y la vejiga urinaria.

uterus *n.* útero, matriz, órgano muscular femenino del aparato reproductivo que contiene y nutre al embrión y feto durante la gestación; **didelphys** ___ / ___ didelfo.

utriculus *n., L.* (*pl.* **utriculi**) utriculus, pequeña bolsa; ___ **of vestibular organ** / ___ del oído o del vestíbulo; ___ **prostaticus** / ___ prostático o uretral.

uvea *n.* úvea, túnica vascular del ojo formada por el iris, el cuerpo ciliar y la coroide.

uveitis *n.* uveítis, infl. de la úvea.

uvula *n.* úvula, *pop.* campanilla, estructura colgante en el centro posterior del paladar blando.

uvulitis *n.* uvulitis, infl. de la úvula.

uvulotomy *n.* uvulotomía, sección total o parcial de la úvula.

U wave *n.* onda U, onda positiva que sigue a la onda T en el electrocardiograma.

V *abbr.* **valve** / válvula; **vein** / vena; **vide (see)** / vea; **vision** / visión; **volume** / volumen.

vaccinate *v.* vacunar, inocular.

vaccination *n.* vacunación, inoculación de una vacuna.

vaccine *n.* vacuna, preparación de microorganismos atenuados o muertos que se introduce en el cuerpo para establecer una inmunidad en contra de la enfermedad específica causada por dichos microorganismos; **BCG** / ___ del bacilo Calmette-Guérin, contra la tuberculosis; **chickenpox** ___ / ___ contra la varicela; **DTP (diptheria, tetanus, pertussis)** ___ / ___ triple contra la difteria, tétano y pertusis (tos ferina); **hepatitis A** ___ / ___ contra la hepatitis A; **hepatitis B** ___ / ___ contra la hepatitis B; **influenza** ___ / ___ contra la influenza; **measles virus, inactivated** ___ / ___ antisarampión, inactivada; **measles virus, live attenuated** ___ / ___ antisarampión de virus vivo, atenuada; **pneumococcal polyvalent** ___ / ___ antineumocócica polivalente; **pneumovax** ___ / ___ neumocócica polisacárida; **poliovirus, live oral trivalent** ___ / ___ antipolio trivalente o de Sabin; **rabies** ___ / ___ antirrábica; **Salk's antipoliomyelitis** ___ / ___ antipoliomielítica de Salk; **smallpox** ___ / ___ antivariolosa, antivariólica; **tetanus** ___ / ___ contra el tétano; **typhus** ___ / ___ antitífica; **typhoid** ___ / ___ contra la tifoidea; ___ **reaction** / reacción a la ___ .

vaccinia *n.* vaccina, virus causante de la viruela bovina del cual se obtiene la vacuna contra la viruela.

vacillating *a.* vacilante, oscilante, fluctuante.

vacuole *n.* vacuola, pequeña cavidad o espacio en el protoplasma celular que contiene líquido o aire.

vacuum *n., L.* vacuum, vacío, espacio desprovisto de materia o aire; *v.* extraer el polvo con una aspiradora; ___ **packed** / envasado-a al vacío.

vagal *a.* vagal, rel. al nervio vago o neumogástrico.

vagina *n.* vagina. 1. conducto en la mujer que se extiende del útero a la vulva; 2. estructura semejante a una vaina.

vaginal *a.* vaginal. 1. que posee forma de vaina; 2. rel. a la vagina; ___ **bleeding** / sangrado ___ , hemorragia ___; ___ **candidiasis** / candidiasis ___; ___ **culture** / cultivo ___; ___**cysts** / quistes vaginales; ___ **discharge** / flujo ___; ___ **drying treatment** / tratamiento de secamiento ___; ___ **itching** / picazón ___; ___ **wall repair** / reparación de la pared de la ___; ___ **smear** / frotis ___; ___ **suppository** / óvulo ___ ; ___ **tumor** / tumor ___ .

vaginismus *L.* vaginismus, contracción dolorosa espasmódica de la vagina.

vaginitis *n.* vaginitis, infl. de la vagina; **bacterial** ___ / ___ bacteriana.

vaginoplasty *n.* vaginoplastia, cirugía plástica de la vagina.

vaginosis *n.* enfermedad de la vagina; **bacterial** ___ / ___ bacteriana.

vagolysis *n.* destrucción quirúrgica del nervio vago.

vagotomy *n.* vagotomía, interrupción del nervio vago.

vagus *n.* vago, nervio neumogástrico.

valgus *n., L.* valgus, doblado o torcido hacia afuera.

validity *n.* validez.

vallecula *n.* valécula, depresión, surco o fisura esp. en referencia a estructuras anatómicas.

valley fever *n.* fiebre del valle. *Syn.* **coccidioidomycosis.**

Valsalva's maneuver *n.* maniobra, experimento de Valsalva, procedimiento para demostrar la permeabilidad de la trompa de Eustaquio o de ajustar la presión del oído medio mediante una espiración forzada con la boca y la nariz tapadas.

valve *n.* (*pl.* **valvae**) válvula, valva, estructura membranosa en un canal u orificio que al cerrarse temporalmente impide el reflujo del contenido que pasa a través de ella; **aortic** ___ / ___ aórtica; **aortic-semilunar** ___ / ___ aórtica semilunar; **atrioventricular left** ___ / ___ auriculoventricular izquierda; **atrioventricular right** ___ , **tricuspid** / ___ auriculoventricular derecha, tricúspide; **bicuspid or mitral** ___ / ___ bicúspide o mitral; **ileocecal** ___ / ___ ileocecal; **pulmonary** ___ / ___ pulmonar; **pyloric** ___ / ___ pilórica.

valvotomy *n.* valvotomía, 1. incision de una válvula; 2. cirugía de una válvula cardíaca para tratar la obstrucción.

valvulae conniventes *n., pl.* válvulas conniventes, pliegues circulares membranosos localizados en el intestino delgado que retardan el paso del contenido alimenticio en el intestino.

valvular *a.* valvular, rel. a una válvula o de su naturaleza; **___ pulmonary stenosis** / estenosis pulmonar **___** .

valvulitis *n.* valvulitis, infl. de una válvula, esp. una válvula cardíaca.

valvuloplasty *n.* valvuloplastia, operación plástica de una válvula.

valvulotome *n.* valvulótomo, instrumento quirúrgico que se usa para seccionar una válvula.

vapor *n.* vapor, gas.

vaporization *n.* vaporización. 1. acción o efecto de vaporizar; 2. uso terapéutico de vapores.

vaporizer *n.* vaporizador, dispositivo para convertir una sustancia en vapor y aplicarla a usos terapéuticos.

variable *n.* variable, factor que puede variar; *a.* que puede cambiar.

variant *n.* variante, objeto esencialmente igual a otro pero que difiere en la forma; *a.* variable, inconstante, que cambia o varía.

varicella *n.* varicela. V. **chickenpox**.

varicocele *n.* varicocele, condición varicosa de las venas del cordón espermático que produce una masa blanda en el escroto.

varicocelectomy *n.* varicocelectomía, operación para corregir un varicocele.

varicose *a.* varicoso-a, rel. a las várices o que se les asemeja; **___ veins** / venas **___** -s.

varicotomy *n.* varicotomía, excisión de una vena varicosa.

variolic, variolous *a.* variólico-a, rel. a la viruela.

varix *n.* (*pl.* **varices**) várice, vena, arteria o vaso linfático aumentado o dilatado.

vascular *a.* vascular, rel. a vasos sanguíneos; **___ ectasia of the colon** / ectasia **___** del colon; **___ purpura** / púrpura **___**; **___ skin changes** / cambios cutáneos vasculares; **___ spasm** / espasmo **___**; **___ system** / sistema **___**, todos los vasos del cuerpo esp. los sanguíneos; **___ tunic** / túnica **___** .

vascular dementia *n.* demencia o deterioro vascular de facultades intelectuales causada por infartos al hemisferio cerebral.

vascularization *n.* vascularización, formación de vasos sanguíneos nuevos.

vasculopathy *n.* vasculopatía, cualquier enfermedad de los vasos sanguíneos.

vas deferens *n., L.* vas deferens, conducto excretor de espermatozoides.

vasectomy *n.* vasectomía, excisión parcial y ligadura de los conductos deferentes para impedir la salida de espermatozoides en el semen, procedimiento gen. usado como contraceptivo.

vasoactive *a.* vasoactivo, que afecta los vasos sanguíneos.

vasoconstrictive *a.* vasoconstrictivo-a, que causa constricción en los vasos sanguíneos.

vasodepression *n.* vasodepressión, aumento en el diámetro de un vaso sanguíneo.

vasodilation *n.* vasodilatación, aumento del calibre de los vasos sanguíneos.

vasodilator *n.* vasodilatador, agente que causa vasodilatación; *a.* vasodilatador-a; que causa vasodilatación.

vasomotor *n.* vasomotora, agente que regula las contracciones y la dilatación de los vasos sanguíneos; *a.* vasomotor-a, que causa dilatación o contracción en los vasos sanguíneos; **___ angina** / angina **___**; **___ rhinitis** / rinitis **___** .

vasopressin *n.* vasopresina, hormona liberada por la pituitaria posterior que aumenta la reabsorción de agua en el riñón elevando la presión arterial.

vasopressor *n.* vasopresor, agente que produce constricción en los vasos sanguíneos; *a.* que tiene efecto vasoconstrictivo.

vasospasm *n.* vasoespasmo; **coronary ___** / **___** coronario e. V. **angiospasm**.

vasotonic *a.* vasotónico, rel. al tono de un vaso.

vasovagal syncope *n.* síncope vasovagal, desmayo súbito breve debido a un trastorno vasomotor y vagal.

Vater's ampulla *n.* ámpula de Vater, punto de entrada en el duodeno de los conductos excretores biliar y pancreático.

vector *n.* vector, portador, organismo microbiano transmisor de agentes infecciosos.

vegan *n.* vegetariano-a, que omite en la dieta toda clase de alimentos de contenido animal.

vegetable *n.* vegetal.

vegetarian *n.* vegetariano-a, persona cuya dieta consiste principalmente en vegetales; *a.* rel. a los vegetales.

vegetarianism *n.* vegetarianismo, método de alimentación que consiste mayormente en una dieta de vegetales y frutas.

vegetation *n.* vegetación, crecimiento anormal de verrugas o excrecencias en una parte del cuerpo tal como se ve en la endocarditis.

vegetative *a.* vegetativo-a. 1. rel. a funciones de crecimiento y nutrición; 2. rel. a funciones corporales involuntarias o inconscientes.

vehicle *n.* vehículo. 1. sustancia sin acción terapéutica que acompaña a un agente activo en una preparación medicinal; 2. agente de transmisión.

veil *n.* velo. 1. membrana o cubierta fina que cubre una parte del cuerpo; 2. parte de la membrana amniótica que cubre la cara del feto; 3. alteración ligera de la voz.

vein *n.* vena, vaso fibromuscular que lleva la sangre de los capilares al corazón; **spider __-s / __** varicosas.

vena cava *n.* vena cava, una de las dos venas mayores, la vena cava inferior y la vena cava superior, que devuelven la sangre desoxigenada a la aurícula derecha del corazón.

venipuncture *n.* venipuntura, punción de una vena.

venereal *a.* venéreo-a, que resulta a consecuencia del acto sexual; **__ disease** / enfermedad __; **__wart** / verruga __ .

venin-antivenin *n.* veninantivenina, suero antídoto contra el veneno de serpientes.

venin, venine *n.* venina, sustancia tóxica del veneno de serpientes.

venoconstriction *n.* venoconstricción, reducción de las paredes venosas.

venogram *n.* venograma, radiografía de las venas usando un medio de contraste; **renal __ / __** renal.

venography *n.* venografía, gráfica e información de un venograma.

venom *n.* veneno, sustancia tóxica.

veno-occlusive *a.* venoclusivo-a, rel. a una obstrucción venosa.

venous *a.* venoso-a, rel. a las venas; **__ blood** / sangre __; **__ congestion /** congestión __; **__ insufficiency /** insuficiencia __; **__ return** / retorno __; **__ sinus** / seno __; **__ thrombo-embolism /** tromboembolismo __; **__ thrombosis** / trombosis __ .

ventilation *n.* ventilación. 1. circulación de aire fresco en una habitación; 2. oxigenación de la sangre; **pulmonary __ / __** pulmonar; 3. expresión franca de conflictos emocionales internos.

ventilator *n.* ventilador; respirador artificial.

ventral *a.* ventral, abdominal, rel. al vientre o a la parte anterior del cuerpo humano.

ventricle *n.* ventrículo, cavidad pequeña esp. una estructura del corazón, el cerebro o la laringe; **fourth __ of the brain** / cuarto __ cerebral; **larynx __ / __** de la laringe; **lateral __ of the brain** / __ lateral del cerebro; **left __ of the heart** / __ izquierdo del corazón; **right __ of the heart** / __ derecho del corazón; **third __ of the brain** / tercer __ del cerebro.

ventricular *a.* ventricular, rel. a un ventrículo; **__ fibrillation** / fibrilación __; **__ puncture** / punción __; **__ septal defect** / defecto septal __; **__ tachycardia** / taquicardia __ .

ventricular septal defect *n.* defecto del tabique ventricular.

ventriculitis *n.* ventriculitis, infl. de un ventrículo.

ventriculotomy *n.* ventriculotomía, incisión de un ventrículo.

venule *n.* vénula, vena diminuta que conecta los vasos capilares con venas mayores.

vermicide *n.* vermicida, vermífugo, agente destructor de vermes (gusanos).

vermiform appendix *n.* apéndice vermiforme.

vermilion border *n.* borde bermellón, el margen rosado expuesto del labio.

vermis *n.*, *L.* vermis. 1. gusano parásito; 2. estructura semejante a un gusano tal como el lóbulo medio del cerebelo.

vernal conjunctivitis *n.* conjuntivitis vernal o primaveral, conjuntivitis bilateral acompañada por intensa picazón y fotofobia o evasión de la luz.

vernix *n.*, *L.* barniz; ___ **caseosa** / unto sebáceo, secreción que protege la piel del feto.

verruca *n.* (*pl.* **verrucae**) verruga; **plantaris (plantar wart)** ___ / ___ plantaris; **seborrheic** ___ / ___ seborreica; ___ **filiformis** / ___ filiforme; ___ **planae juveniles** / ___ planas juveniles; ___ **simples** / ___ simple; **vulgaris** ___ / ___ vulgaris.

verrucous *a.* verrugoso-a.

version *n.* versión. 1. cambio de dirección de un órgano tal como el útero; 2. cambio de posición del feto en el útero que facilita el parto; **bimanual** ___ / ___ bimanual; **bipolar** ___ / ___ bipolar; **cephalic** ___ / ___ cefálica; **combined** ___ / ___ combinada; **external** ___ / ___ externa; **spontaneous** ___ / ___ espontánea.

vertebra *n.* (*pl.* **vertebrae**) vértebra, cada uno de los treinta y tres huesos que forman la columna vertebral; **cervical** ___ / ___ cervical; **coccygeal** ___ / ___ coccígea; **lumbar** ___ / ___ lumbar; **sacral** ___ / ___ sacra; **thoracic** ___ / ___ torácica.

vertebral *a.* vertebral, rel. a las vértebras; ___ **artery** / arteria ___; ___ **canal** / conducto ___; ___ **ribs** / costillas ___ -es.

vertebral-basilar *n.* vertebrobasilar unión de dos arterias localizadas en la base del cráneo que forman la arteria basilar.

vertebrate *n.* vertebrado, que posee columna vertebral o una estructura semejante.

vertebrobasilar *a.* vertebrobasilar, rel. a las arterias vertebral y basilar; ___ **circulatory disorders** / trastornos ___ -es de la circulación; ___ **insufficiency** / insuficiencia ___ ; ___ **system** / sistema ___ .

vertex *n.* (*pl.* **vertices**) vértice. 1. cúspide de una estructura, tal como el punto extremo de la cabeza; 2. punto en que concurren los lados de un ángulo.

vertical *a.* 1. vertical, de posición erecta; 2. rel. al vértice; **-ly** *adv.* verticalmente.

vertigo *n.* vértigo, sensación de rotación en la que se cree que uno gira alrededor del mundo exterior o que éste gira alrededor de uno; **labyrinthine** ___ / ___ laberíntico.

verumontanitis *f.* verumontanitis, infl. del verumontanum.

verumontanum *n.*, *L.* verumontanum, elevación en la uretra en el punto de entrada de los conductos seminales.

vesical *a.* vesical, rel. a una vejiga o semejante a ella.

vesication *n.* vesicación 1. formación de ampollas; 2. una ampolla.

vesicle *n.* vesícula. 1. pequeña ampolla; 2. bolsa pequeña de la capa exterior de la piel que contiene líquido seroso.

vesicovaginal *a.* vesicovaginal, rel. a la vejiga urinaria y la vagina.

vesicular *a.* vesicular, rel. a las vesículas.

vesiculation *n.* vesiculación, presencia de un número de vesiculas.

vesiculitis *n.* vesiculitis, infl. de una vesicula.

vessel *n.* vaso, conducto o canal portador de un fluido tal como la sangre y la linfa; **blood** ___ / ___ sanguíneo; **collateral** ___ / ___ colateral; **great -s** / grandes ___ -s; **lymphatic** ___ / ___ linfático.

vestibular *a.* vestibular, rel. a un vestíbulo; ___ **bulb** / bulbo ___; ___ **nerve** / nervio ___ .

vestibule *n.* vestíbulo, cavidad que da acceso a un conducto.

veterinarian *n.* veterinario-a, persona especializada en veterinaria; *a.* veterinario-a, rel. a la veterinaria.

veterinary medicine *n.* veterinaria, ciencia que trata de la prevención y cura de enfermedades y lesiones de animales, esp. domésticos.

via *n.*, *L.* vía, tracto, conducto.

viable *a.* viable, capaz de sobrevivir, término que se usa gen. en referencia al feto o al recién nacido.

vibrative, vibratory *a.* vibratorio-a, que produce vibración u oscila; ___ **sense** / sentido ___ .

vicious *a.* [ridden by vice] vicioso-a, depravado-a; **-ly** *adv.* viciosamente, malvadamente.

victim *n.* victima.

video *n.* video; ___ **tape** / videocinta.

vigil

vigil *n.* vigilia. 1. estado de respuesta consciente a un estímulo; 2. insomnio.

vigilance *n.* vigilancia, estado alerta o de atención.

vigor *n.* vigor, fortaleza.

vigorous *a.* vigoroso-a; fuerte; **-ly** *adv.* vigorosamente.

villus *n.* (*pl.* **villi**) vellosidad, vello, proyección filiforme que crece en una superficie membranosa; **aracnoid** ___ / ___ aracnoidea; **chorionic** ___ / ___ -es coriónicas; **intestinal** ___ / ___ intestinal.

violet *n.* color violeta; *a.* violeta.

viper *n.* víbora.

viral *a.* viral, rel. a un virus; ___ **arthritis** / artritis ___; ___ **croup** / crup ___; ___ **gastroenteritis** / gastroenteritis ___; ___ **hemorrhagic fever** / fiebre hemorrágica ___; ___ **hepatitis** / hepatitis ___; ___ **pneumonia** / neumonía ___; ___ **replication** / replicación ___; ___ **upper respiratory infection** / infección ___ del sistema respiratorio superior.

viremia *n.* viremia, presencia de un virus en la sangre.

virgin *n.* virgen. 1. sustancia sin contaminación; 2. persona que no ha realizado el acto sexual.

virile *a.* viril, varonil.

virility *n.* virilidad. 1. potencia sexual; 2. estado de poseer características masculinas.

virilization *n.* virilización, masculinización, proceso por el cual se desarrollan en la mujer características masculinas gen. debido a un trastorno hormonal o al suplemento artificial de hormonas masculinas.

virion *n.* virión, partícula viral madura que constituye la forma extracelular infecciosa de un virus.

virology *n.* virología, ciencia que estudia los virus.

virtual *a.* virtual, de existencia aparente, no real.

virulence *n.* virulencia. 1. poder de un organismo de causar determinadas enfermedades en el huésped; 2. cualidad o estado de ser virulento.

virulent *a.* virulento-a, nocivo-a, extremadamente tóxico.

virus *n.* virus, microorganismo ultramicroscópico capaz de causar enfermedades infecciosas; **attenuated** ___ / ___ atenuado; **Cocsackie** ___ / ___ de Cocsackie; **cytomegalic** ___ / ___ citomegálico; **ECHO** ___ / ___ ECHO; **enteric** ___ / ___ entérico; **herpes** ___ / ___ herpético; **pox** ___ / ___ variólico o de Pox; **respiratory syncytial** ___ / ___ sincitial respiratorio; **tumor** ___ / ___ oncogénico.

viscera *n., pl.* vísceras, órganos internos del cuerpo, esp. del abdomen.

visceroptosis *a.* descenso visceral de una posición normal.

viscosity *n.* viscosidad, cualidad de ser viscoso, esp. la propiedad de los líquidos de no fluir libremente debido a la fricción de las moléculas.

viscous *a.* viscoso-a, gelatinoso-a, pegajoso-a.

visible *a.* visible, aparente, evidente; **-ly** *adv.* visiblemente, evidentemente; aparentemente.

vision *n.* visión. 1. sentido de la vista; 2. capacidad de percibir los objetos por la acción de la luz a través de los órganos visuales y los centros cerebrales con que se relacionan. V. cuadro en la página 497.

visiting hours *n.* horas de visita.

visual *a.* visual, rel. a la visión; ___ **acuity** / acuidad ___; ___ **field** / campo ___; ___ **memory** / memoria ___ .

visualization, imagery *n.* visualización, proceso de crear imágenes como ayuda al tratamiento de curación.

visualize *v.* visualizar. 1. crear una imagen visual de algo; 2. hacer visible, tal como copiar la imagen de un órgano en una radiografía.

vital *a.* vital, rel. a la vida o esencial en el mantenimiento de la misma; ___ **capacity** / capacidad ___; ___ **signs** / signos ___ -es; ___ **statistics** / estadística demográfica.

vitality *n.* vitalidad. 1. cualidad de vivir; 2. vigor mental o físico.

vitalize *v.* vitalizar, dar vida; reanimar.

vitamin *n.* vitamina, uno de los compuestos orgánicos que se encuentran en pequeñas cantidades en los alimentos y que son esenciales en el desarrollo y funcionamiento del organismo.

vitiligo *n.* vitiligo, trastorno epidérmico benigno que se manifiesta con manchas blancas en partes expuestas del cuerpo.

vitrectomy *n.* vitrectomía, extirpación de todo o parte del humor vítreo del ojo. Se recomienda a veces en casos

496

Vision	Visión
achromatic	acromática
binocular	binocular
blurred	nublada
central	central
chromatic	cromática
distance	a distancia
double // diplopia	doble // diplopia
in tunnel	en túnel
monocular	monocular
night	nocturna
photopic	fotopsia
stocopic	estocópica

avanzados de retinopatía proliferativa diabética.

vitreous *n.* fluído semejante a gelatina que llena el interior del ojo; vítreo-a, vidrioso-a, casi transparente, hialino; __ **chamber** / cámara __; __ **body** / cuerpo __; __ **humor** / humor __ .

vivisection *n.* vivisección, corte o sección realizada en animales con fines investigativos.

vocal *a.* vocal, oral, rel. a la voz o producido por ella.

vocal cords *n., pl.* cuerdas vocales; órgano esencial de la voz; **false** __ / __ superiores o falsas; **true** __ / __ inferiores o verdaderas.

vocalization *n.* vocalización.

voice *n.* voz.

volatile *a.* volátil, que se evapora fácilmente.

volition *n.* volición, voluntad, poder de determinación.

Volkman's contracture *n.* Volkmann, contractura de, contractura isquémica como resultado de una necrosis irreversible del tejido muscular, vista gen. en el antebrazo y la mano.

volume *n.* volumen. 1. espacio ocupado por una sustancia o un cuerpo; 2. cantidad, intensidad; **blood** __ / __ sanguíneo; **expiratory air reserve** __ / __ de reserva expiratoria o aire de reserva; **heart** __ / __ cardíaco; **residual** __ / __ residual; **stroke** __ / __ sistólico; **tidal** __ / __ de ventilación pulmonar.

voluntary *a.* voluntario-a; __ **muscle** / músculo __ .

volvulus *a.* vólvulo, obstrucción intestinal causada por torsión o anudamiento del intestino en torno al mesenterio.

vomer *n.* vómer, hueso impar que forma parte del tabique medio de las fosas nasales.

vomiting *n.* manifestación de vómitos.

Von Gierke disease *n.* Von Gierke, enfermedad de, almacenamiento anormal de glucógeno.

Von Willebrand's disease *n.* Von Willebrand, enfermedad de, desorden hereditario de la sangre caracterizado por episodios hemorrágicos gen. en las membranas mucosas.

voracious *a.* voraz, que es insaciable al comer.

vortex *n.* (*pl.* **vortices**) vórtice, estructura de forma espiral.

voyeurism *n.* voyeurismo, perversión sexual por la cual la contemplación de actos u órganos sexuales induce erotismo.

vulnerable *a.* vulnerable, propenso a accidentes o enfermedades.

vulva *n.*, *L.* vulva, conjunto de los órganos femeninos externos del aparato genital.

vulvectomy *n.* vulvectomía, excisión de la vulva.

vulvitis *n.* vulvitis, infl. de la vulva.

vulvovaginal *a.* vulvovaginal, rel. a la vulva y la vagina.

vulvovaginitis *n.* vulvovaginitis, infl. de la vulva y la vagina.

W

W *abbr.* water / agua; **weight** / peso.

waddle *n.* marcha tambaleante, andar anserino.

wail *v.* lamentarse; gemir.

waist *n.* cintura; talle.

waistline *n.* talle de la cintura.

waiting *n.* espera; demora; ___ **room** / sala de ___ .

wakefulness *n.* dificultad para dormir, insomnio.

Waldenstrom's macroglobulinemia *n.* Waldenstrom, macroglobulinemia de, síndrome hemorrágico con manifestaciones de anemia y adenomegalia.

walk *n.* paseo; caminata; *v.* caminar, andar; **to ___ up and down** / caminar de un lado a otro.

walker *n.* andador, andaderas, aparato que se usa para ayudar a caminar.

walking *n.* el acto de caminar; ___ **pneumonia** / neumonía errante; ___ **cast** / molde para andar.

wall *n.* pared; **cell ___** / tabique cellular; **chest ___** / tabique del tórax; ___ **tooth** / diente molar.

walled-off *a.* encapsulado-a.

walleye *n.* 1. estrabismo divergente, exotropía; 2. leucoma corneal.

wandering *a.* errante, errático-a; desviado-a; ___ **cell** / célula; ___ **goiter** / bocio móvil; ___ **pain** / dolor ___; ___ **tooth** / diente desviado.

ward *n.* sala de hospital; **isolation___** / sala de aislamiento; ___ **diet** / dieta hospitalaria; ___ **of the state** / bajo custodia, bajo tutela del estado.

warfarin *n.* warfarina, nombre genérico de Coumadin, anticoagulante usado en la prevención de infartos y trombosis.

warm *a.* caluroso-a; caliente; [*lukewarm*] tibio-a; [*character*] afectuoso-a, expresivo-a; *v.* **to be ___** / tener calor, [*not very hot but feverish*] tener destemplanza; [*weather*] hacer calor; **to ___ to** / simpatizar con; **to ___ up** / calentar; **-ly** *adv.* afectuosamente, con entusiasmo.

warm-up *n.* [*physical fitness*] calentamiento.

warning *n.* advertencia; aviso; [*hard lesson*] escarmiento; ___ **signal** / advertencia; señal premonitoria; ___ **symptoms** / síntomas premonitorios.

wart *n.* verruga. V. **verruca**.

warty *a.* verrugoso-a, rel. a verrugas.

wash *n.* lavado, baño, lavadura; **mouth-___** / enjuague; *v.* lavar; **to ___ away** / quitar con una lavadura; [*oneself*] lavarse.

wasp *n.* avispa; ___ **sting** / picadura de ___ .

Wasserman test *n.* prueba de Wasserman, análisis serológico de la sífilis.

waste *n.* desperdicio, residuo, gasto inútil; merma, pérdida; ___ **of time** / pérdida de tiempo *v.* desperdiciar, desgastar, malgastar; **to ___ away** / demacrarse, consumirse.

wastebasket *n.* cesto de basura.

wasted *a.* desgastado-a, malgastado-a; [*person*] demacrado-a; consumido-a.

wasting *n.* agotamiento, consunción, pérdida de funciones vitales.

water *n.* agua, líquidos del cuerpo; infusión; ___**bag** / bolsa de ___; ___ **bed** / cama de, colchón de ___; ___ **blister** / ampolla acuosa; ___**-cooled** / enfriado-a por ___; ___ **faucet** / grifo, pila, llave; ___ **intake** / ingestión o toma de ___; ___ **level** / nivel del ___; ___ **pill** / diurético; ___ **pollution** / contaminación del ___; ___ **purification** / purificación del ___; ___ **-tight** / hermético, impermeable; ___ **-soluble** / soluble en ___, que se disuelve en ___; ___ **supply** / abastecimiento de ___; *v.* **to be in deep ___** / tener dificultades; **to give ___** / ___; **to wash with ___** / lavar con ___ .

water balance *n.* balance hídrico, medida del equilibrio entre los líquidos tomados y la cantidad excretada.

water-electrolyte balance *n.* equilibrio hidroelectrolítico.

Waterhouse-Friderichsen syndrome *n.* Waterhouse-Friderichsen, síndrome de hemorragia aguda en las glándulas suprarrenales asociada con repentino choque bacteriogénico agudo.

water intoxication *n.* intoxicación acuosa, retención excesiva de agua.

watery *a.* acuoso-a, aguado-a, húmedo-a; ___ **eyes** / ojos llorosos.

wave *n.* onda, ondulación; ademán de la mano. 1. movimiento o vibración ondulante que tiene una dirección fija y prosigue en una curva de ondulación; 2. representación gráfica de una actividad tal como la obtenida en un encefalograma; **brain __ -s / __ -s** cerebrales; **electromagnetic __ -s / __ -s** electromagnéticas; **excitation __ / __** de excitación; **high-frequency __ / __** de alta frecuencia; **short __ / __** corta; **ultrasonic __ -s / __ -s** ultrasónicas; ___ **length** / longitud de __; v. hacer señales o ademanes con la mano.

wax n. cera. 1. cera producida por abejas; 2. secreción cerosa; **ear__ / __** del oído; 3. cerumen, sustancia de origen animal, vegetal o mineral que se emplea en preparaciones de pomadas y ceratos; **depilatory__ / __** depilatoria.

way n. vía, camino; pasaje; **by the __ / a** propósito; **in no __ / de** ningún modo; **out of the __ / fuera** de curso, desviado-a; lejano-a; **that __ / por** allí; **the other __ around / por** el contrario; ___ **of life / manera** de vivir; costumbres; ___ **out** / salida; v. **to make __ for** / abrir paso.

weak a. débil, flojo-a, endeble, enclenque; poco fuerte.

weakness n. debilidad, debilitamiento, flojera, flaqueza.

weaning n. destete, terminación de la lactancia.

weanling n. el, la recién destetado-a, desmamado-a.

wear n. uso, gasto, deterioro, deteriorización; vr. usar, llevar puesto; desgastar; **to __ out** / gastar; gastarse; desgastarse.

weary a. cansado-a, fatigado-a.

weather n. [climate] tiempo; ___ **forecasting** / pronóstico del __ .

web n. red, membrana; **pulmonary arterial __ / __ -es de** membranas arteriopulmonares.

webbed n. unido-a por una telilla o membrana.

wedge n. cuña.

weight n. peso; **birth __ / __ al** nacer; ___ **gain** / aumento de __; ___ **loss** / pérdida de __ .

welfare n. bien, bienestar; salud; asistencia; ___**benefits** / beneficios de asistencia social; ___**work** / trabajo de asistencia social; ___**worker** / trabajador-a social.

well a. bueno-a; en buena salud; **well-being** / bienestar adv. bien,

favorablemente, felizmente; **all is __ / todo** va bien.

welt n. verdugón, roncha.

wens n. quiste.

Wertheim operation n. extirpación del útero, los ovaries, las trompas y los tejidos adyacentes.

Western Blot, immunoblot n. Western Blot, "inmunoblot", prueba subsecuente para confirmar la infección por el virus VIH, en pacientes con evidencia de exposición, indicada por un ensayo enzimático inmuno-sorbente (ELISA).

West Nile Virus n. Virus del Nilo Occidental, transmitido a humanos y animales por mosquitos que se infectaron al picar pájaros infectados. Personas con un sistema inmune normal manifiestan si son infectadas, síntomas similares a los del flu benigno. Otras víctimas de un sistema inmune deficiente corren el riesgo de contraer encefalitis y sufrir otros daños severos.

wet a. mojado-a, humedecido-a; v. mojar, humedecer.

wet brain n. hidrocefalia.

wet dream n. emisión seminal nocturna.

Wharton's duct n. conducto de Wharton, conducto excretorio de la glándula submaxilar.

wheal n. roncha.

wheelchair n. silla de ruedas.

wheezing n. respiración sibilante.

whenever adv. cuando quiera; siempre que; ___ **is needed** / siempre que se necesite; ___ **you wish** / siempre que lo desee.

while adv. mientras, un rato, algún tiempo; **for a __ / temporalmente**; **not for a __ / por** ahora no.

whimper n. quejido, lloriqueo; v. sollozar, lloriquear.

whiplash injury n. lesión de latigazo.

Whipple's disease n. enfermedad de Whipple, trastorno causado por la acumulación de depósitos lípidos en los tejidos linfáticos e intestinales.

whisper n. susurro, cuchicheo; v. susurrar, cuchichear.

white matter n. sustancia blanca, tejido nervioso formado en su mayor parte por fibras mielínicas y que constituye el elemento conductor del cerebro y de la médula espinal.

whoop *n.* estridor, sonido que caracteriza la respiración después de un ataque de tos ferina.

whooping cough *n.* tos ferina. V. **pertussis**.

wide *a.* ancho-a; **three feet __** / tres pies de ancho; amplio-a; extenso-a; **__ open** / muy abierto; **-ly** *adv.* ampliamente, extensamente.

widespread *a.* extendido-a; muy difundido-a; general.

widow *n.* viuda.

widower *n.* viudo.

width *n.* anchura, ancho.

wife *n.* esposa.

wig *n.* peluca.

will *n.* voluntad, determinación, deseo; testamento; *v.* querer, ordenar, mandar.

Wilms' tumor *n.* tumor de Wilms, neoplasma del riñón que se desarrolla rápidamente y usu. se manifiesta en la infancia.

Wilson's disease *n.* enfermedad de Wilson, trastorno raro genético, enfermedad del cobre, originando acumulación del metal en el hígado el cual lo libera a otros órganos, tal como el cerebro, produciendo eventualmente demencia y cirrosis.

wind *n.* viento, aire; flato, ventosidad.

windburn *n.* quemadura por el viento.

windpipe *n.* tráquea; *pop.* gaznate.

wink *n.* pestañeo; *v.* pestañear.

wisdom teeth *n.* cordales, muelas del juicio.

wise *n.* cuerdo, prudente.

withdrawal *n.* supresión, retracción; introversión; privación.

withdrawal syndrome *n.* síndrome de privación de una droga adictiva como resultado de la supresión de la misma.

withdrawal treatment *n.* tratamiento de desintoxicación.

within *prep.* dentro de, en el interior de; a distancia de; al alcance de; cerca de; **__ an hour** / **__** una hora.

without *prep.* sin, falto de, fuera de; *adv.* fuera, afuera.

withstand *vi.* resistir, soportar, sufrir.

woman *n.* (*pl.* **women**) mujer.

womb *n.* matriz, útero. V. **uterus**.

wool sorter's disease *n.* enfermedad de los cargadores de lana. anthrax.

work *n.* trabajo, empleo, ocupación; *v.* trabajar.

workshop *n.* laboratorio o taller de trabajo.

workup *n.* 1. preparación del paciente para la aplicación de un tratamiento; 2. obtención de los datos pertinentes a un caso.

worm *n.* lombriz, gusano.

wormlike *a.* vermicular, vermiforme.

worsen *v.* agravarse.

wound *n.* herida, lesión; **contused __** / **__** contusa, lesión subcutánea; **gunshot __** / **__** de bala; **penetrating __** / **__** penetrante; **puncture __** / **__** de punción, con un instrumento afilado; **__ debridement** / desbridamiento de **__** .

wrinkle *n.* arruga; *v.* arrugarse.

wrist *n.* carpo, muñeca. **carpus**; **__ drop** / muñeca caída.

wrong *n.* error, falsedad; *a.* erróneo-a; incorrecto-a; **__ treatment** / el tratamiento equivocado**__**; **the __ side** / el lado afectado, el lado incorrecto; *v.* **to be __** / no tener razón; estar equivocado-a; **to go __** / [*to fail to understand*] interpretar mal; equivocarse; **-ly** *adv.* mal; incorrectamente, equivocadamente.

X *abbr.* **xanthine** / xantina

xanthelasma *n.* xantelasma, manchas o placas amarillentas que aparecen gen. alrededor de los párpados.

xanthic *a.* amarillento-a, rel. a la xantina.

xanthine *n.* xantina, grupo de substancias tales como la cafeína estimulantes del sistema nervioso central y del corazón.

xanthochromia *n.* xantocromía, color amarillento visto en placas de la piel o en el líquido cefalorraquídeo.

xanthoderma *n.* xantoderma, color amarillento de la piel.

xanthoma *n.* xantoma, formación tumoral de placas o nódulos en la piel; **diabetic** ___ / ___ diabético; **disseminated** ___ / ___ diseminado; **eruptive** ___ / ___ eruptivo; **planar** ___ / ___ plano; ___ **tendinosum** / ___ tendinoso; ___ **tuberosum** / ___ tuberoso.

xanthosis *n.* xantosis, descoloración amarillenta de la piel debida a ingestión excesiva de alimentos tales como la zanahoria y la calabaza.

x chromosome *n.* cromosoma x, cromosoma sexual diferencial que determina las características del sexo femenino.

xenograft *n.* xenoinjerto; ___ **rejection** / rechazo de ___ .

xenon *n.* xenón, elemento gaseoso, radioisótopo que se encuentra en pequeñas cantidades en el aire atmosférico.

xenon-133 *n.* xenón 133, radioisótopo de xenón usado en la fotoescanción del pulmón.

xenophobia *n.* xenofobia, temor excesivo o aversión a algo o a alguien extraño o extranjero.

xenotransplant *n.* xenotransplante, proceso de trasplantar un órgano o parte de una especie a otra.

xeroderma *n.* xeroderma, piel excesivamente seca.

xeromammography *n.* xeromamografía, xerorradiografía de la mama.

xerophthalmia *n.* xeroftalmia, sequedad excesiva de la conjuntiva causada por deficiencia de vitamina A.

xeroradiography *n.* xerorradiografía, registro de imágenes electrostáticas por medio de un proceso en seco usando placas cubiertas con un elemento metálico tal como el selenio.

xerosis *n.* xerosis, sequedad anormal presente en la piel, ojos y membranas mucosas.

xerostomia *n.* xerostomía, excesiva sequedad en la boca debida a una deficiencia de secreción salival.

xiphoid *a.* xifoide, en forma de espada, similar al apéndice xifoide o ensiforme.

xiphoid process *n.* apéndice xifoide, formación cartilaginosa que se une al cuerpo del esternón.

X-linked *a.* rel. a caracteres genéticos que se relacionan con el cromosoma x.

x-rays *n.* rayos-x (equis), radiografía. 1. ondas electromagnéticas de alta energía de radiación que se usan para penetrar tejidos y órganos del cuerpo y registrar densidades en una placa o pantalla; 2. placa fotográfica o fluorescente que obtiene la imagen de estructuras internas del organismo.

Y

y

Y *abbr.* **y/o** year-old / de un año de edad.
yaw *n.* lesión primaria de la frambesia.
yawn *n.* bostezo; *v.* bostezar.
yaws *n.* lesión ulcerativa primaria de yaws, (frambesia o pian). Enfermedad tropical no venérea.
Y chromosome *n.* cromosoma Y, cromosoma sexual diferencial que determina las características sexuales del sexo masculino.
year *n.* año; **at the beginning of the ___** / a principios de ___ ; **at the end of the ___** / al final del ___ ; **every ___** / todos los ___ -s; **last ___** / el ___ pasado; **New Year** / Año Nuevo; **once a ___** / una vez al ___; **-ly** *adv.* anualmente.
years of potential life lost *n.* años perdidos de vida potencial. Medida potencial del impacto en un individuo de enfermedades y fuerzas letales sociales. Se tienen en cuenta los años que la persona pudo haber vivido si una muerte prematura debido a heridas mortales, cáncer, enfermedades del corazón, etc. no hubiera ocurrido.
yeast *n.* levadura, hongo diminuto capaz de provocar fermentación que se usa en la nutrición como fuente de vitaminas y proteínas.
yell *n.* grito, alarido; *v.* gritar.
yellow *n.* color amarillo; *a.* amarillo-a.
yellow atrophy of the liver *n.* atrofia amarilla del hígado.
yellow bile *n.* bilis amarilla, uno de los cuatro humores del cuerpo según la antiguedad, que produce irritabilidad.
yellow body *n.* cuerpo amarillo. V. **corpus luteum**.

yellow fever *n.* fiebre amarilla, enfermedad endémica de regiones tropicales debida a un virus que es transmitido por la picadura del mosquito hembra *Aedes Aegypti* y que se manifiesta con fiebre, ictericia y albuminuria.
yellow fibers *n.* fibras amarillas. *Syn.* **elastic fibers.**
yellow hepatization *n.* hepatización de etapa final, en la cual las exudaciones se han convertido virulentas.
yellow jack *n. pop.* fiebre amarilla.
yellow spot *n.* mácula lútea.
yellowish *a.* amarillento-a.
yersinia *n.* yersinia. gene del tipo de especie *Yersinia pestis,* bacteria parasítica en humanos, que no forma esporas y contiene bastoncillos de células ovoides, gramma negativas.
yet *conj.* todavía; no obstante, sin embargo.
yield *n.* rendimiento; producción; *v.* producir, rendir.
ying-yang *n.* concepto de la filosofía china manteniendo el balance entre filofofía y medicina, comparado con el ying y yang, dos entidades opuestas que se complementan. La meta consiste en obtener el balance biológico de ambas entidades.
Y ligament *n.* ligamento iliofemoral.
yoga *n.* yoga, práctica de meditación y autodominio a través del cual se trata de alcanzar un estado de unión entre el yo y el universo.
yolk *n.* 1. yema del huevo; 2. conjunto de sustancias que nutren al embrión.
young *a.* joven; juvenil.
youngster *n.* jovencito-a, muchacho-a.
youth *n.* juventud, mocedad, periodo entre la niñez y madurez.
youthful *a.* juvenil, joven; **to look ___** / parecer joven.

Z

Z *abbr.* **z** zero / cero ; **zone** / zona.
zero balancing *n.* equilibrio cero,
método para producir un estado de
equilibrio en el organismo
alineando la energía con el uso de
manipulación de selectas partes del
cuerpo.
zero population growth *n.*
crecimiento cero de población,
condición demográfica que existe en un
período de tiempo determinado en el
cual la población permanece estable,
sin aumentar ni disminuir.
zinc *n.* zinc, elemento metálico cristalino
de propiedad astringente; __ **oxide** /
óxido de __; __ **peroxide** / peróxido
de __; __ **sulfate** / sulfato de __.
zinc ointment *n.* pomada de
zinc.
Zollinger-Ellison syndrome *n.*
síndrome de Zollinger-Ellison,
condición manifestada por
hipersecreción gástrica, hiperacidez y
ulceración péptica del estómago e
intestino delgado.

zona *n.* zona. 1. área o capa específica;
2. herpes zóster.
zone *n.* zona, estructura anatómica en
forma de banda; **comfort** __ / __ de
bienestar; **equivalence** __ / __ de
equivalencia; **gliding** __ / __ de
deslizamiento; **respiratory** __ / __
respiratoria; **transition** __ / __ de
transición; __ **radiata** / __ radiada.
zoogenous *a.* zoógeno-a, que se
adquiere o deriva de animales.
zoograft *n.* zooinjerto, injerto que
proviene de tejido animal.
zoophobia *n.* zoofobia, ansiedad y
miedo irracional hacia los animales.
zootoxin *n.* zootoxina, sustancia
venenosa que procede de un animal
como el veneno de la serpiente.
zoster *n.* zóster. V. **herpes zóster,
shingles**.
zoster ophthalmicus *n.* zóster
oftálmico, infección herpética del ojo,
que afecta esp. el nervio óptico.
zygoma *n.* cigoma, zigoma,
prominencia ósea que forma un arco en
la unión del hueso malar y el temporal.
zygomatic *a.* cigomático-a, rel. al
cigoto; __ **arch** / arco __; __ **bone** /
hueso __; __ **egg** / óvulo __ .
zygote *n.* cigoto, óvulo fertilizado,
célula fecundada por la unión de dos
gametos.

Appendix A
- ## Questioning the Patient
- ## Specialties
- ## Medical Phrases

Apéndice A
- ## Preguntas al paciente
- ## Especialidades
- ## Frases médicas

QUESTIONING THE PATIENT / PREGUNTAS AL PACIENTE

Interrogative Words	Palabras interrogativas
ENGLISH	**SPANISH**
whom?	¿a quién, a quiénes?
which?	¿cuál, cuáles?
when?	¿cuándo?
how many? how much?	¿cuánto?, ¿cuántos?, ¿cuántas?
where from?	¿de dónde?
whose?	¿de quién, de quiénes?
where?	¿dónde?
why?	¿por qué?
what?	¿qué?
when?	¿cuándo?
where?	¿dónde?
where to?	¿adónde?
where from?	¿de dónde?
who?	¿quién?, ¿quiénes?
whom?	¿a quién?, ¿a quiénes?
which?	¿cuál?, ¿cuáles?
whose?	¿de quién?, ¿de quiénes?
why?	¿por qué?

Personal Data

ENGLISH

The questions are followed by one or more possible answers, other than ___**Yes** ___ **No** and the patient is to choose the one more appropriate or the one corresponding to him or her.

Datos personales

SPANISH

Las siguientes preguntas están seguidas de dos o más posibles respuestas fuera de ___ **Si** ___ **No** y el/la paciente debe escoger la más apropiada o la que mejor le corresponda a él/ella.

Personal Data	**Datos personales**
Name _____	nombre _____
Age ___	edad ___
Address _____	dirección _____
Family Members _____	familiares _____

ENGLISH	SPANISH
1. Are you the patient?	1. ¿Es usted el/la paciente?
2. Who is the patient? ___ I am. ___ She is. ___ My mother is the patient.	2. ¿Quién es el/la paciente? ___ Soy yo. ___ Es ella. ___ Mi madre es la paciente.
3. What is your name? My name is ___ John, ___ Linda.	3. ¿Cómo se llama usted? Me llamo ___ Juan, ___ Linda.
4. How old are you? I am ___ twenty, ___ thirty, ___ seventy-five years old.	4. ¿Cuántos años tiene? Tengo ___ veinte, ___ treinta, ___ setenta y cinco años.
5. How old is the patient? He/she is ___ forty, ___ fifty, ___ seventy-five years of age.	5. ¿Cuántos años tiene el/la paciente? El/Ella tiene ___ cuarenta, ___ cincuenta, ___ setenta y cinco años.
6. What is your telephone number? It is 323-4197 (three, two, three, four, one, nine, seven).	6. ¿Cuál es su número de teléfono? Es 323-4197 (tres, dos, tres, cuatro, uno, nueve, siete).
7. What is your address? My address is 43 N. (forty-three North) Elm.	7. ¿Cuál es su dirección? Mi dirección es 43 N. (cuarenta y tres Norte) Elm.
8. Is this your permanent address?	8. ¿Es ésta su dirección permanente?
9. What is your present address? It is 789 S. (seven, eight, nine, South) Paseo del Monte.	9. ¿Cuál es su dirección actual? Es 789 S. (siete, ocho, nueve, Sur) Paseo del Monte.
10. How long have you lived at the present address? ___ three months ___ one year ___ five years	10. ¿Qué tiempo hace que vive en su dirección actual? ___ tres meses ___ un año ___ cinco años
11. Are your parents living? ___ My mother is living. ___ My father is deceased.	11. ¿Sus padres viven? ___ Mi madre vive. ___ Mi padre murió.
12. What is your father's name? Peter Smith.	12. ¿Cómo se llama su padre? Pedro Smith.

Personal Data / Datos personales

ENGLISH	SPANISH
13. What is your mother's name? ___ Her name is Rose. ___ My mother's name is Rose.	13. ¿Cómo se llama su madre? ___ Su nombre es Rosa. ___ Mi madre se llama Rosa.
14. Are you ___ single? ___ married? ___ divorced? ___ separated? ___ living with partner? ___ a widow? ___ a widower?	14. ¿Es usted ___ soltero-a? ___ casado-a? ___ divorciado-a? ___ está separado-a? ___ convive con alguien? ___ viudo-a?
15. What is your spouse's name? ___ His name is Henry Pritchard. ___ Her name is Sylvia Pritchard.	15. ¿Cómo se llama su esposo-a? ___ Su nombre es Enrique Pastor. ___ Ella se llama Silvia Pastor.
16. Do you have children? How many? I have ___ one child, ___ three children.	16. ¿Tiene hijos? ¿Cuántos? Tengo ___ un hijo, ___ tres hijos.
17. Do they live with you?	17. ¿Viven con usted?
18. Do you live alone?	18. ¿Vive solo-a?
19. Can you give us the name, address, and telephone of a person that can be notified in case of an emergency?	19. ¿Nos puede dar el nombre, dirección y teléfono de alguien a quien podamos notificar en caso de emergencia?

Financial Facts

- medical insurance
- occupation
- paying the bill

Finanzas y pagos

- seguro médico
- occupación
- pago de la cuenta

ENGLISH	SPANISH
1. What is your occupation? ___ teacher ___ mechanic ___ dentist ___ painter ___ doctor	1. ¿Cuál es su trabajo o profesión? ___ maestro-a ___ mecánico ___ dentista ___ pintor ___ doctor
2. Where do you work? ___ at home ___ in a garage ___ in a warehouse ___ in an office	2. ¿Dónde trabaja? ___ en mi casa ___ en un garaje ___ en un almacén ___ en una oficina
3. What is the name and address of your employer? ___ His name is Mark Smith and his address is 3967 E. (three, nine, six, seven East) Swan.	3. ¿Cuál es el nombre y dirección de la persona para quien trabaja? ___ Es el señor Marcos Smith y su dirección es 3967 E. (tres, nueve, seis, siete Este) Swan.
4. What is your Social Security number? ___ It is 457-55-5462 (four, five, seven, five, five, five, four, six, two).	4. ¿Cuál su número de Seguro Social? ___ Es el 457-55-5462 (cuatro, cinco, siete, cinco, cinco, cinco, quarto, seis, dos).
5. Do you receive any workman's compensation?	5. ¿Recibe alguna compensación laboral?
6. Are you self-supporting?	6. ¿Se mantiene con sus propios recursos?
7. Do you have medical insurance?	7. ¿Tiene seguro médico?
8. Do you have Medicare?	8. ¿Tiene Medicare?
9. Do you have supplementary insurance?	9. ¿Tiene seguro suplementario?
10. May I have your insurance cards in order to copy them? ___ I don't have them with me.	10. ¿Me permite sus tarjetas de seguro médico para copiarlas? ___ No las tengo conmigo.
11. How would you like to pay your bill? ___ by cash ___ by check ___ with a credit card	11. ¿Cómo quiere pagar su cuenta? ___ en efectivo ___ con cheque ___ con tarjeta de crédito
12. Will you pay for this bill in a lump sum or would you like to make other arrangements? ___ I would like to pay the full amount. ___ I need to make other arrangements.	12. ¿Va a pagar esta cuenta en su totalidad o quiere hacer otros arreglos? ___ La voy a pagar en su totalidad. ___ Tengo que hacer otros arreglos.

AN APPOINTMENT WITH THE DOCTOR / UNA CONSULTA CON EL MÉDICO

ENGLISH	SPANISH
1. Please indicate if you have seen the doctor before.	1. Por favor indique si ha visto al doctor antes.
2. Please fill out this form.	2. Por favor, llene esta planilla.
3. Please sit down, and we will call you shortly.	3. Siéntese, por favor, y le llamaremos dentro de poco.
4. Follow me, please.	4. Sígame, por favor.
5. Please get on the scale.	5. Por favor, súbase a la balanza.
6. Now I am going to take your blood pressure.	6. Ahora le voy a tomar la presión arterial.
7. Please undress and put on this gown.	7. Por favor, desvístase y póngase esta bata.
8. Would you like to use the bathroom?	8. ¿Quiere usar el baño?
9. The doctor will be here shortly.	9. El doctor vendrá dentro de poco.
10. Breathe ___ normally ___ deeply ___ hold your breath	10. Respire ___ normalmente ___ profundamente ___ aguante la respiración
11. Cough lightly.	11. Tosa ligeramente.
12. Does it hurt here when I touch you?	12. ¿Le duele aquí cuando le toco?
13. Show me where it hurts.	13. Indíqueme donde le duele.
14. You may get dressed now.	14. Ya se puede vestir.
15. The doctor would like to see you in ___ a week ___ a month ___ 6 months ___ a year	15. El doctor lo quiere ver dentro de: ___ una semana ___ un mes ___ 6 meses ___ un año
16. You can make an appointment now.	16. Puede hacer una cita ahora.
17. You may take care of your bill now.	17. Puede pagar su cuenta ahora.

CHIEF COMPLAINT / QUEJA PRINCIPAL

▶ PRESENT ILLNESS
▶ DATE AND TIME OF ONSET OF ILLNESS
▶ CHARACTERISTICS OF ILLNESS
▶ FREQUENCY OF ILLNESS

▶ ENFERMEDAD ACTUAL
▶ COMIENZO DE LA ENFERMEDAD
▶ CARACTERÍSTICAS DE LA ENFERMEDAD
▶ FRECUENCIA DE LA ENFERMEDAD

ENGLISH	SPANISH
1. What brings you here? ___ My yearly check-up. ___ I have not been feeling well. ___ This is a follow-up appointment.	1. ¿Cuál es la causa de su visita? ___ Mi chequeo anual. ___ No me he estado sintiendo bien. ___ Esta es una visita de seguimiento.
2. How do you feel right now? ___ not well ___ not too good	2. ¿Cómo se siente en este momento? ___ no me siento bien ___ no muy bien
3. When did this problem begin? ___ It began about a month ago. ___ It has been going on for quite a while.	3. ¿Cuando comenzó este problema? ___ Empezó hace como un mes. ___ Empezó hace bastante tiempo.
4. Have you lost any weight recently? ___ some	4. ¿Ha bajado de peso recientemente? ___ algo
5. Is this problem preventing you from working? ___ sometimes ___ once in a while	5. ¿Este trastorno (problema o condición) le impide trabajar? ___ algunas veces ___ de vez en cuando
6. Is this problem affecting your regular activities? ___ up to a point	6. ¿Este problema afecta sus actividades diarias? ___ hasta cierto punto
7. Are you able to do housework? ___ only light chores	7. ¿Puede hacer los quehaceres de la casa? ___ solamente los más simples
8. Have you had this problem (symptom or discomfort) before?	8. ¿Ha tenido este malestar, (síntoma, trastomo) antes?
9. Did it start suddenly or gradually? ___ suddenly, ___ gradually	9. ¿Le empezó de pronto o gradualmente? ___ de pronto, ___ gradualmente
10. Do you have this problem constantly? ___ when I get up in the morning ___ after meals	10. ¿Tiene este trastorno continuamente? ___ cuando me levanto en la mañana ___ después de las comidas
11. Every day? ___ almost every day ___ not every day, but very frequently	11. ¿Todos los días? ___ casi todos los días ___ no todos los días, pero muy frecuentemente
12. How many times a day? ___ once a day ___ a few times a day ___ when I get up ___ in the afternoons	12. ¿Cuántas veces al día? ___ una vez al día ___ varias veces al día ___ cuando me levanto ___ por las tardes
13. When do you feel worse? ___ in the evenings	13. ¿Cuándo se siente peor? ___ por la noche

ENGLISH	SPANISH
14. Does it make you feel ___ weak? ___ tired?	14. ¿Le hace sentirse ___ débil? ___ cansado-a?
15. Do you have a fever?	15. ¿Tiene fiebre?
16. Are you in pain now? ___ Not at this time. ___ I am in a lot of pain.	16. ¿Tiene dolor ahora? ___ No en este momento. ___ Tengo mucho dolor.
17. Have you seen a doctor since you became ill?	17. ¿Ha visto a algún doctor desde que se enfermó?
18. Is your family aware of this problem?	18. ¿Está su familia al tanto de su problema?
19. Are you taking medication now? ___ only pain killers	19. ¿Está tomando alguna medicina ahora? ___ solamente pastillas para el dolor
20. Have you taken or done anything that seems to help you? ___ I take aspirin.	20. ¿Ha hecho o tomado algo que le mejore? ___ Tomo aspirina.
21. Have you ever been hospitalized on account of this problem?	21. ¿Ha tenido que ingresar alguna vez al hospital debido a este problema?

MEDICAL HISTORY / HISTORIA CLÍNICA

General Questions	Preguntas generales
ENGLISH	**SPANISH**
1. Have you gained weight recently? ___ a little bit, some	1. ¿Ha aumentado de peso últimamente? ___ un poco
2. Have you lost weight recently?	2. ¿Ha bajado de peso recientemente?
3. Do you have any pain?	3. ¿Tiene dolor?
4. How long have you had this pain? ___ for about two months ___ for about a week ___ since my last period	4. ¿Cuánto tiempo hace que tiene el dolor? ___ hace como dos meses ___ hace como una semana ___ desde mi última menstruación
5. Where does it hurt? ___ here ___ in the neck ___ in the chest	5. ¿Dónde le duele? ___ aquí ___ en el cuello ___ en el pecho
6. Is the pain ___ sharp? ___ severe? ___ mild? ___ dull?	6. ¿Es el dolor ___ agudo? ___ fuerte? ___ leve? ___ sordo?
7. Do you tire easily? ___ sometimes	7. ¿Se cansa fácilmente? ___ algunas veces
8. Do you feel dizzy?	8. ¿Se siente mareado-a?
9. Do you generally sleep well? ___ pretty well	9. ¿Duerme bien generalmente? ___ bastante bien
10. How many hours do you sleep? ___ I sleep about three, five, seven hours.	10. ¿Cuántas horas duerme durante la noche? ___ Duermo como tres, cinco, siete horas.
11. Do you sleep during the day? ___ once in a while	11. ¿Duerme durante el día? ___ a veces
12. Do you take any pills to help you to sleep?	12. ¿Toma alguna pastilla para dormir?

Family History; Past Medical History

Historia familiar; historia clínica previa

ENGLISH	SPANISH
1. Do you have any children?	1. ¿Tiene hijos?
2. How old were you when you had your first child? I was ___ twenty-one, ___ thirty-three, ___ forty years old.	2. ¿Cuántos años tenía cuando nació su primer/a hijo/a? Yo tenía ___ veintiún, ___ treinta y tres, ___ cuarenta años.
3. Do your children live with you?	3. ¿Viven sus hijos con usted?
4. Are your parents living?	4. ¿Viven sus padres?
5. Are they in good health? ___ fair	5. ¿Tienen buena salud? ___ regular
6. Is your father living?	6. ¿Vive su padre?
[*if the answer is Yes*] 7. What is his health like? ___ good ___ fair	[*Si la respuesta es sí*] 7. ¿Cómo está de salud? ___ bien ___ regular
[*if the answer is No*] 8. What did he die from? ___ from a stroke ___ from surgery complications	[*Si la respuesta es no*] 8. ¿De qué murió? ___ de una embolia cerebral ___ de complicaciones de una cirugía
9. How old was he when he died? He was ___ sixty-two, ___ seventy, ___ eighty-two years old.	9. ¿Qué edad tenía cuando murió? Tenía ___ sesenta y dos, ___ setenta, ___ ochenta y dos años.
10. Is your mother living?	10. ¿Vive su madre?
11. What is her health like? ___ fair ___ bad	11. ¿Cómo está de salud? ___ regular, más o menos ___ mal
12. What did she die of? ___ from breast cancer	12. ¿De qué murió ella? ___ de cáncer del seno
13. Have you ever been hospitalized?	13. ¿Ha estado hospitalizado-a alguna vez?
14. What for? ___ for surgery ___ to deliver a baby ___ for acute respiratory problems	14. ¿Debido a qué? ___ para operarme ___ por estar de parto ___ por un problema respiratorio agudo
15. For how long? ___ a week ___ fourteen days ___ a month	15. ¿Por cuánto tiempo? ___ una semana ___ catorce días ___ un mes
16. How many times? ___ one ___ two ___ three times	16. ¿Cuántas veces? ___ una ___ dos ___ tres veces

Family History; Past Medical History

Historia familiar; historia clínica previa

ENGLISH	SPANISH

17. Have you or your parents, grandparents, or close relatives ever had any of the following illnesses?
    ___ amebic dysentery
    ___ allergies
    ___ anemia
    ___ appendicitis
    ___ arthritis
    ___ asthma
    ___ cancer
    ___ chicken pox
    ___ chorea
    ___ chronic laryngitis
    ___ chronic tonsilitis
    ___ cirrhosis
    ___ conjunctivitis
    ___ cystitis
    ___ diabetes
    ___ diphteria
    ___ ear infections
    ___ emphysema
    ___ epilepsy
    ___ gallbladder attack
    ___ gallstones
    ___ goiter
    ___ gonorrhea
    ___ hay fever
    ___ heart disease
    ___ hepatitis
    ___ high blood pressure
    ___ jaundice
    ___ measles, German measles, rubella
    ___ mononucleosis
    ___ mumps
    ___ scarlet fever
    ___ syphilis
    ___ tuberculosis
    ___ typhoid fever

17. ¿Han padecido sus padres, abuelos o familiars inmediatos algunas de las enfermedades siguientes?
    ___ disenteria amebiana
    ___ alergias
    ___ anemia
    ___ apendicitis
    ___ artritis
    ___ asma
    ___ cáncer
    ___ varicela
    ___ corea
    ___ laringitis crónica
    ___ amigadalitis crónica
    ___ cirrosis
    ___ conjuntivitis
    ___ cistitis
    ___ diabetes
    ___ difteria
    ___ infecciones de los oídos
    ___ enfisema
    ___ epilepsia
    ___ ataque vesicular
    ___ cálculos en la vejiga
    ___ bocio
    ___ gonorrea
    ___ fiebre del heno
    ___ enfermedad del corazón
    ___ hepatitis
    ___ presión arterial alta
    ___ ictericia
    ___ sarampión, sarampión alemán, rubéola
    ___ mononucleosis
    ___ paperas
    ___ fiebre escarlatina
    ___ sífilis
    ___ tuberculosis
    ___ fiebre tifoidea

---

18. Have you or any of your immediate relatives been addicted to
    ___ alcohol?
    ___ tobacco?
    ___ drugs?

18. ¿Usted o algún familiar cercano ha sido adicto-a a
    ___ alcohol?
    ___ tabaco?
    ___ drogas?

---

19. Has anyone in your family died of a heart attack?

19. ¿Ha muerto algún familiar cercano de un ataque al corazón?

---

20. Have any of your siblings died?

20. ¿Han muerto alguno de sus hermanos -as?

Family History; Past Medical History	Historia familiar; historia clínica previa
ENGLISH	**SPANISH**

21. How old was he/she? He/she was ___ twenty-three, ___ thirty-five, ___ forty years old.	21. ¿Qué edad tenía? Él/ella tenía ___ veintitrés, ___ treinta y cinco, ___ cuarenta años.
22. Where have you lived most of your life? ___ here in the United States ___ abroad ___ in my native country	22. ¿Dónde ha vivido la mayor parte de su vida? ___ aquí en los Estados Unidos ___ fuera del país ___ en mi país natal

SPECIALTIES / ESPECIALIDADES

Eyes, Ears, Nose, and Throat	Ojos, oídos, nariz y garganta
ENGLISH	**SPANISH**
1. Have you noticed any bleeding from your gums or mouth?	1. ¿Ha notado si las encías o la boca le sangran?
2. Does your tongue feel sore? Is any part of your mouth sore?	2. ¿Siente la lengua adolorida? ¿Le duele otra parte de la boca?
3. Do you have swelling or lumps in the mouth?	3. ¿Tiene alguna hinchazón o protuberancia en la boca?
4. Do you have difficulty swallowing?	4. ¿Tiene dificultad al tragar?
5. Do you suffer from sore throats? How frequently? ___ about once a month ___ several times a year	5. ¿Padece de dolor de garganta? ¿Con qué frecuencia? ___ como una vez al mes ___ varias veces al año
6. Do you have any dripping or drainage in the back of the throat?	6. ¿Tiene alguna supuración o flema en la parte posterior de la garganta?
7. Are you often hoarse?	7. ¿Tiene ronquera frecuentemente?
8. Have you noticed any swelling in your neck?	8. ¿Ha notado alguna hinchazón en su cuello?
9. Have you ever had nosebleeds?	9. ¿Ha tenido sangramiento por la nariz?
10. Do you have any difficulty hearing?	10. ¿Tiene alguna dificultad para oír?
11. Do you have ringing in your ears? ___ right ear ___ left ear ___ both	11. ¿Tiene zumbido o tintineo en los oídos? ___ en el derecho ___ en el izquierdo ___ en ambos
12. Have you noticed any secretion from your ears?	12. ¿Ha notado alguna secreción por los oídos?
13. Do you have earaches?	13. ¿Padece de dolor de oído?
14. Have you noticed any change in your vision?	14. ¿Ha notado algún cambio en la vista?
15. Do you wear glasses or contact lenses? ___ for close-up ___ for distance ___ for reading ___ all the time	15. ¿Usa espejuelos o lentes de contacto? ___ para ver de cerca ___ para distancia ___ para leer ___ siempre
16. Have you noticed any redness or swelling in your eyes?	16. ¿Ha notado que sus ojos estén enrojecidos o hinchados?
17. Do you have double vision?	17. ¿Tiene visión doble?
18. Do you see spots or flashes of light?	18. ¿Ve manchas o destellos de luces?
19. Have you had pain in your eyes?	19. ¿Ha tenido dolor en los ojos?
20. Do you have any discharge from your eyes?	20. ¿Le supuran los ojos?

Eyes, Ears, Nose, and Throat

Ojos, oídos, nariz y garganta

ENGLISH	SPANISH
21. Have your eyes ever been affected by any sickness or accident?	21. ¿Ha sido su vista afectada por alguna enfermedad o accidente?
22. Do you have blurred vision?	22. ¿Se le nubla la vista?
23. Do you have a burning feeling in your eyes?	23. ¿Le arden los ojos?
24. Do you have to strain your eyes to see better?	24. ¿Tiene que forzar la vista para ver mejor?
25. When was your last vision test? ___ it has been a year ___ two years ago ___ since I was a child	25. ¿Cuándo fue su último examen de la vista? ___ hace un año ___ dos años atrás ___ desde que esa niño -a

Cardiopulmonary | Cardiopulmonar

ENGLISH	SPANISH
1. Have you ever had an electrocardiogram?	1. ¿Se le ha hecho alguna vez un electrocardiograma?
2. Have you ever noticed rapid heartbeats?	2. ¿Ha notado alguna vez si tiene palpitaciones del corazón?
3. Have you ever had chest pain?	3. ¿Ha tenido alguna vez dolor en el pecho?
4. How long did it last? ___ a couple of hours ___ all day yesterday ___ almost a week	4. ¿Cuánto tiempo le duró? ___ un par de horas ___ todo el día de ayer ___ casi una semana
5. In what part of the chest? ___ the upper chest ___ the lower chest	5. ¿En qué parte del pecho? ___ en la parte superior del pecho ___ en la parte inferior del pecho
6. Does it radiate to any part of your body? ___ arm ___ shoulder ___ neck ___ back	6. ¿Se le corre a alguna parte del cuerpo? ___ al brazo ___ al hombro ___ al cuello ___ a la espalda
7. Do you cough? ___ a little ___ a lot ___ a dry cough	7. ¿Tiene tos? ___ poca tos ___ mucha tos ___ una tos seca
8. Does your chest hurt when you cough?	8. ¿Le duele el pecho cuando tose?
9. Do you have any swelling in your legs or ankles?	9. ¿Tiene hinchazón en las piernas o los tobillos?
10. Do you have high blood pressure?	10. ¿Tiene la presión arterial alta?
11. Do you bleed easily?	11. ¿Tiene tendencia a sangrar?
12. Do you smoke? For how long have you smoked? ___ for one year ___ for a long time	12. ¿Fuma? ¿Cuánto tiempo hace que fuma? ___ un año ___ hace mucho tiempo
13. How many cigarettes per day? ___ five ___ ten ___ a pack a day	13. ¿Cuántos cigarrillos al día? ___ cinco ___ diez ___ un paquete al día
14. Have you tried to stop?	14. ¿Ha tratado de dejar de fumar?
15. Have you ever had lung disease?	15. ¿Ha tenido alguna enfermedad de los pulmones?
16. Do you have frequent colds?	16. ¿Tiene catarros frecuentes?
17. Do you cough up any phlegm?	17. ¿Tose con flema?

Cardiopulmonary

Cardiopulmonar

ENGLISH	SPANISH

18. What does it look like?
   ___ viscous
   ___ bloody
   ___ watery

18. ¿Cómo es la flema?
   ___ viscosa
   ___ sangrienta
   ___ aguada

---

19. What color is it?
   ___ clear
   ___ white
   ___ yellow
   ___ green
   ___ dark
   ___ brown

19. ¿De qué color es la flema?
   ___ clara
   ___ blanca
   ___ amarilla
   ___ verde
   ___ oscura
   ___ marrón

---

20. Have you ever coughed up blood?

20. ¿Alguna vez ha tenido sangre al toser?

---

21. Have you had any trouble breathing?

21. ¿Ha tenido dificultad para respirar?

---

22. Are you short of breath
   ___ at night?
   ___ when you walk?
   ___ even when resting?

22. ¿Le falta la respiración
   ___ por la noche?
   ___ cuando camina?
   ___ aún cuando descansa?

---

23. Have you noticed any particular sound in your breathing?

23. ¿Ha notado algún sonido diferente al respirar?

---

24. Is there any position that makes your breathing
   ___ easier?
   ___ worse?

24. ¿Hay alguna posición que le permite respirar
   ___ mejor?
   ___ peor?

Gastrointestinal | Gastrointestinal

ENGLISH	SPANISH
1. Is there any food that disagrees with you? ___ fried foods ___ acid fruits ___ dairy foods	1. ¿Le cae mal algún alimento? ___ comidas fritas ___ frutas ácidas ___ comidas lácteas
2. Do you have heartburn?	2. ¿Tiene ardor en el estómago?
3. Do you suffer from stomachaches? ___ before eating ___ while eating ___ after eating	3. ¿Padece de dolores del estómago? ___ antes de comer ___ mientras come ___ después de comer
4. Do you suffer from indigestion?	4. ¿Padece de indigestión?
5. Do you drink or eat between meals?	5. ¿Come o toma líquidos entre las comidas?
6. Do you drink coffee? How many cups a day? ___ one ___ two ___ three ___ four cups	6. ¿Toma café? ¿Cuántas tazas al día? ___ una ___ dos ___ tres ___ cuatro tazas
7. Do you eat fried or fatty foods?	7. ¿Come comidas fritas o grasosas?
8. Do you burp a lot?	8. ¿Eructa mucho?
9. How much milk do you drink? What kind? ___ 2% ___ skim ___ whole milk	9. ¿Cuánta leche toma? ¿De qué clase? ___ desnatada ___ natural ___ completa
10. At what time do you eat breakfast?	10. ¿A qué hora desayuna?
11. At what time do you eat your last meal of the day?	11. ¿A qué hora hace su última comida del día?
12. Do you try to eat a balanced meal every day?	12. ¿Trata de comer una comida balanceada todos los días?
13. What kind of food do you generally eat more of? ___ meats ___ vegetables ___ bread and cereals ___ fruits	13. ¿Qué clase de alimentos generalmente come más? ___ carnes ___ vegetales ___ panes y cereales ___ frutas
14. Do you eat a good breakfast every day?	14. ¿Toma un buen desayuno todos los días?
15. Are you constipated?	15. ¿Padece de estreñimiento?
16. Do you have a bowel movement every day?	16. ¿Elimina (obra, está al corriente) todos los días?
17. Are your stools normal?	17. ¿Son normales sus evacuaciones?

Gastrointestinal

Gastrointestinal

ENGLISH	SPANISH
18. What color and consistency are they? ___ normal ___ hard and dark ___ bloody ___ greasy ___ dark and viscous	18. ¿Qué color y consistencia tienen? ___ normal ___ oscuras y duras ___ con sangre ___ grasientas ___ oscuras y viscosas
19. Do you have diarrhea?	19. ¿Tiene diarrea?
20. Have you noticed any blood or mucous in the stools?	20. ¿Ha notado sangre o mucosidad en las heces fecales?

Musculoskeletal — Musculoesquelética

ENGLISH	SPANISH
1. Do you have pain in your joints?	1. ¿Le duelen las articulaciones?
2. Do you have pain in the neck or back?	2. ¿Tiene dolor en el cuello o la espalda?
3. Do your muscles hurt?	3. ¿Le duelen los músculos?
4. Do you feel general muscle weakness?	4. ¿Siente debilidad muscular general?
5. Have you noticed any swelling on a bone?	5. ¿Ha notado hinchazón en algún hueso?
6. Do your bones ache?	6. ¿Siente dolor en los huesos?
7. Have you ever had a fracture or a sprain?	7. ¿Ha tenido alguna vez una fractura o luxación?
8. How long ago? ___ last year ___ five years ago ___ a long time ago	8. ¿Cuánto tiempo hace? ___ el año pasado ___ hace cinco años ___ hace mucho tiempo
9. What bone or part was affected? ___ I fractured my wrist. ___ I broke the femur. ___ I had a hip fracture.	9. ¿Qué hueso o parte le afectó? ___ Me fracturé la muñeca ___ Me partí el fémur ___ Me fracturé la cadera.

Neurological / Neurológica

ENGLISH	SPANISH
1. Do you have any feeling of tingling or numbness?	1. ¿Tiene alguna sensación de hormigueo o entumecimiento?
2. Do you forget things easily?	2. ¿Olvida las cosas con facilidad?
3. Is your memory worse than before?	3. ¿Tiene la memoria peor que antes?
4. Do you have good balance?	4. ¿Tiene buen equilibrio?
5. Do you have any difficulty walking?	5. ¿Tiene alguna dificultad para caminar?
6. Do you have difficulty moving ___ towards the right? ___ towards the left?	6. ¿Tiene dificultad al moverse ___ hacia la derecha? ___ hacia la izquierda?
7. Have you ever lost consciousness?	7. ¿Ha perdido el conocimiento alguna vez?
8. More than once?	8. ¿Más de una vez?
9. Do you walk without difficulty?	9. ¿Camina sin dificultad?
10. Do you need any walking device to maintain your balance? ___ cane ___ walker	10. ¿Necesita alguna ayuda para mantener el equilibrio? ___ bastón ___ caminador
11. Do you feel sometimes like you are going to fall?	11. ¿Siente algunas veces como si fuera a caerse?
12. Have you had any seizures or convulsions?	12. ¿Ha tenido ataques o convulsiones de algún tipo?
13. Is your memory ___ good? ___ bad? ___ not as good as it used to be?	13. ¿Es su memoria ___ buena? ___ mala? ___ no tan buena como antes?
14. Can you feel this?	14. ¿Puede sentir esto?
15. Can you smell this?	15. ¿Puede oler esto?
16. Does any particular food taste different to you?	16. ¿El sabor de algún alimento en particular le parece distinto?

Skin / Piel

ENGLISH	SPANISH
1. Do you have any sores or blisters?	1. ¿Tiene algunas llagas o ampollas?
2. Do you have any mole that is red or itchy?	2. ¿Tiene algún lunar enrojecido o que le pica?
3. Do you have a skin rash?	3. ¿Tiene alguna erupción?
4. Since when have you had this eruption?	4. ¿Desde cuándo ha tenido esta erupción?
5. Have you noticed any change?	5. ¿Ha notado algún cambio?
6. Have you noticed any unusual spots in your skin?	6. ¿Ha notado alguna mancha peculiar en la piel?
7. Do you use any cosmetics that cause redness or swelling to your skin?	7. ¿Usa cosméticos que le causen enrojecimiento o hinchazón en la piel?
8. Have you had any severe burns?	8. ¿Ha tenido alguna vez una quemadura grave?
9. Does anything make you itchy?	9. ¿Hay algo que le da picazón?
10. Is your skin very sensitive to the sun's rays?	10. ¿Es su piel muy sensitiva a los rayos del sol?
11. Do you use any sunblockers (creme or lotion) if you are going to be exposed to the sun?	11. ¿Usa algún bloqueador de sol (crema o loción) si va a estar expuesto-a a los rayos del sol?
12. Have you noticed any discoloration on your skin?	12. ¿Ha notado algún cambio de color en la piel?

Genitourinary

Genitourinaria

ENGLISH

SPANISH

(TO FEMALE PATIENTS)

(PARA LAS PACIENTES FEMENINAS)

1. How old were you when you had your first period?
   I was
   ___ ten
   ___ thirteen
   ___ fourteen years old.

1. ¿Qué edad tenía cuando tuvo la primera regla (periodo)?
   Yo tenía
   ___ diez
   ___ trece
   ___ catorce años de edad.

2. When was your last period?
   ___ one week ago
   ___ three weeks ago
   ___ two months ago
   ___ six months ago

2. ¿Cuándo tuvo la última regla?
   ___ hace una semana
   ___ hace tres semanas
   ___ dos meses
   ___ seis meses

3. Are your periods difficult?

3. ¿Son sus periodos difíciles?
   (¿Es la regla dificultosa?)

4. How long does your period last?
   ___ three to four days
   ___ a week
   ___ eight to nine days

4. ¿Cuántos días le dura el periodo?
   ___ tres o cuatro días
   ___ una semana
   ___ ocho a nueve días

5. Do you ever bleed between periods?

5. ¿Tiene algún sangramiento entre reglas?

6. Do you have any discharge from the vagina?

6. ¿Tiene algún flujo o secreción de vagina?

7. What does it look like?
   ___ viscous
   ___ yellowish
   ___ bloody

7. ¿Cómo es?
   ___ viscosa
   ___ amarillenta
   ___ con sangre

8. Do you have any itching or burning in the genital area?

8. ¿Tiene alguna picazón o ardor en alguna parte privada?

9. Have you ever had a venereal disease?

9. ¿Ha tenido alguna enfermedad venérea?

10. Are you pregnant?

10. ¿Está embarazada (en estado encinta)?

11. Have you ever been pregnant? How many times?
    ___ two
    ___ four
    ___ seven times

11. ¿Ha estado embarazada alguna vez? ¿Cuántas veces?
    ___ dos
    ___ cuatro
    ___ siete veces

12. Have you ever had a miscarriage? How many times?
    ___ one
    ___ two
    ___ three times

12. ¿Ha tenido alguna vez un malparto? ¿Cuántas veces?
    ___ una
    ___ dos
    ___ tres veces

13. Have you ever had an induced abortion? How many times?
    ___ once
    ___ twice

13. ¿Ha tenido alguna vez un aborto inducido? ¿Cuántas veces?
    ___ una vez
    ___ dos veces

Genitourinary

ENGLISH	SPANISH
(TO FEMALE PATIENTS)	**(PARA LAS PACIENTES FEMENINAS)**
14. Do you have any problem during intercourse?	14. ¿Tiene algún problema o dificultad durante las relaciones sexuales?
15. Do you have any pain during intercourse?	15. ¿Tiene dolor durante las relaciones sexuales?
16. Do you use any type of birth control?	16. ¿Usa algún tipo de anticonceptivo?
17. How many live births have you had?	17. ¿Cuántos embarazos se le han logrado?
18. Have you had any stillbirths?	18. ¿Ha tenido algún parto no logrado?

Genitourinaria

(TO MALE PATIENTS)	**(PARA PACIENTES MASCULINOS)**
1. Do you have any discharge from the penis?	1. ¿Tiene alguna secreción por el pene?
2. Do you have pain in the testicles?	2. ¿Tiene dolor en los testículos?
3. Do you have pain or swelling in the scrotum?	3. ¿Tiene dolor o hinchazón en el escroto?
4. Are you unable to have an erection?	4. ¿Se le dificulta tener una erección?
5. Do you have a satisfactory sex life?	5. ¿Está satisfecho con su vida sexual?
6. Have you had any venereal disease?	6. ¿Ha tenido alguna enfermedad venérea?
7. Have you fathered any children?	7. ¿Ha tenido hijos?

Urinary

Urinaria

ENGLISH

SPANISH

1. Do you have any trouble urinating?	1. ¿Tiene dificultad cuando orina?
2. Do you have to get up to urinate during the night? How many times? ___ two ___ three times	2. ¿Tiene que levantarse por la noche a orinar? ¿Cuántas veces? ___ dos ___ tres veces
3. Do you have pain or burning when urinating?	3. ¿Tiene dolor o ardor cuando orina?
4. Is the color of the urine ___ yellow ___ murky ___ milky ___ pale ___ reddish?	4. ¿Es la orina ___ amarilla ___ turbia ___ lechosa ___ sin color ___ rojiza?
5. Do you have blood in the urine?	5. ¿Tiene sangre en la orina?
6. Are you unable to control your urination?	6. ¿No puede controlar la salida de orina?
7. Do you urinate too often?	7. ¿Orina con demasiada frecuencia?
8. Do you pass a little or a lot of urine regularly?	8. ¿Orina mucho o poco regularmente?
9. Do you have difficulty starting to urinate?	9. ¿Tiene dificultad para comenzar a orinar?
10. Do you have difficulty maintaining a continuous flow of urine?	10. ¿Tiene dificultad en mantener el chorro?
11. Do you have any urine leakage?	11. ¿Tiene pérdida de orina?
12. When does it usually occur? ___ when I change positions when I am sitting down ___ when I cough	12. ¿Cuándo ocurre generalmente? ___ cuando cambio de posición mientras estoy sentado-a ___ cuando toso
13. Do you have back or flank pain?	13. ¿Tiene algún dolor en la espalda o en el costado?
14. Have you ever had any kidney problem?	14. ¿Ha padecido de los riñones?
15. Have you ever passed stones?	15. ¿Ha expulsado cálculos?
16. Have you had a vasectomy?	16. ¿Se ha hecho una vasectomía?
17. Do you examine your testicles regularly?	17. ¿Se examina los testículos regularmente?
18. Have you had a PSA test? When? ___ about six months ago ___ I have never had the test.	18. ¿Se ha hecho la prueba del PSA? ¿Cuándo? ___ hace como seis meses ___ Nunca me he hecho la prueba.

AMBULANCE AND EMERGENCY ROOM / AMBULANCIA Y SALÓN DE EMERGENCIA

Questions Addressed Directly to the Patient / **Preguntas directas al paciente**

ENGLISH	SPANISH
1. What is your name?	1. ¿Cómo se llama usted?
2. Where do you live?	2. ¿Dónde vive?
3. Where are you calling from?	3. ¿De dónde está llamando?
4. Are you the person having the problem?	4. ¿Es usted la persona que tiene el problema?
5. Can you describe as best as possible what is the problem?	5. ¿Puede usted describir lo mejor posible cuál es el problema?
6. To what hospital do you wish to go?	6. ¿A qué hospital quiere que lo (la) llevemos?
7. Do you understand what I am saying?	7. ¿Entiende lo que le digo?
8. What is your name?	8. ¿Cómo se llama?
9. What day of the week is it?	9. ¿Qué día de la semana es hoy?
10. Who is your doctor?	10. ¿Quién es su médico?
11. Has someone notified your doctor?	11. ¿Alguién le ha notificado a su médico?
12. Are you in pain?	12. ¿Tiene dolor?
13. Are you having any problem breathing?	13. ¿Tiene alguna dificultad para respirar?
14. Have you fainted or lost consciousness at any time?	14. ¿Se ha desmayado o ha perdido el conocimiento alguna vez?
15. Are you taking any medication?	15. ¿Está tomando alguna medicina?
16. How many pills did you take?	16. ¿Cuántas pastillas tomó?
17. Are you allergic to any medications?	17. ¿Es alérgico-a a alguna medicina?
18. When did the accident occur?	18. ¿Cuándo ocurrió el accidente?
19. Where did it happen?	19. ¿Dónde ocurrió?
20. Have you had a tetanus shot?	20. ¿Se ha inyectado contra el tétano?
21. When was the last time?	21. ¿Cuándo fue la última vez?
22. Have you been hospitalized before? When?	22. ¿Ha sido hospitalizado-a alguna vez? ¿Cuándo?
23. For what reason?	23. ¿Por qué razón?
24. Was it here or somewhere else?	24. ¿Fue aquí o en alguna otra parte?
(to a female patient) 25. Do you know if you are pregnant?	*(a pacientes femeninos)* 25. ¿Sabe usted si está embarazada?

HOSPITALIZATION / HOSPITALIZACIÓN

ENGLISH	SPANISH
1. Do you have the written doctor's orders with you?	1. ¿Tiene las indicaciones del doctor consigo?
2. It is necessary to complete some paper work before you are admitted.	2. Necesitamos obtener cierta información antes de ingresarlo-a.
3. Sit in this wheelchair, please.	3. Siéntese en esta silla de ruedas, por favor.
4. We are taking you to your room.	4. Lo (la) vamos a llevar a su cuarto.
5. We suggest you don't keep any valuables in your room because the hospital is not responsible for lost items.	5. Le aconsejamos que no deje objetos de valor en el cuarto ya que el hospital no se hace responsable por cualquier pérdida de objetos.
6. We need a signed consent for your surgery.	6. Necesitamos una autorización firmada para su operación.
7. Push this button for assistance.	7. Apriete este botón si necesita algo.
8. Call if you need ___ to use the bedpan ___ a sleeping pill ___ something for the pain ___ something to drink ___ an extra pillow or blanket	8. Llame si necesita ___ usar el bacín ___ una pastilla para dormir ___ algo para aliviar el dolor ___ algo para tomar ___ una almohada o una frazada (cobija) adicional
9. You can get out of bed.	9. Puede bajarse de la cama.
10. You must stay in bed.	10. Debe quedarse en la cama.
11. I am the nurse.	11. Soy el (la) enfermero-a.
12. I need to take your ___ pulse ___ temperature ___ blood pressure	12. Tengo que tomarle ___ el pulso ___ la temperatura ___ la presión arterial
13. I am going to take a sample of blood.	13. Voy a tomarle una muestra de sangre.
14. I need to give you a shot.	14. Tengo que ponerle una inyección.
15. I am going to give you an intravenous feeding.	15. Voy a ponerle un suero en la vena.
16. This will not hurt.	16. No le va a doler.
17. Someone will come to take you to ___ the x-ray room ___ the laboratory ___ the rehabilitation room	17. Alguien va a venir a llevarlo-a ___ a la sala de rayos-x ___ al laboratorio ___ a la sala de rehabilitación

Surgery / Cirugía

ENGLISH	SPANISH
1. I am going to prepare you for surgery.	1. Voy a prepararlo-a para la operación.
2. I am going to give you an enema.	2. Voy a ponerle un lavado intestinal.
3. I am going to shave you.	3. Lo (la) voy a rasurar.
4. Your surgery is scheduled for ___ later ___ this afternoon ___ tomorrow morning ___ tomorrow afternoon	4. La cirugía va a ser ___ más tarde ___ esta tarde ___ mañana por la mañana ___ mañana por la tarde
5. The anesthetist will be here to talk to you and ask you some questions ___ later ___ before surgery	5. El (la) anestesista vendrá a hablar con usted y a hacerle algunas preguntas ___ más tarde ___ antes de la operación
6. We will give you a sedative before taking you to the operating room.	6. Le vamos a dar un calmante antes de llevarlo-a a la sala de operaciones.
7. After the operation you will be taken to the recovery room.	7. Después de la operación lo (la) llevarán a la sala de recuperación.
8. When you wake up you may have ___ a tube in your throat to help you breathe ___ a tube in the bladder to help you urinate ___ a tube in the stomach so you will not vomit	8. Al despertarse tal vez tenga ___ un tubo en la garganta para ayudarlo-a a respirar ___ un tubo en la vejiga para que pueda orinar ___ un tubo en el estómago para que no vomite
9. An IV will be inserted before and throughout surgery until you start eating and drinking again.	9. Le van a poner un suero intravenoso antes y durante la cirugía hasta que empiece a alimentarse y tomar líquidos.
10. Your doctor will be here ___ later ___ tomorrow	10. Su médico vendrá a verle ___ más tarde ___ mañana
11. You will be discharged ___ later ___ tomorrow ___ in a week	11. Le van a dar de alta ___ más tarde ___ mañana ___ dentro de una semana
12. Call your doctor's office and make an appointment ___ in a week ___ in ten days	12. Llame a la consulta de su médico y pida turno para dentro de ___ una semana ___ diez días
13. Call us if you need help, but if it is an emergency, call 911 (nine one one).	13. Llame aquí si necesita asistencia, pero si se trata de una emergencia, llame al 911 (nueve uno uno).

Anesthesia / Anestesia

ENGLISH	SPANISH
1. I am the anesthetist.	1. Soy el/la anestesista.
2. I need to ask you some questions.	2. Tengo que hacerle algunas preguntas.
3. Are you allergic to anything? To what?	3. ¿Es alérgico-a a algo? ¿A qué?
4. Are you allergic to any medication? Which?	4. ¿Es usted alérgico-a a alguna medicina? ¿A cuál?
5. Are you taking any medication? Which?	5. ¿Está tomando alguna medicina? ¿Cuál?
6. How long have you been taking it?	6. ¿Cuánto tiempo lleva tomándola?
7. Have you been taking aspirin for any reason?	7. ¿Ha estado tomando aspirina por algún motivo?
8. Are you taking any diuretic?	8. ¿Toma algún diurético?
9. Have you had surgery before?	9. ¿Ha tenido alguna operación anteriormente?
10. What kind of an operation was it?	10. ¿Qué tipo de operación fue?
11. Do you remember what kind of anesthesia you had?	11. ¿Recuerda usted que clase de anestesia le dieron?
12. Did you have any trouble with the anesthesia?	12. ¿Tuvo alguna dificultad con la anestesia?
13. What kind of trouble?	13. ¿Qué tipo de dificultad?
14. Today we are going to give you the following anesthesia.	14. Hoy le vamos a dar la siguiente anestesia.
15. Try to relax.	15. Trate de relajarse.

TRAUMA AND EMERGENCY PROBLEMS / TRAUMA Y PROBLEMAS DE EMERGENCIA

ENGLISH		SPANISH	
Foreign Bodies Penetrating the Body		**Cuerpos extraños que penetran el cuerpo**	
ORGAN OR PART	CAUSE CONSEQUENCES	ÓRGANO O PARTE	CAUSA CONSECUENCIAS
abdomen	splinter	abdomen	astilla, espina
chest	abrasions	tórax	abrasiones
eye, ear,	knives	ojo, oído,	cuchillos
throat	hemorrhage	garganta	hemorragia
extremities	sharp instruments	extremidades	instrumentos afilados
skull	infections	cráneo	infecciones
	bullet		heridas de bala
	projectile wounds		laceraciones por proyectil
	scratches		rasguños

Airway Foreign Bodies		**Cuerpos extraños en el conducto respiratorio**	
VIA	SYMPTOMS	VIA	SÍNTOMAS
penetrating through puncture wounds, by swallowing	cough, chest pain, dyspnea, gasping for air, unable to speak, unable to swallow normally	penetrando a través de heridas de perforación, o al tragar	tos, dolor en el pecho, disnea, estridor, jadeo, dificultad al hablar o al tragar

ENGLISH	SPANISH
Substances Causing Toxic Effects by Inhalation, Ingestion, or by Direct Contact	**Sustancias que causan efectos tóxicos por aspiración, ingestión o por contacto directo**
SUBSTANCE	SUSTANCIA
alcohols (ethanol, methanol)	alcoholes (etanol, metanol)
alkalis (ammonia)	alcalíes (amoníaco)
arsenic	arsénico
boric acid	ácido bórico
carbon monoxide	monóxide de carbono
cleaners (toilet, ovens, pools)	limpiadores (de servicios, hornos, piscinas)
contaminated fish, ciguatera	pescado contaminado, ciguatera
cyanide	cianuro
herbicides	herbicidas
metals (iron, lead)	metales (hierro, plomo)
muriatic acid	ácido muriático
mushrooms	setas (hongos)
overdose of medications (salicylates, neuroleptics, antidepressants, opiates, etc.)	sobredosis de medicamentos (salicilatos, neurolépticos, tranquilizantes, opiáceos, etc.)
paint thinners, antifreeze, etc.	aguarrás, trementina, anticongelante
plants (hemlock, morning glory, daffodil, hyacinth, ivy, oleander)	plantas (cicuta, gloria de la mañana, narciso trompón, jacinto, hiedra venenosa, adelfa)
contaminated shellfish	mariscos contaminados
strong acids	ácidos fuertes

ENGLISH	SPANISH
Intoxication— poisoning	**Intoxicación— envenenamiento**
alkali poisoning – ingestion of an alkali or ammoniac	**ingestión de una sustancia alcalí** – amoníaco, lejía
caffeinism – excessive ingestion of products containing caffeine	**cafeinismo** – envenenamiento por ingestión excesiva de productos con cafeína
carbon monoxide – absorbing carbon monoxide causes a toxic condition that can be lethal	**monóxido de carbono** – envenenamiento por absorción e inhalación de monóxido de carbono puede ser letal
cyanide poisoning – can occur by inhaling smoke or ingesting cyanide industrial chemicals	**envenenamiento de cianuro** puede ocurrir por inhalaciones de humo o ingestión de sustancias químicas industriales
ergotism – ingesting ergot-infected grain products that cause diarrhea, vomiting and even alteration of the heart rhythm	**ergotismo** – consumiendo productos de grano infestado por ergot que pueden causar diarrea, vómitos y hasta causar alteración del ritmo cardíaco
alcohol intoxication – excessive ingestion of alcohol can be habit forming and cause serious physical and psychological problems	**intoxicación alcohólica** – ingestión excesiva de alcohol puede ser adictiva y causar serios problemas físicos y psicológicos
lead poisoning – by ingestion or inhalation of paints that contain lead, or containers of water such as water pipes and water tanks	**envenenamiento por plomo** – por ingestión o absorción causado por pinturas que contienen plomo, o por contenedores de agua tal como tuberías y tanques
mercury poisoning – poisoning by ingesting mercury could cause acute kidney damage, vomiting, and diarrhea that could be lethal	**envenenamiento por mercurio** – puede causar daño severo al riñón, vómito y diarrea que pueden ser letales
nicotine poisoning – inhalation and ingestion of great amounts of nicotine	**envenenamiento por nicotina** – inhalación e ingestión de una gran cantidad de nicotina
overdose of drugs – salicylates, neuroleptics, antidepressants, and opiates prescribed or obtained illegally	**sobredosis de drogas** – salicilatos, neurolépticos, antidepresivos y opiados prescritos u obtenidos ilegalmente
contaminated shellfish	**mariscos contaminados**
ophidism – poisoning by snakes, bees, ants, spiders, producing an injected venom	**ofidismo** – envenenamiento causado por la ponzoña de una abeja, hormiga, avispa, o araña negra o el veneno de una serpiente
strong cleaning substances – mixed with strong acids	**sustancias limpiadoras** – mezcladas con ácidos fuertes

ENGLISH	SPANISH

Burns / Quemaduras

ENGLISH	SPANISH
acid burns	quemaduras por ácido
fire burns	quemaduras por fuego
frostbite	quemadura de frío
radiation burns	quemaduras por radiación
sunburns	quemadura de sol

Chest Pain / Dolor en el pecho

POSSIBLE CAUSES	SYMPTOMS	CAUSA POSIBLE	SÍNTOMAS
myocardial infarction, heart attack	chest pain in the center of the chest behind the sternum; sweating, possible nausea and vomiting	infarto del miocardio, ataque al corazón	dolor en el pecho que puede correrse al cuello, al maxilar y al brazo; sudor y posibles náuseas y vómitos
angina pectoris	chest pain with a sensation of pressure, sweaty brow, pain radiates to the left shoulder, and sometimes to the arm	angina de pecho	dolor en el pecho con sensación de presión, sudores en la frente; el dolor se irradia al hombro izquierdo y a veces al brazo
pericarditis	chest pain, dull or sharp, rapid breathing, cough	pericarditis	dolor sordo o agudo en el pecho, respiración rápida, tos

Loss of Consciousness / Pérdida del conocimiento

CAUSED BY SEIZURES — **DEBIDO A CONVULSIONES**

alcohol or other drug withdrawal	privación de alcohol o de otra droga
drug abuse	adicción a las drogas
epilepsy	epilepsia
febrile convulsions	convulsiones febriles
head trauma	contusión cerebral
metabolic problems	problemas metabólicos

CAUSED BY COMA — **DEBIDO A COMA**

diabetic	diabético
traumatic: head, massive hemothorax	traumático: cerebral, hemotórax masivo
hyperglycemic	hiperglicémico
hypoglycemic	hipoglicémico
drug overdose	sobredosis

ENGLISH	SPANISH

Eye Emergencies / Emergencias de la vista

SYMPTOM	SÍNTOMA
abrasion, scrape	abrasión o desgarramiento
perforating injury	herida con perforación
swelling and pain	hinchazón y dolor
chemical penetration	penetración de una sustancia química
foreign body piercing	penetración de cuerpo extraño
eye discharge with pus and redness	enrojecimiento y supuración del ojo con pus
severe constant pain	dolor constante y fuerte
sudden red or pink colored vision	visión súbita de color rojo o rosada
sudden blindness or double vision	ceguera súbita o visión doble

Other Emergencies / Otras emergencias

cardiopulmonary resuscitation	reanimación cardiopulmonar
overdose	sobredosis
emergency delivery	parto de emergencia
vaginal bleeding	sangramiento vaginal
hypertension	hipertensión
child abuse	niños maltratados
sexual assault	violación sexual
drowning	ahogo
suicide	suicidio

MEDICAL PHRASES / FRASES MÉDICAS

ENGLISH	SPANISH
acquired immunity	inmunidad adquirida
admitting diagnosis	diagnóstico de ingreso
ambulatory care	cuidado ambulatorio
attending physician	médico de cabecera
blind study	estudio con anonimato
blood bank	banco de sangre
blood clot	coágulo de sangre
blood count	hemograma
blood culture	hemocultivo
blood donor	donante de sangre
blood transfusion	tranfusión de sangre
care unit	unidad de cuidado
casualty	víctima de un accidente
chemotherapeutic agents	antineoplásticos
chronic illness	enfermedad crónica
collapse of the lung	atelectasia pulmonar
congestive heart failure	colapso o fallo cardíaco
current medications	medicamentos actuales
day of admission	día de ingreso
decreased sperm count	descuento en el esperma
differential blood count	fórmula leucocítica
discharged and sent home	dado de alta y enviado a su casa
disease-free area	zona indemne
distended bladder	distensión vesical
doctor on call	médico de guardia
dosage interval	intervalo de administración de la dosis
electroshock therapy	terapia electroconvulsiva
electrolyte balance	equilibrio hidroelectrolítico
emergency center	centro de emergencia
epileptic seizure	ataque epiléptico
essential hypertension	hipertensión (arterial) idiopática
estrogen replacement therapy	terapia de reemplazo de estrógeno
evaluation of a disorder	evaluación de un trastorno
expected date of delivery	fecha prevista del parto
feeding tube	tubo de alimentación

ENGLISH	SPANISH
fetal movement (quickening)	movimiento fetal (animación)
fever blisters	herpes labial
fluid balance chart	hoja de balance hídrico
fluid depletion	deshidratación
follow-up appointment	consulta de seguimiento
food additives	aditivos alimenticios
full blood count	hemograma completo
gastrointestinal bleeding	sangramiento gastrointestinal
gastrointestinal disorders	trastornos digestivos
general condition	estado general
genital area	zona inguinal
gestational psychosis	psicosis gravídica
gross exam	examen macroscópico
gross findings	resultados del examen macroscópico
gross pathology	anatomía patológica macroscópica
guarded condition	estado de gravedad
health certificate	certificado de salud
health care	atención a la salud
health food	comida saludable
health services	servicios de salud
health services for the aged	cuidado de la salud de los ancianos
heart rate	frecuencia cardíaca
heavy smoker	fumador empedernido
high calorie diet	dieta hipercalórica
high risk	alto riesgo
home health care	cuidado de la salud en el hogar
homologous insemination	inseminación artificial con semen del marido
immune response	respuesta o reacción inmune
impaired lung function	función pulmonar disminuida
impaired short memory	memoria inmediata impedida
impaired thought processes	proceso cognitivo dañado
impaired vision	vista defectuosa
in urgent need of treatment	urgente necesidad de recibir tratamiento
infirmities of old age	achaques de la vejez
initial bleeding	hematuria inicial
inpatient discharge	alta del paciente hospitalizado
intestinal malabsorption	hipoabsorción intestinal

ENGLISH	SPANISH
intracranial pressure monitoring	monitoreo de presión intracraneal
invasive devices	dispositivos invasores
isolation ward	sala de aislamiento
joint motion	movilidad articular
joint pain	dolor en las coyunturas
kidney stone	cálculo renal
labyrinthine concussion	conmoción laberíntica
laboratory findings	datos analíticos del laboratorio
language skills	habilidad lingüística
legal rights	derechos legales
length of stay in hospital	tiempo de hospitalización
life expentancy	expectativa de vida
life threatening	que puede ser mortal
light wound	herida leve
living relative donor transplantation	trasplante de órgano de un pariente vivo
long term care facility	institución de atención médica prolongada
long term memory	memoria distante
low blood pressure	hipotensión arterial
low-grade lymphoma	linfoma de menor grado
low-grade tumor	tumor bien diferenciado
lymphatic spread	diseminación por vía linfática
memory assessment	evaluación de la memoria
mental disorders	trastornos psíquicos
mental impediment	impedimento mental
metabolic defect	trastorno o alteración metabólica
metabolic disturbances	trastornos metabólicos
minor illness	enfermedad leve
mottled skin	piel veteada
narrowing of joint space	reducción del espacio articular
noninvasive diagnostic tool	instrumento diagnóstico no-invasivo
normal disease progression	enfermedad de progresión normal
nurse in charge	enfermero-a jefe, jefe de sala
onset of labor	comienzo del parto
operating surgeon	cirujano a cargo de la operación
outpatient	paciente externo
outpatient clinic	clínica para pacientes externos
over the counter medication	medicamento de venta sin receta
overt hyperglycemia	hiperglucemia franca

ENGLISH	SPANISH
oxygen tent	cámara de oxígeno
packed cells	concentrado de eritrocitos
patient in need of urgent care	paciente con necesidad de atención urgente
patient's care	atención o cuidado del/de la paciente
patient's discharge	alta del/de la paciente
patient's record	expediente del/de la paciente
patient's rights	derechos del/de la paciente
physical assessment	evaluación física
physical changes	cambios físicos
primary diagnosis	diagnosis principal
primary lesion	lesión principal
prolapsed disc	hernia de disco, hernia discal
protein requirements	necesidades proteínicas
public health	salud pública
public health facilities	instituciones de salud pública
recovery room	sala de recuperación
rehabilitation center	centro de rehabilitación
right to receive treatment	derecho a recibir tratamiento
root curettage	raspado radicular
rough murmur	soplo rudo áspero
sexual arousal	excitación sexual
short of breath	falto de aire
short term memory impairment	memoria inmediata impedida
shoulder or thoracic girdle	cintura escapular
signs and symptoms	signos y síntomas
silent bleeding	hemorragia oculta
single all-purpose vaccine	vacuna única polivalente
sore throat	dolor de garganta
speech defect	defecto en el habla
state of mind	estado de ánimo
stuffy nose	nariz tupida (*mex.* tapada)
support group	grupo de apoyo
surgical procedure	procedimiento quirúrgico
temperature range	variación de la temperatura
therapeutic services	servicios terapéuticos
tightness of the chest	opresión en el pecho
to leave against medical advice	salir sin consentimiento médico
to pass a stone	eliminar un cálculo

ENGLISH	SPANISH
to pass out	desmayarse, desvanecerse
to refuse treatment	rehusar tratamiento
to remain in bed	guardar cama, permanecer en cama
traffic accident	accidente de tráfico
treatment and monitoring	tratamiento y monitoreo
triggering point	punto de desencadenamiento
undescended testicle	testículo no descendido
unpredictable behaviour	conducta incierta
unsatisfactory treatment	tratamiento sin resultado positivo
urgent care	tratamiento urgente
uterine curettage	raspado del útero, raspado de la matriz
vaginal examination	tacto vaginal
verbal ability	capacidad verbal
visiting hours	horas de visita
voluntary admission	ingreso voluntario
water pollution	contaminación del agua
water bag	bolsa de agua
white matter	sustancia blanca
withdrawal symptoms	síntomas de abstinencia
X-ray film	radiografía o película radiográfica

Phrases Related to Health Insurance Policy Claims / Frases relativas a reclamos de pólizas de seguro de salud

ENGLISH	SPANISH
accumulation period	días deducibles de beneficio
allocated benefits	beneficios alocados
benefits coordination	coordinación de beneficios
cancellation of insurance	cancelacion de la póliza
claim	reclamación de beneficios
copayment of not covered expenses	pago por la porción de servicios no cubiertos
credit for prior coverage	crédito por gastos deducibles
deductible amount	cantidad deducible
disability insurance	seguro por incapacidad
exclusion of coverage	exclusión de cobertura
explanation of benefits	explicación de beneficios
grace period	tiempo de gracia
group insurance	seguro de grupo
health care provider	entidad suministradora de servicios de salud
hospital insurance	póliza de hospitalización
ID card/identification card	tarjeta de identificación
indemnity insurance plans	plan de póliza de indemnización
indemnity policy	póliza de indemnización
insurance cancellation	cancelación de la póliza
insurance effective date	fecha de comienzo de la póliza
lapsed policy	póliza vencida
lifetime maximum benefit	beneficio máximo de por vida
long-term care	cuidado de salud de largo tiempo
managed care	coordinación de servicios de salud
personal injury	delito de lesiones
policy limit	límite de la póliza
potential benefits	beneficios potenciales
pre-certification	pre-aprobación requerida de servicios
pre-existing condition	condición anterior existente del asegurado
premium	prima de la póliza
short-term medical	cobertura temporal de servicios médicos
to pay by medical insurance	pago por seguro médico
work related accident	accidente de trabajo

THE NEWBORN / EL RECIÉN NACIDO

Characteristics	Características
ENGLISH	SPANISH
full-term	nacido(-a) a término completo
premature	prematuro
body weight at birth	peso al nacer
body length	largo del cuerpo
body temperature at birth	temperatura al nacer
normal breathing	respiración normal
vital signs normal	signos vitales normales
facial features	rasgos faciales
breastfed	(lactante) toma el pecho de la madre
bottle-fed	toma el biberón
normal patterns of sleep	patrones normales de sueño
normal cry	llanto normal
nurses well	toma el pecho bien
crying when hungry or wet	llora cuando tiene hambre o está mojado-a
weight gain normal	aumento de peso normal
normal growth and development	crecimiento y desarrollo normales
weight loss	pérdida de peso
time sleeping	tiempo durmiendo
time awake	tiempo despierto
movements	movimientos
alertness	expresión viva
lifts his/her head	levanta la cabeza
umbilical cord drop	caída del cordón umbilical
taking vitamins with formula	toma vitaminas en la fórmula
suckling well from breast or bottle	toma bien el pecho o chupa bien el biberón

Anomalies / Anomalías

Anomalies	Anomalías
abdominal swelling	inflamación abdominal
blood in the stools	sangre en las deposiciones
cyanosis	cianosis
colic	cólico
constipation	estreñimiento
convulsions	convulsiones
cradle cap	costra láctea
diaper rash	eritema, erupción
diarrhea sudden and explosive	diarrea explosiva y súbita
Down syndrome	síndrome de Down
dry scales	escama seca
excessive crying	llanto excesivo
feeding problems	problemas de alimentación
inadequate gaining	aumento inadecuado de peso
increasing fussiness	mayor intranquilidad
infantile spasms	espasmos infantiles
infections	infecciones
intolerance to lactose	intolerancia a la lactosa
jaundice	ictericia
Marfan's syndrome	síndrome de Marfán
milk allergy	alergia a la leche
nasal congestion	congestión nasal
seborrheic eczema	eczema seborreico
skin irritation	irritaciones en la piel
sudden jerk	contracción brusca
vaginal bleeding	sangramiento vaginal
weight loss	pérdida de peso

Appendix B
- ## Signs and Symptoms
- ## Diagnoses, Tests, Studies, and Medications
- ## Alzheimer's Disease, Breast Cancer, Diabetes, Prostate Cancer

---

Apéndice B
- ## Señales y síntomas
- ## Diagnósticos, pruebas, estudios y medicamentos
- ## Enfermedad de Alzheimer, cáncer del seno, diabetes, cáncer de la próstata

SIGNS AND SYMPTOMS / SEÑALES Y SÍNTOMAS

Signs and Symptoms in Most Common Disorders and Diseases / Señales y síntomas de trastornos y enfermedades más comunes

ENGLISH	SPANISH
abscess in	**absceso**
brain	cerebral
breast	de la mama
kidney	del riñón
throat (tonsilar)	amigdalino (garganta)
abnormal color in feces, stools	**color anormal en las heces fecales o excremento**
black	ennegrecido
pale	pálido
red	rojizo
white	blanquecino
abnormal color in the urine	**cambios anormales en el color de la orina**
coffee	pardo-negrusco
pale	casi sin color
pink, reddish	rosáceo, rojo
yellow-orange	amarillo-anaranjado
abnormal odor in urine	**olor anormal en la orina**
aromatic	aromático
foul	fétido
accummulation of fluids in	**acumulación de líquido en**
abdomen	el abdomen
joints	las articulaciones
tissues	los tejidos
absent periods	**falta de menstruación**
aging, premature	**envejecimiento prematuro**
anxiety	**ansiedad**
apathy	**apatía**
atrophy of muscles	**atrofia muscular**
asphyxiating episodes	**ataques de asfixia**
attention span, limited	**capacidad de atención limitada**
backache	**dolor de espalda**
low	en la parte inferior
bad breath, halitosis	**mal aliento, halitosis**
baldness	**calvicie**
behavior	**conducta**
belligerent	agresiva, violenta
excited	excitada
belching	**eructos, eructación**
black-and-blue marks	**morados, moretones**

Signs and Symptoms in Most Common Disorders and Diseases / Señales y síntomas de trastornos y enfermedades más comunes

ENGLISH	SPANISH
bleeding from	**sangramiento [sangrado de]**
the ear	el oído
the gums	las encías
the mouth	la boca
the nose	la nariz
the vagina	la vagina
under the skin	debajo de la piel (sangrado subcutáneo)
a wound	una herida
blemishes	**manchas**
blindness	**ceguera**
blind spots	**puntos ciegos**
blisters	**ampollas**
blood clot	**coágulo**
blood in	**sangre en**
feces	las heces fecales
urine, spotty	la orina, con manchas
bloodshot eye	**ojo inyectado**
bluish skin	**piel amoratada**
blurring	**vista nublada**
body odor	**olor fuerte a sudor**
boil	**grano, comedón**
bones	**huesos**
calcium loss	pérdida de calcio
deformity	deformidad
fractures	fracturas
spontaneous fractures	fracturas espontáneas
breathing	**respiración**
abnormal breathing	respiración anormal
choking sensation	sensación de ahogo
difficulty in exhaling	dificultad al exhalar
difficulty in inhaling	dificultad al aspirar
bruised body	**contusiones en el cuerpo**
bulbous red nose	**nariz roja y bulbosa**
burning feeling	**ardor; sensación quemante**
cardiac arrhythmia	**arritmia cardíaca**
change in bowel habits	**cambio en el hábito de defecar, obrar**
chapped lips	**labios resecos**
chest pain	**dolor en el pecho**
chills	**escalofríos**
cleft lip	**labio leporino**

ENGLISH	SPANISH
clotting of blood	coagulación de la sangre
clubbed fingers	dedos en maza
coated tongue	lengua pastosa
coldness in extremities	frialdad de manos y pies
collapse	colapso
common cold	catarro, resfriado

constipation
  extended, chronic
	estreñimiento
	  prolongado, crónico

constriction of the penis	constricción del pene
contractions	contracciones
convulsions	convulsiones

cough
  dry
  excessive
  coughing up blood
  coughing up bloody phlegm
	tos
	  seca
	  excesiva
	  expectoración de sangre
	  expectoración de flema sanguinolenta

crack in the corner of the mouth	grieta en la comisura del labio
cracked lips	labios agrietados
cramps	calambre
cyanosis	cianosis
cyst	quiste
deafness	sordera
dehydration	deshidratación
delirium	delirio
depression	depresión
diaper rash	eritema de los pañales
diarrhea	diarrea

difficulty in
  breathing
  defecating
  urinating
  swallowing
	dificultad al
	  respirar
	  defecar, obrar
	  orinar
	  tragar

dilated pupil	pupila dilatada

discharge from
  the ear
  the eye
  the nipples
  the penis
  the vagina
	supuración por
	  el oído
	  el ojo
	  los pezones
	  el pene
	  la vagina

discomfort in passing water	dificultad, molestia al orinar
distended abdomen	abdomen, vientre distendido

Signs and Symptoms in Most Common Disorders and Diseases / Señales y síntomas de trastornos y enfermedades más comunes

ENGLISH	SPANISH
distortion of (visual)	**distorsión visual de**
color	color
size	tamaño
shape	forma
dizziness	**mareo**
double vision	**visión doble**
drowsiness	**amodorramiento**
dry mouth	**boca seca**
dyspepsia	**dispepsia**
earache	**dolor de oído**
edema	**edema**
emaciation	**emaciación, enflaquecimiento**
enlarged	**agrandamiento, engrosamiento**
abdomen	del abdomen
eyeball	del globo del ojo
feet	de los pies
heart	del corazón
lymph nodes	de los nódulos linfáticos
exhaustion	**agotamiento**
eyeball	**globo ocular**
rolled upward	virado hacia arriba
palsied	paralizado
protruding	protuberante
failure to gain weight	**no poder aumentar de peso**
failure to lose weight	**no poder adelgazar**
fainting	**desmayo**
false labor pains	**dolores de parto falsos**
fatigue	**cansancio excesivo**
fever	**fiebre, calentura**
erratic	errática
high	alta
intermittent	intermitente
persistent	persistente
recurrent	recurrente
fissured tongue	**lengua fisurada**
fixed pupil	**pupila fija**
flabby skin	**piel flácida**
flushing	**rubor**
foul breath	**aliento fétido**
foul taste	**sabor (muy) desagradable**

ENGLISH	SPANISH
fragility of bones	fragilidad de los huesos
frigidity	frigidez
frostbite	quemadura de frío, congelación
furred tongue	lengua saburral
growing pains	dolores del crecimiento

hard nodules
   in the face
   in the head
	nódulos endurecidos
	   en la cara
	   en la cabeza

hardening of the skin	endurecimiento de la piel
harelip	labio leporino
headache	dolor de cabeza
hearing loss	pérdida de la audición
heart attack	ataque al corazón

heartbeat
   extra, repeated
   irregular
   skipped
   slow
	latido del corazón
	   extra, repetido
	   irregular
	   intermitente
	   lento

heartburn	ardor en el estómago
heart palpitations	palpitaciónes cardíacas
heavy breasts	senos pesados
height loss	disminución en la estatura
hemorrhage after menopause	hemorragia después de la menopausia
hiccups	hipo
hissing in the ear, ringing	zumbido en los oídos
hoarseness	ronquera
hot flashes	fogaje

incontinence
   of feces
   of urine
	incontinencia
	   de heces focales
	   de la orina

indigestion	indigestión
inflammation	inflamación
insensibility	insensibilidad
insensitivity to heat or cold	insensibilidad térmica al frío o al calor
insomnia	insomnio
intercourse, painful	coito doloroso
irregular periods	menstruación irregular
lack of appetite	falta de apetito

Signs and Symptoms in Most Common Disorders and Diseases / Señales y síntomas de trastornos y enfermedades más comunes

ENGLISH	SPANISH
large	**agrandamiento**
head	de la cabeza
limbs	de las extremidades
tongue	de la lengua
lesion	**lesión**
lethargy	**letargo**
listlessness	**falta de ánimo, apatía**
locked jaw	**mandíbula bloqueada**
locked knee	**rodilla bloqueada**
loss of	**pérdida**
appetite	del apetito
balance	del equilibrio
bladder control	del control de la vejiga
consciousness	del conocimiento
control of muscle tonicity	del control del tono muscular
muscular coordination	de la coordinación muscular
feeling	del sentido del tacto
libido	de la libido
luster in hair	del brillo del pelo
luster in nails	del brillo de las uñas
peripheral vision	de la visión periférica
smell	del olfato
voice	de la voz
lumps in	**bultos, masa en**
breast	el seno, la mama
joints	las articulaciones
neck	el cuello
pubic area	el pubis
magenta tongue	**lengua magenta**
malocclusion	**maloclusión**
memory loss	**pérdida de la memoria**
menstruation problems	**problemas de la menstruación**
mental ability impairment	**deterioro de la habilidad mental**
moles	**lunares**
mouth breathing	**respiración por la boca**
muscular incoordination	**falta de coordinación muscular**
nasal speech	**habla nasal**
night blindness	**ceguera nocturna**
night urination	**micción nocturna**
numbness	**entumecimiento**
oozing	**excreción**

ENGLISH	SPANISH
pain	**dolor**
dull	sordo
fulminant	fulminante
gripping	opresivo, con sensación de agarrotamiento
lancinating	lancinante
intense	intenso, agudo
irradiating	que se irradia, que se corre
mild	leve
persistent	persistente
severe	severo
painful gums	**encías dolorosas**
painful swelling	**hinchazón dolorosa**
paleness	**palidez**
pallor	**palidez**
palpitations	**palpitaciones**
palsy	**parálisis**
paralysis	**parálisis**
peeling of the skin	**peladura, descamación de la piel**
pins and needles sensation	**cosquilleo, hormigueo**
polyps	**pólipos**
postnasal drip	**goteo postnasal**
premature aging	**envejecimiento prematuro**
premature beat	**latido prematuro**
premature ejaculation	**eyaculación prematura**
premature menopause	**menopausia prematura**
premenstrual tension	**tensión premenstrual**
profuse sweating	**sudor excesivo**
prostration	**postración**
protrusion from vagina	**protrusión desde la vagina**
puffiness	**hinchazón, intumescencia, abotagamiento**
of the face	de la cara
of the legs	de las piernas
pulmonary	**pulmonar**
abscess	absceso
edema	edema
embolism	embolia
infarction	infarto
tuberculosis	tuberculosis
rapid heartbeat	**latidos rápidos**
rapid loss of vision	**pérdida precipitada de la visión**
rapid loss of weight	**rápida pérdida de peso**
rapid pulse	**pulso rápido**

Signs and Symptoms in Most Common Disorders and Diseases / Señales y síntomas de trastornos y enfermedades más comunes

ENGLISH	SPANISH
rash	erupción, ronchas
red spots (tiny)	pequeñas manchas rojas
red and swollen joints	articulaciones inflamadas y enrojecidas
restlessness	intranquilidad
retraction of the nipple	retracción del pezón
rigidity	rigidez
ringing in the ears	zumbido en los oídos
salivation, excessive	salivación excesiva
salivation and difficulty in swallowing	salivación y dificultad al tragar
scaled ulcer	llaga con costra
scanty urine	escasez de orina
seizures	ataques, episodios
shock	shock, choque
shortness of breath	falta de respiración
skin	piel
clammy	pegajosa
cold	fría
moist	húmeda
skin discoloration	cambio de color de la piel
ashen	cenicienta
brownish	cetrina
darkening	oscurecida
pale	pálida
pallor (face)	palidez (en la cara)
reddening	enrojecimiento
reddening (flushing)	rubor
yellow-white	blanco-amarillenta
slow clotting blood	coagulación lenta
slow growth	crecimiento retardado
slow loss of vision	pérdida gradual de la visión
slow pulse	pulso lento
slow speech	habla despaciosa
sneezing	estornudo
snoring	ronquido
softening of	reblandecimiento de
the bones	los huesos
the nails	las uñas
soft ulcerating tumor	tumor ulceroso blando

ENGLISH	SPANISH
sore	llaga
sore, hard crusted	llaga de costra dura
sore throat	dolor de garganta
spasm	espasmo
spastic gait	marcha espástica
spasticity	espasticidad
speech difficulties	trastornos del habla
split nails	uñas partidas
stiff neck	cuello rígido
stools	heces fecales
hard and dark	oscuras y duras
clay-colored	de color arcilloso
bulky and greasy	deposición abundante y grasienta
black and tarry	oscuras y viscosas
pencil shaped	largas y finas
persistently bloody	con persistente presencia de sangre
subnormal temperature	temperatura subnormal
swallowing difficulty	dificultad al tragar
swelling	hinchazón
tachycardia	taquicardia
thirst, excessive	sed excesiva
tingling	cosquilleo
total lack of urination	ausencia total de orina
tremor	temblor
tumor	tumor
twitch	sacudida nerviosa, "tic nervioso"
ulcer	úlcera, llaga
unconsciousness	pérdida del conocimiento
urination, frequent	orina frecuente
vaginal bleeding	sangramiento vaginal
vaginal discharge	flujo vaginal
varicose veins	venas varicosas
vertigo	vértigo, vahido
vomiting	vómitos
warts	verrugas
weak muscles	debilidad en los músculos
weakness	debilidad
weight	peso
loss	pérdida de
gain	aumento de

Signs and Symptoms in Most Common Disorders and Diseases / Señales y síntomas de trastornos y enfermedades más comunes

ENGLISH	SPANISH
wheezing	respiración sibilante

worms
    in instestine
    in stool
	gusanos, lombrices, parásitos
	    en el intestino
	    en el excremento

wrist fracture	fractura de la muñeca
yawning	bostezo

Warning Signs of a Heart Attack / Señales de advertencia de un ataque al corazón

ENGLISH	SPANISH
Most heart attacks start slowly, with mild pain or discomfort.	La mayor parte de los ataques al corazón comienzan lentamente, con un dolor leve o malestar.

The mild signs that are ignored in many cases, could be the onset of an imminent heart attack. The *American Heart Association* indicates the importance of these and other signs:	Las señales benignas que son ignoradas en muchos casos pueden señalar el comienzo de un inminente ataque al corazón. La Asociación Americana del Corazón nos indica la importancia de éstas señales y otros síntomas:
▶ **Chest discomfort.** You may feel certain discomfort in the center of the chest that could last more than a few minutes. This symptom could go away and then come back. It will change to feel like a big pressure, squeezing, with feeling of fullness or pain. Some patients describe it as "an elephant sitting on my chest."	▶ **Malestar en el pecho.** Se puede sentir cierto malestar en el centro del pecho que podría durar más de unos pocos minutos. Este síntoma puede desaparecer y volver. Puede sentir una presión irresistible que aprieta el pecho con sensación de llenura o de un dolor. Algunos pacientes lo describen como "un elefante sentado en mi pecho".
▶ Other parts of the upper body could be affected. You may feel discomfort or pain in the stomach, in one or both arms, the back, neck, and the jaw.	▶ Otras partes superiores del cuerpo pueden ser afectadas. Puede sentir malestar o dolor en el estómago, en un brazo o ambos brazos, en la espalda, el cuello y la mandíbula.
▶ **Shortness of breath.** This symptom appears regularly with the chest discomfort although it may occur before the feeling of tightness in the chest.	▶ **Falta de respiración.** Este síntoma se manifiesta con regularidad al mismo tiempo que el malestar en el pecho, aunque puede ocurrir antes de que sienta la presión en el pecho.
▶ **Other Signs:** Nausea and lightheadedness could be other symptoms, accompanied by breaking out in a cold sweat.	▶ **Otras señales:** Náusea o mareo pueden manifestarse acompañados de sudores fríos.

If the above signs are present, it is necessary to call 911 immediately and request an ambulance.	Si las señales antes indicadas se presentan, es necesario llamar al teléfono 911 inmediatamente y pedir una ambulancia.

Stroke Warning Signals / Señales de un derrame cerebral

ENGLISH	SPANISH
The following stroke warning signals are indicated by the American Stroke Association:	La Sociedad Americana de Estudios sobre el Derrame Cerebral indica las siguientes señales de advertencia de una embolia o derrame cerebral:
▶ Sudden numbness or weakness in the face, arm or leg present especially on one side of the body	▶ Entumecimiento o debilidad repentina en la cara, el brazo o la pierna, especialmente en un lado del cuerpo
▶ Sudden confusion and inability to speak coherently, faulty understanding	▶ Confusión repentina, dificultad en hablar coherentemente, confusión mental
▶ Difficulty seeing in one or both eyes	▶ Dificultad para ver con un ojo o ambos ojos
▶ Sudden trouble walking, dizziness, loss of balance or coordination	▶ Dificultad repentina al andar, mareo, pérdida de equilibrio o coordinación
▶ Sudden severe headache with no known cause	▶ Fuerte y repentino dolor de cabeza, sin causa conocida
A person that suffers a stroke is almost totally helpless requiring immediate professional attention. It is extremely important that THE TIME when symptoms started be recorded or remembered by the person attending the victim and he or she communicate it to the paramedics and to the staff at the emergency room.	Una persona que sufre un derrame cerebral está casi en total desvalida y requiere atención profesional inmediata. Es extremadamente importante que la persona que asista a la víctima recuerde con seguridad LA HORA en que se presentaron los síntomas y lo comunique a los paramédicos y al personal de emergencia del hospital.
Sometimes symptoms of a stroke are difficult to identify. Unfortunately, the lack of awareness spells disaster. The stroke victim may suffer severe brain damage when people nearby fail to recognize the symptoms of a stroke. Now doctors say a bystander can recognize a stroke by asking three simple questions: ▶ Ask the individual to SMILE ▶ Ask the person to TALK coherently, to SPEAK A SIMPLE SENTENCE (i.e. It is sunny out today.) ▶ Ask him or her to RAISE BOTH ARMS	A veces los síntomas de un derrame cerebral son difíciles de identificar. Infortunadamente, la falta de advertencia resulta en desastre. La víctima de un derrame cerebral puede sufrir un daño cerebral grave cuando las personas que están cerca no reconocen los síntomas de un derrame cerebral. Ahora los médicos dicen que cualquier persona puede reconocer un derrame cerebral haciendo simplemente tres preguntas: ▶ Pedirle a la víctima que se sonría ▶ Decirle que hable coherentemente, decir una simple frase (hoy hace sol) ▶ Pedirle que levante ambos brazos
▶ The drug TPA (tissue plasminogen activator, a protein used as a thrombolitic agent), is a life saver to stroke victims, as long as it can be successfully administered within three hours of the onset of the stroke. TPA is commonly known as "clog buster."	▶ La droga conocida por TPA (activador de plasminógeno en el tejido, proteína usada como agente trombolítico) es una droga que puede salvar la vida o reducir la posibilidad de invalidez permanente en víctimas de derrame cerebral. El medicamento TPA es comúnmente llamado "estirpador de coágulo."

Stroke Warning Signals / Señales de un derrame cerebral

ENGLISH	SPANISH
If you notice that these symptoms are present, either of a heart attack or stroke, do not waste time, call 911 and request an ambulance. The paramedics will start the necessary help as soon as they arrive, and will continue to do so on the way to the hospital. A patient taken to the hospital by ambulance receives faster care than if he/she is taken by a private car.	Si nota que estos síntomas están presentes, de un ataque al corazón o de un derrame cerebral, no pierda tiempo, llame al teléfono 911 y pida una ambulancia. Los paramédicos comenzarán a atender a la víctima apenas lleguen y continuarán haciéndolo mientras la trasladan al hospital. Una paciente que es transportada al hospital en ambulancia generalmente recibe una atención más rápida que si es llevado en un automóvil particular.

Symptoms Related to Drug Abuse

Síntomas relacionados con la adicción a las drogas

ENGLISH	SPANISH
anxiety	ansiedad
blisters	ampollas
blood vessel constriction	constricción de los vasos sanguíneos
chemical odor on breath	aliento con olor a sustancia química
chronic cough	tos crónica
damage in the brain	daño cerebral
depression	depresión
dilated pupils	pupilas dilatadas
disorientation	desorientación
elevated blood pressure	presión (tensión) arterial alta
excitement	excitación
goose bumps	carne de gallina
heightened sexual sensations	sensaciones sexuales exaltadas
hyperactivity	hiperactividad
in the kidneys	en los riñones
in the liver	en el hígado
in the lungs	en los pulmones
in the nerves	en los nervios
increased heart rate	aumento de la frecuencia cardíaca
increased sensory perception	aumento en la percepción sensorial
increased heart beat	taquicardia
increased sweating	aumento sudorífico
liver failure	fallo hepático
rash around the mouth	erupción alrededor de la boca
rash around the nose	erupción alrededor de la nariz
reduced anxiety	ansiedad disminuída
reduced inhibition	inhibición disminuída
restlessness	inquietud
seizures	convulsiones
tremors	temblores

MEDICAL TESTS / PRUEBAS MÉDICAS

Diagnostic Tests	Pruebas de diagnóstico
ENGLISH	SPANISH
Abdominal computerized tomography	Tomografía computada abdominal
Abdominal ultrasound	Ultrasonido abdominal
Acid-fast stain	Tinción fijada en ácido
AIDS serology	Serología de SIDA
Alpha-fetoprotein test	Prueba fetal de alpha-proteína
Amniocentesis, analysis	Amniocentesis, análisis
ANA titer	Titer anticuerpo antinuclear
Angiography	Angiografía
Antiglobulin test	Análisis de antiglobulina
Arterial blood flow leg studies	Estudio del flujo de sangre arterial en las venas
Arterial blood gases	Tensión de gases en sangre arterial
Barium X-ray examinations	Serie de rayos X con uso de sulfato de bario
Biochemical profile	Pruebas selectivas bioquímicas
Biochemical screening	Análisis bioquímico selectivo
Biopsy of the lung	Biopsia pulmonar
Biopsy of the lymph nodes	Biopsia de los ganglios linfáticos
Biopsy of the skin	Biopsia de la piel
Blood smears	Espécimen sanguíneo
Bone densitometry	Densitometría ósea
Bone marrow aspiration	Aspiración de la médula ósea
Bone scan	Escán óseo
Bone marrow biopsy	Biopsia de la médula ósea
BRCA1, BRCA2 genetic tests	BRCA1, BRCA2 pruebas genéticas
Bronchography	Broncografía
Bronchoscopy	Broncoscopía
CA 125 marker test	CA 125 marcador de cáncer
CBC complete blood count	CBC conteo sanguíneo completo
Cervical smear test	prueba cervical de espécimen
Colonoscopy	Colonoscopía
CT scan	Tomografía axial computada, (escán)
Cholecistography	Colecistografía
Cholescintigraphy, gallbladder scanning	Colescintigrafía, escán de la vesícula biliar
Chorionic Villus Sampling	Muestra de vellocidad coriónica
Chromosome análisis	Análisis de los cromosomas
Electrocardiogram	Electrocardiograma

Diagnostic Tests

Pruebas de diagnóstico

ENGLISH	SPANISH
Electrolyte panel tests	Pruebas en panel de electrolitos
Electrophysiological (EP) heart testing	Electrofisiológica (EP), prueba cardíaca
Endoscopic Cholangiopancreotography	Colangiopancreotografía endoscópica
Enzyme tests	Pruebas enzimáticas
Enzyme-linked immunosorbent (ELISA) assay	Análisis inmunosorbente enzimático (ELISA)
Epstein-Barr antibody	Anticuerpos de Epstein-Barr
ESR erythrocyte sedimentation rate	Índice de eritrosedimentación
Kidneys excretory function	Función excretora de los riñones
Febrile agglutinins	Aglutinantes febriles
Gammagraphy lung	Gammagrafía pulmonar
Gram stain	Tinción de Gram
Gastric aspirate	Aspiración gástrica
Gastroscopy	Gastroscopía
Histoplasmin	Histoplasmina
Holter monitoring	Monitoreo de Holter
Hysterosalpingography	Histersalpingografía
Intravenous pyelography	Pielografía intravenosa
Liver/spleen scanning, nuclear	Escán (nuclear) del hígado, bazo
Lung Scan	Escán del pulmón
Lymphangiography to detect lymphomas	Linfografía para detectar linfomas
Mammography	Mamografía
Measure of clotting ability	Medida de la habilidad de coagulación
Mediastinoscopy	Mediastinoscopía
Mono test	Prueba de aglutinación heterófila
MRA, Magnetic resonance angiography	ARM, Angiografía de resonancia magnética
MRI, Magnetic resonance imaging	IRM, Imagen de resonancia magnética
Needle aspiration biopsy	Biopsia de aspiración con aguja
Needle biopsy of the liver	Biopsia por aguja del hígado
Occult blood (fecal)	Sangre oculta (fecal)
Occult blood of the amniotic fluid	Sangre oculta del líquido amniótico
PSA, Prostate-specific antigen	AEP, Antígeno específico de la próstata
Protein electrophoresis	Electroforesis proteínica
Prothrombin time (PT)	PT, Tiempo de protrombina

ENGLISH	SPANISH
Pleural fluid sampling	Muestra del flujo pleural
Pulmonary function tests	Análisis de la función pulmonar
Respiratory function tests	Análisis de la función respiratoria
Rheumatoid factor	Factor reumatoide
Scan of the liver and the spleen	Visualización del hígado y el bazo
Sedimentation rate	Velocidad de sedimentación
Serosal biopsy	Biopsia sérica
Serum creatinine or BUN	Creatinina sérica o BUN
Serum electrolytes	Electrolitos séricos
Serum potassium	Potasio sérico
Serum protein	Proteína sérica
Skin testing	Pruebas cutáneas
Sonogram	Sonograma
Sputum culture	Cultivo de esputo
Stools for ova, parasites	Defecacíon para óvulos, parásitos
Thyroid function tests	Análisis de la función tiroidea
Thyroid sonogram	Sonograma de la tiroides
Tuberculin test	Análisis de la tuberculina
Ultrasonography	Ultrasonografía
Urynalisis	Análisis de orina
Ventilation-perfusion or (V-Q scan)	Perfusión por ventilación o (escán V-Q)
Venuous ultrasound of the legs	Ultrasonido venoso de las piernas
Wasserman test	Análisis serológico de sífilis
Wright stain	Tinción de Wright

Radiologic Studies

INDICATIONS FOR LABORATORY AND X-RAY EXAMINATION

ENGLISH

1. You cannot drink or eat anything before the test.

2. You can brush your teeth, but do not drink water.

3. Before the test you should not
   ___ eat
   ___ drink water or any other liquid
   ___ smoke
   ___ chew gum
   ___ take any medicine
   ___ suck any pills or candy

4. You should eat at least two hours before taking a cathartic.

5. You should eat a light supper the night before the test (operation).

6. You should not eat any greasy food the day before the test.

7. You must take these tablets which are especially for this test.

8. The tablets contain a substance that we can trace during the test and that will help make a diagnosis.

9. You must follow these directions exactly as you are told.

WHEN YOU ARRIVE FOR YOUR TEST, YOU MAY BE REQUESTED:

1. ___ to indicate what type of test you are there for

2. ___ to give them the written orders of the doctor

3. ___ to indicate if you have had anything to eat or drink that morning

4. ___ to indicate if you ate or drank anything after midnight

5. ___ to indicate if you ever had an x-ray examination that required
   ___ an injection
   ___ swallowing any pills
   ___ special medication
   ___ catheterization
   before the x-ray was taken

6. ___ to tell them if you are allergic to any medication

Estudios Radiológico

INDICACIONES PARA PRUEBAS DE LABORATORIO Y RADIOGRAFÍAS

SPANISH

1. Tiene que estar en ayunas (sin beber ni comer nada) antes de la prueba.

2. Se puede lavar los dientes, pero no tome agua.

3. Antes del examen no debe
   ___ comer
   ___ tomar agua ni ningún otro líquido
   ___ fumar
   ___ masticar chicle
   ___ tomar ninguna medicina
   ___ chupar ninguna pastilla o caramelo

4. Debe comer por lo menos dos horas antes de tomar un purgante.

5. Debe comer una comida ligera la noche antes de la prueba (operación).

6. No debe comer comidas grasosas el día antes del examen.

7. Debe tomarse estas pastillas que son especialmente para esta prueba.

8. Las tabletas contienen una substancia que se puede rastrear durante la prueba y que ayudará a hacer el diagnóstico.

9. Debe seguir estas instrucciones al pie de la letra.

CUANDO USTED LLEGUE PARA HACERSE LA PRUEBA, LE PUEDEN PEDIR:

1. ___ que indique que clase de prueba (análisis) se vino a hacer

2. ___ que les dé la orden escrita del médico

3. ___ que indique si ha comido o bebido algo esa mañana

4. ___ que indique si ha comido o bebido algo después de la medianoche

5. ___ que indique si le han hecho alguna vez una radiografía que haya requerido
   ___ una inyección
   ___ tomar alguna pastilla
   ___ un medicamento especial
   ___ cateterización antes de hacerse la radiografía

6. ___ que les diga es alérgico a algún medicamento

ENGLISH	SPANISH
7. ___ to tell them if you are presently taking any medication	7. ___ que les diga si está tomando actualmente algún medicamento
8. ___ to let them know if you suffer from or have ever suffered from asthma	8. ___ hacerles saber si padece o ha padecido alguna vez de asma
9. ___ to let them know if you suffer from any allergies	9. ___ hacerles saber si padece de alguna alergia

POSSIBLE INDICATIONS DURING THE EXAM | **POSSIBLES INDICACIONES DURANTE LA PRUEBA**

ENGLISH	SPANISH
1. You may use this room to remove your clothes and put on the gown that is on the chair. Tie the gown ___ in the front, ___ in the back.	1. Puede usar este cuarto para desvertirse y ponerse la bata que está en la silla. Amárrese la bata ___ en el frente, ___ por atrás.
2. I have to take an x-ray.	2. Tengo que hacer una radiografía.
3. Breathe deeply.	3. Respire profundamente.
4. Breathe deeply and hold your breath.	4. Respire profundamente y aguante la respiración.
5. You can breathe normally.	5. Puede respirar normalmente.
6. I have to take one more x-ray.	6. Tengo que sacarle una radiografía más.
7. Please wait but do not put on your clothes yet to make sure I don't need to take another x-ray.	7. Por favor, espere un momento pero no se vista todavía para que pueda comprobar si tengo que tomar otra radiografía.
8. We are going to take a series of x-rays.	8. Le vamos a sacar una serie de radiografías.
9. After the first x-rays, we will give you a liquid to drink.	9. Después de las primeras radiografías le daremos un líquido para a tomar.
10. Drink this liquid, please.	10. Tómese este líquido, por favor.
11. After the test, you can have something to eat.	11. Después de la prueba puede comer algo.
12. We are going to give you a barium enema.	12. Le vamos a poner un enema de bario.
13. We are going to turn off the light.	13. Vamos a apagar la luz.
14. This is not going to hurt you, but it may be unpleasant.	14. Esto no le va a causar dolor, pero puede causar cierta molestia.
15. This light is used to examine your intestine.	15. Esta luz es para examinarle el intestino.
16. You can use the bathroom here.	16. Puede usar el servicio (el baño) aquí.
17. I am going to inject this into your vein.	17. Voy a inyectarle esta sustancia en la vena.
18. In this test I am going to take fluid from your spine.	18. En esta prueba le voy a sacar líquido de la columna.
19. This is a cold solution.	19. Esta es una solución fría.

Radiologic Studies

POSSIBLE INDICATIONS DURING THE EXAM

ENGLISH

20. This machine is to take the mucus from your lungs.

21. I am going to insert this tube to
___ take out the phlegm that is bothering you
___ help you void

22. We are going to draw some blood from
___ the vein
___ the finger
___ the ear

23. Leave the cotton (the Band-aid) in place for a few minutes.

24. Call tomorrow to find out the results of the test.

25. We will call to notify you.

Estudios Radiológico

POSSIBLES INDICACIONES DURANTE LA PRUEBA

SPANISH

20. Esta máquina es para extraer el moco de sus pulmones.

21. Voy a ponerle esta sonda
___ para sacarle la flema que le molesta
___ para ayudarle a orinar

22. Le vamos a extraer sangre
___ de la vena
___ del dedo
___ de la oreja

23. Déjese el algodón (la curita) puesto-a por unos minutos.

24. Llame mañana para saber el resultado de la prueba.

25. Le llamaremos para notificarle.

CT Scan

ENGLISH

1. You cannot eat or drink anything 4 to 8 hours before the test.

2. Change into a hospital gown.

3. You will be secured on the table by a strap.

4. You will receive a contrast medium by mouth or by injection.

5. Sometimes you may receive the contrast medium before your test.

6. You will be moved into the scanner; it will scan your body in about 15 minutes.

7. You must remain still to prevent the images from blurring.

8. During the scan you may be asked to hold your breath for a few seconds.

9. You may hear some noises made by the x-ray machine.

10. Remain still. They may need more images to complete the exam.

11. During the test you can usually talk to the technician over an intercom if necessary.

12. If you get nervous and cannot continue the test, you can press a button and let them know and the test will stop.

Tomografía computada

SPANISH

1. No puede comer o beber líquidos de 4 a 8 horas antes del examen.

2. Póngase esta bata.

3. Le ayudarán a sujetarse a la mesa con un cinturón de seguridad.

4. Le administrarán un medio de contraste oralmente por o inyectción.

5. A veces se administra el medio de contraste antes del examen.

6. Pasará al interior del escáner (explorador), el cual explorará su cuerpo en unos 15 minutos.

7. No se mueva para evitar que las imágenes salgan borrosas.

8. Durante la exploración es posible que le indiquen que aguante la respiración por unos segundos.

9. Es posible que oiga los ruidos que hace la máquina de rayos-x.

10. No se mueva. Es posible que necesiten tomar más imágenes para completar el examen.

11. Durante la prueba generalmente puede hablar con el/la técnico-a por el intercomunicador.

12. Si se pone muy nervioso-a y no puede continuar el examen, puede apretar un botón y el examen se descontinuará.

MRI

ENGLISH

▶ The MRI (Magnetic Resonance Image) test is an imaging technique used to produce clear images of the inside of the human body. This test may require signing a consent form.

▶ The MRI personnel has your doctor's orders and will ask you some questions to determine if you can be safely imaged.

▶ The test may require a medication or contrast agent depending on the part of the body that is going to be examined.

▶ When the test begins you will be placed on a table that will slide into the tube-cylinder.

▶ Your position in the tube-cylinder will depend on the part of the body that will be imaged.

▶ If your shoulder, chest, or head is imaged, your feet will not be inside the magnet.

▶ If your feet and knees are imaged, your head will be outside the magnet.

▶ At all times you will be able to press a button located next to your hand to indicate that you want to communicate with the technician.

El IRM

SPANISH

▶ La IRM (Imagen de Resonancia Magnética) es una prueba para reproducir visualmente imágenes de alta calidad del interior del cuerpo humano. Esta prueba puede requerir que el paciente firme un formulario de consentimiento.

▶ El personal del equipo de IRM tiene las indicaciones de su médico y le hará algunas preguntas para determinar si usted puede hacerse la prueba de IRM de manera segura.

▶ Es posible que la prueba requiera que le administren algún medicamento o agente de contraste de acuerdo con la parte del cuerpo que va a ser examinado.

▶ Cuando comience la prueba, lo colocarán en una mesa que se desliza dentro del tubo cilíndrico.

▶ Su posición en el tubo cilíndrico depende de la parte del cuerpo que necesita ser reproducida en la imagen.

▶ Si su hombro, tórax o cabeza van a ser reproducidos en imagen, sus pies no estarán dentro del imán.

▶ Si sus pies y rodillas van a ser reproducidas en la imagen, su cabeza quedará fuera del imán.

▶ En cualquier momento podrá presionar un botón colocado al lado de su mano para indicar que desea comunicarse con el técnico.

DIAGNOSES / DIAGNÓSTICOS

Cardiology Diagnoses	Diagnósticos cardiológico
ENGLISH	**SPANISH**
acute aortic dissection	disección aórtica aguda
acute myocardial infarct	infarto agudo del miocardio
acute pericarditis	pericarditis aguda
aneurismal murmur	soplo aneurismático
angina pectoris	angina del pecho
aortic compression	coartación aórtica
aortic fluid output obstruction	obstrucción de salida del flujo aórtico
aortic leakage	escape aórtico
arrythmogenic right ventricular dysplasia	displasia arritmogénica ventricular derecha
arterial embolism and thrombosis	trombosis y embolismo arterial
atrial fibrillation	fibrilación auricular
atrial flutter	aleteo auricular
atrial myxoma	mixoma auricular
atrial septal defect	comunicación interauricular defectuosa
atrioventricular nodal reentrant tachycardia	taquicardia reentrante nodal auriculoventricular
cardiac arrhythmias	arritmias cardíacas
cardiac hypertrophy	hipertrofía cardíaca
cardiac tamponade	taponamiento cardíaco
chronic alveolar hypoventilation	hipoventilación alveolar crónica
chronic atrial fibrillation	fibrilación auricular crónica
congenital cardiopathy	cardiopatía congénita
congestive heart failure	insuficiencia cardíaca
constrictive pericarditis	pericarditis constrictiva
coronary artery disease	artereopatía coronaria
coronary atherosclerosis	aterosclerosis coronaria
coronary thrombosis	trombosis coronaria
cyanotic congenital heart disease	cardiopatía congénita cianótica
endocarditis	endocarditis
heart failure	fallo cardíaco, paro cardíaco
hyperkalemia	hiperpotasiemia
hyperparatiroidism	hiperparatiroidismo
hypertensive cardiopathy	cardiopatía hipertensiva
left ventricular dilation	dilatación ventricular izquierda
middiastolic murmur	soplo mediodiastólico
mitral stenosis	estenosis mitral

Cardiology Diagnoses	Diagnósticos cardiológico
ENGLISH	**SPANISH**
mitral regurgitation	insuficiencia, reflujo mitral
mitral valve infectious endocarditis	endocarditis infecciosa de la válvula mitral
mitral valve prolapse	prolapso de la válvula mitral
myocardial ischemia	isquemia del miocardio
myocarditis neonatorum	miocarditis del neonato
myocardial infarction	infarto del miocardio
myocardial rupture	ruptura del miocardio
pericardial effusion	efusión pericárdica
pericarditis	pericarditis
peripartum cardiomyopathy	cardiomiopatía peripartum
primary valvular aortic insufficiency	insuficiencia valvular aórtica primaria
right auricle dilation	dilatación auricular derecha
right auricular tumors	tumores auriculares derechos
right ventricular infarction	infarto del ventrículo derecho
stenosis mitral	mitral estenosis
subacute bacterial endocarditis	endocarditis bacteriana subaguda
supraventricular tachycardia	taquicardia supraventricular
tachycardia	taquicardia
tricuspid defficiency	insuficiencia tricuspídea
tricuspid valve disease	enfermedad de la válvula tricúspide
tricuspid stenosis	estenosis de la válvula tricúspide
tromboangiitis	tromboangiitis

Pulmonary Diagnoses

ENGLISH

Diagnósticos pulmonar

SPANISH

ENGLISH	SPANISH
acute bronchitis	bronquitis aguda
bronchiectasis	bronquiectasia
chronic airway disorder	trastorno crónico de las vías respiratorias
atelectasis	atelectasia
congenital atelectasis	atelectasia congénita
coal workers disease	enfermedad de los carboneros
pneumonia	neumonía
walking pneumonia	neumonía migratoria o errante
streptococcal neumonia	neumonía por estreptococos
staphylococcal pneumonia	neumonía estafilocócica
lobar pneumonia	neumonía lobular
legionnaire's disease	enfermedad de los legionarios
silicosis	silicosis
pulmonary embolism	embolismo pulmonar
asthma	asma
pleurisy	pleuresía
respiratory failure	fallo respiratorio
lung abscess	absceso del pulmón
pleural effusion	derrame pleural
allergic bronchopulmonary aspergillosis	aspergilosis pulmonar alérgica
bronchogenic carcinoma	carcinoma broncogénico
dyspnea	disnea
hemoptisis	hemoptisis
paroxysmal nocturnal dyspnea	dispnea nocturna paroxística
adult respiratory distress syndrome	malestar respiratorio en la persona adulta
secondary bacterial supra-infections	suprainfecciones bacterianas secundarias
emphysema	enfisema
chronic bronchitis	bronquitis crónica
acute bronchitis	bronquitis aguda
P. carinii pneumonia	neumonía *P. carinii*
bronchopulmonary aspergillosis	aspergilosis broncopulmonar
pulmonary edema	edema pulmonar

Cancer Diagnoses

ENGLISH

Acute Lymphoblastic leucemia (childhood)	
Adrenal cancer	
Adrenocortical carcinoma	
Anal cancer	
Astrocytoma (cerebral, childhood)	
Betel cancer	
Bile duct cancer	
Bladder cancer (childhood)	
Bone cancer	
Brain cancer	
Brain tumor, ependymoma (childhood)	
Brain tumor, medulloblastoma (childhood)	
Breast cancer	
Bronchial adenoma	
Basal cell carcinoma	
Cancer en cuirasse	
Cancer of the heart	
Cardiac sarcoma	
Central nervous system lymphoma	
Cervical cancer	
Chimney sweep's cancer	
Cholangiosarcoma	
Colorectal cancer	
Ductal carcinoma in situ	
Ductal invasive carcinoma	
Endometrial cancer	
Epithelial cancer	
Epithelial ovarian cancer	
Esophagial cancer	
Eye cancer	
Familial cancer	
Follicular lymphoma	
Follicular thyroid cancer	
Genital cancer	
Glandular cancer	
Hodgkin's lymphoma	
Hypothalamic glioma (childhood)	

Diagnósticos de cáncer

SPANISH

Leucemia linfoblástica aguda (niñez)
Cáncer de las glándulas suprarenales
Carcinoma adrenocortical
Cáncer anal
Astrocitoma (cerebral, niñez)
Cáncer de la mucosa de la mejilla
Cáncer del conducto biliar
Cáncer de la vejiga (niñez)
Cáncer de los huesos
Cáncer del cerebro
Tumor cerebral, ependimoma (niñez)
Tumor cerebral, meduloblastoma (niñez)
Cáncer de la mama, del seno
Adenoma bronquial
Carcinoma de células basales
Cáncer progresivo del tórax
Cáncer cardíaco
Sarcoma cardíaco
Linfoma del sistema nervioso central
Cáncer del cuello uterino
Cáncer del escroto, cáncer ocupacional
Colangiosarcoma
Cáncer colorectal
Carcinoma ductal in situ
Carcinoma ductal invasivo
Cáncer endometrioso
Carcinoma epitelial
Cáncer epitelial ovárico
Cáncer esofágico
Cáncer del ojo, ocular
Cáncer familiar
Linfoma folicular
Cáncer folicular de la tiroides
Cáncer de los genitales
Cáncer glandular
Linfoma de Hodgkin
Glioma hipotalámico (niñez)

Cancer Diagnoses

ENGLISH

Kidney cancer
Larynx cancer
Leptomeningeal cancer
Leukemia
Liposarcoma
Liver cancer
Lobular carcinoma in situ
Lobular invasive carcinoma
Local cancer
Localizad gallbladder cancer
Lung cancer
Lymphoma
Medular cancer
Mesothelioma
Mucinous cancer
Non-Hodgkin's lymphoma
Oral cancer
Ovarian cancer
Penis cancer
Prostate cancer
Rectal cancer
Retinoblastoma
Skin cancer
Small intestine cancer
Throat cancer
Thyroid cancer
Tongue cancer
Tubular cancer
Ureter cancer
Urinary system cancer
Uterine cancer

Diagnósticos de cáncer

SPANISH

Cáncer del riñón
Cáncer de la laringe
Cáncer leptomeníngico
Leucemia, cáncer de la sangre
Liposarcoma
Cáncer del hígado
Carcinoma lobular in situ
Carcinoma lobular invasivo
Cáncer local
Cáncer localizado de la vesícula biliar
Cáncer del pulmón
Linfoma
Cáncer medular
Mesotelioma
Cáncer mucinoso
Linfoma non-Hodgkin's
Cáncer bucal
Cáncer ovárico
Cáncer del pene
Cáncer de la próstata
Cáncer del recto
Retinoblastoma
Cáncer de la piel
Cáncer del intestino delgado
Cáncer de la garganta
Cáncer de la tiroides
Cáncer de la lengua
Cáncer tubular
Cáncer del uréter
Cáncer del sistema urinario
Cáncer uterino

SEXUALLY TRANSMITTED DISEASES (STD) / ENFERMEDADES VENÉREAS

SICKNESS	TRANSMISSION	ENFERMEDAD	CONTAGIO
candidiasis *Candida albicans*, fungus, yeast infection; thick, creamy discharge	sexual contact, use of towels or clothing belonging to an infected person, or caused by a low pH in the vagina	**candidiasis** *Cándida albicans*, infección fungosa caracterizada por flujo cremoso	contacto sexual, uso de toallas o ropa de una persona infectada, o por tener el pH bajo en la vagina
chlamiydia *Chlamydia Trachomatis*, causative agents of urethritis, lymphogranuloma, prostatitis, salpingitis, newborn conjunctivitis	sexual contact; newborns may be infected during childbirth	**clamidia** *Chlamydia Trachomatis*, agente causante de uretritis, linfogranuloma, prostatitis, salpingitis, conjuntivitis del neonato	contacto sexual, o de la madre al feto durante el parto
condyloma acuminatum Venereal warts	by sexual contact or by using towels belonging to an infected person	**condiloma acuminatum** Verrugas venéreas	por contacto sexual o por el uso de toallas de una persona infectada
genital herpes virus type 2 causing blisters and sores on the genitals	anal, oral, vaginal sexual contact at the outbreak of the disease; touching blisters and sores; can be transmitted to the newborn at birth	**herpes de los genitales, virus de tipo 2** causante de ampollas y ulceraciones en los genitales	contacto sexual anal, oral o vaginal; cuando la enfermedad brota; por contacto con ampollas y ulceraciones
gonorrhea *gonococcus Neisseria*, infection invading the genitourinary tract, pharynx, anus	anal, oral, vaginal sexual contact; from mother to child during childbirth; period of incubation from 3 to 5 days	**gonorrea** *gonococo Neisseria*, infección que invade el tracto genitourinario, la faringe y el recto	contacto sexual rectal, oral o vaginal; de la madre a la criatura durante el parto; período de incubación de 3 a 5 días
hepatitis: A-, B-, C-, and D-type viruses inflammation of the liver; other serious disorders are also present	sexual contact, transfusion of contaminated blood; contact through abrasions, tiny cuts, or wounds with the blood of an infected person; or by the mother at childbirth or through breastfeeding	**hepatitis: viruses de tipo A, B, C y D (delta)** inflamación del hígado, manifestándose en otros trastornos serios	por contacto sexual, transfusión de sangre contaminada; contacto a través de heridas o abrasiones con la sangre de una persona infectada; por la madre durante el parto o durante la lactancia

SICKNESS	TRANSMISSION	ENFERMEDAD	CONTAGIO
hepatitis B	usually involves oral-anal sex	**hepatitis B**	generalmente resulta de contacto sexual oral-anal
HPV virus human *papillomavirus*, considered a strong cocarcinogen; generally present with other STD diseases	venereal disease, characterized by warts, can expand by autoinoculation in the genitals and anus	**virus HPV** *papillomavirus* humano, considerado un cocarcinógeno fuerte; generalmente presente con otras enfermedades venéreas	enfermedad venérea, caracterizada por verrugas o condilomas en los genitales y el ano que se expanden por autoinoculación
pubic lice, crabs *pthirus pubis* discomfort produced by itching	sexual contact, transmitted in bed linen, towels, toilet seats	**el piojo púbico** *pthirus pubis*, malestar por intensa picazón	contacto sexual, transmitido en toallas, sabanas de cama y asientos de retrete, (inodoro)
syphilis *Treponema pallidum*, 10 to 90 day incubation period; ulceration, warts in the genital area; invades the bloodstream to different organs	anal, oral, vaginal sexual contact, by sores through mucous membranes or abrasions or by touching a chancre; from mother to child; in pregnancy can cause stillbirth or congenital syphilis	**sífilis** *Treponema pallidum*, de 10 a 90 días de incubación; úlcera primera, verrugas en el área genital; se extiende por la vía sanguínea a diferentes órganos	contacto sexual rectal, oral, vaginal, por contacto con ulceraciones a través de membranas mucosas o abrasiones o al tocar un chancro; durante el embarazo puede causar sífilis congénita o muerte al feto
trichomoniasis *Trichomonas vaginalis*, causes foul-smelling vaginal discharge, itching, burning	sexual activity, infected semen on washcloths, bedclothes	**tricomoniasis** *trichomonas vaginalis*, causa flujo vaginal de olor desagradable, picazón, ardor	actividad sexual, semen infeccioso en toallas o ropa de cama

Testing of HIV should be administered to patients that have genital ulcers caused by *T. palidum* or *H. ducreyi*, which are cases of genital herpes, chancroid and syphilis. When chancroid is diagnosed, testing of HIV would be a precuaution, and 3 months later the patient should be retested for syphilis and HIV if the test of chancroid was negative.

Pruebas del VIH deben ser administradas a los pacientes con úlceras genitales causadas por *T. palidium* o *H. ducreyi* que son casos de herpes genitales de chancro y sífilis. Cuando hay un diagnóstico de chancro las pruebas de VIH se harían como precaución, y tres meses más tarde el paciente debe hacerse pruebas de sífilis y de VIH si la prueba de chancro fue negativa.

STD testing is available for sexually active men and women. / Las pruebas de enfermedades venéreas son accesibles a hombres y mujeres que son sexualmente activos.

► HIV serology / serología de VIH
► syphilis serology / serología de sífilis
► urethral culture or urine test for chlamydia / cultivo uretral o de la orina para clamidia
► pharyngeal culture for gonorrhea and chlamydia / cultivo faríngeo para gonorrea y clamidia
► rectal gonorrhea and chlamidya culture / cultivo rectal de gonorrea y clamidia

HIV AND AIDS / EL VIH Y EL SIDA

Questions and Answers on HIV and AIDS	Preguntas y respuestas sobre el VIH y el SIDA
ENGLISH	**SPANISH**
1. What causes AIDS (*acquired immune deficiency syndrome*)? The retrovirus HIV (*human immunodeficiency virus*)[1] causes AIDS. AIDS is a late manifestation of HIV.	1. ¿Qué causa el SIDA (*síndrome de inmunodeficiencia adquirida*)? El VIH (*virus de la inmunodeficiencia humana*[2]) es el retrovirus causante del SIDA. SIDA es una manifestación tardía de VIH.
2. How does an HIV infection occur? HIV is transmitted through four body fluids: a) blood b) semen c) vaginal fluid d) breast milk	2. ¿Cómo ocurre una infección de VIH? El VIH es transmitido a través de cuatro líquidos corporales: a) sangre b) semen c) secreción vaginal d) leche materna
3. How does HIV attack the body system? The infecting virus HIV attacks the immune system that protects the body against infections. It overpowers the immune cells CD4 and reproduces itself in them, thus debilitating the immune system. This evolution opens the door to "opportunistic" infections that attack a body already low in antibodies. When the body is at its lowest level count of CD4, or T cells, it is vulnerable to AIDS.	3. ¿Cómo ataca el VIH al organismo? El virus VIH ataca el sistema inmunológico que protege el organismo contra las infecciones. Comienza a dominar las células CD4 y se reproduce en ellas; de esta manera debilita el sistema inmune. Esta evolución abre la puerta a infecciones "oportunistas" que atacan un organismo bajo en anticuerpos. Cuando el organismo presenta el nivel más bajo de células CD4, o T, es vulnerable al SIDA.

Questions and Answers on HIV and AIDS

Preguntas y respuestas sobre el VIH y el SIDA

ENGLISH	SPANISH

4. How a transmission occurs:
   a) HIV is transmitted by having intercourse (vaginal or anal) with an infected partner. If one of the partners is infected by HIV, the virus is transmitted to his or her partner during intercourse by introducing the infected semen or vaginal secretion through the mucous membranes or through a small cut or sore hardly visible.
   b) By direct blood contact such as injection with exchanged drug needles and syringes between drug addicts infected by AIDS; in direct transmission by tainted blood transfusions, or by accident if it enters the system through a percutaneous lesion when handling infected blood.[3]
   c) Transmission from hemophiliacs who had been treated with Factor VIII[5] (contaminated platelets) to their sexual partners without knowing that they were carriers.
   d) The transmission of HIV from the infected mother to the fetus (perinatal or vertical transmission)[7] during pregnancy, or during labor and birth to the newborn has approximately 20% probability of transmission if she has not received a drug treatment to reduce this probability.

4. Cómo ocurre una transmisión de VIH:
   a) VIH se transmite por medio del acto sexual (vaginal o anal) con una persona infectada. Si una de las personas está infectada por VIH el/ella puede transmitir el virus al otro en el semen o la secreción vaginal a través de las membranas mucosas o una pequeña cortada apenas visible.
   b) Por contacto sanguíneo directo tal como una inyección con agujas y jeringas intercambiadas entre drogadictos infectados por el SIDA; en transfusión de sangre contaminada, o por accidente si sucediera una exposición durante el manejo de sangre infectada[4] a través de una lesión percutánea.
   c) Transmisión por hemofílicos que habían sido tratados con Factor VIII[6] (de plaquetas infectadas) a su pareja sexual sin saber que eran portadores del virus VIH.
   d) La transmisión de la madre infectada por VIH al feto (transmisión perinatal o vertical) durante el embarazo, o en los labores del parto, el bebé tiene una probabilidad de transmisión de aproximadamente un 20% si ella no ha recibido tratamiento para evitar la probabilidad de transmisión.

5. What is done today to avoid PNT/ TMC[8]? Clinical studies have indicated that if the delivery is done by caesarean section before labor begins, it would be possible to reduce the probability of HIV-1 infection to the newborn. This is a procedure that is done in combination with AZT[9] therapy.

5. ¿Qué se ha hecho para evitar la transmision perinatal (TMH)[8]? Estudios clínicos han indicado que si antes de comenzar la labor del parto se realiza una cesárea combinada con un tratamiento de terapia de AZT[10] que se hace durante el embarazo, la transmisión perinatal disminuye considerablemente.

Questions and Answers on HIV and AIDS

Preguntas y respuestas sobre el VIH y el SIDA

ENGLISH	SPANISH

6. What is the HIV transmission probability to an infant through the mother's milk? The infected mother's milk contains HIV-1 virus, which is a viable means of infection with approx. 12% of probability of transmission. If the mother is not following any treatment to avoid transmission during pregnancy, the risk is very high. In 1994 a clinical analysis "076" determined that women who submitted voluntarily to AZT therapy would diminish considerably the probability of HIV infection to their children.

6. ¿Cuál es la probabilidad de un neonato infectarse con VIH a través de la leche materna? La leche infectada de la madre que contiene el virus VIH-1, es una fuente de infección que proporciona un 12% de probabilidad de transmisión. Si la madre no sigue ningún tratamiento para evitar transmisión durante el embarazo, el riesgo es muy alto. En 1994 el análisis clínico "076" determinó que las mujeres que se sometieron voluntariamente a la terapia de AZT disminuyeron considerablemente la probabilidad de infección de VIH a su hijo-a.

7. What recommendations are given to HIV infected pregnant women?

- ▶ To submit voluntarily to a therapy of drug inhibitor's program.
- ▶ To follow a therapeutic regimen of antiretroviral drugs reducers of VIH and perinatal transmission.
- ▶ To keep visits and therapy with their physician as regularly as recommended.
- ▶ To take her medication accordingly
- ▶ To request assistance to monitor the progress of the disease in herself and her baby.
- ▶ To be aware of any drug interaction effect and report it to their doctors.

7. ¿Qué recomendaciones se han dado a mujeres embarazadas infectadas por VIH?

- ▶ Someterse voluntariamente a una terapia de medicamentos de inhibidores de retrovirus.
- ▶ Seguir un régimen terapéutico de fármacos antiretrovíricos reductores de VIH y de la transmisión perinatal.
- ▶ Asistir regularmente a las citas con el médico y seguir con regularidad la terapia recomendada.
- ▶ Pedir asistencia para poder seguir la evolución del virus en ella misma y su bebé.
- ▶ Estar al tanto de cualquier efecto inesperado de las medicinas que tome y reportarlo al personal médico que le atiende.

---

[1] Also called human T-lymphotrophic virus.
[2] También llamado virus T-linfotrófico humano.
[3] There is a very small percentage of health providers who have been infected by accident with HIV.
[4] Existe un porciento muy bajo de asistentes de salud que se han infectado accidentalmente por HIV.
[5] Factor VIII made by donated blood from various donors is now treated to avoid transmission.
[6] El Factor VIII hecho por sangre donada por varios donantes se trata ahora para evitar transmisión.
[7] PNT perinatal transmission / transmisión perinatal.
[8] TMH transmisión de madre a hijo / TMC transmission of mother to child.
[9] An analog inhibitor of replication of HIV virus.
[10] Análogo inhibidor de replicación del VIH.

Observations Related to HIV and AIDS

ENGLISH

Observaciones generales en relación con VIH y el SIDA

SPANISH

HTV *seronegative* means that the test does not show HIV antibodies in the bloodstream.

VIH *seronegativo* quiere decir que la prueba no indica la presencia de anticuerpos VIH en la corriente sanguínea.

---

1. Why should you be tested for HIV?:
   a) you think you may have had any kind of sexual contact with an infected person.
   b) you have used intravenous drugs and exchanged needles or syringes with an infected person.
   c) you had sexual contact with a person who belongs to a *"high risk"* group.
   d) you are pregnant and have doubts about whether your sexual partner belongs to a *"high risk"* group.

1. ¿Cuándo debe usted hacerse la prueba del VIH?:
   a) ha tenido cualquier tipo de contacto sexual con una persona infectada.
   b) ha usado drogas intravenosas o compartido agujas o jeringuillas con personas infectadas.
   c) ha tenido contacto sexual con una persona que pertenece a un grupo de *"alto riesgo"*.
   d) está embarazada y tiene dudas si su compañero está asociado a un grupo de *"alto riesgo"*.

HTV *seropositive* means that there are HIV antibodies in the bloodstream.

VIH *seropositivo* quiere decir que existen anticuerpos de VIH en la corriente sanguínea.

---

2. It is very important to follow a safe sexual conduct.

2. Es sumamente importante evitar una conducta sexual arriesgada.

---

3. You are capable of being infected by the virus even if you are exposed only once.

3. Usted puede ser infectado-a por el virus aunque haya estado expuesto-a una sola vez.

---

4. Does the health laboratory official have the obligation to report the results of the test to the health authorities?
   Yes, it has to be reported to the health authorities and also it has to be registered in the infected person's medical record. Other persons who also have had sexual contact with the infected person should be notified in order to have a serologic test and determine if there is infection.

4. ¿Tiene el profesional de salud o director del laboratorio que reporter resultados de la prueba a las autoridades de salubridad? Sí, se debe reportar a las autoridades los casos de VIH y de SIDA, y también debe ser registrado en el expediente médico de la persona infectada. Otras personas que tuvieron contacto sexual con la persona infectada deben ser notificadas para que se hagan una prueba serológica y puedan determinar si hay contagio.

---

serostatus unknown refers to any person that has never been tested for HIV infection.

seroestado desconocido indica el estado de una persona que nunca se ha hecho una prueba de VIH.

Observationes Related to HIV and AIDS

Observaciones generales en relación con VIH y el SIDA

ENGLISH	SPANISH
5. If the results of your tests are positive, you should be right away under the care of an immunologist or an AIDS knowledgeable health professional.	5. Si el resultado de las pruebas es positivo, usted debe estar en seguida bajo el cuidado de un inmunólogo o profesional de salud con conocimientos del tratamiento del SIDA.
6. It would be helpful if you would join a support group.	6. Sería beneficioso que usted se asociara a un grupo de apoyo.
Note: Concerning questions 4 and 5. All AIDS clinics observe confidentiality, some observe total anonymity; the patient is observed and identified only by a code number. Results of the test are only given to the patient by his doctor.	*Nota:* Respecto a las preguntas 4 y 5. Todas las clínicas de SIDA observan confidencialidad, algunas observan completa anonimidad; el paciente es asistido y se identifica por un número o código. Los resultados de las pruebas son dados solamente al paciente por su médico.

ALZHEIMER'S DISEASE

Dementia is a brain disorder that affects parts of the brain that control thought, memory and language. Alzheimer's disease, AD, is the most common form of dementia in older people, although it may occur in earlier ages as well. It is a severe and devastating disease that impairs the person's ability to carry out activities of daily living. Symptoms continue to increase in severity as the disease progresses, and includes severe loss of memory, confusion, disorientation, incapacity to recognize familiar persons or objects, inability to make coordinated movements, anxiety, and even hallucinations.

Cause

There is still great uncertainty among scientists as to what causes Alzheimer's disease. Dr. Alois Alzheimer, after whom the disease is named, found "clumps" (today called amyloid plaques) and "tangles" in the brain of a patient who died of a severe mental condition. It is believed that the presence of these plaques and tangles is a sign of AD, but it is not clear exactly what role they play in the disease. The presence of plaques and tangles can only be determined after death, but a skilled physician generally can accurately diagnose Alzheimer's disease through other means in about 90% of the cases. As the population in general lives to an older age, and the baby boomer generation starts to reach the critical age for the disease, it is expected that the number of AD patients will greatly increase in the next few years.

It is thought that certain genetic factors may interact with non-genetic ones causing the disease. There is one known genetic factor called alipoprotein E (ApoE) that carries cholesterol in the blood. Although it is found in everyone's body, only about 15% of people carry a form of the gene that is related to AD. Studies to find the presence of other genes that may be Alzheimer-related are ongoing. There is also growing evidence that some disorders such as brain tumors, blood vessel diseases, or diabetes, can increase the risk of AD as well, so it is important to treat these diseases and follow all indications as to diet, exercise, etc.

Diagnosis

The health professional can obtain some important information by questioning the patient or his or her family members about the person's general health, medical history, and ability to carry out activities of daily living. The health professional can also administer tests in language, problem solving, arithmetic, and other matters, as well as physical tests such as blood and urine analysis or a brain scan. Sometimes test results lead to other possible causes for the person's symptoms.

Treatment

There is no cure at this time for AD. However, by treating it through several means, the progress of the disease can be slowed down and/or the patient may find relief from some of the symptoms. Non-drug strategies, such as behavioral techniques and environmental modification (changing the person's environment to resolve challenges and obstacles to comfort, security and ease of mind) should always be tried first.

Some drugs, such as tacrine, donepezil, rivastigmine, or galantamine, have been helpful in preventing some symptoms from becoming worse for a limited time, or in controlling symptoms such as sleeplessness and anxiety. It is important to remember that these medications can only help with some symptoms, and do not cure the disease. Currently, there are a number of new drugs being studied. There is hope that at least one of these drugs will go beyond simply helping, and will actually be able to alter the course of the disease.

Care of the Patient

At the onset of the disease, the patient usually receives day-to-day care from a spouse, companion, or relative. As the disease progresses, the patient becomes more difficult to manage, affecting the family life and mental health of caregivers. It is important for the caregiver to seek help from groups such as the Alzheimer's Association for services, support groups, and education.

Alzheimer's Association
www.alz.org
e-mail: info@alz.org
24/7 Helpline: 1-800-272-3900

LA ENFERMEDAD DE ALZHEIMER

La demencia es un trastorno cerebral que afecta partes del cerebro que controlan el pensamiento, la memoria y el lenguaje. La enfermedad de Alzheimer, AD, es la forma más común de demencia que afecta a personas de edad avanzada, aunque a veces ocurre en personas más jóvenes. Es una enfermedad devastadora que incapacita a la persona a desempeñar las más sencillas actividades cotidianas. Se manifiestan síntomas que aumentan en severidad al progresar la enfermedad, incluyendo la pérdida de la memoria, confusión, desorientación, incapacidad de reconocer a familiares y objetos, falta de coordinación en los movimientos, ansiedad y hasta alucinaciones.

Causa

La presencia de estas anomalías solamente se puede detectar después de la muerte, pero un buen médico generalmente puede diagnosticar la enfermedad correctamente en approximente 90% de los casos. El Dr. Alois Alzheimer, por quien se ha nombrado la enfermedad, informó que después de la muerte de una de sus pacientas de una enfermedad mental severa, había encontrado en el cerebro de la misma ciertos depósitos anormales formados por una proteína amilácea (beta amyloid) y otra anomalía, una acumulación de fibras nerviosas entrecruzadas (neurofibrilary tangles). No hay seguridad hasta ahora que la presencia de estos dos elementos sean una posible causa de la enfermedad.

El diagnóstico de la enfermedad es solamente probable, y en el mejor de los casos, se declara posible. No obstante, en centros especializados, se hacen diagnósticos correctos de los casos en un 90% de ellos. La población en general vive actualmente hasta una edad más avanzada, y con el prospecto del "boomer generation" (la generación nacida después de la Segunda Guerra mundial) de llegar a la edad riesgosa de ser víctima de la enfermedad, se espera que el número de pacientes de AD aumente en los próximos años.

Se cree también que ciertos factores genéticos interactúan con otros factores no genéticos causando esta dura enfermedad. Actualmente se reconoce el factor genético alipoproteína E (ApoE) que conduce el colesterol en la sangre como factor, y aunque este gene se encuentra en todas las personas, sólo cerca de un 15% tienen una forma del gene que se ha relacionado con AD. Se realizan continuos estudios para descubrir la presencia de otros genes que puedan estar relacionados con la enfermedad. Existe una evidencia creciente que algunos trastornos médicos tales como tumores cerebrales, enfermedades vasculares, diabetes, y otras enfermedades pueden aumentar el riesgo de AD, por lo cual es muy importante tratar la enfermedad y seguir todas las indicaciones sobre dietas, ejercicios, y pruebas posibles.

Diagnóstico

El profesional de la salud puede obtener cierta información importante interrogando al paciente o a los miembros de su familia acerca de su salud en general, su historial medico y su habilidad de llevar a cabo actividades rutinarias del diario vivir. El profesional de la salud también puede llevar a cabo pruebas que midan el nivel de lengua o nivel lingüístico del paciente, su capacidad de resolver problemas, sus habilidades matemáticas y de otra índole así como recabar exámenes y análisis médicos tales como los análisis de sangre u orina o llevar a cabo una tomografía axial computarizada del cerebro. A veces el resultado de dichas pruebas y exámenes médicos apuntan a otras causas para explicar la sintomatología del paciente.

Tratamiento

En la actualidad no existe cura conocida para la enfermedad de Alzheimer. Sin embargo, a través de la aplicación de varios tratamientos diferentes, el progreso de la enfermedad puede reducirse y/o el paciente puede obtener alivio de algunos de sus síntomas a través de dichos tratamientos. Las estrategias naturales que no involucran el uso terapéutico de fármacos y drogas tal como las técnicas de cambios de comportamiento y entorno del paciente (el cambiar el medio y el entorno del paciente a fin de resolver los retos y obstáculos que se le presentan en relación a su seguridad, comodidad y tranquilidad) siempre se deben intentar antes que las terapias con medicamentos.

Algunos fármacos tales como la tacrina, el donepezil, la rivastigmina y la galantamina han sido de gran ayuda para prevenir, por un tiempo limitado, que algunos síntomas empeoren o para manejar o controlar otros síntomas tales como la ansiedad y el insomnio. Es importante recordar que dichos medicamentos sólo pueden ayudar con el alivio de algunos síntomas, es decir sus efectos son meramente paliativos y no constituyen, en si mismos, una cura para esta enfermedad. Actualmente, existen una serie de nuevos medicamentos cuyos efectos están siendo estudiados y se tiene la esperanza de que algunos de estos nuevos medicamentos experimentales puedan ser más que simples paliativos y que en un futuro próximo puedan en verdad alterar el curso de esta enfermedad.

Cuidado de los pacientes

Cuando la enfermedad se manifiesta, el/la paciente generalmente recibe asistencia diaria de un ser querido, de una persona acompañante, o de algún familiar. A medida que la enfermedad avanza se hace más difícil el manejo del/la paciente. Es entonces muy importante para quien le esté atendiendo obtener toda la información posible a través de la "Asociación de Alzheimer" y grupos de soporte y educación sobre servicios disponibles para asistir a los enfermos.

Alzheimer's Association
www.alz.org
e-mail: info@alz.org
24/7 Helpline: 1-800-272-3900

Different Stages of Alzheimer Disease / Diferentes fases de la enfermedad de Alzheimer

Phases 1 and 2 / Primera y Segunda fase	Mild dementia that precedes senility may come to an end; forgetfulness, no significant brain change; the patient is able to perform most of his daily activities; most significant early symptom is loss of short-term memory.	Estado leve de demencia que precede a la de senilidad y que puede dejar de avanzar; falta de memoria sin producirse cambios mayores en el cerebro; continuación con las actividades diarias; el síntoma más significativo es la pérdida de la memoria inmediata.
Phase 3 / Tercera fase	Moderate dementia. Still able to perform many of the daily living activities; frustration and anger start to set in as the inability to remember names, facts, and faces becomes progressively more acute; patient is still aware of what is happening to him.	Demencia moderada. El paciente todavía puede desempeñar muchas de las actividades diarias; comienza a sentir frustración e ira al no poder recordar muchos nombres, hechos y caras; todavía está consciente de lo que le está sucediendo.
Phase 4 / Cuarta fase	Mild Alzheimer. The patient is very confused and starts to misplace things as memory is getting worse; difficulty in carrying out daily activities; although patient is aware of a problem, he does not seem to think it is of major concern.	Estado leve de Alzheimer. El paciente está muy confuso y empieza a situar cosas fuera de su lugar común; la memoría se va empeorando; tiene dificultad en llevar a cabo actividades cotidianas; reconoce que existe un problema, pero no le concieme.
Phase 5 / Quinta fase	Moderate Alzheimer. Patient needs custodial care; early dementia will cause him/her to be very disoriented; anger and frustration increase due to severe lapses of memory.	Estado moderado de Alzheimer. El paciente requiere estar bajo custodia; la incipiente demencia le desorienta grandemente; largos lapsos de la memoria aumentan la ira y la frustración.
Phase 6 / Sexta fase	Moderately severe Alzheimer's. The patient has almost a total loss of memory; unable to take care of himself in any way; increased anger, hostility; patient may become combative and develop fear of water.	Alzheimer moderadamente severa. Casi total pérdida de la memoria; el paciente no puede desempeñar las actividades diarias; incremento en la ira y hostilidad; en esta fase se vuelve combativo y muestra fobia al agua.

DIABETES

Diabetes is a serious illness caused by a metabolic disorder that affects the capacity of the body to transform food into energy. Part of what we eat is transformed into a type of sugar called glucose that travels in the blood through the body. The glucose is then stored in the cells in order to be used as energy. But without the hormone insulin, glucose can't get into the cells. The glucose remains in the bloodstream and the cells are starved of their energy source.

Diabetes results when the body does not produce enough insulin. The World Health Organization recognizes three main forms of diabetes: type 1, type 2, and gestational diabetes. Type 1 diabetes is caused by the autoimmune destruction of the cells that produce insulin. In type 2 and gestational diabetes, while the pancreas is still able to produce insulin, either it is not able to produce enough insulin or the cells in the body are insulin resistant. Though not actually a type of diabetes, pre-diabetes is a medical condition that often leads to type 2 diabetes.

General Diabetes Symptoms

blurry vision
extreme hunger
frequent urination
increased fatigue
excessive thirst
irritability
weight loss even with increased appetite

Pre-diabetes

Pre-diabetes occurs when the blood glucose levels are higher than normal, but not to the levels reached in type 2 diabetes. Testing and medical supervision are important to determine the state of pre-diabetes. While pre-diabetes often leads to type 2 diabetes, it is possible to delay or prevent type 2 diabetes from developing by managing your blood glucose, making changes in your diet, and increasing your level of physical activity.

Gestational Diabetes

Gestational diabetes occurs in pregnant women who did not have diabetes before their pregnancy but developed high blood sugar (hyperglycemia) during pregnancy. The hormones during pregnancy cause insulin resistance in women genetically predisposed to develop this condition. It affects the mother in late pregnancy, after the baby's body has been formed, so usually gestational diabetes does not cause the birth defects seen in cases where the woman was diabetic prior to her pregnancy. Nevertheless, if not treated or controlled properly, it can lead to serious problems for the baby and mother. Medical help and supervision are very important. Gestational diabetes is usually resolved at the end of the pregnancy.

Type 1 Diabetes Mellitus

Type 1 diabetes is also known as insulin-dependent or juvenile diabetes because it is usually discovered in children and young adults. It generally appears in people younger than 25. It is a chronic and incurable disease, the exact cause of which is still unknown. There is some certainty that genetics and external factors play a part. The onset of type 1 seems to be triggered by an outside factor such as a viral infection or exposure to certain chemicals or drugs.

In type 1 diabetes, the beta cells of the pancreas produce no insulin. Without a sufficient amount of insulin, the glucose stays in the bloodstream instead of being stored in the cells of the body. As a result, the person may feel hungry even after eating. The build up of glucose in the bloodstream can also cause the afflicted person to be uncommonly thirsty, resulting in increased urination.

Treatment

The onset of type 1 diabetes is rather sudden and severe and the initial treatment may require hospitalization. Beyond that, the patient will probably need weekly visits to the doctor until he or she has good control of their blood glucose level. There are several tests that can be used to diagnose diabetes. Once it is diagnosed, the immediate concern is to treat the ketoacidosis (excess of ketones, acids in the blood) and high blood glucose levels in the body.

Clinically, type 1 diabetes is treated with insulin. Insulin will allow the glucose in the blood to enter the cells causing it to lower the blood sugar. It can be administered by an injection under the skin with a syringe or through an infusion pump that delivers the insulin continuously. Insulin preparations differ and the health care professional should direct the patient as to the type of insulin, the dose required and the correct mode of administration. In addition, the level of glucose in the blood requires constant monitoring through testing. With the help of the health professional, the patient should be able to learn how to do careful self-testing of blood glucose. According to the readings of the blood glucose levels, insulin injections may be needed from 1 to 4 times a day. The amount of carbohydrates and the intake of insulin are highly correlated and the health professional should be able to help the patient establish the right balance.

The external aspects of the treatment consist in proper diet (planning of meals is very important), weight control, and proper exercise. It is also strongly advised that the individual take care of the feet by checking every day for signs of infection, check their vision yearly, visit the dentist twice a year, not smoke, and drink alcohol moderately or not at all.

Type 2 Diabetes Mellitus

Type 2 diabetes, also known as non-insulin dependent, adult-onset diabetes, or obesity-related diabetes, is the most common type of diabetes. It is usually seen in adults over 40 years of age, although an increasing number of younger adults and children are being diagnosed with the disease. In type 2 diabetes, the pancreas does not make enough insulin or the body tissues and muscles become resistant to the insulin. As a result, sugar accumulates in the bloodstream and your cells can become starved for energy.

Like type 1 diabetes, it is a chronic and incurable disease, but it is possible to manage type 2 diabetes without medication. While the exact cause of type 2 diabetes is still unknown, it appears that genetics and external factors such as diet, physical inactivity, and obesity play a part. Unlike type 1 diabetes, people who later develop type 2 diabetes usually have pre-diabetes first. However it is possible for people who have pre-diabetes to delay or prevent type 2 diabetes from developing by making changes in their diet and increasing their level of physical activity.

Treatment

Type 2 diabetes symptoms can be mild and may go unnoticed. Many times it is discovered through routine medical tests. The first apparent symptom can be increased thirst. There are several tests that can be given to properly diagnose type 2 diabetes. Due to its slow development, sometimes damage has already been done to some organs such as the eyes and the kidneys before detection occurs. Controlling the blood sugar is essential to take control of the disease. The health professional should be able to guide the patient to self-monitoring and recording the results, as this is a crucial part of the treatment. Patients with type 2 diabetes usually do not require insulin injections. Type 2 diabetes can often be managed through a combination of oral medications, proper diet and physical activity. Type 2 diabetes is common among overweight, inactive people. Therefore, lifestyle change is a crucial part of controlling the disease.

Although the purpose of oral medications for diabetes is to lower the level of blood sugar, other medications that the patient may be taking for other health disorders may do the opposite, that is, raise the blood sugar. It is very important that the health professional have full knowledge of the medications the patient is taking, so that the proper balance of drugs can be established.

Possible Complications of Types 1 and 2 Diabetes

Besides the symptoms mentioned earlier, diabetes can cause slow-healing sores and infections, swollen and tender gums, and edema in the legs. Some of the more severe increased risks include:

Blindness (retinopathy)
Heart disease (cardiovascular)
Kidney disease (nephropathy)
Foot ulcers

People who have had diabetes for an extended period of time may develop some of these long-term complications. Proper diabetic management can help manage any of these complications.

The goals for the long-term treatment of diabetes are to prolong life, decrease symptoms, and to prevent as long and as much as possible severe complications. The patient should avail himself or herself with as much information as possible and be well educated in so far as the disease is concerned, for the patient is the most important person in managing the diabetes. Although a serious illness, the diabetic patient can live a long, happy, and good-quality life.

Diet

What, how, when, and the amount the patient eats affects the blood sugar level. Diet should be low in fat, salt, and added sugars. Carbohydrates such as whole-grain breads, cereals, vegetables, and fruit will help to control the sugar level, as well as the blood pressure and cholesterol levels. Portions should also be taken into account to maintain a healthy weight. The diet should be regulated to the specific needs under the guidance of the health professional.

Sweeteners

Sweeteners can be classified in two kinds: nutritive sweeteners and non-nutritive sweeteners. Nutritive sweeteners are carbohydrates that provide calories and affect the blood sugar. Non-nutritive sweeteners can satisfy the craving for sweets without the risks of added calories and glucose. Some of the more common are:

NUTRITIVE SWEETENERS	NON-NUTRITIVE SWEETENERS
honey	aspartame (NutraSweet, Equal)
jam, jelly	saccharin (Sweet'N Low)
maple, corn, and malt syrups	sucralose (Splenda)
molasses	

Exercise and Physical Activity

Generally, the more active a person is, the lower their blood sugar level. However not everyone has the same response to exercise, so it is useful to check blood glucose levels before and after exercise. It is recommended that the diabetic patient talk to a medical professional before starting a new exercise regimen in order to determine what activities and level of activity are appropriate.

For further information, visit the American Diabetes Association website: www.diabetes.org.

DIABETES

La diabetes es una enfermedad severa causada por un trastorno metabólico que afecta la capacidad que tiene el cuerpo de convertir la comida en energía. Parte de los alimentos que ingerimos se convierten en un tipo de azúcar llamado glucosa que viaja por el cuerpo a través de la sangre. Posteriormente esta glucosa se almacena en las células para ser usada como energía. Sin embargo, sin la presencia de la hormona llamada insulina, la glucosa no puede hacer contacto con las células. Por lo cual, la glucosa se queda en el torrente sanguíneo y las células agonizan sin su fuente de energía.

La diabetes se produce cuando el cuerpo no produce suficiente insulina. La organización mundial de la salud reconoce tres formas de diabetes: La diabetes tipo 1, la diabetes tipo 2 y la diabetes en el embarazo o diabetes gestacional. La diabetes tipo 1 se produce por la destrucción autoinmune de las células que producen insulina. En la diabetes tipo 2 y la diabetes gestacional a pesar de que el páncreas aún tiene la capacidad de producir insulina, ésta no puede producir suficiente insulina o las células corporales son resistentes a la insulina. Por otro lado, a pesar de que la pre-diabetes no es considerada un tipo de diabetes en si, ésta es una condición médica que puede derivar en diabetes.

Síntomas Generales

visión nublada
padecer demasiada hambre
incontinencia de orina
fatiga excesiva
sed excesiva
irritabilidad
perdida de peso a pesar de un aumento del apetito

Pre-diabetes

La pre-diabetes ocurre cuando el nivel de glucosa en la sangre es más alto que el normal, pero no llega a los niveles de la diabetes tipo 1 y diabetes tipo 2. Para determinar el estado de pre-diabetes es necesario estar bajo supervisión médica y hacerse las pruebas necesarias. Mientras que la pre-diabetes a menudo conduce a la diabetes tipo 2, es posible retrasar o inclusive evitar el desarrollo de esta condición médica controlando su nivel de azúcar en la sangre, llevando a cabo cambios alimenticios en su dieta y aumentando su nivel de actividad física.

Diabetes del embarazo

Este tipo de diabetes ocurre en mujeres embarazadas que no han tenido diabetes antes de su embarazo y que desarrollan un nivel alto de azúcar en la sangre (hiperglucemia). Las hormonas del embarazo crean resistencia a la insulina en mujeres que están predispuestas genéticamente a desarrollar esta condición en una fase tardía del embarazo después que el cuerpo del feto está ya formado. Por esta razón, la diabetes del embarazo no implica generalmente defectos de nacimiento, lo que si puede ocurrir en aquellos casos en que la madre haya sido diabética antes del embarazo. Sin embargo si la Diabetes del embarazo no se controla y atiende debidamente puede llegar a causar problemas serios en la madre y el bebé. La Diabetes del embarazo deja de manifestarse al terminar el embarazo.

Diabetes mellitus tipo 1

A la diabetes tipo 1 también se la conoce como diabetes insulina-dependiente o juvenil porque mayormente se encuentra en niños y jóvenes adultos. Generalmente se presenta en personas menores de 25 años. Es una enfermedad crónica e incurable cuyas causas exactas aún se desconocen. Sin embargo, existe cierta certeza de que la genética y los factores externos juegan un papel en dicha condición médica. El acceso repentino de la diabetes tipo 1 parece ser provocado por un factor externo tal como una infección viral o la exposición a ciertas sustancias químicas o medicamentos.

En la diabetes tipo 1, las células beta del páncreas producen ninguna insulina. Esta insuficiencia ocasiona que las células en vez de almacenarse en las células del cuerpo se almacenen en el flujo sanguíneo, y que aunque el cuerpo tenga la cantidad de insulina necesaria no la pueda consumir. Como resultado, la persona diabética puede tener un hambre excesivo aunque haya acabado de comer. La acumulación de glucosa en la sangre puede causar frecuencia urinaria, razón por la cual la persona diabética experimente mayor sed que de costumbre.

Tratamiento

El acceso de la diabetes tipo 1 es sumamente repentino y severo, por lo que su tratamiento inicial puede requerir la hospitalización. Una vez superada la etapa de la hospitalización, el paciente puede necesitar visitas médicas semanales con su doctor hasta que el o ella aprenda a tener un mejor control sobre su nivel de glucosa en la sangre. Existen varios tipos de pruebas que pueden ser utilizados para detectar la presencia de la diabetes. Una vez que ésta ha sido detectada, la prioridad será la de atacar y tratar la cetoacidosis (exceso cetonas, subproductos del metabolismo de las grasas en el torrente sanguíneo) y de los elevados niveles de glucosa en el cuerpo.

Clínicamente, la diabetes tipo 1 se trata con insulina. La insulina permite que la glucosa en la sangre ingrese a las células lo que permitirá reducir el nivel de azúcar en la sangre. La insulina puede administrarse por medio de una inyección subcutánea o a través de una bomba de insulina que otorga al paciente una infusión subcutánea continua de insulina. Las preparaciones de insulina son de diversos tipos y el profesional de la salud debe aconsejar al paciente sobre el tipo de preparación, la dosis requerida y la forma de administración correcta de dicho medicamento. Asimismo, el nivel de azúcar en la sangre requiere de un monitoreo continuo por medio de pruebas del nivel de azúcar. Con la ayuda del profesional de la salud que le atiende, debería poder aprender como auto administrarse pruebas de detección del nivel de la glucosa en la sangre. Dependiendo de los resultados de dichos análisis o pruebas el paciente puede necesitar de entre 1 a 4 inyecciones de insulina por día. La cantidad de carbohidratos ingeridos y el nivel de insulina tienen una correlación exacta y el profesional de la salud debe poder ayudar al paciente a lograr el equilibrio deseado entre las dos.

El aspecto externo del tratamiento consiste en el seguimiento por parte del paciente de una dieta médica, el control de su peso así como el la cantidad de ejercicio adecuados. También se altamente recomendable que el paciente cuide sus pies estando alerta a posibles síntomas de infección, se haga revisar la vista cada año, visite a su dentista cada dos años y no tome ni fuma, o lo haga con mucha moderación.

Diabetes mellitus tipo 2

La diabetes tipo 2 también conocida como diabetes no insulina-dependiente o diabetes de la obesidad es el tipo de diabetes más común. Usualmente esta presente en los adultos que tienen más de cuarenta años, a pesar de que actualmente un número mayor de jóvenes adultos y niños están siendo diagnosticados con este mal. En la diabetes tipo 2 el páncreas no produce suficiente insulina o los tejidos musculares o corporales se vuelven resistentes a ella. En consecuencia, el azúcar se acumula en el torrente sanguíneo y las células agonizan por la falta de energía que esto genera.

Así como la diabetes tipo 1, el tipo 2 es una enfermedad crónica incurable. La diabetes tipo 2 se puede tratar sin medicamentos. Aunque no se conoce la causa de la enfermedad en este tipo de diabetes parece que factores genéticos y externos tal como la dieta, inactividad física y obesidad son elementos que toman parte en el desarrollo de la enfermedad. Los pacientes que contraen la enfermedad generalmente han tenido pre-diabetes anteriormente.

Pre-diabetes, lo que los difiere de a los pacientes de la diabetes tipo 1. Sin embargo, es posible que los pacientes que tienen pre-diabetes puedan retrasar o prevenir la diabetes tipo 2 si hacen cambios en la dieta y aumentan el nivel de actividad física.

Tratamiento

Los síntomas de Diabetes Tipo 2 pueden ser leves y puede que no se manifiesten. En muchos casos la enfermedad se descubre en pruebas médicas de rutina. El primer síntoma aparente es el aumento de la sed. Existen varias pruebas para detectar y diagnosticar la diabetes. Debido al desarrollo lento, en ciertos casos ya ha ocurrido daño en algunos órganos, tal como en la vista y los riñones, antes que la enfermedad se detectara. Es muy importante el control del azúcar en la sangre para poder controlar la enfermedad. Los profesionales de salud deben ser capaces de guiar al paciente a monitorearse y registrar los resultados, ya que esta operación es una parte esencial del tratamiento. Los pacientes de Diabetes tipo 2 usualmente no requieren inyecciones de insulina. La Diabetes Tipo 2 puede tratarse frecuentemente en combinación con medicamentos tomados oralmente, una dieta balanceada y actividad física. La diabetes Tipo 2 es común en personas que tienen sobrepeso y son inactivas físicamente. Por lo que un cambio en el estilo de vida es una parte esencial del control de la enfermedad.

Aunque el propósito de los medicamentos orales es bajar el nivel del azúcar en la sangre, otros medicamentos que el paciente toma para tratar sus trastornos pueden hacer lo opuesto, esto es, subir el nivel del azúcar. Es sumamente importante que el facultativo que atiende al paciente tenga completo conocimiento de todos los medicamentos del paciente, para poder establecer el balance apropiado de las drogas.

Complicaciones posibles de los tipos de diabetes 1 y 2

Además de los síntomas mencionados anteriormente, la diabetes puede causar infecciones y úlceras, encías inflamadas y sensibles, y edemas en las piernas.
Algunos de los riesgos más severos incluyen:

Ceguera (retinopatía)
Cardiopatía (enfermedad cardiovascular)
Enfermedad renal (nefropatía)
Nervios afectados (neuropatía)
Úlceras en los pies.

Las personas que han padecido de diabetes por largo tiempo pueden llegar a tener estos problemas. Un tratamiento adecuado de la diabetes puede ayudar a tratar cualquiera de estas complicaciones.

La meta de un largo tratamiento de diabetes es de prolongar la vida, disminuir los síntomas y prevenir cuanto más sea posible complicaciones severas. Los pacientes deben tratar de educarse todo lo posible acerca de la enfermedad, ya que cada paciente es la persona más importante en manejar su propia enfermedad. Aunque la diabetes es una enfermedad severa el paciente diabético puede vivir una buena calidad de vida, larga y feliz.

Dieta

Qué, Cómo, Cuándo y Cuanto Come el/la paciente afecta el nivel de azúcar. La dieta debe ser baja en grasa, sal, y aditivos de azúcares. Los carbohidratos tal como panes de grano entero, cereales, vegetales y frutas le ayudarán a controlar el nivel del azúcar lo mismo que el nivel de la presión arterial y del colesterol. Las porciones también se deben tener en consideración para mantener un peso saludable. La dieta debe ser regulada bajo la guía de un profesional de la salud, teniendo en cuenta necesidades específicas del/la paciente.

Edulcorantes

Los edulcorantes se clasifican en dos clases: nutritivos y no-nutritivos. Los nutritivos son carbohidratos que proporcionan calorías y afectan el nivel de azúcar en la sangre. Los no-nutritivos satisfacen las ganas de comer algo dulce sin el riesgo de añadir calorías y glucosa.

EDULCORANTES NUTRITIVOS	EDULCORANTES NO-NUTRITIVOS
miel / honey	aspartame (NutraSweet, Equal)
mermelada, jalea / jam, jelly	sacarina / saccharin (Sweet'N Low)
siropes o jarabes de arce, maíz y malta	sucralosa / sucralose (Splenda)
melasa / molasses	

Ejercicios y actividad física

Generalmente mientras más activa sea una persona, más bajo será el nivel del azúcar en la sangre. Sin embargo, no toda persona diabética tiene el mismo resultado con el ejercicio, así que es necesario comprobar los niveles de glucosa antes y después del ejercicio. Se recomienda que el paciente diabético consulte a un profesional de la salud antes de comenzar un régimen de ejercicios y que determine actividades y el nivel adecuado de las mismas.

Para más información visite en la Internet la Asociación Americana de Diabetes: www.diabetes.org/espanol.

Vocabulary / Vocabularío

ENGLISH	SPANISH
calories	calorías
carbohydrates	carbohidratos
celiac disease	enfermedad celíaca
cholesterol	colesterol
frozen shoulder	hombro tieso
genetic	genético-a
gestational	gestacional
glucose	glucosa
hemochromatosis	hemocromatosis
heredity	herencia
hyperglycemia	hiperglicemia
hypoglycemia	hipoglicemia
insulin	insulina
insulin-resistant	resistente a la insulina
ketoacidosis	quetoacidosis
ketone bodies	cuerpos cetónicos
macrosomia	macrosomia
metabolism	metabolismo
monitoring	monitoreo
nephropathy	nefropatía
neuropathy	neuropatía
pancreatitis	pancreatitis
polydipsia	polidipsia
polyuria	poliuria
retinopathy	retinopatía
weight fluctuation	fluctuación en el peso

BREAST CANCER / EL CÁNCER DEL SENO

▶ Breast cancer has increased alarmingly in the twenty-first century. It is a deadly disease.	▶ El cáncer del seno continúa aumentando en el siglo veintiuno en una manera alarmante.
▶ Breast cancer attacks women in their early twenties, during their forties and fifties or in their old age. Age is no boundary.	▶ El cáncer del seno es una enfermedad grave que ataca a la mujer en sus primeros veinte años, a los cuarenta o cincuenta años o en la vejez. La edad no es un límite en las mujeres que sufren de cáncer.
▶ The incidence percentage in younger women is lower, but their illnesses are usually more severe.	▶ El porcentaje de incidencia del cáncer en la mujer joven es más bajo pero es ésta la edad en la cual el cáncer del seno parece ser más desvastador.
▶ The highest percentage of diagnostic cases is in fifty-and sixty-year-old women.	▶ El mayor porcentaje de casos diagnosticados es en mujeres entre los cincuenta y los sesenta años de edad.

Formation of Breast Cancer

Formación del cáncer del seno

Lobular carcinoma in situ refers to cancerous cells growing out of control in the tissues lining a gland. This type of cancerous cells indicates a pre-cancerous stage of breast cancer. The tumor begins to develop through the proliferation of these abnormal cells.	*Lobular carcinoma in situ* se refiere a un grupo de células cancerosas creciendo sin control en los tejidos de los lóbulos de la mama. El tumor comienza a desarrollarse en células pre-cancerosas y próximas a convertirse en cáncer del seno.
Ductal carcinoma in situ is the proliferation of abnormal cells growing and developing in the ducts of the breast, which connect to the breast nipple. This type of tumor is also considered to be pre-cancerous.	*Ductal carcinoma in situ* se llama así a la proliferación de células anormales creciendo rápidamente en los conductos lácteos, conectores al pezón.
The Latin phrase *in situ* means that the cancer has not spread, remaining where it originated.	La frase en latín *in situ* quiere decir que el tumor no se ha expandido y permanece en el lugar donde se originó.
Both *lobular* and *ductal carcinoma in situ* may become invasive.	El *carcinoma lobular in situ* y el *carcinoma ductal in situ* pueden llegar a ser *invasivos*.

Cancer Stages / Etapas del cáncer

Cancer is characterized by stages, depending on the growth and expansion of the cancer cells. / El cáncer se clasifica en etapas dependiendo del crecimiento del tumor y expansión de las células cancerosas.

STAGE 0	ETAPA 0
This Stage refers to non-invasive breast cancer. Only a 5% to a 10% of the *lobular carcinoma in situ* tumors become invasive. However, even as 75% of the *ductal carcinoma* becomes *invasive,* there is not evidence that any given tumor would necessarily do so. When *lobular carcinoma in situ* and *ductal carcinoma in situ* are not invasive,they are described as a pre-cancerous abnormal lump, tumor or mass *in situ*.	Esta Etapa se refiere a cáncer del seno no-invasivo. Sólo de un 5% a 10% de células clasificadas como *carcinoma lobular in situ* se convierten en *invasivos*. Se calcula que un 75% del *carcinoma ductal* se convierte en *invasivo,* aunque tampoco puede afirmarse que se convierta necesariamente en *invasivo*. Cuando el *carcinoma lobular in situ y el carcinoma ductal* no son *invasivos* se describen como un bulto o masa pre-cancerosa *in situ*.
STAGE I	**ETAPAS I**
Cancer cells have begun to break through or invade adjacent normal tissue, but no lymph nodes are involved. The tumor is about 2 centimeters in diameter. Surgery and radiation are recommended.	Células cancerosas comienzan a invadir tejidos normales adyacentes, sin que haya invasión de los ganglios linfáticos. El tumor tiene cerca de 2 centímetros de diámetro. Se recomienda cirugía y radiación.
STAGE II	**ETAPA II**
In **Stage II**, the cancer has become *invasive*, having moved to the lymph nodes under the same arm of the affected breast. The affected lymph nodes have not stuck to one another or to the surrounding tissues. This is a sign that the cancer has not become a Stage III cancer. The tumor is at least 2 cms., but no more than 5 cms.	En la **Etapa II** el cáncer el cáncer es ya *invasivo*, hacia los ganglios linfáticos debajo de la axila, del mimo lado del seno afectado, pero los ganglios no se han juntado apretadamente entre sí o a los tejidos adyacentes. Esta es una señal que el cáncer no se encuentra aún en la tercera etapa. El tumor mide por lo menos 2 centímetros pero no más de 5 centímetros.
STAGE III	**ETAPA III**
This stage is divided in two subcategories known as **III A** and **III B**.	**Etapa III** comprende dos subcategorías llamadas **III A** y **III B**.
Stage III A tumor can be more than 5 centimeters in diameter or it can spread to the underarm lymph nodes near the breast bone or to other nearby tissues. The lymph nodes are stuck together or to the adjacent tissues. A treatment to remove and destroy the cancer is applied and a systemic or hormonal treatment is usually prescribed to try to diminish the tumor's size.	En la **Etapa III A** el cáncer puede alcanzar más de 5 centímetros de diámetro, o se ha expandido hasta los ganglios linfáticos bajo la axila y los músculos cercanos al esternón, o a otros tejidos adyacentes. Un tratamiento de extirpación del tumor es necesario, generalmente por terapia de radiación y quimioterapia sistémica hormonal para reducir el tumor.

Stage III B includes inflammatory breast cancer, although not common, it is a very aggressive, insidious cancer. The symptoms are an inflammatory breast with a redness, warm feeling, puffiness of the skin, hard sensation, with appearance of "peau d'orange" (similar to the orange peel or cortex), ridges or welts. A mass is present in a few cases.

Etapa III B incluye cáncer del seno con inflamación, aunque no es común es un tipo de cáncer muy agresivo, insidioso, manifiesta el seno enrojecido con entumecimiento, acalorado, y con semejanza a "peau d' orange" (la piel o corteza de una naranja), con ronchas y aspereza. En algunos casos se manifiesta en una masa.

STAGE IV

ETAPA IV

In Stage IV the cancer has metastasized. In other words, it has continued its devastating destruction and is invading other parts of the body in addition to the internal mammary and lymph nodes. A tumor may have spread to the subclavicular lymph nodes, located in the base of the neck, to the lungs, liver or brain. If diagnosed "Metastatic at presentation" it means that the primary breast cancer was not found when it was only inside the breast. This cancer is also considered Stage IV.

In cases of Stage IV, treatment generally consists of chemotherapy and radiation may be given to other parts of the body as well as to the affected breast.

En la Etapa IV el cáncer ha hecho metástasis y ha continuado su destrucción devastadora y ha invadido otras partes del cuerpo en adición al seno y los ganglios linfáticos. El tumor quizás se haya expandido a los ganglios linfáticos subclaviculares localizados en la base del cuello, los pulmones, hígado o cerebro. Si el diagnóstico ha sido "Metástasico en presentación", quiere decir que el cáncer de la mama primario no fue encontrado dentro del seno en su principio. Este cáncer también es considerado de Etapa IV.

En estos casos de esta Etapa IV generalmente se continúa el tratamiento de quimioterapia y radiación aplicada a otras partes del cuerpo al igual que al seno afectado.

Breast Examination

Examen del seno

Women should schedule a breast examination with their doctor before having a mammogram. The examination and the mammography should be done annually.

Toda mujer debe hacer una consulta con su médico para que le examinen el seno antes del mamograma. El examen del seno y la mamografía deben hacerse anualmente.

Every woman should get into the habit of self-examining her breasts by detecting any changes in the breast appearance and feeling each breast systematically and routinely with her fingertips. If a lump is found, it does not necessarily indicate cancer. The lump could be due to other factors, such as the menstrual cycle. However, when a lump is observed or there is a change in the skin, swelling, redness or secretion from the nipple, it is necessary to consult a physician.

Además, toda mujer debe acostumbrarse a auto-examinar los senos palpándose con la yema de los dedos para detectar cambios en la apariencia del seno. Si se encontrase un bulto o se detectase la presencia de una masa abultada en una de las mamas, no se alarme, esto no quiere decir, necesariamente, que usted padece cáncer. El bulto puede deberse a una infinidad de otros factores tales como el ciclo menstrual. Sin embargo, si se detecta un bulto o un cambio en la piel, hinchazón, una coloración rojiza o secreciones del pezón usted debed consultar con un doctor.

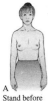

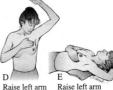

A	B	C	D	E
Stand before mirror	Clasp hands behind and press hands forward	Hands on hips and bow toward mirror as you pull shoulders and elbows forward	Raise left arm (repeat with right)	Raise left arm and lie down (repeat with right)
De pié frente a un espejo	Entrelace las manos detrás del cuello y presiónelas hacia adelante	Con las manos en la cadera inclínese hacia el espejo mientras alza los hombros y los codos hacia adelante	Levante el brazo izquierdo (repita con el derecho)	En posición acostada levante el brazo izquierdo y póngalo debajo del cuello (repítalo con el derecho)

Breast self-examination: standing before a mirror, (A) check both breasts for anything unusual, (B, C); while in the shower, (D) massage breast in circular pattern feeling for any unusual lumps or masses under the skin and squeeze nipple to look for discharge; (E) using the same circular motion in panel D, check again for any unusual lumps or masses while lying down

Auto-examen del seno: de pié frente a un espejo, (A) examine ambos senos para comprobar que no muestran nada extraño, (B, C); mientras toma una ducha, (D) masaje el seno con un movimiento circular mientras palpa el seno en busca de cualquier cambio, un bulto o masa debajo de la piel; exprima el pezón para comprobar si suelta alguna secreción; (E) haciendo el mismo movimiento circular del panel D, compruebe otra vez mientras está acostada si hay bultos

Source: Smeltzer SC, RN, EdD, FAAN & Bare BG, RN, MSN. Brunner & Suddarth's Textbook of Medical-Surgical Nursing, 9th Edition. Philadelphia: Lippincott Williams & Wilkins, 2000.

Early Detection

Mammography of breast cancer tumors is an early detector with findings of 90% positive even when symptoms are not present. In the other 10%, missing the tumors has been attributed to the high density of breast tissues in postmenopausal women who were under hormone replacement treatment for a long time, or due to an extremely small tumor. In such cases the mammogram should be followed by other blood tests and ultrasound.

Detección temprana del cáncer

La mamografía es la prueba de diagnóstico más frecuente con hallazgos de un 90% positivos aún cuando no hay síntomas presente. En el otro 10% la falta de detección se atribuye a la alta densidad de tejidos mamarios en mujeres en la postmenopausia que por largo tiempo se sometieron a un tratamiento de reemplazo de hormona, o debido a un tumor extremadamente pequeño. En dichos casos la mamografía debe ser seguida por pruebas sanguíneas y por una prueba de ultrasonido.

Cancer Markers

There are blood tests that indicate whether or not a cancer is present. A certain kind of protein in the blood known as CA15.3 reveals the presence of breast and ovarian cancer. During chemotherapy the readings of the markers will indicate progression or recurrence of the cancer. However, if the cancer has metastasized, the results given by the markers about the cancer's origin are uncertain making the place of recurrence of the cancer doubtful.

Marcadores de cáncer

Hay pruebas sanguíneas que indican si un cáncer se encuentra en el organismo. La prueba de CA15.3 cierto tipo de proteína en la sangre marca la presencia de un cáncer. Esta proteína es marcadora de cáncer del seno y del ovario. Cuando se administra quimioterapia los resultados de los marcadores indican la progresión o la reincidencia en el tratamiento. Sin embargo cuando el cáncer ha hecho metástasis los resultados de los marcadores son dudosos con respecto al origen y la reincidencia del cáncer.

Risks

There are many factors contributing to a higher risk of breast cancer:

1. Age (including early menarche, and older age at first pregnancy)
2. Late menopause
3. Postmenopausal disorders
4. Use of oral contraceptives
5. Obesity after menopause
6. Use of hormone replacement therapy
7. Family history, inherited genes (If a mother, daughter, or sister has or had breast cancer)

Riesgos

Hay varios factores que contribuyen a un alto riesgo de cáncer del seno:

1. Edad (pubertad temprana, embarazo tardío)
2. Menopausia tardía
3. Trastornos postmenopausal
4. Uso de contraceptivos orales
5. Obesidad después de la menopausia
6. Uso de terapia de reemplazo de hormona
7. Historia médica familiar, genes heredados (Si la madre, hermana o hija tienen o han tenido cáncer de la mama.)

Treatments and Surgery

Lumpectomy
Removal of cancer tissues and a rim of
normal tissues.

Mastectomy
Removal of entire breast and lymph
nodes under the arm.

Radical Mastectomy
Removal of entire breast, lymph nodes
under the arm and underlying chest wall
muscle.

Radiation Therapy
After surgery: destroying cancer cells
that may remain; before surgery:
reducing the tumor's size.

Systemic therapy
Chemotherapy and hormone therapy
combined.

Biological therapy
Use of Herceptin, against HER2

Hormone therapy
Testing for positive estrogen in
postmenopausal women with breast
cancer who were given an antiestrogen.

Tratamientos y cirugía

Tumorectomía
Extirpación de células cancerosas y un
borde de tejidos normales.

Mastectomía
Extirpación completa de la mama y
ganglios linfáticos debajo de la axila.

Mastectomía radical
Extirpación completa del seno, los
ganglióos linfáticos bajo la axila y el
músculo subyacente a la pared del tórax.

Terapia de radiación
Después de la cirugía: destruye todas las
células cancerígenas que quedaron; antes
de la cirugía: reduce el tamaño del tumor.

Terapia sistémica
Quimioterapia y terapia hormonal
combinadas.

Terapia biológica
Uso de Herceptin, against HER2.

Terapia hormonal
Pruebas para estrogeno positivo en mujeres
con cáncer del seno que después de la
menopausia recibieron un antiestrógeno.

Vocabulary

Vocabulario

Vocabulary	Vocabulario
Abnormal cells	Células anormales
Adenoma – a tumor of glandular origin	Adenoma – tumor de origen glandular
Alopecia – loss of hair	Alopecia – pérdida del cabello
Antiemetic – medication to combat nausea	Antiemético – medicamento que evita la náusea
Axillary dissection	Excision de los nódulos debajo de la axila
Benign breast disease	Enfermedad benigna de la mama
Benign tumor	Tumor benigno
Biopsy – procedure to remove sample tissue	Biopsia – procedimiento para extraer muestra de tejido
Blood analysis	Análisis de sangre
Blood plasma	Plasma sanguíneo
Bone marrow	Médula ósea
Bone scan	Escán óseo
Breast self-examination	Auto-examen del seno
Breast tissue	Tejido de la mama
CA15.3 – protein marker for breast and ovarian cancer	CA15.3 – marcador de proteína para el cáncer en el seno y el ovario
CA125 – protein marker for ovarian and breast cancer recurrence	CA125 – marcador de proteína indica la recurrencia del cáncer ovárico o del seno
Cancer cells	Células cancerosas
Carcinembrionic antigen, CEA	Antígeno carcinoembriónico, CEA
Cauterize – burn by application of heat or electricity	Cauterizar – quemar aplicando calor o electricidad
Chemotherapy – treatment by use of chemical agents	Quimioterapia – tratamiento usando agentes químicos
CT or CAT scan	TA o CAT escán
Cyst – sac or pouch containing fluid or semifluid matter	Quiste – bolsa que contiene líquido o materia semilíquida
Deep-seated mass	Masa de asiento profundo
Drainage	Drenaje, secreción
Ductal carcinoma – carcinoma originating in the mammary ducts	Carcinoma ductal – cáncer que se origina en los conductos lácteos del seno
Ducts – connectors to the nipple	Conducto mamario
Early detection – when the cancer is detected as it begins by a mammogram, ultrasound or palpation	Detección temprana del cáncer por medio de mamografía, ultrasonido o palpación.
Estrogen	Estrógeno
Genetic factor	Factor genético
HER2 – helper gene to control the growth and repair of cells	HER2 – Gene ayudante en el control del crecimiento y la reparación de las células
Hidden cancer	Cáncer oculto – no detectado a simple vista

Vocabulary	Vocabulario
Hormone receptor	Receptor hormonal
Hormone therapy	Terapia hormonal
Host defenses – primary and secondary defenses against attacking illness	Defensas – primaria y secundaria del organismo de resistencia contra una enfermedad que ataca
Inflammatory carcinoma	Carcinoma inflamatorio
Inverted nipple	Pezón invertido
Lobe – 15 to 20 portions of the mammary gland	Lóbulo – de 15 a 20 porciones de las glándulas mamarias
Immune defense system – resistance created by the body to defend against sickness	Sistema inmunológico – Resistencia creada por el organismo en contra de una enfermedad atacante
Lobular carcinoma *in situ* (LCS)	Carcinoma lobular *in situ* (CLIS)
Lobular carcinoma *invasivo* (LCI)	Carcinoma lobular *invasivo* (CLI)
Lump	Bulto, masa, bolita
Lumpectomy – removal of a tumor excluding the lymph nodes and adjacent tissues	Tumorectomía – excision de un tumor con exclusíon de ganglios y tejidos adyacentes
Lymph glands	Glándulas linfáticas
Lymph node areas	Áreas de ganglios linfáticos
Lymphedema – swelling as a result of obstruction in the lymph nodes	Linfedema – inflamación como resultado de una obstrucción en los ganglios linfáticos
Malignant tumor	Tumor canceroso, maligno
Mammary glands	Glándulas mamarias
Mastectomy – plastic surgery of the breast	Mastectomía – cirugía plástica del seno
Mastodynia – breast pain	Mastodinia – dolor en el seno
Negative RE – type of cancer that does not have estrogen receptors	ER negativo – tipo de cáncer que no tiene receptores de estrógeno
Positive RE – cancer type having estrogen receptors	ER positivo – tipo de cáncer que tiene receptores de estrógeno
Nipple	Pezón
Node – ganglion	Ganglio, nódulo
Oncologist	Oncólogo, oncóloga

PROSTATE CANCER

The prostate is a gland about the size of a large walnut that is part of the male reproductive system. It surrounds the urethra, the tube through which urine flows, and is located in front of the rectum and under the bladder. This location is the reason why prostate diseases often affect the functions of defecation, ejaculation, and urination.

Like all other parts of the body, the prostate is made up of cells. These cells follow the normal cycle of growing, dividing, and producing more cells to keep the body functioning the right way. When the process malfunctions, the cells of the prostate mutate and begin multiplying in an uncontrolled manner. These uncontrolled cells form a mass of tissue becoming a growth or tumor. Growths or tumors can be benign or malignant.

Prostate cancer is the result of a malignant tumor forming in the tissue of the prostate. Metastasis in prostate cancer occurs when malignant cancer cells break away, entering the bloodstream or the lymphatic system and traveling to other parts of the body, especially to the bones and lymph nodes.

Cause and Risk Factors

The exact causes for prostate cancer are not known, but there are certain risk factors that may increase the likelihood of developing the disease. Some studies done on prostate cancer point strongly to the following risk factors:

▶ Age: It is the main risk factor. The average age of the individual at the time of diagnosis is 70 years old. Prostate cancer is rare in men younger than 45.
▶ Family history: Men whose close relatives (father, uncle, or brother) have suffered or suffer from the disease are more likely to have the disease. However, no single gene has been found to be the cause of prostate cancer; rather, there seem to be multiple genes implicated.
▶ Race: White males seem to be at less risk than African American or Hispanic men.
▶ Diet: Men who follow a diet high in animal fat or meat are at higher risk than men who have a diet rich in fruit and vegetables.

Other factors such as medications, medical condition of the individual, obesity, and smoking are also linked to prostate cancer.

Risk factors such as family history cannot be avoided, but other factors such as exercise, a healthy diet, routine checks with a specialist, and annual testing are preventive measures that are recommended.

Symptoms

There are usually no symptoms manifested in early stages of prostate cancer. This is the main reason why the majority of cases are not detected until the cancer has spread beyond the prostate.

The most common symptoms of the disease are:

▶ Difficulty starting urination
▶ Urgency of urination
▶ Frequent urination and increased urination at night
▶ Pain during urination
▶ Intermittent urine flow
▶ Blood in the urine
▶ Difficulty achieving erection or painful ejaculation

Sometimes a dull pain in the lower pelvic area and general pain in the lower back, hips, or upper thighs can occur, usually after the early stage, and generally followed by appetite and weight loss.

Screening

Prostate cancer is a slow growing cancer, in most cases never growing to the point of causing symptoms. The purpose of annual screening is to detect the cancer at its earliest stages before any symptoms are detected. If prostate cancer is detected at an early stage through screening, it can usually be treated very effectively. Screening can initially be done at the doctor's office through two tests:

▶ PSA (prostate-specific antigen blood test)
▶ DRE (digital rectal exam)

PSA is a protein produced by the prostate and released in very small amounts into the bloodstream. If there is any abnormality shown such as a cancer, PSA is released in greater amounts and the levels of the PSA in the blood become an indicator of some problem in the prostate. PSA levels under 4 are considered "normal", above 10 are considered "high," and between 4 and 10 "intermediate". PSA can show a "high" level due to other factors than cancer, such as infection of the prostate. With additional testing, such as a biopsy, the presence of any cancer can be determined.

DRE is a physical exam in which the physician examines the prostate by introducing a gloved and lubricated finger into the rectum and examines the prostate for irregularities in size, shape, or texture. Although DRE evaluates only the back of the prostate, a large percentage of the prostate cancers are formed in this area. Usually a cancer detected through DRE is an advanced cancer.

The American Cancer Society recommends that both tests should be done annually, beginning at age 50. Men at high risk should begin testing at age 45. Treating any prostate cancer earlier offers more options to the patient as to the possible treatments. It is very important that patient and doctor discuss carefully the benefits of diagnostic procedures and treatments before making a decision.

Treatment

Once cancer is found in the prostate, the physician determines at what stage of growth the cancer is and if it has spread to other parts of the body. If it has spread, it must be determined to where in order to decide the most advantageous treatment. This is done using imaging tests such as MRI (magnetic resonance imaging) and blood tests.

Four stages describe the development of prostate cancer:

▶ Stage 1: the cancer is too small to be detected and is usually found during surgery treating another problem such as an enlarged prostate.
▶ Stage 2: the cancer is still within the prostate but involves more tissue. Usually detected through DRE or a biopsy that has been indicated because of a high PSA.
▶ Stage 3: the cancer has spread to nearby tissues.
▶ Stage 4: the cancer has spread and metastasize to the lymph nodes or other parts of the body.

There are many ways to treat prostate cancer. The patient should learn as much as possible about options, risks, and benefits of each treatment and then discuss the matter with his physicians, a urologist, a radiation oncologist, and a medical oncologist before making a decision. The stage of the disease is at times a determining factor.

Treatment options include:

▶ Active Surveillance: also called watchful waiting, it involves careful observation and monitoring without using invasive treatment. Usually recommended in cases of early or slow-growing cancers or when other serious medical conditions that may shorten the life span of the patient are present.
▶ Surgery: usually indicated in cases where the cancer is confined to the prostate. It is used to remove all or part of the prostate.
▶ Radiation therapy: consists in killing cancer cells in the prostate and surrounding tissues through ionizing radiation.
▶ Hormone therapy: used to stop testosterone from being released or preventing the hormone from acting on the prostate cells, as testosterone serves as the main fuel for their growth.

► Chemotherapy: based on the use of chemicals to stop the growth or kill the cancer cells. Usually administered in cases where there is advanced metastasis of the cancer.

Other approaches recently have been applied are cryotherapy, which consists of freezing the prostate cells and tumors through a probe inserted into the prostate via the perineum, and high-intensity focused ultrasound.

Scientists and researchers continue to identify new drugs, new regimens, and new treatments with the hope of halting the progression of the disease, alleviating side effects, and offering the afflicted patient a good-quality life.

For further information, visit the National Cancer Society website: www.cancer.gov.

CÁNCER DE LA PRÓSTATA

La próstata es una glándula del tamaño más o menos de una nuez grande que es parte del sistema reproductivo masculino. Rodea a la uretra, el tubo de salida de la orina, situada en frente del recto y debajo de la vejiga. Debido a su ubicación, las enfermedades de la próstata pueden afectar las funciones de defecar, eyacular y orinar.

Al igual que todas las otras partes del cuerpo, la próstata se compone de células. Estas células siguen el ciclo normal al crecer, dividirse y producir más células para mantener las funciones normales del cuerpo. Cuando este proceso deja de funcionar normalmente, las células comienzan a hacer mutaciones multiplicándose sin control y forman una masa de tejido o tumor. Los tumores pueden ser benignos o malignos. El cáncer de la próstata resulta de un tumor maligno. La metástasis en el cáncer de la próstata ocurre cuando las células se desprenden del tumor y entran en el flujo sanguíneo o en el sistema linfático y viajan a otras partes del cuerpo especialmente los huesos y los nódulos linfáticos.

Causa y Factores de Riesgo

Las causas exactas que producen el *cáncer de la próstata* se desconocen, pero hay ciertos factores de riesgo que pueden causar la enfermedad. Varios estudios indican los siguientes factores de riesgo:

► La edad: Es el factor de mayor riesgo. La edad media del paciente de *cáncer de la próstata* es de 70 años. No es común encontrar la enfermedad en individuos menores de 45 años.
► Historial médico: Los pacientes con familiares cercanos, un padre, un hermano, un tío, que padecieron o padecen de la enfermedad son más susceptibles a contraer la enfermedad. No obstante, no se ha encontrado un gene específico que cause el cáncer; más bien, parecen encontrarse más de uno.
► Raza: Hombres de la raza blanca parecen tener menos riesgo que hombres afroamericanos o hispanos.
► Dieta: Hombres que mantienen una dieta alta en grasa de animal o de carne tienen mayor riesgo que los que mantienen una dieta más abundante en frutas y vegetales.

Existen otros factores tales como drogas, el estado general de salud del individuo, la obesidad y la adicción a fumar que se relacionan con el cáncer de la próstata. Algunos factores tal como el historial médico, no pueden evitarse, pero otros factores preventivos pueden adoptarse como ejercicio, una dieta saludable, cheques de rutina con un especialista y prueba anual.

Síntomas

En la fase temprana de la enfermedad generalmente no hay síntomas. Esta es la razón principal por la cual algunos casos no se detectan hasta después de que el cáncer ya se ha extendido más allá de la próstata. Una vez que los síntomas empiezan a presentarse, los más comunes son:

► dificultad en empezar a orinar
► urgencia urinaria
► dolor durante el acto de orinar
► flujo intermitente de orina

▶ sangre en la orina
▶ frecuencia urinaria nocturna
▶ dificultad en lograr una erección o eyaculación dolorosa

Algunas veces el paciente siente un dolor sordo en el área de la pelvis o un dolor generalizado en la parte baja de la espalda, las caderas o en la parte superior de los muslos que generalmente sucede después de la fase más temprana de la enfermedad. Seguidamente pueden presentarse falta de apetito y pérdida de peso.

Escrutinio

El cáncer de la próstata es un cáncer de crecimiento lento y en muchos casos no alcanza la fase de manifestar síntomas. El propósito de hacer un escrutinio es detectar el cáncer en su comienzo, la fase más temprana cuando aún no se han presentado los síntomas. Cuando el cáncer se detecta por medio de un escrutinio generalmente se puede tratar con mucha efectividad. El escrutinio se puede hacer inicialmente en la consulta del médico aplicando dos pruebas:

▶ PSA (antígeno específico prostático, prueba de sangre)
▶ DRE (examen rectal digital)

PSA es una proteína producida por la próstata que se libera en la sangre en pequeñas cantidades. Si hay alguna irregularidad en la próstata tal como un cáncer, la cantidad de PSA que se libera en la sangre aumenta y los niveles elevados de PSA en la sangre pueden indicar algún problema presente en la próstata. Los niveles de PSA bajo 4 se consideran "normales", sobre 10 se consideran "altos" y entre 4 y 10 "intermedios". La prueba de PSA puede indicar a veces un nivel "alto" debido a otros factores que no sean cáncer, como por ejemplo una prostitis (infección de la próstata). Este resultado puede dar una sobre indicación para determinar la presencia de cáncer con una biopsia u otro tipo de prueba.

DRE es un examen físico en el cual el médico examina la próstata introduciendo un dedo (con un guante lubricado) en el recto para detectar el tamaño, forma y textura de la próstata. El examen DRE evalúa solamente la parte posterior de la próstata, área donde se forman la mayoría de los cánceres. Generalmente un cáncer que se detecta por medio de este examen está en una fase más adelantada de desarrollo.

La American Cancer Society recomienda que ambas pruebas se ofrezcan anualmente a partir de los 50 años. Recomienda comenzar a los 45 años a hombres que se consideran como alto riesgo. Encontrando y tratando el cáncer en una fase temprana, dándole más opciones al paciente para elegir el tratamiento que prefiera. Es sumamente importante que el paciente y el médico consideren detalladamente antes de tomar una decisión los beneficios de los procedimientos, diagnósticos y tratamientos.

Tratamiento

Una vez que el cáncer se descubre en la próstata, el profesional médico debe determinar en que fase de crecimiento está el cáncer, si se ha extendido a otras partes del cuerpo, y que partes son, para poder decidir el tipo de tratamiento más efectivo. Esto se hace por medio del uso de pruebas de sangre y de imágenes tales como MRI (imágenes por resonancia magnética.) Hay cuatro fases o estadías en el desarrollo del cancer:

▶ Primera estadía: el cáncer es demasiado pequeño para ser detectado y generalmente se descubre durante una cirugía para tratar otro problema, como por ejemplo, una próstata agrandada.
▶ Segunda estadía: el cáncer está todavía circunscrito a la próstata pero ya cubre más tejido. Generalmente, se detecta a través de un examen DRE o una biopsia que ha sido indicada como resultado de una prueba PSA "alta."
▶ Tercera estadía: el cáncer se ha extendido a tejidos cercanos.
▶ Cuarta estadía: el cáncer ha hecho metástasis extendiéndose a los nódulos linfáticos o a otras partes del cuerpo.

Hay más de una manera de tratar el cáncer de la próstata y es muy importante que el paciente se informe sobre las posibles opciones, riesgos y beneficios de cada tratamiento y después trate su caso con sus médicos, el urólogo, el oncólogo y el oncólogo de radiación antes de tomar una decisión. La estadía de la enfermedad es en muchos casos un factor determinante.

Tipos de tratamiento:

► Vigilancia activa: también llamada espera vigilante, implica observación y monitoreo sin el uso de un tratamiento invasivo. Se recomienda generalmente, a) en casos de cáncer en una fase temprana o de desarrollo lento; b) cuando existen otras condiciones médicas apremiantes que puedan acortar la vida del paciente.

► Cirugía: indicada por lo general en casos en que el cáncer está circunscrito a la próstata. Se emplea para extirpar toda o parte de la misma.

► Terapia de radiación: consiste en matar las células cancerosas en la próstata y en los tejidos circundantes por medio de radiación ionizante.

► Terapia hormonal: se emplea para evitar la liberación de la testosterona, o prevenir que la hormona actúe sobre las células prostáticas, ya que la testosterona determina el crecimiento de las mismas.

► Quimioterapia: se basa en el uso de elementos químicos que detengan el crecimiento de las células cancerosas o matarlas. Generalmente, se emplea en casos de matástasis.

Otros tipos de tratamiento empleados son la crioterapia que consiste en matar las células prostáticas y tumores congelándolos por medio de una sonda insertada en la próstata a través del perineo, y ultrasonido enfocado de alta intensidad (high-intensity focused ultrasound).

Los científicos e investigadores continúan identificando nuevas drogas, nuevos regímenes y tratamientos con la esperanza de detener la progresión de la enfermedad, aliviar los efectos secundarios y ofrecer al paciente una buena calidad de vida.

Para más información visite en la Internet www.cancer.gov/espanol.

MEDICATIONS / MEDICAMENTOS

Types of Medications — Tipos de medicamentos

MEDICATION	MAIN USE	MEDICAMENTO	USO PRINCIPAL
ENGLISH		SPANISH	
adrenergenic	to dilate the pupil; increase heart rate; strengthen heart beat	adrenérgicos	para dilatar la pupila; dar fuerza a los latidos del corazón
aminosalicylates	to help treat inflammation	aminosalicilatos	para tratar inflamaciones
anesthetics	to reduce sensation of pain	anestésicos	para aliviar el dolor
antiarrythmics	to treat arrythmia	antiarrítmicos	para tratar la arritmia
antibiotics	to treat bacterial infections	antibióticos	para tratar infecciones bacterianas
anticholinergics	to increase heart rate	anticolinérgicos	para aumentar la frecuencia cardíaca
anticoagulants	to prevent blood clotting	anticoagulantes	para prevenir la coagulación sanguínea
anticonvulsants	to prevent or treat convulsions	anticonvulsivos	para prevenir o tratar convulsiones
antidepressants	to treat depression	antidepresivos	para tratar la depresión
antidiarrheal	to treat diarrhea	antidiarreicos	para tratar la diarrea
antiemetics	to prevent nausea or vomiting	antiemético	para prevenir o tratar la náusea o vómitos
antihistaminics	to block histamine receptors	antihistamínicos	para bloquear los receptores de histamina
antihypertensives	to lower blood pressure	antihipertensivos	para bajar la presión arterial
anti-inflammatory	to reduce inflammation	antiinflamatorio	para reducir la inflamación
anti-leukotrienes	to treat allergies	anti-leucotrienes	para tratar alergias
antilipidemics	to reduce concentration of lipids in the serum	antilipidémicos	para reducir la concentración de lípidos en el suero
antioncotics	to treat tumefaction	antioncóticos	para tratar la tumefacción
antipruritics	to reduce itching symptoms	antipruríticos	para tratar síntomas de picazón
antiseptics	to inhibit infection or putrefaction	antisépticos	para impedir infección o la putrefacción
antitussive	to relieve or reduce cough	antitusivos	para aliviar o reducir la tos

MEDICATION	MAIN USE	MEDICAMENTO	USO PRINCIPAL
ENGLISH		**SPANISH**	
barbiturics	to relieve anxiety or insomnia	barbitúricos	para reducir la ansiedad o el insomnio
bronchodilators	to expand the air passages or dilate bronchi	broncodilatador	para ampliar los conductos respiratorios o dilatar los bronquios
cathartics	to treat constipation	catárticos, purgantes	para tratar el estreñimiento
corticosteroids	to treat swelling, or glands deficiency	corticosteroides	para tratar la inchazón o la deficiencia glandular
decongestants	to reduce congestion or swelling	descongestionantes	para reducir la congestión o la hinchazón
diuretics	to increase urine production	diuréticos	para aumentar la producción de orina
emetics	to cause vomiting	eméticos	para promover el vómito
expectorants	to promote expectoration	expectorantes	para promover la expectoración
hypnotics, soporifics	to induce sleep and treat anxiety	hipnóticos o soporíficos	para inducir el sueño y tratar la ansiedad
laxatives	to prevent or treat constipation	laxantes	para prevenir o tratar el estreñimiento
stimulants	to stimulate or produce a reaction	estimulantes	para estimular o producir una reacción
tranquilizers	to treat stress and anxiety	tranquilizantes	para tratar el estrés y la ansiedad
vasodilators	to cause vasodilation	vasodilatador	para causar la vasodilatación

A medication may be prescribed to:

Se puede recetar una medicina para:

ENGLISH	SPANISH
1. Prevent or diagnose a disease.	1. Prevenir o diagnosticar una enfermedad.
2. Relieve a physical pain or mental problem.	2. Aliviar un dolor físico o un problema mental.
3. Destroy bacteria in the organism.	3. Destruir bacterias en el organismo.
4. Add to the body a substance that is not produced naturally anymore.	4. Añadir al cuerpo una sustancia que no produce ya naturalmente.
5. Create antibodies as a helper to the immune system.	5. Como una ayuda al sistema inmunológico para crear anticuerpos.

Dosage and Manipulation

ENGLISH	SPANISH
All medications must be safely discarded when it is outdated.	Todo medicamento debe ser desechado en un lugar seguro cuando está pasado de fecha.
If you forget to take the medication do not take a double dose; wait until the next indicated time.	Si se le olvida tomar la medicina no tome una dosis doble; tome la dosis regulada en el próximo tiempo indicado.
The dosage of your medication has been regulated according to your needs; do not give your medication to another person.	La dosis de su medicina se ha graduado de acuerdo con sus necesidades; no ofrezca su medicina a otra persona.
Keep antibiotics refrigerated.	Mantenga los antibióticos refrigerados.
Make sure they are discarded safely.	Cuando los deseche hágalo con precaución.
Always shake the bottle well.	Siempre agite bien la botella.
Certain medicines should be kept at room temperature, below 86 degrees F, or 30 degrees C, away from heat, moisture, and light.	Ciertas medicinas deben guardarse a una temperatura ambiental, de no más de 86 grados F, o 30 grados C, lejos del calor, la humedad y la luz.

Dosage / Dosis

Dosage	Dosis
drops	gotas
half teaspoon	media cucharadita
one tablespoon 1 tbsp	una cucharada 1 cda.
one teaspoon 1 tsp	una cucharadita 1 cdta.
one drop	una gota
5 (five) milligrams (mg.)	5 (cinco) miligramos (mg.)
50 (fifty) milligrams (mg.)	50 (cincuenta) miligramos (mg.)
120 (one hundred and twenty) milligrams	120 (ciento veinte) miligramos
240 (two hundred and forty) milligrams	240 (doscientos cuarenta) miligramos
500 (five hundred) milligrams	500 (quinientos) miligramos
1 cubic centimeter (cm^3)	1 (un) centímetro cúbico (cm^3)
1 (one) ounce	1 (una) onza

Appendix C
- ## Weights and Measures, Time, Numbers
- ## Nutrition, Physical Fitness
- ## Verbs

Apéndice C
- ## Pesos y medidas, El tiempo, Números
- ## Nutrición, Acondicionamiento físico
- ## Verbos

WEIGHTS AND MEASURES / PESOS Y MEDIDAS

All equivalents are approximate. / Todas las equivalencias son aproximadas.

Liquid Measure doses	Líquidos: Capacidad dosis (sistema métrico)
1 quart / cuarto = 0.946 liter / litro	1000 cc.[a]
1 pint / pinta = 0.0473 liter / litro	500 cc.
8 fluid ounces / onzas	240 cc.
3.5 fluid ounces / onzas	100 cc.
1 fluid ounce / onza	30 cc.
4 fluid drams / dracmas	4 cc.
15 minims, drops / gotas	1 cc.
1 minim, drop / gota	0.06 cc.
1 teaspoonful / cucharadita de café	4 cc.
1 tablespoonful / cucharada sopera	15 cc.
1 teacupful / media taza	120 cc.
1 cup / taza	240 cc.

a. cc. *abbr.* cubic centimeters / centímetros cúbicos

Solids	Sólidos
1 pound / libra	373.24 grams / gramos
1 ounce / onza	30 grams / gramos
4 drams / dracmas	15 grams / gramos
1 dram / dracma	4 grams / gramos
60 grains / granos = 1 dram / dracma	4 grams / gramos
30 grains / granos = 0.5 dram / dracma	2 grams / gramos
15 grains / granos	1 gram / gramo
10 grains / granos	0.6 grams / gramos
1 grain / grano	60 milligrams / miligramos
$3/4$ grain / grano	50 mg.[a] $1/2$ grain / grano
$1/2$ grain / grano	30 mg.
$1/4$ grain / grano	15 mg.
$1/10$ grain / grano	6 mg.

[a] mg. *abbr.* milligrams / miligramos

Weights and Measures / Pesos y medidas

Other Liquid Measures	Otras medidas líquidas
1 barrel / barril	119.07 liters /litros
1 gallon / galón = 8 pints / pintas (*Ingl.*) 3.785 L[a]	4 quarts / cuartos 3.785 L
1 liter / litro	2.113 pints / pintas
1 quart / cuarto	0.946 L
1 pint / pinta	0.473 L

a. L *abbr.* liter / litro.

Avoirdupois Weights	Peso avoirdupois (comercio)
1 ton / tonelada	1016 kilograms / kilos
1 hundredweight = 112 pounds / libras	50.80 kilograms / kilos
2.20 pounds / libras	1 kilogram / kilo
1 pound / libra = 16 ounces / onzas	0.453 kilograms / kilo
1 ounce / onza	28.34 grams / gramos

Length	Longitud
1 mile / milla	1.60 kilometers / kilómetros
1 yard / yarda = 3 feet / pies	0.914 meters / metros
1 foot / pie = 12 inches / pulgadas	0.304 meter / metro
1 inch / pulgada	25.4 millimeters / milímetros
0.04 inch / pulgada	1 millimeter / milímetro
0.39 inch / pulgada	1 centimer / centímetro
39.37 inches / pulgadas	1 meter / metro

NUMERALS / NÚMEROS

Cardinal Numerals	Números cardinales
0 cero / zero	30 treinta / thirty
1 uno (un, una) / one	40 cuarenta / forty
2 dos / two	50 cincuenta / fifty
3 tres / three	60 sesenta / sixty
4 cuatro / four	70 setenta / seventy
5 cinco / five	80 ochenta / eighty
6 seis / six	90 noventa / ninety
7 siete / seven	100 ciento, cien / one hundred
8 ocho / eight	101 ciento uno / one hundred and one
9 nueve / nine	110 ciento diez / one hundred and ten
10 diez / ten	200 doscientos / two hundred
11 once / eleven	300 trescientos / three hundred
12 doce / twelve	400 cuatrocientos / four hundred
13 trece / thirteen	500 quinientos / five hundred
14 catorce / fourteen	600 seiscientos / six hundred
15 quince / fifteen	700 setecientos / seven hundred
16 diez y seis, dieciséis / sixteen	800 ochocientos / eight hundred
17 diez y siete, diecisiete / seventeen	900 novecientos / nine hundred
18 diez y ocho, dieciocho / eighteen	1,000 mil / one thousand
19 diez y nueve, diecinueve / nineteen	1,010 mil diez / one thousand and ten
20 veinte / twenty	1,500 mil quinientos / one thousand five hundred
21 veinte y uno, veintiuno / twenty-one	2,000 dos mil / two thousand
	1,000,000 un millón / one million

Note: **Uno and ciento** and its multiples are the only cardinal numbers that change form. **Uno** drops the -o when it precedes a masculine singular noun (one liter of water / **un litro de agua**) but it does not drop the -o in one out of ten / **uno de cada diez**. **Ciento** changes to **cien** before nouns and before **mil** and **millón**: one hundred cases / **cien casos**; one hundred thousand cases / **cien mil casos**.

Multiples of **ciento** agree in gender and number with the nouns they modify: two hundred cases / **doscientos casos**; two hundred pills / **doscientas píldoras**.

Ordinal Numerals / Números ordinales

ENGLISH	MASCULINE	FEMININE
first	1° primero	1ª primera
second	2° segundo	2ª segunda
third	3° tercero	3ª tercera
fourth	4° cuarto	4ª cuarta
fifth	5° quinto	5ª quinta
sixth	6° sexto	6ª sexta
seventh	7° séptimo	7ª séptima
eighth	8° octavo	8ª octava
ninth	9° noveno	9ª novena
tenth	10° décimo	10ª décima

Primero and **tercero** drop the -o before masculine singular nouns.

the first year / **el primer año**
the third day / **el tercer día**

Note: If a cardinal number and a numeral are used to qualify the same noun, the cardinal always precedes the ordinal.

the first three patients / **los tres primeros pacientes**
Take the first two pills now. / **Tome las dos primeras pastillas ahora.**

In reference to dates, the ordinal **primero** is used for the first day of the month; the cardinal is used for the other dates.

Fractions / Fracciones

$\frac{1}{2}$	a, one half / medio, la mitad
$\frac{1}{3}$	a, one third / un tercio, una tercera parte
$\frac{1}{4}$	a, one fourth / un cuarto, una cuarta parte
$\frac{1}{5}$	a, one fifth / un quinto, una quinta parte
$\frac{1}{6}$	a, one sixth / un sexto, una sexta parte
$\frac{1}{8}$	a, one eighth / un octavo, una octava parte
$\frac{1}{10}$	a, one tenth / un décimo, una décima parte
$\frac{3}{5}$	three fifths / tres quintos
$\frac{5}{8}$	five eighths / cinco octavos
$\frac{7}{10}$	seven tenths / siete décimos
0.1	a, one tenth / un décimo
0.01	a, one hundredth / un centésimo
0.001	a, one thousandth / un milésimo

TEMPERATURE / TEMPERATURA

Celsius (centigrade) and Fahrenheit Temperatures / Temperaturas de grados Celsius (centígrados) y grados Fahrenheit

Degrees Celsius / Grados Celsius	Degrees Fahrenheit / Grados Fahrenheit
36.0	96.8
36.5	97.7
37	98.6
37.5	99.5
38	100.4
38.5	101.3
39	102.2
39.5	103.1
40	104
40.5	104.9
41	105.8
41.5	106.7
42	107.6

Converting F° to C° Subtract 32, then divide by 1.8	**Converting C° to F°** Multiply by 1.8, then add 32
Convertiendo F° a C° Réstese 32, divídase por 1,8	**Convertiendo C° a F°** Multiplíquese por 1,8, agréguese 32

Common Temperatures in Fahrenheit and Celsius / Temperaturas comunes en grados Celsius y grados Fahrenheit

	FAHRENHEIT	CELSIUS
Freezing point of water / Punto de congelación del agua	32	0
Refrigerator temperature / Temperatura del refrigerador	35–46	2–8
Room temperature / Temperatura ambiente	59–86	15–30
Incubator temperature / Temperatura de la incubadora	98.6	37
Body temperature / Temperatura corporal	98.6	37
Boiling point of water / Punto de ebullición del agua	212	100

TIME / EL TIEMPO

Days of the Week   Días de la semana

Monday	lunes
Tuesday	martes
Wednesday	miércoles
Thursday	jueves
Friday	viernes
Saturday	sábado
Sunday	domingo

You must return on Monday. / **Debe volver el lunes.**
On Thursdays the office is closed. / **Los jueves la consulta está cerrada.**
The test will be next Friday. / **La prueba será el próximo viernes.**

Note: Days of the week and months of the year are not capitalized in Spanish. / **En inglés los días de la semana y los meses del año se escriben con mayúscula.**

Seasons and Months of the Year / Estaciones y meses del año

SPRING	PRIMAVERA
March	marzo
April	abril
May	mayo

Your operation will be in May. / **Su operación será en mayo.**

SUMMER	VERANO
June	junio
July	julio
August	agosto

It is very hot in the summer. / **Hace mucho calor en el verano.**

AUTUMN	OTOÑO
September	septiembre
October	octubre
November	noviembre

I saw the patient last September. / **Vi al paciente el pasado mes de septiembre.**

WINTER	INVIERNO
December	diciembre
January	enero
February	febrero

Do you have many colds in the winter? / **¿Tiene muchos resfriados en el invierno?**

618

Time of Day | La hora

Time of Day	La hora
What time is it?	¿Qué hora es?
At what time?	¿A qué hora?
It is ...	Es la... (Son las...)
At	a la, a las
in the morning	por la mañana
in the afternoon	por la tarde
in the evening (at night)	por la noche

Es la una.	**A la una** tomo la medicina. / I take the medication **at one.**
Son las dos.	**A las dos** llegaré al hospital. / I will arrive at the hospital **at two.**
Son las dos y media.	**A las dos y media** tengo una consulta. / I have an appointment **at two-thirty.**
Son las cuatro.	**A las cuatro** voy a la farmacia. / I am going to the pharmacy **at four.**
Son las once.	**A las once** hablé con la enfermera. / I spoke to the nurse **at eleven.**
Son las doce.	**Al mediodía** como el almuerzo. / I eat lunch **at noon.**

Expressions of Time / Expresiones de tiempo

GENERAL TERMS	TÉRMINOS GENERALES	GENERAL TERMS	TÉRMINOS GENERALES
night	noche	daily	diario, diariamente
midnight	medianoche	2 weeks	dos semanas, quince días
mid-morning	media mañana	annual	anual
evening	tardecita	bimester	bimestre
sunset	atardecer	century	siglo
morning	mañana	date	fecha
day	día	decade	década
sunrise, dawn	amanecer, aurora	monthly	mensual, mensualmente
afternoon	tarde	trimester	trimestre
night	noche	twice a day	dos veces al día
noon	mediodía	weekly	semanal, semanalmente
after lunch	después del almuerzo	at bedtime	al acostarse
at dinner time	a la hora de la cena	before breakfast	antes de desayunar
during meals	durante las comidas	one week from today	en una semana, en siete días

Timing Tests and Medications / Tiempo marcado en pruebas y medicinas

liquid intake 24 hours	toma líquida de 24 horas
first morning specimen	espécimen de primera hora en la mañana
timed specimen	espécimen de tiempo marcado
fasting blood test	prueba sanguínea en ayunas
one teaspoon every three hours	una cucharadita cada tres horas
one pill a day	una pastilla al día

PHYSICAL FITNESS / ACONDICIONAMIENTO FÍSICO

What is physical fitness?

Physical fitness is the ability of an individual to carry out everyday activities in a manner that enables him or her to perform optimally in work or sports.

¿Qué es acondicionamiento físico?

Acondicionamiento físico es la habilidad de un individuo de desempeñar las actividades diarias en forma óptima ya sea en su trabajo o en deportes.

What is considered physical activity?

Physical activity is any movement of the body that uses energy. For health benefits, physical activity should be moderate to vigorous. Walking, gardening, dancing, or playing tennis can be considered moderate activities, but not doing light household chores or the amount of walking one does while shopping. The moderate or vigorous activity should add up to at least thirty minutes per day.

¿Qué se considera actividad física?

Actividad física es cualquier movimiento del cuerpo que usa energía. Para que sea beneficiosa para la salud, la actividad física debe ser de moderada a vigorosa. Caminar, hacer trabajo de jardinería, bailar o jugar al tenis se pueden considerar actividades moderadas, pero no caen en esa categoría hacer trabajos simples de la casa o caminar como se hace mientras se va de compras. La actividad ya sea moderada o vigorosa se debe mantener por treinta minutos por lo menos.

Vocabulary	Vocabulario
aerobic	aeróbico
cardiovascular	cardiovascular
cool down	enfriamiento
dancing	bailar
endurance	resistencia
equipment	equipo
exercise	ejercicio
flexibility	flexibilidad
gardening	jardinería
hiking	caminar
lifting weights	levantamiento de pesas
muscle tone	tonicidad muscular
strenghthening	fortalecimiento
strength training	programa de fortalecimiento
stretching out	estiramiento
treadmill	rueda de andar
warm-up	calentamiento
workout	régimen de ejercicio

To avoid pain or injury as a result of exercising, it is important to perform some warming-up and cooling-down exercises before and after engaging in any strenuous physical activity.

Para evitar dolor o alguna lesión debido a un esfuerzo físico, es conveniente hacer algunos ejercicios de calentamiento y enfriamiento antes y después de hacer un esfuerzo físico riguroso.

Warming-up and Cooling-down Exercises	Ejercicios de calentamiento y de enfriamiento
arm circles	rotación de los brazos
breathing deeply	respirar profundamente
making a fist	abrir y cerrar el puño
neck stretches	estiramiento del cuello
raising and lowering the shoulders	alzar y bajar los hombros
raising on toes	pararse de puntillas
rotating the ankles	rotación de los tobillos
rotating the neck	rotación del cuello
stretching the calves and arms	estiramiento de las pantorrillas y brazos
waist bends	doblamiento de la cintura

Physical Activities and Sports	Actividades físicas y deportes
MODERATE	**MODERADOS**
bicycling at a moderate pace	ciclismo a una velocidad moderada
golf	jugar al golf
hiking	caminar
lifting weights (light workout)	levantar pesas (régimen ligero)
VIGOROUS	**VIGOROSOS**
aerobics	aerobic
bicycling (vigorously)	ciclismo (acelerado)
running / jogging (at a fast pace)	correr rítmicamente (a paso acelerado)
swimming	natación

Estimated Daily Calorie Needs / Estimado de calorías diarias necesarias

Calorie Range / Escala de calorías		
	Sedentary / Sedentarios	Active / Activos
Children / Niños		
2–3 years / años	1,000	1,400
Females / Mujeres		
4–8 years / años	1,200	1,800
9–13	1,600	2,200
14–18	1,800	2,400
19–30	2,000	2,400
31–50	1,800	2,200
51+	1,600	2,200
Males / Hombres		
4–8 years / años	1,400	2,000
9–13	1,800	2,600
14–18	2,200	3,200
19–30	2,400	3,000
31–50	2,200	3,000
51+	2,000	2,800

U.S. Department of Agriculture, Center for Nutrition Policy and Promotion, April 2005

Sedentary means a lifestyle that includes only the light physical activity associated with typical day-to-day life.

Sedentario-a se refiere a un estilo de vida que incluye solamente las actividades cotidianas.

Active means a lifestyle that includes physical activity equivalent to walking more than 3 miles per day at 3 to 4 miles per hour, in addition to the light physical activity associated with typical day-to-day life.

Activo-a se refiere a actividad física equivalente a caminar más de 3 millas al día a un paso de 3 a 4 millas por hora, además de las actividades cotidianas.

General Observations and Recommendations / Observaciones y recomendaciones generales

General Observations and Recommendations	Observaciones y recomendaciones generales
Exercise helps in many ways.	El ejercicio es beneficioso de muchas maneras.
It keeps the lungs and heart healthy.	Mantiene los pulmones y el corazón saludables.
It helps the blood flow in the body.	Ayuda la circulación de la sangre.
It improves muscle tone.	Aumenta la tonicidad muscular.
It alleviates arthritic pain.	Alivia el dolor artrítico.
It strengthens bones and stimulates the production of hormones.	Fortalece los huesos y estimula la producción de hormonas.
It helps keep weight down.	Ayuda a mantener un buen peso.
It makes one feel good.	Le hace sentirse bien.
Do exercises that you like.	Haga ejercicios que le gusten.
Exercise a few times a week.	Haga ejercicios varias veces a la semana.
Talk to your doctor about a good exercise program for you.	Consulte con su médico sobre un programa de ejercicios que sea beneficioso para usted.

Taking Care of Your Back / El cuidado de la espalda

Taking Care of Your Back	El cuidado de la espalda
Maintain a good posture.	Mantenga una postura correcta.
When lifting, allow the legs to do the work.	Cuando levante algún peso, deje que las piernas hagan el esfuerzo.
Bend your knees, not your back.	Doble las rodillas, no la espalda.
Don't stand or sit in the same position for long periods of time.	No mantenga la misma posición, sentado-a o parado-a, por largo tiempo.
Sleep on your side with legs pulled in towards the chest.	Duerma sobre el costado con las piernas dobladas hacia el pecho.
Watch your weight.	Mantenga un buen peso.
Talk to your doctor about a good exercise program for you.	Consulte a su médico sobre un programa de ejercicios que sea adecuado para usted.

NUTRITION / NUTRICIÓN

For a long time, the prevention of diseases was based on keeping the body healthy, which was thought to be necessary to have a healthy mind. Nowadays, it has been proven that many diseases are caused by either an excess or a deprivation of nutrients, or by a metabolic imbalance of food intake. Malnutrition can produce chronic diseases such as marasmus. Excessive nutrients can cause gross weight gain at an early age leading to chronic vascular disease, diabetes, and injuries to the gastrointestinal system, manifested in obesity. Lack of vitamins and minerals in daily nutrient intake may also do major harm to the mental and physical development of a child and the well-being of persons of any sex and age. A balanced diet and physical activity are recognized as key to maintaining good health.

Por varios años la prevención de enfermedades se basaba en el aforismo "cuerpo sano, mente sana". En nuestros días, se prueba que muchas enfermedades se deben a la falta de una buena alimentación por la privación el excese de elementos nutritivos o al desequilibrio metabólico causado por los alimentos ingeridos. La malnutrición produce enfermedades crónicas tales como el marasmo. La ingestión inconmensurable de alimentos puede causar un aumento excesivo de peso a una edad temprana y causar trastornos vasculares, diabetes y daños al sistema gastrointestinal que se manifiestan en obesidad. La falta de vitaminas y minerales en la ingestión de nutrientes puede ocasionar trastornos en el desarrollo mental y físico de los niños y en general, al bienestar de personas de cualquier edad y sexo. Una dieta balanceada y la actividad física se reconocen como claves para mantener un buen estado de salud.

In 2005, the Center for Nutrition Policy revised its "Daily Food Pyramid" and replaced it with "MyPyramid, Steps to a Healthier You," a new plan for healthy Americans age 2 and over.

En el año 2005, el Centro de Regulación Alimenticia revisó su "Pirámide Alimentaria Diaria" y la reemplazó con "MiPirámide, Pasos Hacia una Mejor Salud", un nuevo plan para americanos saludables de 2 o más años de edad.

MYPYRAMID OBJECTIVES

► Make smart choices from every food group.
► Find your balance between food and physical activity.
► Get the most nutrition out of your calories.
► Stay within your daily calorie needs.

OBJETIVOS DE MIPIRÁMIDE

► Realizar elecciones inteligentes de cada grupo alimenticio.
► Encontrar un equilibrio entre la alimentación y la actividad física.
► Obtener la mejor nutrición de las calorías consumidas.
► Permanezca diariamente dentro de sus calorías necesarias.

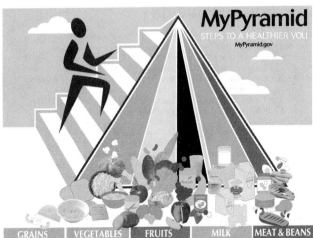

MyPyramid
STEPS TO A HEALTHIER YOU
MyPyramid.gov

GRAINS Make half your grains whole	VEGETABLES Vary your veggies	FRUITS Focus on fruits	MILK Get your calcium- rich foods	MEAT & BEANS Go lean with protein
Eat at least 3 oz. of whole-grain cereals, breads, crackers, rice, or pasta every day. 1 oz. is about 1 slice of bread, about 1 cup of breakfast cereal, or 1/2 cup of cooked rice, cereal, or pasta.	Eat more dark-green veggies like broccoli, spinach, and other dark leafy greens. Eat more orange vegetables like carrots and sweet potatoes. Eat more dry beans and peas like pinto beans, kidney beans, and lentils.	Eat a variety of fruit. Choose fresh, frozen, canned, or dried fruit. Go easy on fruit juices.	Go low-fat or fat-free when you choose milk, yogurt, and other milk products. If you don't or can't consume milk, choose lactose-free products or other calcium sources such as fortified foods and beverages.	Choose low-fat or lean meats and poultry. Bake it, broil it, or grill it. Vary your protein routine – choose more fish, beans, peas, nuts, and seeds.

For a 2,000-calorie diet, you need the amounts below from each food group.
To find the amounts that are right for you, go to MyPyramid.gov.

Eat 6 oz. every day	Eat 2 1/2 cups every day	Eat 2 cups every day	Get 3 cups every day; for kids 2 to 8, it's 2	Eat 5 1/2 oz. every day

Find your balance between food and physical activity
- Be sure to stay within your daily calorie needs.
- Be physically active for at least 30 minutes most days of the week.
- About 60 minutes a day of physical activity may be needed to prevent weight gain.
- For sustaining weight loss, at least 60 to 90 minutes a day of physical activity may be required.
- Children and teenagers should be physically active for 60 minutes every day, or most days.

Know the limits on fats, sugars, and salt (sodium)
- Make most of your fat sources from fish, nuts, and vegetable oils.
- Limit solid fats like butter, margarine, shortening, and lard, as well as foods that contain these.
- Check the Nutrition Facts label to keep saturated fats, *trans* fats, and sodium low.
- Choose food and beverages low in added sugars. Added sugars contribute calories with few, if any, nutrients.

Source: The Center for Nutrition Policy and Promotion, U.S. Department of Agriculture

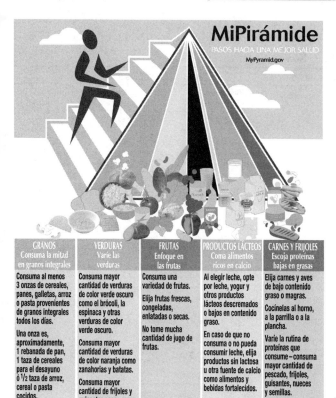

MiPirámide
PASOS HACIA UNA MEJOR SALUD
MyPyramid.gov

GRANOS Consuma la mitad en granos integrales	VERDURAS Varíe las verduras	FRUTAS Enfoque en las frutas	PRODUCTOS LÁCTEOS Coma alimentos ricos en calcio	CARNES Y FRIJOLES Escoja proteínas bajas en grasas
Consuma al menos 3 onzas de cereales, panes, galletas, arroz o pasta provenientes de granos integrales todos los días. Una onza es, aproximadamente, 1 rebanada de pan, 1 taza de cereales para el desayuno ó 1/2 taza de arroz, cereal o pasta cocidos.	Consuma mayor cantidad de verduras de color verde oscuro como el brócoli, la espinaca y otras verduras de color verde oscuro. Consuma mayor cantidad de verduras de color naranja como zanahorias y batatas. Consuma mayor cantidad de frijoles y guisantes secos como fríjoles pinto, colorados y lentejas.	Consuma una variedad de frutas. Elija frutas frescas, congeladas, enlatadas o secas. No tome mucha cantidad de jugo de frutas.	Al elegir leche, opte por leche, yogur y otros productos lácteos descremados o bajos en contenido graso. En caso de que no consuma o no pueda consumir leche, elija productos sin lactosa u otra fuente de calcio como alimentos y bebidas fortalecidos.	Elija carnes y aves de bajo contenido graso o magras. Cocínelas al horno, a la parrilla o a la plancha. Varíe la rutina de proteínas que consume – consuma mayor cantidad de pescado, frijoles, guisantes, nueces y semillas.

En una dieta de 2,000 calorías, necesita consumir las siguientes cantidades de cada grupo de alimentos.
Para consultar las cantidades correctas para usted, visite MyPyramid.gov.

Coma 6 onzas cada día	Coma 2 1/2 tazas cada día	Coma 2 tazas cada día	Coma 3 tazas cada día; para niños edades 2-8, 2 tazas	Coma 5 1/2 onzas cada día

Encuentre el equilibrio entre lo que come y su actividad física

- Asegúrese de mantenerse dentro de sus necesidades calóricas diarias.
- Manténgase físicamente activo por lo menos durante 30 minutos la mayoría de los días de la semana.
- Es posible que necesite alrededor de 60 minutos diarios de actividad física para evitar subir de peso.
- Para mantener la pérdida de peso, se necesitan al menos entre 60 y 90 minutos diarios de actividad física.
- Los niños y adolescentes deberían estar físicamente activos durante 60 minutos todos los días o la mayoría de los días.

Conozca los límites de las grasas, los azúcares y la sal (sodio)

- Trate de que la mayor parte de su fuente de grasas provenga del pescado, las nueces y los aceites vegetales.
- Limite las grasas sólidas como la mantequilla, la margarina, la manteca vegetal y la manteca de cerdo, así como los alimentos que los contengan.
- Verifique las etiquetas de Datos Nutricionales para mantener bajo el nivel de grasas saturadas, grasas trans y sodio.
- Elija alimentos y bebidas con un nivel bajo de azúcares agregados. Los azúcares agregados aportan calorías con pocos o ningún nutriente.

Source: The Center for Nutrition Policy and Promotion, U.S. Department of Agriculture

MyPyramid Food Intake Pattern Calories Levels /
MiPirámide Patrón de Ingestión, Nivel de Calorías

Men / Hombres

AGE / EDAD	ACTIVITY LEVEL / NIVEL DE ACTIVIDAD		
	Sedentary / Sedentaria*	Mod. Active / Mod. Activa*	Active / Activa*
2	1,000	1,000	1,000
3	1,000	1,400	1,400
4	1,200	1,400	1,600
5	1,200	1,400	1,600
6	1,400	1,600	1,800
7	1,400	1,600	1,800
8	1,400	1,600	2,000
9	1,600	1,800	2,000
10	1,600	1,800	2,200
11	1,800	2,000	2,200
12	1,800	2,220	2,400
13	2,000	2,200	2,600
14	2,000	2,400	2,800
15	2,200	2,600	3,000
16	2,400	2,800	3,200
17	2,400	2,800	3,200
18	2,400	2,800	3,200
19–20	2,600	2,800	3,000
21–25	2,400	2,800	3,000
26–30	2,400	2,600	3,000
31–35	2,400	2,600	3,000
36–40	2,400	2,600	2,800
41–45	2,200	2,600	2,800
46–50	2,200	2,400	2,800
51–55	2,200	2,400	2,800
56–60	2,200	2,400	2,600
61–65	2,000	2,400	2,600
66–70	2,000	2,200	2,600
71–75	2,000	2,200	2,600
76+	2,000	2,200	2,400

United States Department of Agriculture, Center for Nutrition Policy and Promotion, April 2005.

Females / Mujeres

AGE / EDAD	ACTIVITY LEVEL / NIVEL DE ACTIVIDAD		
	Sedentary / Sedentaria*	Mod. Active / Mod. Activa*	Active / Activa*
2	1,000	1,000	1,000
3	1,000	1,200	1,400
4	1,200	1,400	1,400
5	1,200	1,400	1,600
6	1,200	1,400	1,600
7	1,200	1,600	1,800
8	1,400	1,600	1,800
9	1,400	1,600	1,800
10	1,400	1,800	2,000
11	1,600	1,800	2,000
12	1,600	2,000	2,200
13	1,600	2,000	2,200
14	1,800	2,000	2,400
15	1,800	2,000	2,400
16	1,800	2,000	2,400
17	1,800	2,000	2,400
18	1,800	2,000	2,400
19–20	2,000	2,200	2,400
21–25	2,000	2,200	2,400
26–30	1,800	2,000	2,400
31–35	1,800	2,000	2,200
36–40	1,800	2,000	2,200
41–45	1,800	2,000	2,200
46–50	1,800	2,000	2,200
51–55	1,600	1,800	2,200
56–60	1,600	1,800	2,200
61–65	1,600	1,800	2,000
66–70	1,600	1,800	2,000
71–75	1,600	1,800	2,000
76+	1,600	1,800	2,000

United States Department of Agriculture, Center for Nutrition Policy and Promotion, April 2005.

*Calorie levels are based on the Estimated Energy Requirements (EER) and activity levels from the Institute of Medicine Dietary Reference Intakes Macronutrients Report, 2002.
Los niveles de calorías se basan en los Requisitos de Energía Estimados (EER, por sus siglas en inglés) y en los niveles de actividad del Informe de nutrientes macro de consumo de referencia dietario del Instituto de Medicina (Institute of Medicine Dietary Reference Intakes Macro nutrients Report) de 2002.

SEDENTARY = less than 30 minutes a day of moderate physical activity in addition to daily activities.
SEDENTARIA = menos de 30 minutos diarios de actividad física moderada además de las actividades diarias.

MOD. ACTIVE = at least 30 minutes up to 60 minutes a day of moderate physical activity in addition to daily activities.
MOD. ACTIVA = por lo menos 30 a 60 minutos por día de actividad física moderada además de las actividades diarias.

ACTIVE = 60 or more minutes a day of moderate physical activity in addition to daily activities.
ACTIVA = 60 minutos o más por día de actividad física moderada además de las actividades diarias.

Food Groups	Grupos de alimentos	Suggestions	Sugerencias
Fruits: juice, fresh, dry, canned or frozen, sliced, or cut for salads or stewed.	**Frutas:** jugo (zumo), frescas, enlatadas o congeladas, cortadas para ensaladas o cocidas.	Consume fruit juice from fresh fruits, rich in potassium, fiber, vitamin C, low in calories and sodium.	Consumir jugo (zumo) de frutas frescas, frutas ricas en potasio, fibra, vitamina C, bajas en calorías y sodio.
Vegetables: includes vegetable juices, natural, canned, frozen; vegetables dry, cooked, steamed, on the grill or baked.	**Verduras:** incluya jugos de vegetales frescos, en lata o congelados; verduras secas y congeladas; cocinadas al vapor, en parrilla o asadas.	Consume vegetable juice with fresh vegetables, use with other vegetables in stews, soups and gravies; decorate serving dishes with baby spinach or parsley with fish, lean meat and poultry to enhance their appearance.	Consumir jugo (zumo) de verduras frescas, en ensaladas cocidas, sopas y salsas; decorar sirviendo platos con espinacas o perejil con pescado, carne magra y aves para una mejor apariencia.
Grains: wheat, corn, barley, oats, foods made with integral flour, barley, corn flour and popcorn and their refined products are part of a balanced diet.	**Granos:** trigo, maíz, cebada, avena, alimentos hechos con harina integral, avena, harina de maíz, palomitas de maíz, y productos de granos refinados, que son parte de una dieta balanceada.	Consume at least half of the food made from whole grain wheat, rice, oats, cornmeal, such as bread, pasta and cereals.	Consumir por lo menos la mitad de los alimentos granos integrales: como pan integral, arroz, avena, harina de maíz, pan, pasta y cereales.
Lean meats: poultry, chicken, turkey, fish, dry beans, eggs, and nuts, such as peanuts, hazelnuts, almonds, sunflower and sesame seeds.	**Carnes magras :** aves, pollo, pavo, pescado, frijoles, huevos y nueces tales como cachuetes, avellanas, almendras, semillas de girasol y de sésamo.	Meals prepared with lean meats low in fats, poultry, beans and more frequently fish; use nuts and dry beans; fish rich in Omega-3, mixed with vegetables in salads, sauces, cooked on the grill or steamed.	Consumir comidas hechas con carne magra; aves con poca grasa en cocidos; frijoles y con más frecuencia pescados, nueces y frijoles preparados y agregados a ensaladas y ricos en Omega-3 mezclados con vegetales en ensaladas, salsas, o cocinados a la braza o al vapor.

Milk products: liquid milk and foods that retain their calcium made with low fat milk, avoid products with trans fats and products low in calcium.	**Productos lácteos**: leche líquida y alimentos que retienen el calcio hechos con leche desgrasada, evite productos con grasas trans y productos bajos en calcio.	Liquid milk low in fat mixed with chocolate or strawberry; cheeses: cheddar, mozzarella, Swiss and parmesan, mixed with pastas, salads; pizza and yogurt; puddings, breads, avoiding trans fat products low in calcium.	Leches líquidas de poca grasa mezcladas con chocolate o fresa; quesos tal como cheddar, mozzarella, suizo o parmesano combinados con pastas, ensaladas, pizza; yogur; pudines y panes; evitar productos ricos en grasa trans bajos en calcio.
Vegetable oils: canola, corn oil, olive oil, safflower oil, soybean oil, sunflower seeds, oil from fish, avocados.	**Aceites de vegetales:** canola, aceite de maíz, de oliva, de alazor, de soya, de semillas, de girasol y aceites de pescado y aguacates.	Oils are generally used for cooking or in salads for adding flavor to sauces and with spices in the preparation of meats, fish and poultry.	Los aceites se usan generalmente para cocinar o en ensaladas, para dar sabor en salsas y con especias en la preparación de carnes, pescado y aves.

Food Vocabulary / Vocabulario de los alimentos

FOODS: fruits, vegetables, fish and seafood, grains (beans, nuts), milk products, breads and beverages.

ALIMENTOS: frutas, verduras, carnes (pescado y mariscos), granos (frijoles y nueces) productos lácteos, panes y bebidas.

FRUITS	FRUTAS	FRUITS	FRUTAS
avocado	aguacate	mango	mango
apple	manzana	melon	melón
apricot	albaricoque	nectarine	nectarina
banana	plátano	orange	naranja
blueberry	mora azul	papaya	papaya
blackberry	zarzamora	peach	durazno, melocotón
cantaloupe	cantalú (melón)	pear	pera
coconut	coco	pineapple	piña
cranberries	arándano	plum	ciruela
cherry	cereza	prune	ciruela pasa
date	dátil	raisins	pasas
fig	higo	raspberry	frambuesa
grape	uva	strawberry	fresa
guava	guayaba	tangerine	mandarina
grapefruit	toronja	watermelon	sandía
lemon	limón		

Fruits are rich in potassium, carbohydrates, fiber, and vitamins A and C. / Las frutas son ricas en potasio, carbohidratos, fibra y vitaminas A y C.

VEGETABLES	VERDURAS	MEATS	CARNES
asparagus	espárrago	beef	res, carne de vaca
basil	albahaca	chicken, hen	pollo, gallina
beans	frijoles	mutton, lamb	carnero, cordero
beets	remolacha, betabel	pork	cerdo, puerco
broccoli	bróculi	veal	ternera
kale	col rizada	turkey	pavo
leek	puerro	duck	pato
lettuce	lechuga	fish	pescado
mushrooms	hongos, champiñones	geese	ganso
olives	aceitunas	ham	jamán
carrots	zanahoria	game	carner de cara
celery	apio	bison	bisonte
onions	cebollas	rabbit	conejo
parsley	perejil	deer	venado
peas	guisantes, arvejas		
potato	papas, patatas		
rice	arroz		
rosemary	romero		
spinach	espinaca		
squash	calabaza		
sweet potato	camote, boniato, batata		
tomato	tomate		
yam	ñame		
watercress	berro		

SHELLFISH	MARISCOS	FISH	PESCADOS
lobster	langosta	cod	bacalao
clams	almejas	flounder	platija
shrimp	camarón	herring	arenque
crab	cangrejo	salmon	salmón
squid	calamar	sea bass	lubina
prawns	gambas	hake	merluza
mussels	mejillones	snapper	pargo
oysters	ostra	sword fish	pez espada
octopus	pulpo	trout	trucha
		tuna	bonito, atún
		monkfish	rape
		croaker	corvina

BREADS AND CEREALS	PANES Y CEREALES
barley	cebada
buttermilk bread	pan de suero
cheese bread	pan de queso
cookies	galleticas
cornbread	pan de maíz
crackers	galletas
egg bread	pan de huevo
oat bran	salvado de avena
French bread	pan francés
potato bread	pan de papas
rolls	panecitos
sweet rolls	panecitos dulces
tortillas	tortillas
white bread	pan blanco
whole-grain bread	pan de grano entero
whole-wheat toast	pan de trigo, pan negro

MILK PRODUCTS	PRODUCTOS LÁCTEOS	LIQUID MILK	LECHE LÍQUIDA
cottage cheese	requesón	whole milk	leche completa
cream	crema	condensed milk	leche condensada
yogurt	yogur	skim milk	leche descremada
butter	mantequilla	milk 2% fat	leche descremada 2%
cheese	queso	fat-free milk	leche desgrasada
ice cream	helado	evaporated milk	leche evaporada
margarine	margarina	cream	nata
milk	leche	whipped cream	nata batida

Nutrition / Nutrición

BEVERAGES	BEBIDAS
beer	cerveza
bouillon	caldo claro de carne
broth	caldo
carbonated drinks	sodas
chocolate	chocolate
coffee	café
consommé	consomé
fruit juices	jugos de fruta
gelatin	gelatina
ice	hielo
lemonade	limonada
mineral water	agua mineral
sherbet	sherbet
tea; herbal tea	té negro; té de hierbas
thirst-quencher beverages	bebidas que matan la sed
water (mineral)	agua mineral
water (spring)	agua de manantial
wine	vino

FOOD QUALITIES	CUALIDADES DE LOS ALIMENTOS	FOOD QUALITIES	CUALIDADES DE LOS ALIMENTOS
light	ligero	nutritious	nutritivo
highly priced	muy caro	washed	lavado
liquified	licuado	kneaded	amasado
acid	ácido	strained	escurrido
bitter	amargo	soft	blando
bloody	algo crudo, con sangre	rich	rico
cold	frío	savory	sabroso, apetitoso
dry	seco, escurrido	seasoned	sazonado
enough	suficiente	rare	algo crudo, poco hecho
healthy	saludable	sour	agrio
spoiled	dañado, contaminado	sticky	pegajoso
fresh	fresco	strong	fuerte
frozen	congelado	sweet	dulce
ground	molido	tasty	sabroso, de buen gusto

Vitamins / Vitaminas

Vitamin A: fish, liver, egg yolk, butter, yellow fruits.

Vitamin D: fish liver oils, liver, egg yolk, butter.

Vitamin E: vegetable oil, wheat germ, leafy vegetables, margarine, egg yolk, legumes.

Vitamin K, K1, K2: pork, liver, vegetable oils.

Vitamin B6 group: spinach, organ meats, fish, legumes, whole-grain cereals, sweet potatoes, avocado.

Vitamin B12: liver, meats, egg yolk, milk and dairy products.

Vitamin C (ascorbic acid): citric fruits, tomatoes, green peppers, cabbage.

Fatty Acids: vegetable oils (sunflower, corn, canola), margarine.

Folic Acid: fresh green vegetables, fruits, gizzards, kidneys, liver.

Biotin: legumes, liver, nuts, cauliflower, egg yolk.

Niacin (niacinamide, nicotinic acid): dried yeast, liver, meat, fish, legumes, whole grain cereal.

Thiamine (vitamin B1): potatoes, legumes, pork, liver, enriched cereals.

Riboflavin (Vitamin B2): milk, cheese, liver, eggs, enriched cereals.

Potassium: bananas, apricots, peaches, prunes, raisins, milk.

Calcium: milk, milk products, meat, fish, eggs, beans, fruits, vegetables.

Copper: liver, shellfish, whole grains, nuts, poultry.

Magnesium: dark green vegetables, dairy products, nuts, meat, whole grain cereals.

Phosphorus: dairy products, meat, fish, poultry, legumes, grains, nuts.

Iron: meats, spinach, radishes.

Sodium: beef, pork, cheese, olives, sauerkraut.

Zinc: dairy products, liver, wheat bran, shellfish.

Vitamina A: pescado, hígado, yema de huevo, mantequilla, frutas amarillas.

Vitamina D: aceite de hígado de pescado, yema de huevo, mantequilla.

Vitamina E: aceite vegetal, germen de trigo, hojas vegetales, margarina, yema de huevo, legumbres.

Vitamina K, K1, K2: cerdo, hígado, aceites vegetales.

Grupo de B6: espinaca, pescado, cereales de integrales, legumbres, boniato, aguacate.

Vitamina B12: hígado, carnes, yema de huevo, leche y derivados.

Vitamina C (ácido ascórbico): frutas cítricas, tomate, pimiento verde, repollo.

Acidos grasos: aceites vegetales (de maíz, girasol, canola), margarina.

Acido fólico: vegetales frescos, frutas, molleja de ave, hígado, riñones.

Biotina: legumbres, hígado, nueces, coliflor, yema de huevo.

Niacina (niacinamida, ácido nicotínico): levadura en polvo, hígado, carne, pescado, legumbres, cereales integrales.

Tiamina (vitamina B1): papas, legumbres, cerdo, hígado, cereales enriquecidos.

Riboflavina (vitamina B2): leche, queso, huevos, cereales enriquecidos.

Potasio: plátanos, albaricoque, durazno (melocotón), ciruelas pasas, pasas, leche.

Calcio: leche y sus derivados, carnes, pescado, huevos, frijoles, vegetales, frutas.

Cobre: mariscos, hígado, granos integrales, carne de ave.

Magnesio: verduras verdes oscuro, productos lácteos, nueces, carne, cereales de granos integrales.

Fósforo: productos lácteos, carne, pescado, carne de ave, legumbres, granos integrales, nueces.

Hierro: carnes, espinaca, rábanos.

Sodio: carne de res, cerdo, queso, aceitunas, col agria.

Zinc: productos lácteos, hígado, salvado, mariscos.

WHY VITAMINS ARE ESSENTIAL?

Vitamin A: helps to have good vision, healthy hair, skin and nails; fights infection

Vitamin D: calcium absorbent, helps to maintain healthy bones and teeth

Vitamin E: important in the formation of red blood cells, and building tissues and muscle development

Vitamin K, K1, K2: intervenes in the formation of prothrombin and other coagulation factors

Vitamin B6 group: of great importance in the metabolism and absorption of proteins

Vitamin B12: effective in pernicious anemia, aids in formation of genetic materials (DNA and RNA)

Vitamin C (ascorbic acid): aids in the formation of collagen, helps prevent infection and bleeding of the gums

Fatty Acid: precursors of prostaglandins, builders of many lipids

Folic Acid: maturation of red blood cells, helpful to prevent anemia, intervenes in the formation of genetic material

Biotin: aids in body growth, amino acid and fatty acid metabolism

Niacin (niacinamide, nicotinic acid): helps in carbohydrates metabolism

Thiamine (vitamin B1): aids in peripheral and central nerve cell functions, and to metabolize carbohydrates into energy

Riboflavin (Vitamin B2): aids to metabolize carbohydrates, proteins and fats

Potassium: necessary to keep acid-base balance, muscle activity, water retention

Calcium: blood coagulation, bone and teeth formation, transmission of nerve impulses

Copper: necessary in the synthesis of hemoglobin, component of digestive enzymes

Magnesium: aids to synthesize protein, formation of bones and teeth

¿POR QUÉ SON ESENCIALES LAS VITAMINAS?

Vitamina A: ayuda a tener buena visión y pelo, piel y uñas saludables; combate infecciones

Vitamina D: absorbente del calcio, ayuda a mantener saludables los huesos y dientes.

Vitamina E: importante en la formación de glóbulos rojos y en el desarrollo de los tejidos y desarrollo muscular

Vitamina K, K1, K2: intervienen en la formación de protrombina y otros factores de coagulación

Grupo de B6: de gran importancia en el metabolismo y en la absorsión de las proteínas

Vitamina B12: efectiva en la anemia perniciosa, ayuda a la formación de materiales genéticos (ADN y ARN)

Vitamina C (ácido ascórbico): ayuda a la formación de colágeno, ayuda a prevenir infecciones y sangramiento de las encías

Acidos grasos: precursores de prostaglandinas, constructores de varios lípidos

Acido fólico: maturación de glóbulos rojos, ayuda a prevenir la anemia, necesario en la formación de elementos genéticos

Biotina: ayuda al crecimiento, metabolismo de aminoácidos y ácidos grasos

Niacina (niacinamida, ácido nicotínico): ayuda en el metabolismo de carbohidratos

Tiamina (vitamina B1): ayuda en la funciones de las células nerviosas centrales y periféricas, y en la conversión de carbohidratos en energía

Riboflavina (vitamina B2): ayuda a metabolizar carbohidratos, proteínas y grasas

Potasio: necesario al balance ácido-básico, a la actividad muscular, en la retención de agua

Calcio: coagulación de la sangre, formación de dientes y huesos, transmisión de impulsos nerviosos

Cobre: necesario en la síntesis de hemoglobina, componente de enzimas digestivas

Magnesio: ayuda en la síntesis de las proteínas, formación de huesos y dientes

Phosphorus: aids metabolism of calcium, protein and glucose, formation of bones and teeth
Sodium: acid-base balance, blood pH, muscle activity
Iron: needed to maintain the correct level of hemoglobin in the blood

Zinc: aids metabolism of proteins

Fósforo: ayuda a metabolizar el calcio, las proteínas y la glucosa, esencial en la formación de huesos y dientes
Sodio: balance ácido básico, actividad muscular, pH sanguíneo
Hierro: necesario para mantener el nivel correcto de hemoglobina en la sangre
Zinc: ayuda en el metabolismo de las proteínas

POSITIONS AND BODY MOVEMENTS / POSITIONES Y MOVIMIENTOS DEL CUERPO

ENGLISH	SPANISH
1. Stand here.	1. Párese aquí.
2. Stand here and do not move.	2. Párese aquí y no se mueva.
3. Sit on the table.	3. Siéntese sobre la mesa.
4. Lie down on the table ___ on your back ___ face down ___ on your right side ___ on your left side	4. Acuéstese sobre la mesa ___ boca arriba ___ boca abajo ___ sobre el lado derecho ___ sobre el lado izquierdo
5. Put your knees against your chest and let your chin touch your chest.	5. Acerque las rodillas al pecho lo más posible y deje que la barbilla toque el pecho.
6. Put your arms around this machine.	6. Ponga los brazos alrededor de esta máquina.
7. Do not get up, remain lying down.	7. No se levante, quédese acostado-a.
8. Raise your head.	8. Levante la cabeza.
9. Raise your hands.	9. Levante las manos.
10. Raise your right hand.	10. Levante la mano derecha.
11. Raise your left hand ___ higher ___ lower	11. Levante la mano izquierda ___ más hacia arriba ___ más hacia abajo
12. Open your hand.	12. Abra la mano.
13. Close your hand. Make as first.	13. Cierre la mano. Cierre el puño.
14. Extend your fingers.	14. Extienda los dedos.
15. Close your fingers one at a time.	15. Cierre uno por uno los dedos.
16. Lift your right leg.	16. Levante la pierna derecha.
17. Lift your left leg.	17. Levante la pierna izquierda.
18. Can you move the leg?	18. ¿Puede mover la pierna?
19. Bend over.	19. Dóblese.
20. Bend over backwards.	20. Dóblese hacia atrás.
21. Raise your buttocks (hips).	21. Levante las nalgas (las caderas).
22. Put your hands behind your head.	22. Ponga las manos detrás de la cabeza.
23. Extend your arms, and bringing them towards the front, touch the tips of your index fingers together.	23. Extienda los brazos, trayéndolos hacia el frente, toque las puntas de los dedos índice.
24. Bend your arm.	24. Doble el brazo.
25. Extend your arm.	25. Extienda el brazo.
26. Squeeze my hand as hard as you can.	26. Apriéteme la mano lo más fuerte que pueda.

VERBS / VERBOS

List of Useful Verbs / Lista de verbos útiles

ENGLISH	SPANISH
to abort	abortar, acortar, impedir
to abstain, to refrain	abstenerse de
to accelerate, to speed up	acelerar
to accept	aceptar
to accompany, to go with	acompañar
to accumulate, to gather	acumular
to ache, to hurt	doler (ue)[a]
to acquire	adquirir (ie)
to add	añadir, agregar
to admit	admitir
to advise	aconsejar
to age	envejecer
to affect	afectar
to aggravate	empeorar, empeorarse, agravarse, agravar
to aid	ayudar
to alleviate	aliviar
to amputate	amputar
to approve	aprobar (ue)
to arrange	arreglar
to arrive; to arrive on time	llegar; llegar a tiempo
to ask for (*to request*)[b]	pedir (i)
to ask for (*to question*)[b]	preguntar
to aspirate	aspirar
to assimilate	asimilar
to associate	asociar
to assure	asegurar
to attack	atacar
to attend	asistir, cuidar
to bathe	bañarse
to be	estar; ser
to be able, can	poder (ue)
to be afraid	tener miedo
to be born	nacer
to be hot, cold [*body temperature*][b]	tener calor, tener frío
to be hot, cold [*weather*][b]	hacer calor, hacer frío
to be hungry	tener hambre

ENGLISH	SPANISH
to be in a hurry	tener prisa
to be quiet	callarse
to be sick	estar enfermo -a
to be sleepy	tener sueño
to be . . . years old	tener . . . años
to become (*adj.*)	hacerse; ponerse (+ *adj.*)
to begin	empezar (ie), comenzar (ie)
to behave	portarse
to believe	creer
to bend, to flex	doblar, doblarse
to bite	morder (ue)
to blame	culpar
to bleed	sangrar
to blink	parpadear
to bother, to annoy	molestar
to break	romper; quebrar
to breast-feed	amamantar; dar el pecho
to breathe	respirar
to bring	traer
to buy	comprar
to bruise	magullarse; amoratarse
to brush	cepillar
to burn	quemar; quemarse
to burp	eructar
to call	llamar
to calm down	calmarse
to carry, to wear	llevar
to cause	causar
to change (one's clothes)	cambiarse (de ropa)
to chat	charlar
to choke	atragantarse; ahogar; sofocar
to choose	escoger; elegir (i)
to clean	limpiar
to climb	subirse
to close	cerrar (ie)

List of Useful Verbs / Lista de verbos útiles

ENGLISH	SPANISH
to come	venir
to complain (of, about)	quejarse (de)
to complete	completar
to conceive	concebir (i)
to consider	considerar
to contact	contactar
to contain	contener
to continue	continuar, seguir (i)
to convalesce	convalecer; recuperarse
to cost	costar (ue)
to count	contar (ue)
to cough	toser
to cry	llorar
to cut	cortar
to deliver [to give birth]	dar a luz; estar de parto; pop. aliviarse
to deny	negar (ie)
to develop	desarrollar; [a photo] revelar
to die	morir (ue, u)
to diet	estar a dieta; hacer una dieta
to discharge [secretion]	tener secreciones
to discharge [a patient]	dar de alta
to disinfect	desinfectar
to do, to make	hacer
to doubt	dudar
to dream	soñar (ue)
to dress [with clothes]	vestir; vestirse (i)
to drink	beber; tomar
to earn	ganar
to eat	comer
to eat breakfast	desayunar
to eat dinner	cenar
to eat lunch	almorzar (ue)
to ejaculate	eyacular
to enter	entrar

Verbs / Verbos

ENGLISH	SPANISH
to examine	examinar
to exercise	hacer ejercicio
to expect	esperar
to explain	explicar
to fall asleep	dormirse (ue, u)
to fall down	caerse
to fear	temer; tener miedo
to feel	sentir (ie, i)
to follow	seguir (i)
to forget	olvidar
to fracture	fracturar; quebrar; romper
to function	funcionar
to gargle	hacer gárgaras
to get	obtener, conseguir (i)
to get angry	enfadarse, enojarse
to get better	mejorarse
to get up	levantarse
to get well	curarse, sanarse, ponerse bien
to give	dar
to go	ir; salir
to go away	irse
to go to bed	acostarse (ue)
to grow	crecer
to hand over	entregar
to have	tener; *aux.* haber
to hear	oír
to help	ayudar
to hope	esperar
to hurry	apurarse, darse prisa
to hurt	doler (ue); lastimar
to improve	mejorar
to incline	inclinar, inclinarse
to increase	aumentar
to inform	informar
to inject	inyectar
to insert	insertar, introducir, meter
to kill	matar
to know	saber; [*to be acquainted with*] conocer

List of Useful Verbs / Lista de verbos útiles

ENGLISH	SPANISH
to lack	faltar
to leak	gotear
to lean on	apoyarse en
to learn	aprender
to leave	salir
to let	dejar, permitir
to lie	mentir (ie, i)
to lie down	acostarse (ue)
to lift	levantar, alzar
to like	gustar
to listen	escuchar, atender (ie)
to live	vivir
to look at	mirar
to look for	buscar
to lose	perder (ie)
to love	amar; querer (ie)
to lower [arm, leg]	bajar
to marry	casarse
to masturbate	masturbarse
to menstruate	menstruar
to miscarry	abortar
to move	mover (ue)
to need	necesitar
to nurse [a baby]	amamantar
to nurse [the sick]	cuidar
to obtain	conseguir (i), obtener
to obstruct	obstruir
to open	abrir
to order	ordenar, mandar
to palpate	palpar
to participate	participar
to pay	pagar
to penetrate	penetrar
to permit	permitir, dejar
to plan	planear
to practice	practicar
to prefer	preferir (ie)

ENGLISH	SPANISH
to prescribe	recetar; prescribir
to promise	prometer
to push [*downward*]	pujar
to put	poner
to put in	poner; meter
to put on [*clothing*]	ponerse
to raise	levantar
to react	reaccionar
to read	leer
to receive	recibir
to recuperate	recuperar; recobrar
to relax	relajar; aflojar
to release	soltar (ue); librar; desprender
to relieve	aliviar; mejorar
to remain	quedar
to remember	recordar (ue)
to remove, take off	quitar; quitarse
to repeat	repetir (i)
to reply	contestar; responder
to respond	responder
to rest	descansar
to return	volver (ue)
to run	correr
to say	decir
to scratch	arañar
to see	ver
to send	mandar
to serve	servir (i)
to shake	agitar
to show	mostrar (ue); señalar; enseñar
to sit down	sentarse (ie)
to smoke	fumar
to sneeze	estornudar
to speak	hablar
to spend	gastar; [*time*] pasar
to spit	escupir
to sprain	torcer; torcerse
to stand up	levantarse

List of Useful Verbs / Lista de verbos útiles

ENGLISH	SPANISH
to stimulate	estimular
to study	estudiar
to suck	chupar, absorber
to suffer	sufrir
to swallow	tragar
to sweat	sudar
to sweeten	endulzar
to swell	hinchar, hincharse
to take	tomar, tomarse
to take off [clothes]	quitar, quitarse [la ropa]
to talk	hablar
to teach	enseñar
to tell	decir
to think	pensar (ie)
to tighten	apretar, ajustar
to try	tratar de; probar (ue)
to turn	virar; virarse
to turn around	dar vuelta; voltearse
to urinate	orinar
to use	usar, emplear
to visit	visitar
to vomit	vomitar
to wait	esperar
to wake up	despertarse (ie)
to want	querer (ie), desear
to wheeze	respirar con ruido sibilante
to wish	querer (ie), desear
to work	trabajar
to write	escribir

[a] Vowels in parentheses indicate root-changing verbs.
[b] Brackets clarify the meaning of the verb. Parentheses indicate a synonym.

INFINITIVE / INFINITIVO	PRETERIT / PRETÉRITO	PAST PARTICIPLE / PARTICIPIO PASADO
to arise / levantarse	arose	arisen
to awake / despertarse	awoke	awoke, awoken
to be / ser, estar	was, were	been
to become / volverse, hacerse	became	become
to begin / empezar	began	begun
to bend / inclinarse, doblarse	bent	bent
to bite / morder	bit	bit, bitten
to bleed / sangrar	bled	bled
to break / romper, quebrar	broke	broken
to bring / traer	brought	brought
to burn / quemar	burnt, burned	burnt, burned
to burst / reventar	burst	burst
to buy / comprar	bought	bought
can (*defectivo, aux.*) / poder	could	---
to choose / escoger, elegir	chose	chosen
to come / venir	came	come
to cost / costar	cost	cost
to cut / cortar	cut	cut
to deal with / tratar de, resolver	dealt with	dealt with
to dream / soñar	dreamt, dreamed	dreamt, dreamed
to drink / beber, tomar	drank	drunk
to drive / manejar, conducir	drove	driven
to eat / comer	ate	eaten
to fall / caerse, desprenderse	fell	fallen
to feed / alimentar, dar de comer	fed	fed
to feel / sentir, palpar	felt	felt
to fight / pelear	fought	fought
to find / encontrar, hallar	found	found
to forget / olvidar	forgot	forgot, forgotten
to forgive / perdonar	forgave	forgiven
to freeze / congelar	froze	frozen
to get / obtener	got	got, gotten
to give / dar	gave	given

INFINITIVE / INFINITIVO	PRETERIT / PRETÉRITO	PAST PARTICIPLE / PARTICIPIO PASADO
to grow / crecer, madurar	grew	grown
to have / tener, haber	had	had
to hear / oír, escuchar	heard	heard
to hide / esconder(se)	hid	hid, hidden
to hit / pegar	hit	hit
to hold / aguantar	held	held
to hurt / lastimar, doler	hurt	hurt
to keep / guardar	kept	kept
to know / saber, conocer	knew	known
to lay / poner, colocar	laid	laid
to leave / irse, dejar	left	left
to let / permitir, dejar	let	let
to lie / acostarse	lay	lain
to light / encender	lit, lighted	lit, lighted
to lose / perder	lost	lost
to make / hacer	made	made
may / poder	might	---
to meet / conocer, encontrarse	met	met
must (*defectivo; aux.*) / deber de, tener que	---	---
ought to (*defectivo; aux.*) / deber de	---	---
to pay / pagar	paid	paid
to put / poner	put	put
to read / leer	read	read
to run / correr	ran	run
to say / decir	said	said
to see / ver	saw	seen
to sell / vender	sold	sold
to send / enviar	sent	sent
to shake / agitar, temblar	shook	shaken
to show / mostrar	showed	shown, showed
to sit / sentarse	sat	sat
to sleep / dormir(se)	slept	slept
to speak / hablar	spoke	spoken
to spend / gastar	spent	spent
to spill / botar, derramar	spilled, spilt	spilled, spilt
to spin / dar vueltas	spun	spun

Verbs / Verbos

INFINITIVE / INFINITIVO	PRETERIT / PRETÉRITO	PAST PARTICIPLE / PARTICIPIO PASADO
to spit / escupir	spit, spat	spit, spat
to stand / pararse	stood	stood
to stick / punzar, picar	stuck	stuck
to sting / picar, pinchar	stung	stung
to swell / hincharse	swelled	swollen, swelled
to swim / nadar	swam	swum
to take / tomar	took	taken
to teach / enseñar	taught	taught
to tear / rasgar, desgarrar	tore	torn
to tell / decir, contar	told	told
to think / pensar	thought	thought
to throw / tirar	threw	thrown
to understand / comprender, entender	understood	understood
to undo / deshacer	undid	undone
to visualize / visualizar	visualized	visualized
to wake / despertar	woke, waked	waked, woken
to wear / usar, llevar	wore	worn
to wet / mojar, humedecer	wet, wetted	wet, wetted
to win / ganar	won	won
to withstand / soportar, resistir	withstood	withstood
to write / escribir	wrote	written

For more information on Irregular Spanish verbs consult the *Spanish-English, English-Spanish Medical Dictionary,* third edition, Lippincott, Williams and Wilkins.

Spanish Verbs with Irregular Past Participles /
El verbo español con participios pasado irregulares*

INFINITIVE / INFINITIVO	PAST PARTICIPLE / PARTICIPO PASADO
SPANISH / ENGLISH	**SPANISH / ENGLISH**
abrir / to open	**abierto** / opened
atender / to attend	**atento** / attended
componer / to fix	**compuesto** / fixed
corregir / to correct	**correcto** / corrected
cubrir / to cover	**cubierto** / covered
decir / to say, to tell	**dicho** / said
descubrir / to discover	**descubierto** / discovered
despertar / to awake	**despierto** / awaken
disolver / to dissolve	**disuelto** / dissolved
escribir / to write	**escrito** / written
exponer / to expose	**expuesto** / exposed
hacer / to do, to make	**hecho** / done, made
juntar / to join	**junto** /joined
poner / to put	**puesto** / put
pudrir / to rot	**podrido** / rotten
revolver / to turn over	**revuelto** / turned over
romper / to break	**roto** / broken
satisfacer / to satisfy	**satisfecho** / satisfied
sujetar / to hold	**sujeto** / held
ver / to see	**visto** / seen
volver / to return, turn around	**vuelto** /returned

Note: Past participles compuesto, correcto, cubierto, escrito, hecho, puesto, and vuelto serve as models for the derivate compound forms that do not appear in this list. / Los verbos en **negrita** sirven de modelo para las formas derivadas que no aparecen en esta lista.

*The list includes some past participles that have regular forms as well, and are used in compound tenses with the forms of the verb *haber* as well as with *ser* and *estar*. / La lista incluye varios participios de pasado que tienen también un participio regular usado con los tiempos compuestos del verbo *haber.*

For more information on Irregular Spanish verbs consult the *Spanish-English, English-Spanish Medical Dictionary,* third edition, Lippincott, Williams and Wilkins.

Perfect Tenses / Tiempos Perfecto

INDICATIVE / INDICATIVO

Present perfect: present of **haber** + past participle of the conjugated verb.	**He tomado**
Past perfect: imperfect of **haber** + past participle of the conjugated verb.	**Había comido**
Preterit perfect: preterit of **haber** + past participle of the conjugated verb.	**Hube venido**
Future perfect: future of **haber** + past participle of the conjugated verb.	**Habré dormido**

Note: In spoken Spanish the simple preterit replaces the preterit perfect.

SUBJUNCTIVE / SUBJUNTIVO

Present perfect: present of **haber** + past participle of the conjugated verb.	**Yo haya tomado**
Past perfect: imperfect of **haber** + past participle of the conjugated verb.	**Yo hubiera comido**

CONDITIONAL / CONDICIONAL

Conditional perfect: conditional form of **haber** + past participle of the conjugated verb.	**Yo habría dormido**

IRREGULAR VERBS / VERBOS IRREGULARES

Changes in the Root (Present Tenses Indicative, Subjunctive, and Commands)

1. e to **ie** in some infinitive ending in **–ar** and **–er: cerrar:** (present tense, *sing.* and 3rd person *pl.*) conjugated as atender, pensar, entender
2. o to **ue** some infinitive ending in **–ar** and **–er: mover** (present tense, *sing.* and 3rd person *pl.*) conjugated as **mover:** contar, doler, probar
3. e to **ie** and **i** in verbs ending in **–ir** as in **sentir** (present tense, *sing* (ie) and preterit 3rd person *sing pl.* to **i**) conjugated as **sentir:** herir; hervir; mentir
4. o to **ue** and **u** in verbs ending in **–ir** as in **dormir** (present tense, *sing* (ie) and preterit 3rd person *sing pl.* to **u**) conjugated as morir,
5. e to **i** The e of some **–ir** verbs as in **pedir** becomes **i** (present tense, *sing* (ie) and preterit 3rd person *sing pl.* to **i**) conjugated as repetir, competir

verb: CERRAR / *to close*

	SINGULAR			PLURAL		
Tense	1st person	2nd person	3rd person	1st person	2nd person	3rd person
PRES. IND.	cierro	cierras	cierra	cerramos	cerráis	cierran
PRES. SUBJ.	cierre	cierres	cierre	cerremos	cerréis	cierran
IMPERATIVE		cierra	cierre			

verb: MOVER / *to move*

	SINGULAR			PLURAL		
Tense	1st person	2nd person	3rd person	1st person	2nd person	3rd person
PRES. IND.	muevo	mueves	mueve	movemos	movéis	mueven
PRES. SUBJ.	mueva	muevas	mueva	movamos	továis	muevan
IMPERATIVE		mueve	mueva			

verb: SENTIR / *to feel*

	SINGULAR			PLURAL		
Tense	1st person	2nd person	3rd person	1st person	2nd person	3rd person
PRES. IND.	siento	sientes	siente	sentimos	sentís	sienten
PRES. SUBJ.	sienta	sientas	sienta	sintamos	sintáis	sientan
IMPERATIVE		siente	sienta			
PRET. IND.	sentí	sentiste	sintió	sentimos	sentisteis	sintieron
IMP. SUBJ.	sintiera	sintieras	sintiera	sintiéramos	sintierais	sintieran

verb: DORMIR / *to sleep*

	SINGULAR			PLURAL		
Tense	1st person	2nd person	3rd person	1st person	2nd person	3rd person
PRES. IND.	duermo	duermes	duerme	dormimos	dormís	duermen
PRES. SUBJ.	duerma	duermas	duerma	durmamos	durmáis	duerman
IMPERATIVE		duerme	duerma			
PRET. IND.	dormí	dormiste	durmió	dormimos	dormisteis	durmieron
IMP. SUBJ.	durmiera	durmieras	durmiera	durmiéramos	durmierais	durmieran

verb: PEDIR / *to request*

	SINGULAR			PLURAL		
Tense	1st person	2nd person	3rd person	1st person	2nd person	3rd person
PRES. IND.	pido	pides	pide	pedimos	pedís	piden
PRES. SUBJ.	pida	pidas	pida	pidamos	pidáis	pidan
IMPERATIVE		pide	pida			
PRET. IND.	pedí	pediste	pidió	pedimos	pedisteis	pidieron
IMP. SUBJ.	pidiera	pidieras	pidiera	pidiéramos	pidierais	pidieran

For more information on Irregular Spanish verbs consult the *Spanish-English, English-Spanish Medical Dictionary,* third edition, Lippincott, Williams and Wilkins.

Ortographic Changes

1. **c** to **zc** in some verbs ending in **–cer** as in **conocer** (first person singular, present tense) **conozco** (I am acquainted with)
   Changing the last syllable of the first person of the PRES. IND. and PRES. SUBJ. preserving the sound of the infinitive root.
2. Verbs ending in **–car** change the **c** to **q** before **e** the preterit; buscar busqué conjugated as: aplicar, appliqué
3. Verbs ending in **–gar** change **g** to **gu** before **e** to preserve the guttural sound of the **g**; llegar, pagar have the same conjugation.
4. Verbs ending in **–zar** change the **z** to **c** before **e** in the PRET. IND. and in the PRES. SUBJ.; comenzar, organizar

verb: BUSCAR / *to search*

	SINGULAR			PLURAL		
Tense	1st person	2nd person	3rd person	1st person	2nd person	3rd person
PRES. SUBJ.	busque	busques	busque	busquemos	busquéis	busquen
PRET. IND.	busqué	buscaste	buscó	buscamos	buscasteis	buscaron

verb: LLEGAR / *to arrive*

Tense	SINGULAR			PLURAL		
	1st person	2nd person	3rd person	1st person	2nd person	3rd person
PRES. IND.	llego	llegas	llega	llegamos	llegáis	llegan
PRES. SUBJ.	llegue	llegues	llegue	lleguemos	lleguéis	lleguen
IMPERATIVE		llega	llegue			
PRET. IND.	llegué	llegaste	llegó	llegamos	llegasteis	llegaron

verb: COMENZAR / *to begin*

Tense	SINGULAR			PLURAL		
	1st person	2nd person	3rd person	1st person	2nd person	3rd person
PRES. IND.	comienzo	comienzas	comienza	comenzamos	comenzáis	comienzan
PRES. SUBJ.	comience	comiences	comience	comencemos	comencéis	comiencen
IMPERATIVE		comienza	comience			
PRET. IND.	comencé	comenzaste	comenzó	comenzamos	comenzasteis	comenzaron

For more information on Irregular Spanish verbs consult the *Spanish-English, English-Spanish Medical Dictionary,* third edition, Lippincott, Williams and Wilkins.

Only tenses that have irregular forms are listed. Preterit forms of the verbs tener, poder, saber, hacer, querer, traer and decir are listed separately.

verb: ANDAR / *to walk* (andando, andado)

Tense	SINGULAR			PLURAL		
	1st person	2nd person	3rd person	1st person	2nd person	3rd person
PRET. IND.	anduve	anduviste	anduvo	anduvimos	anduvisteis	anduvieron
IMP. SUBJ.	anduviera	anduvieras	anduviera	anduviéramos	anduvierais	anduvieran

verb: CABER / *to fit* (cabiendo, cabido)

Tense	SINGULAR			PLURAL		
	1st person	2nd person	3rd person	1st person	2nd person	3rd person
PRES. IND.	quepo	cabes	cabe	cabemos	cabéis	caben
PRES. SUBJ.	quepa	quepas	quepa	quepamos	quepáis	quepan
FUT. IND.	cabré	cabrás	cabrá	cabremos	cabréis	cabrán
PRET. IND.	cupe	cupiste	cupo	cupimos	cupisteis	cupieron
IMP. SUBJ.	cupiera	cupieras	cupiera	cupiéramos	cupierais	cupieran

verb: CAER / to fall (cayendo, caído)

Tense	SINGULAR			PLURAL		
	1st person	2nd person	3rd person	1st person	2nd person	3rd person
PRES. IND	caigo	caes	cae	caemos	caéis	caen
PRES. SUBJ.	caiga	caigas	caiga	caigamos	caigáis	caigan
PRET. IND.	caí	caíste	cayó	caímos	caísteis	cayeron
IMP. SUBJ.	cayera	cayeras	cayera	cayéramos	cayerais	cayeran

verb: DAR / to give (dando, dado)

Tense	SINGULAR			PLURAL		
	1st person	2nd person	3rd person	1st person	2nd person	3rd person
PRES. IND	doy	das	da	damos	dais	dan
PRES. SUBJ.	dé	des	dé	demos	deis	den
PRET. IND.	di	diste	dio	dimos	disteis	dieron
IMP. SUBJ.	diera	dieras	diera	diéramos	dierais	dieran

verb: DECIR / to say, tell (diciendo, dicho)

Tense	SINGULAR			PLURAL		
	1st person	2nd person	3rd person	1st person	2nd person	3rd person
PRES. IND.	digo	dices	dice	decimos	decís	dicen
PRES. SUBJ.	diga	digas	diga	digamos	digáis	digan
FUT. IND.	diré	dirás	dirá	diremos	diréis	dirán
IMP. SUBJ.	dijera	dijeras	dijera	dijéramos	dijerais	dijeran

verb: ESTAR / to be (estando, estado)

Tense	SINGULAR			PLURAL		
	1st person	2nd person	3rd person	1st person	2nd person	3rd person
PRES. IND.	estoy	estás	está	estamos	estáis	están
PRES. SUBJ.	esté	estés	esté	estemos	estéis	estén
IMP. SUBJ.	estuviera	estuvieras	estuviera	estuviéramos	estuvierais	estuvieran

verb: HACER / to do, make (haciendo, hecho)

Tense	SINGULAR			PLURAL		
	1st person	2nd person	3rd person	1st person	2nd person	3rd person
PRES. IND.	hago	haces	hace	hacemos	hacéis	hacen
PRES. SUBJ.	haga	hagas	haga	hagamos	hagáis	hagan
IMPERATIVE		haz	haga		haced	
FUTURE	haré	harás	hará	haremos	haréis	harán
IMP. SUBJ.	hiciera	hicieras	hiciera	hiciéramos	hicierais	hicieran

verb: IR / to go (yendo, ido)

Tense	SINGULAR			PLURAL		
	1st person	2nd person	3rd person	1st person	2nd person	3rd person
PRES. IND.	voy	vas	va	vamos	vais	van
PRES. SUBJ.	vaya	vayas	vaya	vayamos	vayáis	vayan
IMPERATIVE		ve	vaya		id	
IMP. IND.	iba	ibas	iba	íbamos	ibais	iban
IMP. SUBJ.	fuera	fueras	fuera	fuéramos	fuerais	fueran

verb: OÍR / to hear (oyendo, oído)

Tense	SINGULAR			PLURAL		
	1st person	2nd person	3rd person	1st person	2nd person	3rd person
PRES. IND.	oigo	oyes	oye	oímos	oís	oyen
PRES. SUBJ.	oiga	oigas	oiga	oigamos	oigáis	oigan
IMPERATIVE		oye	oiga		oíd	
IMP. IND.	oía	oías	oía	oíamos	oíais	oían
IMP. SUBJ.	oyera	oyeras	oyera	oyéramos	oyerais	oyeran

verb: PODER / to be able (pudiendo, podido)

Tense	SINGULAR			PLURAL		
	1st person	2nd person	3rd person	1st person	2nd person	3rd person
PRES. IND.	puedo	puedes	puede	podemos	podéis	pueden
PRES. SUBJ.	pueda	puedas	pueda	podamos	podáis	puedan
FUT. IND.	podré	podrás	podrá	podremos	podréis	podrán
IMP. SUBJ.	pudiera	pudieras	pudiera	pudiéramos	pudierais	pudieran

verb: PONER / to put (poniendo, puesto)

Tense	SINGULAR			PLURAL		
	1st person	2nd person	3rd person	1st person	2nd person	3rd person
PRES. IND.	pongo	pones	pone	ponemos	ponéis	ponen
PRES. SUBJ.	ponga	pongas	ponga	pongamos	pongáis	pongan
IMPERATIVE		pon	ponga		poned	
FUT. IND.	pondré	pondrás	pondrá	pondremos	pondréis	pondrán
IMP. SUBJ.	pusiera	pusieras	pusiera	pusiéramos	pusierais	pusieran

verb: QUERER / to wish, to want (queriendo, querido)

Tense	SINGULAR			PLURAL		
	1st person	2nd person	3rd person	1st person	2nd person	3rd person
PRES. IND.	quiero	quieres	quiere	queremos	queréis	quieren
PRES. SUBJ.	quiera	quieras	quiera	queramos	queráis	quieran
FUT. IND.	querré	querrás	querrá	querremos	querréis	querrán
IMP. SUBJ.	quisiera	quisieras	quisiera	quisiéramos	quisierais	quisieran

verb: SABER / to know (sabiendo, sabido)

Tense	SINGULAR			PLURAL		
	1st person	2nd person	3rd person	1st person	2nd person	3rd person
PRES. IND.	sé	sabes	sabe	sabemos	sabéis	saben
PRES. SUBJ.	sepa	sepas	sepa	sepamos	sepáis	sepan
FUT. IND.	sabré	sabrás	sabrá	sabremos	sabréis	sabrán
IMP. SUBJ.	supiera	supieras	supiera	supiéramos	supierais	supieran

verb: SALIR / to get out (saliendo, salido)

Tense	SINGULAR			PLURAL		
	1st person	2nd person	3rd person	1st person	2nd person	3rd person
PRES. IND.	salgo	sales	sale	salimos	salís	salen
PRES. SUBJ.	salga	salgas	salga	salgamos	salgáis	salgan
FUT. IMP.	saldré	saldrás	saldrá	saldremos	saldréis	saldrán
IMP. SUBJ.	saliera	salieras	saliera	saliéramos	salierais	salieran

verb: TRAER / *to bring* (trayendo, traído)

	SINGULAR			PLURAL		
Tense	1st person	2nd person	3rd person	1st person	2nd person	3rd person
PRES. IND.	traigo	traes	trae	traemos	traéis	traen
PRES. SUBJ.	traiga	traigas	traiga	traigamos	traigáis	traigan
FUT. IND.	traeré	traerás	traerá	traeremos	traeréis	traerán
IMP. SUBJ.	trajera	trajeras	trajera	trajéramos	trajerais	trajeran

verb: VENIR / *to come* (viniendo, venido)

	SINGULAR			PLURAL		
Tense	1st person	2nd person	3rd person	1st person	2nd person	3rd person
PRES. IND.	vengo	vienes	viene	venimos	venís	vienen
PRES. SUBJ.	venga	vengas	venga	vengamos	vengáis	vengan
IMPERATIVE		ven	venga		venid	
FUT. IND.	vendré	vendrás	vendrá	vendremos	vendréis	vendrán
IMP. SUBJ.	viniera	vinieras	viniera	viniéramos	vinierais	vinieran

verb: TENER / *to have* (teniendo, tenido)

	SINGULAR			PLURAL		
Tense	1st person	2nd person	3rd person	1st person	2nd person	3rd person
PRES. IND.	tengo	tienes	tiene	tenemos	tenéis	tienen
PRES. SUBJ.	tenga	tengas	tenga	tengamos	tengáis	tengan
IMPERATIVE		ten	tenga		tened	
FUT. IND.	tendré	tendrás	tendrá	tendremos	tendréis	tendrán
IMP. SUBJ.	tuviera	tuvieras	tuviera	tuviéramos	tuvierais	tuvieran

verb: VER / *to see* (viendo, visto)*

	SINGULAR			PLURAL		
Tense	1st person	2nd person	3rd person	1st person	2nd person	3rd person
PRES. IND.	veo	ves	ve	vemos	veis	ven
PRES. SUBJ.	vea	veas	vea	veamos	veáis	vean
IMP. SUBJ.	viera	vieras	viera	viéramos	vierais	vieran

*See the preterit of **ver** in the list of irregular preterits.

verb: **VALER** / *to be worth* **(valiendo, valido)**

	SINGULAR			PLURAL		
Tense	**1st person**	**2nd person**	**3rd person**	**1st person**	**2nd person**	**3rd person**
PRES. IND.	valgo	vales	vale	valemos	valéis	valen
PRES. SUBJ.	valga	valgas	valga	valgamos	valgáis	valgan
IMPERATIVE		vale	valga		valed	
FUT. IND.	valdré	valdrás	valdrá	valdremos	valdréis	valdrán

Conditional Forms

The conditional forms of tener, haber, salir, valer, saber, poder, and poner use the same root that they have in the future of the indicative. Note: The endings of the conditional are the same endings of the verbs of infinitive endings (-er and -ir) of the imperfect indicative.

Tener—tendr + endings of the conditional added to all: -ía, -ías, ía, -íamos, -íais, ían. Tendría, tendrías, tendría, tendríamos, tendríais, tendrían

Haber—habr: habría, habrías, habría; habríamos, habríais, habrían

Salir—saldr: saldría, saldrías, saldría, saldríamos, saldríais, saldrían

Valer—valdr: valdría, valdrías, valdría, valdríamos, valdríais, valdrían

Saber—sabr: sabría, sabrías, sabría, sabríamos, sabríais, sabrían

Poder—podr: podría, podrías, podría, podríamos, podríais, podrían

Poner—pondr: pondría, pondrías, pondría, pondríamos, pondríais, pondrían